YOUMANS

Neurological Surgery

YOUMANS
Neurological Surgery

SIXTH EDITION

H. Richard Winn, MD

Professor and Director of Neurosurgery
Lenox Hill Hospital
New York, New York;
Hofstra University
Hempstead, New York;
Adjunct Professor
Department of Neurological Surgery
University of Iowa
Iowa City, Iowa;
Clinical Professor
Weill Cornell Medical College
Columbia University
Mount Sinai School of Medicine
New York, New York;
Visiting Professor of Surgery (Neurosurgery)
Tribhuvan University Teaching Hospital
Kathmandu, Nepal

VOLUME 1

ELSEVIER
SAUNDERS

ELSEVIER
SAUNDERS

1600 John F. Kennedy Blvd.
Ste 1800
Philadelphia, PA 19103-2899

YOUMANS NEUROLOGICAL SURGERY

ISBN: 978-1-4160-5316-3
Vol 1 PN: 9996059006
Vol 2 PN: 9996059065
Vol 3 PN: 999605912X
Vol 4 PN: 9996058948

Notices

Knowledge and best practice in this field are constantly changing. As new research and experience broaden our understanding, changes in research methods, professional practices, or medical treatment may become necessary.

Practitioners and researchers must always rely on their own experience and knowledge in evaluating and using any information, methods, compounds, or experiments described herein. In using such information or methods they should be mindful of their own safety and the safety of others, including parties for whom they have a professional responsibility.

With respect to any drug or pharmaceutical products identified, readers are advised to check the most current information provided (i) on procedures featured or (ii) by the manufacturer of each product to be administered, to verify the recommended dose or formula, the method and duration of administration, and contraindications. It is the responsibility of practitioners, relying on their own experience and knowledge of their patients, to make diagnoses, to determine dosages and the best treatment for each individual patient, and to take all appropriate safety precautions.

To the fullest extent of the law, neither the Publisher nor the authors, contributors, or editors assume any liability for any injury and/or damage to persons or property as a matter of products liability, negligence or otherwise, or from any use or operation of any methods, products, instructions, or ideas contained in the material herein.

Chapter 16, "Neuropsychological Testing" by Jordan Grafman, is in the public domain.
Chapter 31, "Thorascopic Surgery of the Spine" by Rudolf Beisse: Rudolf Beisse retains copyright to his original video.
Chapter 242, "Secondary Procedures for Brachial Plexus Injuries" by Huan Wang, Alexander Y. Shin, Allen T. Bishop, and Robert J. Spinner: Mayo Foundation retains copyright to their original artwork.
Chapter 321, "Osteoporotic Fractures: Evaluation and Treatment with Vertebroplasty and Kyphoplasty" by R. Webster Crowley, H. Kwang Yeoh, M. Sean McKisic, Rod J. Oskouian Jr, and Aaron S. Dumont: Michael McKisic retains copyright to his original illustrations.

Library of Congress Cataloging-in-Publication Data

Youmans neurological surgery / [edited by] H. Richard Winn.—6th ed.
    v. ; cm.
    Includes bibliographical references and index.
    ISBN 978-1-4160-5316-3 (4 vol. set : hardcover)
    1. Nervous system—Surgery. I. Youmans, Julian R., 1928- II. Winn, H. Richard. III. Title: Neurological surgery.
    [DNLM: 1. Neurosurgical Procedures. 2. Nervous System Diseases—surgery. 3. Neurosurgery—methods. WL 368 Y671 2011]
    RD593.N4153 2011
    617.4'8—dc22

2009034477

Acquisitions Editor: Rebecca Gaertner
Senior Developmental Editor: Jennifer Shreiner
Publishing Services Manager: Anne Altepeter
Team Manager: Radhika Pallamparthy
Senior Project Manager: Doug Turner
Project Manager: Preethi Kerala Varma
Designer: Louis Forgione

Printed in the People's Republic of China

Last digit is the print number: 9 8 7 6 5 4 3 2 1

To my wife and family, and to my residents who have carried the message

Section Editors

Ron L. Alterman, MD
Professor
Department of Neurosurgery;
Director
Functional and Restorative Neurosurgery
Mount Sinai School of Medicine
New York, New York
  Functional Neurosurgery

Henry Brem, MD
Harvey Cushing Professor and Chair
Department of Neurosurgery;
Professor
Department of Neurosurgery, Ophthalmology and Oncology
  and Biomedical Engineering;
Director
Hunterian Neurosurgical Laboratory
Department of Neurosurgery
Johns Hopkins University School of Medicine;
Neurosurgeon-in-Chief
The Johns Hopkins Hospital
Baltimore, Maryland
  Oncology

M. Ross Bullock, MD, PhD
Professor
Department of Neurosurgery
University of Miami;
Director
Neurotrauma
Jackson Memorial Hospital
Miami, Florida
  Trauma

Kim J. Burchiel, MD
John Raaf Professor and Chairman
Department of Neurological Surgery;
Professor
Department of Anesthesiology and Perioperative Medicine
Oregon Health & Science University
Portland, Oregon
  Pain

E. Antonio Chiocca, MD, PhD
Chairman
Department of Neurological Surgery
Dardinger Family Professor of Oncologic Neurosurgery
Physician Director
OSUMC Neuroscience Signature Program;
Co-Director
Dardinger Center for Neuro-oncology and Neurosciences;
Co-Director
Viral Oncology Program of the Comprehensive Cancer Center
James Cancer Hospital and Solove Research Institute
The Ohio State University Medical Center
Columbus, Ohio
  Oncology

E. Sander Connolly Jr, MD
Bennett M. Stein Professor and Vice-Chair
Department of Neurological Surgery
College of Physicians and Surgeons
Columbia University
New York, New York
  Vascular

William T. Couldwell, MD, PhD
Professor and Chair
Department of Neurosurgery
University of Utah School of Medicine
Salt Lake City, Utah
  General Neurosurgery

Aaron G. Filler, MD, PhD, FRCS
Medical Director
Institute for Nerve Medicine
Santa Monica, California
  Peripheral Nerve

William A. Friedman, MD
Professor and Chair
Department of Neurosurgery
University of Florida
Gainesville, Florida
  Radiation

Saadi Ghatan, MD, FACS
Florence Irving Assistant Professor of Neurological Surgery
Columbia University College of Physicians and Surgeons
New York, New York
Pediatrics

David A. Hovda, PhD
Professor
Departments of Neurosurgery and Molecular and Medical
    Pharmacology
David Geffen School of Medicine at UCLA
University of California, Los Angeles
Los Angeles, California
Trauma

Matthew A. Howard III, MD
Professor and Head
Department of Neurosurgery
University of Iowa
Iowa City, Iowa
Epilepsy

David G. Kline, MD
Emeritus Chairman and Boyd Professor
Department of Neurosurgery
Louisiana State University Health Sciences Center
New Orleans, Louisiana
Peripheral Nerve

Peter D. LeRoux, MD, MB, ChB
Associate Professor
Department of Neurosurgery
University of Pennsylvania School of Medicine
Philadelphia, Pennsylvania
Introduction and Basic Science

Andres M. Lozano, MD, PhD, FRCSC, FRS
Professor and Chairman of Neurosurgery
University of Toronto;
RR Tasker Chair in Functional Neurosurgery
Toronto Western Hospital
Canada Research Chair in Neuroscience
Toronto, Canada
Functional Neurosurgery

L. Dade Lunsford, MD, FACS
Lars Leksell and Distinguished Professor
Department of Neurological Surgery
University of Pittsburgh School of Medicine;
Director
Center for Image Guided Neurosurgery
University of Pittsburgh Medical Center
Pittsburgh, Pennsylvania
Radiation

Pierre Magistretti, MD, PhD
Professor of Neurosciences
Brain Mind Institute
École Polytechnique Fédérale de Lausanne (EPFL);
Director
Center for Psychiatric Neurosciences
Department of Psychiatry, CHUV-UNIL
University of Lausanne
Lausanne, Switzerland
Introduction and Basic Science

Guy M. McKhann II, MD
Florence Irving Associate Professor of Neurological Surgery
Columbia University College of Physicians
New York Presbyterian Hospital
New York, New York
Epilepsy

Fredric B. Meyer, MD, FACS
Professor and Chair
Department of Neurological Surgery
Mayo Clinic
Rochester, Minnesota
Vascular

Edward H. Oldfield, MD
Crutchfield Professor of Neurosurgery
Professor of Internal Medicine
Department of Neurological Surgery
University of Virginia School of Medicine
Charlottesville, Virginia
Introduction and Basic Science

T. S. Park, MD
Shi H. Huang Professor of Neurological Surgery
Washington University School of Medicine;
Neurosurgeon-In-Chief
St. Louis Children's Hospital
St. Louis, Missouri
Pediatrics

Bruce E. Pollock, MD
Professor
Departments of Neurological Surgery and Radiation Oncology
Mayo Clinic College of Medicine
Rochester, Minnesota
Radiation

Raymond Sawaya, MD
Professor and Chairman
Department of Neurosurgery
Baylor College of Medicine;
Professor and Chairman
Department of Neurosurgery
The University of Texas M. D. Anderson Cancer Center
Houston, Texas
Oncology

R. Michael Scott, MD
Professor of Surgery
Department of Neurosurgery
Harvard Medical School;
Neurosurgeon-in-Chief
The Children's Hospital, Boston
Boston, Massachusetts
Pediatrics

Christopher I. Shaffrey, MD, FACS
Harrison Distinguished Professor
Departments of Neurological and Orthopaedic Surgery
University of Virginia School of Medicine
Charlottesville, Virginia
Spine

Volker K. H. Sonntag, MD
Vice Chairman, Emeritus
Barrow Neurological Institute
Phoenix, Arizona
Spine

Robert F. Spetzler, MD
Director and J. N. Harber Chair of Neurological Surgery
Barrow Neurological Institute
Phoenix, Arizona;
Professor
Department of Surgery
Section of Neurosurgery
University of Arizona College of Medicine
Tucson, Arizona
Vascular

Dennis G. Vollmer, MD
Neurosurgeon
Colorado Brain and Spine Institute
Englewood, Colorado
Spine

Eric L. Zager, MD, FACS
Professor
Department of Neurosurgery
University of Pennsylvania School of Medicine
Philadelphia, Pennsylvania
Peripheral Nerve

Video Editors

Robert E. Harbaugh, MD, FACS, FAHA
Director
Institute of the Neurosciences
University Distinguished Professor and Chair
Department of Neurosurgery;
Professor
Department of Engineering Science & Mechanics
Chair
Department of Neurosurgery Penn State University College of
    Medicine
Penn State Milton S. Hershey Medical Center
Hershey, Pennsylvania

Dong Gyu Kim, MD, PhD
Professor
Department of Neurosurgery;
Director
Gamma Knife Center;
Chairman
Clinical Research Institute
Seoul National University Hospital
Seoul National University College of Medicine
Seoul, Korea

Contents

†Deceased.

Contributors

Bizhan Aarabi, MD, FACS, FRCSC
Associate Professor
Department of Neurosurgery
University of Maryland School of Medicine;
Director
Neurotrauma Service
R. Adams Cowley Shock Trauma Center
Baltimore, Maryland
Ch. 336: Traumatic and Penetrating Head Injuries

Rick Abbott, MD
Professor
Department of Clinical Neurosurgery
Albert Einstein College of Medicine;
Senior Attending
Montefiore Medical Center
Bronx, New York
Ch. 221: Management of Intramedullary Spinal Cord Tumors in Children

Saleem I. Abdulrauf, MD, FACS
Neurosurgeon-in-Chief
Saint Louis University Hospital;
Professor
Department of Neurological Surgery;
Director
Saint Louis University Center for Cerebrovascular and Skull Base Surgery
Saint Louis University School of Medicine
St. Louis, Missouri
Ch. 131: Meningiomas

Frank L. Acosta, Jr, MD
Director
Spine Deformity
Department of Neurosurgery
Cedars-Sinai Medical Center
Los Angeles, California
Ch. 273: Diagnosis and Management of Diskogenic Lower Back Pain
Ch. 287: Adult Thoracolumbar Scoliosis

John R. Adler Jr, MD
Dorothy and T. K. Chan Professor
Department of Neurosurgery
Stanford University School of Medicine
Stanford, California
Ch. 257: Image-Guided Robotic Radiosurgery: The CyberKnife

Nzhde Agazaryan, PhD, DABR
Associate Professor
Department of Radiation Oncology and Biomedical Physics Graduate Program
David Geffen School of Medicine at UCLA
University of California, Los Angeles
Los Angeles, California
Ch. 255: Linear Accelerator Radiosurgery: Technical Aspects

Manish Aghi, MD, PhD
Assistant Professor
Department of Neurological Surgery
University of California, San Francisco
San Francisco, California
Ch. 253: Interstitial and Intracavitary Irradiation of Brain Tumors

Edward S. Ahn, MD
Assistant Professor
Department of Neurosurgery and Plastic Surgery
Johns Hopkins University School of Medicine
Baltimore, Maryland
Ch. 219: Achondroplasia and Other Dwarfisms

Ali Alaraj, MD
Assistant Professor
Department of Neurosurgery
University of Illinois at Chicago
Chicago, Illinois
Ch. 354: Extracranial Vertebral Artery Diseases

Gregory W. Albert, MD
Resident Physician
Department of Neurosurgery
University of Iowa Hospitals and Clinics
Iowa City, Iowa
Ch. 289: Acquired Abnormalities of the Craniocervical Junction

Leland Albright, MD
Professor
Departments of Neurosurgery and Pediatrics
University of Wisconsin Health Center
Madison, Wisconsin
Ch. 226: Intrathecal Baclofen Therapy for Cerebral Palsy
Ch. 228: Dystonia in Children

Felipe C. Albuquerque, MD
Assistant Director
Endovascular Neurosurgery
Department of Neurological Surgery
Barrow Neurological Institute
Phoenix, Arizona
  Ch. 374: Endovascular Approaches to Intracranial Aneurysms
  Ch. 375: Endovascular Coiling of Intracranial Aneurysms:
  Evidence Supporting Their Use

Tord D. Alden, MD
Assistant Professor
Department of Neurosurgery
Northwestern University Feinberg School of Medicine;
Attending Neurosurgeon
Children's Memorial Hospital
Chicago, Illinois
  Ch. 222: Spine Tumors in Children

Michael J. Alexander, MD, FACS
Professor and Clinical Chief
Department of Neurosurgery;
Director
Neurovascular Center
Cedars-Sinai Medical Center
Los Angeles, California
  Ch. 353: Nonatherosclerotic Carotid Lesions

Andrei V. Alexandrov, MD
Professor and Director
Comprehensive Stroke Center
University of Alabama Hospital
Birmingham, Alabama
  Ch. 347: Transcranial Doppler Ultrasonography and
  Neurosonology

Ossama Al-Mefty, MD
Director of Skull Base Surgery
Department of Neurosurgery
Brigham and Women's Hospital
Boston, Massachusetts
  Ch. 131: Meningiomas

Ron L. Alterman, MD
Professor
Department of Neurosurgery;
Director
Functional and Restorative Neurosurgery
Mount Sinai School of Medicine
New York, New York
  Ch. 71: Introduction
  Ch. 82: Deep Brain Stimulation for Dystonia

Lázaro Álvarez, MD
Clinic of Movement Disorders
International Center for Neurological Restoration
Havana, Cuba
  Ch. 81: Subthalamotomy in Parkinson's Disease: Indications and
  Outcome

Nduka M. Amankulor, MD
Chief Resident
Department of Neurosurgery
Yale University School of Medicine
New Haven, Connecticut
  Ch. 100: Molecular Genetics and the Development of Targets for
  Glioma Therapy

Peter S. Amenta, MD
Resident
Department of Neurosurgery
Thomas Jefferson University Hospital
Philadelphia, Pennsylvania
  Ch. 316: Pathology of the Cervicothoracic Junction: Evaluation
  and Treatment

Christopher P. Ames, MD
Director
UCSF Spine Center
University of California, San Francisco
San Francisco, California
  Ch. 273: Diagnosis and Management of Diskogenic Lower Back
  Pain
  Ch. 287: Adult Thoracolumbar Scoliosis

Sepideh Amin-Hanjani, MD, FACS, FAHA
Associate Professor and Program Director;
Co-Director
Neurovascular Surgery Section
Department of Neurosurgery
University of Illinois College of Medicine at Chicago
Chicago, Illinois
  Ch. 354: Extracranial Vertebral Artery Diseases

Mario Ammirati, MD, MBA
Professor
Departments of Neurosurgery and Radiation Oncology
The Ohio State University College of Medicine;
Director
Skull Base Neurosurgery and Stereotactic Radiosurgery
Department of Neurological Surgery
The Ohio State University Medical Center
Columbus, Ohio
  Ch. 139: Overview of Skull Base Tumors

Carryn Anderson, MD
Assistant Professor
Department of Radiation Oncology
University of Iowa;
Assistant Professor
Department of Radiation Oncology
University of Iowa Hospitals and Clinics
Iowa City, Iowa
  Ch. 248: Principles of Radiation Therapy

Richard C. E. Anderson, MD, FACS, FAAP
Assistant Professor
Department of Neurological Surgery
Columbia University College of Physicians and Surgeons
Morgan Stanley Children's Hospital of New York
New York, New York
  Ch. 214: Myelomeningocele and Myelocystocele

Paul H. Chapman, MD
Distinguished Nicholas T. Zervas Professor of Neurosurgery
Departments of Neurosurgery and Radiation Oncology
Massachusetts General Hospital
Harvard Medical School
Boston, Massachusetts
 Ch. 254: Proton Radiosurgery

Fady T. Charbel, MD
Professor and Head
Department of Neurosurgery
University of Illinois at Chicago
Chicago, Illinois
 Ch. 348: Neurovascular Imaging
 Ch. 354: Extracranial Vertebral Artery Diseases

Patrick Chauvel, MD
Neurophysiologic and Neuropsychological Service
Hôpital de la Timone (Timone University Hospital)
Neurophysiologic and Neuropsychological Laboratory
INSERM, Faculty of Medicine
Marseille, France
 Ch. 68: Radiosurgical Treatment of Epilepsy

Grace Chen, MD
Assistant Professor
Department of Anesthesiology
School of Medicine
Oregon Health & Science University
Portland, Oregon
 Ch. 158: Management of Pain by Anesthetic Techniques

Boyle C. Cheng, PhD
Assistant Professor
Department of Neurosurgery
Drexel University Allegheny General Hospital Campus;
Director
Department of Neurosurgery Spine and Biomechanics
 Research Laboratory
University of Pittsburgh
Pittsburgh, Pennsylvania
 *Ch. 295: Nucleoplasty and Posterior Dynamic Stabilization
Systems*

Joseph S. Cheng, MD, MS
Associate Professor
Department of Neurological Surgery
Director
Neurosurgery Spine Program
Co-Director
Comprehensive Spine Center
Vanderbilt University Medical Center
Nashville, Tennessee
 *Ch. 292: Bone Graft Options, Bone Graft Substitutes, and Bone
Harvest Techniques*

Joshua J. Chern, MD
Chief Resident
Department of Neurosurgery
Baylor College of Medicine
Houston, Texas
 Ch. 126: Medulloblastoma

E. Antonio Chiocca, MD, PhD
Chairman
Department of Neurological Surgery
Dardinger Family Professor of Oncologic Neurosurgery
Physician Director
OSUMC Neuroscience Signature Program;
Co-Director
Dardinger Center for Neuro-oncology and Neurosciences;
Co-Director
Viral Oncology Program of the Comprehensive Cancer Center
James Cancer Hospital and Solove Research Institute
The Ohio State University Medical Center
Columbus, Ohio
 Ch. 95: Brain Tumors: General Considerations
 Ch. 107: Gene- and Viral-Based Therapies for Gliomas

Ondrej Choutka, BMBCh, Oxon
Chief Resident
Department of Neurosurgery
University of Cincinnati College of Medicine
Cincinnati, Ohio
 Ch. 177: Dandy-Walker Syndrome

Shakeel A. Chowdhry, MD
Resident Physician
Department of Neurosurgery
University Hospitals Case Medical Center;
Case Western Reserve University
Cleveland, Ohio
 Ch. 187: Infantile Posthemorrhagic Hydrocephalus

Cindy W. Christian, MD
Chair
Child Abuse and Neglect Prevention
Children's Hospital of Philadelphia;
Associate Professor
Department of Pediatrics
University of Pennsylvania School of Medicine
Philadelphia, Pennsylvania
 Ch. 210: Child Abuse

Kathy Chuang, MD
Researcher
Department of Physical Medicine and Rehabilitation
Harvard University;
Resident
Department of Neurology
Massachusetts General Hospital;
Brigham and Women's Hospital
Boston, Massachusetts
 Ch. 342: Rehabilitation of Patients with Traumatic Brain Injury

Jan Claassen, MD, PhD
Assistant Professor
Departments of Neurology and Neurosurgery
Division of Critical Care Neurology
Columbia University College of Physicians and Surgeons
New York, New York
　Ch. 54: Continuous Electroencephalography in Neurological-
　Neurosurgical Intensive Care: Applications and Value

Richard E. Clatterbuck, MD, PhD
Department of Neurosurgery
Hattiesburg Clinic
Hattiesburg, Mississippi
　Ch. 151: Sarcoidosis, Tuberculosis, and Xanthogranuloma

Elizabeth B. Claus, MD, PhD
Professor
Yale University School of Medicine
New Haven, Connecticut;
Attending Neurosurgeon
Brigham and Women's Hospital
Boston, Massachusetts
　Ch. 149: Scalp Tumors

Daniel R. Cleary, MS
Neuroscience Graduate Student
Department of Neurological Surgery
School of Medicine
Oregon Health & Science University
Portland, Oregon
　Ch. 154: Anatomy and Physiology of Pain

Robert J. Coffey, MD
Medical Advisor
Medtronic, Inc.
Minneapolis, Minnesota
　Ch. 165: Evidence Base: Neurostimulation for Pain

Alan R. Cohen, MD, FACS, FAAP
Professor
Departments of Neurological Surgery and Pediatrics
Case Western Reserve University School of Medicine;
Surgeon-in-Chief and Chief
Department of Pediatric Neurological Surgery
University Hospitals Rainbow Babies and Children's Hospital
Cleveland, Ohio
　Ch. 191: Neuroendoscopy

Andrew J. Cole, MD, FRCP(C)
Associate Professor
Department of Neurology
Harvard Medical School;
Director
MGH Epilepsy Service and Epilepsy Research Laboratory
Massachusetts General Hospital
Boston, Massachusetts
　Ch. 56: Evaluation of Patients for Epilepsy Surgery

E. Sander Connolly Jr, MD
Bennett M. Stein Professor and Vice-Chair
Department of Neurological Surgery
College of Physicians and Surgeons
Columbia University
New York, New York
　Ch. 346: Circulatory Arrest with Deep Hypothermia
　Ch. 369: Microsurgery of Distal Anterior Cerebral Artery
　Aneurysms
　Ch. 387: Endovascular Management of Arteriovenous
　Malformations for Cure

Patrick J. Connolly, MD
Assistant Professor
Department of Neurosurgery
Temple University School of Medicine
Philadelphia, Pennsylvania
　Ch. 65: Topectomy and Multiple Subpial Transection

Anne G. Copay, PhD
Associate Director
Research
Spinal Research Foundation
Reston, Virginia
　Ch. 266: Biomaterials and Biomechanics of Spinal Arthroplasty

Jeroen R. Coppens, MD
Department of Neurosurgery
University of Utah
Salt Lake City, Utah
　Ch. 30: Advantages and Limitations of Cranial Endoscopy

James J. Corbett, MD
Professor
Departments of Neurology and Ophthalmology
University of Mississippi Medical Center
Jackson, Mississippi
　Ch. 13: Neuro-ophthalmology

Daniel M. Corcos, PhD
Professor
Department of Kinesiology
University of Illinois at Chicago
Chicago, Illinois
　Ch. 91: Management of Spasticity by Central Nervous System
　Infusion Techniques

Domagoj Coric, MD
Chief of Neurosurgery
Carolinas Medical Center;
Carolina Neurosurgery and Spine Associates
Charlotte, North Carolina
　Ch. 294: Lumbar Arthroplasty: Total Disk Replacement and
　Nucleus Replacement Technologies

Garth Rees Cosgrove, MD
Chair
Department of Neurosurgery
Warren Alpert Medical School of Brown University;
Chief of Neurosurgery
Miriam Hospital
Rhode Island Hospital
Providence, Rhode Island
    Ch. 56: Evaluation of Patients for Epilepsy Surgery
    Ch. 86: A History of Psychosurgery

William T. Couldwell, MD, PhD
Professor and Chair
Department of Neurosurgery
University of Utah
Salt Lake City, Utah
    Ch. 30: Advantages and Limitations of Cranial Endoscopy

Stirling Craig, MD
Resident
Department of Plastic Surgery
Yale-New Haven Hospital
New Haven, Connecticut
    Ch. 29: Incisions and Closures

Neil R. Crawford, PhD
Associate Staff Scientist
Spinal Biomechanics
Barrow Neurological Institute
Phoenix, Arizona
    Ch. 291: Basic Principles of Spinal Internal Fixation

Peter B. Crino, MD, PhD
Associate Professor
Department of Neurology
University of Pennsylvania School of Medicine;
Director
Penn Epilepsy Center
Hospital of the University of Pennsylvania
Philadelphia, Pennsylvania
    Ch. 51: Malformations of Cortical Development

R. Webster Crowley, MD
Chief Resident
Department of Neurosurgery
University of Virginia
Charlottesville, Virginia
    Ch. 26: Positioning for Cranial Surgery
    *Ch. 321: Osteoporotic Fractures: Evaluation and Treatment with
    Vertebroplasty and Kyphoplasty*

Bradford A. Curt, MD
Pediatrician
Bristol Park Medical Group
Irvine, California
    *Ch. 272: Differential Diagnosis and Initial Management of
    Spine Pathology*

Marek Czosnyka, PhD
Reader in Brain Physics
Departments of Neurosurgery and Clinical Neurosciences
University of Cambridge
Cambridge, United Kingdom
    Ch. 34: Clinical Evaluation of Adult Hydrocephalus

Zofia Czosnyka, PhD
Senior Research Associate
Departments of Neurosurgery and Clinical Neurosciences
University of Cambridge
Cambridge, United Kingdom
    Ch. 34: Clinical Evaluation of Adult Hydrocephalus

Vladimir Y. Dadashev, MD
Chief Resident
Department of Neurosurgery
Emory University School of Medicine
Atlanta, Georgia
    *Ch. 278: Treatment of Disk and Ligamentous Diseases of the
    Cervical Spine*

Andrew T. Dailey, MD
Associate Professor
Department of Neurosurgery
University of Utah
Salt Lake City, Utah
    *Ch. 304: Posterior, Transforaminal, and Anterior Lumbar
    Interbody Fusion: Techniques and Instrumentation*

Deepa Danan, BA
Columbia University College of Physicians and Surgeons
New York, New York
    Ch. 170: Diagnosis and Management of Painful Neuromas

Shabbar F. Danish, MD
Director
Department of Stereotactic and Functional Neurosurgery
Robert Wood Johnson Medical School
New Brunswick, New Jersey
    Ch. 32: Cranioplasty

Shervin R. Dashti, MD, PhD
Co-Director
Division of Cerebrovascular and Endovascular Neurosurgery
Norton Neuroscience Institute
Louisville, Kentucky
    *Ch. 395: Classification of Spinal Arteriovenous Lesions:
    Arteriovenous Fistulas and Arteriovenous Malformations*

Carlos A. David, MD
Assistant Professor
Department of Neurosurgery
Tufts University School of Medicine
Boston, Massachusetts;
Director
Cerebrovascular and Skull Base Surgery
Lahey Clinic
Burlington, Massachusetts
    Ch. 355: Intracranial Occlusive Disease

David J. David, MD, AC, FRACS, FRCS, FRCSEd, FRCST (hon)
Clinical Professor
Department of Craniomaxillofacial Surgery
University of Adelaide;
Head
Australian Craniofacial Unit
Women's and Children's Hospital
Adelaide, Australia
  Ch. 339: Craniofacial Injuries

Arthur L. Day, MD
Professor
Program Director
Department of Neurosurgery
The University of Texas Medical School at Houston
Houston, Texas
  Ch. 366: Microsurgery of Paraclinoid Aneurysms

Antonio A. F. De Salles, MD, PhD
Professor
Department of Neurosurgery;
Head
Division of Stereotactic Surgery
David Geffen School of Medicine at UCLA
University of California, Los Angeles
Los Angeles, California
  Ch. 20: Molecular Imaging of the Brain with Positron Emission Tomography
  Ch. 255: Linear Accelerator Radiosurgery: Technical Aspects

Amir R. Dehdashti, MD
Director
Cerebrovascular and Skull Base Surgery
Department of Neurosurgery
Geisinger Neurosciences Institute
Danville, Pennsylvania;
Assistant Professor
Temple University School of Medicine
Philadelphia, Pennsylvania
  Ch. 367: Intracranial Internal Carotid Artery Aneurysms

Oscar H. Del Brutto, MD
Coordinator
Stroke Unit
Hospital-Clínica Kennedy
Guayaquil, Ecuador
  Ch. 46: Parasitic Infections

Johnny B. Delashaw Jr, MD
Professor and Neurosurgeon
Department of Neurological Surgery
School of Medicine
Oregon Health & Science University
Portland, Oregon
  Ch. 140: Chordomas and Chondrosarcomas

Bradley Delman, MD
Associate Professor
Department of Radiology
Mount Sinai School of Medicine
New York, New York
  Ch. 19: Physiologic Evaluation of the Brain with Magnetic Resonance Imaging

Mahlon R. DeLong, MD
Professor
Department of Neurology
Emory University School of Medicine
Atlanta, Georgia
  Ch. 73: Rationale for Surgical Interventions in Movement Disorders

Franco DeMonte, MD
Professor and Mary Beth Pawelek Chair
Department of Neurosurgery
The University of Texas M. D. Anderson Cancer Center
Houston, Texas
  Ch. 142: Neoplasms of the Paranasal Sinuses

Sanjay S. Dhall, MD
Spine Fellow
University of California, San Francisco
San Francisco, California
  Ch. 293: Cervical Arthroplasty

Mark S. Dias, MD
Professor
Department of Neurosurgery
Penn State University College of Medicine;
Vice Chair
Department of Clinical Neurosurgery;
Director
Department of Pediatric Neurosurgery
Penn State Milton S. Hershey Medical Center
Hershey, Pennsylvania
  Ch. 175: Normal and Abnormal Embryology of the Brain

Curtis A. Dickman, MD
Associate Chief
Spine Section
Barrow Neurological Institute
Phoenix, Arizona
  Ch. 291: Basic Principles of Spinal Internal Fixation
  Ch. 297: Anterior Cervical Instrumentation
  Ch. 306: Thoracoscopic Approaches to the Spine

W. Dalton Dietrich, PhD
Professor
Department of Neurological Surgery
University of Miami Miller School of Medicine
Miami, Florida
  Ch. 329: Current Concepts of Hypothermia in Traumatic Brain Injury

Paul A. Gardner, MD
Assistant Professor
Co-Director
Cranial Base Surgery
Department of Neurosurgery
University of Pittsburgh Medical Center
Pittsburgh, Pennsylvania
Ch. 147: Tumors of the Orbit

Mark Garrett, MD
Resident
Department of Neurosurgery
Barrow Neurological Institute
Phoenix, Arizona
Ch. 280: Anterior Approach for Cervical Spondylotic Myelopathy

Hugh Garton, MD, MHSc
Associate Professor
Department of Neurosurgery
University of Michigan Health System
Ann Arbor, Michigan
Ch. 11: Neurosurgical Epidemiology and Outcomes Assessment

Cormac G. Gavin, MB, BCh, BAO, FRCS(I), FRCS
Specialist Registrar
Victor Horsley Department of Neurosurgery
National Hospital for Neurology and Neurosurgery
London, United Kingdom
Ch. 383: Pathobiology of True Arteriovenous Malformations

Alisa D. Gean, MD
Professor
Departments of Radiology and Biomedical Imaging
Adjunct Professor
Departments of Neurology and Neurological Surgery
University of California, San Francisco;
Brain and Spinal Injury Center (BASIC)
San Francisco General Hospital
San Francisco, California
Ch. 330: Imaging of Traumatic Brain Injury

Thomas A. Gennarelli, MD, FACS
Professor
Department of Neurosurgery
Medical College of Wisconsin
Milwaukee, Wisconsin
Ch. 324: Biomechanical Basis of Traumatic Brain Injury

Venelin Gerganov, MD
Associate Neurosurgeon
Department of Neurosurgery
International Neuroscience Institute
Hannover, Germany
Ch. 116: Basic Principles of Skull Base Surgery

Anand V. Germanwala, MD
Assistant Professor
Division of Neurological Surgery
University of North Carolina at Chapel Hill School of
    Medicine
Chapel Hill, North Carolina
Ch. 368: Anterior Communicating Artery Aneurysms

Massimo Gerosa, MD
Professor
Department of Neurosurgery
University of Verona;
Chairman
Department of Neurosurgery
Ospedale di Borgo Trento
Verona, Italy
Ch. 141: Glomus Tumors

Elizabeth R. Gerstner
Assistant Professor
Department of Neurology
Harvard University;
Assistant in Neurology
Massachusetts General Hospital
Boston, Massachusetts
Ch. 129: Central Nervous System Lymphoma

Peter C. Gerszten, MD, MPH, FACS
Professor
Departments of Neurological Surgery and Radiation Oncology
University of Pittsburgh Medical Center
Pittsburgh, Pennsylvania
*Ch. 263: Radiosurgery for Benign Spine Tumors and Vascular
    Malformations*

Saadi Ghatan, MD, FACS
Florence Irving Assistant Professor of Neurosurgery
Department of Neurosurgery
Columbia University College of Physicians and Surgeons
New York, New York
Ch. 176: Encephalocele

Samer Ghostine, MD
Director, Neurosurgery Spine;
Department of Neurosurgery
Assistant Professor
Department of Clinical Neurosurgery
University of California, Irvine
Irvine, California
Ch. 283: Treatment of Thoracic Disk Herniation

Steven Giannotta, MD
Professor
Department of Neurological Surgery
University of Southern California Keck School of Medicine
Los Angeles, California
Ch. 372: Basilar Trunk Aneurysms

Paul R. Gigante, MD, BS
Resident
Department of Neurological Surgery
Columbia University Medical Center
New York, New York
> Ch. 27: *Patient Positioning for Spinal Surgery*
> Ch. 346: *Circulatory Arrest with Deep Hypothermia*

Frank Gilliam, MD, MPH
Professor
Department of Neurology
Weill Cornell Medical College
Cornell University
New York, New York
> Ch. 52: *Diagnosis and Classification of Seizures and Epilepsy*

Holly Gilmer-Hill, MD
Department of Neurological Surgery
University of California, Davis Medical Center
Davis, California
> Ch. 238: *Piriformis Syndrome, Obturator Internus Syndrome, Pudendal Nerve Entrapment, and Other Pelvic Entrapments*

Albert Gjedde, MD, DSc, FRSC
Professor
Department of Neurobiology and Pharmacology;
Chair
Department of Neuroscience and Pharmacology
University of Copenhagen
Copenhagen, Denmark
> Ch. 7: *Cellular Mechanisms of Brain Energy Metabolism*

Roberta P. Glick, MD
Professor
Departments of Neurosurgery and Anatomy and Cell Biology
Mount Sinai Hospital;
Rush University Medical Center;
University of Illinois at Chicago
Chicago, Illinois
> Ch. 97: *Brain Tumor Immunology and Immunotherapy*

Ziya L. Gokaslan, MD, FACS
Professor
Departments of Neurosurgery, Oncology, and Orthopaedic Surgery
Donlin M. Long Professor of Neurosurgery
Vice-Chair and Director
Spine Center
Department of Neurosurgery
Johns Hopkins University School of Medicine
The Johns Hopkins Hospital
Baltimore, Maryland
> Ch. 310: *Evaluation and Management of Spinal Axis Tumors: Benign and Primary Malignant*

Yakov Gologorsky, MD
Senior Resident
Department of Neurosurgery
Mount Sinai Hospital
New York, New York
> Ch. 396: *Endovascular Treatment of Spinal Vascular Malformations*

Kiarash Golshani, MD
Fellow
Neurosurgery and Neurointerventional Radiology
Duke University Medical Center
Durham, North Carolina
> Ch. 382: *Traumatic Cerebral Aneurysms Secondary to Penetrating Intracranial Injuries*

Nestor R. Gonzalez, MD
Assistant Professor
Departments of Neurosurgery and Radiology
David Geffen School of Medicine at UCLA
University of California, Los Angeles
Los Angeles, California
> Ch. 380: *Revascularization Techniques for Complex Aneurysms and Skull Base Tumors*

James Tait Goodrich, MD, PhD, DSci
Professor
Departments of Clinical Neurosurgery, Pediatrics, and Plastic and Reconstructive Surgery
Albert Einstein College of Medicine;
Director
Division of Pediatric Neurosurgery
Leo Davidoff Department of Neurological Surgery
Children's Hospital at Montefiore
Bronx, New York
> Ch. 1: *Historical Overview of Neurosurgery*
> Ch. 180: *Craniopagus Twins*

Tessa Gordon, PhD
Emeritus Professor and Senior Scientist
University of Alberta
Edmonton, Canada;
Senior Scientist
Hospital for Sick Children
University of Toronto
Toronto, Canada
> Ch. 230: *Pathophysiology of Surgical Nerve Disorders*

Alessandra A. Gorgulho, MD, MSc
Director of Research
Adjunct Instructor
Division of Stereotactic Surgery
Department of Neurosurgery
David Geffen School of Medicine at UCLA
University of California, Los Angeles
Los Angeles, California
> Ch. 255: *Linear Accelerator Radiosurgery: Technical Aspects*

Liliana C. Goumnerova, MD
Associate Professor of Surgery (Neurosurgery)
Harvard Medical School;
Director
Clinical Pediatric Neurosurgical Oncology
Children's Hospital/Dana Farber Cancer Institute
Boston, Massachusetts
> Ch. 203: *Brainstem Glioma*

M. Sean Grady, MD
Professor and Chair
Department of Neurosurgery
University of Pennsylvania School of Medicine
Philadelphia, Pennsylvania
    Ch. 32: Cranioplasty
    *Ch. 333: Initial Resuscitation, Prehospital Care, and Emergency
    Room Care of Traumatic Brain Injury*

Jordan Grafman, PhD
Chief
Cognitive Neuroscience Section
National Institute of Neurological Disorders and Stroke
Bethesda, Maryland
    Ch. 16: Neuropsychological Testing

Sylvie Grand, MD
Assistant Professor
Joseph Fourier University
Grenoble, France
    *Ch. 80: Subthalamic Deep Brain Stimulation for Parkinson's
    Disease*

Gerald A. Grant, MD
Associate Professor
Department of Pediatric Neurosurgery
Duke University School of Medicine
Durham, North Carolina
    Ch. 8: Blood-Brain Barrier
    *Ch. 194: General Approaches and Considerations for Pediatric
    Brain Tumors*
    Ch. 337: Blast-Induced Neurotrauma

Gregory P. Graziano, MD
Associate Professor
Department of Orthopaedic Surgery
Chief
Orthopaedic Spine Division
Department of Orthopaedic Surgery
University of Michigan Health System
Ann Arbor, Michigan
    *Ch. 281: Spondyloarthropathies (Including Ankylosing
    Spondylitis)*

Benjamin Greenberg, MD, PhD
Associate Professor
Department of Psychiatry and Human Behavior
Warren Alpert Medical School at Brown University;
Butler Hospital
Providence, Rhode Island
    Ch. 88: Surgery for Obsessive-Compulsive Disorder

James Guest, MD
Associate Professor
Department of Neurological Surgery
University of Miami Miller School of Medicine
Miami, Florida
    *Ch. 267: Principles of Translation of Biologic Therapies in Spinal
    Cord Injury*

Abhijit Guha, MSc, MD, FRCSC, FACS
Professor of Surgery (Neurosurgery)
University of Toronto;
Alan and Susan Hudson Chair in Neuro-oncology
University Health Network;
Senior Scientist and Co-Director
Arthur and Sonia Labatt Brain Tumour Center Research
    Centre
Hospital for Sick Children
Toronto, Canada
    Ch. 101: Growth Factors in Glial Tumors
    *Ch. 245: Surgery for Malignant Peripheral Nerve Sheath
    Tumors*

Murat Günel, MD
Nixdorff-German Professor
Chief
Yale Neurovascular Surgery Program
Co-Director
Yale Program on Neurogenetics
Departments of Neurosurgery and Genetics
Yale University School of Medicine
New Haven, Connecticut
    Ch. 393: Genetics of Cerebral Cavernous Malformations

Gaurav Gupta, MD
Chief Resident
Department of Neurological Surgery
University of Medicine and Dentistry of New Jersey–New
    Jersey Medical School
Newark, New Jersey
    *Ch. 245: Surgery for Malignant Peripheral Nerve Sheath
    Tumors*

Nalin Gupta, MD, PhD
Associate Professor
Departments of Neurological Surgery and Pediatrics
University of California, San Francisco;
Chief
Division of Pediatric Neurosurgery
University of California, San Francisco
Benioff Children's Hospital
San Francisco, California
    Ch. 193: Shunt Infections and Their Treatment

Jorge Guridi, MD, PhD
Assistant Professor
Department of Neurological Surgery
Clínica Universitaria
Navarra University
Pamplona, Spain
    *Ch. 81: Subthalamotomy in Parkinson's Disease: Indications and
    Outcome*

Barton L. Guthrie, MD
Professor
Division of Neurosurgery
Department of Surgery
University of Alabama at Birmingham
Birmingham, Alabama
    *Ch. 132: Meningeal Sarcoma and Meningeal
    Hemangiopericytoma*

Georges F. Haddad, MD, FRCS(C)
Clinical Associate Professor
Division of Neurosurgery
American University of Beirut
Beirut, Lebanon
    Ch. 131: Meningiomas

Michael M. Haglund, MD, PhD
Professor and Program Training Director
Departments of Neurosurgery and Neurobiology
Division of Neurosurgery
Department of Surgery
Duke University Medical Center
Durham, North Carolina
    Ch. 57: Motor, Sensory, and Language Mapping and Monitoring for Cortical Resections

Regis W. Haid Jr, MD
Medical Director
Piedmont Spine Center
Neuroscience Service Line
Piedmont Hospital;
Atlanta Brain and Spine Care
Atlanta, Georgia
    Ch. 293: Cervical Arthroplasty

Stephen J. Haines, MD
Lyle A. French Chair, Professor and Head
Department of Neurosurgery
University of Minnesota
Minneapolis, Minnesota
    Ch. 11: Neurosurgical Epidemiology and Outcomes Assessment
    Ch. 42: The Use and Misuse of Antibiotics in Neurosurgery

Clement Hamani, MD, PhD
Assistant Professor
Division of Neurosurgery
Toronto Western Hospital
University of Toronto
Toronto, Canada
    Ch. 89: Surgical Treatment of Major Depression
    Ch. 165: Evidence Base: Neurostimulation for Pain

Bronwyn E. Hamilton, MD
Associate Professor of Radiology
Director
Magnetic Resonance Imaging
School of Medicine
Oregon Health & Science University
Portland, Oregon
    Ch. 357: Cerebral Venous and Sinus Thrombosis

D. Kojo Hamilton, MD
Assistant Professor
Department of Neurosurgery
University of Maryland School of Medicine
Baltimore, Maryland
    Ch. 288: Flat Back and Sagittal Plane Deformity

Todd C. Hankinson, MD, MBA
Assistant Professor
Department of Neurosurgery
The Children's Hospital of Denver
University of Colorado Denver
Aurora, Colorado
    Ch. 214: Myelomeningocele and Myelocystocele

Leo T. Happel, PhD
Emeritus Professor Neurology, Neurosurgery, Physiology and Neuroscience
Department of Neurosurgery
Louisiana State University Health Sciences Center
New Orleans, Louisiana
    Ch. 234: Operative Neurophysiology of Peripheral Nerves

Ihtsham Ul Haq, MD
Assistant Professor
Department of Neurology
Wake Forest University Baptist Medical Center
Winston Salem, North Carolina
    Ch. 75: Clinical Overview of Movement Disorders

Raqeeb Haque, MD
Resident
Department of Neurological Surgery
Columbia University Medical Center
New York, New York
    Ch. 377: Endovascular Hunterian Ligation

Robert E. Harbaugh, MD, FACS, FAHA
Director
Institute of the Neurosciences
University Distinguished Professor and Chair
Department of Neurosurgery;
Professor
Department of Engineering Science & Mechanics
Chair
Department of Neurosurgery Penn State University College of Medicine
Penn State Milton S. Hershey Medical Center
Hershey, Pennsylvania
    Ch. 349: Carotid Occlusive Disease: Natural History and Medical Management

Ciara D. Harraher, MD, MPH
Clinical Instructor
Department of Neurosurgery
Stanford University Medical Center
Stanford, California
    Ch. 149: Scalp Tumors

Leo Harris, PA
Physician's Assistant
Department of Neurological Surgery
University of Miami
Jackson Memorial Hospital in Florida
Miami, Florida
    Ch. 335: Surgical Management of Traumatic Brain Injury

Geoffrey T. Manley, MD, PhD
Professor and Vice Chairman
Department of Neurological Surgery
University of California, San Francisco;
Chief of Neurosurgery and Co-Director
Brain and Spinal Injury Center
San Francisco General Hospital
San Francisco, California
    Ch. 23: Intracranial Pressure Monitoring

Daniel Marchac, MD
Professor
Collège de Médecine des Hôpitaux de Paris;
Chirurgie Plastique Reconstructrice et Esthétique
Chirurgie Cranio-Faciale
Paris, France
    Ch. 183: Syndromic Craniosynostosis

†Anthony Marmarou, PhD
Professor
Virginia Commonwealth University Medical College
Richmond, Virginia
    Ch. 10: Physiology of the Cerebrospinal Fluid and Intracranial Pressure

Joseph C. Maroon, MD
Professor and Vice Chairman
Department of Neurosurgery
Heindl Scholar in Neuroscience
University of Pittsburgh Medical Center;
Team Neurosurgeon
The Pittsburgh Steelers
Pittsburgh, Pennsylvania
    Ch. 147: Tumors of the Orbit
    Ch. 332: Mild Traumatic Brain Injury in Adults and Concussion in Sports

Lawrence F. Marshall, MD
Distinguished Professor of Neurosurgery
Chair Emeritus
UCSD Medical Center
San Diego, California
    Ch. 38: Medical and Surgical Management of Chronic Subdural Hematomas
    Ch. 341: Traumatic Cerebrospinal Fluid Fistulas

Neil A. Martin, MD
W. Eugene Stern Professor and Chairman
Department of Neurosurgery
David Geffen School of Medicine at UCLA
University of California, Los Angeles;
Ronald Reagan UCLA Medical Center
Los Angeles, California
    Ch. 380: Revascularization Techniques for Complex Aneurysms and Skull Base Tumors

Timothy J. Martin, MD
Associate Professor
Department of Surgical Sciences/Ophthalmology and Neurology
Wake Forest University School of Medicine
Winston Salem, North Carolina
    Ch. 13: Neuro-ophthalmology

Alexander M. Mason, MD
Neurological Surgery
Boulder Neurosurgical Associates
Boulder, Colorado
    Ch. 370: Surgical Management of Middle Cerebral Artery Aneurysms

Marlon S. Mathews, MD
Resident
Department of Neurological Surgery
University at Buffalo
State University New York
Buffalo, New York
    Ch. 160: Trigeminal Neuralgia: Diagnosis and Nonoperative Management

Helen S. Mayberg, MD
Professor
Departments of Psychiatry and Neurology
Dorothy C. Fuqua Chair in Psychiatric Neuroimaging and Therapeutics
Department of Psychiatry
Emory University School of Medicine
Atlanta, Georgia
    Ch. 89: Surgical Treatment of Major Depression

James P. McAllister II, PhD
Professor and Director
Basic Hydrocephalus Research
Primary Children's Medical Center;
Professor
Departments of Bioengineering and Physiology
Department of Neurosurgery
Division of Pediatric Neurosurgery
University of Utah
Salt Lake City, Utah
    Ch. 189: Experimental Hydrocephalus

J. Gordon McComb, MD
Professor and Head
Division of Neurosurgery
Children's Hospital Los Angeles;
Department of Neurological Surgery
University of Southern California Keck School of Medicine
Los Angeles, California
    Ch. 188: Cerebrospinal Fluid Physiology

Paul C. McCormick, MD, MPH
Herbert and Linda Gallen Professor of Neurological Surgery
Columbia University College of Physicians and Surgeons
New York, New York
  Ch. 27: Patient Positioning for Spinal Surgery
  Ch. 279: Posterior Approach to Cervical Degenerative Disease
  Ch. 300: Anterior Thoracic Instrumentation
  Ch. 309: Spinal Cord Tumors in Adults

Ian E. McCutcheon, MD
Professor
Department of Neurosurgery
The University of Texas M. D. Anderson Cancer Center
Houston, Texas
  Ch. 44: Meningitis and Encephalitis
  Ch. 148: Skull Tumors

Michael W. McDermott, MD
Professor and Vice Chairman
Department of Neurological Surgery
University of California, San Francisco
San Francisco, California
  Ch. 251: Fractionated Radiation Therapy for Benign Brain Tumors
  Ch. 253: Interstitial and Intracavitary Irradiation of Brain Tumors

Cameron G. McDougall, MD, FRCSC
Director
Endovascular Neurosurgery
Lou and Evelyn Grubb Endowed Chair for Neurovascular Research
Barrow Neurological Institute
Phoenix, Arizona
  Ch. 374: Endovascular Approaches to Intracranial Aneurysms
  Ch. 375: Endovascular Coiling of Intracranial Aneurysms: Supporting Evidence

Matthew McGehee, MD
Medical Director
Pain Management Program
Progressive Rehabilitation Associates
Portland, Oregon
  Ch. 158: Management of Pain by Anesthetic Techniques

Cameron C. McIntyre, PhD
Associate Professor
Department of Biomedical Engineering
Cleveland Clinic
Cleveland, Ohio
  Ch. 83: Deep Brain Stimulation: Mechanisms of Action

Guy M. McKhann II, MD
Florence Irving Associate Professor of Neurological Surgery
Columbia University College of Physicians
New York Presbyterian Hospital
New York, New York
  Ch. 48: Epilepsy Surgery Overview
  Ch. 49: Electrophysiologic Properties of the Mammalian Central Nervous System
  Ch. 58: Auditory Language Mapping

M. Sean McKisic, MD
Resident
Department of Neurosurgery
University of Virginia
Charlottesville, Virginia
  Ch. 26: Positioning for Cranial Surgery
  Ch. 321: Osteoporotic Fractures: Evaluation and Treatment with Vertebroplasty and Kyphoplasty

David F. Meaney, PhD
Professor
Department of Bioengineering
University of Pennsylvania School of Engineering and Applied Science
Philadelphia, Pennsylvania
  Ch. 324: Biomechanical Basis of Traumatic Brain Injury

Minesh P. Mehta, MD, FASTRO
Professor
Department of Radiation Oncology
Northwestern University Feinberg School of Medicine
Chicago, Illinois
  Ch. 250: Fractionated Radiation Therapy for Malignant Brain Tumors

Vivek Mehta, MD, MSc (Epid), FRCSC, FACS
Assistant Professor
Department of Neurosurgery
University of Alberta
Edmonton, Canada
  Ch. 135: Craniopharyngioma in Adults

William P. Melega, PhD
Professor
Department of Molecular and Medical Pharmacology
David Geffen School of Medicine at UCLA
University of California, Los Angeles
Los Angeles, California
  Ch. 20: Molecular Imaging of the Brain with Positron Emission Tomography

Arnold H. Menezes, MD
Professor and Vice Chairman
Department of Neurosurgery
University of Iowa Carver College of Medicine;
Professor of Neurosurgery
University of Iowa Hospitals and Clinics
Iowa City, Iowa
  Ch. 218: Developmental Abnormalities of the Craniocervical Junction
  Ch. 289: Acquired Abnormalities of the Craniocervical Junction
  Ch. 308: Tumors of the Craniovertebral Junction

Patrick Mertens, MD, PhD
Professor of Anatomy
Department of Neurosurgery Chairman
Hôpital Neurologique P. Wertheimer
Claude-Bernard Lyon 1 University
Lyon, France
  Ch. 90: Ablative Surgery for Spasticity

Fredric B. Meyer, MD, FACS
Professor and Chair
Department of Neurological Surgery
Mayo Clinic
Rochester, Minnesota
Ch. 343: *Cerebral Blood Flow and Metabolism and Cerebral Ischemia*
Ch. 350: *Carotid Endarterectomy*
Ch. 381: *Multimodality Management of Complex Cerebrovascular Lesions*
Ch. 390: *Carotid-Cavernous Fistulas*

Scott A. Meyer, MD
Resident
Mount Sinai School of Medicine
New York, New York
Ch. 133: *Acoustic Neuroma*
Ch. 379: *Infectious Intracranial Aneurysms*

Philip M. Meyers, MD
Associate Professor
Departments of Radiology and Neurological Surgery
Columbia University College of Physicians and Surgeons;
Clinical Director
Neuroendovascular Service
New York-Presbyterian Hospital
New York, New York
Ch. 386: *Adjuvant Endovascular Management of Arteriovenous Malformations*
Ch. 387: *Endovascular Management of Arteriovenous Malformations for Cure*

Costas Michaelides, MRCP (UK)
Clinical and Research Fellow in Epilepsy and Clinical Neurophysiology
Massachusetts General Hospital
Harvard Medical School
Boston, Massachusetts
Ch. 56: *Evaluation of Patients for Epilepsy Surgery*

Karine Michaud, MD
Clinical Instructor and Fellow
Department of Neuro-oncology
University of California, San Francisco
San Francisco, California
Ch. 112: *Principles of Chemotherapy*

Rajiv Midha, MD, MSc, FRCS(C)
Chief
Division of Neurosurgery
Professor
Department of Clinical Neurosciences
University of Calgary
Calgary, Canada
Ch. 230: *Pathophysiology of Surgical Nerve Disorders*
Ch. 231: *Peripheral Nerve Examination, Evaluation, and Biopsy*
Ch. 239: *Techniques and Options in Nerve Reconstruction and Repair*

Vincent J. Miele, MD
Department of Neurosurgery
UHC Neurosurgery and Spine Center
Clarksburg, West Virginia
Ch. 265: *Concepts and Mechanisms of Spinal Biomechanics*

Jonathan Miller, MD
Assistant Professor
Department of Neurological Surgery
Case Western Reserve University School of Medicine;
Director
Department of Functional and Restorative Neurosurgery
University Hospitals Case Medical Center
Cleveland, Ohio
Ch. 163: *Microvascular Decompression for Trigeminal Neuralgia*

Matthew L. Miller, MD
Resident
Department of Neurosurgery
Medical College of Wisconsin
Milwaukee, Wisconsin
Ch. 299: *Posterior Subaxial and Cervicothoracic Instrumentation*

Neil R. Miller, MD
Professor
Departments of Ophthalmology, Neurology, and Neurosurgery
Frank B. Walsh Professor of Neuro-Ophthalmology
Johns Hopkins University School of Medicine
Baltimore, Maryland
Ch. 150: *Pseudotumor Cerebri*

John Mitrofanis, PhD
Professor of Anatomy
Associate Dean (Curriculum)
Department of Anatomy and Histology
University of Sydney
Sydney, Australia
Ch. 80: *Subthalamic Deep Brain Stimulation for Parkinson's Disease*

Kevin Y. Miyashiro
Department of Pharmacology
Department of Psychiatry
University of Pennsylvania School of Medicine
Philadelphia, Pennsylvania
Ch. 3: *Molecular Biology Primer for Neurosurgeons*

J. Mocco, MD, MS
Assistant Professor
Departments of Neurologic Surgery and Radiology
College of Medicine
University of Florida
Gainesville, Florida
Ch. 351: *Carotid Artery Angioplasty and Stenting*

Michael T. Modic, MD
Professor of Radiology
Cleveland Clinic Lerner College of Medicine of Case Western
    Reserve University;
Chairman
Neurological Institute
Cleveland Clinic
Cleveland, Ohio
    Ch. 18: Radiology of the Spine

Parham Moftakhar, MD
Resident in Neurosurgery
Cedars-Sinai Medical Center
Los Angeles, California
    Ch. 353: Nonatherosclerotic Carotid Lesions

Avinash Mohan, MD
Assistant Professor
Departments of Neurosurgery and Pediatrics
New York Medical College;
Assistant Professor
Departments of Neurosurgery and Pediatrics
Westchester Medical Center
Maria Farreri Children's Hospital
Valhalla, New York
    Ch. 195: Optic Pathway Hypothalamic Gliomas
    Ch. 212: Birth Head Trauma

Stephen J. Monteith, MD
Resident
Department of Neurosurgery
University of Virginia
Charlottesville, Virginia
    Ch. 162: Stereotactic Radiosurgery for Trigeminal Neuralgia

Jacques J. Morcos, MD, FRCS(Eng), FRCS(Ed)
Professor
Department of Neurological Surgery and Otolaryngology
University of Miami Miller School of Medicine
Miami, Florida
    Ch. 358: Nonlesional Spontaneous Intracerebral Hemorrhage

**Michael Morgan, MD, PhD (Honorary), BS, MMedEd,
FRACS**
Professor and Dean
Australian School of Advanced Medicine
Macquarie University
Sydney, Australia
    Ch. 385: Therapeutic Decision Making

David E. Morris, MD
Associate Professor
Department of Radiation Oncology
Director
UNC Cyberknife Program
Lineberger Comprehensive Cancer Center
University of North Carolina at Chapel Hill
Chapel Hill, North Carolina
    Ch. 257: Image-Guided Robotic Radiosurgery: The CyberKnife

S. David Moss, MD
Associate Professor
Department of Neurosurgery
University of Arizona
Tucson;
Director
Pediatric Neurosurgical Training
Cardon Children's Hospital
Mesa, Arizona
    Ch. 185: Plagiocephaly

J. Paul Muizelaar, MD, PhD
Professor
Department of Neurological Surgery
University of California, Davis
Sacramento, California
    Ch. 331: Clinical Pathophysiology of Traumatic Brain Injury

Karim Mukhida, MD
Resident
Division of Neurosurgery
University of Toronto
Toronto, Canada
    *Ch. 84: Emerging and Experimental Neurosurgical Treatments
    for Parkinson's Disease*

Praveen V. Mummaneni, MD
Associate Professor
Department of Neurosurgery
University of California, San Francisco;
Co-Director
UCSF Spine Center
San Francisco, California
    Ch. 293: Cervical Arthroplasty
    Ch. 296: Spinopelvic Fixation
    *Ch. 304: Posterior, Transforaminal, and Anterior Interbody
    Fusion: Techniques and Instrumentation*

Gregory J. A. Murad, MD
Assistant Professor
Department of Neurosurgery
University of Florida
Gainesville, Florida
    Ch. 258: Radiosurgery for Malignant Tumors

Karin Muraszko, MD
Julian T. Hoff Professor and Chair
Department of Neurosurgery
University of Michigan Health System
Ann Arbor, Michigan
    Ch. 124: Primitive Neuroectodermal Tumors

Antônio C. M. Mussi, MD, PhD
Staff Neurosurgeon
Hospital de Caridad
Hospital Governador Celso Ramos
Florianópolis, Brazil
    Ch. 2: Surgical Anatomy of the Brain

Imad Najm, MD
Director
Basic Sciences
Cleveland Clinic Lerner College of Medicine of Case Western
    Reserve University;
Director
Cleveland Clinic Epilepsy Center
Cleveland Clinic
Cleveland, Ohio
    Ch. 62: Standard Temporal Lobectomy

Peter Nakaji, MD
Director
Neurosurgery Residency Program
Barrow Neurological Institute
Phoenix, Arizona
    Ch. 119: Endoscopic Approaches to Brain Tumors

Sandra Narayanan, MD
Fellow
Interventional Neuroradiology
Emory University Hospital
Atlanta, Georgia
    *Ch. 391: Treatment of Other Intracranial Dural Arteriovenous
    Fistulas*

David W. Newell, MD
Executive Director
Swedish Neuroscience Institute
Seattle, Washington
    *Ch. 347: Transcranial Doppler Ultrasonography and
    Neurosonology*

M. Kelly Nicholas, MD, PhD
Director
Neuro-oncology Service
University of Chicago
Chicago, Illinois
    Ch. 45: Acquired Immune Deficiency Syndrome

Yasunari Niimi, MD, DMSc
Professor
Departments of Clinical Radiology and Neurosurgery
Albert Einstein College of Medicine;
Attending Physician
Roosevelt Hospital and Beth Israel Medical Center
New York, New York
    Ch. 208: Vein of Galen Aneurysmal Malformation

Shahid M. Nimjee, MD, PhD
Neurosurgery Resident
Division of Neurosurgery
Duke University Medical Center
Durham, North Carolina
    Ch. 8: Blood-Brain Barrier

Ajay Niranjan, MD, MBA
Associate Professor
Department of Neurological Surgery
University of Pittsburgh;
Director
Brain Mapping Center
University of Pittsburgh Medical Center
Pittsburgh, Pennsylvania
    Ch. 256: Gamma Knife Radiosurgery

Richard B. North, MD
Neurosurgeon
Berman Brain and Spine Institute;
Professor (Retired)
Departments of Neurosurgery, Anesthesiology, and Critical
    Care Medicine
Johns Hopkins University School of Medicine
Baltimore, Maryland
    Ch. 164: Neurosurgical Management of Intractable Pain

Josef Novotny, Jr, MSc, PhD
Assistant Professor and Medical Physicist
Department of Radiation Oncology
University of Pittsburgh Medical Center
Pittsburgh, Pennsylvania
    Ch. 256: Gamma Knife Radiosurgery

Turo Nurmikko, MD, PhD
Professor
Department of Pain Science
Faculty of Health and Life Sciences
University of Liverpool;
Honorary Consultant in Pain Relief
Walton Centre for Neurology and Neurosurgery NHS Trust;
Pain Research Institute
Liverpool, United Kingdom
    *Ch. 159: Evidence-Based Approach to the Treatment of Facial
    Pain*

Samuel E. Nutt, BS
Department of Neurological Surgery
University of Washington
Seattle, Washington
    Ch. 5: Stem Cell Biology in the Central Nervous System

W. Jerry Oakes, MD
Professor
Division of Neurosurgery
University of Alabama at Birmingham
Children's Hospital
Birmingham, Alabama
    Ch. 179: Chiari Malformations

José A. Obeso
Department of Neurology
Clínica Universitaria and Medical School of Navarra
Neuroscience Centre (CIMA)
University of Navarra
Navarra, Spain
    *Ch. 81: Subthalamotomy in Parkinson's Disease: Indications and
    Outcome*

Alfred T. Ogden, MD
Assistant Professor
Department of Neurological Surgery
Neurological Institute of New York
Columbia University Medical Center
New York, New York
>   Ch. 307: *Minimally Invasive Techniques for Lumbar Disorders*
>   Ch. 309: *Spinal Cord Tumors in Adults*

Lissa Ogieglo, MD
Resident
Department of Neurosurgery
University of Saskatchewan
Saskatoon, Canada
>   Ch. 142: *Neoplasms of the Paranasal Sinuses*

Christopher S. Ogilvy, MD
Director
Endovascular and Operative Neurovascular Surgery
Massachusetts General Hospital;
Robert G. and A. Jean Ojemann Professor of Neurosurgery
Harvard Medical School
Boston, Massachusetts
>   Ch. 371: *Microsurgery of Vertebral Artery, Posterior Inferior Cerebellar Artery, and Vertebrobasilar Junction Aneurysms*

David O. Okonkwo, MD, PhD
Chief
Division of Neurotrauma
University of Pittsburgh Medical Center
Pittsburgh, Pennsylvania
>   Ch. 318: *Diagnosis and Management of Thoracic Spine Fractures*

Michael S. Okun, MD
Associate Professor
Department of Neurology and Neurosurgery
Co-Director
Movement Disorders Center
McKnight Brain Institute
University of Florida
Gainesville, Florida
>   Ch. 75: *Clinical Overview of Movement Disorders*

Edward H. Oldfield, MD
Crutchfield Professor of Neurosurgery
Professor of Internal Medicine
Department of Neurological Surgery
University of Virginia School of Medicine
Charlottesville, Virginia
>   Ch. 9: *Cerebral Edema*
>   Ch. 128: *Hemangioblastomas*
>   Ch. 397: *Spinal Vascular Malformations*

Alessandro Olivi, MD
Professor
Departments of Neurosurgery and Oncology
Director
Division of Neurosurgical Oncology
Department of Neurosurgery
Johns Hopkins University School of Medicine
Baltimore, Maryland
>   Ch. 111: *Brain Tumors during Pregnancy*
>   Ch. 114: *Frame and Frameless Stereotactic Brain Biopsy*

Stephen E. Olvey, MD
Associate Professor
Department of Clinical Neurology and Neurosurgery
University of Miami Miller School of Medicine;
Director
Neuroscience Intensive Care Unit
Jackson Memorial Hospital
Miami, Florida;
Founding Fellow
FIA Institute for Motor Sport Safety
Paris, France
>   Ch. 324: *Biomechanical Basis of Traumatic Brain Injury*

David Omahen, MD, FRCS(C)
Department of Clinical Neurosciences
Foothills Medical Centre
Calgary, Canada
>   Ch. 101: *Growth Factors in Glial Tumors*

Brent O'Neill, MD
Department of Neurosurgery
Allegheny General Hospital
Pittsburgh, Pennsylvania
>   Ch. 37: *Pathophysiology of Subdural Hematomas*

Rod J. Oskouian Jr, MD
Co-Director
Spine Fellowship
Swedish Neuroscience Specialists
Swedish Neuroscience Institute
Seattle, Washington
>   Ch. 288: *Flat Back and Sagittal Plane Deformity*
>   Ch. 321: *Osteoporotic Fractures: Evaluation and Treatment with Vertebroplasty/Kyphoplasty*

Robert Owen, MD
Assistant Professor
Department of Neurosurgery
University of Kentucky
Kentucky Children's Hospital
Lexington, Kentucky
>   Ch. 211: *Growing Skull Fracture*

Koray Özduman, MD
Assistant Professor
Department of Neurosurgery
Acibadem University School of Medicine
Istanbul, Turkey
>   Ch. 144: *Trigeminal Schwannomas*

Ali Kemal Ozturk, MD
Resident Physician
Department of Neurosurgery
Yale University School of Medicine
New Haven, Connecticut
> Ch. 393: *Genetics of Cerebral Cavernous Malformations*

M. Necmettin Pamir, MD
Professor and Chairman
Department of Neurosurgery
Acibadem University School of Medicine
Istanbul, Turkey
> Ch. 144: *Trigeminal Schwannomas*

Dachling Pang, MD, FRCS(C), FACS
Chief
Department of Pediatric Neurosurgery
Regional Center for Pediatric Neurosurgery
Kaiser Permanente Hospitals, Northern California
Oakland;
Professor of Pediatric Neurosurgery
Department of Neurological Surgery
University of California, Davis
Sacramento, California
> Ch. 224: *Pediatric Vertebral Column and Spinal Cord Injuries*

Jamie Pardini, PhD
Assistant Professor
Department of Orthopedic Surgery
University of Pittsburgh School of Medicine;
Neuropsychologist
Sports Concussion Program
University of Pittsburgh Medical Center
Pittsburgh, Pennsylvania
> Ch. 332: *Mild Traumatic Brain Injury in Adults and Concussion in Sports*

Andrew D. Parent, MD
Professor
Department of Neurosurgery
University of Mississippi Medical Center
Jackson, Mississippi
> Ch. 206: *Skull Tumors and Fibrous Dysplasia*

T. S. Park, MD
Shi H. Huang Professor of Neurological Surgery
Washington University School of Medicine;
Neurosurgeon-in-Chief
St. Louis Children's Hospital
St. Louis, Missouri
> Ch. 213: *Birth Brachial Plexus Injury*
> Ch. 227: *Selective Dorsal Rhizotomy for Spastic Cerebral Palsy*

Michael D. Partington, MD
Pediatric Neurosurgeon
Gillette Children's Specialty Healthcare
St. Paul, Minnesota
> Ch. 175: *Normal and Abnormal Embryology of the Brain*

Aman B. Patel, MD
Associate Professor
Departments of Neurosurgery and Radiology
Mount Sinai School of Medicine;
Director of Neuro-endovascular Surgery
Mount Sinai Hospital
New York, New York
> Ch. 396: *Endovascular Treatment of Spinal Vascular Malformations*

Parag G. Patil, MD, PhD
Assistant Professor
Departments of Neurosurgery, Anesthesiology, and Biomedical Engineering
University of Michigan Medical School
Ann Arbor, Michigan
> Ch. 92: *Treatment of Intractable Vertigo*

Nicola Pavese, MD
Senior Investigator Scientist
Honorary Clinical Senior Lecturer in Neurology
MRC Clinical Sciences Centre
Centre for Neuroscience
Division of Experimental Medicine
Imperial College
London, United Kingdom
> Ch. 77: *Functional Imaging in Movement Disorders*

Richard D. Penn, MD
Professor
Department of Neurology
University of Chicago
Chicago, Illinois
> Ch. 91: *Management of Spasticity by Central Nervous System Infusion Techniques*

Noel I. Perin, MD
Director
Division of Spine Surgery
St. Luke's-Roosevelt Hospital
New York, New York
> Ch. 320: *Sacral Fractures*

John A. Persing, MD
Professor and Chief
Plastic and Reconstructive Surgery
Yale University School of Medicine;
Attending Physician
Yale-New Haven Hospital
New Haven, Connecticut
> Ch. 29: *Incisions and Closures*
> Ch. 149: *Scalp Tumors*
> Ch. 182: *Craniosynostosis*

Erika A. Petersen, MD
Department of Neurological Surgery
The University of Texas Southwestern Medical School
Dallas, Texas
> Ch. 157: *Pharmacologic Treatment of Pain*

Anthony L. Petraglia, MD
Resident Physician
Department of Neurosurgery
University of Rochester Medical Center
Rochester, New York
Ch. 70: Epilepsy Surgery: Outcome and Complications

Brigitte Piallat, PhD
Assistant Professor
Grenoble Institute of Neuroscience
University of Grenoble I
INSERM U836
Grenoble, France
Ch. 80: Subthalamic Deep Brain Stimulation for Parkinson's Disease

Joseph H. Piatt, MD, FAAP
Professor
Department of Pediatrics
Drexel University College of Medicine;
Chief
Section of Neurosurgery
St. Christopher's Hospital for Children
Philadelphia, Pennsylvania
Ch. 182: Craniosynostosis

John D. Pickard, MA, MB, MChir, FRCS, FMedSci
Professor
Department of Neurosurgery
University of Cambridge;
Professor of Neurosurgery
Divisional Director
Neurosciences
Addenbrookes Hospital
Cambridge, United Kingdom
Ch. 34: Clinical Evaluation of Adult Hydrocephalus

Joseph M. Piepmeier, MD
Nixdorff/German Professor
Department of Neurosurgery
Yale University School of Medicine
New Haven, Connecticut
Ch. 123: Unusual Gliomas

Webster H. Pilcher, MD, PhD
Frank P. Smith Professor and Chairman of Neurosurgery
Department of Neurosurgery
University of Rochester Medical Center
Rochester, New York
Ch. 70: Epilepsy Surgery: Outcome and Complications

José Pineda, MD
Assistant Professor
Department of Pediatrics and Neurology
Washington University School of Medicine
St. Louis, Missouri
Ch. 174: Neurocritical Care in Children

Joseph D. Pinter, MD
Associate Professor
Department of Pediatrics (Pediatric Neurology)
Oregon Health & Science University
Portland, Oregon
Ch. 4: Neuroembryology

Mary L. Pisculli, MD, MPH
Clinical Instructor
Harvard Medical School;
Associate Physician
Division of Infectious Disease
Department of Medicine
Brigham and Women's Hospital
Boston, Massachusetts
Ch. 40: Postoperative Infections of the Head and Brain

Thomas Pittman, MD
Professor
Department of Neurosurgery
University of Kentucky
Kentucky Children's Hospital
Lexington, Kentucky
Ch. 211: Growing Skull Fracture

Ian F. Pollack, MD
Professor
Department of Neurosurgery
Vice Chair for Academic Affairs
University of Pittsburgh School of Medicine;
Chief
Department of Pediatric Neurosurgery
Children's Hospital of Pittsburgh
University of Pittsburgh Medical Center
Pittsburgh, Pennsylvania
Ch. 204: Intracranial Germ Cell Tumors

Pierre Pollak, MD
Professor and Chairman
Department of Neurology
University Hospital of Geneva
Geneva, Switzerland
Ch. 80: Subthalamic Deep Brain Stimulation for Parkinson's Disease

Bruce E. Pollock, MD
Professor
Departments of Neurological Surgery and Radiation Oncology
Mayo Clinic College of Medicine
Rochester, Minnesota
Ch. 260: Radiosurgery for Intracranial Vascular Malformations
Ch. 381: Multimodality Management of Complex Cerebrovascular Lesions

Prakash Sampath, MD
Department of Neurological Surgery
Johns Hopkins University School of Medicine
Baltimore, Maryland
Ch. 151: Sarcoidosis, Tuberculosis, and Xanthogranuloma

Srinath Samudrala, MD, FACS
Director
The Spine Institute
Glendale Adventist Medical Center
Glendale, California
Ch. 283: Treatment of Thoracic Disk Herniation

Nader Sanai, MD
Director
Department of Neurosurgical Oncology
Division of Neurological Surgery
Barrow Neurological Institute
Phoenix, Arizona
Ch. 121: Low-Grade Gliomas: Astrocytoma, Oligodendroglioma, and Mixed Glioma
Ch. 378: Microsurgical Management of Giant Intracranial Aneurysms

Robert A. Sanford, MD
Professor
Department of Neurosurgery
The University of Tennessee
Memphis, Tennessee
Ch. 198: Pediatric Craniopharyngioma

Paul Santiago, MD
Associate Professor
Departments of Neurological and Orthopaedic Surgery
Washington University School of Medicine
St. Louis, Missouri
Ch. 290: Congenital Abnormalities of the Thoracic and Lumbar Spine

Teresa Santiago-Sim, PhD
Assistant Professor
Department of Neurosurgery
The University of Texas Health Science Center at Houston
Houston, Texas
Ch. 361: Pathobiology of Intracranial Aneurysms

Harvey B. Sarnat, MS, MD, FRCPC
Professor
Departments of Paediatrics, Pathology (Neuropathology), and
  Clinical Neurosciences
University of Calgary Faculty of Medicine;
Alberta Children's Hospital
Calgary, Canada
Ch. 4: Neuroembryology

Raymond Sawaya, MD
Professor and Chairman
Department of Neurosurgery
Baylor College of Medicine;
Professor and Chairman
Department of Neurosurgery
The University of Texas M. D. Anderson Cancer Center
Houston, Texas
Ch. 95: Brain Tumors: General Considerations
Ch. 130: Metastatic Brain Tumors
Ch. 136: Epidermoid, Dermoid, and Neurenteric Cysts

W. Michael Scheld, MD
Professor
Department of Medicine
Clinical Professor
Department of Neurosurgery
University of Virginia
Charlottesville, Virginia
Ch. 39: Basic Science of Central Nervous System Infections
Ch. 43: Brain Abscess

Wouter I. Shirzadi, MD
Professor
Department of Neurosurgery
Director of Vascular Neurosurgery
Cedars-Sinai Medical Center
Los Angeles, California
Ch. 359: Genetics of Intracranial Aneurysms

Nicholas D. Schiff, MD
Professor
Department of Neurology and Neuroscience
Weill Cornell Medical College
New York, New York
Ch. 12: Altered Consciousness

Clemens M. Schirmer, MD
Assistant Professor
Department of Neurosurgery
Tufts University School of Medicine
Boston, Massachusetts;
Director
Cerebrovascular and Neuroendovascular Surgery
Baystate Medical Center
Springfield, Massachusetts
Ch. 203: Brainstem Glioma

David Schlesinger, PhD
Assistant Professor
Department of Radiation Oncology
University of Virginia
Charlottesville, Virginia
Ch. 249: The Radiobiology and Physics of Radiosurgery

Meic H. Schmidt, MD, FACS
Ronald Apfelbaum Endowed Chair in Spine Surgery
Associate Professor
Chief of Spine Surgery
Department of Neurosurgery
University of Utah
Salt Lake City, Utah
  Ch. 41: Postoperative Infections of the Spine

Joost W. Schouten, MD
Neurosurgeon
Erasmus Medical Center Rotterdam
Rotterdam, The Netherlands
  Ch. 323: Epidemiology of Traumatic Brain Injury

Johannes Schramm, MD
Professor and Chairman
Department of Neurosurgery
Bonn University Medical Center
Bonn, Germany
  Ch. 66: Hemispheric Disconnection Procedures

Thomas C. Schuler, MD, FACS
Chief Executive Officer
Virginia Spine Institute
Spinal Research Foundation
Reston, Virginia
  Ch. 266: Biomaterials and Biomechanics of Spinal Arthroplasty

James M. Schuster, MD, PhD
Associate Professor
Department of Neurosurgery
University of Pennsylvania
Philadelphia, Pennsylvania
  Ch. 301: Posterior Thoracic Instrumentation

Theodore H. Schwartz, MD, FACS
Professor
Departments of Neurosurgery, Otolaryngology, Neurology,
  and Neuroscience
Weill Cornell Medical College;
New York-Presbyterian Hospital
New York, New York
  Ch. 309: Spinal Cord Tumors in Adults

Judith A. Schwartzbaum, PhD
Associate Professor
Division of Epidemiology
College of Public Health
The Ohio State University
Columbus, Ohio
  Ch. 106: Epidemiology of Brain Tumors

Patrick M. Schweder, MD
Department of Neurosurgery
The Royal Melbourne Hospital
Parkville, Australia
  Ch. 86: A History of Psychosurgery

R. Michael Scott, MD
Professor of Surgery
Department of Neurosurgery
Harvard Medical School;
Neurosurgeon-in-Chief
The Children's Hospital, Boston
Boston, Massachusetts
  Ch. 207: Moyamoya Disease

Eric Seigneuret, MD
Neurosurgery Department
Grenoble University Hospital
Grenoble Institute of Neuroscience
Grenoble, France
  *Ch. 80: Subthalamic Deep Brain Stimulation for Parkinson's
  Disease*

Nathan R. Selden, MD, PhD
Mario and Edith Campagna Professor
Department of Neurological Surgery
Oregon Health & Science University
Portland, Oregon
  Ch. 216: Split Spinal Cord

Warren R. Selman, MD
Director
The Neurological Institute
University Hospitals Case Medical Center;
Harvey Huntington Brown Jr Professor and Chairman
Department of Neurological Surgery
Case Western Reserve University School of Medicine
Cleveland, Ohio
  Ch. 345: Intraoperative Cerebral Protection

Christopher I. Shaffrey, MD, FACS
Harrison Distinguished Professor
Departments of Neurological and Orthopaedic Surgery
University of Virginia School of Medicine
Charlottesville, Virginia
  Ch. 223: Thoracolumbar Spinal Disorders in Pediatric Patients
  Ch. 264: Overview and Historical Considerations
  Ch. 286: Pediatric Spondylolisthesis
  Ch. 288: Flat Back and Sagittal Plane Deformity
  Ch. 303: Posterior Lumbar Instrumentation
  *Ch. 317: Transient Quadriparesis and Athletic Injuries of the
  Cervical Spine*

Manish N. Shah, MD
Resident
Department of Neurological Surgery
Washington University School of Medicine
St. Louis, Missouri
  *Ch. 290: Congenital Abnormalities of the Thoracic and Lumbar
  Spine*

Kiarash Shahlaie, MD, PhD
Assistant Professor
Department of Neurological Surgery
University of California, Davis
Sacramento, California
  Ch. 331: Clinical Pathophysiology of Traumatic Brain Injury

G. Alexander West, MD, PhD
Neurosurgeon
Colorado Brain and Spine Institute
Swedish Medical Center
Englewood, Colorado
  Ch. 382: *Traumatic Cerebral Aneurysms Secondary to Penetrating Intracranial Injuries*

Nicholas M. Wetjen, MD
Assistant Professor
Departments of Neurologic Surgery and Pediatrics
Mayo Clinic College of Medicine;
Senior Associate Consultant
Pediatric Neurosurgeon
Mayo Clinic
Rochester, Minnesota
  Ch. 178: *Arachnoid Cysts*
  Ch. 220: *Cervical Spine Disorders in Children*

Robert G. Whitmore, MD
Resident
Department of Neurosurgery
Hospital of the University of Pennsylvania
Philadelphia, Pennsylvania
  Ch. 32: *Cranioplasty*

Louis A. Whitworth, MD
Associate Professor
Departments of Neurological Surgery and Radiation Oncology
The University of Texas Southwestern Medical Center
Dallas, Texas
  Ch. 157: *Pharmacologic Treatment of Pain*

Thomas Wichmann, MD
Professor
Department of Neurology
Emory University School of Medicine
Atlanta, Georgia
  Ch. 73: *Rationale for Surgical Interventions in Movement Disorders*

Joseph L. Wiemels, PhD
Associate Professor
Department of Epidemiology and Biostatistics
University of California, San Francisco
San Francisco, California
  Ch. 106: *Epidemiology of Brain Tumors*

Eelco F. M. Wijdicks, MD, PhD, FACP
Professor
Department of Neurology
Chair
Division of Critical Care Neurology
Mayo Clinic College of Medicine
Mayo Clinic
Rochester, Minnesota
  Ch. 24: *Principles of Neurocritical Care*

Adam C. Wilberger, BS
Department of Neurosurgery
Allegheny General Hospital
Pittsburgh, Pennsylvania
  Ch. 37: *Pathophysiology of Subdural Hematomas*

Jack Wilberger, MD, FACE
Professor and Chairman
Department of Neurosurgery
Allegheny General Hospital
Drexel University College of Medicine;
Vice President
Graduate Medical Education
Allegheny General Hospital
Western Pennsylvania Hospital Medical Education Consortium
Pittsburgh, Pennsylvania
  Ch. 37: *Pathophysiology of Subdural Hematomas*

David M. Wildrick, PhD
Surgery Publications Program Manager
Department of Neurosurgery
The University of Texas M. D. Anderson Cancer Center
Houston, Texas
  Ch. 130: *Metastatic Brain Tumors*

Jason Wilson, MD, MS
Skullbase Fellow
Goodman and Campbell Brain and Spine
Indianapolis, Indiana
  Ch. 345: *Intraoperative Cerebral Protection*

Christopher J. Winfree, MD
Assistant Professor
Department of Neurological Surgery
Columbia University College of Physicians and Surgeons;
Neurological Institute of New York
Columbia University Medical Center
New York, New York
  Ch. 170: *Diagnosis and Management of Painful Neuromas*

H. Richard Winn, MD
Professor and Director of Neurosurgery
Lenox Hill Hospital
New York, New York;
Hofstra University
Hempstead, New York;
Adjunct Professor
Department of Neurological Surgery
University of Iowa
Iowa City, Iowa;
Clinical Professor
Weill Cornell Medical College
Columbia University
Mount Sinai School of Medicine
New York, New York;
Visiting Professor of Surgery (Neurosurgery)
Tribhuvan University Teaching Hospital
Kathmandu, Nepal
  Ch. 8: Blood-Brain Barrier
  Ch. 337: Blast-Induced Neurotrauma
  Ch. 360: The Natural History of Cerebral Aneurysms
  *Ch. 362: Surgical Decision Making for the Treatment of
  Intracranial Aneurysms*
  Ch. 365: Surgical Approaches to Intracranial Aneurysms

Christopher Wolfla, MD
Associate Professor
Department of Neurosurgery
Medical College of Wisconsin
Milwaukee, Wisconsin
  Ch. 299: Posterior Subaxial and Cervicothoracic Instrumentation

Eric T. Wong, MD
Associate Professor
Department of Neurology
Harvard Medical School;
Co-Director
Brain Tumor Center
Director
Neuro-Oncology Unit
Beth Israel Deaconess Medical Center
Boston, Massachusetts
  *Ch. 104: Angiogenesis and Brain Tumors: Molecular Targets
  and Molecular Scalpels*

Peter J. Wormald, MD, MBChB, FRACS, FCS(SA), FRCS
Chairman
Department of Otolaryngology Head and Neck Surgery
Universities of Adelaide and Flinders
Adelaide, Australia
  Ch. 341: Traumatic Cerebrospinal Fluid Fistulas

Margaret Wrensch, PhD
Professor
Department of Neurological Surgery
University of California, San Francisco
San Francisco, California
  Ch. 106: Epidemiology of Brain Tumors

Neill M. Wright, MD
Herbert Lourie Professor of Neurological Surgery
Associate Professor
Departments of Neurological and Orthopaedic Surgery
Washington University School of Medicine
St. Louis, Missouri
  Ch. 298: Occiput, C1, and C2 Instrumentation

Zachary Wright, MD
Resident
Department of Neurosurgery
Allegheny General Hospital
Pittsburgh, Pennsylvania
  Ch. 58: Auditory Language Mapping

David Yam
Resident
Department of Neurosurgery
The University of Tennessee
Memphis, Tennessee
  Ch. 198: Pediatric Craniopharyngioma

Shinya Yamada, MD
Department of Neurosurgery
Tokai University Oiso Hospital
Kanagawa, Japan
  Ch. 188: Cerebrospinal Fluid Physiology

Yoshiya Yamada, MD, FRCPC
Associate Attending Physician
Department of Radiation Oncology
Memorial Sloan-Kettering Cancer Center
New York, New York
  *Ch. 262: Stereotactic Radiosurgery for the Treatment of Spinal
  Metastases*

Isaac Yang, MD
Resident
Department of Neurological Surgery
University of California, San Francisco
San Francisco, California
  Ch. 68: Radiosurgical Treatment of Epilepsy

Victor X. D. Yang, MD, MASc, PhD
Resident
Department of Neurosurgery
University of Toronto
Toronto, Canada
  *Ch. 269: Intraoperative Monitoring of the Spinal Cord and
  Nerve Roots*

Tom Yao, MD
Co-Director
Cerebrovascular and Endovascular Neurosurgery
Co-Director
Stroke Program
Norton Neuroscience Institute
Louisville, Kentucky
  *Ch. 292: Bone Graft Options, Bone Graft Substitutes, and Bone
  Harvest Techniques*

Chun-Po Yen, MD
Fellow
Division of Neuro-oncology
Department of Neurosurgery
University of Virginia
Charlottesville, Virginia
Ch. 249: The Radiobiology and Physics of Radiosurgery

H. Kwang Yeoh, MD
Resident
Department of Neurosurgery
Thomas Jefferson University Hospital
Philadelphia, Pennsylvania
Ch. 321: Osteoporotic Fractures: Evaluation and Treatment with Vertebroplasty and Kyphoplasty

Yasuhiro Yonekawa, MD
Professor Emeritus
University of Zurich;
Consultant
Im Park Clinic
Zurich, Switzerland
Ch. 356: Adult Moyamoya Disease

Alice Yoo, MD
Surgical Pathologist
Swedish Medical Center
Englewood, Colorado
Ch. 382: Traumatic Cerebral Aneurysms Secondary to Penetrating Intracranial Injuries

David M. Yousem, MD, MBA
Director
Division of Neuroradiology
Vice Chairman of Program Development
Russell H. Morgan Department of Radiology and Radiological Sciences
The Johns Hopkins Health System
Baltimore, Maryland
Ch. 109: Radiologic Features of Central Nervous System Tumors

Eric C. Yuen, MD
Associate Director of Clinical Research
Department of Clinical Neuroscience
Merck Research Laboratories
West Point, Pennsylvania
Ch. 232: Electrodiagnostic Evaluation of Peripheral Nerves: Electromyography and Nerve Conduction Studies

Joseph M. Zabramski, MD
Chief
Section of Cerebrovascular Surgery
Division of Neurological Surgery
Barrow Neurological Institute
Phoenix, Arizona
Ch. 392: Natural History of Cavernous Malformations

Andrew C. Zacest, MBBS
Abbie Simpson Clinical Fellow
University of Adelaide;
Neurosurgeon
Royal Adelaide Hospital
Adelaide, Australia
Ch. 63: Selective Amygdalohippocampectomy
Ch. 153: Pain: General Historical Considerations

J. Christopher Zacko, MD
Fellow
Department of Neurological Surgery
University of Miami Miller School of Medicine
Miami, Florida
Ch. 327: Neurochemical Pathomechanisms in Traumatic Brain Injury
Ch. 335: Surgical Management of Traumatic Brain Injury

Gabriel Zada, MD
Clinical Instructor and Resident Supervisor
Department of Neurological Surgery
University of Southern California Keck School of Medicine
Los Angeles, California
Ch. 25: Surgical Planning: Overview
Ch. 372: Basilar Trunk Aneurysms

Ross Zafonte, DO
Earl P. and Ida S. Charlton Professor of Physical Medicine and Rehabilitation
Harvard Medical School;
Vice President
Medical Affairs
Spaulding Rehabilitation Network;
Chief
Department of Physical Medicine and Rehabilitation
Massachusetts General Hospital
Boston, Massachusetts
Ch. 342: Rehabilitation of Patients with Traumatic Brain Injury

Eric L. Zager, MD, FACS
Professor
Department of Neurosurgery
University of Pennsylvania School of Medicine
Philadelphia, Pennsylvania
Ch. 236: Distal Entrapment Syndromes: Carpal Tunnel, Cubital Tunnel, Peroneal, and Tarsal Tunnel
Ch. 237: Thoracic Outlet Syndrome

Hasan A. Zaidi, MD
Resident
Division of Neurosurgery
Barrow Neurological Institute
Phoenix, Arizona
Ch. 98: Brain Tumor Stem Cells

Hekmat Zarzour, MD
Clinical Fellow
Department of Radiology
Brigham and Women's Hospital
Boston, Massachusetts
Ch. 139: Overview of Skull Base Tumors

Vasilios A. Zerris, MD, MPH, MMSc
Vice-Chairman and Chief
Department of Neurosurgery
Texas A & M University Medical Center
Scott and White Hospital
College Station, Texas
Ch. 94: Neuroprosthetics

Justin A. Zivin, MD, PhD
Professor
Department of Neurosciences
University of California, San Diego;
Staff Neurologist
Department of Neurology
San Diego Veterans Affairs Medical Center
San Diego, California
Ch. 344: Acute Medical Management of Ischemic/Hemorrhagic Stroke

John G. Zovickian, MD, FACS
Attending Pediatric Neurosurgeon
Department of Pediatric Neurosurgery
Regional Center for Pediatric Neurosurgery
Kaiser Permanente Hospitals, Northern California
Oakland, California;
Clinical Instructor
Department of Neurological Surgery
University of California, Davis
Sacramento, California
Ch. 224: Pediatric Vertebral Column and Spinal Cord Injuries

Alexander Y. Zubkov, MD, PhD, FAHA
Director
Stroke Center
Fairview Southdale Hospital
Minneapolis Clinic of Neurology
Edina, Minnesota
Ch. 24: Principles of Neurocritical Care

Marike Zwienenberg-Lee, MD
Assistant Clinical Professor
Department of Neurosurgery
Pediatric Neurosurgeon
University of California, Davis
Davis, California
Ch. 331: Clinical Pathophysiology of Traumatic Brain Injury

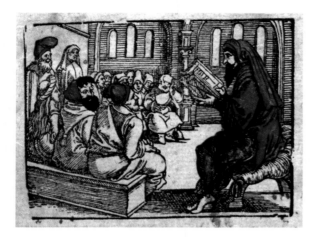

FIGURE 1-12 Constantine the African lecturing at the School of Salerno.

Constantinus Africanus—*magister orientis et occidentis* (1020-1087).[42] Constantine, a *Magistri Salernitani*, provided an important bridge in medicine by introducing the scholarship of Islamic/Arabic medicine there and eventually to all of Europe. Constantine received his medical education in Baghdad, where he learned the prevalent views of Islamic medicine. He moved to a monastery at Monte Cassino, where in the tradition of this period he translated Arabic manuscripts into Latin. Modern scholars believe that his translations included inaccuracies and introduced errors into the medical literature. Recent studies suggest that Constantine was a plagiarist and unreliable translator. Nonetheless, one cannot underestimate his contributions by providing the earliest transfer of Arabic/Islamic medical literature to Europe.

In looking back, what we see are Greek texts originally translated into Arabic and now being translated into Latin, with the legacy of Galen and other early writers remaining firmly entrenched as dogma. Rather than providing or developing new ideas, the classical texts in medicine remained fully in control of medical dogma. One can only imagine how much medical and surgical knowledge was lost or distorted by inaccuracies in these successive translations. Constantine did make a key contribution to medieval medicine when he reintroduced anatomic dissection with an annual dissection of a pig, but the findings were compared with those recorded in the Greek classics. If the prosector's findings did not match the ancient texts, they were simply ignored! Constantine was clearly a learned man, but his style of teaching became typical of the Medieval Ages; extensive compilations and translations were undertaken, but original thought or advances in knowledge were absent. In the Middle Ages the School of Salerno lead the way and was followed by the great medical schools at Naples, Bologna, Paris, and Montpellier, the early pillars of medieval medicine.

An unusual and remarkable book was produced during this period—*Regimen Sanitatis Salernitum*, a work that first appeared in the 12th century and was later republished in 140 different editions extending well into the 19th century.[41] This book summarizes the Salernitan school directions for maintenance and care of patients in medicine. In Europe a strong educational system was being developed, but medicine remained cloaked in the literature of the classical Greeks and Islamic writing; for the most part, surgical education and surgical practice continued to be treated as an avocation limited to uneducated barber-surgeons and apprentices. However, there were talented surgeons who escaped the norm and produced original surgical works and practices.

Roger of Salerno (Ruggiero Frugardi, fl. 1170) is considered the first learned medieval European writer on surgery (Figs. 1-14

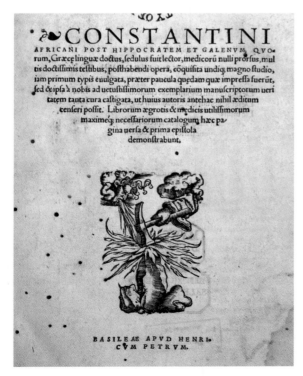

FIGURE 1-13 Title page from a collection of the works of Constantine the African—1536. (*From Constantinus Africanus. Constantini Africani Post Hippocratem et Galenum. Basel: Henricus Petrus; 1536.*)

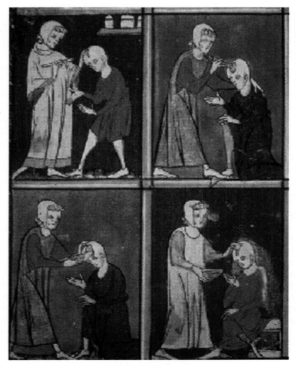

FIGURE 1-14 Roger of Salerno's demonstration of brain and skull surgery. (*From the Sloane manuscript, 1977—Courtesy of the British Museum.*)

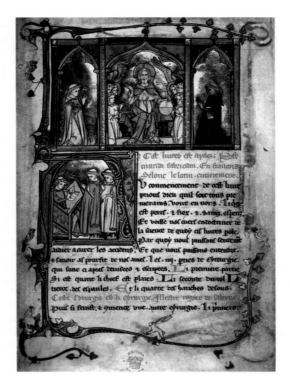

FIGURE 1-15 An early medieval manuscript on the writings of Roger of Salerno in which is demonstrated the "professor and student," a reflection of the educational style of this period. *(From the Sloane manuscript, 1977—Courtesy of the British Museum.)*

and 1-15). Roger was educated in the Salerno tradition and followed many of its teachings. His book on surgical practice, *Practica Chirurgiae*,[43] offers techniques of interest to neurosurgeons. An example was his technique for checking for a tear of the dura and leakage of CSF in a patient with a skull fracture. To detect a leak, Roger would have the patient hold his breath and strain (i.e., Valsalva maneuver) and then look for air bubbles around the fracture site, a clear sign of a leak. He was a pioneer in the techniques of managing peripheral nerve injury. In a severed nerve, he argued for reanastomosis of the nerve ends with close attention paid to their alignment. In dealing with the large bleeding veins of the neck, he urged direct ligation with suture rather than cautery. Several chapters of his text are devoted to the treatment of skull fractures. Much of the technique described mirrors the views of earlier classical writers, but the style is clearer and more succinct. An example of this style is seen in this short description of the management of various skull fractures:

When a fracture occurs it is accompanied by various wounds and contusions. If the contusion of the flesh is small but that of the bone great, the flesh should be divided by a cruciate incision down to the bone and everywhere elevated from the bone. Then a piece of light, old cloth is inserted for a day, and if there are fragments of the bone present, they are to be thoroughly removed. If the bone is unbroken on one side, it is left in place, and if necessary elevated with a flat sound (spatumile) and the bone is perforated by chipping with the spatumile so that clotted blood may be soaked up with a wad of wool and feathers. When it has consolidated, we apply lint and then, if it is necessary (but not until after the whole wound has become level with the skin), the patient may be bathed. After he leaves the bath, we apply a thin cooling plaster made of wormwood with rose water and egg.[43,44]

A 12th century manuscript owned by Harvey Cushing and attributed to Roger of Salerno has recently been translated. It contains an early description of a soporific for pain relief for use in surgery. Roger was particularly fond of citing the writings of Albucasis and Paul of Aegina. He strongly favored therapeutic plasters and salves but was not a strong advocate of the popular application of grease to injuries of the dura. He advocated the use of trephination for the treatment of epilepsy, although he is not clear why this technique would work. Chapters 1 to 13 (capita 1-13) detail contemporary surgical treatment of scalp wounds and fractures of the skull. One of his most significant errors in surgical practice was the concept that provoking suppuration of pus in a wound encouraged healing. This introduced the concept of "laudable pus" in wound healing and delayed good wound care until Lister and 19th century antisepsis.

An unusually talented and inventive medieval surgeon from Bologna was Theodoric of Cervia (Borgognoni, 1205-1298). In contrast to Roger of Salerno, Theodoric was a pioneer in the use of aseptic technique—not what we would refer to as the "clean" aseptic technique of today but rather a method based on avoidance of "laudable pus." Theodoric thought that he had found the ideal principles for good wound healing, which included control of bleeding, removal of contaminated or necrotic material, avoidance of dead space, and careful application of a wound dressing bathed in wine, the last providing a degree of antisepsis. He also argued for primary closure of all wounds when possible and avoiding "laudable pus."

For it is not necessary, as Roger and Roland have written, as many of their disciples teach, and as all modern surgeons profess, that pus should be generated in wounds. No error can be greater than this. Such a practice is indeed to hinder nature, to prolong the disease, and to prevent the conglutination and consolidation of the wound.[45,46]

Theodoric's surgical work, which was first written in 1267, provides one of the best reviews of contemporary medieval surgery.[45] He is also remembered as one of the earliest writers to include illustrations of his techniques. His recommendations called for meticulous (almost Halstedian) techniques with gentle handling of surgical tissues. Theodoric believed that aspiring surgeons should train only under competent masters. In the field of head injury, he argued that parts of the brain could be removed through a wound with little effect on the patient. In the treatment of skull fractures, he strongly argued for elevating depressed fractures. He advocated avoiding punctures of the dura because they could lead to abscess, convulsions, and bad outcomes. For pain relief during surgery, he developed his own "soporific sponge" that contained opium, mandragora, hemlock, and other less important ingredients applied to the nostrils, and once the patient fell asleep, he began surgery. Opium was probably the key ingredient.

William of Saliceto (Guglielo da Saliceto, 1210-1277) was a uniquely skilled Italian surgeon of the 13th century and a professor at the University of Bologna. His book on surgery, *Chirurgia* (or *Cyrurgia*), was completed in 1275, and in it we find highly original concepts that are not totally based on previous classical writings but in which the influence of Galen and Avicenna are clearly present.[47] This book was written by William for his son Bernardino. The observations offered are based on his own surgical cases. Book IV contains the earliest known treatise on surgical and regional anatomy. His most significant contribution for this era was probably his decision to replace cautery with the surgical knife.

De anathomia in communi et de formis membrorum et figures que sunt considerande in incision et cauterizatione.[47]

He describes interesting and unique techniques for primary peripheral nerve suture repair. In this pre-Harvey era he distinguished arterial from venous bleeding by the "spurting" of blood. He also put forth interesting neurological concepts, such as that the cerebrum governs voluntary motion and the cerebellum involuntary function.

Leonard of Bertapalia (1380?-1460) was a prominent 15th century Italian surgeon and writer. Leonard established an extensive and lucrative practice in the area of Padua and in neighboring Venice. At a time when anatomic dissection was rarely practiced in Europe, he became one of the earliest proponents of the study of anatomy. In 1429 he offered a course of surgery that included the dissection of an executed criminal. He devoted a third of his book to surgery on the nervous system and head injuries.[48,49] He considered the brain the most precious of organs and regarded it as the source of voluntary and involuntary functions. In reviewing his treatment of skull fractures, he would always avoid materials that might generate pus. He argued for never placing a compressive dressing that might drive bone into the brain and proposed that if a piece of bone pierces the brain, the surgeon should remove it.

Leonard put together a set of rules to guide the practice of 15th century surgeons that have modern tones—rules still applicable 5 centuries later.

> To be the perfect surgeon, you must always bear in mind these eight notations, and remembering them you will be preferred to others.
>
> The first task to become a good surgeon should be to use his eyes.
>
> Second, you must accompany and observe the qualified physician, seeing him work before you yourself practice.
>
> Third, you must command the most gentle touch in operating and treating lest you cause pain to the patient.
>
> Fourth, you must insure that your instruments be sharp and unrusted whenever you cut anywhere.
>
> Fifth, you must be courageous in operating and cutting but timid to cut in the vicinity of nerves, sinews and arteries, and, so as not to commit error, you should study anatomy, which is the mother of this art perform your surgery cleverly and never operate on human flesh as if you were working on wood or leather.
>
> Sixth, you must be kind and sympathetic to the poor, for piety and humility greatly augment your reputation and the sick will more freely commit themselves to your care.
>
> Seventh, you must never refuse anything brought you as a fee, for the sick will respect you more.
>
> Eighth, you must never argue about fees with the sick, or indeed demand anything unless it be previously agreed upon, for avarice is the most ignoble of vices and should you be so inflicted, you will never achieve the reputation of a good doctor.[49]

Lanfranchi of Milan (d. 1306) was a pupil of William of Saliceto and often referred to as the father of French surgery. Lanfranchi advocated his teacher's use of the knife in place of the burning cautery. Although born and educated in Italy, he had to leave Italy for France to avoid political strife. In his *Cyrugia Parva* we find a number of interesting surgical techniques. Lanfranchi perfected the use of suture for primary wound repairs.[50] He was among the first to relate the direct effect of head injury to brain function. Hippocrates was the first to articulate the concept of *commotio cerebri*, but it is to Lanfranchi that we owe the first modern characterization of what is now called a *cerebral concussion*. For surgeons he developed a series of guidelines for trephination in skull fractures and "release of irritation" of the dura. Because of the dangers of skull surgery, Lanfranchi argued for using the trephine only when absolutely necessary; otherwise, he evoked the skills of the "Holy Ghost" to provide cure. Among his innovative surgical techniques was the development of esophageal intubation during surgery, a technique not commonly practiced until the 19th century. As an educated surgeon and a "Surgeon of the Long Robe" (i.e., academic), he attempted to elevate the art and science of surgery above the mediocre level of the menial barber-surgeon ("Surgeons of the Short Robe"). Lanfranchi also argued against the separation of surgery and medicine, advocated since the time of Avicenna, for he thought that a good surgeon should also be a good physician.

After Lanfranchi came another important figure in the history of French medicine and surgery—Henri de Mondeville (d. 1317). Educated in Paris and Montpellier, Henri later went on to become a professor at Montpellier. He was strongly motivated to elevate the profession of the surgeon and clearly detested the barber-surgeon: "Most of them were illiterates, debauchees, cheats, forgers, alchemists, courtesans, procuresses, etc."[46]

In 1306 Henri undertook the task of developing a new treatise on surgery for the education of his students at Montpellier. Unfortunately, because of tuberculosis and ill health, the manuscript was never completed. Ironically, the edited portions were not published until 1892, when Professor Julius Pagel of Berlin completed the task.[51] Henri adopted and followed a number of the views of Lanfranchi. He was a believer in clean wounds and avoiding "laudable pus." Unfortunately, Henri would be the last surgeon in this era to argue for avoiding "laudable pus"; after him, surgeons returned to the older belief of pus developing in a wound being a good sign of healing. Henri offered originality in wound management by advocating for healing by primary intention—*"modus novus noster."* In the surgical treatment of wounds, he encouraged the removal of foreign bodies and the use of wine dressings in wound care. Henri was clever in designing a number of surgical instruments. He is remembered for the design of a needle holder and also a forceps-type instrument for extraction of arrowheads. He argued against elevating skull fractures if there was no injury to the overlying soft tissues. He believed that nature would do a better job at healing the fracture by natural union. It was his opinion that unnecessary exploration and probing of the wound would only cause more injury than natural healing—in retrospect a rather brilliant insight into wound care (Fig. 1-16).[46]

No history of surgery can be complete without a discussion of the contributions of Guy de Chauliac (1300-1368) (Fig. 1-17).[52] This surgeon was clearly the most influential European surgeon of the 14th and 15th centuries. He was so highly

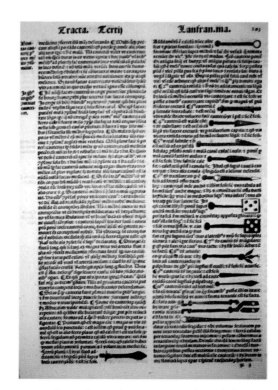

FIGURE 1-16 Surgical instruments designed by Lanfranchi are illustrated here in this early 1519 book. (*From Lanfranchi of Milan. Chirurgia. In: Guy de Chauliac Cyrurgia et Cyrurgia Bruni, Teodorici, Rolandi, Lanfranci, Rogerii, Bertapalie. Venice: Bernardinus Venetus de Vitalibus; 1519.*)

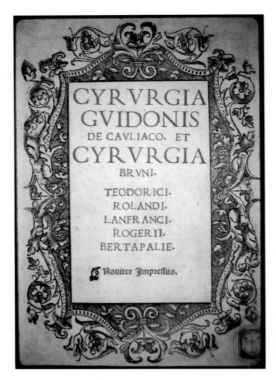

FIGURE 1-17 Title page from collected works dealing with the surgical writings of a number of medieval surgeons, including Guy de Chauliac. (*From Guy de Chauliac. Chirurgia magna. In:* Guy de Chauliac Cyrurgia et Cyrurgia Bruni, Teodorici, Rolandi, Lanfranci, Rogerii, Bertapali. *Venice: Bernardinus Venetus de Vitalibus; 1519. See also Leonardo, RA: History of Surgery. New York, Froben Press, 1943:116.*)

respected that he became the physician for three popes at Avignon (Pope Clement VI, Innocent VI, and Urban V) and leading surgeon and educator at the school of Montpellier. Guy was educated at Toulouse, Paris, Montpellier, and Bologna. He was an early proponent of anatomic dissection of a human cadaver. He states: "In these two ways we must teach anatomy on the bodies of men, apes, swine, and divers other animals, and not from pictures, as did Henri de Mondeville who had 13 pictures for demonstration of anatomy."[53] His writings were popular and continued to exert an influence on surgery until well into the 17th century. His principal didactic surgical text was scribed in 1363 and titled the *Collectorium Cyrurgie*.[53] There are 34 known manuscripts of this work, with the first printed edition appearing in 1478, and more than 70 editions followed. In promoting surgeons as more skilled individuals (versus "mechanics," i.e., barbersurgeons), he stated four conditions that must be satisfied for a practitioner to be a good surgeon: (1) the surgeon should be learned; (2) he should be an expert; (3) he must be ingenious; and (4) he should be able to adapt himself (from the introduction of *Ars Chirurgica*). For the modern neurosurgeon, Guy provides an interesting discussion of techniques that he devised for the treatment of head injuries. Before beginning surgery the head needs to be shaved. Shaving of the hair will prevent hair from getting into the wound and interfering with primary healing. For depressed skull fractures, Guy preferred to put wine-soaked cloths into the injured site to assist healing. He categorized head injuries into seven types and discussed the management of each in detail. Scalp wounds required only cleaning and débridement, whereas a compound depressed skull fracture must be treated by means of trephination and elevation. Skin closure was done by primary repair and for which he claimed good results. To help control excessive bleeding and provide hemostasis, he used egg albumin.

As England was moving away from the barbarian invasions and into the Middle Ages, university education in England began to become comparable to the European model. The leading surgeon of this period in England was John of Arderne (Arden, 1307-1380), who trained as a military surgeon and saw much war experience. In 1370 he came to London and joined the Guild of Military Surgeons. He adopted the phase "*chirurgus inter medicos*," or a surgeon among physicians. His manuscript on surgery was written about 1412.[54] This manuscript, *De Arte Phisicali et de Cirurgia*, was translated into English by D'Arcy Power in 1922, a valuable addition to the English literature on early surgery.[55] His writings suggest that he was a skilled surgeon and had a number of practical insights into what could or could not be done surgically. He was a firm believer in clean hands and well-shaped nails for surgery, although some writers have thought that this was more for social reasons than for surgery.[56] In addition, he would bathe his open wounds with an irrigation fluid that contained turpentine, a useful surgical antiseptic for keeping wounds clean. Most importantly, John of Arderne was a firm believer in education and learning. The surgeon must also "always be sober during any surgery as drunkenness destroys all virtue and brings it to naught."[46]

In reviewing the late Byzantine/Islamic and Medieval period we see an era of great misguided intellectual activity, an era of innovative somnolence where originality of thought is concerned. Clearly, the educators had more faith in the teachings of antiquity. From the fall of the Roman Empire until the beginning of the 16th century, anatomy and the practice of surgery, with rare exceptions, lay dormant, chained to a staunch Galenic and Hippocratic orthodoxy. The transliteration of medical manuscripts from Latin, Greek, and Hebrew into Arabic and back into Latin resulted in many errors of translation and interpretation. The combination of a lack of anatomic knowledge and poor surgical outcomes naturally led physicians to recommend against operating on the brain, except in simple cases. A review of the work done by the surgical personalities described previously reveals that despite a period of intellectual paralysis, there still existed a number of prominent personalities who did make advances. Monastic recluses in often-inaccessible mountain retreats carefully guarded medical knowledge, yet some surgeons nonetheless succeeded in mastering their art in the midst of intellectual darkness.

The history of medicine consists of a successive series of intellectual movements proceeding from different centers and each engulfing its predecessor.[57]

ORIGINS OF NEUROSURGICAL PRACTICE IN THE RENAISSANCE

With the origins of the Renaissance came innovations in surgical concepts and techniques. Beginning in the mid-15th century, physicians and surgeons introduced basic investigative techniques to learn human anatomy and physiology. Of enormous significance was the introduction of routine anatomic dissection in medical schools. Moving away from subservience to the medievalists, great figures such as Leonardo da Vinci, Berengario da Carpi, Nicholas Massa, Andreas Vesalius, and others explored the human body without being encumbered by the erroneous writings of earlier authors. Codified anatomic errors, many ensconced since the Greco-Roman era, were now being corrected. A better understanding of human anatomy led to a change in epistemological presuppositions and in turn resulted in a great surge of interest in surgery. Putting the teachings of antiquity aside, surgeons went forward with great vigor and enthusiasm to unravel the human fabric. This shift from the somber and somnolent

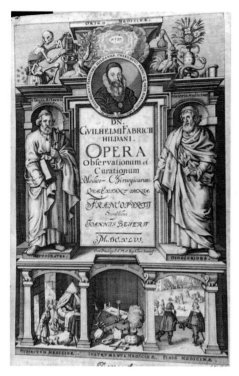

FIGURE 1-40 Allegorical title page from Fabry's collected works. (*From Fabry W. Observationum et Curationum Chirurgicarum Centuriae. Basle: Frankfurt, & Lyons, 1606-1641. A later collected works also contains a number of neurosurgical cases. Opera Observation et Curationum. Frankfurt: Joannis Beyerj; 1646.*)

techniques for bullet extraction, along with original designs for field surgical instruments. He describes operations for intracranial hemorrhage (with cure of insanity), vertebral displacement, congenital hydrocephalus, and an occipital tumor of the newborn (probably an encephalocele). Fabricius carried out trephinations for the treatment of a brain abscess and cure of an old aphasia. He even removed a splinter of metal from the eye with a magnet, a cure that greatly enhanced his reputation.

A monograph in which early and skillfully designed neurosurgical instruments appear is a work by Johann Schultes (Scultetus) of Ulm (1595-1645). With *Armamentarium Chirurgicum XLIII*, Scultetus, also known as Schultes, provides unique and graphic details of neurosurgical instruments, clearly the finest to appear since those published by Berengario in 1518 and Croce in 1573.[37] The illustrations (Figs. 1-42 and 1-43) graphically reveal surgical techniques for treating fractures and dislocations, as well as a variety of bandaging techniques for wounds. The popularity of this surgical work led it to be translated into many languages, including English, and it had a considerable influence on surgery throughout Europe for more than 2 centuries. In reviewing the surgical plates and various operations we find exacting details described, including concepts from antiquity to the present. Interestingly, many of the instruments illustrated by Scultetus remain in use today. His details of surgical operations for injury to the skull and brain are remarkable plebiscite.

Neurosurgical practice continued to evolve in the 17th century. A surgeon who offered interesting technical advances on developing neurosurgical operating skills was John Woodall (ca. 1556?-1643). Woodall was a military surgeon by training and surgeon-general for the East India Company. For the surgeons of the East India Company he compiled a surgical monograph called the *Surgeon's Mate* (1617).[87] In his collected works, published in 1639, he provided a list of surgical instruments and sound advice for a surgical practice.[88] He fabricated a trephine

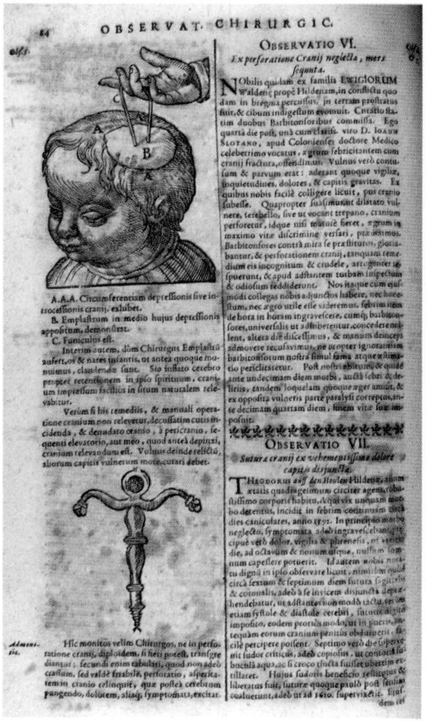

FIGURE 1-41 Illustrations from Fabry's collected works showing a technique for elevating a depressed skull fracture in a child.

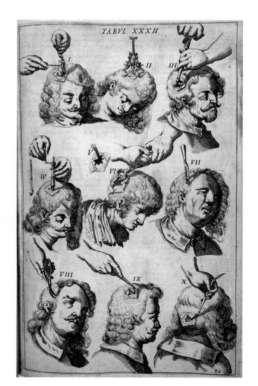

FIGURE 1-42 Surgical techniques designed by Scultetus for trephining the skull. (*From Scultetus J. Χειροπλοθηκη. Armamentarium Chirurgicum XLIII. Ulm: Balthasar Kühnen; 1655.*)

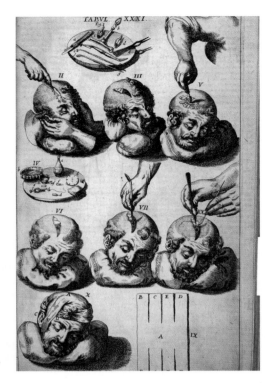

FIGURE 1-43 Scultetus' techniques for dealing with skull fractures. (*From Scultetus J.* Χειροπλοθηκη. Armamentarium Chirurgicum XLIII. *Ulm: Balthasar Kühnen; 1655.*)

with the unique design of a crown that included a center pin, an innovation that prevented the crown from slipping on a bloody skull (Fig. 1-44). This trephine had a brace added that could be placed against the surgeon's chest for additional support and driving force. This allowed the surgeon to drive the trephine with one hand while the other held the head, all of which could be accomplished on a rolling ship's deck. Woodall, recognizing the ignorance of his contemporary German surgical colleagues, believed that a surgeon should practice trephining on sheep or calf skulls first before performing one on a human head. He comments:

> The Germane Surgeons use no Trapan, that ever I could see my eight years living among them, though they both speak and write of it. But for as much as it is apparent, the work of a Trapan is very good, I therefore would advise a young Artist to make some experience first upon a calves head, or a sheep's head, till he can well and easily take out a piece of the bone; so shall he the more safely do it to a man without error when occasion is [see page 4].[88]

An Englishman and Plymouth naval surgeon, James Yonge (1646-1721) was among the first to argue emphatically that "*wounds of the brain are curable*"; Galen had earlier announced, "I have seen the wounded brain heal."[27] Yonge's first surgical text was a small monograph titled *Wounds of the Brain Proved Curable*.[89] He provides a surgical account of a brain operation on a 4-year-old child with extensive compound fractures of the skull from which brain tissue issued forth. The surgery was successful and the child survived, which led Yonge to publish the account. Yonge also reported on more than 60 cases of brain wounds cured that he was able to locate in the older literature, beginning with Galen. The bibliography records the earlier cases that he was able to locate. He comments that this work was written in defense of surgery on the skull and the brain. From the preface,

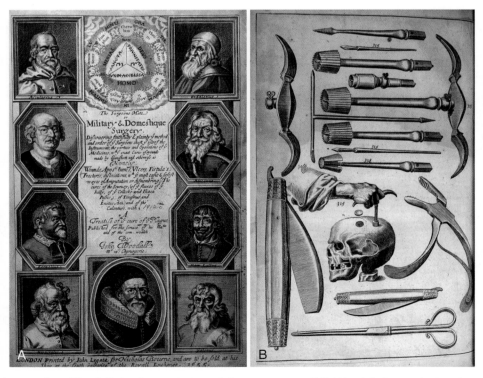

FIGURE 1-44 A, Title page from Woodall's book on military and domestic surgery.[87] **B,** Woodall designed a hand trephine with a series of interchangeable burs along with bone rongeurs. The trephine center pin, Woodall's design, was especially useful on a rolling ship deck when applied to a bloody skull. (*From Woodall J.* The Surgeons Mate. *London: E. Griffin; 1617.*)

I had the good fortune to be a successful chirurgeon to the child, whose case is contained in the following narrative: but I had scarcely wiped my instruments, and put up my plaister-box, before a physician of this town, sneakingly and maliciously endeavor to stifle [my] reputation insinuating that it was impossible to [cure brain wounds] because Wounds of the brain were absolutely mortal.[89]

Yonge is clearly a protagonist of trephination and operating on the skull and brain and demonstrated that it could be done safely.

Other technical innovations for treating head injuries also occurred in this period. Augustin Belloste (1654-1730) describes a technique for repairing "holes in the head" as a result of trauma or trephination with the use of lead plates. Keeping the brain from being exposed to "corrupt air" led to better outcomes in brain surgery.[90]

The 17th century, "the insurgent century," clearly brought a number of advances to the field of brain surgery. Neuroanatomy became an area of intense investigation. Physiologic experimentation, along with the introduction of scientific societies, allowed wide dissemination of the new investigations and scholarly disagreement. Along with this came surgeons with adventurous personalities, individuals who realized that in certain cases brain surgery could be performed safely; not all patients died if you opened the dura mater.

EIGHTEENTH CENTURY—AN ENLIGHTENED PERIOD FOR NEUROSURGERY

The 17th century clearly provided a sound scientific and anatomic basis for neurosurgery and the neurosciences. The 18th century continued this trend and was a period of intense activity in the medical and scientific world. Chemistry as a true science was being propelled forward in the works of Priestley, Lavoisier, Volta, Watt, and others. Clinical bedside medicine, essentially lost since the Byzantine and Islamic era, was reintroduced by Thomas Sydenham (1624-1689), William Cullen (1710-1740), and Herman Boerhaave (1668-1738). With bedside examination came a number of original and new tools for diagnostic examination. Of particular note are the contributions of Leopold Auenbrugger's (1722-1809) introduction of percussion of the chest, William Withering's (1741-1799) pharmacologic introduction of use of digitalis for cardiac problems, and William Jenner's (1749-1823) use of cowpox inoculation for smallpox, which helped eliminate a world scourge. In addition, for the first time the focus for the surgeon is switching from the skull to the brain. This new direction and change in approach to the neurological status of the patient marked a major paradigm shift that represented a very important step toward the origins of a separate surgical discipline of neurosurgery

Judgment in distinguishing, and ability in treating diseases, are not to be attained by a transient cursory view of them; merely running round an Hospital for a few months, or reading a general system of surgery, will not form a compleat practitioner: the man, who aims at that character, must take notice of many little things, which the inattentive pass over, and which cannot be remarked by writers; he must accustom himself to see, and to think for himself; and must regard the rules laid down by authors, as the outlines only of a piece, which he is to fill up and finish: books may give general ideas, but practice, and medication, must make him adroit and discerning; without these, his reading may possibly keep him clear of very gross blunders, but he will still remain injudicious, and inexpert [from preface x-xi, Observations, London 1760].[91]

One of the giants in surgery was Percivall Pott (1714-1788), considered by many historians to be the greatest English surgeon of the 18th century. His list of contributions, several of which apply to neurosurgery, is enormous. His work *Remarks on That Kind of Palsy of the Lower Limbs Found to Accompany a Curvature*

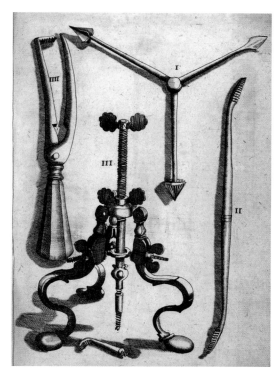

FIGURE 1-45 Pott's trephine for elevating a depressed skull fracture.

of the Spine (London, 1779) describes the disease entity now known as Pott's disease (i.e., tuberculous caries of the spine).[92] His clinical descriptions clearly describe the gibbus and tuberculous infection of the spine. Surprisingly, Pott failed to associate the relationship between the deformity and paralysis. An osteomyelitic infection of the scalp and skull in which pus collects under the pericranium is now called *Pott's puffy tumor*. Pott argued that these lesions should be opened and drained (Figs. 1-45 and 1-46).

Eighteenth century surgeons generated much discussion over the surgical practice of trephination. *To trephine or not to trephine*—Pott was a strong proponent of intervention. In his classic work on head injury (London, 1760), he clearly appreciated that the clinical findings of head injury were due to injury to the brain and not the skull.[93] Pott studied head injuries and began to

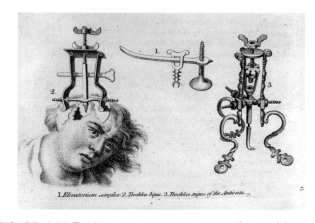

FIGURE 1-46 Trephination instrumentation as designed by Pott. (*From Pott P.* Remarks on That Kind of Palsy of the Lower Limbs Found to Accompany a Curvature of the Spine. *London: J. Johnson; 1779.*)

differentiate between "compression" and "concussion" injury of the brain. The following clinical description from his head injury book outlines some of his views:

> The reasons for trepanning in these cases are, first, the immediate relief of present symptoms arising from pressure of extravasated fluid; or second, the discharge of matter formed between the skull and dura mater, in consequence of inflammation; or third, the prevention of such mischief, as experience has shown may most probably be expected from such kind of violence offered to the last mentioned membrane.
>
> In the mere fracture without depression of bone, or the appearance of such symptoms as indicate commotion, extravasation, or inflammation, it is used as a preventative, and therefore is a matter of choice, more than immediate necessity.[93]

Pott clearly developed his outstanding reputation by his astute clinical observations and bedside treatment. His management of head injuries makes him the first of the modern neurosurgeons. His caveats, presented in the preface to his work on head injury, hold today.

The most significant development in 18th century writings on neurosurgical topics was the gradual recognition of the effects of trauma on brain function rather than just the skull. Several French surgeons drew a clear-cut distinction between the loss of consciousness accompanying a blow to the head and the drowsiness that appeared later. The former came to be recognized as a direct result of cerebral concussion, and the latter, after a lucid interval, came to be accepted as being due to a collection of blood producing compression of the brain. This idea was introduced by Jean Louis Petit (1674-1750), the leading surgeon in Paris in the first half of the 18th century, in a series of lectures that he gave in Paris.[94] The realization that delayed loss of consciousness could serve as an indication for surgical intervention is one of the epochal events that mark the origins of neurosurgery as a discipline dealing with alterations in brain function and not just superficial injuries to the skull. It was a major conceptual change in an approach that had been followed for 2000 years and marks an important turning point in surgical thinking.

One of the earliest descriptions of the "lucid interval" in head injury was provided by Henri Francosi Le Dran (1685-1770). Le Dran was both an anatomist and surgeon who amassed a large surgical experience by serving as the chief surgeon to the French Army. Le Dran established a very popular school of anatomy in Paris that attracted students from all over Europe. *Observations de Chirurgie* [95] (Fig. 1-47) reveals a skilled surgeon with a wide variety of surgical talents. This work became Le Dran's most popular surgical text and was reprinted several times and translated into English in 1749. It is a broad review of surgery, but most important to us are his views on surgery on the head. Le Dran details the concept of the "lucid interval" after a head injury and then attributes it most commonly to an epidural hematoma.

A remarkable and talented figure in English medicine and surgery and a student of Percivall Pott's was John Hunter (1728-1793). Many writers consider Hunter equally as skilled as Pott, but his additional work in anatomy, pathology, physiology, and surgery led him to make a number of important contributions.[96] Hunter, often referred to as the founder of experimental and surgical pathology, spent most of his career at St. George's Hospital in London. He was trained in the apprentice style and had minimal formal education. He began his training under his older brother William Hunter and spent time with William Cheselden, talented mentors. As a surgeon, Hunter was an atypical figure for this time in that he approached the field of surgery in a more practical manner and at the same time added a bench side experimental touch. In *A Treatise on the Blood, Inflammation, and Gun-Shot Wounds* (London, 1794),[97] Hunter drew on his years of military experience and wrote an important work on the management of gunshot wounds. He did not offer much on neurosur-

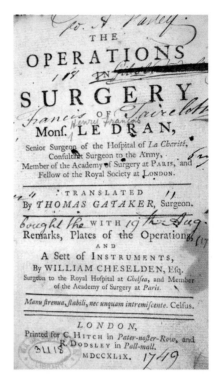

FIGURE 1-47 The title page from the English edition of Le Dran's textbook on surgery, Paris 1749.

gery; the section on skull fractures occupied only one paragraph. In understanding vascular disorders, Hunter described the concept of collateral circulation. His circulation studies were conducted on a buck whose carotid artery was tied off to see the effect on the antler, but no ill effect was noted; the explanation was the development of collateral circulation, which he had now determined anatomically. Hunter later applied these concepts to the treatment of popliteal aneurysms, previously treated by amputation; he tied off the artery and realized that collateral circulation would develop. He was adroit at posing questions raised by his clinical experience, performing animal experiments to answer the questions, and integrating his clinical and scientific results into the best available treatment. He anatomically dissected a case of craniopagus parasiticus, a set of twins from India in which one child was fully formed and the other twin had only the head. The incomplete twin would show emotion and move the lip and mouth during eating (Fig. 1-48).[98] Hunter is also remembered as a devoted student of anatomic curiosities and would go to great lengths, sometimes nefariously, to obtained specimens. The most famous case was an Irish giant whom Harvey Cushing later determined had acromegaly. The Irish giant knew of Hunter's interest in him and went to great lengths to avoid his laboratory after death. However, the Irish giant became part of the Hunterian museum, which contained more than 13,000 specimens and is now part of the Royal College of Surgeons pathologic collection, a direct donation by Hunter.

Following Hunter was a pupil of his, John Abernethy (1764-1831), who was also a talented anatomist and surgeon. For American surgeons, Abernethy is remembered for publishing the first book in America devoted to a neurosurgical topic.[99] So popular was Abernethy as a lecturer that the governors of St. Bartholomew's Hospital built an anatomic theater for him, a place of training sought out by the brighter students of the period. Abernethy eventually went back to Scotland, his country of birth,

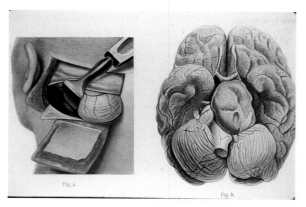

FIGURE 1-65 From Krause's monograph on brain surgery showing one of the earliest cerebellopontine angle approaches for an acoustic neuroma. Both the surgical approach and the anatomy of the tumor in relation to the seventh and eighth cranial nerves are clearly outlined. (*From Krause F. Surgery of the Brain and Spinal Cord Based on Personal Experiences. Translated by H. Haubold and M. Thorek. New York: Rebman Co; 1909-1912.*)

provided him with a strong foundation in neurological diagnosis (Fig. 1-67). Working closely with Charles McBurney (1845-1913), a New York City general surgeon, he came to the realization that not only could brain surgery be done safely but also was clearly necessary in the treatment of certain neurological problems.[149-151] Starr summarized his views in the preface:

Brain surgery is at present a subject both novel and interesting. It is within the past five years only that operations for the relief of epilepsy and

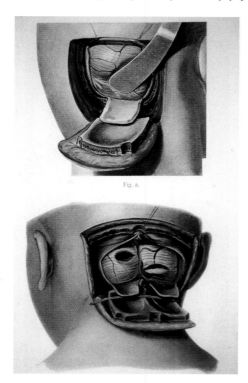

FIGURE 1-66 Krause was an advocate of the "osteoplastic" flap in which the bone was removed with the overlying muscle and scalp. In these images Krause outlines a unilateral and a bilateral craniotomy to expose the cerebellum. (*From Krause F. Surgery of the Brain and Spinal Cord Based on Personal Experiences. Translated by H. Haubold and M. Thorek. New York: Rebman Co; 1909-1912.*)

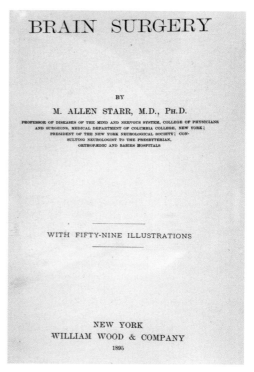

BRAIN SURGERY

BY

M. ALLEN STARR, M.D., Ph.D.

PROFESSOR OF DISEASES OF THE MIND AND NERVOUS SYSTEM, COLLEGE OF PHYSICIANS
AND SURGEONS, MEDICAL DEPARTMENT OF COLUMBIA COLLEGE, NEW YORK;
PRESIDENT OF THE NEW YORK NEUROLOGICAL SOCIETY; CON-
SULTING NEUROLOGIST TO THE PRESBYTERIAN,
ORTHOPÆDIC AND BABIES HOSPITALS

WITH FIFTY-NINE ILLUSTRATIONS

NEW YORK
WILLIAM WOOD & COMPANY
1893

FIGURE 1-67 A neurologist, not a neurosurgeon, authored the first monograph on brain surgery published in the United States. Allen Starr, a neurologist, was one of the earliest and strongest advocates of exploration of the brain based on a thorough neurological examination at the bedside. (*From Starr MA. Brain Surgery. New York: William Wood and Co; 1893.*)

of imbecility, for the removal of clots from the brain, for the opening of abscesses, for the excision of tumors, and the relief of intra-cranial pressure have been generally attempted. Brain surgery has as its essential basis the accurate diagnosis of cerebral lesions, which was impossible until the localization of cerebral functions had been determined. And this diagnosis must be made by the physician before the surgeon is called in to remove the disease. It is the object of this book to state clearly those facts regarding the essential features of brain disease which will enable the reader to determine in any case both the nature and situation of the pathological process in progress, to settle the question whether the disease can be removed by surgical interference, and to estimate the safety and probability of success by operation. The facts have been reached by a careful study of the literature of the subject and by a considerable personal experience. It is my hope that this work may aid the physician to diagnosticate brain diseases with more accuracy, and to select such cases as are properly open to surgical treatment by trephining, and also that may enable the surgeon to perform his delicate task with more precision and with a fuller knowledge of those principles of local diagnosis which should form this constant guide.[149]

Harvey William Cushing (1869-1939) was the founder of American neurosurgery (Figs. 1-68 and 1-69). Cushing had the good fortune to be alive and in training during the formative years of neurosurgery. Educated at Johns Hopkins under one of the premier general surgeons, William Halsted (1852-1922), Cushing learned meticulous surgical technique from his mentor. As was standard then, Cushing spent time in Europe; he worked in the laboratories of Theodore Kocher in Bern, where he investigated the physiology of CSF. These studies led to his important monograph in 1926 on the third circulation.[152] It was during this period of experimentation that the cerebral phenomenon of increased intracranial pressure in association with hypertension and bradycardia was defined; it is now referred to as the *Cushing*

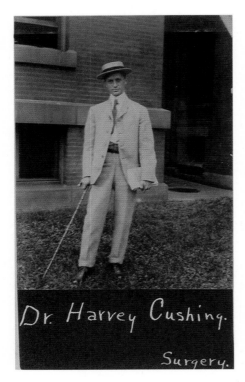

FIGURE 1-68 Photograph of a young dapper Cushing taken during his early period at Johns Hopkins. This portrait comes from a rare album issued in the early part of the 20th century that illustrated some of the prominent figures of the Johns Hopkins University and Hospital. Cushing's personality is evident in this early image of him.

pituitary gland published in 1932.[154] In a monograph written with Percival Bailey in 1926, Cushing introduced the first rational approach to the classification of brain tumors.[155] Cushing's monograph on meningioma, written in collaboration with Louise Eisenhardt in 1938, remains the standard for the profession.[156]

Cushing retired as Moseley Professor of Surgery at Harvard in 1932. When he completed his 2000th brain tumor operation, he had unquestionably made one of the most important contributions to the field of neurosurgery—a contribution comprising meticulous, innovative surgical techniques and a career-long attempt to understand brain function from both a physiologic and a pathologic perspective.[157] An ardent bibliophile, Cushing spent his final years in retirement as Sterling Professor of Neurology at Yale, where he put together his extraordinary monograph on Andreas Vesalius.[158] Cushing's life was faithfully recorded by his close friend and colleague John F. Fulton (1946)[159] and in a recent biography by Michael Bliss.[160]

If Harvey Cushing is the father of American neurosurgery, his prodigal son is Walter Dandy (1886-1946) (Fig. 1-70), who trained under Cushing at Johns Hopkins Hospital. Dandy made a number of important contributions to neurosurgery. Using the serendipitous finding of Luckett,[161] the presence of air in the ventricles after a skull fracture, Dandy developed the technique of pneumoencephalography (PEG).[162-164] The introduction of PEG provided the neurosurgeon, for the first time, the opportunity to localize a tumor by analyzing the displacement of air in the ventricles. Dandy was an innovative neurosurgeon, considerably more aggressive in style and technique than Cushing. Dandy was the first to show that acoustic neuromas could be removed in their totality.[165,166] He devoted much effort to the treatment of hydrocephalus.[167,168] He first introduced the technique of ablating and removing the choroid plexus to reduce the production of CSF.[169] Dandy was among the first to surgically deal with

phenomenon. While traveling through Europe, he met several important surgical personalities, including Macewen and Horsley. These individuals provided the impetus for Cushing to consider neurosurgery as a full-time endeavor.

Cushing's contributions to the literature of neurosurgery are too extensive for this brief chapter. Among his most significant is a monograph on pituitary surgery published in 1912.[153] This monograph was to inaugurate a sterling career in pituitary studies. Cushing's syndrome was defined in his final monograph on the

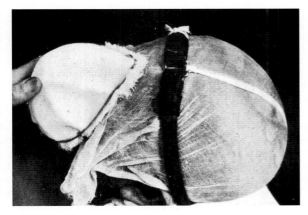

FIGURE 1-69 A key to Cushing's success as a surgeon was a number of inventive techniques designed to reduce morbidity and mortality during neurosurgical procedures. Illustrated here is one of Cushing's numerous innovations, a pneumatic tourniquet placed on the scalp before skin incision to reduce blood loss.

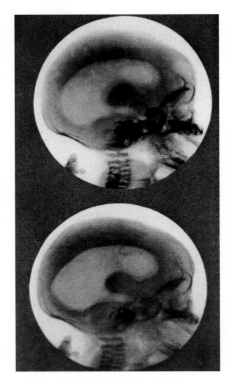

FIGURE 1-70 One of the landmark contributions to neurosurgery made by Dandy (and Blackfan), introduction of the pneumoencephalogram—a technique in which air was introduced into the ventricles and with a radiograph the ventricular system could be seen in outline.

cerebral aneurysms by obliterating them with snare ligatures or metal clips.[170] His monograph on the third ventricle and its anatomy remains a textbook standard to this day, with illustrations that are among the best ever produced.[171]

In the field of spine surgery, two important American figures appeared in the first quarter of the 20th century: Charles Elsberg (1871-1948), professor of neurosurgery at the New York Neurological Institute, and Charles Frazier (1870-1936), professor of surgery at the University of Pennsylvania. Work in the 19th century by J. L. Corning (1885) had shown that lumbar puncture can be safely performed.[172] This procedure was popularized by H. Quincke, who used it for the treatment of hydrocephalus, and from this procedure spine surgery developed.[173,174] When Charles Frazier's book on spine surgery appeared in 1918, the most comprehensive work on spine surgery yet to be written became available.[175] Frazier summarized much of the spine surgery literature to that point. He established that spine surgery could be performed with minimal morbidity and mortality. Frazier's experience in World War I led him to devote his career to neurosurgery. A gracious person, he followed a heavy work schedule. It was not uncommon for Frazier to sweep the operating room at the completion of a case just to relax his shoulder muscles, only then discussing the operation just completed with his colleagues.

Charles Elsberg (1871-1948), a pioneer in spine surgery, had surgical technique that was described as impeccable and consistently led to excellent outcomes. In 1912 Elsberg published a landmark paper in which he reported on a series of 43 laminectomies.[176] In 1916 he published the first of what were to be three monographs on surgery on the spine.[177] One of Elsberg's seminal contributions was a staged technique to allow the delivery of an intramedullary spinal cord tumor.[176] It consisted of first a myelotomy, which in theory allowed an intramedullary tumor to deliver itself over time into the laminectomy. Then at a second operation the tumor could be removed after having extruded through myelotomy. Elsberg was known as a driven worker who approached the practice of neurosurgery with a fierce intensity, always looking for new techniques. Working with Cornelius Dyke (1900-1943), a neuroradiologist at the New York Neurological Institute, he treated spinal glioblastomas with directed radiation in the operating room after the tumor had been exposed! Procedures such as these were performed with the patients receiving only local anesthesia. During the ½-hour therapy, while the radiation was being delivered, the surgeon and assistants stood off in the distance behind a glass shield.[178]

CONCLUSION

The 19th century brought the introduction of anesthesia, antisepsis, and cerebral localization. The later half of the 19th century produced strong surgical personalities, surgeons adventurous enough to perform surgery on the formidable cranial vault and spine. In the first half of the 20th century, formalization of the field of neurosurgery occurred. Besides the pioneering techniques of Dandy, Cushing, and others, a number of diagnostic techniques were introduced that made it easier for the neurosurgeon to localize lesions. One technique, myelography with opaque substances, was brought forward by Jean Athanase Sicard (1872-1929).[179] Using radiopaque iodized oil, the spinal cord and its elements could be outlined on radiographs. Antonio Caetano de Egas Moniz (1874-1955), professor of neurology in Lisbon, Portugal, perfected arterial catheterization techniques and the cerebral angiogram in animal studies.[180,181] This procedure, in combination with PEG, offered the neurosurgeon a detailed view of the intracranial contents. Moniz was awarded the Nobel Prize in 1949 for his work on prefrontal lobotomy for psychiatric disorders.

In 1929 Alexander Fleming (1881-1955) published a report on the first observation of a substance that appeared to block a bacterium from growing.[182] This substance, identified as penicillin, introduced a new era of medicine and surgery. With the World War II experience, antibiotics for the treatment of bacterial infection were perfected, thereby even further reducing the risk for infection during brain and spine surgery.

As a result of our surgical forebearers, surgeons can now complete a neurosurgical procedure with the patient suffering no pain and minimal risk for infection. Our 19th century ancestors provided us pioneering techniques in cerebral localization that have led to the introduction of frameless guidance systems. The surgical fear of operating on the wrong area is no longer an issue; for this we can thank our historical giants, on whose shoulders and studies the field of neurosurgery has developed.

SUGGESTED READINGS

Bakay L. *An Early History of Craniotomy. From Antiquity to the Napoleonic Era.* Springfield. Ill: Charles C Thomas; 1985.

Bakay L. *Neurosurgeons of the Past.* Springfield, III: Charles C Thomas; 1987.

Castiglioni A. *A History of Medicine. Translated from the Italian and Edited by E.B. Krubhaar.* 2nd ed, revised and enlarged. New York: A.A. Knopf; 1947.

Clarke ES, Dewhurst K. *An Illustrated History of Brain Function.* Oxford; 1972. Reprinted in 1992 by Norman Publishing, San Francisco.

Clarke E, O'Malley CD. *The Human Brain and Spinal Cord. A historical study illustrated by writings from antiquity to the twentieth centry.* Berkeley: University of California Press; 1968. Reprinted in 1992 by Norman Publishing, San Francisco.

DeJong RN. *A History of American Neurology.* New York: Raven Press; 1982.

Garrison FH. *An Introduction to the History of Medicine.* 4th ed, revised and enlarged. Philadelphia: Saunders; 1929.

Gurdjian ES. *Head Injury from Antiquity to the Present with Special Reference to Penetrating Head Injury.* Springfield, III: Charles C. Thomas; 1973.

Haymaker W, Schiller F. *The Founders of Neurlogy.* 2nd ed. Springfield, III: Charles C. Thomas; 1970.

Leonardo RA. *History of Surgery.* New York: Froben Press; 1943.

McHenry LC. *Garrison's History of Neurology Revised and Enlarged with a Bibliography of Classical, Original and Standard Works in Neurlogy.* Springfield, III: Charles C. Thomas; 1969.

Mettler CC, ed. *History of Medicine. A Correlative Text, Arranged According to Subjects.* Philadelphia: Blakiston; 1947.

Meyer A. *Historical Aspects of Cerebral Anatomy.* London: Oxford University Press; 1971.

Norman JM, ed. *Norton's Medical Bibliography.* 5th ed. Cambridge, UK: Scholar Press; 1991.

Poynter FNL, ed. *The History and Philosophy of Knowledge of the Brain and its Functions.* Springfield, III: Charles C. Thomas; 1958.

Rose FC, Bynum WF. *Historical Aspects of the Neurosciences. A Festschrift for Macdonald Critchley.* New York: Raven Press; 1982.

Sachs E. *The History and Development of Neurological Surgery.* New York: Paul Hoeber; 1952.

Soury J. *Le Système Nerveux Centrale Structure et Fonctions. Histoire Critique des Théories et des Doctrines.* Paris: Georges Carré & Naud; 1899.

Spillane JD. *The Doctrine of the Nerves. Chapters in the History of Neurology.* London: Oxford University Press; 1981.

Walker AE. *A History of Neurological Surgery.* Baltimore, Md: Williams and Wilkins; 1951.

Wilkins RH. *Neurosurgical Classics. Compiled by Robert H. Wilkins.* New York: Johnson Reprint Co; 1965.

Full references can be found on Expert Consult @ www.expertconsult.com

Basic Science

CHAPTER 2

Surgical Anatomy of the Brain

Hung Tzu Wen ■ Albert L. Rhoton Jr. ■ Antônio C. M. Mussi

It is our belief that observation of the anatomy of the brain from different angles is the key to assemble an authentic tridimensional knowledge. As important as knowledge of the surface anatomy, or the anatomy of deeply located structures, is establishment of correlation between them. Such correlation will empower us to have "x-ray" vision that will enable us to "see" the depths of the brain through its surface.

In this chapter, the surgical anatomy of the neural and vascular structures of both the cerebrum and cerebellum is reviewed in stepwise dissection by following the logical sequence based on the three surfaces that each one of them presents.

CEREBRUM

Lateral Surface: Neural Structures

Superficial Anatomy

The cerebrum is arbitrarily divided into five lobes: frontal, parietal, temporal, occipital, and the hidden insula. On the lateral surface, they are limited by the central sulcus, the posterior ramus of the sylvian fissure, the lateral parietotemporal line (from the impression of the parieto-occipital sulcus to the preoccipital notch), and the temporo-occipital line (from the posterior end of the posterior ramus of the sylvian fissure to the midpoint of the lateral parietotemporal line). The cerebrum has four main sulci that are 100% continuous—the sylvian fissure and the callosal, parieto-occipital, and collateral sulci—and two almost continuous (92%) sulci—the central and calcarine sulci. There are two 100% interrupted sulci: the precentral and inferior temporal sulci.[1] The central sulcus starts from the medial surface of the hemisphere above the cingulate sulcus and extends on the lateral surface of the hemisphere in a medial-to-lateral, superior-to-inferior, and posterior-to-anterior direction. It does not usually intercept the posterior ramus of the sylvian fissure and leaves a "bridge" connecting the precentral to the postcentral gyrus, known as *pli de passage frontoparietal inferior, opercule rolandique,* or the *subcentral gyrus* (Fig. 2-1A).

Frontal Lobe

The two main sulci are the superior and inferior frontal sulci, which are anteroposteriorly oriented and extend from the precentral sulcus to the frontal pole. At their posterior end, these two sulci are intercepted perpendicularly by the precentral sulcus, which has a direction very similar to that of the central sulcus. The precentral sulcus forms the anterior limit of the precentral gyrus. These two frontal sulci divide the lateral surface of the frontal lobe into three gyri: the superior, middle, and inferior frontal gyri (Fig. 2-1A). The anterior horizontal, the anterior ascending, and the posterior rami of the sylvian fissure divide the inferior frontal gyrus into three parts: the pars orbitalis, triangularis, and opercularis. The apex of the pars triangularis is usually retracted superiorly and leaves a space in the sylvian fissure that is generally the largest space in the superficial compartment of the sylvian fissure. The apex of the pars triangularis is directed inferiorly toward the junction of three rami of the sylvian fissure; this junctional point coincides with the anterior limiting sulcus of the insula in the depth of the sylvian fissure. It marks the anterior limit of the basal ganglia and the location of the anterior horn of the lateral ventricle. At the intercepting point between the superior frontal and precentral sulci, the precentral gyrus often has the morphology of the Greek letter "Ω" (omega), with its convexity pointing posteriorly. This is the most easily identifiable landmark of the motor strip and corresponds to the hand area (Fig. 2-1B).

Parietal Lobe

The parietal lobe is limited anteriorly by the central sulcus, medially by the interhemispheric fissure, inferolaterally by the sylvian fissure and the temporo-occipital line, and posteriorly by the lateral parietotemporal line. Its two main sulci are the postcentral and intraparietal sulci. The postcentral sulcus is very similar to the central sulcus, except for its variable continuity. The postcentral sulcus is the posterior limit of the postcentral gyrus, and it can sometimes be double. The intraparietal sulcus starts at the postcentral sulcus and is directed posteriorly and inferiorly toward the occipital pole; its direction is often parallel and 2 to 3 cm lateral to the midline. The bottom of the intraparietal sulcus is related to both the roof of the atrium and the occipital horn. The intraparietal sulcus divides the lateral surface of the parietal lobe into two parts: the superior and inferior parietal lobules. The superior parietal lobule, which is the superomedial and smaller part, continues as the precuneus on the medial surface of the parietal lobe. The inferior parietal lobule is constituted by the supramarginal and angular gyri. The supramarginal gyrus, the posterior continuation of the superior temporal gyrus, turns around the posterior ascending ramus of the sylvian fissure. The

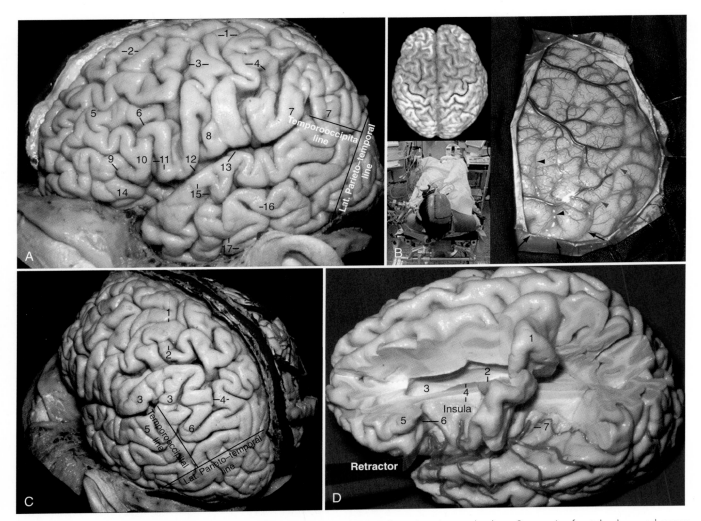

FIGURE 2-1 A, Lateral view of the left hemisphere. 1, "Omega" (motor hand area) and central sulcus; 2, superior frontal sulcus and gyrus; 3, precentral sulcus and gyrus; 4, postcentral sulcus and gyrus; 5, middle frontal gyrus; 6, inferior frontal sulcus; 7, supramarginal gyrus; 8, pli de passage; 9, anterior horizontal ramus; 10, pars triangularis; 11, ascending ramus and pars opercularis; 12, posterior ramus; 13, Heschl's gyrus; 14, pars orbitalis; 15, superior temporal gyrus and sulcus; 16, middle temporal gyrus; 17, inferior temporal sulcus and gyrus. **B,** *Upper left,* "omega"sign. *Lower left,* surgical positioning. *Right,* the *arrows* indicate the "omega," the *black arrowheads* indicate the superior frontal sulcus, and the *blue arrowheads* indicate the central sulcus. **C,** Posterolateral view of the left hemisphere. 1, Central sulcus; 2, postcentral gyrus and sulcus; 3, supramarginal gyrus; 4, intraparietal sulcus and superior parietal lobule; 5, superior temporal gyrus; 6, angular gyrus. **D,** Superolateral view of the left hemisphere. 1, Precentral gyrus; 2, foramen of Monro; 3, frontal horn; 4, head of the caudate nucleus and the superior limiting sulcus (insula); 5, pars orbitalis; 6, anterior limiting sulcus (insula); 7, inferior limiting sulcus (insula).

angular gyrus is the posterior continuation of the middle temporal gyrus and turns superiorly and medially behind the posterior ramus of the sylvian fissure up to the intraparietal sulcus; it is sometimes limited between the two posterior terminations of the superior temporal sulcus, the angular and anterior occipital rami (Fig. 2-1C).

The postcentral and intraparietal sulci and the superior parietal lobule are a "mirror image" of the precentral and superior frontal sulci and the superior frontal gyrus, with the central sulcus being the "mirror."

Temporal Lobe

The temporal lobe is limited superiorly by the posterior ramus of the sylvian fissure and posteriorly by the temporo-occipital and lateral parietotemporal lines. It has two main sulci, the superior and inferior temporal sulci, that divide the lateral surface of the temporal lobe into three gyri, the superior, middle, and inferior

temporal gyri. The inferior temporal gyrus occupies the lateral and basal surfaces of the cerebrum. The superior and inferior temporal gyri converge anteriorly to form the temporal pole (Fig. 2-1A).

Occipital Lobe

The occipital lobe is located behind the lateral parietotemporal line and is composed of a number of irregular convolutions that are divided by a short horizontal sulcus, the lateral occipital sulcus, into the superior and inferior occipital gyri.

The "x-ray" vision concept can be demonstrated by the precentral gyrus, which begins on the medial surface of the cerebrum, above the level of the splenium of the corpus callosum, and passes above the body of the lateral ventricle, thalamus, posterior limb of the internal capsule, and posterior part of the lentiform nucleus to reach the sylvian fissure approximately midway between the anterior and posterior limits of the insula (Fig. 2-1D).

Sylvian Fissure

The sylvian fissure is the space between the frontal, parietal, and temporal opercula and the insula and extends from the basal to the lateral surface of the brain. It is composed of a superficial and a deep part. The superficial part has a stem and three rami; the stem extends medially from the semilunar gyrus of the uncus to the lateral end of the sphenoid ridge, where the stem divides into the anterior horizontal, anterior ascending, and posterior rami (Fig. 2-1A). The deep part is divided into a "sphenoidal compartment" and an "operculoinsular compartment." The sphenoidal compartment, which arises in the region of the limen insulae lateral to the anterior perforated substance (APS), is a narrow space posterior to the sphenoid ridge between the frontal and temporal lobes that communicates medially with the carotid cistern, also called *sylvian vallecula* (see Fig. 2-4D).[2] The operculoinsular compartment is formed by two narrow clefts, the opercular cleft between the opposing lips of the frontoparietal and temporal opercula and the insular cleft, which has a superior limb located between the insula and the frontoparietal opercula

and an inferior limb between the insula and the temporal operculum (Fig. 2-2A).[3] The gyri that constitute the frontal and parietal opercula of the sylvian fissure are, from posterior to anterior, the supramarginal, postcentral, and precentral gyri and the pars opercularis, triangularis, and orbitalis (see Fig. 2-1A); the gyri that constitute the temporal operculum of the sylvian fissure are, from posterior to anterior, the planum temporale, Heschl's gyrus, and the planum polare (Fig. 2-2B, *left*). Each gyrus of the frontoparietal operculum is related to its counterpart on the temporal side; the supramarginal gyrus is in contact with the planum temporale, the postcentral gyrus is in contact with Heschl's gyrus, and the precentral gyrus and pars opercularis, triangularis, and orbitalis are related to the planum polare. The site on the posterior ramus of the sylvian fissure where the postcentral gyrus meets Heschl's gyrus is projected in the same coronal plane as the external acoustic meatus. The medial wall of the sylvian fissure is the insula or island of Reil, which can be seen only when the lips of the sylvian fissure are widely separated. The insula has the shape of a pyramid with its apex directed inferiorly and has an anterior and a lateral surface.

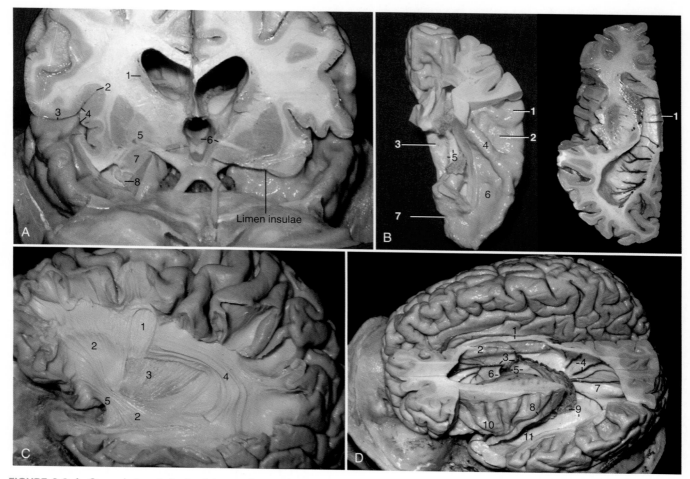

FIGURE 2-2 A, Coronal view. 1, Body of the caudate nucleus; 2, superior limiting sulcus; 3, opercular compartment; 4, insular compartment; 5, globus pallidus; 6, floor of the third ventricle and anterior commissure; 7, amygdala; 8, head of the hippocampus. **B,** *Left,* Anterosuperior view of the left temporal lobe. 1, Posterior transverse temporal gyrus; 2, middle transverse temporal gyrus; 3, parahippocampal gyrus; 4, Heschl's gyrus; 5, fornix and dentate gyrus; 6, planum polare; 7, rhinal incisura. *Right,* Basal view of the roof of the lateral ventricle. 1, Septum pellucidum. The veins of the roof of the lateral ventricle drain toward the midline. **C,** Fiber dissection of the left hemisphere. 1, Corona radiata; 2, inferior occipitofrontal fascicle; 3, putamen; 4, superior longitudinal fascicle; 5, uncinate fascicle. **D,** Lateral view of the left lateral ventricle. 1, Corpus callosum; 2, septum pellucidum; 3, anterior septal and superior choroidal veins; 4, bulb of the callosum and medial atrial vein; 5, thalamostriate vein and thalamus (anterior tubercle); 6, column of the fornix and foramen of Monro; 7, calcar avis; 8, central sulcus of the insula; 9, choroid plexus and atrium; 10, apex of the insula; 11, temporal horn.

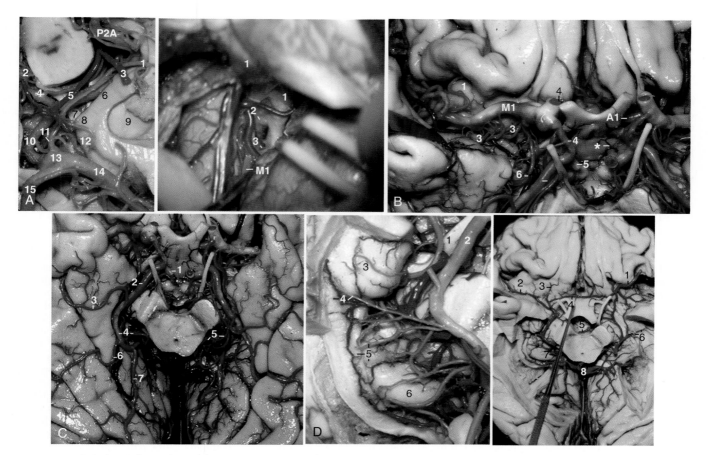

FIGURE 2-6 A, *Left,* 1, Inferior choroidal point; 2, posterior perforating arteries; 3, inferior ventricular vein; 4, P1 and medial posterior choroidal artery; 5, basal vein; 6, uncus (posterior segment); 7, oculomotor nerve; 8, uncus (apex); 9, hippocampus (head); 10, posterior communicating artery; 11, anterior choroidal artery; 12, uncus (anterior segment); 13, internal carotid artery; 14, M1; 15, A1. *Right,* Left trans-sylvian approach. 1, Supraclinoid carotid artery; 2, fetal posterior communicating artery; 3, anterior choroidal artery. **B,** Basal view. 1, Insula; 2, supraclinoid carotid artery; 3, lateral lenticulostriate arteries; 4, posterior communicating artery; 5, P1; 6, anterior choroidal artery; 7, P2A; *, premamillary artery. **C,** Basal view. 1, P1; 2, P2A; 3, anterior inferior temporal artery; 4, P2P and long circumflex arteries; 5, short circumflex arteries; 6, middle inferior temporal artery; 7, posterior inferior temporal artery. **D,** Basal view. *Left,* 1, Optic tract; 2, P2A; 3, uncus (inferior surface); 4, hippocampal artery and dentate gyrus; 5, lateral posterior choroidal artery, fornix, and lateral geniculate body; 6, thalamus (pulvinar). *Right,* Basal view. 1, Fronto-orbital vein; 2, deep middle cerebral vein; 3, olfactory vein; 4, anterior cerebral vein; 5, peduncular vein; 6, inferior ventricular vein and inferior choroidal point; 7, posterior mesencephalic segment; 8, vein of Galen. The choroid plexus separates the roof of the temporal horn from the thalamus.

surface of the uncus, and laterally by the limen insulae. Medially, the APS extends above the optic chiasm to the interhemispheric fissure. The APS and the carotid bifurcation can be identified intraoperatively by following the olfactory tract posteriorly. The APS can be considered the "floor" of the anterior half of the basal ganglia (Fig. 2-5C, *right*).

Basal Surface: Arterial Relationships

The *internal carotid artery* is divided into five parts: the cervical, petrous, cavernous, clinoid, and supraclinoid portions. The supraclinoid portion has been divided into three segments based on the origin of its major branches: the *ophthalmic segment* extends from the origin of the ophthalmic artery to the origin of the posterior communicating artery (PCom), the *communicating segment* extends from the origin of the PCom to the origin of the anterior choroidal artery (AChA), and the *choroidal segment* extends from the origin of the AChA to the bifurcation of the ICA (Fig. 2-5D). The *ophthalmic artery* arises under the optic nerve, usually from the medial third of the superior surface of the ICA, passes anteriorly and laterally to become superolateral to

the carotid, and enters the optic canal and the orbit. The perforating arteries from this segment arise from the posterior, medial, or posteromedial aspect of the ICA and are distributed to the stalk of the pituitary gland, the optic chiasm, and less commonly the optic nerve, premamillary portion of the floor of the third ventricle, and the optic tract. The *superior hypophysial arteries,* which can range from 1 to 5 in number, pass medially to supply the pituitary stalk and the anterior lobe of the pituitary gland. The *inferior hypophysial artery* from the meningohypophysial trunk of the cavernous ICA supplies the posterior lobe. The *infundibular arteries* are another group of arteries that arise from the PCom and supply the same area as the superior hypophysial artery. The PCom arises from the posteromedial or the posterior or posterolateral aspect of the ICA and passes posteromedially to join the posterior cerebral artery (PCA) (Fig. 2-6A, *left*). In the embryo, the PCom continues as PCA, but in adults the PCA becomes part of the basilar system. If the PCom remains the major origin of the PCA, the configuration of the PCom is termed *fetal* (Fig. 2-6A, *right*). In 60% of individuals there are no perforating arteries arising from the communicating segment of the ICA; when present, the perforating arteries from the PCom range from 4 to 14 in number, arise predominantly from the proximal half of the artery, course superiorly, and terminate in the floor of the third ventricle. The largest branch from the PCom is the *premamillary artery* or "*anterior thalamoperforating artery*" (Fig. 2-6B).

The *anterior choroidal artery* arises from either the posterolateral or posterior aspect of the ICA. The AChA courses posteriorly below the optic tract toward the temporal horn by passing through the choroidal fissure (Fig. 2-6A, *left*). The AChA sends off branches to the optic tract, crus cerebri, lateral geniculate body, and uncus and supplies the optic radiation, globus pallidus, midbrain, thalamus, and the retrolenticular and posterior portions of the posterior limb of the internal capsule.

The choroidal segment of the ICA is the most frequent site of perforating arteries (range, one to nine) arising from the posterior aspect of the ICA. They terminate in the posterior half of the central region of the APS, optic tract, and uncus.[16]

The anterior perforating arteries are those arising from the ICA, MCA, AChA, and ACA, and they enter the brain through the APS (Fig. 2-6B).

The M1, or *sphenoidal segment* of the MCA, extends from the bifurcation of the ICA to the limen insulae. It courses first in the carotid cistern and then continues in the sphenoidal compartment. The proximal half of M1 is related posteriorly and inferiorly to the anteromedial surface of the uncus, anteriorly to the lesser wing of the sphenoid, and superiorly to the APS; the distal half is related inferiorly to the planum polare, anteriorly to the lesser wing of the sphenoid, and superiorly and posteriorly to the insular pole. M1 has two types of branches: the lateral lenticulostriate arteries, which arise mostly from the superior or posterosuperior aspect of M1 and penetrate the middle and posterior portions of the lateral half of APS, and the early branches, which course toward the temporal lobe to supply the temporal pole. The bifurcation of the MCA occurs before the limen insulae in 86% of individuals (see Figs. 2-4D and 2-6B and C).[3]

Embryologically, the *posterior cerebral artery* arises as a branch of the ICA, but up to birth its most frequent origin is the basilar artery.[17] The PCA is divided into four segments: *P1* extends from the basilar bifurcation to the site where the PCom joins the PCA. *P2* extends from the PCom to the posterior aspect of the midbrain. P2 is further divided into *P2A (anterior)* and *P2P (posterior) segments*. P2A begins at the PCom and courses around the crus cerebri, inferior to the optic tract, AChA, and basal vein and medial to the posteromedial surface of the uncus, up to the posterior margin of the crus cerebri. P2P begins at the posterior margin of the crus cerebri; runs lateral to the tegmentum of the midbrain within the ambient cistern, parallel and inferior to the basal vein, inferolateral to the geniculate bodies and pulvinar, and medial to the parahippocampal gyrus; and enters the quadrigeminal cistern. *P3* begins under the posterior part of the pulvinar in the lateral aspect of the quadrigeminal cistern and ends at the anterior limit of the anterior calcarine sulcus. P3 often divides into its major terminal branches, the calcarine and parieto-occipital arteries, before reaching the anterior limit of the anterior calcarine sulcus. The point where the PCAs from each side are closer to each other is called the *collicular* or *quadrigeminal point*. It marks the posterior limit of the midbrain on angiograms (see Fig. 2-14A). The *P4 segment* is the cortical branches of the PCA (Fig. 2-6C).

The main branches arising from the PCA are the posterior thalamoperforating, the direct perforating, the short and long circumflex, the thalamogeniculate, the medial and lateral posterior choroidal, the inferior temporal, the parieto-occipital, the calcarine, and the posterior pericallosal arteries. The *posterior thalamoperforating arteries*, which arise from P1 and enter the brain through the posterior perforated substance, interpeduncular fossa, and medial crus cerebri, supply the anterior and part of the posterior thalamus, hypothalamus, subthalamus, substantia

nigra, red nucleus, oculomotor and trochlear nuclei, oculomotor nerve, mesencephalic reticular formation, pretectum, rostromedial floor of the third ventricle, and the posterior portion of the internal capsule. The *direct perforating arteries* to the crus cerebri arise mainly from the P2A segment and supply the crus cerebri. The *short* and *long circumflex arteries* to the brainstem arise mainly from P1 and less frequently from P2A; the short circumflex artery courses around the midbrain and terminates at the geniculate bodies, whereas the long circumflex artery courses around the midbrain and reaches the colliculi. The *thalamogeniculate arteries* arise equally from the P2A or P2P segments, perforate the inferior surface of the geniculate bodies, and supply the posterior half of the lateral thalamus, posterior limb of the internal capsule, and the optic tract (Fig. 2-6C). The *medial posterior choroidal arteries* (MPChAs) arise mainly from P2A and less frequently from the P2P and P1 segments, course around the midbrain medial to the main trunk of the PCA, turn around the pulvinar of the thalamus and proceed superiorly at the lateral side of the colliculi and pineal gland, enter the roof of the third ventricle through the velum interpositum, and finally course through the foramen of Monro to enter the choroid plexus in the lateral ventricle (see Figs. 2-3A, *right*, and 2-5D). The MPChA supplies the crus cerebri, tegmentum, geniculate bodies (mainly the medial one), colliculi, pulvinar, pineal gland, and medial thalamus. Angiographically on a lateral projection, the MPChA describes the shape of the number "3." The inferior curve of the "3" is the point where it turns around the pulvinar, and the superior curve is the point where it contours the colliculi before entering the roof of the third ventricle (Fig. 2-14B). The *lateral posterior choroidal arteries* (LPChAs) arise mainly from P2P and less frequently from the P2A segment and pass laterally and enter the ventricular cavity directly through the choroidal fissure to supply the choroid plexus in the atrium and the temporal horn. It anastomoses with the AChA (see Figs. 2-4D and 2-6D, *left*). The *inferior temporal arteries* are distributed to the basal surface of the temporal and occipital lobes. They include the hippocampal artery and three groups of temporal arteries, namely, the anterior, middle, and posterior temporal arteries (Fig. 2-6C). The anterior temporal artery arises mainly from P2A, whereas the middle and posterior temporal arteries arise mainly from the P2P segment. The *parieto-occipital* and *calcarine arteries* are usually terminal branches of the PCA; they arise predominantly from P3 but may sometimes also arise from the P2P segment and course into the parieto-occipital and calcarine fissures, respectively. As the calcarine fissure reaches laterally and bulges into the medial wall of the atrium and the occipital horn, the calcarine artery also follows laterally into the depth of the calcarine fissure (see Fig. 2-4D). The *splenial* or *posterior pericallosal artery* supplies the splenium of the corpus callosum and arises from the parieto-occipital artery in 62% of individuals, but it can also arise from the calcarine artery, MPChA, posterior temporal artery, P2P, P3, and LPChA.

Basal Surface: Venous Relationships

The inferior frontal veins drain the basal surface of the *frontal lobe*; they either drain anteriorly to the superior sagittal sinus (anterior group) or drain posteriorly to join the deep sylvian vein in the sylvian fissure (posterior group). The *anterior group* is composed of the anterior fronto-orbital and frontopolar veins, whereas the *posterior group* is composed of the olfactory and the posterior fronto-orbital veins. The inferior temporal veins drain the *temporal lobe*; they are divided into a lateral group that drains into the sinuses in the anterolateral part of the tentorium and a medial group that empties into the basal vein. The *lateral group* is composed of the anterior, middle, and posterior temporobasal veins. The temporobasal veins appear to radiate from the preoccipital notch across the inferior surface of the temporal lobe. The *occipital lobe* is drained by the *occipitobasal vein*, which courses anterolaterally toward the preoccipital notch and frequently joins the posterior temporobasal vein before emptying into the lateral tentorial sinus.

The most important deep venous channel on the basal surface is the basal vein of Rosenthal. The *basal vein* originates below the APS and is divided into three segments (Fig. 2-6D, *right*): the *first*, or *anterior* or *striate segment*, originates from the junction of the anterior cerebral, inferior striate, olfactory, fronto-orbital, and deep middle cerebral veins under the APS and runs posteriorly under the optic tract, medial to the anterior portion of the crus cerebri. This point corresponds to the most medial (before its termination into the vein of Galen) and usually most inferior part of the basal vein and laterally indicates the location of the apex of the uncus. The *second*, or *middle* or *peduncular segment*, starts from the most medial point in the course of the basal vein, usually corresponding to the site where the peduncular vein joins the basal vein. It runs laterally between the upper part of the posteromedial surface of the uncus and the upper part of the crus cerebri and under the optic tract to reach the most lateral part of the crus cerebri, which corresponds to the most lateral point of the vein as it turns around the crus cerebri, generally where the inferior ventricular vein joins the basal vein; this is called the *anterior peduncular segment* by Huang and Wolf.[18] It then turns medially, superiorly, and posteriorly to the plane of the lateral mesencephalic sulcus behind the crus cerebri to constitute the posterior peduncular segment. The main tributaries of the second segment are the peduncular or interpeduncular, inferior ventricular, inferior choroidal, hippocampal, and anterior hippocampal veins. The *third*, or *posterior* or *posterior mesencephalic segment*, runs medially, superiorly, and posteriorly from the lateral mesencephalic sulcus and under the pulvinar of the thalamus to penetrate the quadrigeminal cistern and generally drains into the vein of Galen. The main tributaries of the third segment are the lateral mesencephalic, posterior thalamic, posterior longitudinal hippocampal, medial temporal, and medial occipital veins. Sometimes, the precentral cerebellar, superior vermian, internal occipital, splenial, medial atrial, and direct lateral and lateral atrial subependymal veins may drain into the third segment of the basal vein. In the angiographic frontal view, the overall shape of both basal veins resembles the legs of a frog lying on its back with its toes directed anterolaterally. The foot corresponds to the striate segment and is related superiorly to the APS, laterally to the anterior segment of the uncus, medially to the optic tract, and inferiorly to the contents of the carotid cistern. The ankle corresponds posteriorly to the anterior aspect of the crus cerebri, laterally to the apex of the uncus, and superiorly to the optic tract; the leg corresponds to the anterior peduncular segment and is related superiorly to the optic tract, laterally to the upper portion of the posteromedial surface of the uncus, and medially to the upper portion of the crus cerebri. The knee corresponds to the most lateral aspect of the crus cerebri and to the posterior edge of the posterior segment of the uncus. It is related laterally to the inferior choroidal point, superiorly to the optic tract just before it reaches the lateral geniculate body, and inferiorly to the contents of the ambient cistern. The thigh, which includes the posterior peduncular and the posterior mesencephalic segments, is related medially to the tegmentum of the midbrain, laterally to the parahippocampal gyrus, superiorly to the medial aspect of the pulvinar of the thalamus, which is the roof of the wing of the ambient cistern, and inferiorly to the contents of the wing of the ambient cistern (see Fig. 2-6D).[17] In the angiographic lateral view, the basal and the internal cerebral veins delimit the thalamus and hypothalamus (Fig. 2-7A; also see Fig. 2-13D).

Medial Surface: Neural Relationships

The medial surface of the cerebrum contains the sulci and gyri of the frontal, parietal, occipital, and temporal lobes. The general organization of the gyri of the frontal, parietal, and occipital lobes on this surface can be compared with that of a three-layer roll: the inner layer is represented by the corpus callosum, the intermediate layer by the cingulate gyrus, and the outer layer by the medial frontal gyrus, paracentral lobule, precuneus, cuneus, and lingual gyrus. The cingulate gyrus is separated inferiorly from the corpus callosum by the callosal sulcus and superiorly from the outer layer by the cingulate sulcus. Several secondary rami ascend from the cingulate sulcus in a radiating pattern and divide the outer layer into several sections. There are two secondary rami of particular importance: the *paracentral ramus*, which ascends from the cingulate sulcus at the level of the midpoint of the corpus callosum and separates the medial frontal gyrus anteriorly from the paracentral lobule posteriorly, and the *marginal ramus*, which ascends from the cingulate sulcus at the level of the splenium of the corpus callosum and separates the paracentral lobule anteriorly from the precuneus posteriorly. The *marginal ramus* intercepts the postcentral gyrus in almost 100% of individuals and is an important landmark to determine the location of the sensory or motor areas in the lateral convexity on midsagittal magnetic resonance images. The parieto-occipital sulcus separates the precuneus superiorly from the cuneus inferiorly, and the calcarine sulcus separates the cuneus superiorly from the lingual gyrus inferiorly. The paracentral ramus and the marginal ramus form the *paracentral lobule*, which is concerned with movements of the contralateral lower limb and perineal region and is involved in voluntary control of defecation and micturition. The paracentral lobule comprises the anterior portion of the postcentral and precentral gyri and the posterior portion of the superior frontal gyrus. The *precuneus* and the part of the paracentral lobule behind the central sulcus form the medial part of the parietal lobe; the precuneus corresponds to the superior parietal lobule on the lateral surface. The precuneus presents the *subparietal sulcus*, a vaguely H-shaped sulcus where the vertical arm of the H tends to align with the marginal ramus, and the parieto-occipital sulcus, which separates the precuneus above from the cingulate gyrus below (Fig. 2-7A). The parieto-occipital and calcarine sulci define the *cuneus*; the cuneus and medial part of the lingual gyrus are the medial portion of the occipital lobe. The *calcarine sulcus* starts at the occipital pole and is directed anteriorly; it has a slightly curved course with a characteristic upward convexity. The calcarine sulcus joins the parieto-occipital sulcus (only superficially) at an acute angle behind the isthmus of the cingulate gyrus and continues anteriorly to intercept the isthmus of the cingulate gyrus. The portion of the calcarine sulcus anterior to the junction is called *anterior calcarine sulcus*; it is crossed by a buried *anterior cuneolingual gyrus* and bulges into the medial wall of the atrium of the lateral ventricle as the calcar avis. It contains the visual cortex only on its lower lip. The part of the calcarine sulcus posterior to the union is called the *posterior calcarine sulcus* and includes the striate (visual) cortex on its upper and lower lips (Fig. 2-7A and B). Anteriorly, the cingulate and medial frontal gyri wrap around the genu and rostrum of the corpus callosum. At the inferior end of these two gyri, under the rostrum of the corpus callosum and in front of the lamina terminalis, is a narrow triangle of gray matter, the *paraterminal gyrus*, separated from the rest of the cortex by a shallow *posterior paraolfactory sulcus*. Slightly anterior to this sulcus, a short vertical sulcus may occur, the *anterior paraolfactory sulcus*; the cortex between the posterior and anterior paraolfactory sulci is the *subcallosal area* or paraolfactory gyrus. Frequently, two anteroposteriorly directed sulci, the *superior* and *inferior rostral sulci*, which are parallel to the floor of the anterior fossa, divide the inferior portion of the medial frontal gyrus into three parts. Posteriorly, the cingulate gyrus continues inferiorly with the parahippocampal gyrus through the isthmus of the cingulate gyrus. The *mesial portion of the temporal lobe* contains intraventricular and extraventricular elements. The intraventricular

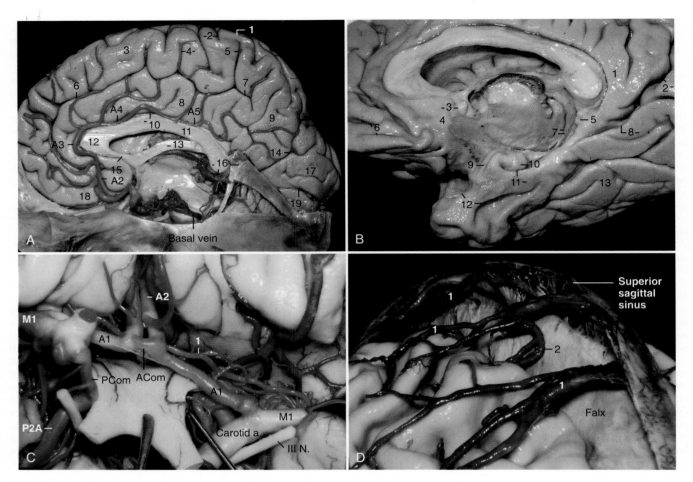

FIGURE 2-7 A, Medial view. 1, Postcentral gyrus; 2, precentral gyrus and central sulcus; 3, medial frontal gyrus; 4, paracentral ramus and para-central lobule; 5, marginal ramus; 6, cingulate sulcus; 7, intraparietal sulcus; 8, cingulate gyrus; 9, precuneus; 10, corpus callosum (body) and callosal sulcus; 11, corpus callosum (isthmus); 12, corpus callosum (genu); 13, fornix and internal cerebral vein; 14, parieto-occipital sulcus; 15, corpus callosum (rostrum); 16, corpus callosum (splenium), vein of Galen, and straight sinus; 17, cuneus; 18, rectus gyrus; 19, posterior calcarine sulcus and lingual gyrus. **B,** Medial view. 1, Cingulate gyrus (isthmus); 2, parieto-occipital sulcus and cuneus; 3, anterior commissure and subcal-losal area; 4, paraterminal gyrus; 5, dentate gyrus; 6, superior and inferior rostral sulci; 7, choroidal fissure and fornix; 8, anterior calcarine sulcus and lingual gyrus; 9, uncus (anterior segment); 10, uncus (posterior segment); 11, uncal notch; 12, rhinal incisura and rhinal sulcus; 13, fusiform gyrus. **C,** Basal view. 1, Recurrent artery. ACom, anterior communicating artery; III n., cranial nerve III, PCom, posterior communicating artery; **D,** Anterolateral view of the right parasagittal area. 1, Vein from the lateral surface; 2, vein from the medial surface.

elements are the hippocampus, fimbria, amygdala, and choroidal fissure; the extraventricular elements are the parahippocampal gyrus, uncus, and dentate gyrus. The *parahippocampal gyrus* extends anteriorly to posteriorly, and at its anterior extremity, it deviates medially and bends posteriorly to constitute the uncus. Posteriorly, just bellow the splenium of the corpus callosum, the parahippocampal gyrus is often intersected by the anterior calca-rine sulcus, which divides the posterior portion of the parahip-pocampal gyrus into the isthmus of the cingulate gyrus superiorly and the parahippocampal gyrus inferiorly; the parahippocampal gyrus continues posteriorly as the lingual gyrus. Superiorly, the parahippocampal gyrus is separated from the dentate gyrus by the hippocampal sulcus. Laterally, the parahippocampal gyrus is limited by the collateral sulcus posteriorly and the rhinal sulcus anteriorly. The rhinal sulcus marks the lateral limit of the ento-rhinal area of the parahippocampal gyrus; the parahippocampal gyrus is separated from the inferior surface of the posterior segment of the uncus by the *uncal notch.* Medially, the parahip-pocampal gyrus is related to the edge of the tentorium and to the contents of the ambient cistern. The various components of the parahippocampal gyrus are the subiculum, presubiculum, parasu-biculum, and entorhinal area; the subiculum is the medial round

edge of the parahippocampal gyrus. The name *uncus* means "hook." It is formed by the anterior portion of the parahippo-campal gyrus, which has deviated medially and folded posteri-orly. Inferiorly, the uncus is separated from the parahippocampal gyrus by the uncal notch. Anteriorly, the uncus continues with the anterior portion of the parahippocampal gyrus without a sharp boundary; superiorly, the uncus is continuous with the globus pallidus. At the basal surface, the uncus is separated later-ally from the temporal pole by the rhinal sulcus, and its medial part is normally herniated medially to the edge of the tentorium. When viewed from its basal surface, the uncus has the shape of an arrowhead with its apex pointing medially; it features an apex, an anterior segment, and a posterior segment (see Fig. 2-3D). The anterior segment of the uncus has one surface, the antero-medial surface, whereas the posterior segment has two surfaces, the posteromedial and inferior surfaces. Both segments converge superiorly at the junction between the amygdala and the globus pallidus. The uncus is composed of five small gyri and a small part of the entorhinal area, which occupies the anterior portion of the anteromedial surface. *The anterior segment* or *anteromedial surface* is part of the parahippocampal gyrus and contains the semilunar and ambient gyri. The semilunar gyrus occupies the lobule), the declive (simple lobule), and the folium (part of the superior semilunar lobule). The primary fissure is located between the quadrangular and simple lobules; the most prominent fissure, the postclival fissure, is located between the simple and superior semilunar lobules. The tentorial surface contains the *cerebellomes-encephalic* or *precentral cerebellar fissure*, which is situated between the cerebellum and the midbrain. Posteriorly, it is limited by the culmen and quadrangular lobule above and the central lobule and its wing below. Anteriorly, it is limited from midline to laterally by the lingula and the superior and middle cerebellar peduncles. The *interpeduncular* or *interbrachial sulcus*, which separates the superior from the middle cerebellar peduncles, ascends from the bottom of the cerebellomesencephalic fissure toward the lateral aspect of the pons, where it is joined by the pontomesencephalic sulcus and proceeds superiorly as the lateral mesencephalic sulcus to the medial geniculate body; the *lateral mesencephalic sulcus* separates the crus cerebri from the tegmentum (see Fig. 2-9B).

Among the cerebellar nuclei (fastigial, globose, emboliform, and dentate), the *dentate nucleus* is the most laterally located and the largest one. The majority of fibers that constitute the superior cerebellar peduncle arise from the dentate nucleus, which is located at the posterior projection of the superior cerebellar peduncle. The dentate nucleus can be considered the roof of the superolateral recess. The superior pole of the tonsils, covered by the inferior medullary velum, is the floor of the superolateral recess.

Suboccipital Surface of the Cerebellum and Fourth Ventricle

The suboccipital surface of the cerebellum and the fourth ventricle are located below the transverse sinuses and between the sigmoid sinuses. Therefore, for better visualization of this surface either during surgery or for anatomic studies, the head has to be bent forward.

The suboccipital surface contains the posterior cerebellar incisura and the vermohemispheric or paravermian fissure, which separates the inferior vermis from the cerebellar hemisphere. The components of the inferior vermis and its hemispheric counterparts are the folium (superior semilunar lobule), tuber (inferior semilunar lobule), pyramid (biventral lobule), uvula (tonsil), and nodule (flocculus). In the anatomic position, the most inferior part of the inferior vermis is the pyramid. The most prominent fissure on the suboccipital surface is the *great horizontal fissure*, which is a circumferential fissure that begins in the posterior cerebellar notch between the folium and the tuber and runs forward and slightly downward on the suboccipital surface, between the superior and inferior semilunar lobules, and then onto the petrosal surface as the petrosal fissure. The *secondary fissure* is located between the tonsils and the biventral lobule (Fig. 2-9C).

After removal of the tonsils, the inferior portion of the roof of the fourth ventricle comes into view (Fig. 2-9D). After removal of the inferior portion of the roof of the fourth ventricle, the floor of the fourth ventricle is exposed.

The *floor of the fourth ventricle* has a rhomboid shape and consists of a strip between the lower margin of the cerebellar peduncles and the site of attachment of the tela choroidea; called the *junctional part*, this strip is formed by the medullary striae, which extend into the lateral recesses. The junctional part divides the floor of the fourth ventricle into two unequal triangles: the superior and larger one, with its apex directed toward the aqueduct, is the pontine part, and the inferior and smaller one, with its apex directed toward the obex, is the medullary part of the floor. These three parts of the floor are also divided longitudinally into two symmetrical halves by the median sulcus. The sulcus limitans, another longitudinal sulcus, divides each half of the floor into a raised median strip called the *median*

eminence and a lateral strip called the *area vestibularis*. The motor nuclei of the cranial nerves are located medial to the sulcus limitans, and the sensory nuclei are situated lateral to it. The pontine part is characterized by two rounded prominences, the *facial colliculi*, located on the median eminence, one on each side of the median sulcus. The facial colliculi are limited laterally by the superior fovea, a dimple formed by the sulcus limitans. The medullary part has the configuration of a feather, or pen nib, and is called the *calamus scriptorius*, with three triangular areas overlying the hypoglossal and vagus nuclei (hypoglossal and vagal trigones) and the area postrema; just lateral to the hypoglossal trigone, the sulcus limitans has another dimple called the *inferior fovea*. At the junctional part the sulcus limitans is discontinuous (Fig. 2-10A).

Veins of the Posterior Fossa

The posterior fossa venous system is divided into three groups: the anterior or petrosal group, which drains into the superior and inferior petrosal sinuses; the superior or galenic group, which drains into the vein of Galen; and the posterior or tentorial group, which drains into the sinuses near the torcula.[22] There is a tendency for the veins to drain into the nearest draining system.

The veins running on the *petrosal surface* of the cerebellum and the anterior surface of the brainstem tend to drain into the petrosal sinuses via the superior petrosal vein, except for the veins running on the surface of the midbrain, which drain into the galenic system. The superior petrosal vein is usually formed by the junction of the transverse pontine and pontotrigeminal (brachial) veins and the vein of the cerebellopontine fissure (great horizontal fissure) (Fig. 2-10B).

The *tentorial surface* and the posterior aspect of the brainstem are served by three draining systems: the midline portion of the cerebellomesencephalic fissure, the veins near the central lobule and culmen (superior vermian veins), and the veins draining the intermediate portion of the wing of the central lobule and the quadrangular lobule (superior hemispheric veins, anterior group), which tend to drain into the vein of Galen. The veins draining the lateral portion of the wing of the central, quadrangular, and simple lobules and the tentorial part of the superior semilunar lobule (superior hemispheric veins, lateral group) tend to drain into the superior petrosal sinus. The veins draining the declive, folium (declival vein), and the intermediate portion of the simple and superior semilunar lobules (superior hemispheric veins, posterior group) tend to drain into the torcula or transverse or tentorial sinus in the tentorium cerebelli (Fig. 2-10C).

The posterior inferior hemispheric veins drain the *suboccipital surface* of the cerebellar hemispheres. Drainage of the inferior vermis is via the inferior vermian veins, which are formed by the junction of the superior and inferior retrotonsillar veins running in the retrotonsillar space (Fig. 2-10D).

The inferior portion of the roof of the fourth ventricle and the lateral recess are drained by the vein of the lateral recess of the fourth ventricle, also called the *vein of the cerebellomedullary fissure*. It courses laterally under the lateral recess toward the cerebellopontine angle, passes above or below the flocculus, joins the vein of the middle cerebellar peduncle or the vein of the cerebellopontine fissure, and finally empties into the superior petrosal sinus via the superior petrosal vein. The vein of the lateral recess of the fourth ventricle can also anastomose with the retrotonsillar veins at the retrotonsillar space to establish communication between the petrosal and the tentorial groups of venous drainage (Fig. 2-10D).

The brachial veins running in the cerebellomesencephalic fissure can also establish communication between the petrosal and galenic groups via the pontotrigeminal and precentral cerebellar veins (Fig. 2-10C).

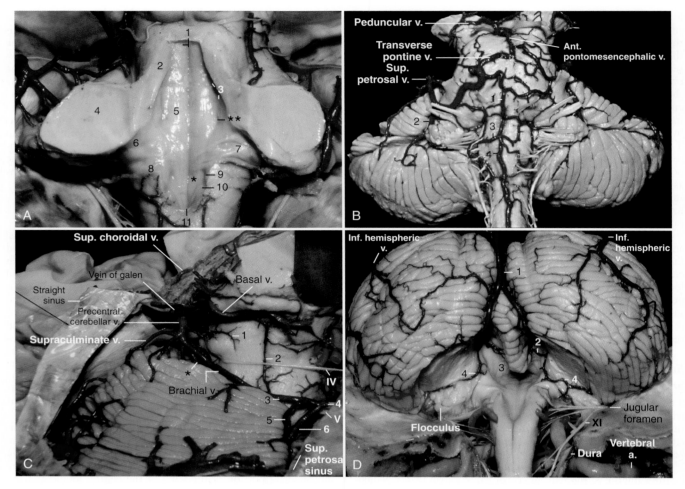

FIGURE 2-10 A, Floor of the fourth ventricle. 1, Median sulcus and median eminence; 2, superior cerebellar peduncle; 3, sulcus limitans and vestibular area; 4, middle cerebellar peduncle; 5, facial colliculus; 6, cochlear area; 7, striae medullaris; 8, inferior cerebellar peduncle; 9, inferior fovea; 10, vagal trigone; 11, obex and area postrema; *, hypoglossal trigone; **, superior fovea. **B,** Frontal view. 1, Anterior pontomesencephalic vein; 2, vein of the great horizontal fissure; 3, transverse medullary vein; 4, anterior medullary vein. **C,** Right posterolateral view of the tentorial surface. 1, Tectal veins; 2, lateral mesencephalic vein; 3, pontotrigeminal vein; 4, superior petrosal vein; 5, superior hemispheric vein; 6, vein of the great horizontal fissure; *, vein of the cerebellomesencephalic fissure. **D,** Suboccipital view. 1, Inferior vermian vein; 2, superior retrotonsillar vein; 3, superior cerebellar peduncle; 4, vein of the lateral recess of the fourth ventricle.

The veins of the posterior fossa can be differentiated into the petrosal group, the superior or galenic group, and the posterior or tentorial group (see Figs. 2-14D and 2-15A to C):

The *petrosal group* may be divided into (1) veins related to the anterior aspect of the brainstem—the anterior pontomesencephalic, transverse pontine, lateral pontine, anterior medullary, and parenchymal perforating veins; (2) veins in the wing of the precentral cerebellar fissure—the brachial veins; (3) veins on the superior and inferior surfaces of the cerebellar hemispheres—the superior and inferior hemispheric veins, including the veins of the great horizontal fissure; (4) veins on the cerebellar side (the medial tonsillar vein) and medullary side (the retro-olivary vein and vein of the inferior cerebellar peduncle of the cerebellomedullary fissure); and (5) the vein of the lateral recess of the fourth ventricle.

The *superior* or *galenic group* includes (1) the mesencephalic tributaries—the median anterior pontomesencephalic, lateral anterior pontomesencephalic, lateral pontomesencephalic, lateral mesencephalic, peduncular, posterior mesencephalic, and tectal veins—and (2) the cerebellar tributaries—the precentral cerebellar vein and its variants and the superior vermian vein.

The *posterior* or *tentorial group* includes the inferior vermian vein and its superior and inferior retrotonsillar tributaries and the superior and inferior hemispheric veins.

Arteries of the Posterior Fossa

The *vertebral artery* (VA) arises from the subclavian artery, enters the transverse foramen of C6, and then ascends through the transverse foramina of the upper cervical vertebrae up to C2. After exiting from the transverse foramen of C2, the VA deviates laterally and enters the laterally placed transverse foramen of C1. The VA then turns behind the lateral mass and above the posterior arch of C1, courses medially and superiorly, and pierces the dura at the foramen magnum. At this level the VA usually gives off the posterior spinal and posterior meningeal arteries. The intradural segment of the VA is divided into lateral medullary and anterior medullary segments before joining its contralateral mate to form the basilar artery (Figs. 2-10D and 2-11B; also see Fig. 2-12B).

The lateral medullary segment of the VA extends from its entrance into the posterior fossa to the preolivary sulcus. From its entrance the VA courses anteriorly, medially, and superiorly

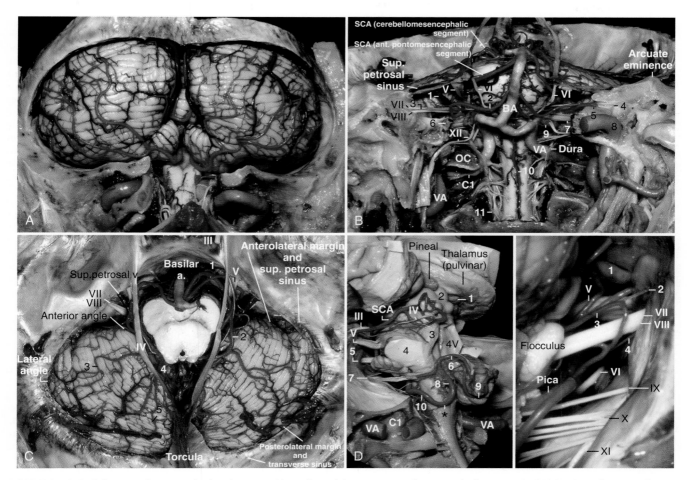

FIGURE 2-11 A, Suboccipital view to display the cortical branches of the posterior inferior cerebellar artery (PICA). **B,** Frontal view. 1, Superior petrosal vein; 2, anterior inferior cerebellar artery (AICA); 3, internal auditory artery; 4, internal acoustic meatus; 5, meatal loop of the AICA; 6, inferior petrosal sinus; 7, vagus nerve; 8, petrous carotid artery; 9, PICA; 10, anterior spinal artery; 11, triangular process of the dentate ligament. BA, basilar artery; OC, occipital condyle; SCA, superior cerebellar artery; VA, vertebral artery. **C,** Superior view of the tentorial surface. 1, Anterior pontomesencephalic segment of the SCA; 2, lateral pontomesencephalic segment of the SCA; 3, superior hemispheric branches of the SCA; 4, cerebellomesencephalic segment of the SCA; 5, superior hemispheric branches of the SCA. **D,** *Left,* Posterolateral view. 1, Medial geniculate body; 2, superior colliculi; 3, superior cerebellar peduncle; 4, middle cerebellar peduncle; 5, AICA, VII and VIII; 6, PICA (supratonsillar segment); 7, jugular foramen; 8, PICA (retrotonsillar segment); 9, PICA (pyramidal loop); 10, PICA (lateral medullary segment); *, caudal loop. *Right,* Retromastoid view of the cerebellopontine angle. 1, Superior petrosal vein; 2, subarcuate artery (AICA); 3, AICA; 4, internal auditory artery.

through the lower cranial nerve rootlets, lateral to the medulla, to reach the preolivary sulcus. The anterior medullary segment begins at the preolivary sulcus, courses in front of or between the hypoglossal rootlets, and crosses the pyramid to join with the other VA at or near the pontomedullary sulcus to form the basilar artery. The main branches of the VA are the posterior spinal artery, anterior spinal artery, PICA, and anterior and posterior meningeal arteries. The VA also sends off branches to supply the lateral and anterior parts of the medulla along its way around the medulla (see Figs. 2-11B, 2-12B, and 2-14A).

The *posterior inferior cerebellar artery* arises from the VA and supplies the medulla, the inferior vermis, the inferior portion of the fourth ventricle, the tonsils, and the inferior aspect of the cerebellum. The "regular" PICA has the most complex and variable course of the cerebellar arteries and is divided into five segments.[23] The *anterior medullary segment* lays in front of the medulla and extends from the origin to the level of the inferior olive. The *lateral medullary segment* courses beside the medulla and extends from the inferior olive to the origin of the glossopharyngeal, vagus, and accessory nerves. The *tonsillomedullary*

or *posterior medullary segment* begins at the level of the nerves and loops below the inferior pole of the cerebellar tonsil and upward along the medial surface of the tonsil toward the inferior medullary velum (caudal loop). The *telovelotonsillar* or *supratonsillar segment* courses in the cleft between the tela choroidea and the inferior medullary velum rostrally and the superior pole of the cerebellar tonsil caudally. It begins below the fastigium, where the PICA turns posteriorly over the medial side of the superior pole of the tonsil. This segment forms the "cranial loop." It sometimes passes posteriorly before reaching the superior pole of the tonsil, thus giving the cranial loop a variable relationship to the fastigium. The junction of the posterior medullary and supratonsillar segments is called the *choroidal point.* The fifth segment is the *cortical segment;* after a short distance distal to the apex of the cranial loop, the PICA continues posteriorly downward in the retrotonsillar fissure, where it usually bifurcates into the tonsillohemispheric branch, which supplies the under aspect of the cerebellar hemisphere, and the inferior vermian branch, which lies on the lower aspect of the inferior vermis and forms a convex loop around the

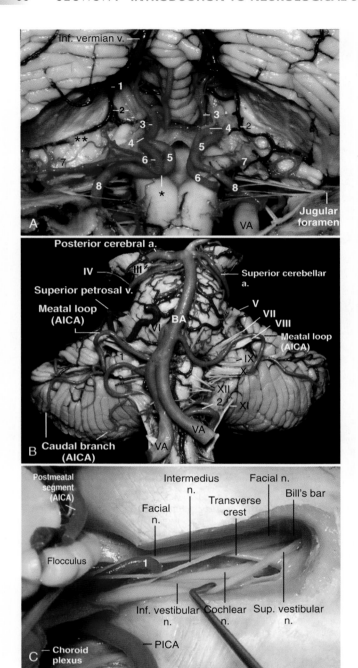

FIGURE 2-12 A, Suboccipital view. The tonsils and the biventral lobule have been removed. 1, Superior retrotonsillar vein; 2, vein of the lateral recess of the fourth ventricle and inferior medullary velum; 3, posterior inferior cerebellar artery (PICA, vermian branch); 4, PICA (supratonsillar segment, cranial loop); 5, PICA (posterior medullary segment); 6, PICA (tonsillohemispheric branch); 7, PICA (choroidal branches); 8, PICA (lateral medullary segment); VA, vertebral artery; *, caudal loop; **, peduncle of the flocculus. **B,** Anterior view. 1, Flocculus; 2, PICA (anterior medullary segment); AICA, anterior inferior cerebellar artery; BA, basal artery. **C,** Posterior view of the contents of the right internal acoustic meatus. 1, AICA (meatal segment).

The *anterior inferior cerebellar artery* and the PICA are defined according to their origin rather than by the portions of cerebellum that they supply. The AICA arises more frequently from the lower third and less frequently from the middle third of the basilar artery. It courses posteriorly, laterally, and usually downward on the belly of the pons, in contact with either the superior or inferior aspect of the abducens nerve. In this course it supplies the lateral aspect of the lower two thirds of the pons and the upper medulla. Either immediately before or after crossing the roots of the facial, intermedius, and acoustic nerves within the cerebellopontine angle, the AICA bifurcates into its two major branches, the *rostrolateral* and the *caudomedial* arteries. The main or *rostrolateral trunk* has been divided into three segments according to their relationship to cranial nerves VII and VIII[24]: the premeatal, meatal, and postmeatal segments. The *premeatal segment* begins at the basilar artery and courses around the brainstem to reach cranial nerves VII and VIII and the region of the meatus, usually anteroinferior to the nerves. Seventy-seven percent of internal auditory arteries and 49% of recurrent perforating arteries to the brainstem arise from this segment. The *meatal segment* is located in the vicinity of the internal auditory meatus, where the nerve-related vessels turn toward the brainstem; this segment often forms a laterally convex loop, the meatal loop, directed toward or through the meatus. It usually stays medial to the meatus, but it sometimes protrudes into the canal. The *postmeatal segment* begins distal to the nerves and courses medially to supply the brainstem and the cerebellum. The subarcuate artery generally arises from this segment (see Figs. 2-11B and D, *right*; 2-12B; 2-14A and C; 2-15C; 2-16A and B).

The *caudomedial artery* originates on the lateral aspect of the pons in the vicinity of the sixth nerve and courses posterosuperiorly toward the pontomedullary sulcus; it has a caudal loop on the lateral aspect of the pons and medulla. This lateral loop can course on the anteroinferolateral aspect of the flocculus or on the petrosal aspect of the biventral lobule. Multiple small arteries to the choroid plexus of the lateral recess often arise from the inner aspect of this lateral loop. Distal to the loop, the biventral segment turns posteroinferiorly on the lateral edge of the inferior surface of the biventral lobule or within the cerebellomedullary fissure to reach the posterior surface of the cerebellum, where it anastomoses with branches of the PICA (Fig. 2-12B).

The *superior cerebellar artery* is the most rostral of the infratentorial vessels, and it arises near the apex of the basilar artery and encircles the pons and the lower midbrain. It supplies the tentorial surface of the cerebellum, the upper brainstem, the deep cerebellar nuclei, and the inferior colliculi. The SCA is divided into four segments. The *anterior pontomesencephalic segment* courses laterally under the oculomotor nerve on the anterior aspect of the upper pons, often in an arcuate convex curve inferiorly; the configuration of the anterior pontomesencephalic segment is related to the height of the basilar bifurcation. With a low basilar bifurcation (anterior to the pons), this segment tends to pass upward, whereas with a high basilar bifurcation (anterior to the midbrain), this segment pursues an anterior and inferior course. The *lateral pontomesencephalic segment* begins at the anterolateral margin of the brainstem and follows caudally onto the lateral side of the upper pons in the infratentorial portion of the ambient cistern, where it terminates at the anterior margin of the cerebellomesencephalic fissure; it is related medially to the brainstem, laterally to the wing of the central lobule, and inferiorly to the middle cerebellar peduncle. The anterior part of this segment is often visible above the free edge of the tentorium, whereas its caudal loop projects toward and often reaches the root entry zone of the trigeminal nerve. Bifurcation of the SCA into rostral and caudal trunks often occurs in this segment; the rostral trunk supplies the vermis and a variable portion of the adjacent tentorial surface, and the caudal trunk supplies the surface lateral to the area supplied by the rostral trunk. The *cerebellomesencephalic*

copula pyramidis (pyramidal loop). The most anterior point of the pyramidal loop is called the *copular point*. The terminal portion of the vermian branch curves around the tuber in the posterior cerebellar notch (see Figs. 2-11A and B; 2-11, *left*; 2-12A; 2-14A and B; 2-15C and D; 2-16A and B).

CHAPTER 3

Molecular Biology Primer for Neurosurgeons

Kevin Y. Miyashiro ■ James Eberwine

Commenting on the structure and connections of neurons during his acceptance speech for the Nobel Prize in Medicine, Ramon y Cajal proposed that

These fibres, ramifying several times, always proceed towards the neuronal body, or towards the protoplasmic expansions around which arise plexuses or very tightly bound and rich nerve nests [these] morphological structures, whose form varies according to the nerve centres being studied, confirm that the nerve elements possess reciprocal relationships in contiguity but not in continuity. It is confirmed also that those more or less intimate contacts are always established, not between the nerve arborizations alone, but between these ramifications on the one hand, and the body and protoplasmic processes on the other.

With these observations in support of the neuron doctrine in 1906, so began one of the most abiding lines of scientific pursuit in biology—understanding the principal mechanisms by which the fate of central neurons are specified during development at the correct time and place to facilitate the quadrillion synaptic connections that are established, maintained, and remodeled. These arrays of neural networks codify our perceptions and other cognitive functions. To do so, synapses bring together in apposition specialized morphologic structures of the presynaptic, usually axonal, and postsynaptic, typically dendritic, subcellular neuronal domains often ensheathed by the end-feet of astrocytes. The precision and strength of these connections rely on the pinpoint placement of gene products in each of these cellular compartments. Our understanding of neuroscience in these molecular terms has been one of the fundamental challenges in the past several decades but has been complicated by the varying intrinsic properties of neurons—including morphology, types of neurotransmitter release, projection targets, and basic input/output characteristics—that exist along a wide spectrum of neuronal phenotypes even within the same neuroanatomic region.

Over the past several decades, neuroscientists have embraced a rapidly evolving set of molecular biologic techniques to gain insight into understanding these dynamics of gene expression. These findings have been critical in understanding not only the mechanistic underpinnings of normal development but also the role that some genes play in neurological diseases from the developmental to the degenerative. Our purpose here is to introduce a series of core methods in the contemporary molecular neuroscientist's toolbox. We do so in the broader context of the traditional candidate gene approach and the more recent rise of functional genomics.

THE CANDIDATE GENE APPROACH

Lacking any biochemical basis that would aid in purifying gene products associated with a disease state, the candidate gene approach was largely an outgrowth of the efforts of positional cloning strategies in the early 1980s. Using linkage analysis to look at differences in chromosome structure in diseased versus nondiseased individuals often in tandem with linkage disequilibrium mapping to define broad (i.e., <10 centimorgans) and much finer respective chromosomal intervals associated with a priori

knowledge of their etiologic role in a disease state enabled molecular geneticists to narrow the number of candidate causative genes. Before completion of the Human Genome Project, identifying these loci was an incredibly arduous and time-consuming task, in large part because of the lack of high-resolution genetic and physical chromosomal maps. The unprecedented efforts to surmount these struggles were most famously recorded in the midst of the pioneering work of Louis Kunkel and Ronald Worton[1] in identifying dystrophin as the gene responsible for Duchenne's muscular dystrophy. In the past several decades, numerous genes with high relative risk for similar "simple" mendelian diseases have been successfully identified with these methods. More than 30% of mendelian disease has neurological manifestations.[2] By applying the tools of molecular biology to a gene or the small set of candidate genes identified within a quantitative trait loci it has become possible to facilitate a systematic approach to answering some very basic questions about the organization of a gene and the expression of its gene products.

Emerging from the sequence of methods conceptualized first by Sol Spiegelman[3] and most effectively by Edwin Southern,[4] molecular biologists have exploited the now well-worn principle of molecular hybridization in which a single-stranded nucleic acid probe (or primer) forms a stable hybrid molecule, as a result of nucleotide complementarity, with a single-stranded target sequence immobilized on a solid support (i.e., nitrocellulose or nylon membranes) or in solution (Fig. 3-1). Under the appropriate experimental conditions, the stability and biochemical kinetics of the hybrid are directly proportional to the length and degree of nucleotide complementarity.

As first applied in Southern blotting whereby genomic DNA was separated according to size by agarose gel electrophoresis, transferred to nitrocellulose, and annealed to complementary DNA probes labeled with a detectable tag hybridized to target genomic DNA, the dosage or deletion analysis, or both, of candidate genes was affirmed. Indeed, Southern blot analysis of the dystrophin gene has identified duplications as well as mapped various exon deletion mutants. Recently, variation in the copy number of genes has received new consideration inasmuch as several new genomic disorders have been shown to be manifested in a gene dosage–dependent manner.[5] Such disorders include dup7 (q11.23) syndrome, methyl-CPG-binding protein 2 (MECP2), and adult-onset autosomal dominant leukodystrophy. By reducing the stringency of hybridization conditions, however, differences in hybridization patterns may reveal the existence of certain fragments that are not able to hybridize to the probe under the most stringent hybridization conditions. These data are often the first clues that the gene is part of a larger multigene family that shares significant but not complete nucleotide sequence identity. By using a modification of the Southern blotting method to screen a complementary DNA library at moderate stringency, the dystrophin-like sequence utrophin was identified.[6]

Traditional Southern blotting has largely been supplanted by the advent of polymerase chain reaction (PCR) protocols. The ability to replicate short fragments of DNA with an enzymatic

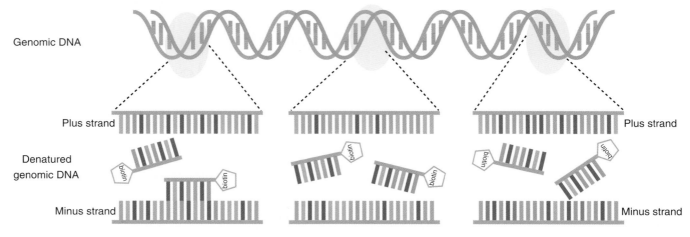

Genomic DNA

Plus strand

Denatured genomic DNA

Minus strand

Plus strand

Minus strand

Technique	Hybridization	Maximum sensitivity	Target sequence	Probe selection	Uses
Southern blot	Solid support	~ 0.5–1.0 pg	DNA	DNA/oligonucletode	Chromosomal mapping, copy number variation, multigene families, gene mutants
Northern blot	Solid support	~ 25 pg	RNA	RNA	Messenger RNA abundance, degradation, and stability, alternative mRNA splicing
RNAse protection assay	Solution	~ 0.1–1.0 pg	RNA	RNA	Messenger RNA abundance
Polymerase chain reaction	Solution	~ 1.0 pg	DNA	DNA	Cloning, messenger RNA abundance, genotyping
In situ hybridization	Solid support (cell matrix)	~ 1–10 copies/cell	RNA	RNA/DNA/oligonucleotide	Subcellular localization
	Solid support (chromosomes)		DNA	DNA/oligonucleotide	Chromosomal mapping, karyotype analysis

FIGURE 3-1 The fundamental tools of molecular biology are based on molecular hybridization. A cartoon schematic of molecular hybridization shows the basic principle in practice illustrated with a portion of genomic DNA. When genomic DNA is transferred to a solid-phase support such as nylon or nitrocellulose in a Southern blot, the DNA is denatured so that labeled probes may hybridize to the single-strand genomic DNA sequence. We highlight three representative areas of the genomic DNA, each having a different sequence. The length of these sequences, as well as the probes, is not drawn to scale and would contain many more base pairs than depicted. A probe, labeled here with biotin, that has nucleotide complementarity to the genomic sequence will bind with specificity. Using this principle in some form, a table of the basic tools of molecular biology is given to provide a cursory overview of the methods and their uses. The maximal sensitivity of the technique is not ordinarily the success that will be found with every experiment; it is the best observed sensitivity.

assay first described by Kleppe and colleagues[7] and transformed by Mullis and associates' use of a thermostable DNA polymerase[8,9] has dramatically reduced lead times in comparison to conventional Southern blotting methods. As with Southern blotting, there must be some knowledge of the target DNA sequence for PCR. In practice, PCR typically requires two primers, one of which is complementary to the 5′ DNA region of interest and the other to the 3′ end of the DNA region. The DNA regions can be any part of a gene, exonic or intronic, although amplifications longer than 10 kilobases become increasingly difficult to isolate. Replication of the DNA fragment, or amplicon, occurs processively as part of a series of 20 to 40 repeated temperature cycles in which one cycle consists of denaturation of the DNA target, annealing of the primers to the single-stranded DNA, and enzymatically catalyzed elongation of complementary DNA by a thermostable DNA polymerase. One noteworthy improvement in the past 15 years has been the addition of thermostable DNA polymerases with separate 3′ to 5′ exonuclease proofreading

activity, which has resulted in higher sequence fidelity of the amplified product. Among the multiple variants of the basic PCR methodology that have been developed, identification of allele-specific, single nucleotide polymorphisms (SNPs)[10] and foci of methylated CpG islands[11] in genomic DNA are just two. Because of the dependability and efficiency of amplifying a specific locus within the genome, PCR and its basic multiplex versions, which can amplify several amplicons simultaneously,[12] continue to be workhorses for the preparation of genomic samples.

A parallel set of approaches for studying expression of the primary products of gene transcription that involve messenger RNA (mRNA) has enabled neuroscientists to assign critical spatiotemporal information to gene function. The first technique developed to do so, the Northern blot,[13] differs from the Southern blot in that the target molecules separated according to size by agarose gel electrophoresis under denaturing conditions and transferred to a membrane support for hybridization consist of RNA, whether total RNA or poly A⁺ mRNA. At the organ or tissue level, it remains unmatched in its ability to provide an accurate size of the transcript and quantifiable patterns of gene expression during development or disease states, or both. Furthermore, differences in the size of the transcript within or among samples suggest any number of possibilities, including but not limited to alterative splicing, alternative start sites, or differences in polyadenylation. Typically, medium- and high-abundance messages are readily visualized with labeled probes. However, low-abundance messages can be difficult to detect.

The low-throughput methodology, long lead times, and limits of detection dictated by RNA immobilization on solid-phase supports have largely been overcome by the development of solution-based hybridization techniques that provide at least an order of magnitude more sensitive for detecting mRNA transcripts. Detection of mRNA in its native state by the ribonuclease protection assay adapts the Northern blot approach by hybridizing a labeled complementary RNA probe (usually 100 to 500 base pairs) with high specific activity to unlabeled cellular RNA that is freely suspended in solution.[14] The resulting RNA duplexes, which are highly stable, are protected from digestion by single-strand–specific ribonucleases and separated by polyacrylamide gel electrophoresis (PAGE). Detection of signal by the isotopic or nonisotopic labels offer sensitive and reliable detection and quantitation of mRNA that is up to 50 times more sensitive than Northern blotting.[15] A second solution-based alternative requires conversion of the native mRNA to complementary DNA by reverse transcriptase followed by PCR. Although gene-specific primers can be used for the reverse transcription, a polythymidine oligonucleotide (oligo-dT), random hexamers, or combination of them are most frequently used. Oligo-dT primers readily hybridize to the translationally important poly A+ tails present in most mRNA and thereby bias the start site of reverse transcription toward the 3′ end of the mRNA. Conversely, random hexamers are often used when attempting to obtain a target template closer to the 5′ end of long mRNA sequences. Detection of the target sequence can be achieved by standard PCR protocols, whereas multiplex PCR protocols allow the simultaneous detection of several amplicons.[12] However, when quantitation is required, quantitative real-time PCR (qRT-PCR) protocols are necessary.[16,17] qRT-PCR requires primers with specific design characteristics and amplicons with no more than 250 base pairs. Before quantitation, it is essential that the primers be exhaustively tested with the target template to ensure that the gene of interest is amplified and is the expected size. Two versions of qRT-PCR are now in use. The most simple qRT-PCR methodology uses a fluorescent dye that emits short wavelengths of ultraviolet spectrum light as a function of the number of amplicons created during each successive cycle when it intercalates with the double-stranded DNA formed during the thermocycling process. The generation of nonspecific, double-stranded PCR products, often referred to as primer-dimers, can interfere with or completely prevent quantitation. A more reliable but more expensive qRT-PCR route uses the addition of a separate sequence-specific RNA- or DNA-based probe modified with a fluorescence reporter at one end of the molecule and a quencher of fluorescence at the other end. In this version of qRT-PCR, the fluorescent reporter probe anneals to the target template somewhere in the target amplicon between the qRT-PCR primers. In intact reporter probes, the fluorescence is quenched. Detection and quantitation occur only as signal is emitted because the fluorescent reporter is physically cleaved from the quencher by the 5′-3′ exonuclease activity of the thermostable polymerase during the elongation step. To ensure accuracy with any of these solution-based mRNA quantitation assays, it is necessary to normalize expression of the target transcript with a stably expressed control gene. These methods are most favored when dealing with low-abundance transcripts and when the cellular RNA material is limited or, in a worst-case scenario, partially degraded.

In the past several years there has been a renaissance in Northern blotting methods for detecting a specific set of small RNA molecules, microRNAs (miRNAs). miRNAs are abundant, single-stranded, 21- to 23-nucleotide RNA molecules processed from endogenous 70-nucleotide pre-miRNAs by two enzymes, Drosha and Dicer.[18-20] These small noncoding RNAs are recruited to unique ribonucleoprotein complexes, RNA-induced silencing complexes,[21,22] where they mediate the translational suppression or degradation of nascent mRNA transcripts bearing homologous antisense sequence in their 3′ untranslated regions.[23] miRNA function appears to have an essential role in neuronal development,[24,25] and recent indications suggest that dysregulation of miRNA networks contributes to neurodegenerative disease.[26-28] As an analytic tool, the popularity of the Northern blot lies in its continued accuracy in estimating the size of the mature miRNA molecule and the ability to detect the pre-miRNA product simultaneously. Enhanced detection advances consisting of cross-linking small RNA molecules (<100 nucleotides) to nylon membranes,[29] as well as the use of locked nucleic acids,[30,31] to increase probe specificity are among the most recent contributions.

Gene expression observations at the organ or tissue level provide only an aggregate view of gene expression because the robust, cell-specific controls that create numerous subpopulations of individual neurons and nonneuronal cell types with considerable heterogeneity in mRNA expression phenotypes within the same anatomic region are lost. In addition, de novo expression, induction, and repression are rarely observed in the mature nervous system, so the dynamic range of expression is often modest. To determine the cellular resolution of gene expression, in situ hybridization is most often used. As a method for detecting and localizing specific mRNA transcripts in morphologically preserved tissue or cells, in situ hybridization uses a single-stranded complementary DNA or RNA probe that hybridizes to the target endogenous mRNA transcripts. Detecting mRNA transcripts within the cellular cytoarchitecture presents a unique balancing act. Because the mRNA population has not been diluted by mRNA from other cell types, the target mRNA of interest is present at its individual steady-state level. Many times, it is present at higher levels of abundance in specific subpopulations of neurons than one would detect within the whole tissue. However, mRNAs within the normal cellular matrix are but one constituent of a multi-megadalton ribonucleoprotein complex, and consequently their primary sequence is often masked or sterically inaccessible to a probe. Thus, one must fix the mRNA in place while balancing the ability to permeabilize the architecture so that the DNA probes, which are typically oligonucleotides of 20 to 50 bases, PCR-generated probes of several hundred bases, or complementary RNA probes (i.e., riboprobes) that can be routinely made with in vitro transcription kits up to one kilobase long, have access to the target mRNA sequences. However, care must be taken when using longer complementary riboprobes because cross-hybridization with similar sequences in other genes may occur. It is important to isolate gene-specific sequences to use as riboprobes. Typically, two or three separate gene-specific complementary DNA probes or riboprobes targeting the same transcript are used to cross-validate the subcellular distribution. There are two usual controls for specificity. The primary control is a competition control with excess unlabeled probe hybridization followed by labeled probe hybridization and subsequent detection. The DNA probes or riboprobes are complementary to the target mRNA transcripts and thus antisense. Sense controls are also used to show the degree of nonspecific background.

Originally, detection schemes for in situ hybridization used isotopic labels (^{33}P or ^{35}S) incorporated into the complementary probes. Quantitative methods for converting radioactive signal with silver grain density via photographic emulsion have been widely used since the mid-1990s.[32] Nonisotopic detection methods have multiplied over the past 2 decades because they take a considerably shorter time, can have greater signal resolution, and allow the simultaneous detection of multiple different targets by combining various detection methods. Complementary probes labeled with biotin or digoxigenin allow a number of different detection options. Some use colorimetric substrates consisting of horseradish peroxidase or alkaline phosphatase conjugated to streptavidin beads or primary antidigoxigenin antibodies to facilitate detection. Data from the Allen Brain Atlas use just such a colorimetric detection strategy, which provides an increasingly comprehensive data set of expressed gene at the cellular level.[33] One continuing technical concern with enzyme-linked amplification schemes is diffusion of the colorimetric signal from the site of localization. Research laboratories have used fluorescence detection schemes within the past several decades that involve new generations of fluorophores with long-term photostability, such as Alexa dyes or quantum dot (Qdot) nanocrystals; these fluorophores have been key components in illuminating the trafficking dynamics of mRNA molecules within the subcellular compartments of dendrites[34] and axons[35,36] via conventional epifluorescent microscopy or single-photon confocal laser scanning microscopy. Quantitative data analysis of these fluorescent images requires the use of image acquisition and analysis software such as Metamorph or IP Lab. In a typical sample, the total fluorescence intensity for a region of interest, normalized against background noise and any differences in the area of the region of interest, is compared across experiments or among samples and subjected to statistical analysis. In contemporary molecular cyto-

genetics, fluorescence in situ hybridization (FISH)-based karyotyping and banding methods refer to a rubric of techniques used for both clinical genetics and tumor cytogenetics that can simultaneously characterize several chromosomes or chromosomal subregions (Box 3-1).

As intermediaries in the continuum between genotype and phenotype, levels of mRNA should be taken as a surrogate for corresponding protein expression or their functional activity with caution. Early data sets attempting to establish a correlation between protein and mRNA levels found varying degrees of concordance. Although a significant positive correlation has been observed in human transitional cell carcinomas,[57] more marginal grading was observed in a comparative examination of 19 genes in the human liver.[58] Conversely, in a more limited study of three matrix metalloproteinase–related genes expressed in benign and neoplastic prostate tissue,[59] no correlative relationships were identified. When these data are placed in the context of the vast regulatory networks that monitor the various posttranscriptional events, this wide variability is not entirely unexpected. A nearly universal theme among the traditional tools for assaying protein expression is the use of affinity between an antibody and an epitope on the target protein to facilitate protein detection. The specificity of the primary antibody is the central determinant in the accuracy of protein recognition. Much like assays for detecting nucleic acids, methods to identify protein expression can be accomplished with the use of blots, free in solution or in situ.

Box 3-1 Array of Fluorescence In Situ Hybridization–Based Methods in Molecular Cytogenetics

Over the past several decades, G-banding has served as one of the routine standards for chromosome banding. It relies on successful culture of the tissue of investigation, often fetal or tumor tissue, and preparation of metaphase cells. It should be noted that product-of-conception samples in particular suffer relatively high rates of failure (10% to 40%) during the tissue-culturing process[37] and poor chromosome morphology.[38] Monochrome changes in the visible karyotype of morphologically optimal samples produced by Giemsa staining can provide low but sufficient chromosomal resolution to distinguish changes in chromosome number and large structural rearrangements whether translocations or macrodeletions. Chromosomes with small translocations, cryptic aberrations, microdeletions, and inversions or more complex karyotypes are often beyond the limits of conventional G-banding analysis.[39] As a result, complementary fluorescence in situ hybridization (FISH)-based karyotyping and banding methods have been developed to overcome the intrinsic morphologic and technical obstacles in karyotyping associated with G-banding protocols.

In its most basic form, FISH-based karyotyping uses DNA probes hybridizing to a specific gene or chromosome locus in metaphase or, less commonly, interphase chromosome preparations for the straightforward detection of deletion/duplication syndromes and gene fusions or rearrangements. In contrast to metaphase FISH, interphase FISH does not require the growth of viable cells for the preparation of a chromosomal spread. Interphase FISH makes use of preserved tissue and cellular material such as that found in paraffin-embedded biopsy samples. Perhaps the most significant advance in the past decade or so has been the development of multicolor FISH-based karyotyping and banding techniques (Fig. 3-2). The various iterations of multicolor FISH karyotyping methods are all based on the availability of chromosome-specific probe sets developed from degenerate oligonucle-

otide–primed polymerase chain reaction of flow-sorted chromosomal libraries[40,41] labeled in tandem with four to seven spectrally separable fluorochrome labels[42] that simultaneously "paint" and distinguish each whole chromosome.[43,44] Chromosome painting with chromosome-specific probes can be done combinatorially (e.g., multiplex FISH or spectral karyotyping) or by using an additional ratiometric approach[45] (i.e., combined binary ratio–FISH) and has proved to be a powerful adjunct to conventional cytogenetic techniques in the diagnostic analysis of interchromosomal events and characterization of the cytogenetic evolution of tumors, even in complex aberrations. The sensitivity (i.e., whether a translocation can be detected) and specificity (i.e., whether it can classified with assurance) of the analysis are vitally dependent on the fluorochrome combinations used in the target chromosomes.[46] The resolution of these whole chromosome–painting techniques is limited by the lack of any additional spatial delineation within a chromosome. For this reason, multicolor karyotyping alone is often not sensitive enough to precisely determine chromosomal breakpoints, subtle chromosome rearrangements, or intrachromosomal aberrations (e.g., inversions, duplications, terminal deletions). Differential hybridization signals obtained with other FISH-based karyotype techniques, such as comparative genomic hybridization, have similar resolving capabilities.[47] Efforts to improve the resolution of these assays have used chromosome arm–specific,[44,48] region-specific,[49,50] centromeric,[51] and subtelomeric probes.[52,53] To address the latter issue of intrachromosomal aberrations, FISH-based banding patterns obtained by using differentially labeled and pooled subregional DNA probes were designed to produce high-resolution chromosomal karyotypes with identifiable fluorescent banding patterns within a single chromosome via spectral color banding,[54] cross-species color banding[49,55] or multicolor banding.[50,56]

sets of siRNA are used and the potency of this siRNA. The most attractive potential of RNAi is the flexibility that it allows in controlling the spatial and temporal effects of inhibition. With the development of inducible siRNA whose expression is controlled by tetracycline- or doxycycline-regulated promoters,[105-109] photoactivated versions of "caged" siRNA,[110] and focal transfection methods,[111] stepwise advances to this promise are being realized. Although the low to moderate concentrations of siRNA typically used to produce significant knockdown tend to evade interferon response–mediated changes in global gene expression,[112,113] a secondary effect has on occasion been noted.[114,115] A more acute concern is the possibility of an siRNA modulating the expression of a closely related sequence[116-118] and resulting in observable changes in phenotype.[119] Chemical modifications of the siRNA can mitigate some of these off-target effects,[120] but the exact nature of siRNA specificity remains unclear (see Elbashir and colleagues[121] and Miller and associates,[122] but compare with Semizarov and coworkers[123]). Until a better consensus of siRNA specificity is reached, current siRNA design suggests allowing for at least two nucleotide mismatches with all off-target genes. A recent editorial suggests that the ideal control is to rescue the siRNA phenotype by using an siRNA-resistant gene with a silent mutation in the 3′ nucleotide of a codon in the middle of the siRNA binding site.[124]

THE RISE OF FUNCTIONAL GENOMICS

Candidate gene studies take advantage of two lines of evidence that dovetail to increase success: the increased efficiency of association studies in selected population-based samples and an a priori understanding of the clinical phenotypes and how it might be affected by candidate gene function. However, this approach has met with mixed success when assessing complex diseases in which multiple genes, as well as their sequence and functional variants, probably initiate small individual contributions and relative risk for a cumulative phenotype that varies in the severity of symptoms and age at onset and evolves over time. Lacking the tools of scale to perform the simultaneous analyses required, continuing efforts toward miniaturization and scalability epitomize the new "omics" technologies that are transforming nervous system studies by allowing data-rich and detailed characterization of the molecular mechanisms underlying cell physiology. Ironically, it does so by using the very same methods of biochemistry, molecular biology, and cell biology worked out decades earlier. At its core, functional genomics aspires to integrate data from the study of different molecular strata—the genome, transcriptome, proteome, metabolome, and their regulatory mechanisms—into a systems-level model of cell biology. The ostensible goal is to obtain a richly detailed, global understanding of the nervous system's emergent properties through the interactions among all its constituent elements.[125] In so doing, it promises to expand our insight into the root problems of complex diseases and transform the current predictive power of our diagnostic and therapeutic regimens.[126]

Transcriptomics

Evolving technologic innovations fostering miniaturization, increased scalability and efficiency, and decreased cost born from the Human Genome Project now exploit this wealth of genomic data. Gene expression profiling[127,128] is the most widely used functional genomics technology due in equal parts to its early development and the ease with which it can be performed. High-density DNA microarrays anchor cDNA[129] or oligonucleotides[130,131] of different genes in massively parallel arrays of up to approximately 10,000 spots/cm² and greater than 1,000,000 spots/cm², respectively, on a glass surface. Using the principle of molecular hybridization, several micrograms of fluorescently labeled RNA or

cDNA probes hybridize with the target DNA and are analyzed with high-resolution scanners that optically detect the strength of fluorescent signal from the bound probes. Raw data are normalized and processed through a series of statistical approaches to determine whether any gene is differentially expressed. The probes are constructed from abundant sources of high-integrity mRNA, which is reverse-transcribed in the presence of fluorophore-coupled deoxyribonucleoside triphosphates (dNTPs) or amino-allyl–labeled dNTPs that can be coupled to a fluorophore such as Cy3 or Cy5. In postmortem tissue, even with extended postmortem intervals of up to 30 hours, high-integrity mRNA can be isolated for microarray sample preparation. However, it is not the postmortem interval inasmuch as it is the pH of the tissue (great than 6.25) that determines mRNA integrity.[132] Alternatively, when confronted with small amounts of starting material, it may be necessary to amplify the mRNA population so that there will be enough material to drive the hybridization reaction when labeled without skewing the complexity of the original mRNA population.[16] Because exponential amplification techniques, such as PCR, do not offer this capability, a linear amplification technique, aRNA amplification, enzymatically converts the mRNA population into a single-stranded cDNA with reverse transcriptase by using a specialized oligo-dT primer containing a 3′ T7 RNA polymerase promoter sequence. When a complementary second strand is synthesized, it serves as a transcription template for T7 RNA polymerase to produce RNA oriented in the antisense direction, which can be labeled directly or converted into labeled cDNA as a probe. Amplification of mRNA by manual harvesting of individual live neurons[128,133,134] or dendrites,[135,136] as well as neurons in fixed tissue,[137,138] has been equally as successful as automated approaches such as laser capture microdissection.[139]

Experimental artifacts can be introduced by sample preparation (e.g., differences in the integrity of mRNA or in the efficiency of labeling), the array (e.g., DNA spotting or printing errors), or processing (e.g., variable fluorescence scanner performance). Careful experimental design (e.g., checking the integrity of the mRNA before use, dye swaps and parallel processing of samples to control for labeling efficiency, quality control experiments for each lot of custom and commercial microarrays) can largely eliminate these issues. Reducing systemic biases in the results requires the optical data to be normalized at the global level to facilitate comparisons across microarray experiments and at the local level to account for individual variations in signal intensity that are unique to the surface of that microarray.[140,141] Common approaches on how best to apply these normalization procedures to distribution of the data are available in the form of open source and open development software offered by the Bioconductor project. When analyzing data, the most conservative treatment of it uses a Bonferroni correction to reduce possible false-positive errors. However, this correction for multiple measurements can also lead to increases in the number of false-negative errors. Various data analysis software packages try to balance the discovery rates of these two types of errors. As with all high-throughput assays, these data should be verified with other techniques. Although the current generation of high-throughput, low-cost cDNA or oligonucleotide microarrays is the primary laboratory workhorse for quantifying the transcriptome, next-generation technology is already on the horizon (Box 3-3).

There are two principal areas where highly paralleled mRNA expression technology has proven utility. One is as a comparative expression profile or signature profile. This genome-wide molecular fingerprint provides a distinctive pattern of gene expression that can be used as a comprehensive framework for assessing differences in classes of neurons[134] and astrocytes,[152] during development in myoblasts,[153] and in genetic mutants in model systems.[154] It has also been used to evaluate the secondary effects

Box 3-3 Next-Generation Technology for mRNA Gene Expression

Sources of noise within the experiment can be controlled, in part, by the normalization techniques discussed earlier. However, there are several notable technical limitations of DNA microarrays at present: high background levels as the result of cross-hybridization by multiple targeting probes[142] and low concordance (≈30% to 40%) of transcript detection between platforms.[143-145] In the former circumstance, the probe will normally bind with high specificity to an arrayed target sequence. Off-target effects such as cross-hybridization occur when a flanking, unbound sequence of the same probe binds weakly to an adjacent arrayed sequence. The resulting background noise contributes to the relatively small dynamic range (≈2 orders of magnitude) of signal detection in microarrays, although in the latter circumstance the weak overlap in mRNA expression profiles across different microarray platforms is a consequence of unpredictable intramolecular folding events in some long probes[146] and hybridization differences driven by the use of different sequences for the same target gene on various platforms. The cross-platform differences can be improved by using the RefSeq database for gene matching[147] and still further when expression patterns are analyzed only when target sequences between platforms overlap.[148]

Next-generation technologies determine the identity of the mRNA transcript with the use of highly paralleled, direct sequencing methods.[149] Although expensive at the moment, RNA sequencing (RNA-Seq) has several clear advantages over the current array-based methods, including low background noise, a large dynamic range (up to ≈3.5 orders of magnitude), and single–base pair resolution, which allows the ability to distinguish different isoforms (i.e., splice variants) and allelic expression (i.e., single nucleotide polymorphisms or structural variants, including insertion-deletions and copy number variations) of the same mRNA without subsequent need for any specialized normalization. Briefly, the total or poly A⁺ mRNA population is converted into a library of short, adaptor-modified cDNA (200 to 500 base pairs) that is compatible with deep-sequencing instrumentation. In the case of a population enriched in poly A⁺ mRNA, there are two general paths for processing. The poly A⁺ mRNA can be fragmented first, usually by hydrolysis or nebulization, and then ligated to adaptors and reverse-transcribed into cDNA. Conversely, the poly A⁺ mRNA can be ligated to the adaptor, reverse-transcribed into cDNA, and then fragmented with DNAse I or sonication. When fragmented at the RNA level, there is limited bias over the length of the transcript.[150] However, fragmentation at the cDNA level greatly biases the readable sequence toward the 3′ end.[151] Depending on the amount of input mRNA, amplification of the population may or may not be necessary. These libraries can generate millions of short reads that typically vary from 30 to 250 base pairs by 454, Solexa, or SOLid sequencing and can be compared against the genomic sequence or the coding sequencing of a gene.

genes expressed in the central nervous system to be approximately 25,000 to 30,000.[158] However, alternative splicing, which is thought to occur in 92% to 94% of genes[159] and is often subverted in disease,[160,161] generates further heterogeneity in the mature mRNA population from a single pre-mRNA transcript.[162] The patterns of expression of alternative splice forms are strongly correlated across different tissues, thus suggesting the presence of tissue-specific regulatory mechanisms.[159,163,164] Because classic microarray designs do not incorporate this additional level of mRNA complexity, filling this gap in signature profile data is a series of new alternative splicing arrays[165-167] with promising insight into transformation of Hodgkin's lymphomas[168] and gliomagenesis.[169] Adaptations of DNA oligonucleotide microarray methods have also been made to signature-profile the expression of miRNA in low-density microarrays.[170,171]

Most highly paralleled gene expression studies make no a priori hypotheses about which individual genes are regulated among comparison sample sets. It is done within the framework of a systems biology approach in which it is assumed that transcription occurs with a finite set of resources. Thus, a change in the mRNA transcription of one gene will have collateral, sometimes seemingly stochastic influences on other mRNA. A second application of gene expression attempts to mine the comparative expression profiles for information on transcriptional regulatory networks. Data mining of signature profile results can identify clusters of mRNA to be transcriptionally active or silent. The genomic sequences of this mRNA are then analyzed for the presence of shared promoter elements that might contribute to the levels of expression. This sequence analysis is usually paired with direct analysis of promoter occupation by the suspected transcription factor via chromatin immunoprecipitation (ChIP).[172,173] In a typical ChIP assay, the DNA-protein interaction is crosslinked by formaldehyde in situ to fix the interaction, although this step can be omitted when analyzing histone-DNA interactions (referred to as a native-ChIP). The DNA is then fragmented into approximately 500–base pair stretches by sonication or enzymatic digestion. The cross-linked transcription factor is used as an epitope to immunoprecipitate the complex. Antibodies for this purpose are often prequalified by commercial suppliers because they must be of very high quality. The cross-linking in the isolated complex is reversed wherein the DNA sequence of the chromatin fragment is identified by direct sequencing (ChIP-seq), a PCR-based method (ChIP-display),[174] or most commonly, hybridization to a tiling array (ChIP-on-chip or ChIP-chip) for genome-wide detection. Tiling arrays are a relatively recent variation of microarrays with many design considerations that contain short (≈25 base pairs) oligonucleotides, or tiles, of non-repetitive regions of genomic sequences that are arrayed linearly (i.e., contiguous sequence end to end or separated by five nucleotides) or with a fractional offset (i.e., overlapping genomic sequence tiles) for higher resolution studies.[175] One important adjunctive function of ChIP-chip studies is the ability to establish the presence of the possible epigenetic effects of histone modifications and, by extension, nongermline DNA methylation.[176-178] It is important to note that these descriptive studies of transcription factor occupancy alone do not indicate the efficacy of the interaction on transcription. However, when integrated with mRNA expression profiling, it is possible to identify functional regulatory network motifs, which is the aim of the ENCODE (Encyclopedia of DNA Elements) Project.[179]

This type of analysis, often enhanced by expression profile comparisons with genetic methods (Box 3-4) that create overexpression or null mutation phenotypes of the transcription factors that bind to the promoter loci, are more likely to reveal the presence of multitiered regulatory networks. A good example of this is maintenance of a human embryonic stem (ES) cell phenotype. ES cells maintain their pluripotency and ability to self-renew by maintaining a feedforward transcriptional regulatory network

of drug compounds on regulation of gene expression.[155] Signature profile comparisons of cells under different stimulation conditions[141] or environmental influences[156] that expand the complexity of the mRNA populations, or "expression space," have colloquially been referred to as "exercising the genome."[157] The Human Genome Project estimated the total number of human

Box 3-4 Genetic Tools for Modifying Gene Function

RNA INTERFERENCE

The processing of hairpin microRNA (miRNA) or plasmid-derived short-hairpin RNA by the enzymes Drosha and Dicer leads to the generation of small interfering RNA (siRNA)—short, double-stranded 21– to 23–base pair RNA with symmetrical 2- to 3-nucleotide 3′ overhangs. Synthetic siRNA gains functional activity by an endogenous kinase that modifies the 5′ hydroxyl groups to phosphate groups. These RNA duplexes are recruited into the RISC complex, where they are guided to endogenous mRNA. On base pairing, the transcript is translationally silenced or cleaved by the catalytic component of the RISC. Although commonly used in cell culture models to reduce gene expression, it has been applied in embryonic stem cells to inactivate genes in a heritable fashion, but without the complete functional reduction in gene expression.

INSERTIONAL MUTAGENESIS

In contrast to chemical mutagenesis, insertional mutagenesis is a transposon-based technique for generating gene disruptions by inserting a molecular tag randomly[180] or, more recently, by using targeted methods that combine the transposon with a DNA-binding domain.[181] In the randomized version, mapping the site of insertion is required to determine where it occurred and whether the insertion site will generate any dysfunction and, if so, the severity of dysfunction in protein activity.

HOMOLOGOUS RECOMBINATION

This most precise and elegant method for altering gene function requires a DNA construct to align with the targeted gene of interest, by mechanisms still poorly understood but probably similar to the alignment of homologous chromosomes during meiosis and mitosis (Fig. 3-5). The recombination event, which is most efficient in yeast and mice but much less common than random insertion events, takes place anywhere in the flanking homologous sequence. The DNA construct contains both a positive (i.e., neomycin) and a negative (i.e., thymidine kinase gene) selection marker to select for homologous recombination events and against nonhomologous recombination, respectively. The neomycin selectable marker by itself, in traditional knockout strategies, causes a significant disturbance in gene function when introduced into an intron. Over the past decade,

site-specific recombinase (SSR) systems have allowed geneticists to conditionally express or silence targeted genes, which can be exogenously engineered transgenes encoding reporter, sensor, or effector molecules.[91,182] In approximately 15% of conventional transgenics, embryonic lethality is an issue. The basic concept of conditional transgenes evolved from this obstacle. The most commonly used SSRs are Cre (causes recombination of the bacteriophage P1 genome) and Flp (named for its ability in *Caenorhabditis elegans* to invert a gene). Three versions of Flp are currently in use (e.g., enhanced Flp, Flp-wt, and low-activity Flp) and have a dynamic range of activity across them of more than 1 order of magnitude. Each of the SSRs catalyze recombination events at specific DNA target motifs built into the DNA construct before homologous recombination. For Cre, that site is *loxP*. The cognate site for wild-type Flp or any of its variants is *FRT*. These SSRs possess a combination of fortuitous characteristics: neither of their DNA target motifs are found naturally in mice, and they catalyze the recombination between these target sequences with efficiency and reliability and do so without the need for any additional cofactors. In traditional gene-targeting deletions, the neomycin marker can interfere with the phenotype by influencing the expression of nearby genes.[183] Removal of the selectable marker is one of the most obvious applications of the SSR system and requires only inserting *loxP* sites flanking the neomycin cassette.[184,185] Conditional transgenesis can remove or repair the gene of interest. In the former, a single SSR strategy has *loxP* sites that remove both the neomycin selectable marker and the exon to be deleted. Partial Cre excision occurs by transient expression of the recombinase in recombinant cells after selection, thereby leaving a conditional null allele. The same situation can be accomplished by using both the Cre and Flp recombinases in tandem. For repairing gene functions, we show two hypothetical approaches. The relative strength of perturbing gene function with a neomycin cassette can be enhanced significantly when the cassette is oriented in the reverse direction of the target gene. Excision of the reverse-orientation neo[r] marker is accomplished by flanking *loxP* sites. An alternative tactic uses a synthetic stop sequence and a positive selection marker placed between the 5′ untranslated region and the start codon[186] with dual SSRs.

that requires the OCT4-SOX2 complex to autoregulate its own expression, as well as initiate expression of NANOG.[187,188] These transcription factors interact to maintain ES cells in the undifferentiated state by repressing the activation of a host of other transcription factors, including key homeodomain proteins, while activating the transcription of another set of transcription factors, including REST, SKIL, and STAT3.[189]

Although these types of analysis were most easily performed with microarray-based signature profiles in model systems such as yeasts early on,[190-192] these methods have gained traction in mammalian models for identifying transcriptional regulatory networks in dopaminergic neurons of the midbrain[193] and in ES cells of neural[194,195] and hematopoietic[196] origin. Additionally, a recent publication has illustrated the power of next-generation RNA-Seq technology when applied to this analysis.[197]

Some epigenetic modifications (i.e., genomic imprinting) or other genetic variations, such as SNPs, that are potential sources of variation in transcript abundance are not likely to be accounted for. Because sequencing results of the human genome estimate that SNPs are the most prevalent class of common genetic variations (i.e., variants with a minor allele frequency of >1%), they

may require additional consideration. Although the vast majority of these genetic variants introduce silent mutations and neutral phenotypes, there has been much focus on determining the relative ratio of neutral, near-neutral,[198] and non-neutral SNPs within populations of different ancestry.[199-201] These genetic polymorphisms are naturally occurring, evolutionarily stable differences thought to confer a predisposition, susceptibility, or resistance to disease and influence individual responses to curative regimens, perhaps by altering the three-dimensional local DNA topography.[202]

There are a number of highly paralleled methods for assaying SNPs across the genome.[203,204] Both the mass spectrometry (MS)-based assay and fluorescence polarization–based assay are allele-specific primer extension methods in which the genomic region is amplified by PCR and used as a template for the annealing of an oligonucleotide primer immediately upstream of the polymorphism. A DNA polymerase then adds only a single nucleotide, because chain-terminating dideoxynucleotide triphosphates (ddNTPs) are used, as dictated by the target DNA sequence at the polymorphic site. Multiplex MS versions rely on the natural differences in molecular weight of the DNA for detection by

Traditional Targeted Gene Deletion

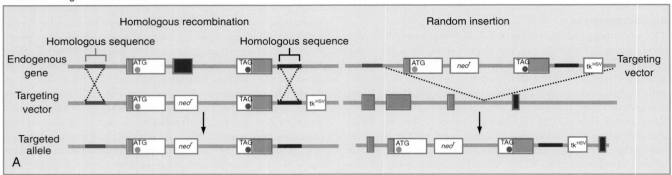

Site-Specific Recombinase Approaches

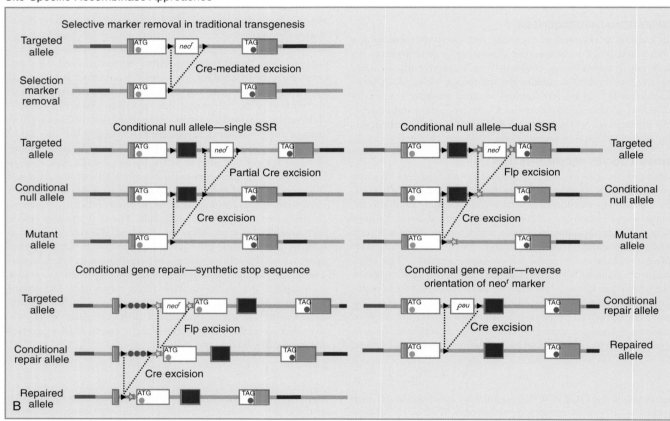

FIGURE 3-5 Mechanism of homologous recombination and the utility of site-specific recombinase approaches. **A,** Homologous recombination uses the presence of both a positive (neomycin [neo^r]) and a negative (herpes simplex virus thymidine kinase gene [tk^{HSV}]) selection marker to identify recombinant cells. Recombinant cells in which one allele is disrupted are conferred resistance to G-418 as a result of the neo^r marker. Unlike its mouse counterpart, tk^{HSV} can convert the nucleotide analogue ganciclovir. Nonhomologous insertions will include the tk^{HSV} gene, thus making only these cells sensitive to ganciclovir. Untranslated regions are represented in *orange boxes* before the start codon (ATG) or after the termination codon (TAG). An intervening exon is denoted in *red* and targeted for replacement with the neo^r cassette. **B,** Various site-specific recombinase strategies are shown starting with the structure of the targeted allele after a homologous recombination event. These strategies entail removing the selection marker cassette used during normal knockout transgenesis, as well as genetic manipulation to allow the conditional disruption or repair of gene function. *Arrowheads* represent *loxP* sites, whereas *stars* represent *FRT* sites.

matrix-assisted laser desorption/ionization (MALDI) time-of-flight (TOF) MS for efficiently assigning genotype.[205] In the fluorescence polarization–based version,[206] the ddNTPs are labeled with different fluorophores. For detection, the labeled ddNTP is incorporated into the primer, which causes it to rotate more slowly within the plane of laser polarization and thereby emit more signal than the unincorporated ddNTPs, which rotate

more quickly. A more robust fluorescence polarization assay uses PCR with a universal fluorescence resonance energy transfer (FRET) reporter system for detection of SNPs.[207] An alternative set of highly multiplexed SNP assays incorporate universal PCR. One example of this is the molecular inversion probe assay,[208] in which a single oligonucleotide simultaneously binds a complementary genomic DNA sequence that flanks either side of the

TABLE 4-1 Known Gene Mutations Causing Human Central Nervous System Malformations

MALFORMATION	INHERITANCE	CHROMOSOMAL LOCATION	GENE OR TRANSCRIPTION PRODUCT	REFERENCES
Cerebrohepatorenal syndrome (Zellweger's)*	AR	Xq22.3-q23	DCX	9
Hemimegalencephaly	AR	Xq28	L1CAM	10
Holoprosencephaly†	AD; AR	7q36-qter	SHH	11-13
Holoprosencephaly	AR; sporadic	13q32	ZIC2	14
Holoprosencephaly	AR; sporadic	2q21	SIX3	15
Holoprosencephaly	AD; sporadic	18p11.3	TGIF	16
Kallmann's syndrome	XR	Xp22.3	KAL1	17, 18
Lissencephaly type 1 (isolated and Miller-Dieker syndrome)	AR	17p13.3	LIS1	19-21
Lissencephaly (Fukuyama's congenital muscular dystrophy)	AR	9q31	FCMD, fukutin	22
Lissencephaly with cerebellar hypoplasia	AR	7q22	RELN	23
Midbrain agenesis and cerebellar hypoplasia	?AR; sporadic	7q36	EN2	24
Periventricular heterotopia	XD	Xq28	FLNA, filamin	25, 26
Rett's syndrome	XD	Xq28	MECP2	27
Sacral agenesis‡	AD	7q36.1-qter	SHH	28-30
Schizencephaly	AR	10q26.1	EMX2	31
Septo-optic pituitary dysplasia	AR; sporadic	3p21.1-p21.2	HESX1	32
Subcortical laminar heterotopia (band heterotopia; double cortex)	XD	Xq22.3-q23	DCX	33-35
Tuberous sclerosis	AD	9q34.3	TSC1, hamartin	36-38
		16p13.3	TSC2, tuberin	39-41
X-linked hydrocephalus (X-linked aqueductal stenosis and pachygyria)	XR	Xq28	L1CAM	42-44

*The DCX (doublecortin) mutation is primary in subcortical laminar heterotopia but is also described in Zellweger's syndrome, although it is probably only a secondary defect in this lysosomal disease associated with major neuroblast migratory defects; DCX is localized on the X chromosome, and Zellweger's syndrome is an autosomal recessive condition.

†Holoprosencephaly is associated with many chromosomal defects in addition to those listed, but the gene products associated with the others have not been identified.

‡Sacral agenesis (autosomal dominant form) maps to the same locus at 7q36 as one form of holoprosencephaly and is associated with defective SHH expression, the same genetic defect expressed at opposite ends of the neural tube. Sacral agenesis and holoprosencephaly also occur with a high incidence in infants born to mothers with diabetes mellitus. Agenesis of more than two vertebral bodies is generally associated with dysplasia of the spinal cord in that region during fetal development, fusion of the ventral horns, and a deformed central canal with heterotopic ependyma, consistent with defective neural induction. A second gene with a locus at 1q41-q42.1 has been identified as another cause of autosomal dominantly transmitted sacral agenesis.

AD, autosomal dominant; AR, autosomal recessive; CAM, cell adhesion molecule; SHH, Sonic Hedgehog; XD, X-linked dominant; XR, X-linked recessive.

Adapted from Sarnat HB. Central nervous system malformations; locations of known human mutations. *Eur J Paediatr Neurol.* 2000;4:289-290.

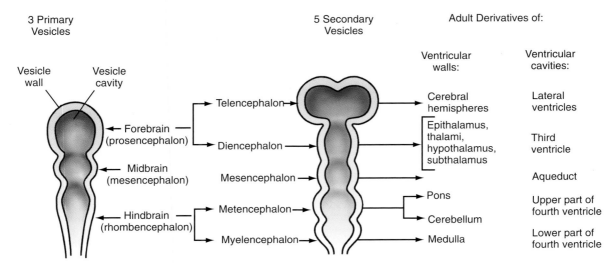

FIGURE 4-1 Embryonic vesicles and their adult derivatives are shown schematically in the progression from three primary vesicles (i.e., neuromeres) during the fourth week of gestation (just after neural tube formation) to five secondary vesicles in the fifth week. (From Jinkins JR. *Atlas of Neuroradiologic Embryology, Anatomy, and Variants.* Philadelphia: Lippincott Williams & Wilkins; 2000:9.)

Along with careful work over the past several decades that resulted in this embryonic staging system, similar analysis of the development of the cerebral vasculature led to a staging system usually referred to as *Padgett stages*.[47-49] Knowledge of how the vascular system evolves leads to a clearer understanding of vascular malformations and common vascular anomalies (covered elsewhere in this book) and the patterns of secondary embryonic and fetal brain injuries and malformations. The arterial system essentially achieves an adult pattern by the end of the embryonic period, whereas the venous system develops much later in the fetal period. Although neither the seven stages of arterial evolution developed by Padgett (and still used) nor cerebral venous development will be considered further here, more information can be found in any of several excellent reviews of vascular development.[50-53]

DEVELOPMENTAL ORGANIZATION: STAGES, GENES, AND REGULATORY FACTORS

Gastrulation

Gastrulation is the birthday of the nervous system. It is not only the time that bilateral symmetry and the three axes are established in the body of all vertebrates but also the time when a neuroepithelium can first be identified and distinguished from primitive germinal tissues. The traditional concept of three germ layers dates from gastrulation as well, but the convenient conception of all mature tissues having been derived from one of the three layers is probably more arbitrary than biologic because the neural crest forms tissues assigned to all three germinal layers and the expression of many families of genes does not respect these germinal boundaries and mediates the development of structures corresponding to all three.

In simple chordates, such as *Amphioxus* and amphibians, gastrulation is the invagination of a spherical blastula. In birds and mammals, the blastula is collapsed as a flattened, bilayered disk, and gastrulation appears not as an invagination but as a groove between two ridges on one surface of this disk, called the *primitive streak* on the *epiblast*. In each embryo, the primitive streak establishes the basic body plan of all vertebrates: a midline axis, bilateral symmetry, rostral and caudal ends, and dorsal and ventral surfaces.

As the primitive streak extends forward, cells aggregate at one end, a collection designated the *primitive node* or *Hensen's node*. Hensen's node defines rostral. Cells of the epiblast on either side move toward the primitive streak, stream through it, and emerge beneath it to pass into the narrow cavity between the two sheets of cells, with the epiblast above and the hypoblast below; these migratory cells give rise to the mesoderm and endoderm internally, and some then replace the hypoblast.[54]

After extending about halfway across the blastoderm (epiblast), the primitive streak with Hensen's node reverses the direction of its growth and retreats, moving posteriorly as the head fold and neural plate form anterior to Hensen's node. As the node regresses, a *notochordal process* develops in the area rostral to it, and somites begin to form on either side of the notochord, with the more caudal somites differentiating first and successive ones differentiating anterior to the somites already formed. The notochord induces epiblast cells to form neuroectoderm (see "Induction"). Several genes essential in creating the fundamental architecture of the embryo and its nervous system are already expressed in the primitive node,[55] and many reappear later to influence more advanced stages of ontogenesis.

Induction

Induction refers to the influence of one embryonic tissue on another such that both the inducer and the induced differentiate

as different mature tissues. In the case of the nervous system, neural tube development may be defined in terms of gradients of inductive influences. Induction usually occurs between germ layers, as with the notochord (mesoderm) inducing the floor plate of the neural tube (ectoderm), although induction also may occur within a single germ layer. An example is the optic cup (neuroectoderm) inducing the formation of a lens and cornea from the overlying epithelium (surface ectoderm) that otherwise would have differentiated as more epidermis. *Neural induction* is the differentiation or maturation of neural structures from undifferentiated ectodermal cells as a result of the influence of surrounding embryonic tissues.

Induction was discovered in 1924, when Hans Spemann and Hilde Mangold demonstrated that the dorsal lip of the newt gastrula was capable of inducing the formation of an ectopic second nervous system when transplanted to another site in a host embryo, into another individual of the same species, or to a ventral site of the same embryo.[56] This *dorsal lip* of the amphibian gastrula, also called the *Spemann organizer*, is homologous with the *Hensen node* of embryonic birds and mammals.

The first gene isolated from the Spemann organizer was *Gsc* (goosecoid), which encodes a *homeodomain* protein (see the later section "Transcription Factors and Homeoboxes") able to recapitulate transplantation of the dorsal lip tissue when injected into an ectopic site. It also normally induces the prechordal mesoderm and contributes to prosencephalic differentiation.[55,57,58] In Hensen's node in the chick, even before the primitive streak is fully formed, *Wnt8c* is expressed and is essential for the regulation of axis formation and later for hindbrain patterning in the region of the future rhombomere 4 (r4).[59] The regulatory gene *Cnot*, with major domains in the primitive node, notochord, and prenodal and postnodal neural plate, is also involved in the induction of prechordal mesoderm and in formation of the notochord in particular.[60]

The specificity of induction lies not in the inductive molecule but rather in the receptor in the induced cell. This distinction is important because foreign molecules similar in structure to the natural inductor molecule may sometimes be erroneously recognized by the receptor as identical; such foreign molecules may act as teratogens if the embryo is exposed to such a toxin. Induction occurs during a very precise temporal window; the period of responsiveness of the induced cell is designated its *competence*, and the cell is incapable of responding before or after that precise time.[61]

Induction receptors are not necessarily in or on the plasma membrane of the cell but may be in the cytoplasm or in the nucleus. Retinoic acid is an example of a nuclear inducer. In some cases, the stimulus acts exclusively at the plasma membrane of target cells and does not require actual penetration of the cell.[61,62] The receptors that represent the specificity of induction are also genetically programmed. *Notch* is a particularly important gene in regulating the competence of a cell to respond to inductive cues from within the neural tube and from surrounding embryonic tissues.[63] Some mesodermal tissues, such as smooth muscle of the fetal gut, can act as *mitogens* on the neuroepithelium by increasing the rate of cellular proliferation,[64,65] but this phenomenon is not true neural induction because the proliferating cells do not differentiate or mature. Some organizer and regulatory genes of the nervous system, such as *Wnt1*, also exhibit mitogenic effects,[66] and *insulin-like growth factor* and *basic fibroblast growth factor* act as mitogens as well.[67-69]

Early formation of the neural plate is not accomplished exclusively by mitotic proliferation of neuroepithelial cells; surrounding cells are also converted to a neural fate. In amphibians, a gene known as *Xash* (achaete-scute) is expressed very early in the dorsal part of the embryo from the time of gastrulation and acts as a molecular switch to change the fate of undifferentiated cells to become neuroepithelium rather than surface ectodermal or mesodermal tissues.[70] Some cells differentiate as specific types because they are actively inhibited from differentiating into others. All ectodermal cells are preprogrammed to form neuroepithelium, and neuroepithelial cells are preprogrammed to become neurons if not inhibited by genes that direct them along a different lineage, such as epidermal, glial, or ependymal.[71-73]

The neural tube induces craniofacial development and mediates it through the neural crest, which migrates rostrally from the prosencephalon, at the dorsal part of the lamina terminalis, and from the dorsal midline of the mesencephalon. The prosencephalic neural crest migrates as a vertical sheet of cells in the midline of the future nose and forehead and forms, among other structures, the intercanthal ligament that hold the orbits together so that the eyes are directed forward in the face instead of being located at the sides of the head. This program is genetically determined in some families of mammals, including primates, felines, canines, bears, and koalas, as well as in one family of birds only, the owls. Other animals have laterally placed eyes, which provide better panoramic, but not stereoscopic vision.

Neurulation

Bending of the neural placode to form the neural tube requires extrinsic and intrinsic mechanical forces in addition to dorsalizing and ventralizing genetic influences, which are discussed in detail later in this chapter.

These forces arise in part from growth of the surrounding mesodermal tissues on either side of the neural tube, the future somites (Table 4-2).[74] After surgical removal of mesoderm and endoderm from one side of the neuroepithelium in experimental animals, the neural tube still closes, but it is rotated and becomes asymmetric.[75] The mesoderm appears to be important for orientation but not for closure of the neural tube. Expansion of the surface epithelium of the embryo is the principal extrinsic force for folding of the neuroepithelium to form the neural tube.[76] Cells of the neural placode are mobile and migrate beneath the surface ectoderm, which causes the lateral margins of the placode to become raised toward the dorsal midline. Growth of the whole

---

TABLE 4-2 Factors Involved in Closure of Neuroepithelium to Form the Neural Tube

Extrinsic mechanical forces
  Surrounding mesodermal tissues
  Surface epithelium
Intrinsic mechanical forces
  Wedge shape of floor plate cells
  Differential growth in the dorsal and ventral zones
  Adhesion molecules
  Orientation of mitotic spindles of the neuroepithelium
  Large fetal central canal
Molecular genetic programming
  Induction of the floor plate by Sonic Hedgehog
  Ventralizing gene transcription products
  Dorsalizing gene transcription products
  Genetic transcription products that regulate axonal guidance
    (attraction and repulsion) across the midline and in the
    longitudinal axis
  Separation of the neural crest

From Menkes JH, Sarnat HB. *Child Neurology*, 6th ed. Philadelphia: Lippincott Williams & Wilkins; 2000:289.

---

embryo itself does not appear to be an important factor because neurulation proceeds equally well in anamniotes (e.g., amphibians), which do not grow during this period, and in amniotes (e.g., mammals), which grow rapidly at this time.[77]

Among the intrinsic forces of the neuroepithelium, the cells of the floor plate have a wedge shape—narrow at the apex and broad at the base—that facilitates bending.[78] Although the width of the floor plate is small, its site in the ventral midline is crucial and sufficient to allow a significant influence. It represents yet another aspect of induction of the floor plate by the notochord, apart from its influence on the differentiation of neural cells.[79] The ependymal cells that form the floor plate are the first neural cells to differentiate, and they induce growth of the parenchyma of the ventral zone more than the dorsal regions.[80,81] This mechanical effect may also facilitate curving of the neural placode. The direction of proliferation of new cells in the mitotic cycle, determined in part by the orientation of the mitotic spindle, becomes another mechanical force shaping the neural tube.[77,78] Adhesion molecules are also probably an important mechanical factor for neurulation. In later stages, the ependymal cell–lined central canal, which is much larger in the fetus than in the newborn, may have a role in exerting a centrifugal force to create the tubular shape, although in early spinal cord development the central canal is a tall, narrow, midline slit and only later in fetal life does it assume a rounded contour as seen in transverse sections.[80]

Neuroepithelial cells of the neural placode or plate downregulate the polarity of their plasma membrane so that the apical and basilar surfaces are not as distinct before neural tube closure. Cell differentiation in general involves such changes in cell polarity.[82] The rostrocaudal orientation of most mitotic spindles of the neuroepithelium and the direction in which they push by the mass of daughter cells that they form also influence the shape of the neural tube (Fig. 4-2).[83]

The neural tube closes in the dorsal midline first in the cervical region, with the closure then extending rostrally and caudally such that the anterior neuropore of the human embryo closes at 24 days and the posterior neuropore closes at 28 days, with the distances from the cervical region being unequal. This traditional view of a continuous zipper-like closure is an oversimplification. In the mouse embryo, the neural tube closes in the cranial region at four distinct sites, with the closure proceeding bidirectionally or unidirectionally and in general synchrony with somite formation.[84,85] An intermittent pattern of anterior neural tube closure involving multiple sites has also been described in human embryos.[86] In this closure pattern, the principal rostral neuropore closes bidirectionally[87] to form the lamina terminalis, an essential primordium of the forebrain.[80]

Bending of the neural plate to form the neural tube is termed *primary neurulation*. Failure of the anterior neuropore to close by 24 days results in anencephaly. Because the lamina terminalis does not form, its derivatives (including the basal ganglia and other forebrain structures) do not develop. The lack of forebrain neuroectoderm results in failure of induction of the overlying mesoderm, and the cranium, meninges, and scalp fail to close in the midline.[88] The term *secondary neurulation* refers only to the most caudal part of the spinal cord (i.e., conus medullaris), which develops from neuroepithelium caudal to the site of posterior neuropore closure. More details on abnormalities that occur because of problems with secondary neurulation are offered in other chapters in this textbook.

Neural crest cells arise from the dorsal midline of the neural tube at or shortly after the time of closure and migrate extensively along prescribed routes through the embryo to differentiate as the peripheral nervous system. This includes the dorsal root and sympathetic ganglia, adrenal medulla and carotid body chromaffin cells, melanocytes, and a few other cell types of ectodermal and mesodermal origin.[89,90]

FIGURE 4-2 Primary neurulation: schematic illustration of formation of the neural tube during the third and fourth weeks of gestation. (From Cowan WM. The development of the brain. *Sci Am.* 1979;241:113.)

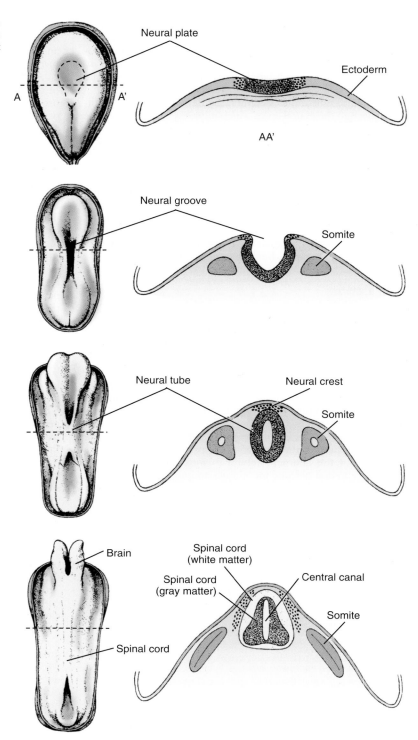

Segmentation and Regionalization

Segmentation of the neural tube creates intrinsic compartments that restrict the movement of cells by physical and chemical boundaries between adjacent compartments. These embryonic compartments are known as *neuromeres*. The spinal cord has the appearance of a highly segmented structure; however, it is not intrinsically segmented in the embryo, fetus, or adult but rather corresponds in its entirety to the most caudal of the eight neuromeres that create the hindbrain. The apparent segmentation of

the spinal cord results from clustering of nerve roots imposed by true segmentation of surrounding tissues derived from the mesoderm, tissues that form the neural arches of the vertebrae, somites, and associated structures. Neuromeres of the hindbrain are designated *rhombomeres*.[91-94] The entire cerebellar cortex, vermis, flocculonodular lobe, and lateral hemispheres develop from rhombomere 1 (r1), with a small contribution to the anterior vermis from the mesencephalic neuromere, but the dentate and other deep cerebellar nuclei are formed in rhombomere 2 (r2).[95,96] The rostral end of the neural tube forms a *mesencephalic neuromere* and probably six forebrain neuromeres (i.e., two diencephalic and four telencephalic prosomeres), although these may be subdivided further.[97-99] The segmentation of the human embryonic brain into neuromeres is summarized in Table 4-3.

The segments of the embryonic neural tube are distinguished by physical barriers formed by processes of early specializing cells that resemble the radial glial cells that appear later in development[100,101] and by chemical barriers from secreted molecules that repel migratory cells. Cell adhesion is increased in the boundary zones between rhombomeres, which also contributes to the creation of barriers against cellular migration in the longitudinal axis. Limited mitotic proliferation of the neuroepithelium occurs in the boundary zones between rhombomeres. Although cells still divide in this zone, their nuclei remain near the ventricle during the mitotic cycle and do not move as far centrifugally within the elongated cell cytoplasm during the interkinetic gap phases as they generally do.[101] The rhombomeres of the brainstem may also be visualized as a series of transverse ridges and grooves on the dorsal surface, the future floor of the fourth ventricle; these ridges are gross morphologic markers of the hindbrain compartments.[94,102]

The first evidence of segmentation is a boundary that separates the future mesencephalic neuromere from r1 of the hindbrain. More genes play a role in this initial segmentation of the neural tube than in any boundaries that subsequently form to separate other neuromeres. The mesencephalic-metencephalic region appears to develop early as a single, independent unit or "organizer" for other neuromeres rostral and caudal to that zone.[103,104] The organizer genes recognized at the mesencephalic-metencephalic boundary for this earliest segmentation of the neural tube include *Pax2, Wnt1, En1, En2, Pax5, Pax8, Otx1, Otx2, Gbx2, Nkx2-2,* and *Fgf8*.

The earliest known gene with regional expression in the mouse is *Pax2*, and it is expressed even before the neural plate forms. It is the earliest gene recognized in the presumptive region of the midbrain-hindbrain boundary.[105,106] In invertebrates, *Pax2* is important for the activation of *Wg* (wingless) genes; this relationship is relevant because the first gene definitely associated with an identified midbrain-hindbrain boundary in vertebrates is *Wnt1*, a homologue of *Wg*. Regulation of *Wnt1* may be divided into two phases. In the early phase (1 or 2 somites), the mesencephalon broadly expresses the gene throughout; in the later phase (15 to 20 somites), expression is restricted to the dorsal regions, the roof plate of the caudal diencephalon, the mesencephalon, the myelencephalon, and the spinal cord, but it is also expressed in a ring that extends ventrally just rostral to the midbrain-hindbrain boundary and in the ventral midline of the caudal diencephalon and mesencephalon.[107-109] *Wnt1* is essential in activating and preserving the function of the mouse engrailed genes *En1* and *En2*. *En1* is coexpressed with *Wnt1* at the 1-somite stage in a domain only slightly caudal to *Wnt1*, which includes the midbrain and r1, the rostral half of the pons, and the cerebellar cortex but excludes the diencephalon.[110] Activation of *En2* begins at the 4-somite stage, and its function in mesencephalic and r1 development is similar, with differences in some details, particularly their roles in cerebellar development.[111,112] The homeobox gene *Otx2* appears early in the initial boundary zone of the midbrain-hindbrain, and as with *Wnt1*, it appears to be essential for the later expression of *En1, En2,* and *Wnt1*.[113,114]

The creation of neuromeres allows the development of structures within regions of the brain without the wandering of neuroblasts that form these nuclei to other parts of the neuraxis where they would not be able to later establish their required synaptic relationships. The interaction of genes with one another is a complexity that makes analysis of single-gene expression more difficult in interpreting programmed malformations of the brain.

Patterning of the Neural Tube

Development of the basic characteristics of the body plan is called *patterning*.[91] These patterns are the anatomic expression of the genetic code within the nuclear DNA of every cell, but they may also result from signals from neighboring cells carried by molecules that are secretory translation products of various families of organizer genes, each in a highly precise and predictable temporal and spatial distribution.

Early development of the CNS in all vertebrates, even before closure of the neural placode or plate to form the neural tube, requires the establishment of a fundamental body plan of bilateral symmetry, with cephalization, or the identity of head and tail ends, and determination of the dorsal and ventral surfaces. These axes of the body itself and the CNS require the expression of genes that impose gradients of differentiation and growth. The genes that determine the polarity and gradients of the anatomic axes are called *organizer genes*. Many express themselves in the CNS and in other organs and tissues.[54,109] The bilateral symmetry of many organs and programmed asymmetries, probably including neural structures such as the different targets of the left and right vagal nerves and left-right asymmetries in the cerebral cortex, is determined in large part by *Pitx2*, a gene expressed as early as in the primitive node.[115] Some genes function to stimulate or inhibit the expression of others, or there is an antagonism or equilibrium between certain families of genes, as exemplified by those that exert dorsoventral or ventrodorsal gradients. The difference between an organizer gene and a regulator gene is its function, and the same gene often subserves both roles at

TABLE 4-3 Segmentation of the Neural Tube

NEUROMERE	DERIVED STRUCTURES IN MATURE CENTRAL NERVOUS SYSTEM
Rhombomere 8 (r8)	Entire spinal cord; caudal medulla oblongata; cranial nerves XI, XII
Rhombomere 7 (r7)	Medulla oblongata; cranial nerves IX, X; neural crest
Rhombomere 6 (r6)	Medulla oblongata; cranial nerves VIII, IX
Rhombomere 5 (r5)	Medulla oblongata; cranial nerves VI, VII; no neural crest
Rhombomere 4 (r4)	Medulla oblongata; cranial nervess VI, VII; neural crest
Rhombomere 3 (r3)	Caudal pons; cranial nerve V; no neural crest
Rhombomere 2 (r2)	Caudal pons; cranial nerves IV, V; cerebellar nuclei
Rhombomere 1 (r1)	Rostral pons; cerebellar cortex
Mesencephalic neuromere	Midbrain; cranial nerve III; neural crest
Diencephalic prosomere 2	Dorsal diencephalons
Diencephalic prosomere 1	Ventral diencephalon
Prosencephalic prosomere 2	Telencephalic nuclei; olfactory bulb
Prosencephalic prosomere 1	Cerebral cortex; hippocampus; corpus callosum

From Menkes JH, Sarnat HB. *Child Neurology*, 6th ed. Philadelphia: Lippincott Williams & Wilkins; 2000:280.

TABLE 4-4 Programs of Developmental Genes

ORGANIZER GENES

Cell proliferation

Identity of organs or tissues (e.g., neural, renal)

Axes of polarity and growth

Ventrodorsal

Dorsoventral

Rostrocaudal

Mesiolateral

Segmentation

Left-right symmetry or asymmetry

REGULATOR GENES

Differentiation of structures within organs

Cell lineage: differentiation and specialization of individual cells

Inhibition of other genetic programs to change a cell lineage

From Menkes JH, Sarnat HB. *Child Neurology*, 6th ed. Philadelphia: Lippincott Williams & Wilkins; 2000:281.

different stages of development. The definitions and programs of these two groups are summarized in Table 4-4.

Transcription Factors and Homeoboxes

Transcription factors are proteins expressed by regulatory genes that bind to the regulatory regions of other genes and control transcription. These transcription factors are essential for functional expression of the gene, and several different protein structural motifs have been discovered to be highly evolutionarily conserved. One such motif is the *basic helix-loop-helix* structure, which is so fundamental to the evolution of life that it appears for the first time in certain bacteria even before evolution of a cell nucleus to concentrate the DNA.[116]

The *zinc finger* is another DNA-binding, gene-specific transcription factor motif. It consists of 28 amino acid repeats with pairs of cysteine and histidine residues and with each sequence folded around a zinc ion.[117] *Krox20* (this gene name is applied to the mouse; the human form is designated *EGR2*) is a zinc finger gene expressed in alternating rhombomeres, especially r3 and r5; neural crest tissue does not differentiate from these two rhombomeres, although it does in adjacent segments, including r4.[118] *Krox20* serves an additional function in the peripheral nervous system, where it regulates myelination by Schwann cells,[119] and it also regulates the expression of some other genes, most notably those of the *Hox* family.[118,120-123] Another developmentally important zinc finger gene is *PLZF* (human promyelocytic zinc finger). Studies of mouse and chick homologues of this gene have revealed that it is expressed in a restricted zone surrounding hindbrain rhombomere boundaries, thus suggesting an important functional role for it and other zinc finger genes in vertebrate hindbrain regionalization.[124]

Some transcription factor genes include *homeoboxes*. These restricted DNA sequences of 183 base pairs of nucleotides encode a class of proteins sharing a common or very similar 60–amino acid motif called the *homeodomain*.[91] Homeoboxes or *homeotic genes* are classified into various families with common molecular structures and similar general expression during ontogenesis. They are especially associated with genes that program segmentation and the rostrocaudal gradients of the neural tube. Some of the families of homeobox genes important in development of the vertebrate nervous system are *Gsc, Hox, En, Wnt, Shh, Nkx, Lim,* and *Otx.*

Growth factors may also influence the pattern of the neural tube by behaving biologically as transcription factors: *basic fibroblast growth factor* behaves as an auxiliary inductor of the longitudinal axis with a rostrocaudal gradient during formation of the neural tube.[125]

Developmental Gene Families of the Central Nervous System

The genes that program the axes and gradients of the neural tube may be classified as *families* based on their similar nucleic acid sequences and their similar general functions, although important differences occur within a family in the site or neuromere where each gene is expressed and the anatomic structures that they form. A dorsalizing gene has a dorsal territory of expression and causes the ventral parts of the neural tube to differentiate as dorsal structures if influences from ventralizing genes do not antagonize them sufficiently and vice versa. In development of the somite, the sclerotome (which forms the cartilage and bone of the vertebral body) is normally situated ventral to the myotome (which forms muscle cells) and the dermatome. Ectopic cells of the floor plate or notochord implanted next to the somite of the chick embryo cause ventralization of the somite such that excess cartilage and bone are formed and there is a deficiency of muscle and dermis.[126,127] The floor plate, or notochord in this instance, is the ventralizing inductor of the mesodermal somite, and this is caused by expression of *Shh* (Sonic Hedgehog), which also serves as a strong ventralizing gradient force in the neural tube.[128-131] If a section of notochord is ectopically implanted dorsal or lateral to the neural tube, a second floor plate forms opposite the notochord, and motor neurons differentiate on either side of it despite the presence of a normal floor plate and motor neurons in the normal position.[132] *Shh*, which is expressed as early as in the primitive node, induces ventralization of a dorsal region of the neural tube or duplicates the neural tube. Such an influence in the human fetus, the so-called split notochord, could be an explanation for the rare cases of diplomyelia or diastematomyelia.[80] Excessive *Shh* expression, particularly its amino-terminal cleavage product, upregulates floor plate differentiation at the expense of motor neuron formation[129] and may induce duplication of the neuraxis. *Shh* exerts a strong influence on differentiation of the ventral and medial structures of the prosencephalon,[133] and defective expression of this gene has been found to be one molecular basis of human holoprosencephaly.[134]

To establish an equilibrium with genes with ventralizing influence, other genes exercise a dorsalizing influence. The *Pax* family is an example of genes that cause differentiation of the dorsal structures of the neural tube.[135,136] The *Wnt* family is also dorsalizing in the hindbrain; in situ hybridization shows its transcription products to be expressed diffusely only in the early neuroepithelium and to be restricted to dorsal regions as the neural tube develops.[137] The zinc finger gene *Zic2* has a dorsalizing gradient in the forebrain. The rostrocaudal axis of the neural tube and segmentation, or the formation of neuromeres, are directed in large part by a family of 38 homeobox genes that are divided into four groups called *Hox* genes.[92,93,138-141] Each of 13 *Hox* genes is expressed in certain rhombomeres and not in others (Table 4-5). *Hox* genes are not expressed in the forebrain. In addition to their functions in establishing the compartments or rhombomeres of the brainstem and effecting the differentiation of certain anatomic structures, *Hox* genes guide the growth cones forming the long descending and ascending pathways between the brain and spinal cord.[158]

Genes that direct the specific differentiation of structures are called *regulator genes*, and in many cases they have served as organizer genes in an earlier period. The most important families for development of the brainstem and midbrain in vertebrates are

TABLE 4-5 Organizer and Regulator Genes of the Embryonic and Fetal Nervous System

GENE*	REGIONS	FUNCTIONS	REFERENCES
Ash3a, Ash3b (Xenopus homologues of Drosophila achaete-scute)	Epiblast	Changes the fate of undifferentiated cells to form neuroepithelium	70
Bmp4 (bone morphogenetic protein)	Hensen's node; neural plate	Inhibits cells from forming neural tissue; dorsalizing to the neural tube; in the TGF-β family	72, 73
Cart1	Head mesenchyme	Organizes head mesoderm before arrival of the neural crest	142
Cnot	Hensen's node	Induces the primitive node to form the notochordal process; induces the neural placode	60
Delta		Antagonizes Notch; inhibits neural differentiation	
Dab1 (disabled-1)	Laminated cortices	Acts downstream of Reln for terminal neuroblast migration and cortical lamination	143
Dkk1 (dickkopf-1)	Primitive node	Head induction	144
Dlx1, Dlx2 (distal-less)	Prosomeres; ventral thalamus; anterior hypothalamus; corpus striatum	Subcortical neuroblast migration; interneuron migration from the basal forebrain to the neocortex	145
Dsl1 (dorsalin-1)	Neural tube	Dorsalizing; in the TGF-β family	146
DCX (doublecortin)	Telencephalon	Neuroblast migration; Xq22.3-q23 locus; defective in subcortical laminar heterotopia (band heterotopia, double-cortex syndrome)	147-149
EMX1	Telencephalon	Cell proliferation; corrects errors in cortical lamination	
EMX2	Telencephalon	Neuroblast migration; defective in schizencephaly	150
En1, En2 (engrailed)	Mesencephalon, r1	Formation of the mesencephalon and metencephalon, including the entire cerebellar cortex	95, 96, 103, 107, 109-112, 151-153
FLNA (previously FLN1 [filamin-1])	Telencephalon	Neuroblast migration; defective in X-linked dominant periventricular heterotopia	154, 155
Foxb1 (previously Fkh5, forkhead)	Mesencephalon, r1-r7	Lamination of the superior colliculus; somatic afferent zone of the hindbrain; dorsalizing gradient	156
Gbx2 (unplugged)	r1-r3	Specification of the anterior hindbrain; contributes to formation of the cerebellum, motor trigeminal nerve	104
Gsc (goosecoid)	Hensen's node, neural plate	Induces the prechordal mesoderm and prosencephalon; ectopically duplicates the neural tube	56-58
HESX1	Prosencephalon	Defective in septo-optic dysplasia	32
Foxa2 (previously Hnf3b, winged helix)	Notochord	Regulates floor plate development; suppresses the dorsalizing influence of Pax3	157
Hox 1.5	r3, r5	Segmentation; formation of the parathyroid, thymus	93, 94
Hox 1.6 (Hoxa1)	r4-r7	Rostrocaudal gradient and segmentation	92-94, 138, 140, 141, 158
Hox 2.1	r8	Rostrocaudal gradient of the spinal cord	
Hox 2.6	Border r6/7-r8	Rostrocaudal gradient and segmentation	
Hox 2.8	Border r2/3-r8	Rostrocaudal gradient and segmentation; regulates axonal projections from r3	
Hox 2.9 (Hoxb1)	r4	Formation of the neural crest	122, 138
Islet1	Ventral neural tube	Motor neuroblast differentiation	159
Islet3	Neural plate	Floor plate differentiation; regulates development of the optic vesicle and tectal and cerebellar primordia	160, 161
EGR2 (Krox20)	r3, r5	Zinc finger; neural crest formation in r3 and r5; regulates expression of HOX genes; regulates myelination by Schwann cells	118-123
L1CAM	Mesencephalon; telencephalon	Formation of the aqueduct; cerebral neuroblast migration and corticospinal axon guidance; defective in X-linked hydrocephalus with aqueductal stenosis and also reported in hemimegalencephaly	162-164

Continued

TABLE 4-5 Organizer and Regulator Genes of the Embryonic and Fetal Nervous System—cont'd

GENE*	REGIONS	FUNCTIONS	REFERENCES
Lhx2	Prosomeres	LIM family homeobox; development of the hippocampus and cellular proliferation for neocortex; development of the eye before formation of the optic cup	165
Lhx9	Subplate neurons of the cortical plate; cerebellar nuclei	Expressed in pioneer axons of the cerebral cortex and in cerebellar nuclei	166
Lim	Neural plate; prechordal mesenchyme	Organizer of cephalic mesenchyme before migration of the neural crest; organizer of the neural placode	160, 161, 167-171
Lis1	Cortical plate	Neuroblast migration; 17p13.3 locus; defective in lissencephaly type 1	172-176
Mash1	Telencephalon; neural crest	Regulates differentiation of the ventral telencephalon; in achaete-scute family; requires Phox2 for expression	177
Math1 (human homologue is ATOH1)	r1, cerebellum	Differentiation of cerebellar granule cells	178
Math5 (human homologue is ATOH7)	Optic cup	Retinal differentiation	179
Mnr2	Motor neuroblasts	Motor neuron identity	180-187
Neuro D	Ectodermal cells	Neuronal differentiation; three subtypes on human chromosomes 2, 5, 17; related to gene regulating transcription of insulin; retinal development	188-190
Ngn1 (neurogenin)	Ectodermal cells	Neuronal differentiation in the central and peripheral nervous systems; expressed earlier than Neuro D; interacts with Delta and Notch; family of subtypes	191
Nkx2-1	Prosomeres	Differentiation of the hypothalamus; induced by Shh	191, 192
Nkx2-2	All neuromeres	Specifies diencephalic neuromeric boundaries; interacts with Dlx1 and transcription factor Ttf1 for prosencephalic differentiation	191
Nkx6-1	Diencephalon–r8; motor neurons	Induced by Shh and repressed by Bmp7; coexpressed with Islet-1 in motor neurons	191
Nkx6-2	Diencephalon–r8	Glial cell differentiation	72, 73, 193, 194
Nog (noggin)	Hensen's node	Inhibits Bmp4 to allow neural plate differentiation	193, 195, 196
Notch	Neural plate; neuroepithelium	Regulates the competence of cells to respond to inductive signals; differentiation of neural placode; asymmetric distribution in cytoplasm during mitotic cycle; Notch3 mutation in CADASIL syndrome in adults	193, 197
Numb	Neural plate; fetal neuroepithelium	Antagonizes Notch by preventing neural differentiation	
Otx1 (orthodenticle)	Mesencephalon/r1 boundary; telencephalon; sensory nerves	Onset of neuromere formation; corticogenesis; sense organ development	113, 114
Otx2 (orthodenticle)	Prestreak blastomere; neural plate	Gastrulation; specification and maintenance of anterior neural plate	
Pou1f1 (previously Pit1, pituitary specific)	Adenohypophysis	Differentiation of anterior pituitary	198-201
Ptc (patched)	Cerebellar cortex	Regulates granule cell proliferation; tumor suppressor gene	103, 105-107, 136
Pax2 (paired)	Primitive streak; r2-r8; prosomeres	Dorsalizing polarity gradient; segmentation regulated by the notochord and floor plate; formation of the ventral half of the optic cup, retina, and optic nerve; overlaps and partially redundant with PAX5	202
Pax3 (paired)	r1; r8	Identity of Bergmann glia; active spinal cord dorsalizing gradient; Waardenburg's syndrome	136

TABLE 4-5 Organizer and Regulator Genes of the Embryonic and Fetal Nervous System—cont'd

GENE*	REGIONS	FUNCTIONS	REFERENCES
Pax5 (paired)	r1	Partially redundant with PAX2 for differentiation of the cerebellar cortex; dorsalizing gradient	136, 202
Pax6 (paired)	r1; r8; prosomeres	Identity of cerebellar granule cells; active in the spinal cord as a dorsalizing gradient; neuroblast migration to the cerebral cortex and deep telencephalic nuclei; iris	135, 136
Arix (Phox2a, Phox2b)	Neural crest	Differentiation of autonomic ganglia; in achaete-scute family	173-176
Pitx	Primitive streak	Determines right-left asymmetries of internal organs	115
RELN (reelin)	Laminar cortices	Extracellular matrix glycoprotein product secreted by Cajal-Retzius neurons and cerebellar granule cells; essential for terminal neuroblast migration and laminar architecture	143, 146, 203-205
RhoB	Dorsal neural tube	Delamination of neural crest cells; expression induced by BMP products	206
SHH (Sonic Hedgehog)	Notochord; floor plate; prechordal mesoderm	Induces floor plate; ventralizing influence of the neural tube; ventral midline of the prosencephalon; induction of motor neurons; mitogen to cerebellar granule cells	127-131, 133, 134, 198, 199, 207
SIX3	Prechordal mesoderm	Differentiation of the rostral neural plate and retina; 2p21 locus; mutation in humans is one cause of holoprosencephaly; overexpression causes ectopic retinas	208, 209
SMN (survival motor neuron)	Motor neuroblasts	Arrests apoptosis of motor neuroblasts	210, 211
TSC1, TSC2	Neuraxis	Encode the proteins hamartin (TSC1 at the 9q34 locus) and tuberin (TSC2 at 16p13); defective in tuberous sclerosis	212-217
Twist	Hensen's node	Organizer of cephalic mesenchyme before migration of the neural crest; cranial neural tube morphogenesis	218
Toad64 (unc33)	Growth cones	Promotes axonal outgrowth	219
Wnt1 (wingless)	r1, r3-r8	Formation of the mesencephalic-metencephalic boundary; formation of the mesencephalon, rostral pons, and cerebellum; essential for expression of EN1; weak dorsal polarizing influence in r3-r8; mitogen	95, 103, 107, 110, 137, 220-222
Wnt3 (wingless)	Mesencephalon; r1; r3-r8	Overlaps and redundant with WNT1 in the mesencephalic neuromere and r1; strong dorsal polarizing influence in r3-r8, including the spinal cord; differentiation of brainstem nuclei; identity of Purkinje cells	137, 223
Wnt7 (wingless)	Prosomeres	Differentiation of structures of the diencephalon and telencephalon	99
Wnt8 (wingless)	Epiblast; primitive streak; r1-r8	Primitive streak formation; segmentation	59
Zic1	Cerebellum	Zinc finger; differentiation of granule cells	224, 225

*An *organizer gene* is one that programs differentiation of the neural placode and axes, gradients, and segmentation of the neural plate and neural tube; a *regulator gene* is one that programs the differentiation of specific structures and cellular types in the developing nervous system, conserves their identity, and mediates developmental processes such as neuroblast migration or synaptogenesis. The genes are listed alphabetically rather than by function because many of the same genes serve various functions at different stages, such as being organizer genes in early ontogenesis and regulator genes at later periods. Developmental genes recognized in invertebrates such as *Drosophila*, but for which the vertebrate homologue has not yet been identified, are excluded. CADASIL, cerebral autosomal dominant arteriopathy with subcortical infarcts and leukoencephalopathy; r1, rhombomere 1; TGF-β, transforming growth factor-β.

Modified from Menkes JH, Sarnat HB. *Child Neurology*, 6th ed. Philadelphia: Lippincott Williams & Wilkins; 2000:283-285.

En, *Wnt*, *Hox*, *Krox*, and *Pax*. Table 4-5 summarizes the sites of expression and functions of selected important organizer and regulator genes. Many regulatory genes change their territories of expression in different stages of development; they can increase their territory to include more rhombomeres or have broader expression early in development and more restricted domains later. Sometimes, expression of a gene in the wrong neuromere, called *ectopic expression*, interferes with normal development (see Table 4-5).

Function of Retinoic Acid

Retinoic acid, the alcohol of which is vitamin A, is a hydrophobic molecule secreted by the notochord and by ependymal floor plate cells.[226] Retinoid-binding proteins and receptors are already strongly expressed in mesenchymal cells of the primitive streak and in the preoptic region of the early developing hindbrain.[227] Ependymal cells other than those of the floor plate and neuroepithelial cells have retinoic acid receptors but do not secrete this compound. Retinoic acid diffuses across the plasma membrane without requiring active transport and binds to intracellular receptors; it then enters the nucleus, where it binds to a specific nuclear receptor protein, changes the structural configuration of that protein, and thereby enables it to attach to a specific receptor on a target gene, where the complex formed by retinoic acid and its receptor then functions as a transcription factor for neural induction.[228,229]

Retinoic acid functions as a polarity molecule for determining the anterior and posterior surfaces of limb buds and, in the nervous system, is important in segmentation polarity. It produces a strong rostrocaudal polarity gradient.[54,230,231] Excessive retinoic acid acts on the neural tube of amphibian tadpoles to transform anterior neural tissue to a posterior morphogenesis, which results in extreme microcephaly and suppression of optic cup formation.[229] In vertebrates, optic cup formation may fail because of suppression of retinoic acid by genes of the *Lim* family, such as *Islet3* and *Lim1*.[160,165] Retinoic acid upregulates homeobox genes, those of the *Hox* family and *Krox20* in particular, and can cause ectopic expression of these genes in rhombomeres where they are not normally expressed.[122,232] An excess of retinoic acid, whether endogenous or exogenous (i.e., excess maternal intake of vitamin A or analogues during early gestation), results in severe malformations of the hindbrain and spinal cord. A single dose of retinoic acid administered intraperitoneally to maternal hamsters on embryonic day 9.5 results in the Chiari II malformation and frequently meningomyelocele in the fetuses.[233-235] In cell cultures of cloned CNS stem cells from the mouse, retinoic acid enhances neuronal proliferation and astroglial differentiation.[236]

FLEXURES AND SULCI OF THE BRAIN

The neural tube begins development as a straight structure, but further growth of surrounding structures exerts an external physical force that causes bending at precise points. The pontine and cervical flexures thus form. At 6 weeks' gestation the telencephalic hemisphere is oval shaped, but ventral bending then occurs to create the operculum and eventually the sylvian fissure (Fig. 4-3). Because both the dorsal (frontal lobe) and ventral (temporal lobe) lips of the sylvian fissure correspond to the ventral surface of the primitive telencephalon, disorders of this region, such as schizencephaly and perisylvian syndromes of polymicrogyria at the lips of the sylvian fissure, follow a ventrodorsal genetic gradient in the vertical axis, and both lips are involved in these malformations.[237]

The lateral ventricle within the primitive telencephalon bends with the hemisphere so that the original posterior pole of the

hemisphere becomes not the occipital pole of the mature brain but the temporal pole. New diverticula or recesses of the lateral ventricles create the occipital horns of the ventricle. Because the occipital horns are the most recent development of the fetal brain, they remain the most variable part of the ventricular system; only 25% of normal subjects have symmetrical occipital horns.

There are five fissures of the human forebrain: (1) the interhemispheric fissure, which creates two telencephalic hemispheres by sagittal splitting of the prosencephalon at 4.5 weeks' gestation; (2) the choroidal fissure at 5 weeks' gestation; (3) the hippocampal fissure, which forms after rotation of the hippocampus from a dorsal to a ventral position at 5 to 6 weeks' gestation; (4) the sylvian fissure, which is derived from the telencephalic flexure at 7 to 8 weeks' gestation; and (5) the calcarine fissure on the medial side of the occipital lobe, which forms at 9 weeks' gestation. If the occipital horns are asymmetric, the calcarine fissure on the side of the smaller occipital horn is generally shallower than that on the other side, but which is primary and which is secondary is uncertain.

Gyri form in the cerebral cortex not as a result of external forces, as with the fissures, but because of internal physical forces created by increasing volume of the neuropil as a result of the development of neurites and glial processes, the increased number of glial cells, and growth in size and volume of the neurons. Gyri are not detected at the surface of the cerebral cortex, either by MRI or by gross neuropathologic inspection, until about 22 to 24 weeks' gestation, but careful microscopic examination shows the early formation of sulci separating new gyri as early as 15 weeks. More than 30 sulci form in the cerebral cortex, and the pattern of their development is temporally and spatially precise.

Folia form in the cerebellar cortex, similar to sulci and gyri of the cerebral cortex. They develop first in the vermis and are simple but recognizable at midgestation, whereas the surface of the lateral cerebellar hemispheres at midgestation is smooth. Folia form in these lateral hemispheres from about 22 weeks' gestation, earliest in the medial (paravermal) parts.

DEVELOPMENTAL PATTERNS AND DISORDERS

Holoprosencephaly

Holoprosencephaly (HPE) results from noncleavage of the midline ventral forebrain at approximately 33 days' gestation and is classified by the degree of failure of hemispheric separation. This ventral failure of induction also leads to a wide spectrum of craniofacial defects ranging from cyclopia to milder defects such as iris colobomas, cleft palate, and single central incisors.[238] In most cases, the severity of the brain abnormality parallels that of the face.[239,240] Neuropathologic studies suggest that the correlation of severity between brain malformation and midfacial hypoplasia may be due to abnormalities in the expression of key developmental genes along their rostrocaudal gradients, which extend as far as the mesencephalic neuromere. These abnormally expressed genes may interfere with formation, migration, or apoptosis of the mesencephalic neural crest, which forms the membranous bones of the face, orbits, nose, and parts of the eyes.[241] In alobar HPE, the most severe form, there is a single midline forebrain ventricle and a cerebral holosphere, with no separation at all into cerebral hemispheres. The interhemispheric fissure and corpus callosum are completely absent. In semilobar HPE, the defect is localized more anteriorly, and some portion of the posterior interhemispheric fissure and variable amounts of the splenium of the corpus callosum are present (Fig. 4-4). In lobar HPE, the mildest form, there is separation of most of the

The telencephalic flexure that forms the sylvian fissure

Dorsal

Lateral

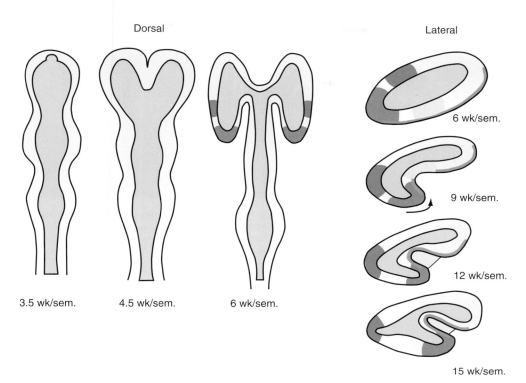

3.5 wk/sem.   4.5 wk/sem.   6 wk/sem.

6 wk/sem.

9 wk/sem.

12 wk/sem.

15 wk/sem.

FIGURE 4-3 Schematic diagram showing the telencephalic flexure in the human fetus at various gestational ages. The original posterior pole of the primitive telencephalic hemisphere becomes the temporal, not the occipital pole of the mature brain. The occipital horn of the lateral ventricle is a new recess that forms after folding of the telencephalon. The flexure forms the sylvian fissure, but both the dorsal (frontal) and ventral (temporal) lips of the fissure are derived from the ventral part of the primitive telencephalon; hence, ventrodorsal genetic gradients in the vertical axis can affect both lips, as in schizencephaly. The insula is an infolding of tissue secondary to bending of the hemisphere. (Reproduced from Sarnat HB, Flores-Sarnat L. The telencephalic flexure and developmental disorders of the Sylvian fissure. 2010, submitted for publication.)

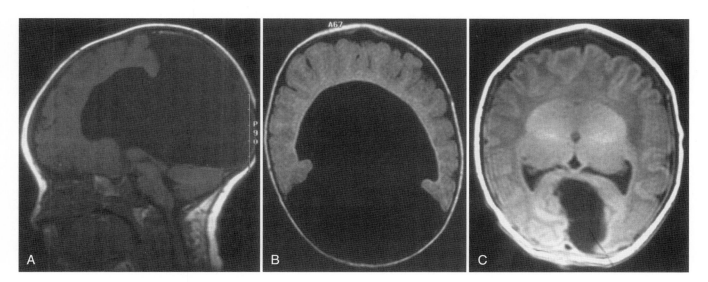

FIGURE 4-4 Holoprosencephaly. **A,** Midsagittal, T1-weighted magnetic resonance imaging (MRI) of a child with alobar holoprosencephaly shows a pancake of brain anteriorly, with the single, midline ventricle leading into a large, dorsal cyst. The corpus callosum is absent. **B,** Axial, T1-weighted MRI of the same child shows the lack of any separation of the brain into hemispheres and the crescent-shaped holoventricle leading into the dorsal cyst. **C,** Axial, T1-weighted MRI of a child with semilobar holoprosencephaly shows a smaller dorsal cyst. Notice the failure of cleavage of the frontal lobes and basal ganglia and the separation into hemispheres posteriorly. (Courtesy of Joseph Pinter, M.D., Children's Hospital and Regional Medical Center, Seattle, WA.)

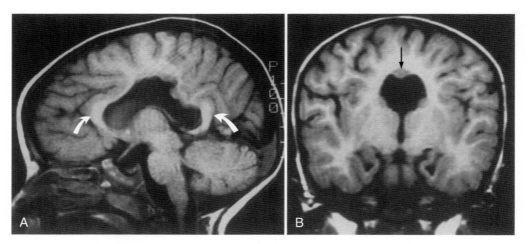

FIGURE 4-5 Middle interhemispheric variant of holoprosencephaly. **A,** Sagittal, T1-weighted magnetic resonance imaging (MRI) shows a grossly normal callosal genu and splenium (*arrows*) but absence of the midportion of the corpus callosum. **B,** Coronal, T1-weighted MRI reveals the absence of an interhemispheric fissure and a continuous band of subcortical white matter crossing the midline. The heterotopic gray matter (*arrow*) at the roof of the ventricle is a common finding in this variant. (From Barkovich AJ. *Pediatric Neuroimaging*, 3rd ed. Philadelphia: Lippincott Williams & Wilkins; 2000:324.)

cerebral hemispheres, with only the most rostral aspects remaining noncleaved. The corpus callosum is absent in the region affected.

The middle interhemispheric variant, once thought to be rare,[242] has in later large studies been identified quite frequently (Fig. 4-5).[243] Radiologic studies have also revealed that HPE is much more variable than the simple classification system described earlier would suggest. There is greater variability in the pattern and degree of noncleavage of the deep gray nuclei than previously appreciated, with almost universal involvement of the hypothalamus.[244] Thalamic noncleavage is correlated with the presence of a dorsal cyst, thus supporting the idea that the cyst arises because of blockage of rostral flow of cerebrospinal fluid, which then egresses dorsally.[245,246]

Human HPE is often seen as part of trisomy 13, but it has also been mapped to several other chromosomes.[238] *SHH* was the first gene identified to cause HPE in humans.[134] The active cleavage product of secreted Shh is covalently bound to cholesterol and then binds to its receptor Ptc (patched), which stops inhibiting the constitutive signaling activity of Smo (smoothened). Binding activates a cascade of molecular events that culminate in the transcription of dorsalizing genes such as *Wnt* and *Bmp*, which encode transcription factors. The *Shh* pathway normally keeps ventralizing and dorsalizing influences in appropriate balance. Interference with this complicated pathway explains why certain toxins cause HPE in animals.[247] Mutations in two other genes, *SIX3* and *TGIF*, can cause HPE through distinct signaling pathways.[15,16] Mutations in the *ZIC2* gene also cause HPE.[14] *ZIC2* promotes embryonic roof plate differentiation in the dorsal midline of the neural tube after closure. In mice, roof plate–specific properties such as an increased apoptotic rate and decreased mitotic rate are critical to formation of the interhemispheric fissure. Compromise of roof plate differentiation could therefore lead to HPE, and one patient with the middle interhemispheric variant has been shown to have this mutation.[243]

Because the telencephalic flexure fails to form in HPE, the hippocampus remains a dorsal structure and has the form of a U-shaped cord that extends across the midline and posteriorly to the caudal poles of the malformed forebrain.[237]

Neuronogenesis

Normal Proliferation of Neuroblasts

The neuroblast is histologically indistinguishable from other stem cells but is identified by its location in the primitive neural plate. After formation of the neural tube, neurons and glial cells are generated by proliferation of neuroepithelial cells in the ventricular zone with mitoses at the ventricular surface. The rate of division is greatest during the early first trimester in the spinal cord and brainstem and during the late first and early second trimester in the forebrain. Within the ventricular zone of the human fetal telencephalon, 33 mitotic cycles provide the total number of neurons required for the mature cerebral cortex. Most mitotic activity in the neuroepithelium occurs at the ventricular surface, and the orientation of the mitotic spindle determines the subsequent immediate fate of the daughter cells. If the cleavage plane is perpendicular to the ventricular surface, the two daughter cells become equal neuroepithelial cells preparing for further mitosis. If, however, the cleavage is parallel to the ventricular surface, the two daughter cells are unequal (i.e., asymmetric cleavage), and the one at the ventricular surface becomes another neuroepithelial cell, whereas the one away from the ventricular surface is separated from its ventricular attachment and becomes a postmitotic neuroblast ready to migrate to the cortical plate. These asymmetric cleavages are mediated by the products of two proteins that determine cell fate, *Notch1* and *Numb*, which are localized to the basal and apical regions, respectively, of the neuroepithelial cell. With symmetrical cleavage, both daughter cells receive the same amount of each, but with asymmetric cleavage, the cells receive unequal ratios of each, thereby resulting in a migratory neuroblast (Fig. 4-6).[195,197,248]

Disorders of Neuronogenesis

Destructive processes may destroy so many neuroblasts that regeneration of the full complement of cells is impossible. This happens when the insult persists for a long time or is repetitive, with each subsequent generation of dividing cells being destroyed.

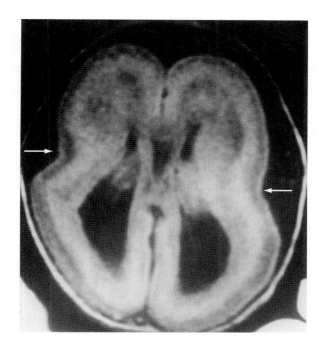

FIGURE 4-12 Lissencephaly. Axial, T1-weighted magnetic resonance imaging shows the thin, outer cortical layer separated from a deep layer of arrested neurons. The sylvian fissures (*arrows*) are open laterally, thus giving the brain a typical figure-of-eight appearance. (From Barkovich AJ. *Pediatric Neuroimaging*, 3rd ed. Philadelphia: Lippincott Williams & Wilkins; 2000:303.)

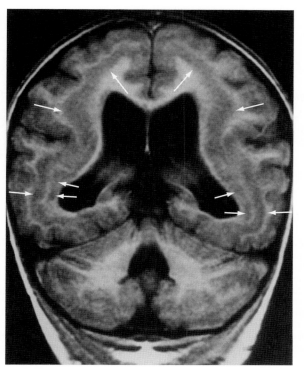

FIGURE 4-13 Subcortical laminar heterotopia (also known as *band heterotopia, double cortex*). Coronal, T1-weighted magnetic resonance imaging shows a single band in the parietal lobes (*top two white arrows*) and two bands (*large* and *small white arrows*) in the temporal lobes. (From Barkovich AJ. *Pediatric Neuroimaging*, 3rd ed. Philadelphia: Lippincott Williams & Wilkins; 2000:311).

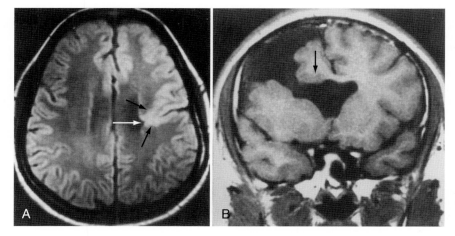

FIGURE 4-14 Schizencephaly. **A,** Axial, spin-echo 2500/20 magnetic resonance imaging (MRI) shows abnormal gray matter (*black arrows*) from the cortex to the ventricular surface (*white arrow*) in the closed-lip form. **B,** Coronal, T1-weighted MRI shows a large cleft in continuity with the lateral ventricle in the open-lip form. Gray matter lines the entire cleft, and heterotopic gray matter occurs along the roof of the lateral ventricle (*arrow*). (From Barkovich AJ. *Pediatric Neuroimaging*, 3rd ed. Philadelphia: Lippincott Williams & Wilkins; 2000:290.)

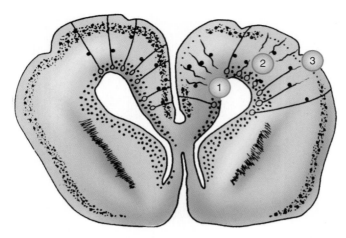

FIGURE 4-15 Diagram of a coronal section of the cerebral hemi-spheres of a third-trimester fetus (or preterm infant) indicating three sites where lesions such as infarcts or hemorrhages may disrupt radial glial fibers and interfere with neuroblast migration: (1) the periventricular region, where radial glial cells may be destroyed; (2) the deep hemispheric white matter, where crossing radial glial fibers may be damaged; and (3) the pial surface, where injury may cause retraction of radial glial fibers and the subsequent development of heterotopic collections of neurons. (From Sarnat HB. *Cerebral Dysgenesis.* New York: Oxford University Press; 1992:263.)

TABLE 4-6 Myelination Cycles in the Human Central Nervous System Based on Myelin Tissue Stains

PATHWAY*	BEGINS†	COMPLETED†
FETAL ONSET		
Spinal motor roots	16 wk	42 wk
Cranial motor nerves III, IV, V, VI	20 wk	28 wk
Spinal sensory roots	20 wk	5 mo
Medial longitudinal fasciculus	24 wk	28 wk
Acoustic nerve	24 wk	36 wk
Ventral commissure, spinal cord	24 wk	4 mo
Trapezoid body and lateral lemniscus	25 wk	36 wk
Inferior cerebellar peduncle (inner part)	26 wk	36 wk
Inferior cerebellar peduncle (outer part)	32 wk	4 mo
Superior cerebellar peduncle	28 wk	6 mo
Middle cerebellar peduncle (pontocerebellar)	42 wk	3 yr
Habenulopeduncular tract	28 wk	34 wk
Dorsal columns, spinal cord	28 wk	36 wk
Ansa reticularis	28 wk	8 mo
Medial lemniscus	32 wk	12 mo
Optic nerve	38 wk	6 mo
Corticospinal (pyramidal) tract	38 wk	2 yr
Optic radiations (geniculocalcarine)	40 wk	6 mo
Acoustic radiations (thalamocortical)	40 wk	3 yr
POSTNATAL ONSET		
Fornix	2 mo	2 yr
Thalamocortical radiations	2 mo	7 yr
Corpus callosum	2 mo	17 yr
Ipsilateral intracortical association fibers, frontotemporal and frontoparietal	3 mo	32 yr
Mamillothalamic tract	8 mo	6 yr

*Myelination as determined by light microscopy using Luxol fast blue and other myelin stains.
†Gestational age is stated in weeks; postnatal age is stated in months and years.
From Sarnat HB. *Cerebral Dysgenesis: Embryology and Clinical Expression.* New York: Oxford University Press; 1992:61.

do. Neocortical synaptogenesis is indirectly reflected in maturation of the electroencephalogram in preterm infants but represents large fields of thousands of synapses. In tissue sections of fetal and neonatal brain at autopsy, an immunocytochemical marker of the synaptic vesicle protein synaptophysin can be used to demonstrate this process in individual neurons.[262] Synaptophysin is nonspecific for the type of synapse—excitatory or inhibitory, axodendritic or axosomatic—or the type of neurotransmitter that the vesicles contain but shows the overall pattern of synapse formation and can be combined with other immunoreactivities to define this specificity. Synaptogenesis requires the terminal axonal projection with mature synaptic vesicles, a postsynaptic membrane with receptors to respond to the chemical stimulus of depolarization, and maturity of the energy-producing Na^+,K^+-ATPase system to maintain a resting membrane potential and electrical excitability of the plasma membrane.

Myelination

Myelination is the process of acquiring a specialized myelin membrane around axons, which is elaborated from the plasma membranes of adjacent oligodendrocytes in the CNS and Schwann cells in the peripheral nervous system (Tables 4-6 and 4-7). As with the other processes of nervous system development, programming of differentiation of these myelin-producing cells and myelin formation is under precise genetic regulation.[263,264] Myelination cycles are specific for each tract and occur during precise time windows. The overall period for myelination is very long; it begins as early as 16 weeks' gestation and continues in some areas past 30 years of age.

Chronic hypoxia in premature infants is probably the most common cause of delayed myelination and contributes to delays in clinical neurological maturation.[265] Unlike disorders of neuroblast migration, delay in myelination is not necessarily irreversible, and if the insult is removed, the process may catch up to the appropriate level of maturity over time.

CONCLUSION

Our growing understanding of the molecular genetic details of normal and abnormal brain development has made it clear that classification systems for disorders based on morphology or genetic mutations are inadequate. They should instead incorporate patterns of gene expression and detailed radiologic and clinical information.[266,267] It is our hope that such approaches will foster collaborations among clinicians and scientists that will lead to a better understanding of brain malformations and creation of the tools to prevent, treat, and cure them.

TABLE 4-7 Appearance of Myelination by Magnetic Resonance Imaging

ANATOMIC REGION	T1WI (BRIGHT)*	T2WI (DARK)
Middle cerebellar peduncle	Birth	Birth-2 mo
Cerebellar white matter	Birth-4 mo	3-5 mo
Posterior limb, internal capsule		
Anterior portion	Birth-1 mo	4-7 mo
Posterior portion	Birth	Birth-2 mo
Anterior limb, internal capsule	2-3 mo	7-11 mo
Genu, corpus callosum	4-6 mo	5-8 mo
Splenium, corpus callosum	3-4 mo	4-6 mo
Occipital white matter		
Central	3-5 mo	9-14 mo
Peripheral	4-7 mo	11-15 mo
Frontal white matter		
Central	3-6 mo	11-16 mo
Peripheral	7-11 mo	14-18 mo
Centrum semiovale	2-6 mo	7-11 mo

*From birth to 3 months, the pattern on T1-weighted imaging (T1WI) is opposite that of the adult brain (gray matter appears brighter than white matter). The adult pattern is achieved by 2 years of age. It is not clear why myelination changes on T1WI and T2-weighted imaging (T2WI) occur at different times. T1WI is most useful for assessing myelination in the first year. Myelination generally progresses from caudad to cephalad, from dorsal to ventral, and from central to peripheral. The changes in signal reflect mainly increased bound water in myelin, which results in shortening of T1 (increased brightness on T1WI).
From Barkovich AJ. *Pediatric Neuroimaging*, 3rd ed. Philadelphia: Lippincott Williams & Wilkins; 2000:39.

SUGGESTED READINGS

Back SA, Volpe JJ. Cellular and molecular pathogenesis of periventricular white matter injury. *Ment Retard Dev Disabil Res Rev.* 1997;3:96-107.
Barkovich AJ, Kuzniecky RI, Jackson GD, et al. Classification system for malformations of cortical development: update 2001. *Neurology.* 2001;57:2168-2178.
Barkovich AJ, Quint DJ. Middle interhemispheric fusion: an unusual variant of holoprosencephaly. *AJNR Am J Neuroradiol.* 1993;14:431-440.
Chao MV, Bothwell M. Neurotrophins: to cleave or not to cleave. *Neuron.* 2002;33:9-12.
Chong SS, Pack SD, Roschke AV, et al. A revision of the lissencephaly and Miller-Dieker syndrome critical regions in chromosome 17p13.3. *Hum Mol Genet.* 1997;6:147-155.
Clark GD. Cerebral gyral dysplasias: molecular genetics and cell biology. *Curr Opin Neurol.* 2001;14:157-162.
de la Rosa EF, de Pablo F. Cell death in early neural development: beyond the neurotrophic theory. *Trends Neurosci.* 2000;23:454-458.
DeMyer W, Zeman W, Palmer CG. The face predicts the brain: diagnostic significance of median facial anomalies for holoprosencephaly (arhinencephaly). *Pediatrics.* 1964;34:256-263.

Dobyns WB, Truwit CL, Ross ME, et al. Differences in the gyral pattern distinguish chromosome 17-linked and X-linked lissencephaly. *Neurology.* 1999;53:270-277.
Eksioglu YZ, Scheffer IE, Cardena P, et al. Periventricular heterotopia: an X-linked dominant epilepsy locus causing aberrant cerebral cortical development. *Neuron.* 1996;16:77-87.
Flores-Sarnat L, Sarnat HB. Axes and gradients of the neural tube for a morphological/molecular genetic classification of central nervous system malformations. In: Sarnat HB, Curatolo P, eds. *Handbook of Clinical Neurology. Vol. 87: Malformations of the Nervous System.* London: Elsevier; 2008:4-11.
Hong SE, Shugart YY, Huang DT, et al. Autosomal recessive lissencephaly with cerebellar hypoplasia is associated with human RELN mutations. *Nat Genet.* 2000;26:93-96.
Incardona JP, Roelink H. The role of cholesterol in Shh signaling and teratogen-induced holoprosencephaly. *Cell Mol Life Sci.* 2000;57:1709-1719.
Kobayashi K, Nakahori Y, Miyake M, et al. An ancient retrotransposal insertion causes Fukuyama-type congenital muscular dystrophy. *Nature.* 1998;394:388-392.
Kuan CY, Roth KA, Flavell RA, et al. Mechanisms of programmed cell death in the developing brain. *Trends Neurosci.* 2000;23:291-297.
Lemke G. The molecular genetics of myelination: an update. *Glia.* 1993;7:263-271.
Lo Nigro C, Chong SS, Smith ACM, et al. Point mutations and an intragenic deletion in LIS1, the lissencephaly causative gene in isolated lissencephaly sequence and Miller-Dieker syndrome. *Hum Mol Genet.* 1997;6:157-164.
Miller FD, Kaplan DR. Neurotrophin signalling pathways regulating neuronal apoptosis. *Cell Mol Life Sci.* 2001;58:1045-1053.
Mione MC, Cavanaugh JF, Harris B, et al. Cell fate specification and symmetrical/asymmetrical divisions in the developing cerebral cortex. *J Neurosci.* 1997;17:2018-2029.
O'Rourke NA, Sullivan DP, Kaznowski CE, et al. Tangential migration of neurons in the developing cerebral cortex. *Development.* 1995;121:2165-2176.
Rakic P. Radial versus tangential migration of neuronal clones in the developing cerebral cortex. *Proc Natl Acad Sci U S A.* 1995;92:11323-11327.
Ross ME, Walsh CA. Human brain malformations and their lessons for neuronal migration. *Annu Rev Neurosci.* 2001;24:1041-1070.
Roth KA, D'Sa C. Apoptosis and brain development. *Ment Retard Dev Disabil Res Rev.* 2001;7:261-266.
Sarnat HB, Benjamin DR, Siebert JR, et al. Agenesis of the mesencephalon and metencephalon with cerebellar hypoplasia: putative mutation in the EN2 gene—report of 2 cases in early infancy. *Pediatr Dev Pathol.* 2002;5:54-68.
Sarnat HB, Curatolo P, eds. *Handbook of Clinical Neurology.* Vol. 87. Series 3: Malformations of the Nervous System. Edinburgh: Elsevier; 2009.
Sarnat HB, Flores-Sarnat L, Trevenen CL. Synaptophysin immunoreactivity in the human hippocampus and neocortex from 6 to 41 weeks of gestation. *J Neuropathol Exp Neurol.* 2010;69:234-235.
Sarnat HB, Flores-Sarnat L. The telencephalic flexure and developmental disorders of the Sylvian fissure. 2010, submitted.
Sarnat HB, Flores-Sarnat L. Neuropathologic research strategies in holoprosencephaly. *J Child Neurol.* 2001;16:918-931.
Simon EM, Barkovich AJ. Holoprosencephaly: new concepts. *Magn Reson Imaging Clin N Am.* 2001;9:149-164, viii-ix.
Simon EM, Hevner RF, Pinter JD, et al. The middle interhemispheric variant of holoprosencephaly. *AJNR Am J Neuroradiol.* 2002;23:151-156.
Simon EM, Hevner RF, Pinter JD, et al. The dorsal cyst in holoprosencephaly and the role of the thalamus in its formation. *Neuroradiology.* 2001;43:787-791.
Simon EM, Hevner RF, Pinter JD, et al. Assessment of the deep gray nuclei in holoprosencephaly. *AJNR Am J Neuroradiol.* 2000;21:1955-1961.
Tietjen I, Bodell A, Apse K, et al. Comprehensive EMX2 genotyping of a large schizencephaly case series. *Am J Med Genet.* 2007;143:1313-1316.
Volpe JJ. Neuronal proliferation, migration, organization and myelination. In: *Neurology of the Newborn.* 4th ed. Philadelphia: WB Saunders; 2001:45-99.
Yu WP, Collarini EJ, Pringle NP, et al. Embryonic expression of myelin genes: evidence for a focal source of oligodendrocyte precursors in the ventricular zone of the neural tube. *Neuron.* 1994;12:1353-1362.
Yuan J, Yankner BA. Apoptosis in the nervous system. *Nature.* 2000;407:802-809.

Full references can be found on Expert Consult @ www.expertconsult.com

CHAPTER 5

Stem Cell Biology
in the Central Nervous System

Philip J. Horner ■ Samuel E. Nutt

In a series of papers published in the 1960s, Joseph Altman and colleagues reported that certain regions of the rat brain contained dividing cells capable of generating progeny with a neuronal morphology.[1] Evidence for cell proliferation in the rat and mouse already existed,[2-4] but conventional wisdom at the time was that the adult mammalian brain was completely incapable of regeneration and that neurons were formed only during development. Because technical limitations made verifying the neuronal nature of cells difficult, Altman's discoveries were met with great skepticism. Decades later, continued research and technical progress have led to unambiguous demonstration of adult neurogenesis. This chapter considers the nature of the neural stem cells (NSCs) responsible for the generation of new neurons and glia in the adult central nervous system (CNS), their role in certain tumors, and the potential cell-based therapies that they represent.

STEM CELLS AND PROGENITORS

A stem cell's defining characteristic is that it is specialized to be unspecialized. Rather than commit itself to oxygen transport like an erythrocyte or to antibody production like a plasma cell, a stem cell per se can do two things: self-replicate and differentiate into a cell that is specialized. Self-replication is the basis of stem cells' ability to renew themselves for a long time. Most adult stem cells in the human body remain quiescent or at least slowly dividing until activated by disease or injury. This low proliferation rate allows a dramatic increase when called on, as in wound repair. The decision to self-replicate, differentiate, or do nothing requires conditions specific to the cell to be generated (if any), including intrinsic cues such as gene expression and external factors such as cytokines, cell-to-cell contact, and certain molecules in their particular niche.

Oftentimes, differentiation is not a one-step process from stem cell to fully differentiated cell. Progenitors represent an intermediate cell type along the differentiation spectrum. A progenitor is a lineage-committed cell that is still replicating. Another related intermediate is the transit-amplifying cell, an aptly named cell in that it is a stop on the road (in transit) to full differentiation and divides more frequently (amplify) than less differentiated cells, although for only a limited number of cycles.

NEUROGENESIS: LOCATION AND FUNCTION

NSCs can give rise to the three major cell types of the CNS: neurons, oligodendrocytes, and astrocytes (Fig. 5-1). The two most studied sites of NSC activity are the subventricular zone (SVZ) and the dentate gyrus of the hippocampus. The bulk of our knowledge of neurogenesis comes from rodent studies, but populations of NSCs have been identified and studied in humans, as discussed later.

The Subventricular Zone

In the early 1990s, Reynolds and Weiss discovered cells in the adult mouse brain that proliferated and differentiated into neurons and astrocytes.[5] These cells were also immunopositive for nestin, an intermediate filament of neuroepithelial stem cells prevalent before differentiation. These results led to identification of the SVZ as one of the neurogenic niches present in the adult brain. Within the SVZ is a layer of proliferative cells along the lateral aspect of the lateral ventricle (Fig. 5-2). These cells express glial fibrillary acidic protein (GFAP), a classic marker for astrocytes, and polysialylated neural cell adhesion molecule (PSA-NCAM). Separating the GFAP+/PSA-NCAM+ cells from the ventricular lumen is a layer of ependymal cells, with most of the astrocytes extending minute apical processes that directly contact the ventricle.[6] Astrocytes from the SVZ differentiate into immature neurons called neuroblasts that travel via a migratory pathway to the olfactory bulb, where they differentiate into neurons.[7-9] This pathway is known as the rostral migratory stream (RMS). The astroglial cells of the SVZ also generate astrocytes, oligodendrocyte precursor cells (OPCs, discussed later), and myelinating oligodendrocytes in response to chemical demyelinating lesions.[10-13] This multipotential nature of SVZ astrocytes earns them the classification of NSCs.

Models of the cytoarchitecture of the SVZ have been in a state of flux, but the basic format has been determined. The primary precursors in vivo are the slowly dividing astrocytes mentioned earlier, called type B cells. B cells divide asymmetrically, which means that mitosis results in two different daughter cells. One is an SVZ astrocyte, just like the parent cell. The other is a short-lived transit-amplifying cell called a type C cell. C cells are antigenically distinct from B cells in that C cells express neither GFAP nor PSA-NCAM. After a brief period of increased mitotic activity, C cells ultimately give rise to migrating neuroblasts (type A cells). The neuroblasts travel from the SVZ via the RMS to the olfactory bulb, where they generate two types of inhibitory interneurons: granule cells and periglomerular neurons. C and A cells in the SVZ and subgranular zone (SGZ) can be identified by their expression of the microtubule-associated protein doublecortin[14] and can be used as a marker to reflect levels of neurogenesis.[15] The transcription factor Tbr2 is also expressed in early postmitotic neurons and their intermediate progenitors.[16]

In addition to their lineage relationships (i.e., B cells giving rise to C cells giving rise to A cells), all three types are closely associated spatially. As neuroblasts migrate toward the olfactory bulb, they coalesce to form a network of chains moving rostrally.[17,18] They do so through cellular tunnels consisting mainly of type B cells with occasional C cells interspersed among them.

Newly born neurons in the adult contend with markedly different circumstances than do those of the embryonic brain. Adult neuroblasts migrate through more intricate terrain, frequently over longer distances. They do so first in a tangential fashion toward the olfactory bulb and then radially away from the RMS.[19] To execute this switch, the neuroblasts must detach from the migrating chain, a process regulated by the extracellular matrix protein tenascin-R.[20] Tangential and radial migration combined takes place in less than a week, after which the cells must integrate into fully functional circuits. For this reason, it is likely that the differentiation patterns do not simply recapitulate development.[21]

microenvironment, as discussed previously. These limitations must be considered when developing therapeutic interventions for CNS injury.

EVIDENCE FOR ADULT HUMAN NEUROGENESIS

NSCs reside in the adult human hippocampus,[152] SVZ,[153-155] and even the cortex[156] and subcortical white matter[62] and can generate neuronal and glial progeny in vitro. As in rodents, adult human NSCs (ahNSCs) respond to certain CNS insults by proliferating and differentiating. Ischemic injury induces neurogenesis in the human brain,[157-159] and when transplanted into a demyelinated rodent spinal cord, human ahNSCs may contribute to remyelination.[155] Research on adult human neurogenesis and gliogenesis is still in its infancy, and the relative paucity of data necessitates significant further characterization before ahNSCs can be seriously considered for treatment of disease and injury.

STEM CELLS AND CANCER

Similarities abound between stem cells and tumor cells. Self-renewal is an essential feature of each, and the signaling pathways regulating this process have been implicated in cancers from a variety of organs. The Sonic Hedgehog (Shh)[160] and Notch[161] pathways are involved in NSC maintenance, and both have been implicated in the formation of tumors such as medulloblastoma[162-164] and gliomas, including glioblastoma multiforme.[165-168] These findings can be interpreted in two ways: (1) that cancer cells appropriate mechanisms for self-renewal characteristic of stem cells or (2) that stem cells are in a way predisposed to becoming tumorigenic themselves in that they have this machinery already activated. Because it is possible for transformation of cells anywhere along a given lineage (from stem cell to progenitor to mature cell), it is likely that both processes occur and contribute to cancer.

Other general similarities between stem cells and cancer cells besides proliferation include the ability to generate new (although not necessarily normal) tissues, as well as the ability of both cells to give rise to phenotypically diverse progeny, as manifested by the heterogeneity of cells composing these tissues.[169-172]

It is in part from these similarities that the cancer stem cell hypothesis was born. There is some confusion, however, regarding exactly what the phrase means. At face value, the term "cancer stem cell" seems to imply that there is a stem cell that in and of itself is carcinogenic; that is, a stem cell or progenitor is the cell of origin. Although this may be the case in many tumors (see later), what the term "cancer stem cell" really refers to is that certain tumors contain within their population a self-renewing cell that is capable of renewing not only itself but the tumor as well and thus shares features with stem cells. One demonstrates this by isolating a cell or cells from a tumor and engrafting them into a new host, where they proliferate and form a new lesion.[173] Thus, the "stemness" of the cell is not that it can renew itself and also differentiate into mature cell types (the classic criteria for stem cells) but rather that it is capable of perpetuating the cancer-forming ability of the growth. Researchers also hypothesize that cancer stem cells are required for growth and metastasis of the tumor and that elimination of this population is necessary for cure.[174]

There remains a question whether the presence of progenitors in gliomas necessarily implicates them in the neoplastic process. A comparison of ahNSCs and cells from grade II astrocytoma or glioblastoma multiforme revealed significant differences with respect to proliferation, differentiation properties, and tumorigenic capacity.[175] An alternative explanation is that NSCs have been drawn into the lesion microenvironment by growth factors, cytokines, chemokines, and other substances and are able to thrive there. These genetically normal progenitors, although not tumorigenic per se, once recruited will then proliferate and contribute significantly to growth of the tumor and thus enhance whatever mass effect the neoplasm may have.

This is not to say that stem cells are incapable of being tumorigenic. Several studies have shown that stem cells are capable of transformation, infiltration, and ultimately, generation of malignant growths. These changes often occur in the context of mutations in tumor suppressor genes such as *Pten* or *p53* or in genes for growth factor receptors such as that for epidermal growth factor receptor (*EGFR*). Even nontumorigenic stem cells transiently display glioma characteristics such as aneuploidy, loss of inhibition by growth and contact, insensitivity to growth factors, and alterations in cell cycle. Stem cell–specific markers such as nestin and CD133 can be used to predict the clinical outcome of glioma patients.

Cells displaying classic OPC features, including NG2, PDGFR-α, or A2B5 expression (or any combination of these markers), have been found in a wide range of neoplasms, most commonly gliomas such as astrocytomas, mixed astrocytomas, and oligodendrogliomas.[176-180] There are probably two events that would need to occur for a stem cell to become tumorigenic: (1) loss of cell cycle control, frequently because of mutation in a gene such as *Pten* or *p53*, and (2) acquired insensitivity to differentiation signals such that stem cells and progenitors proliferate excessively but never fully mature.

STEM CELL–BASED THERAPIES

Stem cells constitute a potential resource for the treatment of a wide variety of conditions seen by neurosurgeons. Putative therapies include treatments that modulate the behavior of endogenous stem cell behavior, as well as transplantation of exogenous cells (Fig. 5-4).

Stimulation of Endogenous Mechanisms of Repair

Although some spontaneous neurogenesis does occur after brain injury, it is often insufficient to generate functional recovery. Thus, approaches are being developed to augment endogenous repair. There are many steps in neurogenesis that can be targeted, including survival, proliferation, migration, and differentiation. Candidate molecules include bFGF, EGF, bone-derived neurotrophic factor (BDNF), noggin, erythropoietin (EPO), vascular endothelial growth factor (VEGF), and many more. Some single cytokines can target multiple components of functional neurogenesis. For example, investigators have used transforming growth factor-α (TGF-α) to induce neural stem cells to proliferate, migrate, and differentiate into neurons in an animal model of Parkinson's disease.[181] In other cases, combinatorial approaches consisting of cocktails of two or more cytokines, either simultaneously or sequentially, may be used.[182,183] It is worth noting that many of these compounds will have effects independent from those on NSCs, and parsing the multiple functions of molecules used for cytokine-mediated regeneration is a continuing challenge.

An important consideration when modulating endogenous regenerative responses is the age of the subject. Neurogenesis in both the SVZ and the hippocampus decreases dramatically with age. However, this may be attributable more to changes in the neurogenic niche than to NSCs themselves.[184] The levels of many cytokines important for NSC function (e.g., FGF2, insulin-like growth factor I [IGF-I], VEGF, and EGF) decline with age.[185,186]

Putative therapies must take into account safety issues as well, most notably the potential for tumor genesis when pursuing augmentation of stem cell proliferation.

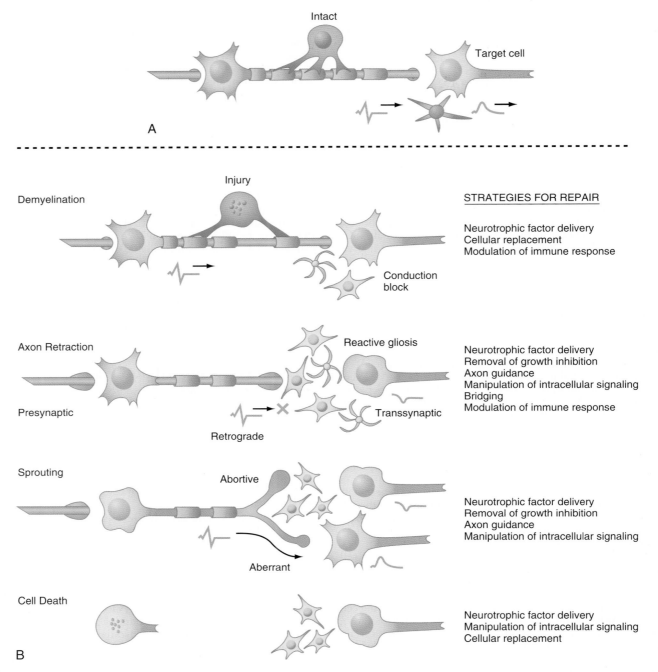

FIGURE 5-4 Potential strategies for repair of central nervous system injury or disease. **A,** Representation of the intact nervous system. Axons are myelinated and forming functional synapses with the correct target cell. **B,** When neurons and glia are injured or lost, there are several potential targets for therapy through endogenous means or transplantation strategies, including but not limited to remyelination, axon guidance, trophic support, and cell replacement.

Transplantation of Stem Cells

A more commonly considered application of stem cells is for the replacement of cells lost to injury or disease. Stem cells can be transplanted in their undifferentiated state if multiple cell types are needed to repopulate the damaged tissue, or they can be differentiated in vitro if there is a specific cell type that is selectively lost, as in Parkinson's disease or amyotrophic lateral sclerosis. Choosing one or the other will depend on the injury or disease and the goal of the treatment. Other potential parameters to be tailored to the patient include timing, route of administration, and immunosuppression.

Many studies have shown that NSCs strongly trend toward differentiation into glial cells, especially astrocytes, after transplantation into the CNS despite proficient capacity to generate neurons in vitro and in neurogenic regions in vivo.[187-189] This lineage restriction has significant implications for the therapeutic outcome with stem cell therapy. In keeping with the theme of the importance of the microenvironment in NSC behavior, modulation of the site into which cells are transplanted may be important. In fact, artificial niches for the transplantation of ahNSCs have been developed for this purpose.[190]

Stem cells can also be engineered to deliver therapeutic compounds (e.g., growth factors, immune system modulators, axon guidance molecules) to a targeted area. Strategies to do so take advantage of the inherent tropism of stem cells to injured or diseased regions of the brain. For example, NSCs show a strong selective tumor tropism that is probably mediated by VEGF.[191] A human NSC line has been engineered to express cytosine deaminase, which converts the prodrug 5-fluorocytosine into the anticancer agent 5-fluorouracil. These cells have been used in animal models to target and reduce volumes of breast cancer and melanoma brain metastases.[192,193] Similar studies have been done in models of medulloblastoma, glioblastoma, and metastatic neuroblastoma.[194-196]

STEM CELL IMAGING

To better understand the behavior of NSCs and the mechanisms of potential therapeutic benefit, in vivo imaging is required. Contemporary modalities include magnetic resonance imaging (MRI), positron emission tomography (PET), and optical imaging. MRI is often used after labeling cells with iron oxide particles and then tracking their migration in the CNS.[197-200] Optical imaging techniques such as bioluminescence imaging involve genetically engineering NSCs to express a luciferase reporter gene that causes the cells to emit photons. These photons can be collected and analyzed to gather information about cell survival, tumorigenicity, and immunogenicity.[201-204] PET has also been used to monitor stem cell behavior and metabolism, although frequently in combination with MRI.[205,206]

Each technique has its own advantages and disadvantages with respect to such parameters as speed, resolution, label specificity, and label retention, among others. For this reason and because different modalities each provide distinct sets of information, it is likely that multimodal approaches to NSC in vivo imaging will be necessary to comprehensively study NSC biology, as well as to develop and apply therapeutic interventions.

CONCLUSION

Since the first evidence of neurogenesis 45 years ago, CNS stem cell biology, like every scientific field, has answered many questions and generated a plethora of others. The versatility of NSCs allows a wide range of applications for understanding biology and disease, as well as potential treatments, many of which will involve the neurosurgeon.

SUGGESTED READINGS

Aboody K, Najbauer J, Schmidt NO, et al. Targeting of melanoma brain metastases using engineered neural stem/progenitor cells. *Neuro Oncol.* 2006;8:119-126.

Belachew S, Chittajallu R, Aguirre AA, et al. Postnatal NG2 proteoglycan–expressing progenitor cells are intrinsically multipotent and generate functional neurons. *J Cell Biol.* 2003;161:169-186.

Burns CT, Verfaille CM, Low WC. Stem cells for ischemic brain injury: a critical review. *J Comp Neurol.* 2009;515:125-144.

Carleton A, Petreanu L, Lansford R, et al. Becoming a new neuron in the adult olfactory bulb. *Nat Neurosci.* 2003;6:507-518.

Chojnacki AK, Mak GK, Weiss S. Identity crisis for adult periventricular neural stem cells: subventricular zone astrocytes, ependymal cells or both? *Nat Rev Neurosci.* 2009;10:152-163.

Curtis MA, Kam M, Nannmark U, et al. Human neuroblasts migrate to the olfactory bulb via a lateral ventricular extension. *Science.* 2007;315:1243-1249.

Doetsch F. The glial identity of neural stem cells. *Nat Neurosci.* 2003;11:1127-1134.

Eriksson PS, Perfilieva E, Bjork-Eriksson T, et al. Neurogenesis in the adult human hippocampus. *Nat Med.* 1998;4:1313-1317.

Guzman R, Uchida N, Bliss TM, et al. Long-term monitoring of transplanted human neural stem cells in developmental and pathological contexts with MRI. *Proc Natl Acad Sci U S A.* 2007;104:10211-10216.

Horner PJ, Gage FH. Regeneration in the adult and aging brain. *Arch Neurol.* 2002;59:1717-1720.

Horner PJ, Power AE, Kempermann G, et al. Proliferation and differentiation of progenitor cells throughout the intact adult rat spinal cord. *J Neurosci.* 2000;20:2218-2228.

Kempermann G, Kuhn HG, Gage FH. More hippocampal neurons in adult mice living in an enriched environment. *Nature.* 1997;386:493-495.

Lasiene J, Matsui A, Sawa Y, et al. Age-related myelin dynamics revealed by increased oligodendrogenesis and short internodes. *Aging Cell.* 2009;8:201-213.

Levine JM, Reynolds R, Fawcett JW. The oligodendrocyte precursor cell in health and disease. *Trends Neurosci.* 2001;24:39-47.

Liu CY, Westerlund U, Svensson M, et al. Artificial niches for human adult neural stem cells: possibility for autologous transplantation therapy. *J Hematother Stem Cell Res.* 2003;12:689-699.

Merkle FT, Tramontin AD, Garcia-Verdugo JM, et al. Radial glia give rise to adult neural stem cells in the subventricular zone. *Proc Natl Acad Sci U S A.* 2004;101:17528-17532.

Nunes MC, Roy NS, Keyoung HM, et al. Identification and isolation of multipotential neural progenitor cells from the subcortical white matter of the adult human brain. *Nat Med.* 2003;9:439-447.

Obermair FJ, Schroter A, Thallmair M. Endogenous neural progenitor cells as therapeutic target after spinal cord injury. *Physiology (Bethesda).* 2008;23:296-304.

Petreanu L, Alvarez-Buylla A. Maturation and death of adult-born olfactory bulb granule neurons: role of olfaction. *J Neurosci.* 2002;22:6106-6113.

Reier PJ. Cellular transplantation strategies for spinal cord injury and translational neurobiology. *NeuroRx.* 2004;1:424-451.

Reynolds BA, Weiss S. Generation of neurons and astrocytes from isolated cells of the adult mammalian nervous system. *Science.* 1992;255:1707-1710.

Seri B, Garcia-Verdugo JM, McEwen BS, et al. Astrocytes give rise to new neurons in the adult mammalian hippocampus. *J Neurosci.* 2001;21:7153-7160.

Shen Q, Goderie SK, Jin L, et al. Endothelial cells stimulate self-renewal and expand neurogenesis of neural stem cells. *Science.* 2004;304:1338-1340.

Shors TJ. From stem cells to grandmother cells: how neurogenesis relates to learning and memory. *Cell Stem Cell.* 2008;3:253-258.

Varghese M, Olstorn H, Sandberg C, et al. A comparison between stem cells from the adult human brain and from brain tumors. *Neurosurgery.* 2008;63:1022-1033.

Zai LJ, Wrathall JR. Cell proliferation and replacement following contusive spinal cord injury. *Glia.* 2005;50:247-257.

Full references can be found on Expert Consult @ www.expertconsult.com

CHAPTER 6

Neurons and Neuroglia

Bruce D. Trapp ■ Karl Herrup

The nervous system is structurally and functionally the most complicated organ of the human body. Normal brain function depends on the anatomic, biochemical, and physiologic integration of multiple cell types. The neuron is the communicating cell of the nervous system. All sensory, motor, and cognitive activities use circuitries consisting of multiple neurons with complex connections. Neuronal development and function, however, require appropriate interactions with and support from glial cells. The astrocyte serves many functions, including structural support, maintenance of the blood-brain barrier, and regulation of neurotransmitters, ions, and energy metabolism. Oligodendrocytes and Schwann cells insulate axons, facilitate rapid communication between neurons, and provide the extrinsic trophic support that is essential for axonal maturation and survival. The brain is protected by resident immune cells called *microglia*. Cells that give rise to oligodendrocytes during development are another major glial cell population in the adult brain that we know little about.

NEURONS

Webster's dictionary defines a neuron as "the structural and functional unit of the nervous system, consisting of the nerve cell body and all its processes, as the dendrites and axon."[1] One may quibble with the attribution of structural properties to the neuron, but otherwise, this is a relatively concise and accurate definition. The problem of defining the neuron in any more detail is curiously difficult. This difficulty arises because more than any other cell type in the body, there is an enormous diversity of structural and functional characteristics possessed by the various cells that go by this name. Consider as three examples the Purkinje cell, the retinal photoreceptor cell, and the dorsal root ganglion neuron (Fig. 6-1). All three are considered neurons, yet the commonalities among them are difficult to pin down. The Purkinje cell is the most straightforward of the three (Fig. 6-1A). There is a clear cellular domain that is the neuronal dendrite, a prominent cell body, and an obvious single axon. The parts of the retinal photoreceptor (Fig. 6-1B) are less easily categorized. The apical portion serves as a receptor for light, yet it is hardly a normal dendrite. The cell body is apparent, but the axon is unconventional in its thickness and appearance. The dorsal root ganglion neuron (Fig. 6-1C) also diverges from the classic neuronal form. A cell body is clear, but the process that emanates from it bifurcates; one branch connects to a peripheral target, and the other branch connects to a target within the central nervous system (CNS). Functionally, the two branches are distinct, but morphologically, they are nearly identical; under most definitions, however, neither would qualify as a dendrite.

These examples and many others suggest that the definition of a neuron has little to do with morphology. Rather, the properties that argue for all these different cells being classified as a single type are related primarily to function. First, all neurons are polarized cells derived from epithelial origin. This property is significant not only during their adult function but also during cell development. Second, all neurons move information from one point on the cell body to another. It is this property that

empowers these cells to function in such a rich array of computational behavior. Third, the information is carried by electrical (i.e., ionic) means. Transient, local shifts in membrane potential caused by metal and halide ion fluxes across the membrane enable a neuron to transfer a packet of information over micrometers or meters in a fraction of a second.

Neuronal Function

The emphasis in the previous section was on the diversity of nerve cell types. Discussion of the functioning of the adult neuron, however, requires a focus on commonalities. The goal of this section is not to describe the biochemical and biophysical mechanisms that the cell uses to create, store, and transmit electrical signals; this information is provided in Chapter 49. Rather, this section follows a packet of information as it moves through a typical nerve cell in the brain, with the goal of introducing the biology of the cell. Figure 6-2A is a diagram of one typical neuron. Synaptic input occurs on all synaptic spines, as shown in the enlarged spines at the far left. Synaptic spines can receive input from a single (Fig. 6-2B) or multiple (Fig. 6-2C) axons.

The information arrives at the nerve cell at a highly specialized structure known as a synapse. At this site, a process from the previous neuron in the circuit approaches to within a few hundred angstroms of the next cell but does not touch it. The gap between the cells remains continuous with the extracellular space. The presence of the gap requires a specialized mechanism for transferring an electrical signal from the presynaptic to the postsynaptic cell. This transfer is achieved by way of the presynaptic cell secreting a chemical transmitter substance into the gap. The transmitter is usually a small molecule such as acetylcholine or noradrenaline, but it can also be a peptide such as substance P or vasointestinal peptide. Diffusion carries this pulse of chemicals across the gap to the membrane of the postsynaptic cell, which is covered with receptor proteins. These receptors recognize the secreted chemicals and transform the information from the chemical pulse into an electrical event that can be propagated down the neuron. This mechanism is discussed in more detail later. A synapse can occur virtually anywhere on the postsynaptic cell, but the most common location is on the neuronal dendrite. The dendrite is usually the first part of the neuron to initiate an electrical response to a signal from the presynaptic neuron. On many neurons, the dendrites have specialized adornments known as spines, and it is with these structures that the presynaptic neuron forms a synapse. Spines can vary in size and shape, but they are generally no more than a few micrometers in length, with a bulb-like shape at the end of a tapered shaft (see Fig. 6-2). An electrical signal that initiates in a spine travels to the dendritic branch on which it occurs and moves down the dendrite toward the cell body. Although many neuritic processes look similar (especially in culture), a dendrite can usually be distinguished from an axon because it is tapered—decreasing in diameter as distance from the cell body increases. A nerve cell can have a single dendritic shaft emanating from its cell body (as in the Purkinje cell in Fig. 6-1A), or it can have several. A typical

dendrites are usually invisible, so white matter and neuropil are generally clear of stain.

During the 1800s, silver salts were found to have a special avidity for nervous tissue. Because of their binding to neuron-specific classes of intermediate filaments, a variety of protocols were developed that revealed the neuronal axon with great clarity. Among this class of stains, the Bodian and Bielschowsky stains are still commonly used. A special class of silver stain is the Golgi impregnation method. In this procedure, pieces of tissue are incubated for many weeks in heavy metal salts. During this time, a small number of cells take up the salts, with their entire intracellular spaces being filled. The tissue is then embedded and sectioned. When the sections are "developed" in reducing agents, an opaque black precipitate is formed that fills the impregnated cells completely. For unknown reasons, only 1% to 2% of the cells react in this fashion (seemingly at random). The details of an individual cell can be seen against a clear background (Fig. 6-5B). Although the technique reveals the finest details of dendritic structure, axons are more resistant to filling and are commonly invisible in Golgi preparations. The technique is used to best advantage in sections ranging from 80 to 120 µm thick.

In the second half of the 20th century, new technologies dramatically expanded our ability to visualize and analyze the nerve cells of the brain. Beginning in the 1950s and 1960s, the transmission electron microscope led to a quantum leap in the ability to resolve the details of nerve cellular structure. In this method, small pieces of tissue (typically 2 to 3 mm wide) are embedded in plastic and cut with a glass or diamond blade in sections ranging in thickness from tens to hundreds of nanometers. Before embedding, the tissues are usually stained with uranyl acetate, lead citrate, and osmium tetroxide, lipophilic dyes that reveal membrane structure with a high degree of clarity. Phosphotungstic acid is a frequently used stain that has a particular affinity for synapses. The resolution afforded by the electron microscope allows the fine structure of the cell to be revealed, and the organelles of the cell body can be analyzed. The unique advantages of using electron microscopy to view the nervous system include the ability to resolve synaptic structures (see Fig. 6-2B and C) such as synaptic vesicles, details of the presynaptic and postsynaptic membranes, and the material of the synaptic cleft. Axon and dendrite morphology, with their unique collections and arrangements of filaments, can also be seen.

In the 1970s and 1980s, serum antibodies were developed as highly specific stains by using the techniques of immunocytochemistry. Lightly fixed tissue is exposed to an antiserum or monoclonal antibody raised against a particular neuronal epitope. The antibody selectively binds to the neural structure that contains that epitope. Most frequently, this primary antibody is revealed through the application of a secondary antibody that is derivatized to carry a detection molecule—either a fluorescent compound, such as fluorescein or rhodamine, or an enzyme, such as horseradish peroxidase or alkaline phosphatase. In the former case, the location of the antibody is determined by examining the tissue with a fluorescence microscope. In the latter instance, the marker enzyme is localized through the use of a specific substrate whose action deposits an insoluble, chromagenic product. Immunocytochemistry is most commonly used to reveal proteins (e.g., tyrosine hydroxylase, microtubule-associated protein 2 [MAP2], the α_6 receptor of γ-aminobutyric acid [GABA$_A$]), but the location of carbohydrates (e.g., polysialic acid, gangliosides, chondroitin sulfate proteoglycan) can also be determined. Immunocytochemistry can be applied at the electron microscopic level as well, where peroxidase or gold particles are used to reveal the location of the secondary antibody. Figure 6-5C presents an example of immunocytochemistry using an antibody against a neurofilament protein, one of the major cytoskeletal components of neuronal cytoplasm.

In the 1980s and 1990s, advances in molecular biology enabled the detection of messenger RNA for specific proteins through a technique known as in situ hybridization (see Chapter 3). Medium- to high-abundance messages are localized to the cell body transcribing them by exposing lightly fixed tissue to labeled nucleotide probes that are complementary to the message sequence. The labeled probe is detected either because of its radioactivity (^{35}S-labeled nucleotide precursors are commonly used) or because of the presence of other derivatives (such as biotin or digoxigenin attached to nucleotides). In either case, the tissue is treated with proteinase to remove the bound proteins and then hybridized at temperatures that ensure the specificity of the probe-message interaction. If radioactivity is used, the location of the hybridized message is determined by apposing the section to x-ray film or by dipping the section in liquid photographic emulsion, which forms a thin coating and is subsequently fogged wherever the labeled nucleotide is found. If nonradioactive methods are used in the detection protocol, their location is revealed with a secondary probe (derivatized avidin in the case of biotin-labeled probes or antibody to digoxigenin). A digoxigenin-labeled probe hybridized to the message for the Purkinje cell–specific nuclear receptor RORα is shown in Figure 6-5D. An important aspect of the interpretation of such images is that the location of the message marks the cell body where the message is synthesized, not the place where the protein is found. For example, the image shown in Figure 6-5D could represent messenger RNA encoding RORα (a nuclear protein), the δ_2-glutamate receptor (found predominantly in dendritic spines), or synaptophysin (found principally in the presynaptic axon terminal).

Dendritic Structure

The dendrite represents a smooth, tapered extension of the neuronal cell body.[5] The main tapered dendritic shafts have many of the same organelles as the cell body, including mitochondria, microtubules, neurofilaments, smooth endoplasmic reticulum, and ribosomes. The existence of ribosomes is correlated with clear evidence of local protein synthesis, and studies have illustrated that a unique subset of the total population of messenger RNA is transported into the dendrites[6] based on specific sequences contained within the message. Despite this rough similarity to the cell body, the dendritic domain has several unique features that make it identifiable with both light and electron microscopy. Biochemically, the dendrite contains several proteins that are located nowhere else in the nerve cell. These proteins include MAP2, as well as several specific receptor species and channel proteins that differ from cell to cell.

The ultrastructure of the typical dendrite includes a relatively electron-lucent cytoplasm, an ordered parallel array of neurofilaments, and a gently tapering caliber. The branch points of large dendrites have their own unique structure. Specialized channel proteins are localized there, and detailed electrophysiologic studies have shown that the consequences of such morphology occasionally include the cell's ability to generate a self-propagating action potential here.

As outlined earlier, the most typical site of contact between a postsynaptic cell and a presynaptic axon is a dendritic spine (see Fig. 6-2B and C). Spines can be found on the cell body (although this is rare in adults) or on the main dendritic branches, but they are most common on the fine terminal branches of the dendrites. The development of a dendritic spine is heavily influenced by the presence of a presynaptic afferent but does not require it. Studies of several pathologic conditions have shown that well-proportioned spines and their associated ultrastructure can be maintained (and possibly developed) in the absence of any presynaptic element. In this case, the structure is usually ensheathed by a glial cell.

Cell Body Structure

Neurons are synthetically active cells. Although the brain typically makes up only 2% of the weight of the human body, it consumes as much as 25% of the oxygen used by the organism. It has been estimated that more than 50% of human genes are either highly enriched or unique to the nervous system. Alternative splicing of transcripts is also more prevalent in the brain than in any other tissue.[7] The ultrastructure of the nerve cell body reflects a high level of protein translation. The Golgi apparatus and rough endoplasmic reticulum are prominent features of the cell body. When there is a main apical dendrite, the Golgi apparatus and rough endoplasmic reticulum are often located between the nucleus and the emanation point of the dendrite. The concentration of rough endoplasmic reticulum is sufficiently great that the term *Nissl substance* is used to describe its prominent, dark floccular appearance on light microscopic images of basophilic dye preparations. Mitochondria are also in abundance, as might be expected given the high aerobic activity of the neuron. Primary and secondary lysosomes are present, and with aging, these organelles tend to accumulate large quantities of a waxy substance known as lipofuscin.[8] The nucleus of most neurons is oval or spherical, with relatively clear nucleoplasm. In most large neurons there is a single prominent nucleolus, whereas in small neurons, such as the granule cells of the olfactory bulb, hippocampus, and cerebral or cerebellar cortex, there are scattered clumps of heterochromatic material with no nucleolus.

Axonal Structure

The axon leaves the cell body and forms a specialized structure known as the axon hillock. This specialized region has a higher density of sodium ion channels and hence a lower threshold for firing an axon potential. The axonal process then continues without tapering to the target area. Occasionally, the axon branches locally, where it forms an axon collateral, or en route to or at the site of termination. Terminal branching is a common occurrence in the nervous system. The axoplasm is filled with ordered parallel arrays of microtubules that appear on electron microscopy to be linked to each other and to a collection of small vesicles by wispy cross-bridges. Neurofilaments are also prominent features of the axoplasm. Mitochondria and smooth endoplasmic reticulum are commonly observed, but ribosomes and Golgi membranes are absent.

Although it is less prominent than in dendrites, recent work has shown that protein synthesis can also be detected in the axon.[9] Even with this local synthetic source, the topology of the nerve cell presents a significant maintenance problem to neurons when the synaptic terminal is more than a meter away from the cell body. To achieve effective translocation between the protein synthetic machinery in the perikaryon and the axon terminal, the axon uses several mechanisms of transport. In the orthograde direction (cell body to axon terminal), bulk materials tend to flow at a pace of about 0.5 mm/day. Organelles and some proteins, however, are transported by rapid axonal transport, which can achieve rates of 400 mm/day. Material also moves from the axon terminal to the cell body, in the retrograde direction, at half the speed of fast orthograde transport.

Synaptic Structure

The physiology of synaptic function is covered in detail in Chapter 49. Underlying the details of ionic fluxes, however, are a number of crucial elements in the cell biologic structure of the neuron. On the presynaptic side, the axon terminates in a highly specialized presynaptic structure (see Fig. 6-2B and C). The shaft of the axon broadens in diameter and assumes a shallow cup-like form. Although microtubules are a prominent feature of the central axon domain, few extend into the terminal area. Instead, the major structural elements of the presynaptic terminal include neurofilaments and actin filaments. Mitochondria are more abundant than in the axon shaft, and a collection of small vesicles appears near the synaptic cleft itself. These vesicles contain the neurotransmitter substances that will be released on invasion of the terminal by an action potential. The vesicles are polymorphic in appearance. Those at excitatory synapses tend to be round, whereas those at inhibitory synapses are more ovoid or flattened. Synapses that release peptides contain larger vesicles with electron-dense material in their centers. These dense-core vesicles are typical of neurosecretory cells. Well in excess of a dozen proteins have been identified as being crucial to the process, which involves filling of the vesicle with transmitter, docking, fusion of the vesicle with cellular membranes, release, and finally, recycling.

Neurotransmitters are packaged and released from synaptic vesicles clustered in the vicinity of the synapse, where modern electron microscopic techniques suggest that they are interconnected with a meshwork of fine filaments. These vesicles must first be filled with neurotransmitter, a function accomplished by a variety of transport proteins. In an active synapse, the filled vesicles are then moved to a region near the active zone where release occurs—a region of about $0.1\ \mu m^2$. As conditions demand, the vesicles dock on the plasma membrane of the active zone. An adenosine triphosphate (ATP)-dependent process then "primes" the vesicle. In this state, the influx of Ca^{+2} ions that accompanies invasion of the action potential into the nerve terminal triggers a process of vesicle-plasma membrane fusion that releases the contents of the vesicle into the synaptic cleft. Vesicle recycling then occurs, although the precise mechanism of this process is still debated and may be dependent on the specific synapse. In general, an endocytic process recycles the fused vesicular membrane back into the cell. The vesicular and plasma membrane proteins that accomplish this process have been well studied, but a full listing of their identities and functions is beyond the scope of this volume.

The Cell Biology of Neuronal Death

Included among the important physiologic functions of a brain cell is its program of cell death. Cell death was once viewed as a passive process, but our understanding of its biology has advanced to the point where we now appreciate that most cell loss is an active process that involves a well-orchestrated program of gene expression, proteolysis, and rearrangement of cellular organelles.[10-13] The programs of cell death are generally divided into the more active form of cell death known as apoptosis and the more passive form known as necrosis. This duality is oversimplified, however; a more nuanced and probably more accurate characterization is that there are many processes that contribute to cell death. It is the summation of these processes along with the internal protective mechanisms that usually come into play in a neuron under stress that ultimately determines whether a neuron will live or die.

Apoptosis is also referred to as programmed cell death or nuclear cell death. During this process, a sequence of genetic transcription and translation is initiated. At a morphologic level, apoptosis is a process that appears to package the cell for removal without initiating an inflammatory response. The cell membrane blebs as the cell shrinks in size. The nucleus condenses and fragments, and the cell dumps its water as it shrinks, with consequent darkening of the cytoplasm. In the end, there remains only a small, round, membrane-bound corpse that is easily ingested by a local macrophage. Different pathways have been found that produce apoptosis. The intrinsic pathway begins with the breakdown of mitochondrial integrity and massive release of cytochrome C from the mitochondria into the cytoplasm. This catalyzes formation of the protein complex known as the apoptosome, which in turn activates one or more members of a group of cysteine-aspartate proteases known as caspases by proteolytically cleaving their "pro" form to generate the activated form of the caspase. There are currently 11 known caspase enzymes. Their substrates range from other caspases to many important cellular targets, where cleavage can either activate a zymogen or destroy a crucial component of cellular homeostasis. A second apoptotic pathway is known as the extrinsic pathway. It is triggered by binding of a ligand to any of several death receptors such as tumor necrosis factor (TNF) or Fas. The receptors trimerize and position pro-forms of caspase-8 or caspase-10 to be proteolytically activated. In virtually every situation that has been studied, adult neurons that are lost to cell death cannot be replaced from endogenous stem cells or other sources. It is not surprising, therefore, that the progress of apoptosis—both the intrinsic and extrinsic pathways—is regulated by several means. Mitochondrial integrity is regulated by a family of small peptides known as the Bcl2 family, which includes Bcl2, Bax, Bad, and others. These proteins bind to each other, and the dimers can either promote or inhibit cell death. Other factors that work against completion of the final apoptotic pathway include such proteins as inhibitors of apoptosis (IAPs).

Necrosis is often referred to as cytoplasmic cell death and is the opposite of apoptosis. The process is believed to be a largely passive one that is not dependent on participation of the synthetic processes of the cell such as transcription or translation. The ATP stores of the cell drop, thereby starving the cell for the energy that it needs for normal homeostatisis. As a result, the cell takes on water and swells, as do the constituent organelles. The mitochondria swell, and the cytoplasm takes on a dilute appearance. Eventually, the surface membrane of the cell loses its integrity, and the cellular contents are dumped into the extracellular space. This process is most common in the immediate aftermath of brain trauma or during certain types of metabolic imbalance.

Recently, autophagy, a process of bulk cellular waste removal, has been proposed as a distinct mechanism of cell death. The normal function of autophagy is to enable the cell to remove large particles of debris such as aggregates of misfolded proteins from the cytoplasm. It is now suspected that this process can become overactive, overwhelm the protective devices of the cell, and thus cause it to literally eat itself. The morphology of autophagic cell death includes swelling of organelles, loss of cytoplasmic membrane integrity, and vacuolization of the cytoplasm. A role for this form of cell death has been proposed in neurodegenerative disease.

The triggers for these cell death programs are diverse. A common example is that of excitotoxic cell death. If a neuron becomes hyperactive, one unavoidable consequence is the accumulation of abnormally high concentrations of intracellular calcium. This calcium activates a variety of calcium-activated proteases, channels, and pumps that will ultimately initiate a caspase cascade leading to an apoptotic crisis. This type of nerve cell death is common after a seizure (hyperactivity of a neuronal network) or a vascular insult (local depolarization inducing concentrations of various ions). Although excitotoxic cell death appears to largely be apoptotic in nature, it has been suggested that it may in fact represent a fourth uniquely neuronal form of cell death.

Another emerging association with neuronal cell death is loss of cell cycle regulation. This represents an odd situation in that most adult neurons exit the cell cycle during embryogenesis, never to return (see Chapter 4). Nonetheless, in a variety of neurodegenerative conditions, including Alzheimer's disease, Parkinson's disease, amyotrophic lateral sclerosis, and ataxia-telangiectasia, as well as stroke and human immunodeficiency virus–associated dementia, neurons that are known to be at risk for death are found to re-express proteins that are normally found

only in cells that are actively engaged in a cell cycle. These proteins include such cell cycle components as Ki-67, cdk4, cyclin D, p16, proliferating cell nuclear antigen, cyclin B, and cdc2.[14-17] Curiously, the cycle is not a productive one; it is never completed. DNA replication is involved, as studies with DNA hybridization techniques have shown in both Alzheimer's and Parkinson's disease, and chromosome copy number increases, as would be expected during a normal S phase of the cell cycle. The actual mitotic process, however, does not occur; chromosomes do not condense and mitotic spindles are not observed, nor are any forms of cytokinesis. Studies in tissue culture suggest that cell cycle initiation is an early part of the death pathway inasmuch as blocking the cycle blocks the death. In the adult brain, however, the linkage between the two processes is not direct; it is estimated that it can be many months to a year from the time that a neuron intitates a cycle until it finally dies. Whether this is a new type of cell death or merely a precursor or trigger to apoptosis or necrosis is not known.

The idea that entrance into a cell cycle might be lethal for a neuron even while it is restorative for other cells in other tissues highlights the fact that neurons, because of their highly specialized form and function, are vulnerable to a variety of insults. Thus, because they are postmitotic and highly differentiated, they cannot tolerate reinitiation of the cell cycle.[18] Similarly, because they are in a nonmitotic state, repair of DNA damage is a crucial neuroprotective activity. Syndromes that involve disruptions of genes that encode elements of the DNA repair pathways nearly always include neurodegeneration as part of their phenotype.[19] Excitotoxicity also reflects unique neuronal vulnerability. Because its internal calcium concentration is exquisitely sensitive to neurotransmitters, it is highly susceptible to damage from overactive synaptic activity. Oxidative damage is also a common trigger for neurodegenerative disease, and failure of antioxidant strategies of the cell can result in death. In truth, both the triggers of neuronal cell death and the death pathways themselves probably have significant overlap and may represent a continuum rather than distinct and wholly separate events. For example, a regular target of oxidative damage is DNA, a lesion that would trigger both DNA repair and antioxidant responses. Similarly, the processes usually associated with apoptosis can be found in cells that have lost their ATP stores and thus would be considered to be undergoing necrosis.

Neurodegenerative Diseases

There are many types of neurodegenerative disorders that afflict humans in which these processes of neuronal cell death run amok. These disorders vary in their age at onset and the specificity of the affected cell populations. Alzheimer's disease is an example of these conditions. Its disease process not only highlights several features of neuronal cell death but also emphasizes the importance of interaction among the various nervous system cell types. Alzheimer's disease is a progressive dementia that affects millions of individuals in the United States alone. Clinically, the disease is manifested as loss of short-term memory, failure of executive function, and a variety of behavioral disorders such as depression and apathy. The disease is defined by the presence of two pathologic features: extracellular deposits of a peptide fragment known as β-amyloid in a largely insoluble aggregate known as a plaque and twisted configurations of fibrils (made up largely of neurofilaments and filament-associated proteins) known as a neuritic tangle. The course of the illness involves not only neurons but also several non-neuronal cells. In the vicinity of the plaque are reactive astrocytes, as well as activated microglial cells[20,21] (discussed later in this chapter). The astrocytes appear to surround the plaque, as though trying to wall it off from the brain. The microglial cells appear to invade the plaque, as though trying to digest it. Associated with the dementia is loss of the majority of the neurons in several discrete neuronal populations: the hippocampus and entorhinal cortex, the basal nucleus of Meynert, the dorsal raphe, and the locus caeruleus. As the disease progresses, a more diffuse loss of neurons is observed that affects many regions of the frontal cortex and leads to significant atrophy of the brain in the later stages. As of this writing, the exact mechanism of neuronal death is controversial. Because the disease process itself can be many years in duration, only a tiny fraction of 1% of the cells in even the most affected population would be expected to be undergoing cell death at any one time. This slow loss of neurons makes it difficult to find the precise cells that are actively engaged in the process of dying. Perhaps as a consequence of this protracted disease course, no consistent evidence of either apoptosis or necrosis can be found in any of the affected populations. Like many other diseases, it is a condition that affects all the cells of the brain—neurons and non-neurons alike. For example, one probable scenario is that the aggregates of the β-amyloid peptide trigger a reaction in the astrocytes and microglial cells. This produces a complex inflammatory cascade that induces the release of numerous cytokines into the brain environment.[22,23] Vascular deposits of amyloid are also found during the disease, and a role of vascular endothelial cells has additionally been proposed. Thus, this common neurodegenerative condition of the elderly highlights both the severe consequences for the individual of losing neurons in large numbers and emphasizes the integrated nature of the cellular functions of the brain. Neurons may be the long-distance carriers of information in the brain, but in both health and disease, the brain works as an ensemble of multiple different cell types.

NEUROGLIA

The term *neuroglia*, or "nerve glue," was coined by Virchow in 1846 to describe an inactive connective tissue or cement that held neurons of the CNS in place.[24] Although neuronal support is the major if not the only function of neuroglia, they are not passive caretakers of neurons. Neuroglia consist of morphologically and functionally distinct cell populations with irreplaceable structural and metabolic roles during brain development, neuronal function, and brain repair. In the human brain, neuroglia outnumber neurons by a factor of 10 and actively participate in information processing.[25]

How many neuroglial cell types are there? The classic metallic impregnation techniques developed by Cajal initially identified two neuroglial cell components: astrocytes and the "third element of the CNS."[26] Subsequently, del Rio-Hortega divided Cajal's third element into the myelin-forming oligodendrocyte and the CNS resident immune cell, the microglia.[27] Recently, a fourth population of glial cells has been identified in the adult human brain that appears to be as abundant as astrocytes, microglia, and oligodendrocytes.[28] These cells can give rise to oligodendrocytes during brain development and are referred to here as oligodendrocyte progenitor cells (OPCs). As discussed later, however, all or some OPCs in the adult brain may have other functions. A fifth glial cell population in the CNS consists of ependymal cells, which line the ventricular system and central canal. In the peripheral nervous system (PNS), the Schwann cell is the major neuroglial component. With the exception of the ependymal cells, most CNS neuroglia extend multiple processes. The distribution and morphology of neuroglial cells in the adult brain are dictated by the functional requirements of these processes. Although many of these functions are understood, further characterization of the molecular properties of glial cells is needed to fully understand their functions.

Neuroglia are significant players in neurosurgery-based therapies, including axonal regeneration in spinal cord injury, neuronal survival in stroke, diagnosis and treatment of gliomas, glial cell transplantation, and gene therapy. Neuroglia also regulate neurotransmitter and glucose levels in the brain and may contribute to psychopathology. Microglia and astrocytes invariably react to CNS damage, and this reactivity may be beneficial or detrimental to brain function or intended procedures. Thus, understanding the role of neuroglia in the nervous system is as important to the neurosurgeon as understanding the neuron. The following sections describe the morphology, distribution, and function of each neuroglial cell population. Other chapters in this volume describe, in more detail, the role of astrocytes and other neuroglia in nervous system development, function, and disease.

Astrocytes

Astrocytes are the most abundant cell within the CNS. It has been estimated that astrocytes constitute 20% to 50% of the volume of many brain areas. Astrocytes mediate many functions through physical contact between their processes and other CNS components. Therefore, astrocyte distribution, shape, and function reflect in part the distribution of the CNS components that they contact. Many astrocyte functions occur ubiquitously throughout the CNS, whereas others are restricted in location. Astrocyte morphologies range from bipolar to stellate. The major functions of astrocytes are summarized in Figure 6-6 and are related to astrocyte distribution and morphology as presented in the following paragraphs.

How many types of astrocytes are there? Most textbooks identify three major astrocyte subtypes: radial glial, fibrous astrocytes of white matter, and protoplasmic astrocytes of gray matter. Astrocytes could be classified into dozens of subtypes (most found in gray matter) based on the differential expression of a variety of molecules, including ion channels, neurotransmitters, neurotrophin, and other cell surface receptors. Common to all astrocytes is a unique population of intermediate filaments enriched in glial fibrillary acidic protein. Bundles of 10-nm-thick intermediate filaments are a characteristic ultrastructural feature of

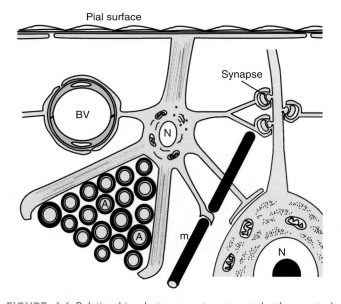

FIGURE 6-6 Relationships between astrocytes and other central nervous system cells. Astrocyte processes surround blood vessels (BV), synapses, nodes of Ranvier, neuronal cell bodies (*blue*), and groups of myelinated axons (A). They form the glial limitans at the pial and ependymal surfaces (not shown). The larger processes contain high concentrations of intermediate filaments. m, myelin; N, nucleus; basal lamina in *orange*.

astrocytes, as is an abundance of glycogen granules.[29] The latter is a reflection of the important role that astrocytes play in brain energy metabolism.

Radial Glia

Transient populations of bipolar-shaped astrocytes are the first glial cells to appear in the developing mammalian brain.[30] Their soma projects a short process to the ventricular surface and an elongated process to the pial surface. These radial glia transversely compartmentalize the developing neural tube and provide supportive scaffolding for the fragile embryonic neural tissue. This scaffolding plays an irreplaceable role in constructing the cytoarchitecture of the CNS by providing the physical substrate for many of the migrating postmitotic neurons that originate in the subventricular zone. These radial glia express a variety of extracellular matrix and adhesion molecules that provide the molecular cues for this neuronal migration. At the end of neuronal cell migration, most radial glia reenter the mitotic cycle and transform into astrocytes of white or gray matter. Radial glia, however, are not the only source of mature astrocytes; many originate from progenitor cells located in the subventricular zone. Bergmann's glia in the cerebellum, cells of Müller in the retina, and tanycytes in the brain and spinal cord retain many characteristics of radial glia in the adult brain.[31]

White Matter Astrocytes

Curiously, no astrocyte functions are unique to white matter. Some functions, however, especially those related to structural support, appear to be more prominent in white matter. Furthermore, because of their high content of intermediate filaments, white matter astrocytes are easier to visualize than their gray matter counterparts. Astrocytes provide the cement or structural support to the adult CNS by extending processes to the ventricles and pial surface, where they form a continuous sheet called the *glial limitans* (see Fig. 6-6). In contrast to bipolar radial glia, most astrocytes that form the glial limitans in the adult brain are multipolar and extend relatively short processes to either the pial or the ventricular surface. Notable exceptions are the large astrocytic processes that form supportive scaffolding for the major white matter tracts and the pial limitans of the spinal cord. In all white matter tracts, smaller astrocytic processes serve as guides for axonal migration during development, secrete growth factors that regulate oligodendrogenesis and angiogenesis, and surround and support bundles of axons projecting to similar locations.

Neuronal communication occurs via chemical and ionic signals that cross the extracellular spaces of the CNS. The extracellular milieu of the CNS, therefore, must be tightly regulated. The astrocyte is the major homeostatic regulator of the CNS microenvironment. Most importantly, the astrocyte restricts the entry of serum factors into the CNS by extending processes that terminate in specialized "end-feet" that surround almost all blood vessels in the CNS. These astrocytic end-feet provide an extrinsic trophic effect that induces and maintains the tight junctions between neighboring endothelial cells, an essential element for formation and maintenance of the blood-brain barrier (see Chapter 8). Astrocytes also buffer the extracellular fluxes of ions and neurotransmitters associated with neuronal electrical activity. In white matter, astrocyte processes cover nodal regions of myelinated axons, where they buffer ionic fluxes associated with saltatory conduction. The "structural" astrocytes in white matter may represent a separate population from the astrocytes that send processes to nodes and vessels. This distinction reflects developmental differences in the timing of their initial appearance and progenitor cell origin. The structural astrocytes appear first, and many originate from radial glia. The structural astrocytes have been referred to as type I astrocytes and those associated with

nodes and vessels as type II. Type II astrocytes are thought to originate from progenitor cells generated in the subventricular zone. In vitro, this progenitor cell may also give rise to oligodendrocytes.[28]

Gray Matter Astrocytes

When compared with white matter astrocytes, gray matter astrocytes are more abundant and project more and shorter processes. Gray matter astrocytes send processes to the pial surface, blood vessels, and nodes of Ranvier and therefore share many functions with white matter astrocytes. Gray matter contains less myelin and more vessels than white matter does, so gray matter astrocytes perform these functions at different proportions. The major difference between white and gray matter astrocytes is that the latter project processes to and ensheathe neuronal cell bodies, dendrites, and synapses (see Fig. 6-6). Ensheathment of synapses helps inactivate and recycle neurotransmitters, such as the excitatory amino acid glutamate. The glutamate and other neurotransmitter transporters are highly enriched in astrocyte processes that ensheathe synapses.[32] Gray matter astrocytes are connected to each other by gap junctions and thereby form a syncytium that permits diffusion of ions and small molecules throughout the brain parenchyma.[33] The potassium ions released from neurons during neurotransmission, for example, are taken up and diffused by astrocytes so that they do not interfere with future synaptic activity. Intercellular calcium waves are also generated from astrocyte to astrocyte in response to neuronal stimulation. Gap junctions have been detected between astrocytes and neurons and, along with astrocytic neurotransmitter receptors, may couple astrocyte and neuronal physiology.[34]

The human brain represents 2% of body weight yet consumes 25% of the body's glucose.[35] Glucose is the obligate energy substrate of the normal human brain and must be obtained from the circulation. The astrocyte is the major regulator of energy metabolism in the brain. One key to understanding this role is the physical connection between astrocytic processes and (1) capillaries, the external source of glucose, and (2) the synapse, a major energy consumer in the brain (see Fig. 6-6). The molecular events that couple synaptic activity, glucose uptake, neurotransmitter pools, and energy substrates can be stoichiometrically directed by synaptic activity. Best understood is the role of glutamate in the excitatory synapse.[35] For each synaptically released glutamate molecule internalized by the astrocytic glutamate transporter, one glucose molecule enters the same astrocyte from the circulation via endothelial cells. From this glucose molecule, 2 ATP molecules are produced by glycolysis, and 2 lactate molecules are released and consumed by the synapse to yield 18 ATP molecules via oxidative phosphorylation (see Chapter 7). This activation also results in astrocytic release of glutamine, which enters the neuron and regenerates the neuronal glutamate pool. One can see from this description that much of brain energy metabolism related to neuronal function at the synapse occurs in astrocytes. Physiologic increases in brain activity visualized by proton emission tomography of ^{18}F-2-deoxyglucose in vivo actually reflect increased blood flow and uptake of the tracer into astrocytes, not direct energy consumption by neurons.

Another important feature of astrocytes is their reaction to CNS pathology induced by trauma, neurotoxicity, neurodegeneration, infection, and inflammation. Astrocytes react by becoming hypertrophic and, in a few cases, hyperplastic. This astrogliosis includes a rapid and marked increase in expression of glial fibrillary acidic protein and intermediate filament formation. Astrocyte processes therefore help stabilize the fragile brain structure caused by destruction of brain tissue. However, reactive astrocytes may also secrete a variety of substances, such as proteoglycans and growth factors, that can inhibit or promote axonal regeneration, brain repair, and neuronal function.

Our classification of astrocytes follows the traditional approach. In older literature, the terms *fibrous astrocyte* and *protoplasmic astrocyte* are also used. This classification reflects a higher intermediate filament content in white matter and reactive astrocytes, but it provides little information regarding specificity of function. As a major cytoskeletal component, intermediate filaments provide structural stability and rigidity to cells and their processes. White matter astrocytes project long processes to stable structures (i.e., pial surface, nodes, and vessels) and thus have more intermediate filaments. In addition to these functions, gray matter astrocytes send processes to neurons, dendrites, and synapses. Because synapses are abundant and often transient structures, gray matter astrocytes are more abundant and their associations with synapses must be dynamic and not restricted by high intermediate filament content. Thus, most astrocytes in normal cerebral cortex contain few intermediate filaments and are not prominently stained by glial fibrillary acidic protein antibodies.

Oligodendrocytes

Rapid electrical communication between the 10^{11} neurons in the human brain controls and integrates the sophisticated mental and motor functions that set us apart from other species. Consider, for example, a complex task such as a 6-ft human dunking a basketball. The motor, sensory, and decision-making circuitry of the brain and peripheral nerves must integrate and coordinate jumping, manipulating the torso, handling the ball, avoiding defenders, and putting the ball in the basket. Millions of coordinated nerve impulses govern this action, and many must travel more than a meter in a fraction of a second. Without rapid nerve conduction, the 10^{11} neurons in the human brain would not be an advantage for function or survival. Two mechanisms have evolved to permit rapid conduction of nerve impulses. In invertebrates, axonal conduction velocity is related to the diameter of the axon.[36] Large-diameter axons conduct at a much faster rate than do small-diameter axons. Although this situation is sufficient for regulating neural function in smaller, less sophisticated organisms, the CNS of humans cannot accommodate the increase in axonal volume required for rapid nerve conduction. For example, the large-diameter motor axons conduct at a velocity of approximately 40 m/sec. If this conduction velocity were regulated solely by axonal diameter, the diameter of this axon would be several millimeters. Multiplying this by the millions of axons in the spinal cord would result in a spinal cord as wide as a telephone pole. Therefore, an additional mechanism evolved to accommodate rapid nerve conduction in the vertebrate brain. Analogous to the conduction of electrical wire, the mammalian nervous system increases the resistance and decreases the capacitance of axonal membrane potentials by surrounding axons with a multilamellar, tightly compacted membrane insulation called *myelin* (Fig. 6-7). Myelin is a specialized extension of the plasma membrane of the oligodendrocyte in the CNS[37] and of the Schwann cell in the PNS.[38] The length of individual myelin segments or myelin internodes varies between several hundred micrometers and 2 mm, with larger diameter axons having longer and thicker (more spiral wraps) myelin internodes. Along each axon, individual myelin internodes are separated from their neighbors by a node of Ranvier, a specialized unmyelinated axonal segment (1 to 5 μm in length) enriched in sodium channels and analogous to the axon hillock or initial axonal segment. Enrichment of voltage-sensitive sodium channels at the node

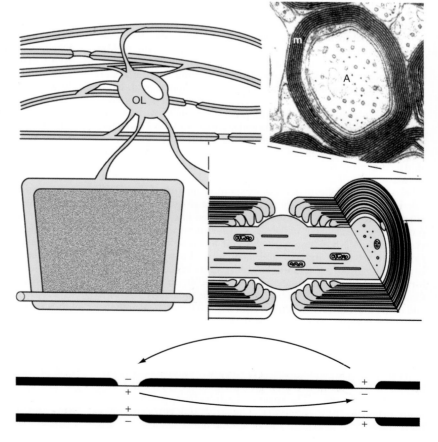

FIGURE 6-7 Oligodendrocytes (OL) in the central nervous system myelinate multiple axons (A). One myelin internode is "unrolled" to depict the continuity between oligodendrocytes and myelin internodes. The compact nature of myelin (m) is shown in the electron micrograph in the *upper right*. Myelin internodes end in paranodal loops at the nodes of Ranvier, depicted in the *cut-away view*. Myelination supports saltatory conduction, in which ion exchange occurs only at the nodes of Ranvier (*lower schematic*). (*From Peters A, Palay SL, Webster HF. The Fine Structure of the Nervous System: Neurons and Their Supporting Cells. 3rd ed. New York: Oxford University Press; 1991.*)

generates ionic impulses only at the node (see Fig. 6-7). The action potential "jumps" from node to node by a process called saltatory conduction (see Chapter 49). Propagation of the action potential is also an energy-dependent process. Saltatory conduction consumes less energy than nonsaltatory conduction does. Therefore, myelin has three general advantages for the function of the human CNS: fast axonal conduction, energy conservation, and space conservation. Myelin is essential for normal neurological function, and a variety of inherited, metabolic, and immune-mediated myelin diseases occur in humans. Axonal degeneration is a consistent and neurologically important phenotype in the brains of individuals with myelin disease,[39] an observation indicating that myelin provides extrinsic trophic support for the survival of axons.[40,41] Similarly, when myelin fails to form developmentally, axons fail to mature. Myelination is therefore essential for the maturation and survival of axons and should be considered an integral part of nerve regeneration paradigms.

The only known function of oligodendrocytes is myelination and axonal support. Consequently, the distribution of oligodendrocytes correlates with the density of axons requiring myelin. Oligodendrocyte-myelin ratios, however, are not directly proportional because different oligodendrocytes can myelinate different numbers of axons.[42] Oligodendrocytes have small, round cell bodies, extend single processes to each myelin internode, and can be identified in tissue sections with a variety of myelin-specific antibodies. As expected, oligodendrocyte density is high in white matter tracts, where the cells often occur in rows oriented parallel to axons. Oligodendrocytes are also present at significant densities in gray matter because many axons terminating on and originating from neurons are myelinated. Oligodendrocyte cell bodies can be found close to neuronal cell bodies in gray matter or close to blood vessels in both gray and white matter. It is not known whether these cells perform functions other than myelination.

Schwann Cells

Myelin is formed by Schwann cells in the PNS, where it serves identical functions as CNS myelin. Schwann cells, however, differ from oligodendrocytes in that they can promote axonal regeneration. Schwann cells form single myelin internodes and surround these internodes with a specialized connective tissue or basal lamina (Fig. 6-8). The basal lamina forms a continuous tube around the entire length of each myelinated fiber. When a PNS axon is transected, the distal axonal segment rapidly degenerates, the myelin is removed, and Schwann cells multiply and form a continuum within each basal lamina tube (Fig. 6-9).[43] The proximal end of the axon, still connected to the neuronal cell body, does not degenerate and can regrow into the Schwann cell tube, which provides a substrate and often direct continuity for

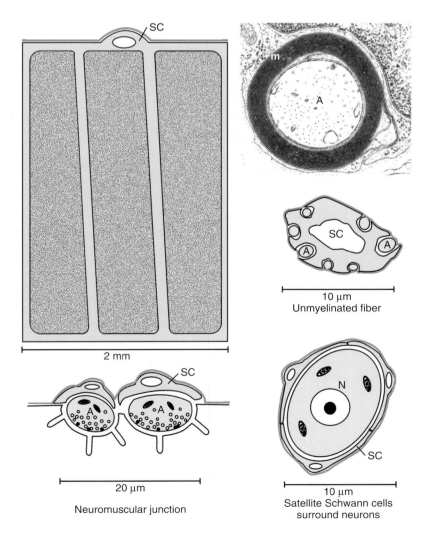

FIGURE 6-8 Schwann cells form single myelin internodes in the peripheral nervous system (PNS). The *upper left schematic* depicts an unrolled myelin internode; the *stippled area* represents compact myelin (m) shown in the electron micrograph. The outer surface of PNS myelin internodes is surrounded by basal lamina (*orange*). Schwann cells (SC) also surround multiple unmyelinated axons (A), neuromuscular junctions, and neuronal perikarya (N) in PNS ganglia. Basal lamina also surrounds these Schwann cells.

SC

2 mm

m

A

10 μm
Unmyelinated fiber

SC

A

A

SC

A

A

20 μm
Neuromuscular junction

N

SC

10 μm
Satellite Schwann cells
surround neurons

FIGURE 6-9 Axonal regeneration after nerve transection in the peripheral nervous system (PNS). After transection of PNS axons (**A**), the distal axon and myelin degenerate (**B**). The proximal axon sprouts and uses the basal lamina (*orange*) as a substrate for regeneration (**C**). Regenerated axons are remyelinated (**D**) by Schwann cells.

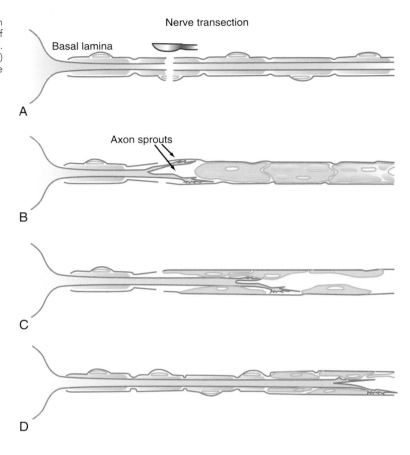

regeneration and reinnervation of appropriate targets. Denervated peripheral nerve segments, as well as Schwann cells isolated and expanded in vitro, have been experimentally transplanted into the CNS or PNS to promote axonal regeneration.[44,45] Although this is a common and often successful method of PNS regeneration in humans, Schwann cell transplantation as a therapy for human spinal cord injury is still under experimental development. Myelination is not the only function of Schwann cells. They also surround the perikaryon of PNS neurons, small-diameter axons, and portions of the neuromuscular junction (see Fig. 6-8). These Schwann cells have a molecular phenotype that differs significantly from myelinating Schwann cells.

Distribution of Microglia and Oligodendrocyte Progenitor Cells

Although the functions of microglia and OPCs are not known to be intimately related, their distribution and morphology are compared here because of their striking similarity. Both cell types are ubiquitous in the normal adult CNS, they project multiple processes from relatively small cell bodies, and each cell occupies distinct domains with little overlap between the processes of neighboring cells (Fig. 6-10). The processes of neighboring microglial cells do not touch; the ends of OPC processes are often closely apposed, and some project to blood vessels. Microglia and OPCs can be distinguished molecularly by immunocytochemistry and to the experienced observer by morphology. Regional variation in the density and shape of each cell type (e.g., white versus gray matter) occurs, however, indicative of the fact that their distribution and shape are regulated by local environments. Based on these morphologic characteristics, both cell

types form a lattice-like network that covers most of the brain parenchyma. They are therefore appropriately positioned to function as homeostatic regulators of normal brain function and as guards ready to respond to brain pathology or neural dysfunction. Although this hypothesis is clearly established for microglia, little is actually known about OPC function in the adult brain.

Function of Microglia

Microglia function as resident immune cells and phagocytes in the CNS. A lineal relationship between microglia and monocytes is supported by the following observations: all antibodies thus far raised against microglia also react with macrophages in peripheral tissues; microglia express activated monocyte markers, including major histocompatibility complex (MHC) class I and II; and microglia can process and present antigens to activated T cells. Microglia also display features not shared by peripheral macrophages and monocytes. Microglia proliferate spontaneously[46] and express a unique ion channel pattern that directs large, inwardly rectifying currents dependent on potassium.[47] Microglia can therefore be considered monocyte-derived cells that have evolved specialized features during their adaptation to the CNS. Although their functions in the normal adult brain are not fully understood, microglia have important roles in CNS development and disease. On the basis of current knowledge, it appears that most microglia originate from bone marrow–derived monocytes that enter the brain during early development. Initially ameboid in shape, these cells help phagocytose degenerating neurons and oligodendrocytes that undergo programmed cell death as part of normal development. They are mitotically active and secrete cytokines and growth factors that may help regulate gliogenesis and angiogenesis. After the early stages of brain

TABLE 7-3 Average Properties of Human Whole Brain and Cerebral Cortex

VARIABLE (UNIT)	WHOLE BRAIN	CEREBRAL CORTEX
CMR_{Glc} (μmol/g/min)	0.25	0.30
$CMRO_2$ (μmol/g/min)	1.40	1.60
CBF (mL/g/min)	0.43	0.50
OGI (ratio)	5.6	5.3
ATP turnover (J_{ATP}, μmol/g/min)	6.25	7.5
Pyruvate turnover (J_{Pyr}, μmol/g/min)	0.5	0.6
Lactate efflux (J_{Lact}, μmol/g/min)	0.035	0.07
LGI (ratio)	−0.14	−0.23

ATP, adenosine triphosphate; CBF, cerebral blood flow; CMR_{Glc}, cerebral metabolic rate of glucose; $CMRO_2$, cerebral metabolic rate of oxygen; LGI, lactate-glucose index; OGI, oxygen-glucose index.
Modified from Kuwabara H, Ohta S, Brust P, et al. Density of perfused capillaries in living human brain during functional activation. *Prog Brain Res.* 1992;91:209-215; Vafaee MS, Meyer E, Marrett S, et al. Frequency-dependent changes in cerebral metabolic rate of oxygen during activation of human visual cortex. *J Cereb Blood Flow Metab.* 1999;19:272-277; and Gjedde A, Johannsen P, Cold GE, et al. Cerebral metabolic response to low blood flow: possible role of cytochrome oxidase inhibition. *J Cereb Blood Flow Metab.* 2005;25:1183-1196.

stage, the total glucose consumption of the human cerebral cortex is about 30 μmol/hg per minute, with an OGI of about 5.5. The 10% nonoxidative metabolism of glucose leads to a rate of lactate production of about 5 to 7 μmol/hg per minute. This lactate flux is about 25% of the maximum transport capacity (T_{max}) of the type 1 monocarboxylic acid transporter (MCT1, see later) in the blood-brain barrier at a tissue lactate concentration of about 1.5 mM (see Table 7-3). The corresponding ATP turnover in humans is unknown because it depends on the average degree of uncoupling of oxidative metabolism in mitochondria.[34,35] In the absence of lactate production and uncoupling in

mitochondria, the theoretical upper limit of ATP generation is 38 mol per molecule of glucose. However, with lactate production and uncoupling in mitochondria, the average gain is about 30 mol per molecule of glucose.[34,36] Brain tissue metabolite stores are as listed in Table 7-4; an oxidative phosphorylation rate of 7.5 μmol/hg per minute represents less than a minute's worth of ATP turnover in the human brain.

Atwell and colleagues evaluated the energy demands imposed by the different mechanisms that contribute to functional activity, commonly known as the brain's energy "budget."[37,38] The main components are the requirements for ion homeostasis and impulse generation. The budget also includes processes such as biosynthesis during functional activity in vivo and neurotransmitter vesicle formation, fusion, and release. In the primate brain, almost all of the energy is spent on the restoration of ion gradients through the action of Na^+,K^+-ATPase. According to the budget, 90% of the energy turnover is devoted to "synaptic" activity and hence maintenance of membrane potential associated with functional activity in the brain. Eighty percent of the turnover occurs in neurons and about 15% in glial cells.[39]

Human brain oxygen consumption may increase to as much as 300 μmol/hg per minute under some physiologic circumstances and be accompanied by increased glucose consumption to as much as 50 μmol/hg per minute.[16,40] These increases are based on magnetic resonance spectroscopic measurements of the total oxidative metabolism of pyruvate, which may increase to as much as 80 to 90 μmol/g per minute in normal human cerebral cortex.

Metabolism Depends on Delivery of Substrate to the Brain

Glucose Transport

Glucose is the source of pyruvate and enters brain tissue, neurons, and astrocytes by means of facilitative insulin and sodium-insensitive diffusion facilitated by several members of the glucose transporter (GLUT) family of membrane-spanning proteins.[41] In brain tissue, the important members of this family are the

TABLE 7-4 Average Metabolites in Human Brain

METABOLITE	CYTOSOL Concentration (mM)	CYTOSOL Content (μmol/g)	GLYCOLYTIC EQUIVALENTS* ATP (μmol/g)	GLYCOLYTIC EQUIVALENTS* Lactate (μmol/g)
PC	5.0	4.0	4.0	
Glycogen	3.0	2.4	3.6	3.6
Glucose	1.2	1.0	2.0	2.0
ATP	2.2	1.7	1.7	
ADP	1.2×10^{-2}	1.0×10^{-2}	5.0×10^{-3}	
AMP	7.1×10^{-5}	5.6×10^{-5}		
Pyruvate	0.16	0.13		0.1
Lactate	2.9 (0.75†)	2.3 (0.6†)		2.3
Total			11.3	8.0

*The "glycolytic equivalent" is the ATP reserve that each metabolite would represent in the case of complete depletion.
†Magnetic resonance spectroscopic measurements generally yield lower values of lactate in vivo (0.5 to 1 mM), but corresponding pyruvate values are not reported and the determination is indirect (From Prichard J, Rothman D, Novotny E, et al. Lactate rise detected by 1H NMR in human visual cortex during physiologic stimulation. *Proc Natl Acad Sci USA.* 1991;88:5829-5831, and Sappey-Marinier D, Calabrese G, Fein G, et al. Effect of photic stimulation on human visual cortex lactate and phosphates using 1H and 31P magnetic resonance spectroscopy. *J Cereb Blood Flow Metab.* 1992;12:584-592).
ADP, adenosine diphosphate; AMP, adenosine monophosphate; ATP, adenosine triphosphate; PC, phosphocreatine.
Data from Olesen J. Total CO_2, lactate, and pyruvate in brain biopsies taken after freezing the tissue in situ. *Acta Neurol Scand.* 1970;46:141-148 and Roth K, Weiner MW. Determination of cytosolic ADP and AMP concentrations and the free energy of ATP hydrolysis in human muscle and brain tissues with 31P nuclear magnetic resonance spectroscopy. *Magn Reson Med.* 1991;22:505-511.

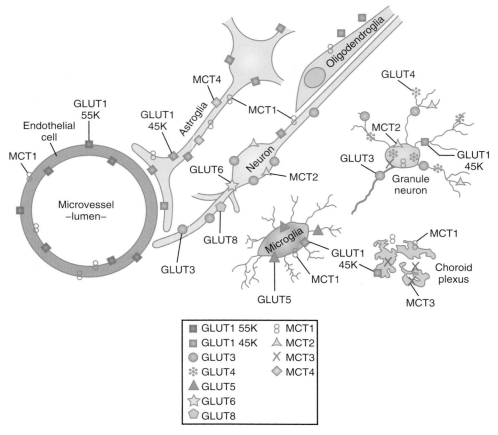

FIGURE 7-2 Distribution of key transporters in mammalian brain as a schematic representation of the cellular localization of glucose transporters (GLUTs) and monocarboxylate transporters (MCTs) in mammalian brain. Note the relative paucity of glucose transporters on glial membranes. *(From Simpson IA, Carruthers A, Vannucci SJ. Supply and demand in cerebral energy metabolism: the role of nutrient transporters. J Cereb Blood Flow Metab. 2007;27:1766-1791.)*

GLUT1 and GLUT3 proteins.[42] The 55-kD GLUT1 protein resides exclusively in the capillary endothelium that constitutes the blood-brain barrier,[43] whereas the alternative 45-kD GLUT1 protein belongs to glial cells, the choroid plexus, and the ependyma but is relatively rare in the end-feet of astrocytes close to the blood-brain barrier. The GLUT3 protein occupies the plasma membranes of neurons.[44] Transport of glucose is nonlinearly proportional to the difference in concentration between blood plasma and cytoplasm, but it is so avid that the glucose concentration is the same substantial fraction of plasma glucose everywhere in brain tissue.[45]

The transport capacity of the GLUT1 protein in the blood-brain barrier is known in some detail, and it has been demonstrated that glucose delivery is rarely rate limiting for brain glucose metabolism.[42,46] The maximum transport capacity, or T_{max}, of the endothelial GLUT1 protein in the blood-brain barrier is about 4 to 8 times the net influx of glucose. This depends on the species, with twice as much glucose being imported as consumed.[42,47] The transport properties of the respective neuronal and glial GLUT3 and GLUT1 proteins are less well known. Simpson and associates summarized the existing information and concluded that the maximum transport capacities of GLUT1 and GLUT3 in the respective cellular compartments were 25% and 5% of the total for GLUT1 in endothelium and interstitial glial membranes and 70% of the total for GLUT3 in neuronal membranes.[47] Thus, total transport capacity is low in the glial compartment in comparison to the 20-fold higher capacity in the endothelial and neuronal compartments.[46] The

interpretation raises the question of compartmentation, which is key to the understanding of homeostasis of glucose and other metabolites in brain tissue. The distribution of glucose transporters is shown in Figure 7-2.[47]

Under normal circumstances, glucose transport is not rate limiting for glycolysis in neurons, but the sufficiency of glucose delivery to glial cells depends on the amount consumed by these cells, which also maintain a reserve of glucose in the form of glycogen. This is the key issue that will be dealt with later: how much of the glucose is consumed by neurons and glial cells, respectively? Blood-brain glucose transport can become rate limiting in pronounced hypoglycemia, and it is in principle possible that it also could be rate limiting in conditions of extreme glycolytic activity unless blood flow keeps pace with glucose demand. In the brains of very active rats, Silver and Erecinska found slight decreases in the extracellular glucose concentration, as determined by means of a glucose-sensitive microelectrode placed in brain tissue.[48] Work by Simpson and coworkers found that at a plasma glucose concentration of 6 mM, the steady-state glucose concentration is less in glial cells (0.9 mM) than in neurons (1.2 mM), which in turn is less than in the interstitium (1.4 mM).[47]

Monocarboxylate Transport

The monocarboxylic acids pyruvate and lactate and the ketone bodies acetoacetate and β-hydroxybuturate[49] cross brain tissue membranes by facilitative proton-dependent transport catalyzed by the MCT family of 14 membrane-spanning proteins.[50-54]

TABLE 7-5 Estimated Saturability of Transporters and Enzymes of Pyruvate and Lactate

TRANSPORTER OR ENZYME	PYRUVATE				LACTATE			
	K_{Mapp} (mM)	V_{max} (mmol/hg/min)	Saturation		K_{Mapp} (mM)	V_{max} (mmol/hg/min)	Saturation	
			0.1 mM	0.5 mM			1 mM	5 mM
MCT4	30		0.003	0.016	30		0.032	0.143
MCT1 (astrocyte)	3.5	2	0.028	0.135	3.5	2	0.222	0.588
MCT1 (BBB)		0.02				0.02		
MCT2	0.7	0.04	0.125	0.417	0.7	0.04	0.588	0.877
mMCT	0.5	0.3	0.167	0.50	0.5	0.3	0.677	0.909
LDH(c)	0.08	20,000	0.556	0.862	1.5/8.6	2,000	0.40/0.104	0.769/0.368
LDH(s)	0.03	10,000	0.769	0.943	1.7/7.8	4,000	0.37/0.114	0.746/0.391

BBB, blood-brain barrier; LDH(c), lactate dehydrogenase in cell bodies; LDH(s), lactate dehydrogenase in synaptosome; MCT, monocarboxylate transporter.

In brain tissue, the important transporters are MCT1, MCT2, and MCT4.[55-57] The low-affinity MCT1 and MCT4 transporters dominate the membranes of the capillary endothelium and astrocytes, whereas the high-affinity MCT2 transporter is specific to neurons, particularly the glutamatergic synapses and postsynaptic densities.[58,59] MCT2 further appears to be regulated by neuronal activity and glycolytic rates, and the MCT4 protein appears to be specific for astrocytes.[57,60] The distribution of MCT is shown in Figure 7-2.[47]

The members of the MCT family are near-equilibrium proton symporters and as such are influenced by cell pH such that symport declines when pH rises. In view of the surface area of neurons and glia, it is probable that exchange of pyruvate and lactate among the compartments of the brain is nearly at equilibrium in steady-state conditions, as it is for glucose. The MCT2 protein has 5-fold higher affinity (0.7 mM) for pyruvate and lactate than the MCT1 protein (3.4 mM) does and 50-fold higher affinity than MCT4 (30 mM) does,[5,7,8,53,61-63] thus indicating that it achieves greater occupancy by lactate at normal concentrations than do the MCT1 and MCT4 proteins (Table 7-5). For this reason, it is likely that lactate's preference for transport by MCT proteins is determined by the lactate concentration in the brain. At higher concentrations, lactate prefers the MCT1 and MCT4 proteins. However, the lower affinities also mean that the transporter turnover numbers are higher, which makes the approach to a new steady-state faster, other factors being equal. None of the isoforms restrict the exchange of pyruvate at the normal low concentration, but the MCT2 isoform may restrict the exchange of lactate between neurons and the extracellular space at higher concentrations. The restriction depends on the maximum transport capacity of MCT2, which may increase in common with glutamate receptors during activation.[64]

The maximum transport capacity (T_{max}) of the MCT1 protein at the blood-brain barrier is 20 µmol/hg per minute,[65] with a Michaelis constant for lactate of about 3 to 5 mM,[53] which is higher than the normal lactate content of brain (see Table 7-4). In brain tissue, the combined transport capacities of the MCT1, MCT4, and MCT2 proteins amount to as much as 2.5 mmol/hg per minute, or 100-fold greater than the blood-brain barrier transport capacity.[58] Because the T_{max} and half-saturation concentrations or Michaelis constants (K_t) of the MCT proteins are about the same for pyruvate and lactate,[66] efflux of lactate and pyruvate across the blood-brain barrier under normal conditions is the rate-limiting step in the lactate and pyruvate tissue distributions. For the same reason, export of pyruvate to the circulation is no more than 10% that of lactate and thus may be ignored in the greater perspective of brain energy metabolism. The transport of lactate across neuronal membranes is close to saturation because of the high affinity of the MCT2 protein, which implies that net transport of lactate or pyruvate across neuronal membranes is prevented.[67]

Both pyruvate and lactate are transported into mitochondria by a specific mitochondrial monocarboxylate transporter (mMCT).[68] The exact nature of the mMCT protein is not known, but the bulk of the evidence suggests that it is related to the high-affinity MCT2 transporter,[53] although identity with the MCT1 protein is also suggested[68,69] because both MCT1 and MCT2 can be found in the inner membrane of neuronal mitochondria. Kinship of the mMCT protein to MCT2 rather than the MCT1 protein is supported by the magnitude of the Michaelis constant of mMCT, which is 0.5 µmol/g, or higher than pyruvate's concentration of 0.1 to 0.2 µmol/g in the cytosol. The T_{max} of 0.3 mmol/hg per minute depends on mitochondrial density,[70,71] but in any case it is fivefold higher than the average flux of pyruvate in human cerebral cortex (60 µmol/hg per minute). Thus, on average the rate of pyruvate entry into mitochondria can rise fivefold as the protein approaches saturation.

It is possible that the mMCT protein may become rate limiting for oxidative metabolism in the brain,[67] as in the heart.[72-74] However, it is more commonly held that the mitochondrial pyruvate concentration saturates the flux-generating pyruvate dehydrogenase (PDH) complex, thus rendering the pyruvate flux independent of the pyruvate concentration and instead a function of PDH and mitochondrial activity.

Oxygen Delivery

Oxygen delivery from blood to brain tissue is limited by its binding to hemoglobin. Other factors, such as specific resistance at the endothelium of brain capillaries,[75,76] may also influence oxygen delivery. A significant fraction of the oxygen transported to brain tissue is extracted during the passage of blood in microvessels in the brain. On average, 40% of the oxygen in blood is extracted, but it may increase to as much as 60%. It appears that oxygen is delivered to the tissue entirely by diffusion and that the large extraction lowers the pressure gradient responsible for diffusion of oxygen. It is possible to calculate the loss of oxygen from the blood that flows through capillaries and hence the decline in oxygen partial pressure, which depends on the extraction fraction. Elevation of blood flow that exceeds the increment in oxygen consumption counters the decline in the pressure gradient, as described by simple one-dimensional models of oxygen diffusion to brain tissue.[77-79] These models explain the nonlinear relationship between changes in blood flow and changes in oxygen consumption, which ensures that the disproportionately elevated blood flow delivers more oxygen during

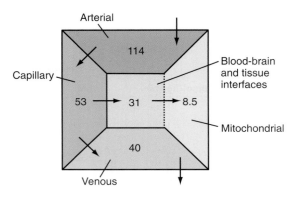

FIGURE 7-3 Compartment model of oxygen tensions in brain. The compartments include arterial, capillary, venous, and mitochondrial spaces. The interface between the capillary and mitochondrial compartments is a diffusion barrier, the exact position of which is not known with certainty, although it may be dominated by the capillary endothelium. The numbers refer to normal oxygen tensions in mm Hg units calculated from the equations for capillary and venous oxygen tensions and for mitochondrial oxygen tension. The oxygen tension of the average tissue compartment or capillary-mitochondrial diffusion interface is a simple linear average. Note that the term *capillary bed* is used for the entire portion of the vascular bed that interacts with the tissue. This portion may include elements of arterial microvessels. (*From Duling BR, Berne RM. Longitudinal gradients in periarteriolar oxygen tension: a possible mechanism for the participation of oxygen in local regulation of blood flow. Circ Res 1970; 27:669-678; Gjedde A. Blood-brain transfer and metabolism of oxygen. In: Dermietzel R, Spray DC, Nedergaard M, eds. Blood-Brain Barriers. New York: Wiley-VCHO; 2006.*)

functional activation. The effect is to maintain mitochondrial oxygen tension relatively constant.

With typical values of the physiologic variables in the equations, the estimated normal distribution of oxygen pressure in the vasculature and tissue compartments is shown in Figure 7-3.[80] Quantitative considerations predict that delivery fails when oxygen extraction reaches 60%, in which case extraction cannot increase further because the low capillary oxygen pressure restricts the diffusion.[40] The neurovascular coupling responsible for the relationship between blood flow, oxygen delivery, and oxygen consumption has been the subject of research for the past 30 years, but no firm conclusions have yet emerged.

HOMEOSTATIC MECHANISMS MAINTAIN CONSTANT ADENOSINE TRIPHOSPHATE

ATP is the energy "currency" of brain cells that links the energy-using and energy-producing processes. This section describes the mechanisms that maintain a constant ATP concentration regardless of the rate of its expenditure. Generally speaking, these processes are glycolysis, or the breakdown of glucose to pyruvate, and oxidative phosphorylation, or the breakdown of pyruvate to carbon dioxide and the reduction of oxygen to water.

At steady state, the normal stoichiometric relationships between the main substrate fluxes are given by the following equations, which ignore the negligible alternative cytosolic glucose and oxygen sinks but do include a degree of uncoupling of mitochondrial activity from ATP production:

$$J_{Pyr} = 2J_{Glc} \qquad (2)$$

$$J_{ATP} = \beta \left(J_{Pyr} + 6J_{O_2} \right) \qquad (3)$$

and

$$J_{Lact} = J_{Pyr} - \frac{1}{3} J_{O_2} \qquad (4)$$

where J_{ATP} is ATP production, β is coupling efficiency (e.g., 75%), J_{Glc} is glucose consumption, J_{Pyr} is the pyruvate generation rate, and J_{Lact} is the lactate production and efflux rate. These relationships apply only to the steady state in which there are no changes in substrate concentrations in the brain and glucose and oxygen do not enter other pathways. The formulation of lactate efflux applies to the tissue as a whole, under the assumption that pyruvate and lactate as monocarboxylic acids are not subject to compartmentation. Thus, the accumulation of lactate is a simple function of the pyruvate concentration and lactate efflux through the blood-brain barrier. Under non–steady-state circumstances, the glucose, glycogen, pyruvate, and lactate concentrations change in complex ways (see later).

Under normal circumstances, brain energy metabolism maintains an approximately constant ATP concentration. Observations in the heart and brain suggest that 2- to 10-fold variations in work rate can be sustained with minimal change in ATP.[81-85] Thus, the processes that maintain this metabolite must be sensitive (directly or indirectly) to increased ATP utilization by feedback or feedforward mechanisms such as monoaminergic and glutamatergic activation of metabotropic receptors.

Several mechanisms potentially explain the remarkable ability of brain tissue to vary energy turnover, blood flow, and metabolic rates manyfold with little change in ATP concentration. The true ADP concentration is much more difficult to ascertain, but it is likely that it undergoes some increase during elevations of metabolism. Enzymes and transporters are among the proteins that subserve the nonequilibrium and near-equilibrium reactions that could contribute to these mechanisms. Near-equilibrium reactions buffer minute changes in the relevant substrates, but flux-generating and flux-directing nonequilibrium reactions adjust the magnitude and direction of metabolism dictated by extrinsic regulators. The main targets of extrinsic regulators include the nonequilibrium hexokinase I (HK-I) and phosphofructokinase-1 (PFK-1) reactions of glycolysis and the nonequilibrium PDH, citrate synthase, and oxoglutarate dehydrogenase reactions of oxidative phosphorylation in mitochondria.

Hydrolysis of Phosphocreatine

Creatine kinase (CK) occupies a pivotal role in early buffering of the ATP concentration.[85] This cytosolic enzyme has tissue-specific isoforms, including the brain-predominant subtype BB-CK and the Mi-CK isoform bound to the inner mitochondrial membrane. The cytosolic CK reaction is in near equilibrium in living human brain.[86,87] The reaction regenerates ATP by transfer of a high-energy phosphate bond from phosphocreatine (PC) to ADP. When the near equilibrium of the cytoplasmic CK reaction is perturbed, it buffers any increase in ADP by increased phosphorylation of ADP. The cytoplasmic PC is replenished by the mitochondrial CK, which in turn is regenerated by hydrolysis of ATP synthesized in mitochondria.[88] The advantage is that PC diffuses an order of magnitude faster through the cytosol than do the adenine nucleotides.[85] Yet under conditions of high metabolic activity, ATP homeostasis may be limited by the speed of the CK transphosphorylation reaction in mitochondria.[88]

Glycolysis

Aerobic glycolysis is the breakdown of glucose to pyruvate under normal aerobic conditions. The overall reaction is the conversion of one part glucose to two parts pyruvate at the expense of the oxidized form of nicotinamide adenine dinucleotide (NAD+), which is converted to the reduced form of NAD (NADH) and ADP, which in turn is phosphorylated to ATP. The gains in

provides an alternative pathway of pyruvate metabolism. In addition, astrocytes have comparatively larger stores of glycogen, and they consume acetate in addition to glucose.[124] The lower affinity MCT1 and MCT4 transporters and the higher affinity LDH4 and LDH5 isozymes together may establish a preference for export of pyruvate rather than conversion to lactate, thus indicating that astrocytes are particularly well equipped for the generation of pyruvate and subsequent oxidative metabolism, either in the astrocytes or after export to other cells.

Import of glutamate stimulates ATP hydrolysis by glutamine synthetase and Na$^+$,K$^+$-ATPase in glial cells.[118,124-126] The neuronal and glial compartments both possess the mechanisms necessary for the completion of glycolysis and oxidative phosphorylation, but the relationship depends on the relative oxidative and glycolytic capacities of the two metabolic compartments.[17,19,127] Although it is certain that pyruvate is metabolized oxidatively in astrocytes,[127-129] the key to the metabolic relationship between the neuronal and glial compartments is the ratio of glycolytic to oxidative activities in the two cell types under different physiologic conditions. Several factors influence the exchange of metabolites between metabolic compartments: the distribution of glycolytic and hexokinase activities among the compartments, the distribution of oxidative capacity among the compartments, and the volumes of the different compartments. These factors in turn determine the number of compartments that must be considered.

When these factors are taken into account, it is likely that at least four different compartments can be discerned. The answer is important because any local imbalance in glycolytic and oxidative capacities necessarily leads to exchanges of pyruvate and lactate among these localities, facilitated as they are by the more or less homogeneous pools of glucose, pyruvate, and lactate that exist in brain tissue. In these pools, glucose is consumed at the sites of phosphorylation in proportion to the hexokinase activity, wherever this is established, whereas pyruvate is consumed in proportion to the local oxidative capacity, with lactate acting as a buffering intermediate among these sites.[129] The current very active discussion of glial metabolism hinges on the relative glycolytic and oxidative capacities of astrocytes and neurons because it remains uncertain whether the metabolic profile of astrocytes not only quantitatively but also qualitatively differs from that of neurons. However, until the advent of high–field strength magnetic resonance spectroscopy,[17] isolated populations of astrocytes and neurons were studied only in vitro, where exchange of metabolites among different cell types is absent.

Distribution of Oxidative Capacities

On the oxidative side, the fraction of total brain oxidative metabolism ascribed to non-neuronal cells is 20%,[16,17,39,126] although it remains a puzzle that a key step in the oxidative metabolism of glucose, the aspartate-glutamate carrier of the malate-aspartate shuttle in mitochondria, in some studies appears to be absent in glial cells, thus rendering them incapable of complete oxidation of pyruvate.[130,131]

Distribution of Glycolytic Capacities

The question of the glycolytic activity of the metabolic compartments in vivo is complicated by the lack of specific glycolytic markers. Some studies suggest that astrocytes are considerably more glycolytic than neurons, but detailed regional measurements in mammalian brain in vivo are still lacking. In a study of both cell types in isolation, Itoh and colleagues found that both release lactate, albeit to different extents.[132] However, the neuronal release of lactate in vitro cannot, of course, be an accurate model of the potential exchanges of pyruvate and lactate under the more active conditions prevailing in vivo. Thus, neurons or

astrocytes, or both, could in principle release pyruvate and lactate at low activity in vitro but still require net uptake of either at high activity in vivo. The significance of this point depends on the individual glycolytic and oxidative capacities of the two cell types and on the extent to which these capacities undergo change during functional activity in vivo. An accurate description of the regional distribution of glycolytic activity, represented by hexokinase, is not available, but there is probably an even distribution of HK-I activity in the cytoplasm of neurons and astrocytes.[133] By complex modeling of known GLUT and MCT transport capacities in rat brain, Simpson and colleagues determined that steady-state neuronal glucose consumption exceeded astrocytic glucose consumption by a factor of 5,[47] which is consistent with the fraction of astrocytic oxidative metabolism. This is the simplest situation in which neurons and glial cells are equally oxidative and glycolytic, but astrocytes have a lower rate of metabolism when their share of the tissue volume is taken into account.

The notion that glial cells are considerably more glycolytic than neurons arises from different experiments. Herrero-Mendez and associates discovered that neurons have low PFK-1 activity because of constitutively regulated degradation of the associated PFK-fb3 (6-phosphofructo-2-kinase/fructose-2,6-bisphosphatase-3) enzyme activity.[134] From these observations, the authors concluded that the glycolytic activity of neurons or parts of neurons must be low and that metabolism of glucose to pyruvate in neurons mainly takes place in the pentose phosphate pathway, which results in the production of reducing equivalents in the form of NADPH. The latter represents the necessary cofactor in the scavenging of reactive oxygen species produced by the high oxidative activity of neurons.[134]

Through a different approach, Silver and Erecinska found 25% to 32% of the ATP production in astrocytoma cells in vitro to be glycolytic.[135] A simple relationship relates the percentage of glycolytic ATP production to the OGI. Indirect studies in vivo also suggest that the proportion of glycolytically generated ATP is close to 20% in astrocytes in vivo.[17,136] The 20% figure is commensurate with an OGI value of 1. The glucose metabolic rate associated with this OGI can be calculated from the oxidative metabolism of the tissue, and the fluxes of ATP and pyruvate and the efflux of lactate in turn can be computed from the glycolytic rate.

Distribution of Volumes among Metabolic Compartments

The volumes that neurons and astrocytes occupy in the cerebral cortex are not known with certainty, in part because extensions from the cell bodies (somata) are intertwined in the cortical neuropil. Recent assessment has shown that the somatic volumes of neurons and astrocytes in human cerebral cortex average 10% and 2% of the total volume, respectively.[137] With an extracellular volume of 17% and a vascular volume of 3%, it is probable that the total neuropil occupies about 70% of the cortical volume. Less recent assessments of the total volume of astrocytes, including the processes from the somata, vary from 20% to 30%,[138,139] which leaves 40% to 50% of the total volume as the neuronal share of the neuropil. The estimation of volumes suggests that at least four compartments are present that correspond to the cell bodies and proximal sites of neurons, cell bodies and proximal sites of astrocytes, distal sites of neurons, and distal sites of astrocytes, with possibly very gradual transitions among the four. These volumes are shown in Figure 7-7A.

Metabolite Cycling

A differential distribution of oxidative capacity can be estimated for the human cerebral cortex by taking into account the relative volumes of neuronal and astroglial somata, the fractions of

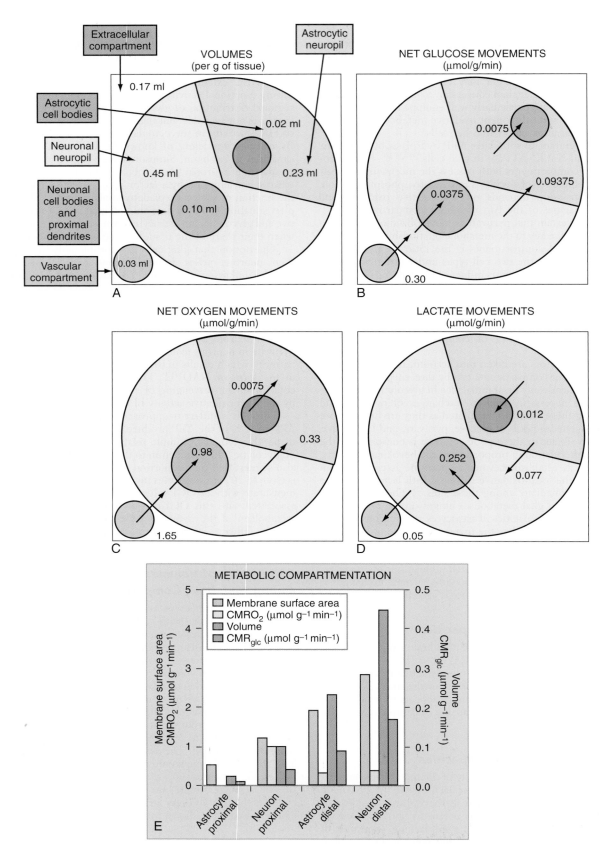

FIGURE 7-7 Estimated glycolytic and oxidative fluxes of glucose, pyruvate, and lactate along with volumes of extracellular fluid and neuronal and astrocytic compartments in the mammalian cerebral cortex. **A,** Volumes. **B,** Net glucose fluxes. **C,** Net oxygen fluxes. **D,** Lactate fluxes. **E,** Histogram of flux relationships. Glucose, pyruvate, and lactate occupy single homogeneous pools encompassing all compartments. Glucose feeds into the pyruvate pool in proportion to the hexokinase capacity of the intracellular compartments, and pyruvate supplies the oxidative metabolism of the two cell types (*green* and *blue*) in proportion to their oxidative capacities.

TABLE 7-7 Average Estimates of Neuronal and Astrocytic Metabolism in Brain

| METABOLITE | FLUX (μmol/g/min) | | | | |
| | ASTROCYTES | | NEURONS | | |
	Proximal	Distal	Proximal	Distal	Total
ATP	0.03	1.4	4.5	1.6	7.5
Glucose	0.0075	0.08625	0.0375	0.1687	0.30
Oxygen	0.0075	0.3225	0.98	0.340	1.65
OGI	1	3.7	26	2.0	5.4
Pyruvate generation	0.015	0.1725	0.075	0.3375	0.60
Pyruvate consumption	0.0030	0.1075	0.3260	0.1135	0.55
Lactate production					0.05

ATP, adenosine triphosphate; OGI, oxygen-glucose index.

neuropil volume assigned to the neuronal and astroglial fractions, the relative density of mitochondria in these fractions, and the fraction of total oxidative metabolism assigned to astrocytes as a whole. By combining the oxidative metabolic rate of astrocytes (20% of the total brain energy metabolic rate) with estimates of the OGI of different parts of astrocytes (Table 7-7) and the average OGI of the cerebral cortex (see Table 3), it appears that the proximal parts of neurons would have an OGI of close to 25, or much greater oxygen than direct glucose use (Table 7-7). This is possible only if these parts of the neurons import the majority of the necessary pyruvate in the form of lactate from sources other than the glucose imported directly by neurons. When other compartments, including the distal parts of neurons and the proximal and distal parts of astrocytes and extracerebral sources of lactate, supply pyruvate to a uniform tissue pool, the proximal elements of neurons draw a sizable portion of their glycolytic needs from this pool. Estimated values of these relationships are provided in Table 7-7 and illustrated in Figure 7-7E. Proximal neuronal sites have the highest oxidative metabolic rate, no less than 9.8 μmol/g neuronal somata per minute, and distal neuronal sites (neuropil) have the next to lowest metabolic rate, no more than 0.76 μmol/g neuronal neuropil per minute. In comparison, distal astrocytic sites (processes) then have the second to highest oxidative metabolic rate of 1.4 μmol/g astrocytic processes per minute (although only 14% of neuronal somata), and proximal astrocytic sites (somata) have the lowest oxidative metabolic rate of 0.375 μmol/g astrocytic somata per minute, as shown in Figure 7-7B to D.

The circumstances listed in Table 7-7 are consistent with a higher rate of production of lactate by astrocytic processes than by neuronal terminals, as demonstrated by Itoh and associates in vitro.[132] The calculation shows that the oxidative capacity of astrocytes is low for two reasons: a higher preference for glycolysis because of low oxidative capacity and a lower rate of total work. Thus, the proximal elements of neurons remain the major sites of oxidative rephosphorylation of ATP, accounting for 60% of the oxidative metabolism but only 12.5% of the glycolytic metabolism of brain tissue,[16,17,132,135,140,141] whereas astrocytes and the neuropil, including the distal elements of neurons, consume 87.5% of the glucose but only 40% of the oxygen.

It is evident that the issue of the rates of glycolysis and oxidative phosphorylation in neurons and glial cells hinges on the mechanisms underlying the estimates of the relative glycolytic and oxidative capacities of the respective cellular compartments, of which there appears to be at least four, including subdivisions of the neuronal and astrocytic populations of cells. The relative capacities arise from the differential activities of hexokinase/phosphofructokinase and cytochrome oxidase in the compartments, which in turn appear to depend on the time constants of the metabolic fluctuations and on the average metabolic activity. Low time constants are likely to favor glycolysis and low average oxidative rates, whereas high time constants favor high oxidative rates, much as in muscle cells.[142-144]

Thus, most evidence indicates that the glycolytic and oxidative rates of metabolism have different proportions in astrocytes and neurons. Under normal physiologic conditions in vivo, a higher share of the glycolytic capacity resides in astrocytes and the neuropil, whereas a higher share of the oxidative capacity relative to volume resides in the proximal elements of neurons, with substantial differences between the proximal and distal parts in both cell types (factor of 5 in astrocytes, factor of 13 in neurons).

Even though neurons and astrocytes differ with respect to metabolite enzyme and transporter distribution, there is no evidence that the pools of glucose, pyruvate, and lactate are compartmentalized inside and outside neurons and glia. Because transport in vivo is entirely passive, it is puzzling that glutamate in vitro inhibits glucose transport into neurons and triggers glucose transport into astrocytes.[145,146] However, there is little direct evidence of a fundamental difference between the ability of neurons and glia to oxidize pyruvate, except for the greater activity of glycolytic enzymes in glia and the neuropil and the greater activity of cytochrome oxidase in the proximal parts of neurons.

Unless pyruvate were strictly compartmentalized (the abundance of MCT1 and MCT2 effectively excludes this), it is kinetically impossible for neurons to prefer pyruvate of non-neuronal origin, whether directly or indirectly imported, over pyruvate of neuronal origin.[147] The evidence suggests that the four compartments of the two populations of cells contribute differentially to joint pyruvate and lactate pools but that the extent of the differential distribution would be a function of the degree of activation of the two cell types.

The simple model of metabolite pathways gleaned from these considerations is shown in Figure 7-6, in which the control points of the differential glycolytic and oxidative capacities are the HK-I/PFK-1 and PDH steps, respectively. The capacities of the separate PDH steps in the subcompartments of neurons and astrocytes are most likely related to the number of calcium-stimulated mitochondria, whereas the capacities of the HK-I/PFK-1 steps are subject to the temporal requirements of glutamate transport and metabolism in astrocytes and glycolysis in neurons. This analysis suggests that the functional ranges of the activities are very different in the two cell types, in keeping with the very different functional contingencies facing the two cell types in normally functioning brain tissue.

The evidence just cited shows that glial energy metabolism in general is somewhat lower than neuronal metabolism in the cerebral cortex, where glial cells occupy 25% of the volume and generate 20% of the ATP and neurons occupy 55% of the volume but generate 80% of the ATP—a twofold difference relative to volume.

ACTIVATION PERTURBS METABOLIC COMPARTMENTS DIFFERENTIALLY

In neuroscience, activation and deactivation are convenient labels for changing brain function. Understanding brain function is the goal of neuroscientific explorations of brain activity, but it is not often clear which specific hypothesis that the explorations are actually testing. To be sure, activation and its opposite represent a range of observations of a change in any number of different physiologic measures of brain activity, such as action potential frequency, local field potentials, membrane polarity, ATP turnover, blood flow, glucose consumption, oxygen consumption, tissue oxygen tension, oxygen extraction fraction, hemoglobin saturation, absolute and relative concentrations and amounts of oxyhemoglobin and deoxyhemoglobin, and blood and vascular volumes, among others. Collectively, these measures can contribute to a comprehensive description of activity in brain tissue, but no single measure can be said to unequivocally represent activation—or even brain function—per se.

At the core of this conundrum is consciousness. The emerging discipline of neuroenergetics focuses on measures of the energy turnover of brain tissue as keys to the functional integrity of brain tissue, including consciousness. The insights gleaned from the accomplishments of this discipline have been limited by the convention that changes in energy turnover are a consequence of or response to changes in brain function rather than the opposite.[148,149]

Thus, it is possible that it is the rate of energy turnover that enables consciousness by means of a phase transition that reorganizes the relevant molecules to such an extent that they cooperate in the service of conscious experiences. Much empirical evidence could be cited in favor of the theory that the unitary experience of consciousness is related to the global level of energy turnover in the brain rather than to the activity in isolated regions of the brain. Among these findings is the correlation between reported magnitudes of global brain energy metabolism and levels of consciousness.[16]

Ion Homeostasis during Activation

The sodium theory explains how neuronal excitation increases the work of the brain by increasing the leakage of ions across cell membranes and how depolarization of neuronal membranes and influx of calcium ions lead to increased oxygen uptake.[12,150] Changes in membrane potential differences occur when ion permeabilities change. The changes in membrane potential reflect changes in both sodium and potassium, or chloride, ion permeabilities. The glucose demand in turn changes to meet the nutrient delivery required to compensate for the increased ATPase activity imposed by oxidative phosphorylation. Figure 7-8 reveals the estimated metabolic consequences of increased sodium and potassium leakage. The glucose supply would have to increase to as much as 60 μmol/hg per minute to fuel an ATP turnover of 2 mmol/hg per minute. In the absence of oxygen (or with no increase in oxygen consumption), the glucose supply would have to increase to as much as 1 mmol/hg per minute, a 30-fold increase, to cover the same need for ATP.

Brain Energy Metabolism during Activation

During maximal excitation of brain tissue in vivo, such as with epileptic seizures, local increases in the metabolism of glucose or oxygen can reach 100% or more of the metabolism of the normal

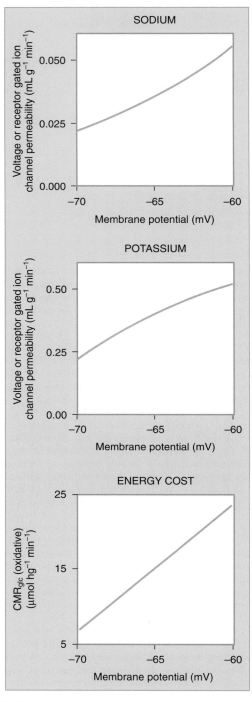

FIGURE 7-8 Energy cost of depolarization. (Top) and (middle) Steady-state neuronal membrane potential change as a function of altered sodium and potassium ion membrane permeabilities at 0.549 mL/g/min constant chloride ion permeability. Ordinates, ion permeability (mL/g/min); abscissae, membrane potential (mV) calculated from the Goldman-Hodgkin-Katz constant field equation. Bottom, Steady-state metabolism permitting membrane depolarization of the magnitude dictated by the increased sodium and potassium permeability. Abscissa, membrane potential (mV) calculated from the Goldman-Hodgkin-Katz constant field equation on the basis of chosen changes in sodium and potassium ion permeability; ordinate, steady-state glucose consumption (μmol/hg/min) calculated from the steady-state ion flux, assuming constant chloride ion permeability. (Redrawn from Gjedde A. The energy cost of neuronal depolarization. In: Gulyas B, Ottoson D, Roland PE, eds. Functional Organization of the Human Visual Cortex. Oxford: Pergamon; 1993:291-306.)

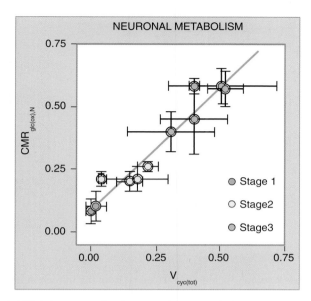

NEURONAL METABOLISM

FIGURE 7-9 Stages of rat brain oxidative metabolism versus the rate of glutamate cycling measured by Sibson et al.,[14] Choi et al.,[254] Henry et al.,[255] de Graaf et al.,[256] Patel et al.,[257] and Oz et al.,[258]. Abscissa, combined neuronal and astrocytic glutamate turnover rate (μmol/g/min); ordinate, oxidative metabolism of glucose in neurons (μmol/g/min). Functional stages were inferred from the type and level of general anesthesia used in each experiment. The slope of the line is 0.97 (unitless), and the y-intercept is 0.09 μmol/g/min. *(Modified from Hyder F, Patel AB, Gjedde A, et al. Neuronal-glial glucose oxidation and glutamatergic-GABAergic function. J Cereb Blood Flow Metab. 2006;26:865-877.)*

TABLE 7-8 Neuronal Activation of Brain Metabolism

STIMULUS	SUPPLY (%)			PRODUCTS (μmol/g/min)	
	ΔJ_{CBF}	ΔJ_{Glc}	ΔJ_{O_2}	ΔJ_{ATP}	ΔJ_{Lact}
Primary	29	19	3.4	0.43	0.089
Secondary and motor	36	38	25	2.89	0.090

ATP, adenosine triphosphate; CBF, cerebral blood flow.
From Gjedde A, Marrett S, Vafaee M. Oxidative and nonoxidative metabolism of excited neurons 644 and astrocytes. *J Cereb Blood Flow Metab.* 2002;22:1-14. Modified on the basis of studies by Roland et al.,[40] Fox and Raichle,[156] Fox et al.,[157] Seitz and Roland,[158] Fujita et al.,[159] Kuwabara et al.,[160] Ginsberg et al.,[161] Raichle et al.,[162] Marrett and Gjedde,[163] Vafaee and Gjedde,[164] Iida et al.,[259] Katayama et al.,[260] Riberio et al.,[261] Roland et al.,[262] and Vafaee and Gjedde.[263]

default state, depending on the intensity of the stimulus.[16,151-153] Under normal circumstances, changes in both blood flow and oxygen consumption tend to be very small, on the order of a few percentage points of the baseline, but the results obtained in experimental conditions vary greatly, depending on the circumstances, some of which may be nonphysiologic.

The experimental evidence for increases in brain energy metabolism during excitation in vivo comes in three different forms: as global steady-state changes brought on by general reductions or increases in brain activity; as localized responses to specific stimulation, mostly the cerebral cortex; and as changes in substrates and metabolites in the circulation and in brain tissue.

Global Steady-State Changes in Energy Metabolism

Average global steady-state changes are presented in Figure 7-9, in which recent magnetic resonance spectroscopic and allied studies in rodent cerebral cortex show a linear relationship between calculated cycling rates of glutamate between the larger (neuronal) and smaller (glial) distal metabolic compartments of the neuropil and calculated turnover rates of the TCA cycle in the combined neuronal compartments. In Figure 7-9, these findings are assigned to the canonic functional stages on the basis of the conditions of the human volunteers and experimental animals. The relationship between glutamate cycling and oxidative glucose metabolism shown in Figure 7-9 is consistent with the oxidative metabolism of 1 mol of glucose for each mole of glutamate released from neuronal terminals and recycled. It is important to note that the functional stages assigned to the global changes reflect major perturbations in consciousness that are not consistent with normal cognition. In fact, normal cognition is not accompanied by significant changes in global cerebral energy

metabolism,[154,155] thus suggesting that any local changes are matched by opposite changes elsewhere or affect regions so small that significance is not achievable.

Local Changes in Energy Metabolism in Response to Stimulation

Focal changes brought on by specific experimental stimulation of cerebral cortex depend on the stimulus but generally tend to be small, which suggests that the awake or conscious cortex normally functions at the same level most of the time. Focal activation responses in a number of stimulation studies of human brain (summarized in Table 7-8) fall into two fundamentally different categories of stimulation.[40,127,156-164] Passive forms of stimulation in which no reaction is required or possible by the subjects generally result in little or no change in oxygen consumption.[156-159,165] During active forms of stimulation, in which a reaction is required or induced, significant increases in oxygen consumption tend to accompany the changes in blood flow, as referenced in Table 7-8 and illustrated in Figure 7-10.

The differences between the two categories of sensorimotor stimulation listed in Table 7-8 suggest that the ultimate increase in oxygen consumption depends significantly on the neuronal pathway mediating the response to the stimulus.[166,167] In brain and in muscle cells, the cytochrome oxidase activity of populations of cells is regulated by signals from mitochondria that reflect the habitual energy requirement, averaged over longer periods.[168-170] In muscle cells, neural input regulates the categorization of muscle cells into types I, IIa, or IIb. Changing the oxidative capacity requires sustained stimulation for an extended period. Thus, brief transient increases in energy metabolism above the habitual level of activity apparently are not accompanied by commensurately increased oxygen consumption. In the brain, this consideration leads to the conclusion that the two categories of response are related to the known differential oxidative and glycolytic responsiveness of the neuronal and glial compartments (see the earlier section "Metabolic Cycling").

Changes in Metabolites during Activation

The changes governing the transient alterations in metabolite pools during activation involve many reactants. Because of their concentrations, ease of measurement, or both, the most commonly reported are glucose, glycogen in glial cells, lactate, and the NAD^+-NADH pair. To make sense and to give an accurate view of the dynamic relationships, the changes must be compared with the influx and efflux measurements of glucose, lactate, and

FIGURE 7-10 Flow–cerebral metabolic rate of oxygen (CMRO₂) and flow-glycolysis coupling during stimulation of comparatively nonoxidative and oxidative cells. The relative increases in glycolysis, blood flow, and oxidative metabolism are estimated for two categories of response to stimulation: passive, primary somatosensory stimulation ("mainly glycolytic") response and demanding, secondary somatosensory or motor ("mainly oxidative") response listed in Table 7-8. Note the similar flow-glycolysis coupling in the two stimulations. Also shown are rates of incremental adenosine triphosphate (ATP) and lactate production during excitation. Stimulus and cells fall into two metabolic categories, one with an average incremental ATP/lactate ratio of less than 10 and one with average ratio of 300. Ordinate: percent increments in the variables listed in the graph. CBF, cerebral blood flow; CMR_{Glc}, cerebral metabolic rate of glucose. (*Modified from Gjedde A, Marrett S, Vafaee M. Oxidative and nonoxidative metabolism of excited neurons and astrocytes. J Cereb Blood Flow Metab. 2002;22:1-14.*)

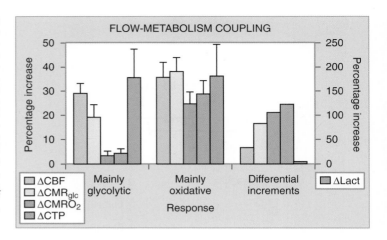

oxygen during the activation. The relationship between the most important metabolites can be reduced to the formula devised by Dienel and Cruz[171]:

$$\Delta[\text{Glc}] + \Delta[\text{Glyc}] + \frac{1}{2}\Delta[\text{Lact}] = \overline{J}_{\text{Glc}}\left(1 + \frac{\overline{\text{LGI}}}{2} - \frac{\overline{\text{OGI}}}{2}\right)\Delta\text{T}$$

(6)

where the right side of the equation is an index of changes in metabolites that can be calculated from vascular measurements of differences in arteriovenous concentration and blood flow and the left side of the equation presents the concurrent changes in major metabolite concentrations in the tissue. Here, $\overline{J}_{\text{Glc}}$ is the net rate of glucose transport across the blood-brain barrier, $\overline{\text{LGI}}$ is the "lactate-glucose index" or ratio of net lactate and glucose transfer across the blood-brain barrier, and $\overline{\text{OGI}}$ similarly is the familiar oxygen-glucose index, in this case the ratio of net rates of oxygen and glucose transfer across the blood-brain barrier, both weighted over the period of observation, shown as ΔT. The equation allows changes in metabolites to be estimated by measurements of the circulation, or vice versa. By taking account of these factors, non–steady states can be properly evaluated during the transients of activation. Two examples of the use of this equation, in rodents and humans, are representative of this approach.

Dienel and Cruz reviewed metabolite and circulatory changes in the rat brain during activation by manual stroking of the rat.[171] These changes were subsequently used in Figure 7-11 to compare the accumulation of metabolites and the value of the measured arteriovenous deficits defined in Equation 6. The comparison shows that metabolites accumulate (particularly glucose and lactate) during the 5-minute activation period and decline (particularly glycogen) in the subsequent 15-minute recovery period. The OGI declined during activation and rose above normal at the subsequent recovery. The changes show that the brains of these rats take up more metabolites than they use during the activation period whereas they use more than they take up during recovery. These changes suggest that the four metabolic compartments are subject to different degrees of activation or undergo differential regulation of their oxidative and glycolytic capacities. Ide and colleagues used measurements of arteriovenous differences across the brain in humans to similarly evaluate metabolite accumulation during and after exercise.[172] The OGI had declined at the end of the exercise period, only to rise above normal at rest. The calculations confirm that metabolites accumulate during exercise and decline slowly toward normal over the next half hour.

Kasischke and coworkers used fluorescence imaging to determine changes in NADH in hippocampal slices exposed to 32-Hz electrical stimuli.[173] The NADH signal from the mitochondria of neurons declined during the first 10 seconds of the 20-second period of stimulation, thus indicating conversion of NADH to NAD⁺, consistent with the increased activity of NADH complex (I) in mitochondria, and then returned to baseline at the end of the 40-second recovery period. Figure 7-12 shows that the NADH signal from the cytosol of astrocytes increased toward the end of the 20-second stimulus and continued to rise for the following 20 seconds of recovery, thus indicating greater generation than metabolism of pyruvate (oxidative as well as nonoxidative) in astrocytes during this period. These findings reveal a failure of oxidative metabolism to increase in parallel with stimulation, beyond the brief initial exhaustion of the putative oxygen reserve

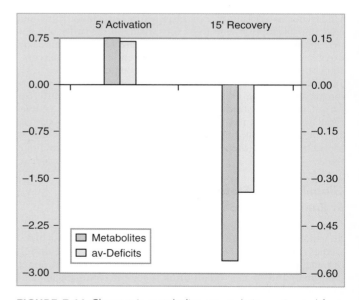

FIGURE 7-11 Changes in metabolite accumulation estimated from arteriovenous (AV) deficits and measured directly during 5 minutes of stimulation and 15 minutes of recovery of rat brain in vivo. Left ordinate, measured changes in metabolites calculated as Δ[Glc] + Δ[Glyc] + Δ[Lact]/2) in units of μmol/g; right ordinate, lactate-glucose (LGI) and oxygen-glucose (OGI) indices calculated as 1 + LGI/2 − OGI/6 The graph shows that metabolites accumulate during stimulation and decline during recovery and that this change is reflected in the AV deficits of glucose and lactate. (*Calculated from a summary published by Dienel GA, Cruz NF. Nutrition during brain activation: does cell-to-cell lactate shuttling contribute significantly to sweet and sour food for thought? Neurochem Int. 2004;45:321-351.*)

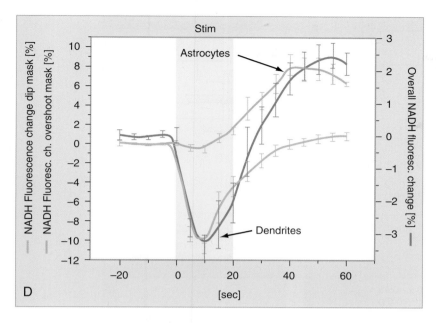

FIGURE 7-12 Biphasic response of the reduced form of nicotinamide adenine dinucleotide (NADH) (*dark purple*, right ordinate) as the sum of two spatially and temporally distinct monophasic metabolic responses, indicative of early oxidative recovery metabolism in dendrites (*light purple curve*, left ordinate), followed by late activation of glycolysis in astrocytes (*red curve*, left ordinate) (n = 8, average ± SEM). (*From Kasischke KA, Vishwasrao HD, Fisher PJ, et al. Neural activity triggers neuronal oxidative metabolism followed by astrocytic glycolysis. Science. 2004;305:99-103.*)

in mitochondria, whether because of limited oxygen delivery to the slice or because of a constitutive inability of mitochondria to match the increased pyruvate generation. The beginning of recovery of NADH in the neuronal (dendritic) mitochondria in the second half of the stimulation is evidence of increased pyruvate oxidation, but it is unclear where this pyruvate is generated. There is no indication of the fate of lactate in the study. Together, the changes in energy metabolism and metabolites show that metabolites accumulate during stimulation and decline during recovery. This paradox implies that oxygen availability declines during stimulation and returns to normal or above normal during recovery.

Substrate Delivery during Activation

The measurements listed in Table 7-8 suggest that the relationship between changes in blood flow and generation of ATP is markedly variable during activation, with relative changes ranging from unity to 20.[174] It is not known which specific aspect of neuronal excitation most critically depends on the increase in blood flow, but surprisingly, the findings suggest that changes in blood flow are unrelated to the immediate satisfaction of increased oxygen requirements. This section describes attempts to identify agents to which blood flow does respond when brain tissue undergoes activation.

Regulation of Microvascular Oxygen

Gjedde and associates considered whether the discrepant glycolytic and oxidative reactions to stimulation can be explained by a failure of blood flow to rise sufficiently to raise oxygen delivery,[75] but during vibrotactile stimulation of human sensorimotor cortex Kuwabara and colleagues found that oxygen consumption remains constant despite significantly increased blood flow and capillary diffusion capacity.[159,160,175] Because oxygen tension rises in the tissue when blood flow rises without a change in oxygen consumption, the experiment indicates that deficient oxygen supply is not the explanation for the limited oxygen consumption.

Possible clues to the discrepant changes in oxygen consumption and blood flow come from studies of the kinetics of oxygen delivery to brain cells.[77,78,176] The diffusion limitation imposed by hemoglobin binding renders oxygen transport, as reflected in the extraction fraction, somewhat insensitive to increases in blood

flow.[177] Therefore, blood flow must increase disproportionately to raise oxygen transport. Perfectly matched flow-metabolism coupling, in contrast, maintains the same capillary oxygen tension profile and extraction fraction and hence cannot raise the oxygen pressure gradient in the absence of capillary recruitment or a decrease in mitochondrial oxygen tension. Kinetic analysis of cytochrome oxidase activity shows that increases in blood flow above the increase in oxygen consumption are needed to deliver more oxygen during excitation.[40]

With the decline in mitochondrial oxygen tension, oxygen consumption increasingly depends on capillary oxygen tension.[178] Brain activation then demands disproportionately increased blood flow to increase mean capillary oxygen tension. The maximum oxygen delivery capacity is the upper limit of oxygen consumption and is reached when mitochondrial oxygen tension drops to the minimum level compatible with sustained cytochrome oxidase activity. The effect of the increase in blood flow is then to raise oxygen consumption. When the rise in blood flow is enough to satisfy the increased need, oxygen extraction declines and the average capillary oxygen tension is raised to a level consistent with the pressure gradient that delivers the necessary oxygen to the mitochondria.[40]

Blood Oxygenation Level–Dependent Changes in Signal during Activation

In the absence of proportionately increased oxygen consumption, increased blood flow leads to higher capillary oxygen tensions and lower extraction fractions and reduces the fraction of deoxygenated hemoglobin in capillary and venous blood (see Figure 7-3). The decline is a measure of the relative increase in oxygenation in cerebral veins when blood flow increases. Deoxyhemoglobin is paramagnetic, and the decline gives rise to a blood oxygenation level–dependent (BOLD) magnetic resonance contrast change during brain activation,[179-182] which primarily is a function of the average extraction of oxygen from the vascular bed.[183] Correlations between changes in metabolism (glucose and oxygen), blood flow, and oxygen extraction fractions and changes in BOLD signal generally support the explanation that changes in BOLD signals reflect the discrepancy between changes in oxygen consumption and blood flow, which are expressed by parallel changes in the oxygen extraction fraction.[184-187] The correlated changes in blood

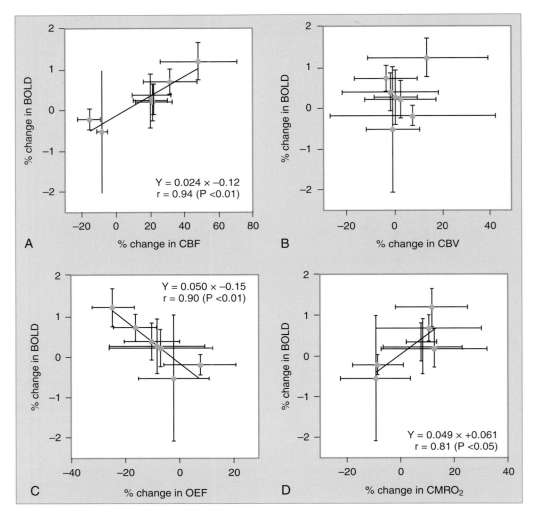

FIGURE 7-13 Relationships between average percent changes in cerebral blood flow (CBF), cerebral blood volume (CBV), oxygen extraction fraction (OEF), and oxygen consumption (CMRO$_2$) and average percent changes in the blood oxygenation level–dependent (BOLD) signal for all regions of interest in seven healthy men performing a simple finger-tapping motor task. Values are means ± SD for each region. **A,** Relationship between average percent changes in CBF and BOLD signal. **B,** Relationship between average percent changes in CBV and BOLD signal. **C,** Relationship between average percent changes in OEF and BOLD signal. **D,** Relationship between average percent changes in CMRO$_2$ and BOLD signal. *(From Ito H, Ibaraki M, Kanno I, eta l. Changes in cerebral blood flow and cerebral oxygen metabolism during neural activation measured by positron emission tomography: comparison with blood oxygenation level–dependent contrast measured by functional magnetic resonance imaging. J Cereb Blood Flow Metab. 2005;25:371-377.)*

flow, BOLD signals, and oxygen extraction fractions observed by Ito and associates are shown in Figure 7-13.[184]

Changes in Tissue Oxygen during Activation

Disproportionate increases in blood flow allow enough oxygen to enter the tissue during functional activation, but the agents responsible for the increase remain uncertain despite decades of research.[188] The minimum oxygen tension in mitochondria can be calculated as the tension that is commensurate with the actual delivery of oxygen, and the commensurate blood flow rate can be estimated for a given arterial oxygen concentration by a form of inverted reasoning in which the mitochondrial oxygen tension must reflect the balance between oxygen delivery and consumption.[80] Hence, tissue oxygen tension depends on, rather than controls, the rate of oxygen consumption.[189,190] Surprisingly, this reasoning describes a compulsory flow limitation that dictates the oxygen consumption associated with a given blood flow rate when other variables such as cytochrome oxidase affinity and capillary recruitment remain constant. Changes in these variables in turn

affect the rate of oxygen consumption. No change in oxygen consumption after a change in blood flow therefore implies a compensatory change in cytochrome *c* oxidase affinity for oxygen or cytochrome *c* or a change in the maximum reaction rate.

Some studies of oxygen supply and delivery suggest that the affinity of cytochrome *c* oxidase for oxygen may change inversely with the oxidative metabolism of a tissue and thus preserve the sensitivity of the cytochrome *c* oxidase reaction to changes in the maximum velocity.[191] Gjedde and colleagues hypothesized that a similar change explains the invariant cerebral oxygen consumption measured during moderate changes in blood flow to the brain.[39] Mason and colleagues speculated that the blood flow modulator nitric oxide (NO) could be the adjustable inhibitor of cytochrome *c* oxidase affinity that competes with access of oxygen to the enzyme.[192] The finding that oxygen tension rises during the phase of blood flow increase and declines below normal when brain energy metabolism increases was demonstrated by Thompson and coworkers, who determined oxygen tensions in the cat visual cortex during stimulation with stripes of varying angles.[193] Oxygen tensions increased during the stimulation, except when

CHAPTER 8

Blood-Brain Barrier

Shahid M. Nimjee ■ Gerald A. Grant ■ H. Richard Winn ■ Damir Janigro

The blood-brain barrier (BBB) is a "neurovascular unit" composed of microvascular endothelium, basement membrane, neurons, and neuroglial structures: astrocytes, pericytes, and microglia. More recently, it has become apparent that in human brain pathology, the BBB also interacts substantially with intravascular signals and circulating blood cells. In this respect, it becomes clear that despite its location at the blood-brain interface, the potential impact and topography of BBB cells are more widespread than initially believed. For example, the interaction of circulating white blood cells infected by human immunodeficiency virus (HIV) has been shown to have an impact on BBB function; in contrast, the BBB in patients with acquired immunodeficiency syndrome seems to act as a reservoir for the virus, thus further extending the reach of this cellular interface.[1,2] The BBB is an active and dynamic organ that ensures adequate concentration of essential compounds such as oxygen and glucose and at the same time protects the brain from deleterious substances in the peripheral circulation. The BBB selectively prevents transportation of substances into brain via tight junctions (TJs), enzymatic reactions, and neurotransmitter signaling and selectively transports small and large molecules by passive and facilitated diffusion and active transport. The synergistic integration of all molecular and structural components gives rise to this functional complex called the *BBB*. Disruption of the BBB is seen in numerous pathologic processes. However, the discriminatory nature of the neurovascular unit also prevents the delivery of therapies to the brain, including chemotherapy agents, antiviral drugs, and beneficial neuromodulators. There are novel methods of circumventing the BBB that may provide novel therapies to treat a variety of neurological disorders. Scientific investigation of the BBB continues to provide insight into this complex and dynamic system and may generate much needed therapies to treat numerous neurological diseases.

HISTORY

Scientific investigation in identifying the BBB dates back to the 19th century. In 1885, Paul Ehrlich, a bacteriologist, observed that aniline dyes intravenously injected into animals colored all organs with the exception of the brain and spinal cord.[3] His interpretation at the time was that there was poor uptake of the dye by the brain. Later, one of Ehrlich's protégés, Edwin Goldmann, injected trypan blue intravenously and was able to visualize the dye in the choroid plexus and meninges but not the brain itself.[4] However, when he injected trypan blue into cerebrospinal fluid (CSF), the dye was present throughout the brain, although it was absent in the rest of the body.[5]

In the 1920s, experiments performed by Stern and Gautier led to greater understanding of the blood-CSF barrier. They studied the transport of substances from blood into CSF. Chemicals such as bromide, bile salts, and morphine injected into the bloodstream were found in CSF, whereas fluorescein and epinephrine were absent, even though they were administered in the same fashion.[6] Moreover, substances that entered the brain affected its

activity and substances that were unable to penetrate the brain had no functional consequence.[7] They coined this semipermeable protection of agents entering the brain "*barrière hématoencéphalique*."

A series of investigations in the 1960s led to the identification of properties of molecular compounds that facilitated transport across the BBB, such as lipid solubility.[8] Moreover, a gradient existed between extracellular fluid in the brain and CSF. This allows substances to be filtered out of the brain through CSF, termed the *sink effect*.[9] More recently, it was shown that molecular transport of substances across the BBB could be determined from their log octanol-water partition coefficients (Fig. 8-1).[10] A plot of log BBB permeability (cm/sec) versus log octanol-water partition coefficient shows that increased lipophilicity directly correlates with increased membrane permeability in that the more lipid soluble a molecule is, the more readily it moves from the aqueous environment of blood across the lipid environment of the endothelial cell (EC) membrane and enters the brain. Compounds subject to active transport will exceed their predicted permeability based on membrane lipophilicity. Counteracting influences that may slow diffusion across the BBB include pH, temperature, and retention in blood because of protein binding. As a general rule, lipid-soluble molecules with a molecular size less than 400 daltons can cross the BBB. Unfortunately, few central nervous system (CNS) diseases respond to small-molecule drugs.

Finally, between 1965 and 1967, a number of scientists identified the structure of the BBB as consisting of a network of capillaries and ECs known as *TJs*.[11-13]

ANATOMY OF THE BLOOD-BRAIN BARRIER

The anatomic BBB is formed by a monolayer of microvascular ECs that line the intraluminal space of brain capillaries. The BBB consists of ECs packed close together and forming TJs. The EC layer has a luminal (inside) and abluminal (outside) compartment separated by 300 to 500 nm of cytoplasm between the blood and brain. The EC layer is composed of TJs, which consist of occludin and claudin; adherent junctions, including cadherin, catenins, vinculin, and actinin; and junctional adhesion molecules (Fig. 8-2).

There are two fundamental morphologic characteristics that differentiate brain ECs from peripheral ECs. The cytoplasm of brain microvascular ECs has rare pinocyte vesicles—fluid-filled cell membrane invaginations that allow compounds to cross the BBB. These ECs also contain a greater concentration of mitochondria. The theory behind this is that there is a greater energy requirement to actively transport nutrients.

In addition to the structural integrity of the BBB, there exists an enzymatic surveillance system that metabolizes drugs and other compounds bypassing the structural barrier. Three main catalytic agents regulate transportation across the BBB: γ-glutamyl transpeptidase (γ-GTP), alkaline phosphatase, and aromatic acid decarboxylase. All are highly concentrated in cerebral vessels.[14]

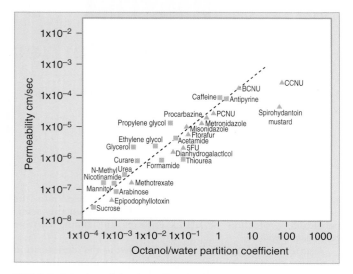

FIGURE 8-1 Plot of the log of octanol-water partition coefficients. The *partition coefficient* is a ratio of concentrations of un-ionized compound between the two solutions (organic solvent, such as octanol, and water) and is a measure of molecular hydrophobicity. Hydrophobic drugs with high partition coefficients are preferentially distributed to hydrophobic compartments such as lipid bilayers of cells, whereas hydrophilic drugs (low partition coefficients) are preferentially found in hydrophilic compartments such as blood serum. The relationship of permeability to octanol-water partition coefficient and molecular weight was found to be predictable for drugs with molecular weights less than 400 daltons. Hydrophobicity affects drug absorption, bioavailability, hydrophobic drug-receptor interactions, metabolism of molecules, and their toxicity. Substances below the dotted *line* penetrate much less than expected from their lipophilicity or are extruded via the P-glycoprotein efflux pump. In contrast, substances that have carrier-mediated uptake mechanisms, such as glucose and amino acids, fall well above the *dotted line.*

There is charge polarity between the abluminal and luminal surface of ECs. This polarity influences permeability of the barrier. Alkaline phosphatase and γ-GTP are concentrated on the luminal compartment, whereas sodium-potassium adenosine triphosphatase (Na^+,K^+-ATPase) and other transporters are clustered on the abluminal side. Other shuttling proteins that contribute to transport polarity include glucose transporter-1 (GLUT-1), which is concentrated at the abluminal membrane,[15] and the drug transporter P-glycoprotein (Pgp), which is concentrated at the luminal membrane.[16]

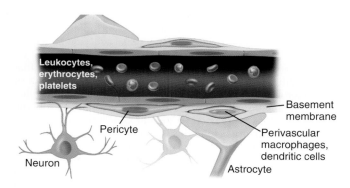

FIGURE 8-2 Schematic of a "neurovascular unit," which consists of endothelial cells, astrocytes, pericytes, macrophages, microglia, neurons, the basement membrane, and the extracellular matrix.

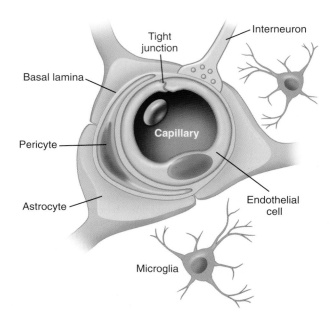

FIGURE 8-3 Schematic of a brain microvascular endothelial cell in cross section.

On the abluminal surface, ECs are enveloped in a basement membrane and separated into regions associated with a pericyte. Pericytes are contractile cells surrounding brain capillaries; they aid in regulating the growth of ECs and serve to modulate the integrity of capillary cells. They also act synergistically with macrophages in controlling substances that cross the BBB by phagocytosis, thereby acting as a secondary barrier to ECs.

The tissue microenvironment is necessary for continued regulation of barrier function. The BBB, also known as the *neurovascular unit,* consists of *astrocytes, pericytes, microglia, neurons,* and the *extracellular matrix* (ECM), all of which play a supportive role in maintaining integrity of the BBB.[17,18] Astrocytes have end-feet that border the basement membrane of vessels of the parenchyma. More than 90% of astrocyte foot processes surround ECs.[19] They are associated with adrenergic and cholinergic nerve terminals, as well as those that respond to peptides (Fig. 8-3).

Astrocytes also densely surround TJs and augment ECs by reducing the size of the gap of TJs.[20] In vitro experiments imply that without astrocytes, the integrity of the BBB is significantly compromised.[20,21] In contrast, other studies indicate that BBB integrity is retained amid degradation of astrocytes,[22] thus suggesting that astrocytes regulate BBB activity indirectly rather than through physical obstruction. Astrocytes are considered to be inducers of both the barrier and permeability properties of the endothelium. Stewart and Wiley in 1981 first demonstrated that newly formed vessels originating from the coelomic cavity display BBB characteristics when placed in contact with grafts of neural tissue.[23] Later, Janzer and Raff first demonstrated that a functional BBB was induced in nonbrain ECs in the anterior chamber of the eye in the presence of astrocytic aggregates.[24]

Pericytes are undifferentiated contractile connective tissue cells that localize to capillary walls and share a common basement membrane with brain ECs. They may not be involved in vessel contraction because they lack a contractile actin subtype.[25] In vitro studies have revealed communication between ECs and pericytes. The proposed mechanism of this communication is through cellular projections, which penetrate the basal lamina and cover 20% to 30% of the microvascular circumference.[25] Pericytes express macrophage functions and are actively involved in the immune response, where they operate as a second line of

TABLE 8-1 *Blood-Brain Barrier Modulation*

DECREASED BLOOD-BRAIN BARRIER PERMEABILITY

Intracellular cyclic adenosine monophosphate (AMP)

Steroids

Adrenomedullin

Noradrenalin

Glial-derived neurotrophic factor (GDNF)

Basic fibroblastic growth factor (bFGF)

Polyunsaturated fatty acids

Transforming growth factor-β (TGF-β)

INCREASED BLOOD-BRAIN BARRIER PERMEABILITY

Bradykinin

HistamineSerotonin (5HT)

Thrombin

Glutamate

Purine nucleotides: adenosine triphosphate (ATP), adenosine
   diphosphate (ADP), AMP

Endothelin-1

Adenosine

Platelet-activating factor

Phospholipase A_2

Arachidonic acid

Prostaglandins

Leukotrienes

Interleukins: IL-1α, IL-1β, IL-6

Tumor necrosis factor-α (TNF-α)

Macrophage inhibitory proteins: MIP-1 and MIP-2

Complement-derived polypeptide: C3a-desArg

Free radicals

Nitric oxide

Adapted from Abbott NJ. Dynamics of CNS barriers: Evolution, differentiation, and modulation. *Cell Mol Neurobiol.* 2005;25:5-23.

defense at the BBB. Pericytes are the most abundant on venules, for which they provide mechanical support and also synthesize ECM proteins such as laminin and fibronectin. Platelet-derived growth factor receptor (PDGFR) is a tyrosine kinase receptor expressed on the surface of pericytes that has been targeted for the treatment of malignant brain tumors. Clinical trials were conducted with imatinib, a PDGFR inhibitor, on patients with glioblastoma multiforme (GBM) who were refractory to chemotherapy and radiation therapy. Patients treated with imatinib and hydroxyurea had a 20% response rate, and the drug combination was reasonably well tolerated in phase II studies.[26,27] Pathologic conditions that increase BBB permeability, such as trauma or hypoxia, result in a significantly decreased pericyte concentration as they migrate away from the site of injury.[28]

Neurons are the building blocks of the CNS. The role of neuronal modulation at the BBB is principally enzymatic (Table 8-1). Functional brain imaging studies, such as positron emission tomography (PET) and functional magnetic resonance imaging (MRI), are based on regional increases in cerebral blood flow and glucose and oxygen consumption, which are associated with regional increases in neuronal activity.[29] Neurons upregulate catalytic factors specific to ECs.[30] Astrocytes and their associated ECs are innervated by noradrenergic,[31] serotoninergic,[32] cholinergic,[33] and GABAergic (transmitting or secreting γ-aminobutyric acid [GABA]) neurons.[34] Lesions of the norepinephrine-

producing locus caeruleus sensitize the BBB to hypertension. In Alzheimer's disease, cholinergic inhibition impairs cerebrovascular blood flow.[33,35]

Microglia serve as surveillance cells for the BBB. They identify foreign compounds that have bypassed the BBB and act as antigen-presenting cells by engulfing these substances and presenting them to activated T cells for destruction. Microglia also secrete cytokines, or proinflammatory molecules, and rapidly proliferate to contain the offending agent.[15]

The ECM provides physical stability to the BBB. It is a critical anchoring site that mediates polarity at the EC-astrocyte interface. Disruption of the ECM predictably impairs the structural integrity of the BBB, which in turn compromises its activity. Structural integrity of the BBB is achieved through interaction with several structural proteins, including laminin, collagen type IV, and integrins.[36] Matrix proteins also upregulate TJ protein expression.[37]

The permeability of the BBB to macromolecules is determined by both TJ-controlled paracellular permeability (through cell-cell junctions) and caveolae-mediated transcellular permeability. Caveolae are sites of endothelial transcytosis, endocytosis, and signal transduction. The relationship between paracellular and transcellular permeability is of crucial importance for the regulation of transendothelial permeability. Using an electron microscope, Majno and colleagues found that carbon particles injected into blood entered the parenchyma after brain tissue had been exposed to histamine.[38] In addition, these authors were able to see gaps between ECs. The concept of osmotic control of the BBB was also based on electron microscope studies, in which it was shown that the nuclei of ECs seemed to have a contracted, raisin-like appearance after exposure to histamine.[39] This method of osmotic regulation of the BBB has since been further described.[40]

The precise vascular localization of the functional term *BBB* might be extended beyond the capillary segments to CNS microvessels (Fig. 8-4). The average total surface area of the brain microvasculature is 20 m^2, whereas the surface area of cerebral capillary endothelium is 100 cm^2/g tissue.[41] The total length is 650 km, the inner capillary lumen is 6 μm, and capillaries are 20 μm apart from one another. The BBB occupies more than 99% of brain capillaries, with the exception of the circumventricular organs, which have a blood-CSF barrier. Circumventricular organs include the median eminence, pituitary gland, choroid plexus, subfornical organ, lamina terminalis, and area postrema. Although not as stringent as the BBB, the blood-CSF barrier prevents blood-borne substances from entering the brain. Other mechanisms of controlling traffic across the BBB besides the structural support include ion channels and transport carriers, which control the traffic of hydrophilic nutrients, metabolites, vitamins and hormones, and ions across the BBB.

In summary, the brain microvascular endothelium differs from peripheral endothelium in three primary ways:

1. Brain lacks fenestrations and is characterized by low pinocytotic activity, both of which markedly impair fluid uptake.[42]
2. TJs are ubiquitous in brain ECs and impede paracellular transport of hydrophobic compounds across the BBB into the brain parenchyma.
3. Mitochondria are present at a much higher concentration, which provides the energy needed for active transport of various proteins and factors required by the brain.

TRANSPORT ACROSS THE BLOOD-BRAIN BARRIER

The biochemical BBB is established by transport systems of the BBB, which can be grouped into four types (Fig. 8-5):

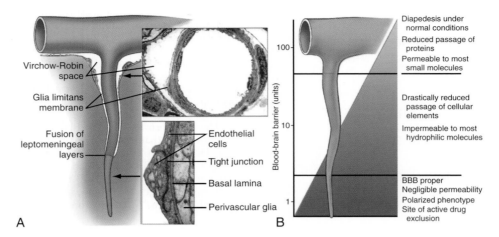

FIGURE 8-4 Schematic of brain pial vasculature showing the permeability gradient as penetrating pial vessels become capillaries and are characterized by the blood-brain barrier phenotype.

1. *Simple diffusion*—transport of solutes occurs down a concentration gradient.
2. *Facilitated diffusion*—solute binds to a specific membrane-spanning protein and, like simple diffusion, travels down a concentration gradient.
3. *Simple diffusion via aqueous channels*—charged ions and solutes are the principal compounds that cross the BBB by this mechanism.
4. *Active transport via protein carriers*—this is the lone mechanism by which solutes are transported against a concentration gradient; a change in affinity of the carrier for solute and expenditure of adenosine triphosphate (ATP) are required for

transport. The vast supply of mitochondria in the ECM is thought to provide these channels with the energy needed for this reaction.

Some critical compounds that are regularly transported across the BBB are essential for brain function. Several independent carrier systems exist at the BBB for transport of hexoses (glucose, galactose); neutral, basic, and acidic amino acids; monocarboxylic acids (lactate, pyruvate); purines (adenine, guanine); nucleosides (adenosine); amines; and ions. Uptake of larger molecules, including insulin and transferrin, occurs via receptor-mediated endocytosis.

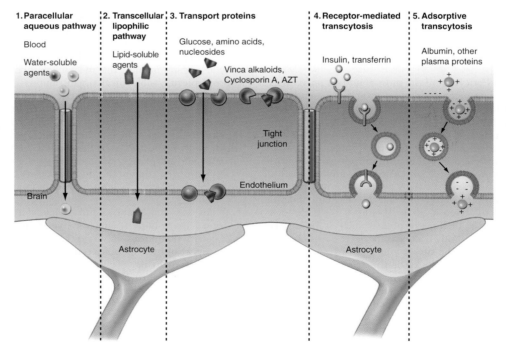

FIGURE 8-5 Schematic demonstrating various transport systems that shuttle molecules across the blood-brain barrier. Tight junctions permit the diffusion of only very small amounts of water-soluble compounds (paracellular), whereas lipid-soluble agents traverse via the transcellular lipophilic pathway. Selective transport systems exist for glucose, amino acids, purine bases, nucleosides, cholines, and other substances, in addition to specific receptor-mediated endocytosis for certain proteins such as insulin and transferrin. AZT, azathioprine.

drugs are believed to cross the BBB as a result of their CNS side effects.[146]

Drug Modifications

Expanding on the initial experiments of Brodie and associates[8] in the 1960s, recent studies have shown that the permeability of most molecules can be predicted by determining their octanol-water coefficients based on their respective nonpolar and polar solubilites.[147,148] Specifically, substances with the greatest ability to pass through the BBB generally have a log octanol-water coefficient between –0.5 and 6.0[149] and a molecular mass of less than 400 to 500 daltons and do not form hydrogen bonds with water.[150] With this understanding, many pharmaceutical researchers have conjugated their bioactive compounds to lipophilic moieties in the hope that they will become sufficiently lipid soluble to passively move through the BBB. Others have masked the hydrophilic groups of the compounds in an effort to increase lipophilicity.[42] Conjugation by esters and disulfide bonds allows enzymes to cleave the lipids from the drug once it has passively entered the CNS, thus making the drug polar and trapping it inside. An example is heroin, an opiate that passes through the BBB 100 times more easily than morphine and is subsequently converted to morphine in the CNS.[141,151] Such prodrugs have proved to be useful, although more research is needed to evaluate their efficacy and safety.[152] Additionally, cleavage to form the active drug may not occur at a sufficient rate and with the necessary accuracy to produce localized therapeutic concentrations of the drug.

Lipophilic conjugation has been used successfully for introduction of the chemotherapeutic agent chlorambucil into the CNS.[153,154] Kitagawa and coworkers[155] evaluated the conjugative properties of adamantine, a compound related to the drug memantine used for the treatment of Parkinson's disease. By conjugating adamantine to [D-Ala2] leu-enkephalin, the opioid gained the ability to pass through the BBB into the CNS. In another experiment, Prokai-Tatrai and colleagues[156] successfully conjugated a different leu-enkephalin analogue to a lipophilic moiety for CNS administration. However, conjugation of drugs may not always be necessary. The simple reduction of hydrogen bonding potential by altering polar side groups has successfully increased permeability of the BBB to some small peptides.[157]

Despite these successes, many difficulties have arisen in the search for successful methods to increase the lipophilicity of pharmacologic compounds. Modification often increases the mass of the drug, and even lipophilic drugs do not cross the BBB effectively when their mass has increased to greater than the 400- to 500-dalton threshold.[42] Increased size of the drugs can affect transport as well. The limit for molecular area appears to be around 80 Å^2, and increases in size to greater than this seem to decrease BBB permeability dramatically.[158] In addition to the physical constraints on lipophilic conjugation, chemical constraints have been demonstrated as well. Conjugation or masking of hydrophilic side groups may make the drug biologically inactive.[152] An increase in lipophilicity can also make the drug susceptible to transport by Pgp and other export proteins despite having little if any susceptibility before the modification. Alternatively, conjugation of some drugs that are already substrates for Pgp can have an added beneficial effect by successfully preventing their export through hindrance of their ability to attach to the Pgp binding site. A derivative of the chemotherapeutic agent paclitaxel has been successfully modified in this fashion while still maintaining cytotoxic action against cells of the breast cancer lineage.[159] Drug modification can alter pharmacokinetic parameters as well. Conjugation may decrease the solubility, plasma protein binding, and liver and reticuloendothelial uptake, thus altering the bioavailability of the drug.[152] New side effects may also be due to increases in drug uptake into other organs as

a result of lipophilic modification and potentially damage the more sensitive organs.

Another strategy of drug modification for bypassing the BBB is conjugation to bioactive molecules, either those that are normally transported into the CNS by specific transport proteins or some that enter the CNS via receptor-mediated endocytosis by cerebrovascular endothelium. Friden and associates[160] successfully conjugated nerve growth factor to an antibody for the transferrin receptor in the rat. Binding of the antibody to the receptor stimulates receptor-mediated endocytosis and provides transcellular passage through the endothelium. Other researchers have successfully conjugated drugs to insulin fragments or antibodies to insulin factor to permit transfer through the BBB.[46,161] Even large molecules, such as the enzyme β-galactosidase, have been successfully transported into the CNS via similar methods of bioactive conjugation.[162]

Exporter Protein Modulation

The most well characterized export protein of the BBB, Pgp, was first described in hamsters in 1976 by Juliano and Ling.[163] As a member of the APT-binding cassette family of transport proteins, Pgp serves to protect the CNS by pumping xenobiotic compounds out of the brain and spinal cord into the vasculature.[164] In general, substrates for Pgp are lipophilic, planar molecules that are either neutral or cationic.[165] Pgp may have developed to remove hydrophobic substances that partitioned into the lipid core of the plasma membrane[166,167] and therefore may be activated by sensing disruptions of the lipid bilayer.[165] Unfortunately, the broad specificity of Pgp, although beneficial in preventing penetration of neurotoxins into the brain and spinal cord, also hinders therapeutic drugs from reaching their targets, thereby creating great difficulty for those researching CNS pharmaceutical design.

The specific location of Pgp in the BBB has recently been a source of debate. Studies have shown that Pgp is expressed in both cerebrovascular ECs and astrocytes in the human brain.[168,169] Many studies suggest that the primary localization of Pgp is on the luminal EC membrane, where it serves to pump compounds directly into the lumen of the microvasculature.[23,170-173] However, some evidence points to localization of Pgp on astrocyte foot processes as well.[168,169] Although Pgp is important in the case of toxin exposure, animal experiments suggest that it may not have any necessary function during normal homeostasis. Mice deficient in the export protein have no changes relative to the wild type unless exposed to drugs that are normally pumped out of the cerebrovascular endothelium by Pgp.[164] In a related experiment, dogs with increased susceptibility to neurotoxicity with the administration of ivermectin were found to be deficient in Pgp as a result of a deletion mutation in the *mdr1* gene.[174]

In the treatment of Parkinson's disease, levodopa is often administered along with carbidopa to increase levels of dopamine in the brain. Carbidopa does not cross the BBB but rather serves to inhibit the peripheral decarboxylases that would convert levodopa to dopamine and thus prevent its entry into the CNS. Similarly, inhibitors of Pgp have been developed to be coadministered with CNS-acting medications for the treatment of a variety of conditions.

Despite its high lipophilicity, cyclosporine was found to ineffectively penetrate the CNS as a result of interactions with Pgp. Studies have shown that cyclosporine inhibits Pgp, but it is not generally used for this purpose because of its immunosuppressive effects.[175-177] The cyclosporine analogue PSC 833 was developed later and maintains the Pgp inhibitory action of its parent drug without the resulting immunosuppression.[178,179] An array of other Pgp inhibitors have since been developed[180-182] and used successfully with a variety of medications.[165] For example, Pgp inhibitors have been shown to enhance delivery of the chemotherapeutic drugs paclitaxel[183,184] and docetaxel to the CNS in animals.[184] Recently, some natural products have been demonstrated to have Pgp inhibitory characteristics as well, including psoralen found in grapefruit,[185,186] ginsenoside Rg₃ from red ginseng,[187] and piperine from black pepper.[188] Clearly a variety of compounds have effects on Pgp, and as knowledge of these substances increases, researchers should be able to develop more effective compounds.

The major drawback of Pgp inhibitors is that historically, many have been toxic in concentrations sufficient for inhibition. However, the toxicologic profiles of the inhibitors have improved in recent years. First-generation inhibitors such as cyclosporine and verapamil were very toxic, whereas second-generation inhibitors such as valspodar and biricodar had improved tolerability.[189] Second-generation inhibitors were later found to have unpredictable interactions when coadministered with chemotherapeutic agents. The recently developed third-generation inhibitors, including tariquidar, zosuquidar, and laniquidar, are very specific for Pgp and have less interaction with coadministered drugs. These new Pgp inhibitors are currently undergoing clinical trials.[190]

Opening of Endothelial Tight Junctions— Osmotic Disruption

Although most vascular ECs contain no TJs, epithelial barriers throughout the body possess these intercellular structures to ensure that the luminal contents remain separate from underlying tissue. TJs between ECs of the cerebral microvasculature seem to be able to separate, effectively open up the BBB, and allow the paracellular passage of water and other molecules. Although the actual mechanism for this type of nonspecific BBB opening remains to be elucidated, a variety of substances appear to alter the permeability of the BBB in this manner. The most common of these techniques used today is osmotic disruption, which involves the injection of hypertonic nonmetabolizable solutes such as mannitol directly into either the internal carotid arteries or the vertebral arteries. The location of injection is important because the permeability of the BBB will be affected only in the vasculature distal to the site of solute injection.[191] CNS drug delivery via this method of BBB opening has been shown to be increased by up to 100-fold.[10]

The predominant hypothesis for the mechanism of osmotic BBB disruption is that shrinking of ECs occurs as a result of hyperosmolarity of the vasculature. This reduction in cell volume causes the TJs to separate and thereby open up the paracellular space for molecular movement.[192,193] However, newer studies suggest that this model may be an oversimplification. Farkas and coworkers[194] have provided evidence of phosphorylation of the multifunctional protein β-catenin during osmotic BBB opening, thus suggesting a more active cell response than passive shrinkage. A calcium-mediated contraction mechanism involving circumferential bundles of actin that interact with a variety of proteins in ECs has been proposed as well.[195,196] Exposure to hypertonic substances appears to increase intracellular calcium in cultured cerebrovascular ECs, which may trigger pathways leading to cell shrinkage itself.[197]

Several studies have demonstrated the benefits of osmotic BBB disruption for the delivery of chemotherapeutic agents to the CNS to treat both primary and metastatic malignancies. Neoplasia represents a unique challenge for administration of pharmaceuticals. The BBB is often more permeable at the core of a tumor, but the brain tissue adjacent to the tumor maintains a high level of BBB integrity.[10,198] Consequently, significantly less drug reaches the periphery and most goes to the center of the tumor.[199] This "sink effect" causes very low levels of drug in the brain tumor periphery, in essence sparing tumor cells and con-

tributing to neoplastic recurrence.[10] Additionally, the surrounding normal brain tissue may contain metastatic seeds that are hidden behind a relatively normal BBB, thus further confounding effective treatment.[133] Evidence also suggests that although the BBB is leaky in the center of tumors, it does not disappear completely in either primary or metastatic lesions.[200,201] In one experiment in mice, Pgp still played a role in the microvasculature of brain tumors despite their increased permeability in comparison to normal brain tissue.[202] The use of osmotic BBB disruption in conjunction with chemotherapy helps maintain a relatively constant level of chemotherapeutic agents throughout the entire region around the tumor, thereby preventing the "sink effect" and exposing any smaller metastatic lesions that would otherwise be inaccessible to the drugs. Osmotic BBB disruption also allows prolonged exposure of tumor to higher localized concentrations of drugs.[203,204]

The first phase I trial of osmotic BBB disruption began in 1979 and used mannitol (25%, 1.37 mol/L) infused via a catheter into the internal carotid artery at 4 to 8 mL/sec for 30 seconds. A transient rise in intracranial pressure occurred in this study, but no clinical sequelae were observed. In a study by Dahlborg and colleagues,[205] 645 osmotic BBB disruptions in conjunction with chemotherapy were performed on 34 patients, and more than 80% showed a partial response and 62% showed a complete response. Kraemer and coworkers[206] found increased survival rates in patients with primary CNS lymphomas who underwent osmotic BBB disruption for delivery of chemotherapeutic drugs. They also identified a positive correlation between patient survival and the number of BBB disruptions. In another study, the estimated 5-year survival rate for patients with non–AIDS-related primary CNS lymphoma treated by osmotic BBB disruption and chemotherapy was 42% with a median survival time of 40.7 months.[207] Such techniques have also been used successfully in pediatric patients.[208]

Despite its increased use in recent years, osmotic BBB disruption is far from perfect. Early hints of potential difficulties with the procedure came from studies in rats in which seizure-like events occurred during BBB modification.[209] Transient increases in intracranial pressure are common during osmotic disruption. In the aforementioned study by Dahlborg and associates,[205] which included 34 patients, one episode of tonsillar herniation occurred with no neurological sequelae, seizures developed in 4% of patients, and sepsis or granulocytopenic fever developed in 3%. In a study by McAllister and coworkers[207] on primary CNS lymphoma, seizures occurred in 6% to 8% of those who underwent osmotic BBB opening. Four of the 74 patients in this study died within 30 days of the procedure, all attributed to infection, with three deaths occurring before the administration of granulocyte colony-stimulating factor. In one case study, expressive aphasia developed in a patient after osmotic BBB disruption but later resolved.[210] Vasospasm is another problem associated with osmotic BBB disruption[211] that can lead to ischemic stroke. Higher relative permeability of the BBB to viruses and proteins also occurs during osmotic BBB disruption.[212,213] Exposure of nervous tissue to protein, specifically serum albumin, may cause astrocyte activation and seizures,[214] although others argue that osmotic BBB disruption does not allow extravasation of serum albumin.[215] Finally, osmotic BBB disruption is a costly and invasive procedure that requires highly trained practitioners to coordinate the treatment effectively.

Opening of Endothelial Tight Junctions— Parasympathetic Stimulation

Although the sympathetic division of the autonomic nervous system is responsible for maintaining and altering vasomotor tone in the body and thus peripheral blood flow, it has little if any effect on cerebral blood flow.[216] This discovery prompted researchers to evaluate alternative pathways for cerebrovascular control. Interestingly, sensory innervation to the circle of Willis travels via the nasociliary nerve, a branch of the ophthalmic nerve, after leaving the cranial cavity through the ethmoidal foramen.[217] Previous studies have shown that substance P–containing pain fibers may also dilate blood vessels via separate branches ending in motor terminals.[218]

Parasympathetic input to the cerebral vasculature was evaluated by Suzuki and associates.[219,220] In this study, the nasociliary nerve was cut to interrupt sensory stimulation, and then the parasympathetic fibers entering the ethmoidal foramen were stimulated, which resulted in a 17% increase in cerebral blood flow. Sectioning the fibers did not affect blood flow, so parasympathetic stimulation also did not contribute to resting levels of vasomotor tone. Moreover, anticholinergic agents such as atropine and scopolamine did not attenuate the increase in cerebral blood flow, thus suggesting that the active neurotransmitter was not acetylcholine. The neurotransmitter mediating this effect was later shown to be NO.[221-223] In another study, stimulation of the rat sphenopalatine ganglion (SPG) increased cerebral blood flow by up to 50% in the ipsilateral parietal cortex.[224-227]

Studies by Mayhan[228,229] showed that both NO donors and histamine increase permeability of the BBB. Yarnitsky and coworkers[230] subsequently hypothesized that stimulation of parasympathetic fibers may increase the permeability of the BBB because parasympathetic fibers release NO. They evaluated the permeability of the BBB by using fluorescein isothiocyanate–labeled dextran in rat parietal cortex exposed by craniotomy. Evans blue–labeled albumin and two chemotherapeutic agents, anti-HER2 monoclonal antibody used for the treatment of breast cancer and etoposide, were used in closed-cranium experiments to evaluate permeability of the BBB as well. All these agents entered through the BBB in significant amounts throughout the ipsilateral brain after stimulation of the postganglionic parasympathetic fibers in the SPG. Some of the contralateral brain was affected as well. Smaller molecules penetrated the BBB more easily than larger ones, thus suggesting that the mechanism of this effect works by opening TJs rather than vesicular transport. No injurious effect on the brain, as measured by nicotinamide adenine dinucleotide (NAD)/reduced NAD (NADH) balance, was found, and no significant brain edema occurred. In another experiment by Yarnitsky and colleagues,[231] SPG stimulation in dogs showed similar effects on the BBB and was also observed to increase BBB permeability of the optic nerve, an extension of the CNS. Unlike the experiments in rodents, however, the effect in dogs and domestic pigs was entirely ipsilateral and only the anterior circulation was affected because the posterior vasculature is innervated by branches from the otic ganglion in these animals. Such findings suggest that SPG stimulation in humans would have similar effects on the ipsilateral anterior cerebral circulation.

Convection-Enhanced Delivery

Chemotherapy is infused into the brain tumor under constant pressure to deliver drug by bulk flow through catheters placed into the tumor bed.[232] Image guidance is used to optimize the accuracy of drug delivery. There are numerous variables that determine whether effective doses of drugs have been delivered to the tumor: the rate of infusion and total volume infused, the molecular weight of the drug agent, the affinity for and concentration in and around the target receptor, and finally, the density of brain tissue.[233] Technical challenges of convection-enhanced delivery include injury to the brain during insertion of the catheter, backflow of infusate, drug infused into the EC space of the CNS, drug efflux by transport mechanisms related to the BBB, premature metabolism of the infusate, and finally, interstitial pressure gradients preventing adequate concentration of drug to remain in the tumor bed.[234]

Local Delivery of Polymer-Infused Chemotherapy

Incorporation of chemotherapy into biodegradable polymers was first developed in 1991[235] and approved for used in 1996 in patients with malignant gliomas. A craniotomy must be performed to implant the drug wafers into the tumor resection cavity. There is variability in the amount of total drug released into the resection cavity, as well as nonuniform release of carmustine into a tumor. This approach relies on passive diffusion of drugs into the brain, unlike convection-enhanced delivery, which forces fluid drugs through the brain.

Targeted Toxin Therapy

This drug delivery system relies on a fusion protein consisting of a protein with affinity for the IL-4 receptor, which is upregulated on tumor cells, and a bacterial toxin that causes apoptosis by inhibiting translation.[236]

Trojan Horse Liposome

An appropriately named therapy, immunoliposomes carry a gene for protein correction gene therapy or small hairpin RNA expressed in plasma to inhibit protein synthesis by RNA interference (RNAi). The molecular Trojan Horse liposome is conjugated to a polyethylene glycol moiety, which increases the circulating half-life of the fusion construct. Polyethylene glycol is a peptidomimetic that binds to BBB transport receptors such as insulin or transferrin to enter the brain parenchyma. Preclinical studies have shown this technique to be a means of gene therapy for treating Parkinson's disease.[237] The most widely characterized receptor-mediated transcytosis system for targeting of drugs to the brain is the transferrin receptor, which mediates cellular uptake of iron bound to transferrin. Drugs targeting the transferrin receptor can be developed either by using an endogenous ligand, transferrin, or by using an antibody directed against the transferrin receptor. The insulin receptor has also been used for targeted delivery of drugs to the brain.

Focused Ultrasound Disruption of the Blood-Brain Barrier

This method uses ultrasound to create lesions in the BBB to increase its permeability. It is monitored closely by MRI thermometry.[238] Vascular penetration was generated without measurable tissue injury by using intravenous contrast dye to visualize disruption of the BBB.[239] Imaging revealed expanded TJs and increased migration across ECs.[240] Preclinical studies with doxorubicin showed increased drug in sites targeted by ultrasound and retained binding of antibodies attached to a chemotherapeutic agent for their ligand.[241]

IMAGING THE BLOOD-BRAIN BARRIER

Neuroimaging technology has advanced to provide insight into the effect of brain tumors on the BBB by enabling clinicians to view the invasiveness of the disease and the effect of the tumor on BBB permeability, as well as to evaluate the efficacy of treatment strategies. Disruption of the BBB by disease processes such as brain tumors can be seen on contrast-enhanced computed tomography (CT) and MRI.[242] Brain tumor lesions have a higher relative cerebral blood volume than normal tissue does, largely because of secretion of VEGF by brain tumors. To assess the relationship between BBB penetration and tumor perfusion, patients with high-grade gliomas underwent MRI screening with a T1-weighted fast spoiled gradient echo technique for

measurement of BBB permeability, followed by dynamic susceptibility contrast-enhanced (DSC) imaging to measure regional
cerebral blood volume. There was a correlation between
T1-weighted and DSC images, which implies a direct relationship between BBB permeability and regional cerebral blood
volume (Fig. 8-7).[242]

Brain MRI has been used to monitor drug delivery and evaluate the success of treatment of CNS tumors.[241] Patients with
intracranial mass lesions underwent MRI before and after corticosteroid therapy. In comparing normal and pathologic brain
tissue, there was a significant difference in T1-weighted contrast
enhancement, as well as a difference between the two groups on
T2-weighted contrast-enhanced images.[243]

More recently, iron oxide nanoparticles have been used for
tumor imaging. When compared with conventional gadolinium
contrast, nanoparticles exhibit superior intravascular retention
and may more accurately delineate brain tumor perfusion.[244]
Advances in PET may help distinguish tumor regrowth from
radiation necrosis and even help stage a tumor.[245]

S-100β: A Peripheral Marker of Blood-Brain Barrier Damage

Opening of the BBB provides molecules normally present in
blood open passage into the CNS. However, this opening, unless
involving specific transporters, does not work in just one direction. Proteins normally present in blood are free to diffuse into
the CNS, and in turn, proteins normally present in high concentration in the CNS are free to diffuse down concentration gradients into blood. These peripheral BBB markers can be detected
in blood to evaluate the permeability characteristics of the BBB

at any given time. In a recent review article, Marchi and associates[246] discussed the ideal properties of a peripheral marker of
BBB disruption. Such proteins should have low or undetectable
plasma levels in normal subjects, be normally present in CSF, and
have a higher normal concentration in CSF than in plasma.
Additionally, the CSF concentration of the protein should
increase in response to insults. The protein should be normally
blocked by the BBB and exhibit flux across the BBB during
barrier disruption. Several proteins, including S-100β, neuron-
specific enolase, and GFAP, have been evaluated for this purpose,
but only S-100β meets the characteristics of having very low
plasma levels with a concentration less than that found in CSF
in normal subjects.

Moore discovered the S-100 protein family in 1965 by isolating a fraction of subcellular material containing proteins from
bovine brain.[247] Moore named the fraction S-100 because its
contents were soluble in 100% saturated ammonium sulfate at
neutral pH. The S-100 family contains more than 15 different
calcium-binding proteins, including S-100β. All of them contain
EF-hand calcium-binding domains and are approximately 10,000
daltons in size,[247] significantly larger than the 400- to 500-dalton
limit for passage through the BBB. Of the proteins in this family,
S-100β is unique in its predominant location in the CNS[248-251]
and is specifically located primarily in both astrocyte end-foot
processes and Schwann cells.[252-254] Although S-100β is found in
several other body tissues, its concentrations in these peripheral
locations are significantly lower than in the CNS.[248,249] The
primary role of S-100β remains to be elucidated, but it interacts
with a number of cytoplasmic proteins with calcium-dependent
actions and thus exerts a variety of influences on cells. It may
exert its effects via a cyclic adenosine monophosphate–related
mechanism.[255]

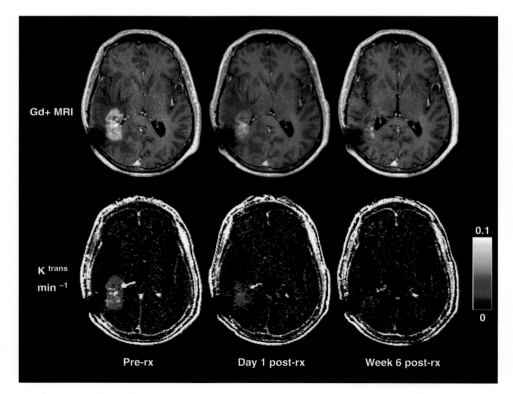

FIGURE 8-7 T1-weighted contrast-enhanced magnetic resonance image (*top*) and K$_{trans}$ permeability maps (*bottom*) in a patient with recurrent glioblastoma multiforme. The *left column* is before treatment, the *middle column* is after a single dose of bevacizumab (Avastin) and irinotecan, and the *right column* is after one course of bevacizumab and irinotecan. (*Courtesy of Dr. Daniel Baboriak, Duke University Medical Center.*)

Plasma levels of S-100β are normally a third of those found in CSF and are nearly undetectable.[256] Several diseases cause an elevation in plasma levels of S-100β, which can be detected and used for both diagnostic and prognostic purposes, as well as for evaluation of disease progression. Plasma S-100β levels increase with cerebral ischemia, with peak levels occurring approximately 3 days after infarction.[257-260] These levels have served as a useful marker of both infarct size and long-term clinical outcome.[257-259,261,262] Traumatic brain injury has also been shown to increase S-100β levels in plasma,[263,264] with a positive correlation between the extent of damage after head injury and elevation in plasma S-100β.[265] Ingebrigtsen and coworkers[266,267] found a negative predictive value of 0.99 for detecting intracranial pathology via serum S-100β levels versus CT studies. The highest S-100β levels in one study of traumatic brain injury were observed in samples taken approximately 2.5 hours after trauma, which is a considerably shorter period than that required for the maximal peak in plasma concentrations during ischemic stroke.[268] A positive correlation was also found between early rises in blood plasma levels, up to 5 hours after trauma, and unfavorable outcome.[262,265,267-270]

Plasma levels of S-100β have also been elevated in patients with hemorrhagic shock,[263] aneurysmal subarachnoid hemorrhage,[271] hypoxia secondary to cardiac arrest,[272] and brain damage subsequent to attempted cardiopulmonary resuscitation.[273] In all these cases, the elevation in S-100β plasma concentration is thought to result from damage to nervous tissue, including both neurons and glial cells. Additionally, depleted ATP levels in the brain during ischemic, hypoxic, and traumatic injury lead to increased adenosine levels,[274-276] which may activate A_1 adenosine receptors and cause release of S-100β from astrocytes. In experiments on cultured astrocytes, Ciccarelli and colleagues[277] observed that adenosine receptor agonists cause the released S-100β to be nearly 160% that of controls. Plasma S-100β has also been elevated during cardiothoracic surgery,[278-280] although these findings remain debatable.[281] Currently, plasma levels of S-100β are predominantly used clinically for the monitoring of melanoma because these malignant cells express the protein. High plasma levels of S-100β correlate with disease progression.[282]

With the exception of melanoma, all the aforementioned disease processes involve some degree of brain damage. Diseases of the CNS that are associated with opening of the BBB do not necessarily cause brain damage or increased adenosine levels, so S-100β plasma levels must rise in response to BBB disruption without coexisting nervous tissue damage. To evaluate this, plasma S-100β levels were determined in patients with primary CNS lymphoma treated by chemotherapy, with intra-arterial infusion of mannitol used for osmotic BBB disruption. Plasma S-100β concentrations increased with mannitol administration. Intra-arterial administration of methotrexate once again caused plasma levels to rise, although patients receiving methotrexate without BBB disruption had no change in plasma S-100β. This elevation in peripheral S-100β levels occurred nearly immediately after BBB disruption, which excludes protein synthesis as a source for the increased S-100β.[283] Intra-arterial infusion of methotrexate with BBB disruption does not appear to damage nervous tissue,[284] thus suggesting that the elevated plasma concentrations reflect release of baseline levels of S-100β protein in the CNS and not release as a result of damaged brain tissue. Further studies have also shown that peripheral S-100β levels rise even in the absence of brain damage.[246,285]

Three hypotheses have been proposed for how the rises in peripheral S-100β occur. CNS concentrations of the protein may increase first because of neuronal damage, with plasma levels rising after subsequent opening of the BBB. Alternatively, the BBB may open first, with subsequent neuronal damage elevating plasma levels. Finally, the rise in peripheral S-100β levels may be due to release of the normal amount of the protein in the CNS

after opening of the BBB. This last hypothesis of plasma S-100β elevation suggests that it is a useful specific marker of BBB permeability. To evaluate the diagnostic utility of S-100β levels, Kanner and associates[285] conducted a prospective study by determining S-100β levels in 51 patients undergoing MRI with and without gadolinium contrast enhancement for diagnostic and volumetric purposes. Normal MRI findings were seen in six patients from this group, and their plasma S-100β levels were found to be close to normal as well. In two patients treated for trigeminal neuralgia, one had a normal MRI study, whereas the other showed lacunar infarcts and related white matter changes. Plasma S-100β levels were elevated in this second patient, probably because of ischemia from the infarcts. All the remaining patients had MRI studies that demonstrated gadolinium enhancement and had significantly elevated basal S-100β levels. No significant differences in S-100β levels were found in patients with metastatic tumors of various origins. Moreover, there was no correlation between tumor size and rise in plasma S-100β concentrations. Primary CNS lymphoma was the only tumor evaluated that did not cause an elevation in S-100β. Immunocytochemical studies showed that this tumor had a uniform cytology devoid of normal astrocytic markers, including GFAP and S-100β, thus explaining the absence of plasma S-100β elevations in these patients.

Based on these studies on the use of peripheral detection of S-100β, Janigro and Marchi published methods to determine plasma levels of S-100β for use in the diagnosis of new conditions, determining the prognosis and progression of various disorders, and providing insight into the permeability characteristics of the BBB for proper drug administration.[286] Research is currently under way to ensure that peripheral S-100β levels correlate well with gadolinium enhancement on MRI. If so, plasma S-100β could be used to screen patients for MRI for the diagnosis of brain tumors. Because BBB disruption can occur transiently for a variety of reasons, elevated plasma S-100β would not necessarily mean that a lesion was present. However, a normal plasma level would suggest that MRI would show no gadolinium enhancement, thus making MRI unnecessary. A simple and inexpensive blood test could be used regularly in place of expensive and time-consuming MRI studies.

Peripheral detection of S-100β also allows unique drug delivery opportunities. Design of a point-of-care system for evaluation of S-100β plasma levels would provide rapid determination of BBB permeability status and allow physicians to administer drugs during periods of some CNS diseases when the BBB is compromised. Moreover, some chronic disorders such as multiple sclerosis may result in alterations in permeability of the BBB that could be detected by measuring plasma S-100β and used for drug administration. Many more potential uses of S-100β measurement may develop as further research is performed on this peripheral marker of BBB disruption.

Blood-Brain Barrier and Neurological Disorders: Epilepsy

A seizure is a paroxysmal event caused by abnormal, excessive, hypersynchronous discharges from an aggregate of CNS neurons. This abnormal electrical activity can be reflected by various clinical/behavioral manifestations ranging from dramatic convulsive activity to experiential phenomena not readily discernible by an observer. Although a variety of factors influence the incidence of seizures, approximately 5% to 10% of the population will have at least one seizure during their lifetime, with the highest incidence occurring in early childhood and late adulthood.

Patients with epilepsy have seizures intermittently, and depending on the underlying cause, many patients are completely seizure free for months or even years. This sporadic appearance of seizures implies that *precipitating factors* induce seizures in patients with epilepsy. Numerous groups have described a number of vascular/blood-related factors that may be tipping the fragile epileptic brain toward seizures.[214,287-294] Seizures are a result of a shift in the normal balance of excitation and inhibition within the CNS. Given the numerous properties that control neuronal activity, it is not surprising that there are many different ways to perturb homeostasis and therefore precipitate seizures. One of the main determinants of neuronal firing rate and synchronicity is the extracellular potassium level. Potassium controls glial and neuronal resting potential, repolarization, ion channel conductance, cerebral blood flow, and Na^+/K^+ pump activity. The complexity of CNS potassium homeostasis underscores its importance in the mammalian brain and also the role of the BBB. The process involves different cell types (neurons, glia, and ECs), several extracellular mechanisms (spatial buffering, cerebral blood flow), and strictly controlled segregation of potassium concentrations between blood (4.0 to 5.0 mM) and brain parenchyma (2.5 to 3.0 mM). Other molecular elements that may either participate in seizure onset or decrease the seizure threshold are brain levels of albumin, antibodies, or drugs.

Systemic pathologies causing BBB failure may also include hypertension, stroke, blood hyperosmolarity, or systemically mediated inflammatory processes (secondary to the production of TNF-α, IL-1β, IL-6, histamine, arachidonic acid, or reactive oxygen species). Furthermore, the normal brain is capable of seizing under the appropriate circumstances if the BBB is transiently breached. Finally, opening of the BBB lowers the threshold for seizures. All these underlying endogenous factors may influence the seizure threshold. Whether these factors are the same in a chronically epileptic patient as those involved in the generation of acute seizures (e.g., in "normal" brain) remains unknown.

Seizures and epilepsy are commonly observed in conjunction with stroke, traumatic brain injury, and CNS infections—all conditions known to compromise BBB function. It remains debatable whether the compromised integrity of the BBB is a factor involved in the etiology of epilepsy or secondary to such pathologies. The etiologic role that the BBB plays in seizures is supported by the fact that BBB disruption after acute head trauma is a well-known pathologic finding in both animal and human studies of S-100β.[294-297] BBB disruption may persist for weeks to years after the injury and may colocalize with abnormal electroencephalographic (EEG) activity. The increased interest in osmotic opening of the BBB as a viable mechanism of increasing drug delivery to the brain provides an opportunity to explore the connection between BBB disruption and seizures in a controlled clinical environment. The marked increase in BBB permeability to intravascular substances (10- to 100-fold for small molecules) after this osmotic disruption procedure is due to both increased diffusion and bulk fluid flow across the TJs. The permeability effect is largely reversed within minutes.[298] In rodents, loss of BBB integrity by intra-arterial administration of hyperosmotic mannitol has been shown to rapidly lead to EEG changes consistent with epileptic seizures (spike/wave complexes interspersed with decreased EEG voltage that persist for several hours after the BBB disruption event).[290,299]

Given these findings, it is not surprising that seizures are the primary complication of osmotic BBB disruption. Indeed, seizures occur in a relatively large number of these patients (13% to 55%). This high incidence was initially attributed to meglumine iothalamate, a known epileptogenic agent used as a contrast agent for CT.[300] However, seizures associated with BBB disruption continued to occur (albeit with decreased frequency) when the disruption was monitored by radionuclide scanning rather than CT. Current research is focused on attempting to establish a correlation between the level of BBB disruption and the probability of a seizure occurring.[290,301]

FUTURE CONSIDERATIONS

The BBB is a dynamic organ that selectively permits essential compounds to enter the brain and also vigorously prevents entry of foreign pathogens by structural, enzymatic, and hormonal control. The properties that shield the brain from deleterious agents are the same properties that prevent drugs from treating disease. Continued effort in basic science research is essential to unravel the intricate pathways of the anatomic, electrochemical, and enzymatic barriers of the neurovascular unit. Developing animal models that recapitulate human disease states of the BBB will facilitate translational research by enabling scientists to rigorously test their hypotheses before proceeding to clinical trials. Finally, further refinement of imaging modalities with increased sensitivity to the BBB and investigating novel stem cell–based strategies of therapy will lead to innovative, effective therapies to treat myriad neurological diseases.

SUGGESTED READINGS

Abbott NJ. Dynamics of CNS barriers: evolution, differentiation, and modulation. *Cell Mol Neurobiol.* 2005;25:5-23.

Agre P, Nielsen S, Ottersen OP. Towards a molecular understanding of water homeostasis in the brain. *Neuroscience.* 2004;129:849-850.

Begley DJ. Delivery of therapeutic agents to the central nervous system: the problems and the possibilities. *Pharmacol Ther.* 2004;104:29-45.

Betz AL, Goldstein GW. Polarity of the blood-brain barrier: neutral amino acid transport into isolated brain capillaries. *Science.* 1978;202:225-227.

Brightman MW. The distribution within the brain of ferritin injected into cerebrospinal fluid compartments. II. Parenchymal distribution. *Am J Anat.* 1965;117:193-219.

Cairncross JG, Macdonald DR, Pexman JH, et al. Steroid-induced CT changes in patients with recurrent malignant glioma. *Neurology.* 1988;38:724-726.

Cervos-Navarro J, Kannuki S, Nakagawa Y. Blood-brain barrier (BBB). Review from morphological aspect. *Histol Histopathol.* 1988;3:203-213.

Davson H. Review lecture. The blood-brain barrier. *J Physiol.* 1976;1-28.

Demeule M, Regina A, Annabi B, et al. Brain endothelial cells as pharmacological targets in brain tumors. *Mol Neurobiol.* 2004;30:157-183.

Dore-Duffy P, Owen C, Balabanov R, et al. Pericyte migration from the vascular wall in response to traumatic brain injury. *Microvasc Res.* 2000;60:55-69.

Fricker G, Miller DS. Modulation of drug transporters at the blood-brain barrier. *Pharmacology.* 2004;70:169-176.

Hanin I. The Gulf War, stress and a leaky blood-brain barrier. *Nat Med.* 1996;2:1307-1308.

Hirase T, Staddon JM, Saitou M, et al. Occludin as a possible determinant of tight junction permeability in endothelial cells. *J Cell Sci.* 1997;110:1603-1613.

Janzer RC, Raff MC. Astrocytes induce blood-brain barrier properties in endothelial cells. *Nature.* 1987;325:253-257.

Kapural M, Krizanac-Bengez L, Barnett G, et al. Serum S-100beta as a possible marker of blood-brain barrier disruption. *Brain Res.* 2002;940:102-104.

Karnovsky MJ. The ultrastructural basis of capillary permeability studied with peroxidase as a tracer. *J Cell Biol.* 1967;35:213-236.

Kroll RA, Neuwelt EA. Outwitting the blood-brain barrier for therapeutic purposes: osmotic opening and other means. *Neurosurgery.* 1998;42:1083-1099; discussion 1099-1100.

Loscher W, Potschka H. Role of drug efflux transporters in the brain for drug disposition and treatment of brain diseases. *Prog Neurobiol.* 2005;76:22-76.

Neuwelt EA. Mechanisms of disease: the blood-brain barrier. *Neurosurgery.* 2004;54:131-140; discussion 141-142.

Oby E, Janigro D. The blood-brain barrier and epilepsy. *Epilepsia.* 2006;47:1761-1774.

Pardridge WM. Molecular biology of the blood-brain barrier. *Mol Biotechnol.* 2005;30:57-70.

Pardridge WM. Blood-brain barrier drug targeting: the future of brain drug development. *Mol Interv.* 2003;3:90-105.

Provenzale JM, Mukundan S, Dewhirst M. The role of blood-brain barrier permeability in brain tumor imaging and therapeutics. *AJR Am J Roentgenol.* 2005;185:763-767.

Reese TS, Karnovsky MJ. Fine structural localization of a blood-brain barrier to exogenous peroxidase. *J Cell Biol.* 1967;34:207-217.

Schinkel AH, Smit JJ, van Tellingen O, et al. Disruption of the mouse mdr1a P-glycoprotein gene leads to a deficiency in the blood-brain barrier and to increased sensitivity to drugs. *Cell.* 1994;77:491-502.

Smith QR. A review of blood-brain barrier transport techniques. *Methods Mol Med.* 2003;89:193-208.

Stewart PA, Wiley MJ. Developing nervous tissue induces formation of blood-brain barrier characteristics in invading endothelial cells: a study using quail-chick transplantation chimeras. *Dev Biol.* 1981;84:183-192.

Tao-Cheng JH, Brightman MW. Development of membrane interactions between brain endothelial cells and astrocytes in vitro. *Int J Dev Neurosci.* 1988;6:25-37.

Thomas H, Coley HM. Overcoming multidrug resistance in cancer: an update on the clinical strategy of inhibiting p-glycoprotein. *Cancer Control*. 2003;10:159-165.

Tontsch U, Bauer HC. Glial cells and neurons induce blood-brain barrier related enzymes in cultured cerebral endothelial cells. *Brain Res*. 1991;539:247-253.

Volk H, Potschka H, Loscher W. Immunohistochemical localization of P-glycoprotein in rat brain and detection of its increased expression by seizures are sensitive to fixation and staining variables. *J Histochem Cytochem*. 2005;53:517-531.

Volk HA, Loscher W. Multidrug resistance in epilepsy: rats with drug-resistant seizures exhibit enhanced brain expression of P-glycoprotein compared with rats with drug-responsive seizures. *Brain*. 2005;128:1358-1368.

Full references can be found on Expert Consult @ www.expertconsult.com

CHAPTER 9

Cerebral Edema

Robert J. Weil ■ Edward H. Oldfield

OVERVIEW AND HISTORICAL BACKGROUND

Cerebral edema represents the accumulation of excess fluid in the intracellular or extracellular spaces of the brain. It can result from a variety of physiologic and pathologic processes and is frequently responsible for much of the morbidity and mortality associated with brain tumors and a variety of other disorders, including trauma, hemorrhage, and infection. A basic conception of the barriers that exist between and among blood, cerebrospinal fluid (CSF), and the brain is required to fully understand cerebral or brain edema. In this chapter we briefly outline the physiology of the blood-brain barrier (BBB) and describe and discuss the principal types and causes of cerebral edema. Several reviews that outline the history of research in this field and recent advances in this area and that provide more detailed summaries beyond the scope of this chapter are cited in the reference section.

Paul Ehrlich was the first to identify a potential barrier between the vasculature and the brain after he observed that intravenous albumin-bound dyes stained all tissues except the brain.[1] Goldmann carried Ehrlich's studies further to demonstrate that dye injected into CSF did not circulate in the systemic circulation.[2] These barriers (Table 9-1), which are rate-limiting steps in the movement of water, ions, solutes, and macromolecules between compartments, help the brain regulate its own environment distinct from the rest of the body. The BBB is an essential component of brain homeostasis.

THE BLOOD-BRAIN BARRIER

The principal component of the BBB is the endothelial cells that line the cerebral microvasculature (Fig. 9-1).[3-10] The tight junctions between adjacent endothelial cells in the brain, which are nonpermissive in comparison to those in the systemic circulation, prevent the paracellular transport of most molecules. Although small substances, such as oxygen and carbon dioxide, and small lipophilic molecules, such as ethanol, may diffuse freely through the lipid membranes that constitute the BBB, larger, bulkier, more complex or hydrophilic molecules require active, transcellular transport mechanisms, potentially on both the luminal (endothelial) and abluminal (brain) membranes, to enter the brain.[11] The active transport mechanisms require energy in the form of adenosine triphosphate (ATP).[11]

Several studies have identified a variety of molecular mechanisms and metabolic barriers that indicate that the BBB is an exceptionally active system.[11-13] For example, endothelial cells contain active peptides, peptidases that inactivate traversing proteins, and numerous intracellular enzymes, such as cytochrome P-450 (1A and 2B isoforms), that inactivate neuroactive and neurotoxic substances.[14,15] In general, to traverse the normal BBB, large or hydrophilic molecules require an active transport mechanism—either receptor-mediated or absorptive-mediated transcytosis. In the cerebral endothelium, these mechanisms are less efficient than in systemic (outside the central nervous system [CNS]) endothelial cells, which enhances the potential BBB. Thus, the BBB contains active and passive features that regulate the passage of substances from the systemic circulation into the brain. Similar versions of these tight junctions and permeability restrictions are found between CSF and the brain (except in the circumventricular organs [area postrema, tuber cinereum, and pineal gland], where the endothelium is penetrated more easily to permit secreted neuropeptides to act systemically; see Table 9-1).[11-16]

The BBB has an extensive surface area—which some researchers have estimated to be approximately 20 m²/1.3 kg of brain. Consequently, no neuron is more than 20 to 25 μm away from a brain capillary, and thus the BBB plays several critical roles in regulation of the brain's microenvironment.[17,18] It manages the entry of nutrients and controls elimination of wastes. The BBB limits distribution and thus contains within the brain generated neuroregulators and neurotransmitters that act centrally while excluding or regulating entry into the brain of similar molecules intended to act peripherally. This reduces or prevents debilitating biochemical crosstalk within the CNS. Finally, the BBB regulates movement of fluid and ions between the circulation and the brain, which permits maintenance of an ideal interstitial fluid that enhances neuronal function. The brain's interstitial fluid has some similarities with plasma but has a lower protein content and lower concentration of calcium (Ca^{2+}) and potassium (K^+) ions and a higher concentration of magnesium (Mg^{2+}), which generates a significant buffering capacity. This limits the effect of fluxes of systemic metabolism, such as occur with exercise, a meal, or starvation.[5,11,19] Continuous turnover of interstitial fluid and CSF, which is regulated by the cerebral endothelium and its barriers (see Table 9-1), is critical to homeostasis of the brain's microenvironment.

MOLECULAR EVENTS IN CEREBRAL EDEMA

Cerebral edema is a common end result of a variety of neurological and systemic disorders. Most classifications of cerebral edema describe four categories (summarized in Table 9-2): *cytotoxic*, or cellular swelling secondary to cell injury; *vasogenic*, which results from vascular leakage through a disrupted BBB and consequently increased fluid and altered concentrations of ions, peptides, and macromolecules in the extracellular space; *interstitial*, which occurs with transependymal flow of CSF in patients with hydrocephalus; and *osmotic*, when the brain is hyperosmolar relative to plasma and thus induces water to flow passively across an intact BBB along its concentration gradient. It may be difficult to separate edema into these distinct classes in every patient because more than one type may be present simultaneously as a result of the nature and timing of the underlying disorder (see Table 9-2). Because interstitial edema and osmotic edema have fewer causes or are uncommon in neurosurgical patients, our principal focus in this chapter is on vasogenic and cytotoxic edema.

Tissue swelling—edema—may be intracellular or extracellular. It has the potential to result in profound shifts in the relative volumes occupied by the cellular and interstitial elements. Continued redistribution of water, ions, peptides, and other neuroactive substances within and between the cells of the CNS (neurons, glia, microglia, and endothelial cells) may exacerbate the primary cause of the edema. These failures lead to a variety of molecular events and cascades that potentiate cerebral and BBB dysfunction, some of which are summarized later and are discussed in greater detail in several recent, specialized monographs.[4,5,20]

TABLE 9-1 Principal Features of the Blood-Brain Neurovascular Unit

INTERFACE	LOCATION OF THE BLOOD-BRAIN JUNCTION	FUNCTIONAL OUTCOME
Blood-brain	Capillary endothelial cell (see Fig. 9-1)	Active transport of most materials. The Na⁺,K⁺-ATPase pump on the apical surface of the capillary endothelium transports materials across high-resistance tight junctions. Tight junctions restrict the entry of hydrophilic materials and high-molecular-weight molecules
Blood–cerebrospinal fluid	Choroid plexus	Ultrafiltration of plasma with active secretion of cerebrospinal fluid; this high-energy process requires ATP. Essential components are ATPase and carbonic anhydrase
Cerebrospinal fluid–venous blood	Arachnoid granulations	Arachnoid granulations transmit cerebrospinal fluid into the cerebral venous sinuses along a pressure gradient

ATP, adenosine triphosphate; ATPase, adenosine triphosphatase.

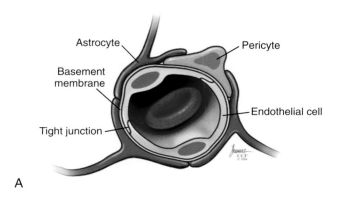

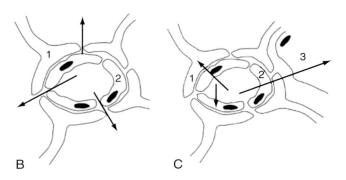

FIGURE 9-1 Microscopic representations of the blood-brain barrier (BBB) and the two most common forms of cerebral edema. **A,** The BBB is created by compact apposition of endothelial cells to create a barrier between the vascular system and the brain parenchyma. This is reinforced by numerous pericytes. A thin basement membrane surrounds the endothelial cells and provides both structural support and a dense physical barrier between the circulation and the microenvironment of the brain. Astrocytes extend cellular processes (astrocytic "foot processes") that cover the basement membrane, which enhances the BBB by limiting the ability of macromolecules or circulating cells to gain access to the central nervous system. **B,** In vasogenic edema, increased permeability of the capillaries, through dehiscent or incompetent tight junctions, leads to exudation of a plasma ultrafiltrate and water into the extracellular space. *Arrows* demonstrate flow through the tight junctions and into the extracellular space. **C,** In cytotoxic edema, depletion of energy and metabolites leads to failure of the sodium-potassium adenosine triphosphatase (Na⁺,K⁺-ATPase) pump and accumulation of sodium within the cells (astrocytes and endothelial cells, as well as neurons); water follows the concentration gradient into the cells, which swell in response. *Arrows* demonstrate the path of water into cells from the vascular space. 1, Astrocytes and astrocytic foot processes; 2, endothelial cells; 3, neurons. (**A,** *Used with permission from the Cleveland Clinic.*)

Vasogenic Edema

Vasogenic edema may share some mechanisms with cytotoxic and other forms of brain edema. However, the principal source of edema formation is abnormal permeability of the BBB.[21] The most common source is a primary or secondary brain tumor, in which case the nascent microvessels are deficient in tight junctions. This "brain-tumor barrier" is an incompetent obstacle that permits leakage of plasma ultrafiltrate into the brain's extracellular space.[18,22,23]

The edema associated with brain tumors results from this passive deficiency and from cellular invasion and migration.[10,24,25] In addition, many tumors have active mechanisms to promote vascular permeability and neovascularity. The most widely studied permeability and angiogenic agent secreted by tumor cells is vascular endothelial growth factor (VEGF), which induces capillary permeability, endothelial proliferation, and migration and organization of new capillaries that lack tight junctions.[26] Additional chemokines, cytokines, growth factors, and inflammatory mediators that play similar or complementary roles in blood-tumor permeability and angiogenesis have been identified. For example, angiopoietin-1, angiopoietin-2, fibroblast growth factor, hepatocyte growth factor/scatter factor, platelet-derived growth factor, interleukin-3 (IL-3), IL-4, IL-8, transforming growth factor-α (TGF-α), TGF-β, a variety of adhesion molecules and proteases such as urokinase plasminogen activator, multiple matrix metalloproteinases, integrins $\alpha_v\beta_3$ and $\alpha_v\beta_5$, and even oncogenes such as mutated *Ras* and tumor suppressor gene products such as Tp53 and vhl protein can affect BBB function. Many of these are discussed elsewhere in this volume.

The most thoroughly studied mechanism that produces cerebral edema is the vasogenic edema mediated by tumor production of a macromolecular protein initially identified as vascular permeability factor (VPF) and later, after its angiogenic activity had been identified, as VEGF. VPF/VEGF was initially identified by Senger and Dvorak in 1983.[27] Their landmark study demonstrated that the ascites caused by the intraperitoneal injection of hepatocarcinoma cells into guinea pigs was a product of excessive permeability of the small vessels that line the peritoneal cavity and, furthermore, that a protein secreted by the tumor and acting on the vessels was responsible for the enhanced vascular permeability. Hepatocarcinoma lines that did not produce the protein did not cause ascites. In addition, in an in vivo biologic assay of cutaneous vascular permeability, the enhanced vascular

TABLE 9-2 Characteristics of the Principal Types of Cerebral Edema

FEATURE	CYTOTOXIC EDEMA	VASOGENIC EDEMA	INTERSTITIAL EDEMA	OSMOTIC EDEMA
Pathophysiology	Osmotic gradient because of metabolic failure of the Na^+,K^+-ATPase pump, with cellular swelling of all elements (neurons, glia, and endothelial cells)	Increased vascular permeability at the level of the blood-brain barrier (or blood-tumor barrier), with extracellular fluid accumulation of an ultrafiltrate of plasma	Transependymal flow of water and solutes into the periventricular extracellular space; caused by hydrocephalus and impaired absorption of cerebrospinal fluid	The brain is hyperosmolar with respect to plasma; water moves along the osmotic gradient
Composition of edema fluid	Net intracellular accumulation of water and sodium	Ultrafiltrate of plasma	Cerebrospinal fluid	Extracellular greater than intracellular
Location of edema	Gray and white matter	White matter principally	Periventricular white matter	White matter
Extracellular fluid volume	Decreased	Increased	Increased	Increased
Typical etiology	Anoxia, diabetic ketoacidosis, hepatic encephalopathy, hypothermia, infarction or ischemia, infection, meningitis, Reye's syndrome, trauma, water intoxication	Brain tumors (primary and metastatic), abscess and encephalitis, infarction in the late stages, lead toxicity, trauma	Hydrocephalus	Hemodialysis, hypertensive crisis, syndrome of inappropriate antidiuretic hormone secretion, water intoxication
Response to therapy	Yes/no	Yes	Yes	Yes/no
Corticosteroids	Not effective	Yes	Not effective	Not effective
Diuretics	Transiently effective	Minimally or not effective	Transiently effective	Not effective
Other	Reversal of primary insult	Reversal of primary insult (e.g., removal of tumor)	Reversal of primary insult (e.g., ventriculoperitoneal shunt or third ventriculostomy)	Reversal of primary insult

ATPase, adenosine triphosphatase.

permeability produced by the protein was blocked by antibodies to the partially isolated protein. Secretion of the same protein was subsequently shown to occur in several systemic and CNS tumors.[28-30] Bruce and colleagues and Heiss and associates demonstrated that vascular permeability is increased by conditioned media from cultures of high-grade gliomas and meningiomas, the types of human brain tumors that most commonly produce clinically significant cerebral edema. In addition, they demonstrated that antibodies to VPF/VEGF block the permeability-enhancing effects of conditioned media from tumor types that produce cerebral edema and showed that glucocorticoids block the permeability-enhancing effects of VPF/VEGF on the vessel wall and inhibit tumor cell production of VPF/VEGF.[29,31] CNS tumors that are frequently associated with marked edema, such as glioblastomas, meningiomas, and metastases, are found to contain high levels of VPF/VEGF gene expression, whereas the types of CNS tumors that are not commonly associated with significant cerebral edema do not usually produce levels of VPF/VEGF mRNA higher than found in normal brain.[30] In clinical studies, the concept that VPF/VEGF is a principal mediator of peritumoral edema is confirmed by the reduction in contrast enhancement (vascular permeability) and surrounding cerebral edema on imaging studies by treatment of glioblastoma patients with bevacizumab, an anti-VEGF antibody (Fig. 9-2).[32,33]

Cytotoxic Edema

Cytotoxic edema occurs after cerebral infarction or ischemia, meningitis, Reye's syndrome, trauma, seizures, and water intoxication. There are several distinct or overlapping mechanisms that

underlie cytotoxic cerebral edema. One common mechanism of cytotoxic edema associated with cerebral ischemia implicates a direct role for excess glutamate.[34-36] After hypoxia, neuronal swelling results from sodium influx through α-amino-3-hydroxy-5-methyl-4-isoxazole propionic acid (AMPA) receptors and kainite receptor activity and from influx of chloride ion and water, which enter passively.[34-36] The glial swelling associated with glutamate toxicity is due to enhanced sodium entry into astrocytes by glutamate transporter hyperactivity.[11,12,17,37] Combined neuronal and astrocytic swelling also involves a variety of additional and complementary mechanisms, including dysfunction of the sodium-potassium adenosine triphosphatase (Na^+,K^+-ATPase) pump, which permits sodium influx, and activation of the Na^+/H^+ and Cl^-/HCO_3^- exchangers and the $Na^+/K^+/2Cl^-$ cotransporter.[11,12,17,37] The altered extracellular potassium ion concentration that occurs, for example, with primary epilepsy or with seizures after ischemia causes swelling through the $Na^+/K^+/2Cl^-$ cotransporter.[38-40] The same transmitter, because it passively allows passage of ammonium ions, has been implicated in the cerebral edema associated with hepatic encephalopathy. Aquaporin-4, a member of the family of aquaporin water channels, is enriched in astroglial end-feet and appears to play a central role in the entry of water into astrocytes.[41-43] Furthermore, the Kir4.1 potassium channel that colocalizes with aquaporin-4 regulates the extracellular potassium concentration. Elevated levels of potassium ions passing through Kir4.1 channels depolarize astrocytes (as they do neurons), which enhances astroglial uptake of sodium and bicarbonate through the Na^+/HCO_3^- cotransporter.[19] This increases intracellular osmolarity and allows water to move passively into the cell through

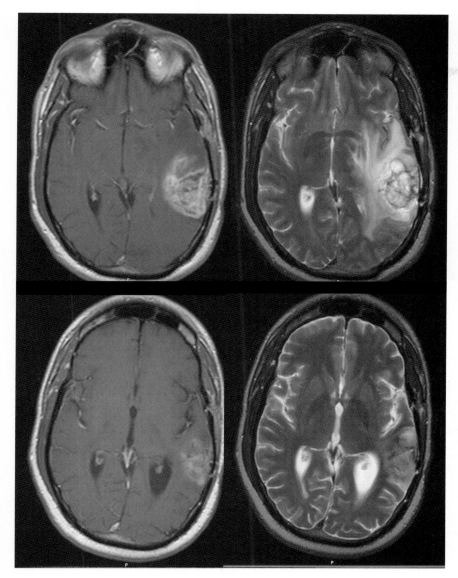

FIGURE 9-2 Effects of treatment with an antibody to vascular endothelial growth factor on the contrast enhancement of a glioblastoma and the surrounding cerebral edema. Magnetic resonance imaging (MRI) in the *upper* set of images was performed before treatment, and MRI in the *lower* set of images was performed 4 weeks after beginning therapy. T1-weighted MRI with contrast enhancement is shown on the *left* and T2-weighted MRI on the *right*. (Courtesy of Dr. David Schiff, Department of Neurology, University of Virginia School of Medicine.)

aquaporin-4 channels. Aquaporin-1 and aquaporin-4 are overexpressed in primary and secondary brain tumors and enhance water uptake.[41-43]

Other mechanisms that lead to or enhance cytotoxic edema occur after hypoxic, ischemic, or traumatic brain injury. Loss of intracellular ATP and glutamate release enhance the influx of calcium ions. Efflux of one calcium ion is associated with the uptake of three sodium ions, which potentiates the osmotic gradient and draws more water into the cell. Excess intracellular calcium ions can initiate apoptosis, activate inflammatory cascades through activation of immediate early genes such as *c-fos* and *c-jun*, and generate the release of a variety of cytokines, free radicals, and proteases that act on surrounding neuronal and glial cells, the extracellular matrix, and the cerebral endothelium.[17,36,37,44-46] Furthermore, nitric oxide (NO), which serves as a vasodilator but may also exert toxic effects through interactions with superoxide anions to generate peroxynitrite anions ($ONOO^-$), may exacerbate cerebral edema in certain circumstances.[47] NO is synthesized by nitric oxide synthase (NOS), which has three distinct forms. Neuronal NOS produces toxic

free radicals early after cytotoxic injury; endothelial NOS produces NO that enhances blood flow through vasodilation; and inducible NOS, produced by macrophages and microglia, can exacerbate injury through generation of NO—and free radicals—24 to 48 hours after the initiating insult has passed.[3,47]

Inflammation may also figure prominently in disruption of the BBB. For example, inflammatory cascades enhance the expression of bradykinin, substance P, leukotrienes, serotonin, and histamine, all of which nonselectively open the BBB to varying degrees.[3,5,48] Lipopolysaccharides, released during infection, induce the production of tumor necrosis factor and reactive oxygen species from microglia with potent effects on BBB permeability and can worsen cytotoxic injury.[3,5,11] Finally, Simard and coworkers recently identified an NCCA, nonselective cation channel or NCCa-ATP channel, that when opened by depletion of ATP, causes cytotoxic edema associated with ischemia. This channel is regulated by sulfonylurea receptor 1, which can be blocked by low doses of glibenclamide and thus provides a potential new approach to treat cerebral edema associated with cerebral infarction and brain trauma.[49-51]

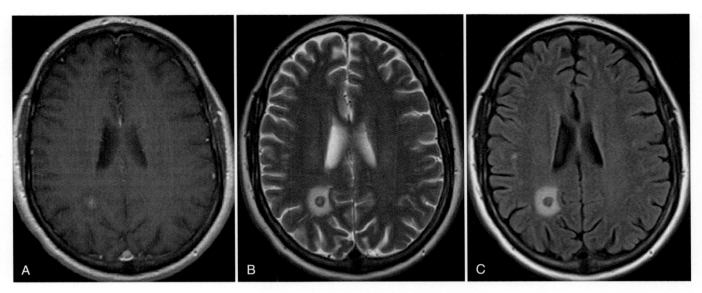

FIGURE 9-3 Imaging of vasogenic edema. **A,** Axial T1-weighted, gadolinium-enhanced magnetic resonance imaging (MRI) showing an enhancing 1-cm-diameter metastatic tumor (lung cancer primary) with surrounding vasogenic edema seen on T2-weighted (**B**) and fluid-attenuated inversion recovery (**C**) MRI.

NEUROIMAGING STUDIES AND CLASSIFICATION OF CEREBRAL EDEMA

The principal types of cerebral edema—cytotoxic, interstitial, and vasogenic—can be characterized in patients, at least to some degree, through neuroimaging studies, especially magnetic resonance imaging (MRI) (Figs. 9-3 to 9-5; see Fig. 9-2).[52-54]

In vasogenic edema (see Figs. 9-2 and 9-3), the edematous tissue is hypodense with respect to normal brain on both non–contrast-enhanced computed tomography and T1-weighted MRI. This feature is highlighted after the administration of contrast material.[53] On imaging, the edema primarily affects the white matter and tends to spare the gray matter, unlike cytotoxic edema. T2-weighted and fluid-attenuated inversion recovery (FLAIR) sequences accentuate the appearance of vasogenic edema and can, in FLAIR sequences, distinguish edema from normal brain water content, such as CSF. FLAIR images, in particular, are also useful to demonstrate the extent of tumor cell migration beyond the enhancing bulk of tumor because these MRI sequences are especially sensitive to the changes in brain water content induced by migrating or invading cells. Because vasogenic edema is primarily extracellular, the interstitial spaces also appear enlarged, a feature that increases the apparent diffusion coefficient (ADC) on diffusion studies.[52,53] MRI perfusion sequences can also demonstrate the enhanced vascularity and permeability associated with tumor angiogenesis, alone or with provocative testing, such as with the administration of dexamethasone.[23] Finally, dynamic, contrast-enhanced MRI can be used to quantify the permeability of the BBB and assess the effects of treatments that target the BBB.[53,54]

Cytotoxic edema, found in patients with ischemic (see Fig. 9-4) or hemorrhagic stroke and traumatic brain injury,[55,56] induces a rapid intracellular influx of water because of energy failure that evolves clinically and neuroradiographically.[52] Within 12 hours, there is loss of the visible gray-white junction and gyral edema, and at 12 to 24 hours, T2-weighted images show hyperintensity. The changes in diffusion-weighted MRI signal intensity may occur rapidly (within minutes after the insult); acute infarcts have a lower ADC than normal brain does, and these ADC maps sensitively indicate early cytotoxic edema.[42]

TREATMENT OF CEREBRAL EDEMA

Most current treatments of cerebral edema are indirect and focused on amelioration of the effects of edema, whereas more specific treatments are directed at the causative disease or condition (see Table 9-2).[21] For cytotoxic, osmotic, and interstitial edema, the main therapeutic intervention is to reverse the cause. In interstitial edema, resolution of transependymal CSF flow requires temporary or permanent diversion of spinal fluid (see Fig. 9-5). In vasogenic edema, the volume of extracellular fluid is a function of the relative rates of production and resorption of extracellular fluid. Higher pressure within the tumor and permeable tumor vessels initiates hydrostatic flow away from the tumor margin and into the extracellular space surrounding it until it reaches (convects to) the ventricles and subarachnoid spaces. There are dynamic limits to resorption: local capillaries absorb extracellular fluid slowly (estimated at 0.0086 mL/hr/cm³), and normal astrocytic cells have a defined capacity to absorb extravasated protein, ions, and water.[5,19,21,57-59] These resorptive mechanisms may often be overwhelmed when the BBB is defective and are not generally capable, without adjunctive methods, of handling the amount of extracellular fluid commonly produced with most tumor types.[58-61]

Several agents, including glucocorticoids, diuretics, and mannitol and other osmotic agents (reviewed in detail elsewhere[21]), have a moderate effect when used to control peritumoral edema. Although ineffective for cytotoxic edema and only modestly but transiently efficacious in the short-term treatment of interstitial edema, glucocorticoids can improve the neurological symptoms and signs caused by vasogenic edema, especially in patients with brain tumors, in whom the clinical features often result from the mass contributed by the peritumoral edema. Experimental evidence indicates that the effects of glucocorticoids are primarily reduced vascular permeability of vessels rather than reduced VEGF production.[26,31] This inhibition of the effects of VPF/VEGF on the vasculature is associated with interference of VEGF's action on vessels and requires the glucocorticoid receptor.[26,31] Thus, the effects of steroids in tumor-induced vasogenic edema is to restrict permeability of the BBB to macromolecules. By contrast, steroids are not effective when the BBB is not functional.[3,26,31,58]

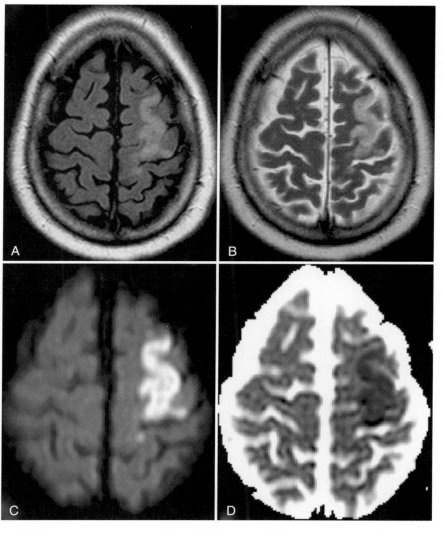

FIGURE 9-4 Imaging of cytotoxic edema. A 55-year-old man suffered an embolic stroke that affected the left cerebral hemisphere. Axial fluid-attenuated inversion recovery (FLAIR) (**A**) and T2-weighted magnetic resonance imaging (MRI) (**B**) demonstrate a small acute cortical infarct in the left superior frontal gyrus that is hyperintense on FLAIR and T2-weighted MRI. **C,** On the diffusion-weighted image, this same tissue is also hyperintense. **D,** The corresponding apparent diffusion coefficient (ADC) map demonstrates that the affected parenchyma has a low ADC, thus indicating that the infarct is acute. The shift of extracellular water to the intracellular space with cytotoxic edema restricts the random diffusion of water molecules into the tissue, hence a low ADC.

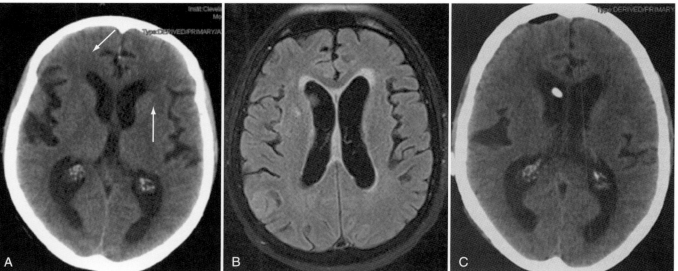

FIGURE 9-5 Imaging of interstitial edema in an adult with hydrocephalus. **A,** Axial, non–contrast-enhanced computed tomography (CT) shows hypodense areas of edematous brain produced by cerebrospinal fluid (CSF) passing into the periventricular white matter. **B,** This is prominently also seen with fluid-attenuated inversion recovery magnetic resonance imaging, where the CSF within the ventricular system is dark and the interstitial brain edema surrounding the ependyma is bright. **C,** Postoperative CT performed the day after placement of a ventriculoperitoneal shunt demonstrates a reduction in the hypodense, periventricular interstitial edema.

Diuretics, such as the loop diuretic furosemide, act by inducing systemic dehydration, which may reverse osmotic flow. This therapeutic effect is limited in time and efficacy.[21] The carbonic anhydrase inhibitor acetazolamide decreases CSF production by reducing hydrogen and bicarbonate production. Like diuretics, acetazolamide's efficacy is modest and short in duration, and systemic metabolic derangements may occur.[21] Osmotic agents such as glycerol, mannitol, hypertonic saline, and urea create an osmotic gradient between the brain and blood, down which extracellular water flows.[21] Because this activity is limited temporally, osmotherapy is generally reserved for settings of acute edema with mass effect and is used as a temporary measure to provide time for the initiation of definitive treatment to eliminate the cause of the edema. Furthermore, prolonged use of osmotic agents can lead to the accumulation of solute (mannitol, glycerol) within the tissues, which can then serve as a "reverse sink" and produce a circumstance in which the edema is refractory to further osmotic therapy. Agents such as mannitol or hypertonic saline may also have other actions, such as vasoconstriction, enhanced cerebral blood flow, and altered rheology, among others, that can alter the content or effect of edema. Many free radical scavengers and neuroprotective agents that have shown promise in the laboratory or in animal models have generally failed in human trials. Whether new agents that modulate the activity of aquaporins, corticotropin-releasing hormone, sulfonylurea receptor 1, or other pathways will prove effective awaits new human trials.[62-64] New agents that can mitigate the secondary neural damage caused by cerebral edema and can do so without the side effects of the current therapies are clearly needed.

SUGGESTED READINGS

Abbott NJ. Astrocyte-endothelial interactions and blood-brain barrier permeability. *J Anat.* 2002;200:629-638.

Abbott NJ, Ronnback, L, Hansson E. Astrocyte-endothelial interactions at the blood-brain barrier. *Nat Rev Neurosci.* 2006;7:41-53.

Al-Okaili RN, Krejza J, Wang S, et al. Advanced MR imaging techniques in the diagnosis of intraaxial brain tumors in adults. *Radiographics.* 2006;26(suppl 1): S173-S189.

Amiry-Moghaddam M, Ottersen OP. The molecular basis of water transport in the brain. *Nat Rev Neurosci.* 2003;4:991-1001.

Ballabh P, Braun A, Nedergaard M. The blood-brain barrier: an overview: structure, regulation, and clinical implications. *Neurobiol Dis.* 2004;16:1-13.

Hawkins BT, Davis TP. The blood-brain barrier/neurovascular unit in health and disease. *Pharmacol Rev.* 2005;57:173-185.

Heiss JD, Papavassiliou E, Merrill MJ, et al. Mechanism of dexamethasone suppression of brain tumor-associated vascular permeability in rats. Involvement of the glucocorticoid receptor and vascular permeability factor. *J Clin Invest.* 1996;98:1400-1408.

Kaal EC, Vecht CJ. The management of brain edema in brain tumors. *Curr Opin Oncol.* 2004;16:593-600.

King LS, Kozono D, Agre P. From structure to disease: the evolving tale of aquaporin biology. *Nat Rev Mol Cell Biol.* 2004;5:687-698.

Manley GT, Fujimura M, Ma T, et al. Aquaporin-4 deletion in mice reduces brain edema after acute water intoxication and ischemic stroke. *Nat Med.* 2000;6:159-163.

Marmarou A, Signoretti S, Fatouros PP, et al. Predominance of cellular edema in traumatic brain swelling in patients with severe head injuries. *J Neurosurg.* 2006;104:720-730.

Merrill MJ, Oldfield EH. A reassessment of vascular endothelial growth factor in central nervous system pathology. *J Neurosurg.* 2005;103:853-868.

Schlageter KE, Molnar P, Lapin GD, et al. Microvessel organization and structure in experimental brain tumors: microvessel populations with distinctive structural and functional properties. *Microvas Res.* 1999;58:312-328.

Seifert G, Shilling K, Steinhauser C. Astrocyte dysfunction in neurological disorders: a molecular perspective. *Nat Rev Neurosci.* 2006;7:194-206.

Senger DR, Galli SJ, Dvorak AM, et al. Tumor cells secrete a vascular permeability factor that promotes accumulation of ascites fluid. *Science.* 1983;219:983-985

Simard JM, Chen M, Tarasov KV, et al. Newly expressed SUR1-regulated NC(Ca-ATP) channel mediates cerebral edema after ischemic stroke. *Nat Med.* 2006;12:433-440.

Strange K. Cellular volume homeostasis. *Adv Physiol Educ.* 2004;28:155-159.

Wolburg H, Lippolt A. Tight junctions of the blood-brain barrier: development, composition, and regulation. *Vasc Pharmacol.* 2002;38:323-337.

Yong VW. Metalloproteinases: mediators of pathology and regeneration in the CNS. *Nat Rev Neurosci.* 2005;6:931-944.

Full references can be found on Expert Consult @ www.expertconsult.com

normal infants have PVIs below 10 mL, and the adult PVI of 25 mL is reached at around 14 years of age.

PVI can be measured clinically by infusion or withdrawal of small boluses of fluid in the CSF space, with concomitant measures of the pressure response. CSF outflow resistance can also be calculated from the rate decay of the pressure peak after a bolus infusion. A complete description of resistance measurement techniques is found in the report of Eklund and colleagues.[53] Methods of continuous PVI measurement have been devised with use of multiple time-averaged small-volume pulses.[54] Although these methods generate less pressure perturbation, they tend to underestimate compliance as measured with the conventional technique.

The compensatory abilities of brain, blood, and CSF at any given point on the pressure-volume curve are dependent on their respective volumes, their ease of egress from the skull, and the level of ICP at which the interactions are occurring, coupled with the rigidity of the skull. Although the brain occupies 80% of the intracranial space, this volume is effectively available for compensation only when increases in V_{OTHER} occur slowly. With more rapid changes, brain shifts and herniations are more likely to occur. Although blood and CSF occupy less of the intracranial space, their total volume can be reduced more rapidly.

These concepts become more complex, as do most models, when they are applied to clinical practice. Although short-term changes cause movement along a single pressure-volume curve, changing intracranial dynamics can create a new pressure-volume curve with time (Fig. 10-6B). Increases in CBV and cerebral edema are also likely to play a role in producing these dynamic pressure-volume interactions.[55] Thus, knowledge of the absolute pressure coupled with some expression of the slope of the ICP volume curve at any given time point provides a more complete description of the stability or instability of ICP.

Effects of Elevated Intracranial Pressure

Under non–steady-state conditions, failure of compensation mechanisms ultimately results in an elevated ICP, the pathologic consequences of which can be severe. First, continued perfusion of the brain relies on a cerebral arteriovenous pressure gradient. ICP is transmitted to the compliant cerebral veins, and therefore the cerebral perfusion pressure (CPP) is defined as the arterial inflow pressure minus ICP. If ICP increases, CPP falls; and if the lower limit of autoregulation is exhausted, CBF will begin to fall.

The autoregulatory reserve may be defined as the difference between the CPP at a given moment and the lower limit of autoregulation. Considering that the lower limit of autoregulation is within the range of 50 to 70 mm Hg, the autoregulatory reserve for a CPP of 90 would be 20 to 40 mm Hg. Thus, a CPP below the autoregulatory threshold exhausts the autoregulatory reserve.[56-60] When CPP decreases, the wall tension of reactive brain vessels decreases, thereby increasing the transmission of the arterial pulse wave to the intracranial contents.[61] Similarly, when a reduction of CPP is caused by increased ICP, brain compliance decreases,[29,62] which also serves to increase pulsatile transmission. Taken in concert, a decrease in CPP results in an increase of both blood pressure and ICP pulsatility. This relationship is highly predictive for fatal outcome[63] because as the ICP pulse amplitude levels off or starts to decrease, it implies that the cerebral vessels are no longer pressure reactive.

By use of these principles, it is clear that the correlation between spontaneous waves of blood pressure and ICP is dependent on the autoregulatory reserve. The correlation coefficient between changes in blood pressure and ICP is defined by Czosnyka[61] as the pressure reactivity index. An example of the use of the pressure reactivity index is illustrated in Figure 10-7. Examples of time-related changes of the pressure reactivity index are shown, in which the index increases from relatively low values

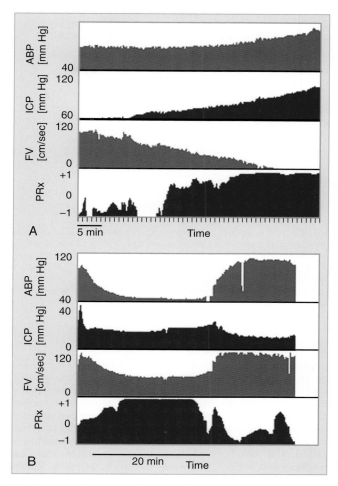

FIGURE 10-7 Examples of the use of the pressure reactivity index to assess autoregulatory reserve and to predict patient outcome. **A,** Mean arterial blood pressure (ABP), ICP, middle cerebral artery flow velocity (FV), and pressure reactivity index (PRx) in a patient with a fatal increase in ICP. The pressure reactivity index rises with ICP increase and remains high. **B,** Comparable data from a patient experiencing a plateau wave in ICP with subsequent recovery. It is notable how the pressure reactivity index falls with recovery and reduction in ICP. *(Courtesy of M. Czosnyka.)*

(no association) to values approaching 1.0 (strong positive association). These values were calculated from a period of 1-hour terminal increase in ICP from 60 to 90 mm Hg in a head-injured patient who died (Fig. 10-7A). Figure 10-7B illustrates a transient change in pressure reactivity index during the period of an ICP plateau wave with rapid recovery when ICP returned to baseline. In summary, the pressure reactivity index provides a practical means of assessing the degree of autoregulation and is useful in elucidating the contribution of the cerebrovasculature to mechanisms causing ICP rise.

Furthermore, in many pathologic cases, autoregulation is disturbed so that the response curve is shifted to the right and is more linear (Fig. 10-8). This reduces the autoregulatory reserve for any given CPP. If the autoregulatory reserve is exhausted, CBF begins to fall, which ultimately causes tissue ischemia. Ischemia creates cytotoxic edema, which, in turn, contributes to the ICP elevation and low CPP. Clearly, a vicious circle of edema and ICP elevation can ensue if treatment attempts do not prevent this. A marked rise in ICP that will not respond to available treatments is called refractory ICP.

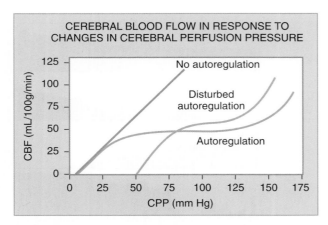

FIGURE 10-8 Cerebral autoregulatory curves. Normal autoregulation maintains cerebral blood flow across a range of mean arterial blood pressure. Disturbed autoregulation causes a shift of the curve to the right and introduces a more linear component (i.e., cerebral blood flow is less stable with rising mean arterial blood pressure). If autoregulation is completely abolished, cerebral blood flow rises linearly with mean arterial blood pressure.

A second problem with increased ICP arises from the generation of pressure gradients.[64,65] CSF will conduct the pressure generated by an increased volume in one region of the brain to others. There are specific anatomic sites where such pressure gradients may cause movement of brain tissue into an abnormal anatomic location—so-called herniation. Several types of herniation have been described, including downward transtentorial (central and uncal), subfalcine, upward transtentorial, and transforaminal.[66] Each syndrome has a characteristic clinical correlate.

Anatomically, in central transtentorial herniation, downward shift of the hemisphere and basal ganglia compresses and displaces the diencephalon through the tentorial incisura. Subsequent displacement of the brainstem will stretch the paramedian branches of the basilar artery, which, in turn, will contribute to the marked diencephalon and brainstem dysfunction. In uncal herniation, the uncus and hippocampal gyrus shift medially into the tentorial notch, which distorts the brainstem and creates significant dysfunction. Subfalcine herniation of the cingulate gyrus is caused by expansion of one hemisphere causing a movement of the cingulate gyrus under the falx cerebri. Cingulate herniation may compress the internal cerebral veins or the ipsilateral anterior cerebral artery. Lesions in the posterior fossa differ slightly in that they may cause upward transtentorial herniation as well as downward transforaminal herniation.

Symptoms and Signs of Elevated Intracranial Pressure

The degree of effect of a given ICP depends greatly on the nature and anatomic location of the underlying pathologic condition. The cardinal symptoms and signs of raised ICP include headache, vomiting, and papilledema. Vomiting without any associated nausea is especially suggestive of intracranial disease. Varying degrees of cranial nerve palsies may arise as a result of pressure on brainstem nuclei (particularly abducens palsies). Papilledema is a reliable and objective measure of raised ICP, with good specificity. However, its sensitivity is observer dependent, and symptoms suggestive of intracranial disease in the absence of papilledema should not be ignored.

Vital signs may also change under conditions of elevated ICP. The Cushing response, defined as arterial hypertension and bradycardia, arises as a result of either generalized central nervous system ischemia or local ischemia due to pressure on the brainstem.[67] Bradycardia is possibly mediated by the vagus nerve and can occur independently of hypertension. Abnormal respiration may also arise,[68] depending in part on the anatomic location of any lesion. Cheyne-Stokes respiration arises from damage to the diencephalic region, and sustained hyperventilation occurs in patients with dysfunction of the midbrain and upper pons.[69] Midpontine lesions cause slow respiration; pontomedullary lesions result in ataxic respirations; upper medullary lesions cause rapid, shallow breathing; and with greater medullary involvement, ataxic breathing predominates.

Herniation Syndromes

Tissue herniation is the most serious complication of raised ICP. Central herniation and uncal herniation cause the central syndrome and the uncal syndrome, respectively.[70] The central syndrome displays progressive dysfunction of structures in a rostral to caudal direction. Diencephalic structures are involved early, which may cause a change in behavior or even loss of consciousness. Diencephalic involvement also alters respiration, causing interruptions of sighing, yawning, or pausing; Cheyne-Stokes respiration may appear. Pupils become small, with a poor reactivity to light. A unilateral lesion can cause contralateral hemiparesis, with ipsilateral paratonia and decorticate responses. With progressive midbrain involvement, respiration becomes tachypneic, and the pupils fall into a midline fixed position. Internuclear ophthalmoplegia may arise, and motor examination will show bilateral decerebrate posturing. As the pons becomes involved, respiration remains rapid and shallow. Motor examination reveals flaccid extremities with bilateral extensor plantar responses. With progressive medullary involvement, respiration slows and becomes irregular with prolonged sighs or gasps. As hypoxia ensues, the pupils dilate, and brain death follows shortly thereafter.

In sharp contrast, the uncal syndrome often begins with a unilaterally dilated and poorly reactive pupil, which can arise even in the presence of a normal conscious level. The pupil will then fully dilate with external oculomotor ophthalmoplegia. If midbrain compression ensues, consciousness may be impaired, followed by contralateral decerebrate posturing. On occasion, posturing or hemiparesis may occur ipsilateral to the lesion as a result of pressure on the contralateral cerebral peduncle on the edge of the tentorium cerebelli.[71] If the uncal syndrome is allowed to progress, extensor plantar response appears bilaterally, along with dilation of the contralateral pupil. Finally, patients will develop hyperpnea, midposition pupils, impaired oculovestibular response, and bilateral decerebrate rigidity. From this point, progression is as for the central syndrome.

Other compression and herniation syndromes may arise, including unilateral hemiparesis and hemianesthesia with compression of cortical structures or compression of the anterior cerebral artery with subfalcine herniation of the cingulate gyrus causing contralateral leg weakness. Although no less distressing for the patient, these symptoms represent a much lesser emergency than either the central or uncal syndrome does.

INTRACRANIAL PRESSURE MONITORING

Several published clinical trials show that monitoring of ICP, under situations in which ICP may be high, either facilitates outcome or promotes aggressive management.[72-74] There is strong clinical evidence that careful control of ICP is important,[75] and maintaining CPP under many different pathologic circumstances is of benefit for outcome.[60] An understanding of the

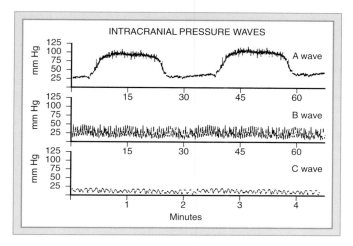

FIGURE 10-9 Lundberg's classification of ICP waves. A waves or plateau waves are prolonged stable increases in ICP that spontaneously recover to a new higher baseline. B waves are short, modest elevations in ICP, and C waves are rapid sinusoidal fluctuations. These waves do not represent part of steady-state ICP dynamics. Their pathologic significance remains to be defined.

indications for initiation of monitoring and the methods by which this can be done is important.

Initial work on direct monitoring of ICP by ventricular puncture was performed by Guillaume and Janny[4] and by Lundberg.[5] In Lundberg's classic report, he described three basic patterns of ICP waveform: A waves (plateau waves), B waves, and C waves (Fig. 10-9).

A waves, or plateau waves, are characterized by increases of ICP that are sustained for several minutes and then return spontaneously to a new baseline, which is usually slightly higher than the preceding one. Lundberg postulated that A waves are a result of an increase in cerebrovascular blood volume due to vasodilation. Rosner[76,77] has postulated that these plateau waves are a normal compensatory response to decreases in CPP, and therefore effective management involves the use of vasopressors. Other more recent studies have suggested that vasopressors may enhance lesion size and edema formation.[78,79] The plateau wave itself is proposed to consist of four phases, called the drift phase, the plateau phase, the ischemic response phase, and the resolution phase.[76] The drift phase is characterized by a decline in CPP, which triggers vasodilation. This vasodilation increases ICP to the plateau level, for the plateau phase. This sudden reduction in CPP causes a degree of cerebral ischemia that triggers brainstem vasomotor centers to mount a Cushing response (ischemic response phase), which, in turn, restores CPP in the resolution phase.

Lundberg B waves are short elevations of a modest nature (10 to 20 mm Hg) that occur at a frequency of 0.5 to 2 Hz and are thought to relate to vasodilation secondary to respiratory fluctuations in $Paco_2$. However, they are seen in ventilated patients, who in theory should have a constant $Paco_2$; therefore, they are of only questionable clinical significance. Transcranial Doppler studies in humans have shown that B waves occur secondary to intracranial vasomotor waves, causing variations in CBF.[80] The physiologic basis for this cyclic change in vasomotor tone is not clear. B waves are believed to reflect increased ICP in a qualitative manner, as is the case with C waves, which are more rapid sinusoidal fluctuations occurring approximately every 10 seconds, corresponding to Traube-Hering-Mayer fluctuations in arterial pressure.

The decision to monitor a patient's ICP is based on the premise that intracranial hypertension reduces CPP both focally and globally and can cause ischemia. The final result of elevated ICP is brain herniation and death, the imminent onset of which can be detected clinically. By monitoring ICP, such problems can be detected and treated much earlier. Furthermore, indiscriminate application of therapy for ICP reduction can be avoided, and if a ventriculostomy is used, there is the added advantage of being able to treat with CSF drainage. These advantages must be weighed against the possible complications of invasive monitoring.

Intracranial hypertension is found in 40% to 60% of severe head injuries and is a major factor in the deaths of 50% of all fatalities.[81] Data from the Traumatic Coma Data Bank have shown that the proportion of hourly ICP recordings above 20 mm Hg is highly significant in predicting outcome.[82] The role of ICP monitoring in adult brain trauma is clear; however, the role in nontraumatic settings depends on the nature and severity of the disease process. Management of intracranial hypertension may be beneficial in Reye's syndrome[83] and other causes of fulminant hepatic failure,[84] although the complication rate is higher in these conditions.[85] In the case of intracranial tumors, ventricular catheters can provide temporary therapeutic ventricular decompression before and after resection of the tumor along with a rational means of testing the reestablishment of normal CSF pathways in the early postoperative period. The role of monitoring in metabolic encephalopathies, cerebral infarction, or diffuse cerebritis is less clear.

After trauma in adults, guidelines for ICP monitoring include a Glasgow Coma Scale score of 3 to 8 and an abnormal computed tomographic scan. In the presence of a normal computed tomographic scan, two or more of the following should prompt monitoring anyway: age older than 40 years, unilateral or bilateral motor posturing, or systolic blood pressure below 90 mm Hg.[86] Patients with a Glasgow Coma Scale score greater than 8 may benefit from ICP monitoring if computed tomographic scans demonstrate significant mass lesions or treatment is required for associated injuries.

METHODS OF INTRACRANIAL PRESSURE MEASUREMENT

Ventriculostomy coupled with a pressure transducer remains the "gold standard" for monitoring of ICP because of accuracy and ease of calibration. Access to CSF for dynamic testing and drainage to control ICP are additional benefits. Disadvantages are that catheter placement can be difficult when the ventricles are small or shifted from the midline, and the risk of infection rises in ventriculostomies after 5 days, although this risk can be lessened by tunneling the catheter under the skin. Current estimates have associated intraventricular monitoring with less than 2% hemorrhagic complications[87] and less than 10% infective complications.[88-91] Changing the catheter at regular intervals does not appear to reduce the infection rate.[89] Parenchymal monitors, in contrast, have less than 1% infective complications.[73]

Alternative methods of monitoring ICP include the subarachnoid bolt,[92] subdural catheter, epidural transducer,[93] and fiberoptic microtransducer.[94] The bolt and epidural transducer, although less invasive, are prone to inaccuracy because of their physical characteristics.[95-97] Fiberoptic catheter-transducers cannot be recalibrated externally; however, their accuracy in practice has proved excellent,[98] they are easy to place, and the complication rate is low because of their small size and lack of fluid coupling. All intraparenchymal monitors may be prone to regional inaccuracy, depending on their placement in relation to the site of any lesion,[99] given that elevated ICP may be regional. The choice of which measurement method to use should be based on the presentation of the patient and the planned treatment. There is no defined reference level for the use of transducers in the intensive care unit; however, the device is typically zeroed at the level of the foramen of Monro, using the external acoustic meatus as an anatomic landmark.

There is no uniform agreement about the critical level of ICP beyond which treatment is mandatory. Saul and Ducker[74] demonstrated benefits by treating ICP above 15 mm Hg compared with a group of patients treated for ICP above 25 mm Hg. Marmarou and colleagues[82] examined data from 428 patients and calculated the ICP threshold most predictive of 6-month outcome by logistic regression. The threshold that correlated best was 20 mm Hg, and this is the current level at which most centers begin treatment. Current opinion now regards CPP as the critical parameter that should be monitored in concert with ICP.

MANAGEMENT OF INTRACRANIAL PRESSURE

Logically, the best therapy for intracranial hypertension is resolution of the cause of the increased pressure. However, when this is not possible, manipulation of the system by other means can lower ICP. No one therapy or series of therapies is appropriate for all cases of elevated ICP, and treatment strategy should be constantly reevaluated in the face of a dynamically changing pathologic condition.

The equation

$$V_{CSF} + V_{BLOOD} + V_{BRAIN} + V_{OTHER} = V_{INTRACRANIAL\ SPACE}$$

provides a conceptual framework by which to consider the components of intracranial volume responsible for non–steady-state ICP situations and allows treatment to be directed in a focused manner (Table 10-2).

V_{CSF}

When hydrocephalus causes intracranial hypertension and its cause cannot be eradicated, temporary or permanent CSF diversion may be necessary. When obstruction of the CSF pathways by a tumor or other mass causes the hydrocephalus, it is usually possible, and indeed preferable, to treat the obstruction in an effort to open the CSF pathways.

If CSF diversion is required, options exist that permit temporary external drainage (ventriculostomy), temporary internal drainage (ventriculosubgaleal shunt), or permanent internal drainage (ventriculoperitoneal shunt, ventriculoatrial shunt, or third ventriculostomy). External ventriculostomy has value as a method for both measuring and controlling ICP, and the technique can be especially helpful in deciding whether a permanent internal drainage procedure will be of benefit. One approach to this includes CSF drainage against minimal resistance early on with eventual elevation of the drip chamber to a level commensurate with physiologic ICP. Pressure is monitored continuously, and CSF is allowed to escape when threshold ICP levels are exceeded. Maintenance of normal ICP and minimal volumes of CSF drainage usually indicate that a permanent shunt will not be needed.

A ventriculosubgaleal shunt provides a closed, temporary method for continuous CSF diversion. It involves placement of a ventricular catheter attached to a reservoir (with or without a valve mechanism) with a short side arm opening into the subgaleal space, which is dissected at the time of surgery. The ventriculosubgaleal shunt provides continuous ventricular decompression for several weeks to months without the need for percutaneous aspiration of the reservoir.

Permanent internal CSF diversion by ventriculoperitoneal shunt is attended by a full array of indications, technical considerations, and risks. Third ventriculostomy by both stereotactic and endoscopic techniques has been repopularized recently.[100] This technique offers an alternative in certain situations without the potential risks inherent in standard ventriculoperitoneal shunting.

When mechanical methods of CSF diversion are not possible or desirable, adjunctive therapy with medications such as acetazolamide, furosemide, and corticosteroids can transiently decrease CSF production. Acetazolamide, which inhibits carbonic anhydrase–mediated CSF production, is used most frequently. Reductions of CSF production by 16% to 66% have been achieved.[24] Synergy has been reported when acetazolamide is combined with furosemide.[101] Acetazolamide also has a cerebral vasodilator effect, which may transiently worsen intracranial hypertension, and so its use is contraindicated in patients with closed head injury.[102]

TABLE 10-2 Therapeutic Modalities for the Reduction of Raised Intracranial Pressure by the Intracranial Compartment of Action*

V_{CSF}	V_{BLOOD}	V_{BRAIN}	V_{OTHER}
Acetazolamide	Hyperventilation	CPP management	Surgical evacuation
Furosemide	Head elevation	Lund protocol	Surgical decompression
Corticosteroids	Barbiturates	Antihypertensives	
External drainage (V)		Fluid resuscitation	
Internal drainage (VPS/VSGS)		Corticosteroids	
		Barbiturates	
		Osmotic agents (M, U, G)	
		Diuretics	
		Hypothermia	

*Although this table provides a conceptual framework, therapies often have multiple methods of action, not all of which can be shown. For example, barbiturates will reduce the metabolic demand of the brain and therefore lower CBF and CBV while reducing energy demand and therefore limiting edema (action at V_{BLOOD} and V_{CSF}).
G, glycerol; M, mannitol; U, urea; V, ventriculostomy; VPS, ventriculoperitoneal shunt; VSGS, ventriculosubgaleal shunt.

V~BLOOD~

The role of V_{BLOOD} in the pathologic process of ICP is complicated. Excess amounts of intracranial blood (hyperemia) can clearly contribute to reduced compliance and elevations in ICP. Other causes of intracranial hypertension, however, can occur at the expense of V_{BLOOD}, which can, in turn, cause ischemia and brain edema. There is no absolute blood volume or CBF that is normal; these parameters are rather defined by the metabolic activity of the brain itself. For example, the mean absolute CBF of 53 mL/100 g per minute in normal subjects may be considered hyperemic in the anesthetized brain or ischemic in a portion of epileptic cortex.

In general terms, most of the CBV resides within the pial vessels and veins; however, the precapillary arterioles control CBF. Relationships among the various factors that reflect the status of CBF are complex and vary according to the timing of measurements, underlying pathologic process, presence or absence of hypoxia or ischemia, systemic blood pressure, ICP, cerebral metabolic rate, and arterial blood gases.

Extremes of CBF, both low and high, have been seen in patients with poor outcome after head injury.[103-106] Bouma and coworkers[107] showed that measurements of CBF performed within 6 hours of severe head trauma (Glasgow Coma Scale score ≤ 8) are reduced (22.5 ± 5.2 mL/l00 g per minute) and correlate well with Glasgow Coma Scale score and eventual outcome. These findings are more common in patients with bilateral diffuse injuries than in patients with mass lesions, who tend to have higher global CBF in the hemisphere of the mass lesion. Between 45% and 65% of head injury victims will exhibit hyperemia in the 12 to 24 hours after injury.[108-110] The increase in CBF is presumably accompanied by increased CBV, which may contribute to intracranial hypertension. Increased CBF and CBV are seen in the acute encephalopathy of Reye's syndrome as well. Clearly, ischemia and hyperemia are not constant phenomena but rather dynamically changing under the influence of several factors. In general, CBF tends to stabilize by 36 to 48 hours after injury.[103,105,108,111]

This complex interplay of factors affecting V_{BLOOD} makes rational treatment difficult. The association among CBF, cerebral metabolic rate of oxygen, arteriovenous oxygen difference, and clinical parameters (ICP, Glasgow Coma Scale score, and outcome) is more easily documented by multivariate analysis than it is explained in terms of physiologic cause and effect. In general terms, as ICP increases, arteriovenous oxygen difference usually rises because of reductions in venous P_{O_2} caused by greater oxygen extraction. CBV increases with vasodilation in response to lowered CPP or a rise in $Paco_2$. Hyperventilation therefore decreases total intracranial blood volume as hypocapnic vasoconstriction moves blood from the pial circulation to the veins and sinuses. Reductions of the cerebral metabolic rate of oxygen are seen after trauma, but these reductions may not reflect the energy demands of the injured brain. Some have attributed these reductions to mitochondrial incapacities or enzymatic deficits that render the neuron incapable of using oxygen.[107,112]

Understanding the role of CBF and CBV in situations of elevated ICP is hindered by difficulties in measuring CBF. Global CBF obtained by the Kety-Schmidt method includes the white matter but lacks anatomic information. Regional CBF determined by the xenon Xe 133 inhalation method largely ignores the contribution of the white matter, and focal areas of ischemia can be missed if they are surrounded by zones of relatively high flow.[113] Magnetic resonance imaging–based measures of cerebral perfusion may yield accurate anatomic information but suffer from a degree of time averaging and lack of widespread availability. A further problem relates to differential sensitivities of structures to reduced flow. For example, the hippocampus may be acutely sensitive to even mild ischemia, whereas diminished

CBF in the brainstem does not correlate with clinical estimates of brainstem function.[58]

Although every effort should be made to prevent cerebral ischemia in the face of intracranial hypertension, treatment of hyperemia or increased CBV may be dangerous until more is understood about these pathophysiologic processes. However, some success has been reported with therapy that reduces CBV.[114,115] The most efficacious methods are hyperventilation and elevation of the head. Hyperventilation causes constriction of pial vessels when blood vessels retain CO_2 responsivity. Pressure autoregulation is frequently lost after head injury; however, CO_2 responsivity can be preserved in the absence of pressure autoregulation, and its prolonged loss is considered a grave sign.[116] In adults, a 1-torr change in $Paco_2$ is associated with a 3% change in CBF. Thus, vasoconstriction reduces CBV and therefore lowers ICP.

In addition to its effects on cerebrovascular tone, hyperventilation induces tissue alkalosis, which can buffer the intracellular and CSF acidosis seen after severe head injury.[117] However, the benefits of hyperventilation may be short-lived, and higher levels can cause vasoconstriction sufficient to produce cerebral ischemia mediated through a mechanism that involves the loss of the CSF bicarbonate buffer.[118,119] In a randomized, prospective trial of head-injured patients, Muizelaar[115] showed that hyperventilation to a $Paco_2$ of 25 ± 2 in patients with a Glasgow motor scale of 4 or 5 resulted in Glasgow outcome scores at 6 months that were significantly worse than those in controls. Consequently, only moderate hyperventilation is necessary (32 to 35 torr), which is thought to be sufficient to avoid ischemic effects.

Some have advanced the concept of "inverse steal" to explain the risk of hyperventilation-induced ischemia. In patients with intact or supersensitive CO_2 responsivity, hypocapnia can lead to shunting of blood from high-resistance, maximally constricted vessels to low-resistance, dilated vessels that lack CO_2 responsivity.[120] These areas may be so severely damaged as to have low oxygen demand; thus, hyperventilation may tend to redistribute blood from viable tissue into nonviable tissue. When possible, these investigators recommend that arteriovenous oxygen difference and CBF be monitored along with ICP[121] and that hyperventilation be performed cautiously in patients with evidence of cerebral ischemia. When hyperventilation is discontinued, it should be tapered during 24 to 48 hours. Abrupt discontinuation can cause vasodilation as the extracellular pH falls, resulting in ICP elevations.[122,123]

Elevation of the head to 30 degrees decreases ICP by facilitating adequate venous drainage and possibly CSF drainage also. This degree of elevation does not alter CPP.[124] Feldman and associates[125] demonstrated the beneficial effects of head elevation on ICP clinically. In this study, CPP and CBF seemed unaffected by head position until the head was elevated to 60 degrees. Rotation of the head or flexion of the neck can also impair jugular venous flow and raise ICP.[126] Therefore, an effort should be made to maintain the head in a neutral position.

An intuitive mechanism by which CBV should be lowered is to lower mean arterial blood pressure and therefore CPP. This principle, coupled with a reduction of hydrostatic forces in damaged capillary beds, underlies the Lund protocol for raised ICP, which advocates reduced CPP, precapillary vasoconstriction with dihydroergotamine, and maintenance of plasma osmolarity with albumin infusion.[127] Initial clinical trials of this approach yielded outcomes no worse than those of more conventional techniques.[128]

This protocol, however, is in stark contrast to the principles of CPP management, which promulgate that low CPP stimulates arteriolar vasodilation, causing increases in both CBV and ICP. By elevation of CPP with vasopressors, the blood vessel will be stimulated by the mechanisms of pressure autoregulation to vasoconstrict, consequently reducing the CBV and ICP.[60] This argument appears to hold only when pressure autoregulation is intact. Rosner also proposes that in many cases in which loss of pressure autoregulation is seen, the mechanism is not lost; rather, the curve is shifted to the right (see Fig. 10-8). By giving pressors, the vessel is manipulated back into a state in which it can autoregulate. If this is true, the real challenge is presented in distinguishing those brains that will benefit from CPP management. The possible risks of pressor therapy in areas in which the blood-brain barrier may be incompetent are unresolved. Several studies have questioned the safety of their use[129] and demonstrated ways in which pathologic changes can be worsened.[78,79]

V~BRAIN~

The third component contributing to ICP is the volume occupied by brain tissue. Increases in V_{BRAIN} occur most frequently as a result of cerebral edema, which is a nonspecific reaction to a variety of processes. Conceptually, treatment of increased ICP due to brain edema is directed toward removal of the cause of edema, control of its propagation, and enhancement of its clearance. Efforts to decrease the formation of vasogenic edema include prevention of cerebrovascular hypertension and appropriate choice of fluid resuscitation.

Control of systemic and cerebrovascular hypertension is especially important when intracranial hypertension exists or when cerebral autoregulation is impaired. The choice of antihypertensive drugs in patients with increased ICP is important. Hirose and coworkers and others showed that nifedipine, chlorpromazine, and reserpine decreased mean arterial pressure and increased ICP, thereby reducing CPP.[130-132] These findings were more pronounced when ICP exceeded 40 mm Hg. In the same studies, thiopental decreased mean arterial pressure and ICP, leaving CPP unchanged, but caused respiratory depression, necessitating intubation and mechanical ventilation. Sodium nitroprusside is commonly used now for rapid control of blood pressure in adult critical care; however, despite its highly efficacious action, prolonged use is not considered safe because of a risk of cyanide ion toxicity.

In a laboratory study using inflated balloons to produce intracranial hypertension, sodium nitroprusside, nitroglycerin, and trimetaphan were used to reduce mean arterial pressure by 20%. All three drugs reduced regional CBF and CO_2 responsivity, leading the authors to recommend caution in their use for blood pressure control in patients with increased ICP. Propranolol has been shown to be superior to hydralazine for control of hypertension in head-injured patients because propranolol decreases both cardiac demands and serum levels of epinephrine and norepinephrine.[133]

The choice of fluid resuscitation in the head-injured patient is critical. Approximately 10% to 15% of head-injured patients are hypotensive because of either the injury itself or associated injuries.[134] Aggressive correction of shock improves survival and clinical outcome; however, the osmolality of the blood has important implications for ICP. Isotonic fluids (e.g., 5% dextrose, 0.45% normal saline, 0.9% normal saline, and lactated Ringer's solution) are in regular use, but hypotonic solutions have the potential to worsen cerebral edema. Hypertonic solutions have been advocated as a possible therapy for elevated ICP. Certainly, bolus doses of hypertonic saline appear to be beneficial[135]; however, fluid replacement therapy with hypertonic saline has been shown to be both beneficial and detrimental for ICP in different studies.[136,137]

Controversy exists as to whether colloids (molecular weight >8000 D) are more beneficial than crystalloids for fluid resuscitation. Some authors have found no difference, whereas Tranmer[138] showed a definite advantage with use of the colloid hetastarch. In a laboratory model of vasogenic edema, treatment with colloid for 2 hours after injury produced no change in ICP, whereas infusions of normal saline and 5% dextrose in water led to elevations in ICP of 91% and 141%, respectively.

In the case of cytotoxic injury, efforts to decrease formation of edema center around correction of the cause of disordered cell function. With toxins, this involves treatment directed toward the causative agent. When anoxia or ischemia is the cause, their reversal may bring improvement if the duration of anoxia and ischemia has not been prolonged.

A second goal of treating ICP is to improve neuronal and axonal function and survival. A variety of agents have been tried,[139-148] some of which were able to influence cerebral edema formation (for review, see Smith and colleagues[149]). Despite reasonable experimental success, no compound has yet been found to be of clinical benefit in limiting edema formation.

Steroids and barbiturates have been widely used for treatment of both vasogenic and cytotoxic edema; however, neither is wholly effective, and both have attendant problems. Steroids are of unquestionable value in the treatment of edema with brain tumors, but no definite benefits have been shown when they are used in patients with head injury.[150-155] A study has also indicated that the newer configurations of steroids, the 21-amino steroids or lazaroids, are also without beneficial effect in traumatic brain injury.[156] The mode of action of steroids in cerebral tumors is not clear, but dramatic effects on both edema[157] and function[158,159] can be seen. Corticosteroids have been shown to have widespread effects on membrane lipid hydrolysis and peroxidation, processes that are thought to be important for development of injury.[160-163]

Use of steroids in subarachnoid hemorrhage has no proven benefit, but angiographically demonstrable vasospasm can be decreased by their use.[164] In cases of cerebral ischemia, steroids worsen outcome either by means of a direct glucocorticoid toxicity or as a consequence of elevated serum glucose levels, which exacerbate ischemic lactic acidosis.[165,166]

Barbiturates are useful in a wide range of situations by decreasing the cerebral metabolic rate of oxygen, thus permitting tolerance of a degree of ischemia or anoxia not otherwise acceptable on the cellular level. This, in turn, lowers demand for CBF, which therefore tends to lower CBV and consequently ICP. Barbiturates seem to have maximal effect in situations in which CBF is greater than metabolism. In addition, Messeter and associates[167] have shown that preservation of cerebral CO_2 responsivity can predict the response of ICP to iatrogenic barbiturate coma. When CO_2 responsivity was normal, barbiturates reduced CBF and normalized ICP in 75% of patients. When this response was reduced or absent, CBF was unchanged or increased, and ICP was reduced in only 20% of patients. Pentobarbital has proved more effective at control of ICP than phenobarbital or thiopental sodium.

Barbiturates are effective at reducing ICP, but in many studies they have not been shown to improve outcome.[168] Even prophylactic use of barbiturates has not improved outcome or led to easier control of ICP.[169] Considering the risks of high-dose barbiturates, their application is most appropriate for patients in whom conventional measures to control ICP have failed. Usually, a bolus of pentobarbital (5 to 10 mg/kg) is administered during 30 minutes, followed by a continuous hourly maintenance infusion of 1 to 5 mg/kg to achieve a serum concentration of 3.5 to 4.5 mg/100 mL[170] or 10 to 20 seconds of burst suppression monitored by bedside electroencephalography. Despite maintenance of normal blood volume and cardiac output, hypotension occurs in 50% of cases and is probably due to decreased peripheral vascular resistance. Volume expansion in addition to dopamine may be necessary to restore systemic blood pressure while maintaining the desired level of suppression. Other potential complications related to high-dose barbiturates include hyponatremia, pneumonia, and cardiac depression.

Barbiturates are anticonvulsant; however, as mentioned before, they should not be used unless all other options have been exhausted. Other prophylactic anticonvulsants, however, should be given. The incidence of seizures is 4% to 25% after injury and 50% after penetrating injuries.[171] Seizures may increase ICP by several factors, including an increased metabolic demand, Valsalva maneuver, and release of excitotoxins.

Finally, V_{BRAIN} can be reduced by increasing the clearance of edema. Both osmotic and loop diuretics are widely used and can treat both vasogenic and cytotoxic edema.[172-174] Osmotic agents increase serum osmolality and create an osmotic gradient between the serum and brain. This effect draws free water from the brain into the intravascular compartment along the osmotic gradient. This is thought both to prevent edema formation and to speed clearance. However, osmotic agents transiently increase CBF independent of their effect on ICP, so their use in the presence of hyperemia and increased CBV may be contraindicated.

The drugs used most commonly for increasing intravascular osmolality are mannitol, urea, and glycerol. Mannitol (20% solution) is usually the agent of choice. Mannitol has a rapid effect on ICP, and it is therefore thought that a second mechanism of action may involve the rheologic characteristics of blood. Mannitol increases plasma volume, decreases hematocrit, and decreases blood viscosity, which can cause a vasoconstriction and a drop in ICP.[175-177]

The dose of mannitol is 0.25 to 1 g/kg, and this can be given as a repeated bolus or, in smaller doses, as a continuous infusion. Complications with osmotic therapy are dehydration, electrolyte imbalance, and, with extreme hyperosmolarity, renal failure. Fluid replacement is aimed at preserving isovolemia while increasing serum osmolality. Osmolality should not exceed 320 mOsm/kg because the renal tubule can be easily injured, especially if other nephrotoxic drugs are used concomitantly. Maintenance of high serum mannitol levels can lead to penetration of mannitol into injured brain,[178] especially in areas of blood-brain barrier deficiency. In this case, the osmolality of brain tissue will tend to draw water into the tissue and worsen edema.[179]

Mannitol is used more commonly than urea (30% solution) and glycerol (10% solution) because plasma and brain concentrations tend to equilibrate more rapidly with urea and glycerol than with mannitol. Glycerol can also cause hemolysis and renal failure when it is administered parenterally.[180] Because glycerol is metabolized, hyperosmolality lasts for less time than with mannitol. In one study comparing mannitol and glycerol, glycerol was less effective in reducing ICP.[181]

Loop diuretics such as furosemide and ethacrynic acid can be used in conjunction with mannitol to control ICP associated with edema.[182,183] Furosemide works synergistically with mannitol to remove free water and is most appropriate in patients with fluid overload. The addition of furosemide increases the likelihood of dehydration and loss of potassium.[102] Although furosemide decreases CSF production, this effect probably does not contribute greatly to lowering of ICP in the acute setting.

Hypothermia was first reported for treatment of brain injury in the mid-20th century.[184-187] Recent reports have suggested a beneficial effect on ICP. Shiozaki and coworkers[187] found a statistically significant reduction in ICP in a group of severely injured patients with intracranial hypertension refractory to other treatment, including barbiturates. Marion and colleagues[188] also demonstrated that hypothermia could lower ICP and improve patient outcome at 3 and 6 months after injury. The ability of hypothermia to lower ICP probably relates to a depression of cerebral metabolic requirements as with barbiturates, coupled with a slowing of injurious cellular events (e.g., lipid peroxidation).

V_OTHER

The most effective treatment of V_{OTHER} consists of removal. When a definable, abnormal mass (e.g., tumors, abscess, or hematoma) is responsible for intracranial hypertension, the mass should be removed. All other therapy should be considered adjunctive and supportive in this case.

It is useful to consider a few rare cases in which the skull limits expansion of the brain. Examples include multisutural craniosynostosis, slit ventricle syndrome, and large depressed skull fractures. This concept should also be extended to some acute settings of severe refractory ICP elevations. In cases of severe ICP elevation, decompressive craniectomy can decrease the incidence of transtentorial herniation; however, formation of edema is enhanced, and residual brain injury may be severe.

PRACTICAL ISSUES

Unfortunately, in most clinical settings, especially trauma, it is not feasible to follow this conceptual approach to the treatment of intracranial hypertension because it is not always clear exactly what is causing the elevated ICP, and indeed there may be multiple causes. The process of placing an ICP monitor and sedating and paralyzing a patient may in itself be sufficient to control the ICP, regardless of cause. In cases in which ICP is still a problem and a specific cause is not readily identifiable, treatment should be approached in a stepwise fashion.

First, CSF can be removed to lower pressure by external drainage. If this maneuver has to be repeated frequently to control ICP, the next step should be directed toward reducing the bulk of the brain by removal of extracellular fluid with use of osmotically active substances. Serum osmolality should be measured frequently, especially when mannitol is given more often than every 6 to 8 hours. In the majority of cases, intracranial hypertension will be successfully managed by the steps outlined before. However, 10% to 15% of patients will require additional treatment, and therapy should be advanced to include vasopressors, hypothermia, and barbiturates.

The key step in the treatment of intracranial hypertension is to recognize a treatment response and not to labor a therapeutic modality that is ineffectual. It is clear that patients respond differently to different therapies.[189] Furthermore, their response may change over time because the pathologic status of the injured brain can alter rapidly. Consequently, the stepwise framework should be followed less than rigidly, and treatment should be primarily tailored around the response of the ICP.

Acknowledgments

This research was supported by NIH/NINDS R01 NS19235.

We also thank Caroline Dermer for her assistance in the preparation of this manuscript.

SUGGESTED READINGS

Avezaat CJ, van Eijndhoven JH, Wyper DJ. Cerebrospinal fluid pulse pressure and intracranial volume-pressure relationships. *J Neurol Neurosurg Psychiatry.* 1979;42:687-700.

Barzó P, Marmarou A, Fatouros P, et al. Contribution of vasogenic and cellular edema to traumatic brain swelling measured by diffusion-weighted imaging. *J Neurosurg.* 1997;87:900-907.

Beaumont A, Marmarou A, Hayasaki K. The permissive nature of blood brain barrier opening in edema formation following traumatic brain injury. *Acta Neurochir Suppl.* 2000;76:125-129.

Czosnyka M, Kirkpatrick PJ, Pickard JD. Multimodal monitoring and assessment of cerebral haemodynamic reserve after severe head injury. *Cerebrovasc Brain Metab Rev.* 1996;8:273-295.

Egnor M, Zheng L, Rosiello A, et al. A model of pulsations in communicating hydrocephalus. *Pediatr Neurosurg.* 2002;36:281-303.

Ekstedt J. CSF hydrodynamic studies in man. 2 . Normal hydrodynamic variables related to CSF pressure and flow. *J Neurol Neurosurg Psychiatry*. 1978;41: 345-353.

Ito J, Marmarou A, Barzó P, et al. Characterization of edema by diffusion-weighted imaging in experimental traumatic brain injury. *J Neurosurg*. 1996;84:97-103.

Madsen JR, Egnor M, Zou R. Cerebrospinal fluid pulsatility and hydrocephalus: the fourth circulation. *Clin Neurosurg*. 2006;53:48-52.

Marion DW, Obrist WD, Carlier PM, et al. The use of moderate therapeutic hypothermia for patients with severe head injuries: a preliminary report. *J Neurosurg*. 1993;79:354-362.

Marmarou A. *Theoretical and experimental evaluation of the cerebrospinal fluid system [PhD thesis]*. Philadelphia: Drexel University, 1973.

Marmarou A, Bergsneider M, Relkin N, et al. Development of guidelines for idiopathic normal-pressure hydrocephalus: introduction. *Neurosurgery*. 2005;57:S1-S3; discussion ii-v.

Marmarou A, Shulman K, Rosende RM. A nonlinear analysis of the cerebrospinal fluid system and intracranial pressure dynamics. *J Neurosurg*. 1978;48:332-344.

Marmarou A, Signoretti S, Fatouros PP, et al. Predominance of cellular edema in traumatic brain swelling in patients with severe head injuries. *J Neurosurg*. 2006;104:720-730.

Maset AL, Marmarou A, Ward JD, et al. Pressure-volume index in head injury. *J Neurosurg*. 1987;67:832-840.

Rosner MJ, Rosner SD, Johnson AH. Cerebral perfusion pressure: management protocol and clinical results. *J Neurosurg*. 1995;83:949-962.

Wagshul ME, Chen JJ, Egnor MR, et al. Amplitude and phase of cerebrospinal fluid pulsations: experimental studies and review of the literature. *J Neurosurg*. 2006;104:810-819.

Full references can be found on Expert Consult @ www.expertconsult.com

CHAPTER 11

Neurosurgical Epidemiology and Outcomes Assessment

Hugh Garton ■ Frederick G. Barker II ■ Stephen J. Haines

In this chapter we focus on the application of statistical and epidemiologic principles to neurosurgical diagnosis, measurement, outcomes assessment and improvement, and critical review skills, which together provide the skill set necessary to develop an evidence-based approach to clinical practice.

To design a rational treatment plan for any patient, a physician must identify that patient's most likely diagnosis, the most likely natural course of events without intervention, the potential risks and benefits of the available therapies, and how this differs from the natural history of the process. Each aspect of this process has strong mathematical and statistical underpinnings. An evidence-based approach then requires the application of experimental clinical data to the individual patient, a concept known as generalization.

These skills are intended to be tools for the practicing clinician and those who perform clinical as opposed to basic science research. Taken together, they are studied academically under the rubric of clinical epidemiology, which differs in scope and purpose from the epidemic investigation and population-based studies of health and disease that characterize the more traditional field of survey epidemiology.

CONCEPTS—SOURCES OF ERROR IN ANALYSIS

Bias

All research must begin with a question. Research design is the process of constructing clinical experiments that provide true answers to the research question. Two types of errors threaten this process: *random* error (noise) and *structural* error (bias). The first of these is a result of the natural variability in subjects in their response to illness or treatment, or both. Random error, given a large enough sample, applies to all groups in a study equally. Usually, although not always, it makes it harder for an experiment to show a difference between experimental and control groups. Adopting the language of radio transmissions, this is the noise that obscures the signal, which is the answer that the investigator or reader is after. This type of error is predictable and, to a certain extent, measurable. Statistical analyses, from simple *t*-tests to complex analyses of variance, are intended to quantify random error.

Structural error, or bias, in contrast, is error that tends to apply specifically to one group of subjects in a study and is a consequence of intentional or unintentional features of the study design itself. This is error designed into the experiment and is not measurable or controllable by statistical techniques, but it can be minimized with proper experimental design. For example, if we are determining the normal head size of term infants by measuring the head size of all such patients born over a 1-week period, we have a high probability of introducing random error into our reported rate because we are considering a small sample. We can measure this tendency of random error in the form of a confidence interval around the reported head size. The larger the confidence interval, the higher the chance that our reported head size differs from the true average head size of our population of interest. We can solve this problem by increasing the sample size without any other change in experimental technique. Conversely, if we choose to conduct our study only in the newborn intensive care unit, with exclusion of the well-child nursery, and reported our measurements as pertaining to newborn children in general, we have introduced a structural error, or bias, into our experimental design. No statistical test that we can apply to our data set will alert us that this is occurring, nor will measures such as increasing the number of patients in our study help solve the problem. In considering the common study designs enumerated later, note how different types of studies are subject to different biases and how the differences in study design arise out of an attempt to control for bias.[1]

Control of Confounding Variables

Common to several of the study methodologies to be noted later is the concept of confounding variables. In studies assessing disease causation, natural history, and treatment efficacy, it is assumed that a number of factors may influence the outcome of interest. The presence of these factors, or confounders, alters the mathematical relationship of the risk factor of interest to the outcome. For example, in a cohort study attempting to assess the impact of smoking on stroke rates, hypertension would be considered a probable confounding variable that might obscure the true relationship between smoking and stroke. There are six basic strategies for dealing with confounders.

Exclusion

One can simply remove all patients with a competing risk factor from the study. This eliminates its effect and provides for a much-simplified analysis. The disadvantage of this approach is that it can miss important interactions between risk factors, reduces sample size, and can limit the degree to which the study findings can be generalized to other settings.

Standardization

Although published rates exist for a particular prognostic factor—disease-outcome pair—it is possible to control for the effect of that factor by considering the expected incidence of disease from published rates as opposed to the observed rate of disease in the study subjects. Age can be handled in this way, with age-specific expected mortality data relatively easy to obtain. Deaths expected because of age alone are then determined by applying the age-specific rates to members of the cohort under study to determine the expected number of total deaths. Obviously, this works only when such specific rates are available and does not permit investigation of the interplay between confounder and the factor of interest.

Stratification

This strategy essentially sets up parallel experiments for patients with and without a risk factor to be controlled. It is commonly used in randomized trials to deal with known, strong predictors of the outcome of interest. In this setting, patients with a risk factor are evenly divided between experimental and control groups by providing separate randomizations for each. In other settings, a separate analysis is performed for each group. The disadvantage is that as earlier, one cannot assess the possibility of interactions among risk factors. In addition, because each group requires a separate analysis or randomization, there is usually a sample size limit on the number of factors that can be controlled inasmuch as each subgroup has a smaller number of patients from which to draw statistical conclusions.

Matching

Similar to stratification and primarily used in case-control studies, this method seeks to assign an equal number of individuals with a risk factor to each group, often matching on an individual patient-by-patient basis. The limitations are the same as for stratification: a confounder's impact cannot be assessed, and trying to match on several factors simultaneously often requires a large sample from which to draw controls.

Modeling

Mathematical models can be constructed that allow various risk factors to be simultaneously considered. These multivariate models are very common in the literature and include generalized linear models and logistic regression. The mathematics behind these methods are complex, and the result of such a multivariate regression is generally an odds ratio for a factor's effect, *all other factors being equal*. Multiple confounders can be considered, although there are sample size limitations. However, these techniques can occasionally lead to results that contradict the unmodeled data, thereby leaving author and reader in somewhat of a quandary.

Randomization

All the aforementioned methods attempt to deal with confounding variables that are known but cannot deal with any that are unknown. One of the principal benefits of randomization is that it allows control of both known *and* unknown variables. The first or second table of most published randomized trials will provide the baseline characteristics of the experimental versus control groups documenting the normally even distribution of most known variables. Most probably, variables unknown to the investigators will also be similarly evenly distributed. Randomization is regularly used in conjunction with both stratification and modeling.

Noise—Statistical Analysis in Outcomes Assessment

The principal role of statistical analysis is to describe and quantify the naturally occurring variations in the world around us. Chance variation in experimentation comes from several sources, but principally from the variability inherent in the study subjects and the variability associated with measurement. The latter can be minimized by choosing the appropriate measurement tool, particularly one with a high degree of clinical agreement associated with its use. Appropriately used statistical analysis answers the question whether the observed differences or relationships seen among groups are beyond what would be expected based on the intrinsic variability in members of each group. The choice of measure used in the analysis depends on the type of data being analyzed, be it continuous or categorical, and whether the underlying population from which the data are drawn can be assumed to have a "normal" or bell-shaped distribution. For continuous data with a normal distribution, *t*-tests and other similar tests are appropriate, whereas for non-normally distributed data, the nonparametric Wilcoxon or Mann-Whitney tests are often used. Categorical data are usually described by using contingency tables, which can be assessed with χ^2 methodology or summarized with odds ratios.

Alpha and Beta Error and Power

In hypothesis testing, two types of statistically rooted error can occur. The first, or type I error, represents the chance that we will incorrectly conclude that a difference exists between groups when it does not. This is traditionally fixed at 5%. That is, in selecting a $P < .05$ value for rejection of the null hypothesis, we understand that 5% of the time a sample from the control population will differ from the population mean by this amount, and we may thus incorrectly conclude that control and experimental groups different by this amount came from different populations. The 5% is an arbitrary value, and the investigator can choose any level that is reasonable and convincing in terms of the study hypothesis.

The second, more common error is a type II or β error.[2] This represents the probability of incorrectly concluding that a difference does not exist between therapies when in fact it does. This is analogous to missing the signal for the noise. Here, the key issue is the natural degree of variability among study subjects, independent of what might be due to treatment effects. When small but real differences exist between groups and there is enough variability among subjects, the study requires a large sample size to be able to show a difference. Missing the difference is a β error, and the power of a study is $1 - \beta$. Study power is driven by sample size. The larger the sample, the greater the power to resolve small differences between groups.

Frequently, when a study fails to show a difference between groups, there is a tendency to assume that there is in fact no difference between them.[3] What is needed is an assessment of the likelihood of a difference being detected, given the sample size and subject variability. Although the authors should provide this, they frequently do not, thereby leaving readers to perform their own calculations or refer to published nomograms.[4,5] Arbitrarily, we say that a power of 80%, or the chance of detecting a difference of a specified amount given a sample size of *n*, is acceptable. If the penalties for missing a difference are high, other values for power can be selected, but the larger the power desired, the larger the sample size required.

Multiple Tests

If the chance that a study or statistical test reports a false-positive result is 1 in 20 (assuming that the level of significance is set at $P > .05$), the chances of at least one of several tests being falsely positive is $[1 - (0.95)^n]$, where *n* is the number of studies performed. Thus, for six comparisons in which $P < .05$ determines rejection of the null hypothesis, there is a 25% chance that at least one false-positive conclusion has been accepted. Several strategies can be used to deal with this problem. Methodologically, protection is afforded by specifying comparisons beforehand, thus reducing the random nature of these comparisons. In other settings, such as secondary data analysis for developing new questions, it is not possible to do this. At a minimum, the bar for rejection of the null hypothesis should be raised. For example, the Bonferroni correction divides the nominal .05 level of significance by the number of tests performed such that for six tests, the value needed for acceptance of any hypothesis is $P < .0083$.

Confidence Intervals

The hypothesis-testing strategy just described is intended to yield an all-or-nothing answer. The null hypothesis is either accepted or rejected. It is often of more use, particularly when describing the relationships between risk factors and outcome, to note the intensity (risk or odds) and direction of the association, as well as the degree to which variability affects the precision of its estimate. This is accomplished in the form of a confidence interval (CI). A 95% CI describes the mean ± 2 standard deviations. Stated another way, given a sample with a mean and a 95% CI, one can be 95% certain that the true population mean falls within the limits given by the CI. In comparing two means, odds ratios, or risk rates, when the 95% CIs of the means do not overlap, there is a 95% chance that they were drawn from different populations, analogous to rejecting the null hypothesis for $P < .05$. The advantage of CIs is that by providing a range of reasonable possible rates, they are easier to incorporate into the clinical setting, where the precision of the research environment may be lacking.

Univariate versus Multivariate Techniques

A comparison between a single risk factor and an outcome is called *univariate analysis* and is often described by odds ratios. Multivariate analysis considers the impact of a variety of potential risk factors on an outcome. Logistic regression is one such technique and is useful when the outcome can be divided into membership in one of two groups, such as failure/success or alive/dead. The interpretation of such models is that a risk factor that is statistically part of the model has an association with the outcome that is independent of the other items in the equation. Multivariate analyses also allow investigation of the interplay between risk factors by demonstrating how the consideration of additional factors influences the associations already present in the model. Regression models can be prone to "overmodeling" the data, or describing patterns that are unique to the particular dataset used in their creation. Determining the validity of the model requires testing the degree to which the model predicts an outcome from risk factors when applied to other datasets not used in development of the model.

Events over Time/Survival Analysis

Frequently, an outcome measure is described as the time to a particular event, such as the time to tumor progression, stroke, or death. Data may best be described in these cases by using Kaplan-Meier or life-table techniques that incorporate both the group membership of the individuals under study and the length of time that they have been part of the group. The graphic reproduction of this analysis is the common survival curve. Survival curves of different cohorts can be compared by using a log-rank test or Breslow-Day statistic. The impact of different factors on a survival curve can be modeled in a multivariate fashion, logically similar to that described for binary outcomes in logistic regression. The Cox proportional hazards model is the most commonly used vehicle for this type of analysis.

STATISTICS AND PROBABILITY IN DIAGNOSIS

The diagnosis of neurosurgical illness, as in other fields, requires the development of a list of possible explanations for the patient's complaints to form a differential diagnosis. As an example, imagine the scenario of a hydrocephalic child with his first shunt placed 3 months earlier who now has a 2-day history of vomiting and irritability. An experienced clinician hearing this story would quickly formulate a list of possible diagnoses, including otitis media, gastroenteritis, constipation, upper respiratory infection, and of course, shunt malfunction. Through a series of additional questions about the medical history and a physical examination, the clinician would be able to narrow this list down considerably to one or two possibilities. Additional tests such as computed tomography (CT) or a shunt tap would then be used to either support or refute particular diagnoses.

Pretest and Posttest Probability— A Bayesian Approach

At the onset, certain quickly ascertainable features about a clinical encounter should lead to the formation of a baseline probability of the most likely diagnoses for the particular clinical findings. In the example just presented, among all children seen by a neurosurgeon within 3 months of initial shunt placement, about 30% will subsequently be found to have shunt malfunction.[6] Before any tests are performed or even a physical examination completed, elements of the history provided allow the clinician to form this first estimate of the likelihood of shunt failure. The remainder of the history and physical findings allow revision of that probability, up or down. This bayesian approach to diagnosis requires some knowledge of how particular symptoms and signs affect the baseline, or the "pretest" probability of an event. The extent to which a particular clinical finding or diagnostic study influences the probability of a particular end diagnosis is a function of its sensitivity and specificity, which may be combined into the clinically more useful likelihood ratio.[7] Estimates of the pretest probability of disease tend to be situation specific; for example, the risk of failure of a cerebrospinal fluid (CSF) shunt after placement is heavily dependent on the age of the patient and the time elapsed since the last shunt-related surgical procedure.[8] Individual practitioners can best provide their own data for this by studying their own practice patterns.

Properties of Diagnostic Tests

Elements of the history, physical examination, and subsequent diagnostic studies can all be assessed to describe their properties as predictors of an outcome of interest. These properties may be summarized as sensitivity, specificity, positive and negative predictive values, and likelihood ratios, as illustrated in Table 11-1.

Sensitivity indicates the percentage of patients with a given illness who have a positive clinical finding or study. In other words, that a straight leg raise test has a sensitivity of 80% for lumbar disk herniation in the setting of sciatic pain means that 80 of 100 patients with sciatica and disk herniation do, in fact, have a positive straight leg raise test.[9] In Table 11-1, sensitivity is equal to $a/(a + c)$. Conversely, *specificity*, equal to $d/(b + d)$ in

TABLE 11-1 The Two-by-Two Table for Diagnosis

	DISEASE PRESENT	DISEASE ABSENT	PREDICTIVE VALUES
Finding present	A (true positives)	B (false positive)	PPV = a/(a + b)
Finding absent	C (false negative)	D (true negative)	NPV = d/(c + d)
	Sensitivity = a/(a + c)	Specificity = d/(b + d)	Prevalence = (a + c)/(a + b + c + d)

NPV, negative predictive value; PPV, positive predictive value.

Table 11-1, refers to the number of patients without a clinical diagnosis who also do not have a clinical finding. Again, using the example of the evaluation of low back pain in patients with sciatica, a positive straight leg raise test has about 40% specificity, which means that of 100 patients with sciatica but without disk herniation, 40 will have a negative straight leg raise test.

Sensitivity and specificity are difficult to use clinically because they describe clinical behavior in a group of patients known to carry the diagnosis of interest. These properties provide no information about performance of the clinical factor in patients who do not have the disease and who probably represent the majority of patients seen. Sensitivity ignores the important category of false-positive results (Table 11-1, B), whereas specificity ignores false-negative results (Table 11-1, C). If the sensitivity of a finding is very high (e.g., >95%) and the disease is not overly common, it is safe to assume that there will be few false-negative results (C in Table 11-1 will be small). Thus, the absence of a finding with high sensitivity for a given condition will tend to rule out the condition. When the specificity is high, the number of false-positive results is low (B in Table 11-1 will be small), and the absence of a symptom will tend to rule in the condition. Epidemiologic texts have suggested the mnemonics SnNout (when sensitivity is high, a negative or absent clinical finding rules out the target disorder) and SpPin (when specificity is very high, a positive study rules in the disorder), although some caution may be in order when applying these mnemonics strictly.[10]

However, when sensitivity or specificity is not as high or a disease process is common, the more relevant clinical quantities are the number of patients with the symptom or study result who end up having the disease of interest, otherwise known as the *positive predictive value* [PPV = a/(a + b)]. The probability of a patient not having the disease when the symptom or study result is absent or negative is referred to as the *negative predictive value* [NPV = d/(c + d)]. Subtracting NPV from 1 gives a useful "rule out" value that provides the probability of a diagnosis even when the symptom is absent or the study result negative.

A key component of these latter two values is the underlying prevalence of the disease. Examine Table 11-2. In both the common disease and rare disease case, the sensitivity and specificity for the presence or absence of a particular sign are each 90%, but in the common disease case, the total number of patients with the diagnosis is much larger, thereby leading to much higher positive and lower negative predictive values. When the prevalence of the disease drops, the important change is the relative increase in the number of false versus true positives, with the reverse being true for false versus true negatives.

The impact of prevalence plays a particularly important role when one tries to assess the role of screening studies in which there is only limited clinical evidence that a disease process is present. Examples include the use of screening magnetic resonance imaging studies for cerebrovascular aneurysms in patients with polycystic kidney disease[11] and routine use of CT for follow-up after shunt insertion[12] and for determining cervical spine instability in patients with Down syndrome,[13] as well as to search for cervical spine injuries in polytrauma patients.[14,15] In these situations, the low prevalence of the disease makes false-positive results likely, particularly if the specificity of the test is not extremely high, and usually results in additional, potentially more hazardous and expensive testing.

Likelihood ratios (LRs) are an extension of the previously noted properties of diagnostic information. LRs express the odds (rather than the percentage) of a patient with a target disorder having a particular finding present as compared with the odds of the finding in patients without the target disorder. An LR of 4 for a clinical finding indicates that it is four times as likely for a patient with the disease to have the finding as those without the disease. The advantage of this approach is that odds ratios, which are based on sensitivity and specificity, do not have to be recalculated for any given prevalence of a disease. In addition, if one starts with the pretest odds of a disease, this may be simply multiplied by the LR to generate the posttest odds of a disease. Nomograms exist to further simplify this process.[16] A number of useful articles and texts are available to the reader for further explanation.[17,18] Table 11-3 gives examples of the predictive values of selected symptoms and signs encountered in clinical neurosurgical conditions.[9,19-24]

Clinical Decision Rules

The preceding examples demonstrate the mathematical consequences of the presence of a single symptom or sign on the diagnostic process. The usual diagnostic process involves the integration of different symptoms and signs, often simultaneous with the process of generating a differential diagnosis. Clinical decision rules or decision instruments allow integration of multiple symptoms or signs into a diagnostic algorithm. The desired properties of such algorithms depend on the disease process studied, the consequences of false-positive and false-negative results, and the risk and cost of evaluation maneuvers. For example, the National Emergency X-Radiography Utilization Study (NEXUS) sought to develop a clinical prediction rule to determine which patients require cervical spine x-ray assessment after blunt trauma.[15]

MEASUREMENT IN CLINICAL NEUROSURGERY

Neurosurgeons have become increasingly aware of the need to offer concrete scientific support for their medical practices. Tradition and reasoning from pathophysiologic principles, although important in generating hypotheses, are not a substitute for scientific method. Coincident with this move toward empiricism has been the recognition that traditional measures of outcome, such as mortality and morbidity rates, are insufficient to capture important changes in functional status. Similarly, traditional outcomes as recorded in the medical record lack precision and reproducibility. Aware that better outcome assessments are required to better provide information on treatment choices, we must ask two important questions. What should we measure? How should we measure it?

TABLE 11-2 The Impact of Prevalence on Positive Study Findings in Diagnosis

	DISEASE PRESENT	DISEASE ABSENT	PREDICTIVE VALUES
COMMON DISEASE			
Finding present	45	5	PPV = 90%
Finding absent	5	45	NPV = 90%
	Sensitivity = 90%	Specificity = 90%	Prevalence = 50%
RARE DISEASE			
Finding present	9	9	PPV = 50%
Finding absent	1	81	NPV = 99%
	Sensitivity = 90%	Specificity = 90%	Prevalence = 10%

NPV, negative predictive value; PPV, positive predictive value.

TABLE 11-5 Common Measurement Instruments in Neurosurgery—cont'd

DISEASE PROCESS/SCALE	FEATURES	REFERENCE
PERIPHERAL NERVE TRAUMA		
Medical Research Council grading system	Scores strength 0-5. Similar to ASIA motor grading	64
DEGENERATIVE SPINE		
North American Spine Society questionnaire	Separate cervical and lumbar instruments. Combines both disease-specific questions and SF-36. Normative data published	65
Oswestry low back pain disability questionnaire	10 Domains, including pain intensity, personal care, lifting, walking, sitting, standing, sleeping, sex life, social life, and traveling; 6-item scale per domain	66
Japanese Orthopedic Association scale	Reported for cervical myelopathy: Scores 0-2 to 0-4 for motor function in arm and leg; sensory function in arm, leg, and trunk; and sphincter dysfunction. Higher scores signify greater function	67
HYDROCEPHALUS		
HOQ (Hydrocephalus Outcome Questionnaire)	51-Question disease-specific multidimensional outcome measure developed and validated for pediatric hydrocephalus. Responses scored to yield overall score from 0 to 1. Can be converted to health utility score	68, 69
CRANIOFACIAL		
Whitaker grade	I: No need for additional surgery II: Minor surgery advisable for soft tissue revision or bone contouring III: Major osteotomy or bone grafting required, although this would be less extensive than the original procedure IV: Major surgery required that equals or exceeds the extent of the original procedure	70
ONCOLOGY		
Karnofsky performance scale	100-Point scale (scored by 10s) from 100 (normal) to 0 (dead) that measures degree of dependence; <70 is no longer independent	71
EORTC QLC 30-	Multidimensional quality-of-life measures used for glioma outcomes	72, 73
University of Toronto	16 Items from Sickness Impact Profile, 13 items specific to brain tumor patients with an overall assessment question, question answered by visual analog–type scale between descriptive extremes	72
FUNCTIONAL		
Functional independence measure (FIM)	7-Point scale from independence to total assistance applied to 6 ADL areas: self-care (eating, grooming, bathing, dressing, and toilet), sphincter control, transfers, locomotion (walking and stairs), communication, and social cognition	74
WeeFIM	Modification of FIM for pediatric patients	75, 76
Barthel index	10-Item (or 15 if the Granger modification version) score addressing ADLs (feeding, transfers, toiletry, etc). Each item scored for dependent vs. independent with several items at intermediate grade. Score of 0-100 (0-20 for modification)	77, 78
PAIN		
McGill Pain Questionnaire	Very common in use. Adjectival description of pain to assess three domains: sensory-discriminative, motivational-affective, and cognitive-evaluative. Adjective selected by patient carries intensity weighting. Several scoring systems exist	79
Visual analog scale	Ruler scale of 0-10 for pain	80
GENERAL/MULTIDIMENSIONAL		
SF-36 and shorter forms	36 Questions. Domains: physical activity, social activity, societal role, pain, mental health, emotions, vitality, and health perceptions. Can be self-administered; current testing involves Web-based applications. Scoring is out of 100 for each of the 8 domains, with higher scores indicating better health. Physical and mental summary scores also available	81
Sickness Impact Profile	136 Questions. Domains/categories: Physical—ambulation, mobility, body care, and movement; Psychosocial—social interaction, communication, alertness behavior, emotional behavior, sleep and rest, eating, home management, recreation and pastimes, employment	82
Nottingham Health Profile	38 Questions. Domains: physical mobility, energy level, pain, emotional reactions, sleep, and social isolation. Can be combined to summary measure	83, 84

ADLs, activities of daily living; ASIA, American Spinal Cord Injury Association; EORTC, European Organization for Research and Treatment of Cancer; NIH, National Institutes of Health; SF-36, short-form health survey (36 items); WFNS, World Federation of Neurological Surgeons.

TABLE 11-6 Study Designs

	EXAMPLE	LIMITATIONS (TYPICAL)
DESCRIPTIVE STUDIES		
Population correlation studies	Rate of disease in population vs. incidence of exposure in population	No link at the individual level, cannot assess or control for other variables. Used for hypothesis generation only
	Changes in disease rates over time	No control for changes in detection techniques
INDIVIDUALS		
Case reports and case series	Identification of rare events, report of outcome of particular therapy	No specific control group or effort to control for selection biases
Cross-sectional surveys	Prevalence of disease in sample, assessment of coincidence of risk factor and disease at a single point in time at an individual level	"Snapshot" view does not allow assessment of causation, cannot assess incident vs. prevalent cases. Sample determines degree to which findings can be generalized
Descriptive cohort studies	Describes outcome over time for specific group of individuals, without comparison of treatments	Cannot determine causation, risk of sample-related biases
ANALYTIC STUDIES		
Observational		
Case control	Disease state is determined first. Identified control group retrospectively compared with cases for presence of particular risk factor	Highly suspect for bias in selection of control group. Generally can study only one or two risk factors
Retrospective cohort studies	Population of interest determined first, outcome and exposure determined retrospectively	Uneven search for exposure and outcome between groups. Susceptible to missing data, results dependent on entry criteria for cohort
Prospective cohort studies	Exposure status determined in a population of interest, then monitored for outcome	Losses to follow-up over time, expensive, dependent on entry criteria for cohort
INTERVENTIONAL		
Dose escalation studies (phase I)	Risk for injury from dose escalation	Comparison is between doses, not vs. placebo. Determines toxicity not efficacy
Controlled nonrandom studies	Allocation to different treatment groups by patient/clinician choice	Selection bias in allocation between treatment groups
Randomized controlled trials	Random allocation of eligible subjects to treatment groups	Expensive. Experimental design can limit generalizability of results
Meta-analysis	Groups randomized trials together to determine average response to treatment	Limited by quality of original studies, difficulty combining different outcome measures. Variability in base study protocols

After Hennekens C, Buring J. *Epidemiology in Medicine.* Boston: Little, Brown; 1987.

explanatory studies have the specific purpose of direct comparison between assembled groups and are designed to yield answers concerning causation and treatment efficacy. Analytic studies may be observational, as in case-control and cohort studies, or interventional, as in controlled clinical trials. In addition to being directed at different questions, different study designs are more or less robust in managing the various study biases that must be considered as threats to their validity (Table 11-7).[1,91]

Descriptive Studies

Case Reports and Case Series

Currently, case reports and case series account for the bulk of the neurosurgical literature. These studies properly have their place in describing new or unusual medical events. In such studies there is an implicit comparison to what is usual or ordinary in clinical practice. They can suggest possible causes and treatments for

events but can offer only limited support for clinical practice patterns and do not provide for hypothesis testing. The main advantage of these types of studies is that they are easy and inexpensive to complete. They can also provide data important in designing subsequent, more complex investigations, particularly if standard outcome measures are used in the analysis.

Cross-Sectional Surveys

These studies attempt to determine the presence of disease and potential exposure causing the disease in individuals at a single point in time. Usually based on interview or questionnaire, such studies can generally be accomplished relatively inexpensively and quickly in comparison to the cohort studies that they mimic. The principal limitation is that because the data are collected at a single point in time, they cannot be used to determine the causal relationship between an exposure and the disease of interest. In addition, the single time assessment does not allow understanding of the course of illness.

TABLE 11-7 Common Biases in Clinical Research

BIAS NAME	EXPLANATION
SAMPLING BIASES	
Prevalence-incidence	Drawing a sample of patients late in a disease process excludes those who have died of the disease early in its course. Prevalent (existing) cases may not reflect the natural history of incident (newly diagnosed) cases
Unmasking	In studies investigating causation, factors that cause symptoms, which in turn cause a more diligent search for the disease of interest. An example might be whether a particular medication caused headaches, which led to the performance of more magnetic resonance imaging studies and resulted in an increase in the diagnosis of arachnoid cysts in patients taking the medication. The conclusion that the medication caused arachnoid cysts would reflect unmasking bias
Diagnostic suspicion	A predisposition to consider an exposure as causative prompts a more thorough search for the presence of the outcome of interest
Referral filter	Patients referred to tertiary care centers are often not reflective of the population as a whole in terms of disease severity and comorbid conditions. Natural history studies are particularly prone to biases of this sort
Chronologic	Patients cared for in previous periods probably underwent different diagnostic studies and treatments. Studies with historical controls are at risk
Nonrespondent/volunteer	Patients who choose to respond or not respond to surveys or follow-up assessments differ in tangible ways. Studies with incomplete follow-up or poor response rates are prone to this bias
Membership bias	Cases or controls drawn from specific self-selected groups often differ from the general population. The result of this bias is the assumption that the group's defining characteristic is the cause of their performance with respect to a risk factor
INTERVENTION BIASES	
Co-intervention	Patients in an experimental or control group systematically undergo an additional treatment not intended by the study protocol. If a treatment were significantly more painful than a control procedure, a potential co-intervention would be increased analgesic use postoperatively. A difference in outcome could be due to either the treatment or the co-intervention
Contamination	When patients in the control group receive the experimental treatment, the potential differences between the groups are masked
Therapeutic personality	In unblinded studies, the belief in a particular therapy may influence the way in which the provider and patient interact and alter the outcome
MEASUREMENT	
Expectation	Prior expectations about the results of an assessment can substitute for actual measurement. In assessments of either diagnosis or therapy, belief in the predictive ability or therapeutic efficacy increases the likelihood that a positive effect will be measured. Unblinded studies and those with a subjective outcome measure are prone to this bias
Recall	In cohort and case-control studies, different assessment techniques or frequencies applied to those with the outcome of interest may increase the likelihood of detection of a risk factor, in particular, asking cases multiple times vs. controls improves chances for recall. This bias applies especially to retrospective studies and is the inverse of the diagnostic-suspicion bias (see earlier)
Unacceptability	Measurements that are uncomfortable, either physically or mentally, may be avoided by study subjects
Unpublished scales	The use of unpublished outcome scales has been shown in certain settings to result in a greater probability of the study finding in favor of experimental treatment[91]
ANALYSIS	
Post hoc significance	When decisions regarding levels of significance or statistical measures to be used are determined after the results are analyzed, it is more likely that a significant result will be found. It is very unlikely that authors would state this in a manuscript, but protection is afforded by publication of the study methods in advance of the study itself
Data dredging	Asking multiple questions of a dataset until something with statistical significance is found. Subgroup analysis, depending on whether preplanned and coherent with the study aims and hypotheses, may also fall into this category

From Sackett DL. Bias in analytic research. *J Chronic Dis.* 32:51, 1979.

Descriptive Cohort Studies

Cohort studies as described more fully later can be primarily descriptive rather than analytic. That is, they can seek to describe events occurring in a defined population over time rather than drawing conclusions about causation, as is usually the case with the classically described cohort study. Simple natural history studies that do not attempt to analyze prognostic factors fit into this category.

Analytic Studies

Case-Control Studies

The aforementioned study methods lack control groups, thus making direct comparisons impossible. Almost always performed retrospectively, a case-control study seeks to make up for this deficiency by selecting a control group of patients who can then be compared with the cases of interest. Originally designed to assess causation in rare diseases in which a cohort would have to be prohibitively large to detect enough cases, the relative simplicity and easy retrospective application of this methodology have made for widespread use. Patients with the disease or outcome of interest are identified first. Then, a control population not showing the disease or outcome of interest is determined, and the two groups are assessed for the presence of particular risk factors. The result is typically an odds ratio, which is the odds of the risk factor in the cases versus the controls. Controls must be selected such that if the disease had developed in them, they would have been eligible to be cases. Controls may be selected at random from a sample, but because such studies are usually small in total number, it is generally important to balance or match the cases and controls for important prognostic factors so that these do not obscure associations between the outcome and the factor of interest. From the standpoint of bias, case-control studies are most susceptible in the choice and assignment of control patients and in the way in which the two groups are screened for the presence of risk factors. Controls are often "historical." Such controls are open to a chronology bias based on changes in practice patterns and the influence of changing technology over time.

The reader will note that a case-control study provides an odds ratio rather than a relative risk. This is because by virtue of the control selection process, a case-control study does not provide information on the actual incidence of a risk factor in a group. A case-control study, because of the nonrandom selection of controls, cannot offer any protection against unknown confounding variables.

Cohort Studies

Cohort studies are primarily used to assess the role of common exposures with modest effects on disease incidence or progression. They can help establish an appropriate temporal relationship between exposure and outcome and can investigate a number of potential risk factors for a disease outcome simultaneously. An important subclass or variant of the cohort study, the natural history study, is discussed more fully later. In the traditional cohort study, investigators assemble a large group of individuals. This group is then assessed for a variety of exposures and monitored, usually by serial assessment over time, to determine the subsequent occurrence of outcome events. Drawing all the members of the cohort from the same setting is one of the ways in which studies of this type try to minimize selection bias. Keys to study design include a constant method of assessment for all members of the cohort regardless of potential exposure and complete follow-up. As opposed to the odds ratios reported in case-control studies, cohort studies report a relative risk because the structure of the study allows a comparative incidence of the outcome to be calculated.

In prospective cohort studies, the outcome events are unknown at the time that the study is started and patients are observed into the future. In retrospective cohort studies, the investigator is looking backward to determine the exposure history for the cohort after the outcome is already known. As always, a prospective study is more robust methodologically because it offers much better protection against assessment biases for the exposure. Retrospective studies are at risk for *diagnostic-suspicion bias* by investigating those with the outcome of interest more closely than those without, thereby biasing the reported relative risks. Prospective studies however, face a greater problem with losses to follow-up.

Diagnosis and Patient Assessment Studies

Studies looking at the discriminatory power of diagnostic tests or strategies ask the general question, "How well do the results of this diagnostic test predict the presence or absence of the sought-after disease?" Most often such studies take on the general form of a cohort study. The group of patients with the suspected disease is the cohort (e.g., all adult patients undergoing major surgery at a particular institution). The cohort is assessed for the presence of a risk factor (positive duplex scan of the lower extremity for clots) and then monitored for an outcome, which is usually the result of the "gold standard" diagnostic test (presence of deep venous thrombosis on venography).[92] Like other cohort studies, studies looking at diagnostic accuracy are susceptible to bias when knowledge of the gold standard result can influence interpretation of the diagnostic study under question, or the reverse. This is similar to recall bias or diagnostic-suspicion bias for the more typical prospective and retrospective cohort studies.

Selection of the cohort under study is of particular importance in studies evaluating diagnosis in terms of the generalizability of the results. The cohort should consist of patients similar in all respects to those to whom the investigator wishes to apply the diagnostic test or algorithm at the conclusion of the study. Any referral filter biases and other typical sampling biases seen in cohort studies must be addressed.

The study methodology should allow assessment of observer agreement or variability, as well as the diagnostic properties of sensitivity, specificity, PPV, and NPV, as described in preceding sections.

Natural History Studies

Usually a variant of a cohort design, natural history studies observe a group of patients drawn from a defined population over time to determine the occurrence of particular outcome events such as mortality, rebleeding rates, stroke rates, and others. In essence, the study seeks to determine how accurately the future outcome can be predicted by a group of know predictors. Studies of this sort occupy a critical place in clinical reasoning because they can provide information about the consequences of a decision not to treat. Natural history studies do not replace a randomized comparison between placebo and treatment, but they are often the starting point for therapy decisions in the absence of such studies and frequently provide the framework for subsequent randomized comparisons. The line between a natural history study and a case series with long-term follow-up may seem a fine one, but the key is in determining the degree to which the study patients are representative of the population as a whole and the degree to which the follow-up investigations are evenly applied. The literature regarding the debate on the hemorrhage rate for unruptured aneurysms smaller than 1 cm provides numerous examples of this type of study and highlights the potential bias in studies of this type.[93-96] Critical in such studies

Approach to the Patient

CHAPTER 12

Altered Consciousness

Nicholas D. Schiff

Altered consciousness after brain injury is associated with several clinical syndromes, including coma, vegetative state (VS), minimally conscious state (MCS), akinetic mutism, and other related conditions. In this chapter a clinically oriented review is presented with emphasis on mechanisms that underlie altered consciousness at the neuronal "circuit" level. A brief taxonomy of altered states of consciousness is presented, followed by a discussion of general strategies to assess patients and formulate a diagnosis and prognosis. The considerable differences in probabilities and time frames of recovery from coma, VS, or MCS can best be understood in the context of the specific factors that underlie the pathophysiology of individual brain injuries and the general mechanisms of forebrain arousal. Finally, the potential contribution of new neuroimaging modalities to the diagnostic assessment of patients with disorders of consciousness is briefly reviewed. Although many challenges currently limit the clinical application of these techniques, greater future roles may be anticipated.

Altered consciousness is a most common finding in patients evaluated by a consulting neurosurgeon or neurologist. The development of a comprehensive differential diagnosis, treatment plan, and prognosis for altered consciousness is well beyond the scope of a single book chapter (instead, see Posner and colleagues[1]). Here, emphasis is placed on conceptualizing neurological disorders of consciousness and formulating an organized and physiologically based approach to the general set of problems. A systematic approach to evaluate patients with altered consciousness requires a foundation of the basic principles that underlie maintenance of the normal wakeful conscious state.

A BRIEF TAXONOMY

Schiff and Plum[2] proposed the following working definition for the normal wakeful conscious state in humans modeled after that of James[3] (1894):

> *At its least, normal human consciousness consists of a serially time-ordered, organized, restricted and reflective awareness of self and the environment. Moreover, it is an experience of graded complexity and quantity.*

Human conscious brain states are characterized by several neuropsychological components, including arousal, attention, intention, memory, awareness, and mood-emotion. A clinically oriented view of global disorders of consciousness suggests a roughly hierarchical organization of these components. The arousal level appears to influence all neuropsychological func-

tions in humans and animals, and absence of an aroused state precludes behavior.[4] Complete loss of patterned arousal is seen only in coma (and in brain death, which is operationally defined and an unambiguous condition equivalent to death[5]). In VS, limited recovery of arousal patterning occurs without evidence of the other neuropsychological components of human consciousness (see discussion later). Fragmentary elements of specific neuropsychological components are evident in these syndromes. For example, fragments of attentional function are evidently preserved in all forms of akinetic mutism, with varying levels of impairment in other components (see later). Similarly, purposeless movements can occur in patients with hyperkinetic mutism or as partially integrated and organized goal-directed sensorimotor activity in those with complex partial seizures or delirium (see Schiff and Plum[2] for a more extended review). Complex brain injuries typically produce a mix of the clinical features observed in these classic syndromes. Here we focus on the classification of global disorders of consciousness most frequently encountered and related to each other as recovery evolves after severe brain injury.

COMA

Coma is an unconscious brain state characterized by the total absence of patterned behavioral arousal or electroencephalographic features of sleep-wake architecture. Comatose patients remain motionless in an eyes-closed state without spontaneous periods of eye opening or change of state with vigorous stimulation. Although effortful stimulation of a comatose patient may produce a grimace in response to painful stimuli or stereotyped withdrawal movements of the limbs generated by spinal reflexes, these movements lack localization of the source of external stimulation and the organized sequence of movements associated with purposeful avoidance. Patients in deep levels of coma typically do not exhibit primitive reflex responses.

By definition, the term *coma* implies that the state has endured for at least 1 hour and in some clinical operational definitions for at least 6 hours. Nonetheless, coma is invariably a transient condition that if uncomplicated by concurrent systemic illness, sedation, or other similar factors, typically does not persist beyond 10 to 14 days. Although some patients quickly pass through coma, many others transition through functional stages of VS and MCS (defined later).

VEGETATIVE STATE

The concept of VS was first introduced in 1972 by Jennett and Plum, who defined the clinical syndrome of the "persistent vegetative state" as being identified by dissociation of an apparent recovery of behavioral wakeful arousal associated with periods of eye opening that alternate with periods of eye closure in patients who show no evidence of awareness of self or their environment.[6] Early use of the term arbitrarily identified VS lasting longer than 30 days as a "persistent vegetative state." However, many organizations and countries have now advocated that the modifier "persistent" not be used because it is often misinterpreted to indicate probable permanence of the VS. The expectation for permanence of the VS can be assessed accurately only by considering the mechanism and elapsed time from the injury (see "Guide to Prognosis" later).

The VS typically follows an initial coma produced by an acute brain insult and most often is associated with patterns of injury that overlap those that produce coma. The two most common causes of VS are severe traumatic brain injury and cardiac arrest. Autopsy studies of patients who remain in VS after both conditions demonstrate a common pattern of extensive loss of thalamic neurons,[7] particularly within the central thalamic intralaminar nuclei and closely adjacent components of thalamic association nuclei.[8] Bilateral injuries restricted to these regions alone can produce coma.[2,9] The severe loss of thalamic neurons reflects widespread disconnection of the corticothalamic system and neuronal death across the cerebrum. Although this finding of extensive thalamic neuronal loss can be seen after both diffuse axonal injury from brain trauma and oxygen deprivation associated with cardiac arrest, widespread neocortical neuronal death is common only with cardiac arrest (64% versus 11%[7]). Significant brainstem damage is not commonly found at autopsy of VS patients, an observation that emphasizes that VS is primarily a disorder of corticothalamic system integration.

Since the original definition of VS, research efforts have typically focused on clinical indicators of permanence and underlying neuropathology (reviewed by Jennett[10]). A small number of early neuroimaging studies of VS patients measured cerebral metabolism with fluorodeoxyglucose-positron emission tomography (FDG-PET) scans. In these studies, VS patients showed a reproducible reduction in resting metabolism to typically 30% to 50% of normal metabolic rates across cerebral structures.[11,12] Comparable reductions in cerebral metabolic rates are found in normal subjects in the pharmacologic coma produced by surgical anesthesia.[13] More recently, several groups have examined functional activation of cerebral networks in response to sensory stimuli in VS patients by using functional neuroimaging methods (^{15}O-PET and functional magnetic resonance imaging [fMRI]). These studies demonstrate widespread failure of functional responses to elementary sensory stimuli in cortical regions remote from the primary sensory cortices in VS patients.[14,15] In some VS patients, unusual behavioral and physiologic variations are correlated with evidence of isolated islands of metabolic activity.[16] In one such VS patient, rare single understandable words were emitted for 20 years without linkage to environmental stimulation. In this patient, the left cerebral structures (including Wernicke's area in the temporal association cortex and Broca's area in the frontal opercular region) demonstrated relatively increased metabolic rates (nearly twice the rates in surrounding brain tissue) and physiologic connections consistent with partial and isolated preservation of brain structures of the human language system.[17] The behavioral fragments more typically identified in chronic VS patients are stereotyped emotional-limbic responses such as grimaces. These emotional displays most probably reflect isolated limbic networks tightly linked to brainstem and basal forebrain structures that operate without functional connection to the thalamocortical systems that are typically severely damaged in VS patients.

MINIMALLY CONSCIOUS STATE

The first level of behavioral recovery beyond VS is operationally defined as MCS. MCS patients show evidence on bedside examination of contingent responses to environmental stimuli or self-initiated behavior that provides unequivocal but inconsistent evidence of awareness of self or the environment[18] (Table 12-1). A wide range of behavioral expressions are currently consistent with the operational criteria for MCS.[19] For example, consistent and sustained visual tracking or fixation may be the only behavioral evidence of responsiveness in an MCS patient. Alternatively, an MCS patient may exhibit intermittent spoken language responses or inconsistent and inaccurate communication with gestural or verbal output. Recovery of functional communication (operationally defined as the ability to consistently and accurately answer simple contextual yes or no questions) defines the upper boundary of MCS. Beyond MCS, varying levels of severe disability are not currently subcategorized.

Even though only subtle findings may distinguish VS and MCS patients at the bedside, a wide separation in underlying functional cerebral substrates associated with the two conditions is indicated by neuroimaging and electrophysiologic and pathologic studies.[20-23] Autopsy studies of patients with clinical histories consistent with MCS demonstrate reduced overall levels of cerebral cell death and, in some MCS patients, no evidence of significant thalamic cell loss or severe diffuse axonal injury—a pattern never observed in VS patients.[23] Neuroimaging studies generally show widespread preservation of distributed cerebral network activation in response to sensory stimuli, including passive language stimuli[20,24] and auditory[15] and somatosensory stimuli.[21] Electrophysiologic studies typically show recovery of a broad range of frequency content on the electroencephalogram and, in some MCS patients, preservation of high-level passive semantic processing of spoken language.[22] Such large-scale integrative network responses that involve cortical association regions are not typically seen in VS patients. The presence of recruitable large-scale cerebral networks in some MCS patients suggests a potential substrate for further recovery in these patients. These

---

TABLE 12-1 Aspen Working Group Criteria for Clinical Diagnosis of the Minimally Conscious State

Evidence of limited but clearly discernible self or environmental awareness on a reproducible or sustained basis, as demonstrated by one or more of the following types of behavior:

1. Simple command following
2. Gestural or verbal "yes/no" responses (independent of accuracy)
3. Intelligible verbalization
4. Purposeful behavior, including movements or affective behavior in a contingent relationship to relevant stimuli; examples include
   a. Appropriate smiling or crying in response to relevant visual or linguistic stimuli
   b. Response to the linguistic content of questions by vocalization or gesture
   c. Reaching for objects in the appropriate direction and location
   d. Touching or holding objects by accommodating to size and shape
   e. Sustained visual fixation or tracking as a response to moving stimuli

From Giacino JT, Ashwal S, Childs N, et al. The minimally conscious state: definition and diagnostic criteria. *Neurology.* 2002;58:349-353.

observations probably underlie the rare, but verified cases of late recovery of spoken language in some severely brain-injured patients with clinical histories consistent with long-standing MCS.[25] In a recent single-subject study, one MCS patient who had demonstrated preserved passive language responses recovered spoken language and consistent verbal and gestural communication with bilateral electrical stimulation of the central thalamus.[26]

AKINETIC MUTISM

The syndrome of *akinetic mutism* includes patients who fulfill the criteria for MCS and patients who can functionally communicate when formally assessed yet demonstrate a severe reduction in spontaneous behavior or extremely slowed interactive responses. Patients with akinetic mutism may appear highly attentive and vigilant with wide eye opening, deliberate visual tracking of the examiner around the room, but no other types of behavior. These patients are included in the MCS spectrum. Other patients sometimes described as akinetic mutes may appear awake but somnolent with apparent psychomotor retardation similar to a variety of subcortical dementias.[27] The patterns of brain injury most commonly associated with these syndromes are bilateral damage to the anterior medial regions of the cerebral cortex, bilateral injury to caudate nuclei (or unilateral dominant hemisphere caudate nucleus), bilateral central thalamic lesions, large basal forebrain injuries, or damage to the mesencephalic reticular formation.[2,28] Akinetic mutism is a classic finding after rupture of an anterior communicating artery aneurysm. Some authors[27] have defined "slow syndrome" to identify this subgroup of patients as a related behavioral phenotype characterized primarily by severe memory loss, severely slowed behavioral responses, and a listless, apathetic appearance sometimes referred to as "abulia."[29] The pattern of focal injuries associated with both akinetic mutism and "slow syndrome" overlaps entirely with those producing acute coma and VS when the lesions are bilateral and larger in rostrocaudal extent.[2]

AN ORGANIZING STRATEGY TO ASSESS DISORDERS OF CONSCIOUSNESS BASED ON ANATOMIC AND PHYSIOLOGIC CONSIDERATIONS

If psychogenic processes are excluded, observed alteration of consciousness in all settings implies one of the following possibilities: (1) diffuse functional impairment of both hemispheres as a result of direct injury and toxic/metabolic alterations associated, for example, with cardiopulmonary dysfunction, infection, poisoning, or a variety of other processes producing bilateral cerebral dysfunction, such as antibody-mediated alteration of neurons or axons, and (2) selective impairment of midline and paramedian upper brainstem and basal forebrain regions containing nuclei associated with ascending arousal input to the anterior forebrain, often damaged in combination with central thalamic nuclei (or isolated to the central thalamus if the lesions are bilateral and relatively large in rostrocaudal extent).[9,30] The severity of a disturbance in consciousness directly reflects the functional disturbance produced in cerebral neurons diffusely or within the relatively restricted network of subsystems involved in forebrain arousal and regulation of arousal.

Although these two classes of mechanisms are well known, applying the general principles to understand altered consciousness in an individual patient is often quite challenging. Broadly speaking, there are three categories of patients with marked alteration of consciousness encountered by the neurosurgical or neurological consultant: (1) patients with overwhelming structural brain injury and known clinical predictors of death or per-

manent VS; (2) patients who show a pattern of early, steady recovery and are predicted to have outcomes better than severe disability with relative certainty; and (3) patients with a mix of structural brain injuries or more diffuse alterations (e.g., hypoxia, infection, inflammation), low-level behavioral responses, and relatively prolonged recovery in which available tools can confirm severe cerebral dysfunction but provide little insight into the patient's future.

Identification of patients in the first category—those with overwhelming structural brain injury—can frequently be done by inspection and clinical judgment (e.g., a patient with complete infarction of the dominant hemisphere and central herniation but not quite meeting brain death criteria). Prospective studies of large numbers of patients in coma have codified a number of strong clinical predictors of death or outcomes limited to permanent VS after the two most common causes: cardiac arrest and severe traumatic brain injury (see Posner and colleagues[1] for a comprehensive review). For example, coma associated with loss of motor response and pupil and corneal reflexes initially and enduring over the first 48 to 72 hours is invariably associated with outcomes no better than permanent VS after cardiac arrest once potential confounding variables are excluded.

The second group of patients, those with early and steady patterns of recovery, are well known but not well characterized in terms of the stages and time frames of their recovery because this is of more scientific than clinical interest. These patients recover consciousness and higher brain function within the first days or weeks after their initial events, and the details of their underlying brain mechanisms of recovery are a secondary concern to clinicians not directly involved in cognitive or motor rehabilitation.

It is the third group of patients who provide a significant challenge to the neurosurgical and neurological consultant. These patients will have sufficient evidence from their clinical history, structural injury to critical brain structures evident on imaging, or electrophysiologic markers of diffuse neuronal dysfunction to raise concern of futility, but they do not demonstrate known clinical or laboratory indicators that predict permanence of their condition. In formulating a clinical judgement in such cases it is important to recognize that all existing indicators are surrogate markers for overwhelming neuronal death and disconnection within the cerebrum. Estimation of the likelihood of further functional recovery and the ultimate functional level of recovery in patients who lack negative predictors presents significant uncertainty. At present, no measurements reliably allow an assessment of whether the underlying remaining brain structures in such patients may allow recovery of consciousness and higher level cognitive functions. Thus, it is most important to have a reasoned and systematic strategy to assess these patients.

An organized approach to this subpopulation of patients with severe brain injury and marked alteration of consciousness begins with an accurate diagnosis. It is absolutely critical to determine whether the patient is in coma, VS, or MCS; this is true whether the assessment is performed in the acute care setting once a comatose patient is stabilized in the emergency room or in more subacute contexts of inpatient units or even nursing facilities. The bedside diagnosis immediately provides an indication of the level of functional integration of cerebral subsystems within the forebrain and should anticipate the results of standard clinical functional assessments such as electroencephalograms, evoked responses, and other tracking measures. For example, comatose patients should show severe diffuse cerebral dysfunction with structural imaging that provides correlative information consistent with the history and cause of the condition. A subtle change in a patient who has remained comatose for 2 weeks (e.g., recovery of intermittent visual fixation when closed eyes are held open) will often correlate with objective findings on electroencephalographic evaluation, such as an increase in the mix of background frequencies or evident reactivity of a still poorly organized record.

When the available information does not support the inference that the patient's functional level is due to overwhelming neuronal death or disconnection, it should prompt consideration of functional disturbances at both the neuronal subcellular and the population ("circuit") level. Many toxic, infectious, inflammatory, and autoimmune processes will alter neuronal function and reduce the capacity of cortical, striatal, and thalamic neurons to maintain firing rates and their functional roles in local networks.[1] Systematic diagnostic evaluations of such mechanisms are currently available, and the clinician should make a judgment about whether the functional level of the patient is well anticipated by the features of the history and structural imaging while recognizing that reversible and irreversible severe cerebral dysfunction will often be functionally indistinguishable. Similarly, mechanisms that underlie neuronal population-level (or "circuit-level") disturbances are not yet well classified but are recognized.[31-33] Among the most important population-level phenomena encountered in the severely brain-injured population is selective vulnerability of the anterior forebrain systems (corticostriatopallidothalamocortical loop systems) to reduced overall background synaptic activity and dopamine levels.[32,34] When not contraindicated, an initial trial of a dopamine agonist (e.g., amantadine) is a reasonable empirical first step in a medically stable patient to see whether behavioral changes can be identified. The most common transitional signs from VS to MCS are visual fixation and visual tracking.[35]

In general, patients who are medically stable and have not recovered past MCS behavioral levels are often quickly transferred out of the care of neurosurgeons and neurologists. Nonetheless, it should be recognized that several observations have demonstrated that severely brain-injured patients may harbor considerable functional integrative capacity despite months and years without clinically evident change.[25] At the least, it can be recommended that time trials of stimulant pharmacologic agents be attempted under the guidance of a physician who can recognize subtle neurological changes on bedside examination and that patients undergo periodic reassessment of their neurological status.[36] Although these are reasonable general recommendations for all patients with persistent alteration of consciousness, it is important to recognize the wide differences in expectation for further recovery in VS and MCS patients over the first 12 months after severe brain injuries.

A GUIDE TO FORMULATING PROGNOSIS IN PATIENTS WITH DISORDERS OF CONSCIOUSNESS

The uncertainty of outcome for an individual patient in coma, VS, or MCS will vary considerably, depending on the details of clinical findings obtained from bedside examinations, time from the initial injury, and the specific cause of the injury. Accordingly, it is not possible to comprehensively review the possible circumstances relevant to formulate a prognosis for an individual patient here (but see Posner and coworkers[1] for an extended review and tabular information specific to etiology, diagnostic category, and time windows). Instead, general principles for organizing information and a guide to develop a prognosis for patients with disorders of consciousness are presented.

It is first important to recognize that coma, VS, and MCS are often transitional states with increasingly long time windows that allow further recovery as each transition is achieved (i.e., coma to VS, VS to MCS). The first step is always to locate the patient temporally within the expected natural history of a disease process

(e.g., VS in the first month after a severe traumatic brain injury is not comparable to VS at 6 months or 1 year). The next step is to identify the cause, but outside of anoxic encephalopathy or severe traumatic brain injury (roughly 80% of coma/VS/MCS causes), there are few specific outcome data.

Coma is an inherently grave illness associated with very high mortality; studies indicate that 40% to 50% of patients in a coma after brain trauma and 54% to 88% of patients comatose after cardiac arrest die. However, if no strong negative clinical predictors are identified, such as bilateral loss of both pupillary and corneal responses at the time of the initial injury, outcome prediction becomes far less certain. Accordingly, most prospective studies of coma outcomes have focused on survival or death as end points. A general conclusion is that comatose patients who suffer traumatic brain injury have a significantly higher likelihood of recovery than do comatose patients after cardiac arrest. The younger age of patients with traumatic brain injury and the delayed mechanisms of neuronal death after brain trauma may contribute to this well-known difference.

The prognosis of VS patients similarly depends on the mechanism that underlies the brain injury. A patient who remains in VS for 3 months after cardiac arrest or other nontraumatic, diffuse brain injury that produces loss of blood flow or brain oxygen is considered to be in a permanent VS. To apply these guidelines beyond patients with known hypoxic-ischemic encephalopathy is risky. For example, patients with encephalitis are difficult to assess with these guidelines. Time frames for recovery after posttraumatic VS are considerably longer, and 1 year is required to expect permanence. After diffuse axonal injury, the widespread neuronal death in thalamic neurons is an indirect result of more delayed transneuronal degeneration, unlike the immediate effects of oxygen deprivation, which induces rapid neuronal death after roughly 6 minutes of oxygen loss. Although a continuum of outcomes after an initial transition from coma to VS is well recognized, the outcomes are not equally distributed across a continuum. Anoxic brain injuries produce relatively sharp cutoffs associated with global neuronal death and frequently lead to VS with an underlying anatomic pathology similar to that of brain death. This underlying mechanistic difference probably controls the much longer time course of recovery and the point beyond which permanence is expected for VS after traumatic brain injury as opposed to cardiac arrest and similar injuries. Recovery after prolonged traumatic coma and VS is well described, and unlike VS after cardiac arrest, unconsciousness for 3 months does not necessarily preclude significant recovery. However, no large studies have continued to monitor patients who remain in VS at 1 year after brain trauma. Some case reports suggest that a small percentage of such patients may show some recovery of conscious awareness past the 1-year time frame.[19]

Prognosis in MCS is the least well characterized because the diagnostic category is relatively new and the available studies suggest that significant further recovery may occur in some patients after 1 year in MCS.[35] Importantly, MCS patients typically show faster changes in the rate of recovery within the first year after injury from either traumatic or nontraumatic injury than do VS patients. In the small cohorts of MCS patients studied, some attain outcomes better than severe disability at 1 year despite remaining in MCS for 1 to 3 months.[35] A recent small prospective cohort study also found a limited correlation between time in MCS and functional outcome at 2 to 5 years.[35] Thus, it is essential that the often small clinical finding that distinguishes VS from MCS be identified on bedside examinations performed within the first few months after injury. Importantly, all verified examples of late recovery of communication in severely brain-injured patients have occurred in the MCS patient population; this indicates the importance of prospective tracking and reassessment of these patients.[36]

EMERGING ROLE OF NEUROIMAGING IN ALTERED CONSCIOUSNESS: OPPORTUNITIES AND LIMITATIONS

Several recent neuroimaging studies of VS and MCS patients suggest that functional imaging tools may become part of the comprehensive assessment of neurological disorders of consciousness.[15,20,25,37]

Owen and colleagues used fMRI to demonstrate unambiguous evidence of command following in a single patient with no visible behavioral response who fit the behavioral criteria for VS.[37] This patient was asked to imagine playing tennis and to imagine walking around her home. The patient's brain activation patterns in the supplementary motor area matched the activity profile of normal subjects who imagined playing tennis. Similar activations of the parahippocampal gyrus and posterior parietal cortex were observed when she imagined spatial navigation through her home. The findings provide evidence that in principle, neuroimaging tools may have the potential to identify false-positive VS diagnoses. Simple command following is an objective criterion for MCS, and the imaging findings are arguably an unambiguous proxy for small movements of a finger, thumb, or eye in response to simple commands.

The patient studied by Owen and associates had remained in VS for 5 months after a severe traumatic brain injury.[37] This time frame provides a nearly 20% chance to recover consciousness at 1 year and a 4% chance to achieve an outcome better than severe disability despite remaining in VS.[10,38] The fMRI measurements in this patient may have measured the early aspects of the natural recovery process inasmuch as visual tracking to a mirror was identified at 11 months and thus provided behavioral evidence of MCS at that time. Although compelling, there are limitations to the findings. First, obtaining reliable fMRI data from severely brain-injured patients is often not possible because of hardware in the brain or skull or uncontrolled patient movement. Second, the signal characteristics in patients in general may be different from those in normal subjects, and simply knowing that it is possible to obtain the result in one patient provides no information about the generalizability and feasibility of using these techniques. This important question, however, has not been systematically studied. Third, it is important to avoid overinterpretation. The evocative picture of carrying out the imagery tasks is suggestive of high-level cognitive function. However, many MCS patients will demonstrate clear and reliable command following by performing small visible movements but cannot establish a communication system to accurately answer simple situational questions. Without further measurements or the use of the imaging tools to assess capacity for communication, the only reasonable conclusion is that the patient's function is at least MCS and not VS.[39]

Another recent and provocative neuroimaging study demonstrated evidence of late structural changes in the brain of an MCS patient.[25] The patient recovered fluent spoken language after 20 years in MCS after a severe traumatic brain injury suffered in a motor vehicle accident. Structural MRI in this patient showed marked diffuse cerebral and subcortical atrophy, particularly brainstem and frontal lobe atrophy. Diffusion tensor imaging (DTI) showed significant reductions in fractional anisotropy across cerebral structures consistent with severe diffuse axonal injury, thus demonstrating that the patient had initially suffered a very severe brain injury. DTI measurements also revealed large regions of increased fractional anisotropy in posterior brain white matter not seen in normal subjects. An 18-month longitudinal study of this patient's brain demonstrated significant changes in fractional anisotropy and left-right directionality of DTI-measured diffusion within the medial posterior parieto-occipital regions and the midline cerebellar white matter. The latter findings correlated with clinical improvements in motor control, including limited recovery of lower extremity and left upper extremity motor control and improved dysarthria. These findings suggest a role of slow structural changes within the patient's white matter in the recovery process. A recent prospective study of a cohort of severely brain-injured patients after traumatic injury also found a correlation of recovery of fractional anisotropy to normal or supernormal levels in areas with early significant reductions and recovery of neurological function.[40]

Although there is promise with advanced neuroimaging tools and although immediate observations in individual patients may provide unanticipated diagnostic information or insight into recovery mechanisms, the challenges to incorporate these methods into the assessment of altered consciousness are immense. Until large numbers of patients are studied with comparable methods at multiple clinical centers, it will not be possible to develop reasonable guidelines to introduce neuroimaging assessments. It is anticipated, however, that such studies and informational databases will be compiled within the next decade and should provide enormous value to clinicians in a wide variety of contexts.

SUGGESTED READINGS

Boly M, Faymonville ME, Peigneux P, et al. Cerebral processing of auditory and noxious stimuli in severely brain injured patients: differences between VS and MCS. *Neuropsychol Rehabil.* 2005;15:283-290.

Coleman MR, Rodd JM, Davis MH, et al. Do vegetative patients retain aspects of language comprehension? Evidence from fMRI. *Brain.* 2007;130:2494-2507.

Fins JJ, Schiff ND, Foley K. Late recovery from the minimally conscious state. *Neurology.* 2007;68:304-307.

Fins JJ, Schiff ND. Shades of gray: new insights into the vegetative state. *Hastings Center Rep.* 2006;36(6):8.

Giacino JT, Whyte J. The vegetative state and minimally conscious state: current knowledge and remaining questions. *J Head Trauma Rehabil.* 2005;20:30-50.

Kotchoubey B, Lang S, Mezger G, et al. Information processing in severe disorders of consciousness: vegetative state and minimally conscious state. *Clin Neurophysiol.* 2005;116:2441-2453.

Lammi MH, Smith VH, Tate RL. The minimally conscious state and recovery potential: a follow-up study 2 to 5 years after traumatic brain injury. *Arch Phys Med Rehabil.* 2005;86:746-754.

Maxwell WL, MacKinnon MA, Smith DH, et al. Thalamic nuclei after human blunt head injury. *J Neuropathol Exp Neurol.* 2006;65:478-488.

Multisociety Task Force on PVS. Medical aspects of the persistent vegetative state. Part 1. *N Engl J Med.* 1994;330:1499-1508.

Owen AM, Coleman MR, Boly M, et al. Detecting awareness in the vegetative state. *Science.* 2006;313:1402.

Posner JB, Saper CB, Schiff ND, et al. *The Diagnosis of Stupor and Coma.* 4th ed. Oxford: Oxford University Press; 2007.

Schiff ND. Modeling the minimally conscious state: measurements of brain function and therapeutic possibilities. *Prog Brain Res.* 2005;150:477-497.

Schiff ND, Plum F. The role of arousal and "gating" systems in the neurology of impaired consciousness. *J Clin Neurophysiol.* 2000;17:438-459.

Schiff ND, Posner JP. Another "awakenings." *Ann Neurol.* 2007;62:5-7.

Schiff ND, Rodriguez-Moreno D, Kamal A, et al. fMRI reveals large-scale network activation in minimally conscious patients. *Neurology.* 2005;64:514-523.

Sidaros A, Engberg AW, Sidaros K, et al. Diffusion tensor imaging during recovery from severe traumatic brain injury and relation to clinical outcome: a longitudinal study. *Brain.* 2008;131:559-572.

Voss HU, Uluç AM, Dyke JP, et al. Possible axonal regrowth in late recovery from the minimally conscious state. *J Clin Invest.* 2006;116:2005-2011.

Full references can be found on Expert Consult @ www.expertconsult.com

CHAPTER 13

Neuroophthalmology

Timothy J. Martin ■ James J. Corbett

Neuroophthalmology is a broad discipline that incorporates important elements of interest to neurosurgeons, neurologists, and ophthalmologists. This chapter offers some clinical tools and examples of common neuroophthalmic disorders, with emphasis on material of importance to neurosurgeons that is not likely to be covered in other chapters of this text. Readers are referred to the authoritative, multivolume *Walsh and Hoyt's Neuro-ophthalmology*[1] and other excellent texts[2-10] for a more detailed discussion of neuroophthalmic conditions.

FROM THE EYE TO THE VISUAL CORTEX: AFFERENT ASPECTS OF VISION

Vision is an extraordinarily complex, psychophysical phenomenon that is difficult to define and measure. *Visual acuity* can be assessed with a Snellen acuity chart, but visual acuity is only one component of visual sensation. Vision encompasses the entire visual field perceived binocularly and incorporates subtleties such as color, contrast, motion, and perception of depth. Clinical tests of vision do not always accurately predict visual function in the real world.

The complexity of treating visual problems is compounded by the fact that many patients have difficulty articulating their visual complaints. Everything from visual field defects to diplopia may be expressed by a patient simply as "blurry vision."

History

Establishing the time course of the patient's visual symptoms is vital. Transient visual obscurations last only seconds and are common with papilledema. Amaurosis fugax may cause loss of vision for minutes, and migraine can cause visual loss for 20 to 30 minutes. Abrupt changes in vision suggest a vascular event, such as anterior ischemic optic neuropathy (AION). Optic neuritis causes a decline in vision over a period of several days, with recovery being slow and taking weeks. A gradual, relentless decline in vision suggests a compressive mechanism (e.g., aneurysm or tumor).

Patients can report their symptoms only from their limited perspective, so the examiner needs to be aware of potential pitfalls in interpreting a patient's history. For example, many patients who have experienced homonymous hemianopic visual field events insist that the problem occurred in only one eye (the eye on the side of the visual field loss).

Accompanying ophthalmic symptoms (e.g., eye pain or redness, diplopia, proptosis, ptosis) and neurological symptoms are important.[11] The time that it takes to perform a thorough neuroophthalmic history is well invested because it often saves the patient (and physician) time, frustration, and health care costs.

Examination

It is key to assess vision in each eye separately. Patients are commonly unaware of or tend to minimize the importance of severe loss of vision in one eye if the opposite one is healthy. Unilateral visual loss may be "discovered" when the sound eye is momentarily covered. Frisén, in his detailed treatise, discusses the techniques for and the inherent difficulties in measuring vision.[12]

Visual acuity is typically measured by using a standard distance chart (Fig. 13-1) and testing one eye at a time with patients wearing their best corrective glasses or contact lenses. A pinhole frequently improves the vision tested at a distance in a patient who does not have the appropriate spectacle correction. A near-vision card is very helpful, as long as the examiner remembers that presbyopic patients (older than 45 years) may need reading glasses.

The *visual field* extends 60 degrees from fixation nasally to 90 degrees temporally. Even the large 20/400 "E" on the Snellen visual acuity chart occupies less than 2 degrees of this 150-degree panorama. Visual acuity alone is therefore insufficient to fully characterize visual function. Assessment of the visual field can be done with tools as simple as the examiner's hands or can be formally plotted with kinetic or static perimetry (Fig. 13-2).[13] Many patients who cannot perform well in "formal perimetry" are capable of providing remarkable diagnostic information with confrontation testing (Box 13-1).[14]

All visual field tests are subjective psychophysical instruments that require a cooperative and reasonably intelligent subject. With increasing sophistication of the various types of perimetry—confrontation, Amsler grid, tangent screen, Goldmann (kinetic), and automated (static) perimetry—the tests become more quantifiable and repeatable, but they are also more difficult for some patients to perform accurately.[15,16] Quantification is essential for the management of disorders in which decision making depends on the time course of visual loss (e.g., sellar masses, optic nerve disease, idiopathic intracranial hypertension [IIH]). Furthermore, formal visual fields are necessary to document the efficacy of treatment.[17]

The *relative afferent pupillary defect* (RAPD) provides an objective comparison of the visual integrity of the two eyes. Its objectivity makes it one of the most important tools in neuroophthalmology (Box 13-2).[18] RAPDs do not cause the pupils to be unequal in size. Unequal pupils (anisocoria) are caused by *efferent* disorders.

Even without a slit lamp, a thoughtful guided penlight examination of the external eye and orbit can be carried out. Dilated, tortuous conjunctival vessels may signal a carotid-cavernous fistula; redness concentrated around the limbus is a sign of intraocular disease such as uveitis or acute glaucoma. Redness of the exposed bulbar conjunctiva within the palpebral fissure zone suggests exposure keratopathy or dry eye syndrome. In contrast, viral conjunctivitis causes a diffuse, nonspecific injection of the eye.

The cornea should show a crisp, clear "point of light" reflex from the penlight. Assessing the cornea is especially important when disorders affect either the trigeminal or the facial nerve, or both. Poor function of the orbicularis oculi that results in incomplete blinking can lead to corneal epithelial defects or corneal ulcers. Decreased corneal sensation can result in a similar fate. *Tarsorrhaphy* is a procedure that surgically apposes a portion of

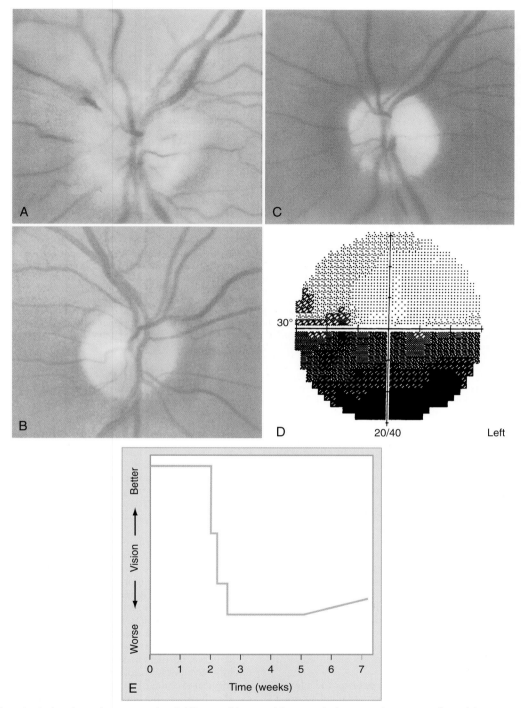

FIGURE 13-6 Anterior ischemic optic neuropathy. A 59-year-old man with systemic hypertension was evaluated because of acute, painless visual loss in his left eye. **A,** Optic nerve. The left optic nerve demonstrates disc edema, more prominent superiorly than inferiorly. **B,** The uninvolved right optic nerve shows a small central cup. This disorder tends to affect patients with small, cupless optic nerves. **C,** Six weeks after the onset of symptoms, the optic disc edema has resolved, with pallor of the superior pole of the optic nerve head being apparent. **D,** Visual field. Although altitudinal visual field defects are common (shown here), virtually any optic nerve–related field defect can be found in patients with ischemic optic neuropathy. **E,** Clinical course. Visual loss is sudden and usually painless. It is often noticed on awakening and may progress initially with stepwise deterioration.

1. Patients who received moderate-dose oral steroids alone had a significantly higher rate of recurrence of optic neuritis than did the other two treatment groups. *Do not treat patients with optic neuritis with moderate-dose prednisone alone.*

2. Patients who had white matter plaques at the onset of optic neuritis identified by contrast-enhanced magnetic resonance imaging (MRI) were more likely than those with a normal MRI result to experience neurological events consistent with MS. The risk for new events in this group was

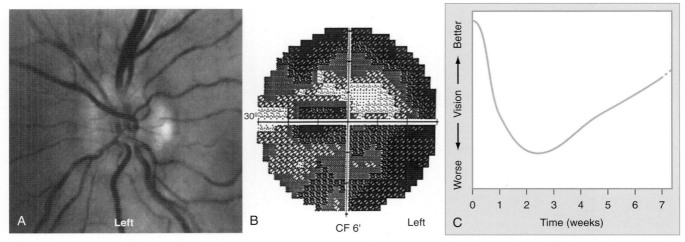

FIGURE 13-7 Optic neuritis. A 34-year-old healthy man experienced a decline in vision in his left eye (to count fingers at 3 ft) over a 4-day period along with retrobulbar pain with eye movement. Ten days after the onset of symptoms, he began to improve. Four months later, the patient had 20/20 vision in his affected eye with a normal visual field. **A,** Disc appearance. This patient demonstrates diffuse disc edema, which is seen in only a third of patients with optic neuritis. The remaining two thirds have a normal disc on evaluation. As the disc edema resolves, optic disc pallor generally appears. **B,** Visual fields. Although central scotomas are common in patients with optic neuritis, any type of optic nerve visual field defect can be seen, including general depression of the visual field, altitudinal visual field defects, and arcuate scotomas. This visual field shows a centrocecal scotoma combined with an inferior nasal step and nonspecific superior field loss. **C,** Clinical course. Vision generally decreases over a week or so, with slow recovery over a period of weeks to months. The patient may recover nearly normal visual acuity and visual fields.

reduced in patients who received high-dose intravenous steroids. However, this effect was evident only for 2 years after the optic neuritis attack. For this reason, MRI with contrast enhancement is helpful in determining treatment options for patients with optic neuritis, and intravenous methylprednisolone should be considered in those with white matter plaques. Because there was no apparent advantage of intravenous steroids beyond 2 years, the decision to perform MRI or treat with intravenous steroids may be individualized.

3. Patients treated with high-dose intravenous steroids improved slightly more quickly than untreated patients did, but all patients improved to the same degree within 6 months to 1 year. Although intravenous steroids offer no long-term advantage for visual recovery, more rapid recovery may be beneficial for patients whose only or better eye is affected.

Many clinicians have modified the original high-dose intravenous regimen (250 mg every 6 hours for 3 days) to make it practical for home intravenous therapy, with 500 mg methylprednisolone administered twice each day or even 1000 mg once daily for 3 to 5 days.[61]

In a high percentage of women with optic neuritis and a lower percentage of men, clinically definite MS is eventually diagnosed in their lifetimes, although some studies did not find a gender predilection.[62] The probability is greatly increased (50% to 80%) when white matter changes are seen on MRI.[58,59]

The discussion regarding long-term treatment options for patients with optic neuritis who are at risk for MS is complex. The Controlled High-Risk Subjects Avonex Multiple Sclerosis Prevention Study (CHAMPS) was one of the first to suggest that patients with isolated optic neuritis (no other neurological symptoms) and white matter lesions on MRI may benefit from initiation of interferon beta-1a. Other clinical studies have added additional information (and complexity) to treatment decisions for potential MS in patients with optic neutitis.[63]

Optic neuritis can occur in response to a viral illness or immunization or may be idiopathic, with clinical findings and a course identical to the optic neuritis associated with MS but without systemic symptoms ever being manifested.

Compressive and Infiltrative Optic Neuropathies

Compression of the optic nerve in the orbit, in the optic canal, or intracranially usually causes slow, progressive loss of vision (Fig. 13-8).[64-68] Common compressive optic neuropathies include optic nerve sheath meningioma and orbital Graves' disease, although any mass lesion adjacent to the optic nerve in the orbit, in the optic canal, or intracranially can be implicated (Fig. 13-E10).

Meningiomas of the optic nerve sheath represent only 5% of all orbital tumors, but because of their anatomic proximity to the optic nerve, they are more likely than other orbital tumors to cause optic nerve compression and loss of vision. Optic nerve sheath meningiomas commonly occur in women (female-to-male ratio of 3:1) in their fourth decade. Optic atrophy and visual loss with opticociliary collateral vessels on the optic disc are characteristic of optic nerve sheath meningiomas.[64,69] Meningiomas can also arise from the intracranial dura and compress the intracranial optic nerve or the chiasm. Sphenoid wing meningiomas frequently have both intraorbital and intracranial components.

Surgical excision of an optic nerve sheath meningioma is indicated only when the tumor is confined to the orbit and the eye is blind because surgical excision of the meningioma invariably strips the vascular supply of the optic nerve and results in blindness. The decision to excise a tumor when intracranial extension is present is complex and depends on whether there is a threat to the contralateral optic nerve or chiasm; the size, location, and growth of the tumor; and the remaining sight in the affected eye. Steroids have only a short-term effect but are often used during radiation therapy.

Observation may be a reasonable initial treatment. The natural history of optic nerve sheath meningiomas is highly variable. They may remain static for many years, or they may progress relatively rapidly. Sequential neuroimaging plus careful monitoring of optic nerve function (sequential visual fields, visual acuity, contrast sensitivity testing, color vision testing, RAPD

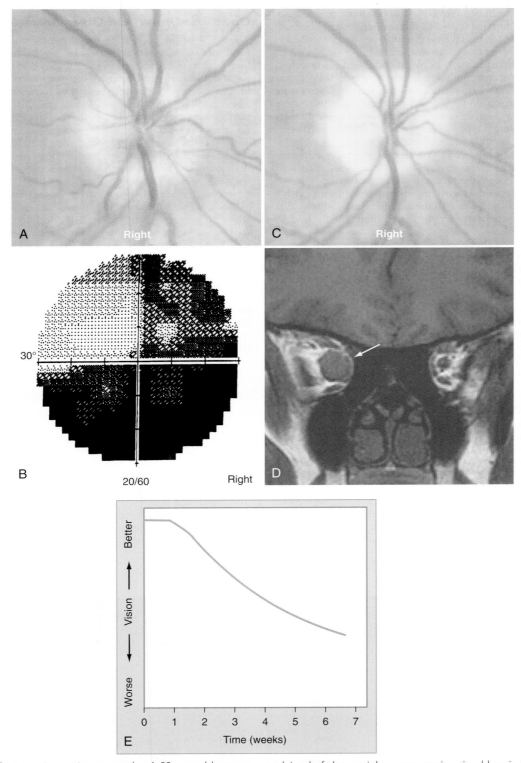

FIGURE 13-8 Compressive optic neuropathy. A 30-year-old woman complained of slow, painless, progressive visual loss in her right eye. An optic nerve sheath meningioma was identified by magnetic resonance imaging and computed tomography. **A,** Optic nerve. Depending on the location of compression, compressive optic neuropathies may be manifested as disc edema, as illustrated here, or as progressive optic disc pallor without edema. **B,** Visual field. Optic nerve compression may cause peripheral or central visual field defects. In this patient, three quadrants were involved, as well as depression of her central vision. **C,** Six months later, this patient's disc edema has partially resolved, but the optic disc pallor remains. **D,** Imaging. Magnetic resonance imaging (coronal view) of the orbit reveals a well-circumscribed orbital optic nerve sheath meningioma (*arrow*). **E,** Clinical course. Slow, progressive visual loss over a period of weeks to months is common.

measurement, and other indicators of optic nerve function) in patients with an optic nerve sheath meningioma is vital because it provides a guide for management. *Conformal radiation therapy is emerging as the most viable treatment option.*[70-73]

Optic nerve gliomas usually occur in childhood (75% before 20 years of age) and are manifested as proptosis, visual loss, strabismus, or nystagmus.[74] About half of optic nerve gliomas arise in the orbital portion of the optic nerve; the remainder arise intracranially. Fifty percent of patients with optic nerve gliomas have neurofibromatosis type 1 (NF1). Fifteen percent of patients with NF1 harbor an optic nerve glioma. These tumors are pilocytic astrocytomas (juvenile type) with a benign cytologic appearance. They enlarge very slowly or may appear inactive.[75] Spontaneous regression of even large, symptomatic optic gliomas can occur, both in patients with and in patients without NF1.[76] By contrast, malignant gliomas of the anterior visual pathway that arise in adulthood behave very differently and rapidly lead to blindness and death.[77,78]

Neuroimaging of childhood gliomas typically reveals a fusiform swelling of the optic nerve or chiasm, or both.[79] Involvement of the chiasm may be associated with endocrine dysfunction and hypothalamic involvement. Children with optic nerve or chiasmal glioma should undergo endocrine evaluation, as well as a thorough search for systemic signs of neurofibromatosis. Most clinicians favor a conservative watch-and-wait approach given the usual static course in children,[75] but surgical resection may be considered in exceptional patients with a blind eye and disfiguring proptosis. The indications for and effectiveness of radiation treatment and chemotherapy for these tumors are controversial and unresolved.

The optic nerve and disc may be directly infiltrated in lymphoproliferative[80-82] or granulomatous (sarcoidosis)[83-87] disorders. Leukemic infiltration with visual loss may respond to urgent radiation treatment (Fig. 13-9).

Infectious agents can affect the optic nerve by direct infiltration, by inciting a local inflammatory response or autoimmune attack on the optic nerve (Fig. 13-E11), by local mass effect from an infectious focus, or by compromise of the vascular supply by vasospasm or vascular occlusion from the products of an inflammatory response. Many agents have been implicated, but syphilis can affect the visual pathway in so many and varied ways that it should always be included in the differential diagnosis of otherwise unexplained optic neuropathy.

Optic Disc Drusen and Other Anomalies

About 1% of the population may have elevated optic discs as a result of *optic nerve head drusen* (Fig. 13-10).[88] In this condition, hyaline material is present in the substance of the optic disc and elevates the axons as they enter the optic nerve head. The rocklike, irregular yellow material is often exposed in older patients.[89] This condition is bilateral in 70% of patients. Peripheral visual field defects may occur, but optic disc drusen typically do not decrease visual acuity.

In young patients, optic disc drusen may be situated deep in the substance of the optic nerve and not be visible with the ophthalmoscope. The elevated appearance of these discs with "buried" drusen can be confused with true optic disc edema. Features that help distinguish these anomalous discs from pathologic optic disc swelling include a "crowded" appearance with no central cup, irregularly scalloped disc margins, anomalous branching of the central retinal artery with many vessels crossing the disc margin, and lack of change over time (Fig. 13-11).

Eyes with a long axial length (i.e., high myopia or nearsightedness) may have an oblique insertion of the nerve into the globe with an apparent elevation of the nasal rim of the disc and an excavation of the temporal aspect: a "tilted" disc. Depression of the retina just temporal to the disc (nasal to the fovea) can cause "refractive" bilateral temporal visual field defects that may simulate chiasmatic lesions.

Toxic and Nutritional Optic Neuropathies

Slow, insidious loss of central vision, often manifested as bilateral central or centrocecal scotoma, suggests a *toxic* (i.e., medication or poison) or *nutritional cause.* Frequently, pallor of the temporal aspect of the optic nerve is present, although the nerve may initially appear normal. The combination of alcohol abuse and poor diet may result in central visual loss. Vitamin supplementation (especially folic acid and thiamine) may dramatically improve these visual deficits. Nutritional and substance abuse consultation may also be needed. Notable toxic substances causing optic neuropathies include ethambutol (slowly progressive central vision loss and disc pallor) and amiodarone (bilateral vision loss and optic disc edema).

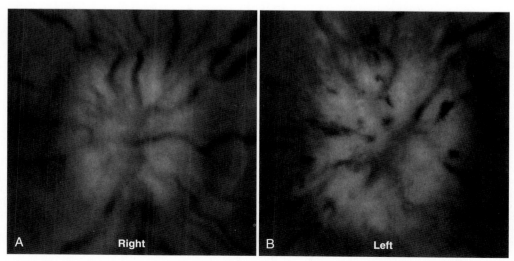

FIGURE 13-9 A and **B,** Infiltrative optic neuropathy. A 17-year-old boy with acute lymphocytic leukemia thought to be in remission experienced sudden loss of vision in his right eye. Marked, pallid edema infiltrating both optic nerves is identified, with hemorrhages present on the left. After an emergency evaluation confirmed the diagnosis, immediate radiotherapy of the optic nerves was instituted.

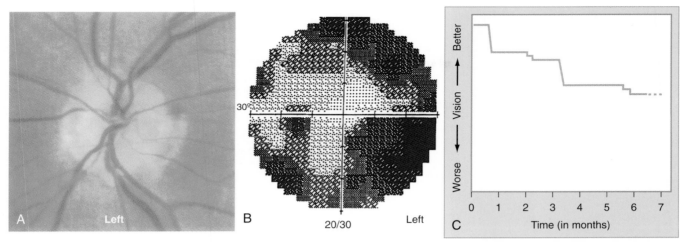

FIGURE 13-10 Disc drusen neuropathy. A 60-year-old woman noticed a stepwise decline in the vision of each eye over the previous year. Optic nerve head drusen were implicated as the cause of her visual loss after an extensive evaluation showed no evidence of other causes. **A,** Optic nerves. In older patients, optic nerve head drusen are often visible as chunks of rock candy–like material poking through the axons of the optic nerve head, as seen in this patient's left optic disc. The right optic disc also showed drusen. **B,** Visual fields. This patient's left visual field demonstrates an inferior nasal step (the right visual field was similar). **C,** Clinical course. Acute, episodic, stepwise decline in the visual field may occur. Transient visual obscurations have also been reported with this entity.

Hereditary Optic Neuropathies

A variety of hereditary optic neuropathies may be manifested as part of a neurological syndrome or appear as isolated findings. *Kjer's dominant optic atrophy* causes relatively mild to moderate central visual loss that may not be noticed until vision-screening examinations at school. The optic discs usually show bilateral temporal pallor, but they may appear relatively normal at the onset of symptoms. The inheritance pattern may not be obvious in the family history because incomplete penetrance is common.[90]

Leber's hereditary optic neuropathy causes rapid, sequential loss of central vision in young men and occasionally in women. Although the disc swelling is rarely impressive, the optic nerves often display fine peripapillary telangiectasia, which gives way to pallor after loss of vision. This disorder is inherited through at least three known mitochondrial DNA mutations and is therefore passed from (usually asymptomatic) women to their children.[91]

Traumatic Optic Neuropathy

Traumatic optic neuropathy may be caused by *direct* trauma to the optic nerve from foreign bodies or bone fragments or by *indirect* trauma, with visual loss resulting from force transmitted to the optic canal by blunt trauma to the brow without fracture.[92,93] The optic disc may appear normal acutely, but pallor inevitably follows in 4 to 8 weeks. High-dose intravenous steroids[94] and surgical decompression of the optic canal[95] have been advocated for the management of acute traumatic optic neuropathy in the past, but the efficacy and safety of these treatments

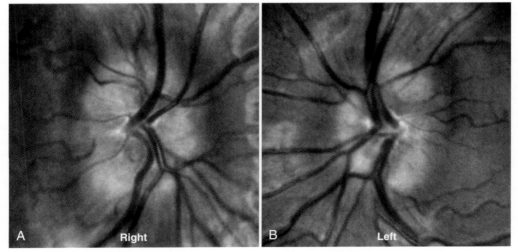

FIGURE 13-11 A and **B,** Congenitally anomalous optic nerves. An asymptomatic 4-year-old boy was referred after a routine ophthalmic examination showed possible disc edema. Five years later, the appearance of the optic disc is identical to that in the initial photographs. As the appearance of this patient's optic disc demonstrates, anomalous optic nerves are frequently "crowded," with no central cup identified. Many vessels cross the disc margin, and many of these optic nerves harbor buried optic disc drusen.

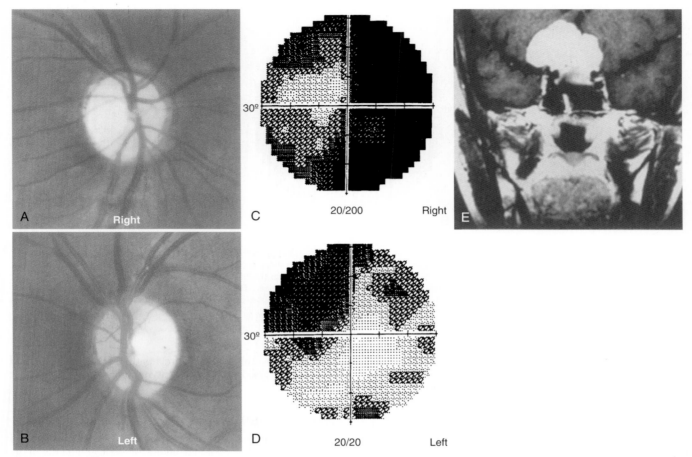

FIGURE 13-12 Chiasmatic compression. A 40-year-old woman noticed a gradual decline in the vision of her right eye over a 6-month period. **A** and **B,** Optic nerves. Pallor of the right optic disc is evident. Mild pallor of the left optic disc is suspected. **C** and **D,** Visual fields. Marked temporal and central field loss can be seen in the right visual field. The asymptomatic left eye had superotemporal visual field loss, which suggested a lesion affecting the chiasm. **E,** Neuroimaging. Magnetic resonance imaging demonstrates a large, enhancing mass in the region of the optic chiasm. Pathologic examination of the surgical specimen confirmed a meningioma.

have been questioned.[96] Retinal detachment, penetrating injuries, and other globe injury must be sought in all cases of visual loss from trauma.[97]

The Chiasm

At the chiasm, axons representing each half of the visual space are routed to their respective optic tracts. Because axons from the nasal hemiretina of each eye decussate, defects in the temporal visual fields of both eyes ("bitemporal hemianopia") result from lesions that affect the central portion of the chiasm (Fig. 13-12). However, chiasmal injury usually arises from mass lesions that do not attack with pinpoint accuracy; the visual fields may reflect damage primarily to one or both optic nerves (optic nerve–related visual field defect), the body of the chiasm (bitemporal field defects), the optic tract (incongruous homonymous field defects), or a combination of these three patterns of visual field loss.[98] Mass lesions arising from the sellar and parasellar region that affect the chiasm include pituitary tumors, meningiomas, craniopharyngiomas, Rathke's cleft cysts, and occasionally, giant aneurysms. The chiasm is located about 1 cm above the sella; thus, tumors arising in the sella (such as pituitary macroadenomas) must be relatively large to compress the chiasm and affect vision. These large pituitary macroadenomas are generally nonsecreting, given that patients with secreting adenomas usually seek medical help for their endocrine dysfunction before the tumor is large enough to compress the chiasm. The prognosis for improvement in visual fields and visual acuity is good (>80%) after transsphenoidal surgery for pituitary adenomas.[99] Rarely, "herniation" of the chiasm into an empty or surgically manipulated sella may affect the body of the chiasm.[100] In addition to mass lesions, conditions that commonly affect the optic nerve are also potential causes of chiasmal dysfunction: demyelination, gliomas, infiltration, vasculitis (Fig. 13-13), and trauma.[101]

Lesions affecting the chiasm almost never cause optic disc swelling but rather result in retrograde axonal atrophy, which with time will result in visible optic disc pallor and loss of nerve fiber layers (Fig. 13-14). An RAPD is often present with chiasmal disease, depending on the density and asymmetry of the visual field loss in each of the two eyes. *The RAPD will be present in the eye with the greatest visual field loss, not necessarily the eye with the worst visual acuity.*

Before modern neuroimaging, visual field testing played a central role in the diagnosis of sellar tumors, with visual field defects identified by perimetry providing neuroanatomic localization. Although the presence and location of tumors in this region can be identified precisely with MRI and computed tomography, visual field testing still plays an important role in the diagnosis and follow-up assessment of patients. Neuroimaging provides a *structural* assessment, which may be difficult to

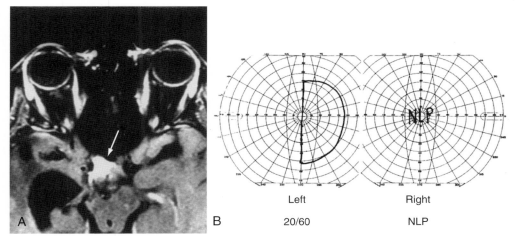

FIGURE 13-13 Chiasmatic radiation vasculitis. A 35-year-old woman underwent surgical resection and subsequent irradiation for a right temporal lobe glioma. She experienced acute visual loss 2 years after radiation therapy. A diagnosis of radiation neuropathy was made after an extensive evaluation had ruled out other causes. **A,** Neuroimaging. Magnetic resonance imaging with gadolinium shows enhancement of the right hemichiasm (*arrow*) involving the right optic nerve and right optic tract. **B,** Visual fields. The patient had no light perception (NLP) in her right eye (right optic nerve lesion), with only her nasal field remaining in the left eye (right optic tract lesion).

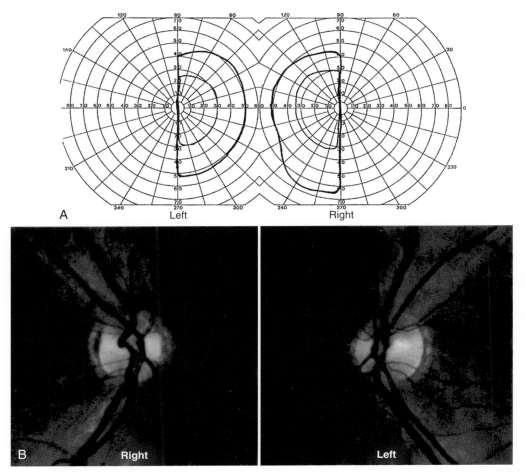

FIGURE 13-14 Chiasmatic trauma. A healthy 7-year-old boy sustained a closed head injury in an automobile accident. **A,** Goldmann visual fields show complete bitemporal hemifield defects. **B,** With time, bilateral "bow-tie" atrophy developed as a result of loss of axons from the nasal hemiretinae (corresponding to the temporal hemifields).

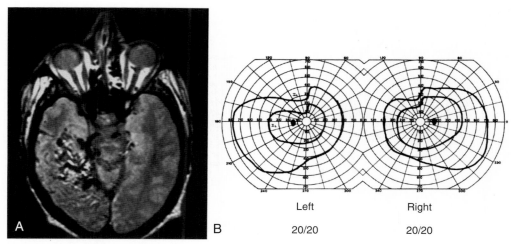

FIGURE 13-15 Temporal lobe arteriovenous malformation. **A,** A right temporal lobe arteriovenous malformation is identified by magnetic resonance imaging. **B,** Visual fields demonstrate a left homonymous superior visual field defect.

interpret in some cases because of postoperative changes. Visual field testing complements neuroimaging by providing a *functional* means of monitoring patients over time to evaluate for recurrence of tumor.

Retrochiasmal Visual Pathways

Lesions of the visual system posterior to the chiasm affect homonymous portions of the visual fields in both eyes. *Optic tract* lesions are caused by the same processes that affect the chiasm. Of 21 patients with tract lesions, 17 were due to tumor or aneurysm.[102] Tract lesions produce relatively incongruous homonymous visual field defects and often produce a specific pattern of optic disc pallor (bow-tie atrophy in the eye with temporal visual field loss, loss of the superior and inferior nerve fiber layer in the eye with nasal field loss). Optic tract lesions may also produce an RAPD because pupillomotor fibers travel in the optic tract before exiting at the brachium of the superior colliculus.[100,103,104] Tract lesions are therefore characterized by contralateral incongruous homonymous visual field defects (Fig. 13-E12) and a small RAPD and optic disc pallor (frequently bow-tie or band atrophy[105]) in the eye contralateral to the lesion.[103]

Axons in the optic tract synapse in the lateral geniculate nuclei. From there, superior retrogeniculate fibers travel directly through the parietal lobe to the occipital cortex and synapse superior to the calcarine fissure. Parietal lesions cause homonymous defects that are denser inferiorly. Inferior fibers take a more indirect route and sweep around the temporal horn of the ventricular system (i.e., Meyer's loop) and through the temporal lobe to neurons in the inferior occipital cortex (see Fig. 13-4). Lesions in the temporal lobe produce homonymous visual field defects that are denser in the superior quadrants (Fig. 13-15). Such superior visual field defects may be created iatrogenically when pallidotomy is performed for Parkinson's disease or temporal lobectomy is performed for seizures.[106]

From the chiasm posteriorly, corresponding axons move closer together as they converge on a single point in the occipital cortex; the more posterior the lesion, the more precise the homonymous defects approximate each other (i.e., greater *congruity*).[107] Occipital lesions tend to be highly congruous (Figs. 13-16, 13-17, and Fig. 13-E13). Complete homonymous visual field defects are said to be nonlocalizing because they can be caused by lesions anywhere from the optic tract to the occipital lobe (Fig. 13-E14). A homonymous hemianopic visual field defect from a

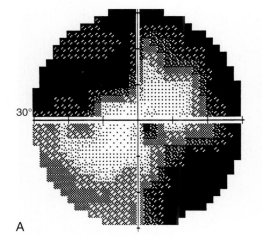

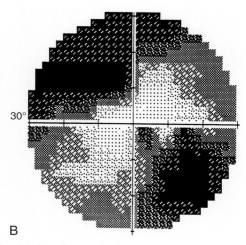

FIGURE 13-16 Checkerboard visual fields. A 60-year-old man noticed a visual deficit after cerebral angiography. His left (**A**) and right (**B**) visual fields demonstrate a right inferior homonymous quadrantic defect and a left superior homonymous quadrantic defect. Magnetic resonance imaging confirmed that this is the result of left superior and right inferior occipital lobe infarcts.

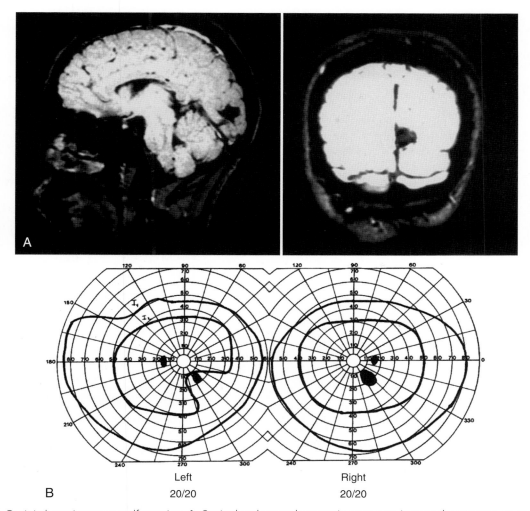

FIGURE 13-17 Occipital arteriovenous malformation. **A,** Sagittal and coronal magnetic resonance images demonstrate an occipital arteriovenous malformation near the surface of the occipital cortex. **B,** Goldmann perimetry demonstrates the corresponding small, but highly congruous homonymous paracentral visual field defects.

unilateral retrochiasmal lesion does not cause decreased visual acuity. However, bilateral retrochiasmal lesions (e.g., bilateral occipital infarcts) can profoundly affect vision in both eyes despite normal findings on ophthalmoscopy and normal pupillary responses (Fig. 13-E15).

OCULAR MOTILITY AND THE PUPIL: THE EFFERENT VISUAL SYSTEM

Anatomy and Pathophysiology

Each orbit contains seven extraocular muscles (including the levator palpebrae) driven by cranial nerves III (oculomotor), IV (trochlear), and VI (abducens). Figure 13-18 reviews the course of these cranial nerves from the brainstem to the orbit.

Both eyes move together to keep an object of regard imaged simultaneously on the fovea of each eye. These two retinal images are not identical because they view the object from slightly different angles. This disparity is processed by the brain to produce the perception of depth, or stereopsis. This "fusion" process can break down if there is a significant problem in the motor (efferent) visual system, with diplopia usually being produced. For example, damage to cranial nerve VI causes a weakness of the

lateral rectus muscle, and as a result the eye turns too far toward the nose. An object viewed with the fovea of the normal eye is also seen by the "crossed" eye but is imaged on the nasal retina and appears to be in the patient's temporal field. The patient has *diplopia*, with the object seen twice when both eyes are open: directly ahead with the fixing eye and in the temporal visual field of the crossed eye. *Confusion* results when there are two different superimposed foveal images or a perception of two different images seen straight ahead.[108,109]

History and Examination

Given the unique wiring diagram for ocular motility, patients' observations about their diplopia can be revealing. The clinician should note whether the diplopia is horizontal, vertical, or oblique and which positions of gaze make it better or worse. Superior oblique (trochlear nerve) palsy often causes diplopia with images that appear tilted with respect to each other. Transient, variable diplopia suggests myasthenia gravis, whereas progressively worsening symptoms suggest cranial nerve compression. The clinician should also ascertain whether the diplopia goes away when the patient closes one eye, as expected for *binocular diplopia*, or when the patient assumes a different head position. The examiner should also discern whether the two images are of

FIGURE 13-18 Anatomy of the motor visual system. Cranial nerves II through VIII are illustrated in this drawing, in which the roof of the right orbit, sphenoid wing, floor of the middle fossa, and petrous ridge have been removed. The cerebellum has been shown retracted to depict the posterior fossa structures. (From Glaser JS. *Neuro-ophthalmology*, 2nd ed. Philadelphia: JB Lippincott; 1990:365.)

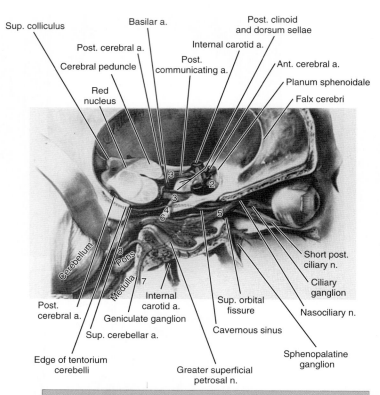

equal quality. A second "ghost" image that is still present when only one eye is viewing suggests corneal disease or cataract causing *monocular diplopia*. Diplopia may simply be reported as "blurred vision" by many patients.

Determining which extraocular muscle or muscles are weak is based on a logical principle: a patient's diplopia, as well as the observed misalignment, should be greatest in the field of action of the weak muscle. Ocular alignment is observed as a patient follows the examiner's fingertip on a prescribed course to test the individual extraocular muscles (Box 13-4).[108,109]

Disorders of the Visual Motor System

Ocular motility disturbances can be caused by lesions anywhere from the orbit to the brain. Orbital processes (e.g., trauma, Graves' disease) can mechanically restrict movement of the globe. Third, fourth, and sixth cranial nerve palsies (i.e., *nuclear and infranuclear* disorders) affect motility in predictable patterns related to the muscles they innervate. *Supranuclear* disorders are the result of intracranial diseases that affect the gaze control centers in the brain and often produce gaze palsies. An *internuclear* disorder affects the interconnecting pathways; the most common of these disorders is internuclear ophthalmoplegia, which is caused by lesions involving the median longitudinal fasciculus and produces an isolated ipsilateral adduction deficit.

In this chapter we primarily address cranial nerve palsies. Table 13-2 shows the causes of isolated and combined cranial neuropathies in a study from the Mayo Clinic in which 4278 cases were reviewed.[110] Tables 13-3 to 13-5 summarize the disorders affecting cranial nerves VI, IV, and III by anatomic location.

Abducens Nerve (Cranial Nerve VI)

In patients with left abducens paresis, there may be no misalignment of right gaze because the left lateral rectus muscle is relaxed in this field of gaze. However, in left gaze, the left lateral rectus muscle cannot fully pull the left eye out, and an esotropia is

---

Box 13-4 How to Examine Ocular Motility

Observe the eyelid position and the pupils for asymmetry with the eyes in the primary position (third cranial nerve or Horner's syndrome) and throughout the examination (aberrant regeneration of the third cranial nerve). Look for nystagmus and smoothness of pursuit by having the patient follow a slowly moving target. Observe horizontal versions to locate weakness or slowness of the adducting eye (intranuclear ophthalmoplegia) or abducting eye (abducents nerve deficit), or both (gaze paresis). Next, examine vertical versions. Straight up-and-down motion gives information about vertical gaze disturbances (dorsal midbrain syndrome) or orbital disturbances (Graves' disease), but isolating the complex, vertically acting muscles requires testing in the vertical plane in right and left gaze. The superior and inferior oblique muscles become the primary vertical muscles when an eye is adducted, and the superior and inferior rectus muscles are most important vertically in abduction. For example, when the left eye looks down and right (adducted), the superior oblique muscle of that eye is being tested (the primary depressor of the abducted right eye is the right inferior rectus). Left trochlear nerve deficiencies are noted in this right and downgaze position (see Fig. 14-20). The patient's report of which positions produce diplopia and determination of the severity of the diplopia in these positions are helpful additions to the examiner's observations. Dissociating the two eyes with a red lens or red Maddox rod over the right eye helps patients report their observations. Ask the patient, "Are the red and white lights further apart when you look here to the right or when I move to the left?" The lens of the Maddox rod produces the image of a red line, which can be oriented to test the patient's vision in a purely vertical or horizontal plane. Additional tests include quantitation of ocular deviations with the prism alternate cover test (which uses known prisms to neutralize the shift in eye position when a cover is moved from eye to eye) and measurement of ocular torsion with the double Maddox rod.

TABLE 13-2 Causes of 4278 Cranial Neuropathies*

CAUSE	ABDUCENS NERVE (%) (n = 1918)	TROCHLEAR NERVE (%) (n = 578)	OCULOMOTOR NERVE (%) (n = 1130)	MULTIPLE NEUROPATHIES (%) (n = 368)	ENTIRE GROUP (%) (n = 4278)
Undetermined	26	32	23	12	25
Neoplasm	22	5	12	35	18
Head trauma	15	29	14	17	17
Aneurysm	3	1	16	9	7
Vascular	13	18	20	4	15
Other	21	15	15	23	18

*Data represent percentages of the total for each cranial nerve column.
Data summarized from Richards BW, Jones FR Jr, Younge BR. Causes and prognosis in 4278 cases of paralysis of the oculomotor, trochlear, and abducens cranial nerves. *Am J Ophthalmol.* 1982;113:489.

TABLE 13-3 Causes and Associated Findings in Patients with Abducens Nerve (Cranial Nerve VI) Paresis by Anatomic Location

LOCATION	POTENTIAL ASSOCIATED FINDINGS*	CAUSE	NOTES
Brainstem			
Nucleus lies on the floor of the fourth ventricle	Ventral pons lesion: V, VII, VIII deficits, Horner's syndrome, and ipsilateral gaze palsy (Foville's syndrome)	Ischemia in the elderly, neoplasm in the young, occasionally demyelination	Nucleus contains interneurons involved in gaze, so nuclear lesions produce ipsilateral gaze palsies
Nerve exits at the pontomedullary junction	Dorsal pons lesion, contralateral hemiparesis (Raymond-Cestan syndrome) with VII deficit, and internuclear ophthalmoplegia (Millard-Gubler syndrome)		Fascicles pass through the ventral brainstem, so isolated palsies are unusual
Subarachnoid space: courses anteriorly along the clivus	Signs of elevated pressure, hearing loss (VIII), and cerebellar signs with cerebellopontine angle masses	Elevated intracranial pressure, hemorrhage, meningitis, inflammation (sarcoidosis), infiltration (lymphoid tumors or carcinoma), compression (chordoma, meningioma)	30% of patients with pseudotumor cerebri have paresis of VI
Petrous apex: enters Dorello's canal	Deafness (VIII), facial pain (V), paresis of VI and VII	Abscess (Gradenigo's syndrome affects V-VIII), petrous bone fracture, arterial-cavernous fistula	VI shares Dorello's canal with the inferior petrosal vein; venous engorgement (arteriovenous fistula) can cause intermittent compression
Cavernous sinus: courses through the middle of the cavernous sinus	Dysfunction of III, IV, V, sympathetics, optic nerve, chiasm, and pituitary gland	Trauma, vascular (ischemia, cavernous aneurysm), neoplastic, inflammatory	Most vulnerable of the cranial nerves in the cavernous sinus
Orbit: innervates the lateral rectus muscle	Proptosis, ocular congestion, mechanical restriction of the globe, dysfunction of III-VI	Tumor, trauma, inflammatory pseudotumor, infection (orbital cellulitis)	
Uncertain	Isolated VI	Postviral, ischemic mononeuropathy	
Other causes of abduction deficits	Vary	Graves' orbitopathy (or other orbital process), myasthenia gravis, traumatic medial rectus entrapment, congenital esotropia, Duane's syndrome, spasm of the near reflex	Resist the urge to call an abduction deficit "VI palsy" until other causes have been ruled out

*Roman numerals refer to the numbered cranial nerves.
Data compiled largely from Bajandas FL, Kline LB. *Neuro-ophthalmology Review Manual*, 3rd ed. Thorofare, NJ: Slack; 1988:77-86.

TABLE 13-4 Causes and Associated Findings in Patients with Trochlear Nerve (Cranial Nerve IV) Paresis by Anatomic Location

LOCATION	POTENTIAL ASSOCIATED FINDINGS*	CAUSE	NOTES
Brainstem			
Nucleus: caudal periaqueductal gray matter	Contralateral Horner's syndrome (because of decussation)	Hemorrhage, infarction, demyelination, trauma (including neurosurgical)	Associated ipsilateral Horner's syndrome suggests cavernous sinus lesion
Fascicles: decussate in the anterior medullary velum			
Subarachnoid space: exits dorsally, long subarachnoid course, passes ventrally and anteriorly	Signs of closed head injury	Trauma, tumor (pinealoma, tentorial meningioma), meningitis, neurosurgical trauma	Longest cranial nerve, vulnerable to trauma
Cavernous sinus: travels in the dura of the lateral wall of the cavernous sinus	Dysfunction of III, VI, V, sympathetics, optic nerve, chiasm, pituitary gland	Trauma, vascular (ischemic, cavernous aneurysm), neoplastic, inflammatory	
Orbit	Proptosis, ocular congestion, mechanical restriction of the globe, dysfunction of III-VI	Tumor, trauma, inflammatory pseudotumor, infection (orbital cellulitis)	
Uncertain		Congenital	

*Roman numerals refer to the numbered cranial nerves.
Data compiled largely from Bajandas FL, Kline LB. *Neuro-ophthalmology Review Manual*, 3rd ed. Thorofare, NJ: Slack; 1988:97-105.

evident. To avoid diplopia, the patient may assume a posture with the head turned to the left. Examination of the function of cranial nerve VI is performed by having the patient look in far right and far left gaze (Fig. 13-19, Video 13-1). Trauma is a common cause of abducens palsy in all age groups (see Table 13-2). Acute, painful abducens paresis in a patient 45 years or older who has hypertension or diabetes suggests an ischemic cranial mononeuropathy. Recovery over a period of 2 to 6 months is the rule. In young patients, abducens palsies may occur as a postviral syndrome, but the clinician must remain alert for the possibility of tumor. Elevation of intracranial pressure can affect the function of one or both sixth cranial nerves (see Table 13-3).

Trochlear Nerve (Cranial Nerve IV)

The trochlear nerve innervates only the superior oblique muscle, but this muscle has a complex action. Because of its redirection at the trochlea and attachment to the globe, the superior oblique muscle intorts, depresses, and abducts the eye. When the globe is adducted, however, the angle of the muscle's insertion minimizes all actions except pure depression. This fact simplifies clinical evaluation of the superior oblique muscle; the clinician looks at how well the right eye can move down in left gaze and how well the left eye moves down in right gaze (Fig. 13-20, Video 13-2). The vital role of the superior oblique muscle in ocular cyclotorsion explains why patients with trochlear palsy often describe diplopia with one image tilted.

Trauma is a common cause of trochlear palsy (also called *superior oblique palsy*). "Decompensation" of congenital fourth cranial nerve palsies is also common but difficult to diagnose convincingly. Neoplasm must be excluded when other causes are not evident (see Tables 13-2 and 13-4).[111,112]

Oculomotor Nerve (Cranial Nerve III)

The oculomotor nerve is complex. It innervates all the extraocular muscles (including the levator palpebrae), except for the lateral rectus and superior oblique muscles. It also carries para-

sympathetic efferent fibers to the pupillary sphincter and ciliary muscle through the ciliary ganglion. *Complete third cranial nerve palsy* produces an eye that is turned down and out (because of remaining function of the superior oblique and lateral rectus muscles) and a dilated pupil with ptosis (Video 13-3). *Partial or incomplete paresis* may present a more confusing picture (Fig. 13-21). The pupillary fibers run superficially in the nerve and are preferentially affected by compression, such as from a posterior communicating artery aneurysm or brainstem herniation. Ischemic cranial mononeuropathy of the vasa nervosum of the third nerve generally shows *relative pupillary sparing*, with the pupil being less affected than motility. Evaluation of the pupil plays a major role in clinical decision making.[113,114] Oculomotor palsy occurring after relatively minor trauma may be the initial sign of a basal intracranial tumor or posterior communicating artery aneurysm.[113] Other causes are outlined in Tables 13-2 and 13-5.

Regeneration after disruption of the axons of the oculomotor nerve may result in misdirection and produce clinical signs of aberrant regeneration: pupillary constriction[115] or lid elevation with attempted adduction or paradoxical motility.[116] *Aberrant regeneration never occurs with an ischemic (diabetic) mononeuropathy* and always implies that the nerve has been injured in such a way that the myelin sheath and perineurium have been broached (i.e., aneurysm, tumor, or trauma).[117] Aberrant regeneration may rarely occur without an antecedent acute third cranial nerve palsy. This is called *primary aberrant regeneration* and occurs as a result of slow-growing cavernous sinus masses, such as a meningioma or aneurysm.

SYMPTOMATIC TREATMENT OF DIPLOPIA

After the cause of a patient's diplopia has been determined and addressed, the remaining symptoms may be treated by occlusion (with a "clip-on" occluder for spectacles or translucent tape over lenses), prisms (using temporary Fresnel prisms or built-in prisms incorporated in the spectacle lenses), or muscle surgery (strabismus). Patients generally prefer to occlude the palsied eye, but

TABLE 13-5 Causes and Associated Findings in Patients with Oculomotor Nerve (Cranial Nerve III) Paresis by Anatomic Location

LOCATION	POTENTIAL ASSOCIATED FINDINGS*	CAUSE	NOTES
Brainstem			
Nucleus: periaqueductal gray matter at level of the superior colliculus	Bilateral ptosis, contralateral superior rectus palsy	Neoplasm (glioma), ischemia, demyelination	Complex subnuclei: the superior rectus subnucleus is contralateral
Fascicles: pass through the red nucleus, medial cerebral peduncle	Superior cerebellar peduncle: ataxia (Nothnagel's syndrome) Red nucleus: contralateral hemitremor (Benedikt's syndrome) Cerebral peduncle: contralateral hemiparesis (Weber's syndrome)	Ischemic, infiltrative (neoplasm), rarely demyelination	
Subarachnoid space: passes between the posterior cerebral and superior cerebellar arteries, runs parallel to the posterior communicating artery	Other signs of aneurysm or uncal herniation	Compression by aneurysm or herniating uncus secondary to intracranial lesion	Pupillary involvement suggests external compression because these fibers run superficially
Cavernous sinus: travels in the lateral wall of the sinus	Dysfunction of IV, V, VI, sympathetics, optic nerve, chiasm, pituitary gland	Trauma, vascular (ischemia, cavernous aneurysm, carotid-cavernous fistula), inflammatory	Aberrant regeneration may result from compression, not ischemia
Orbit	Proptosis, ocular congestion, mechanical restriction of the globe, dysfunction of III-VI	Tumor, trauma, inflammatory pseudotumor, infection (cellulitis)	Superior (superior rectus and levator) and inferior (other muscles) divisions may be affected separately
Other causes			
Ophthalmoplegic migraine	Headache, orbital pain, nausea, vomiting, history of migraine	Vasospasm	Generally in young patients, difficult to exclude compression (aneurysm)
Ischemic mononeuropathy	Ipsilateral pain	Microvascular disease or vasculitis (giant cell arteritis)	Relative pupil sparing in 80% (pupil involved in 95% with compressive cause)

*Roman numerals refer to the numbered cranial nerves.
Data compiled largely from Bajandas FL, Kline LB. *Neuro-ophthalmology Review Manual*, 3rd ed. Thorofare, NJ: Slack; 1988:87-95.

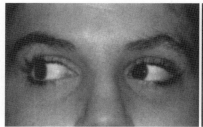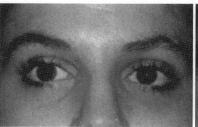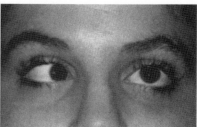

FIGURE 13-19 Abducens palsy in a 20-year-old woman with a traumatic left sixth cranial nerve palsy. Ocular versions are relatively normal on right gaze, but the marked weakness of the left lateral rectus muscle is evident on left gaze.

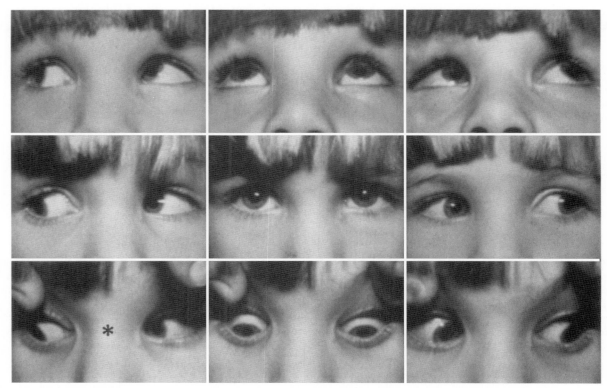

FIGURE 13-20 Superior oblique (trochlear nerve) palsy. This composite of the nine diagnostic positions of gaze demonstrates a left superior oblique palsy. The greatest deviation occurs when the patient looks down and to the right (*asterisk*). In this adducted position, the left superior oblique becomes the major depressor of the left eye, and its weakness is identified as a left hypertropia.

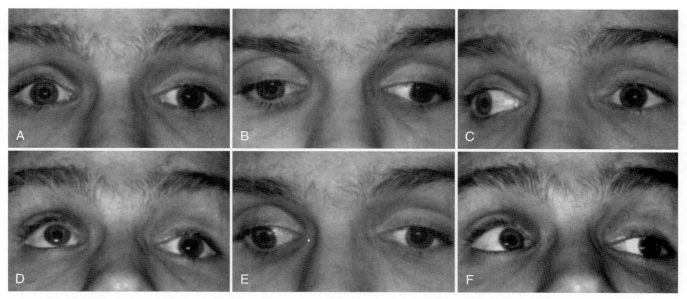

FIGURE 13-21 Oculomotor nerve palsy. In this patient, injury to the left third cranial nerve resulted from closed head trauma. Although motility is only partially affected, the left pupil is fixed and dilated (**A**). In the primary position, a left ptosis (with compensatory right lid retraction) is seen, with the left eye in a "down-and-out" position (**A** and **B**). The affected eye does not adduct (**C**), elevate (**D**), or depress (**E**) well. Notice that abduction (abducens nerve) is intact (**F**).

there may be some merit to alternating occlusion (e.g., when the patient is sedentary) to promote wider excursion and help prevent contracture of antagonist muscles, especially in those with sixth cranial nerve palsies. Translucent tape may be selectively placed over a portion of a spectacle lens when diplopia is manifested only in certain gaze positions. Spectacle prisms can help correct a fixed ocular deviation or help with fusion in the primary position (straight ahead) but cannot account for deviations that change with gaze position (e.g., cranial nerve palsies) or with fatigue (e.g., ocular myasthenia). Prisms do not correct for torsion, which frequently exists in patients with fourth cranial nerve palsies. Strabismus muscle surgery should be considered only after there is no hope of spontaneous recovery, usually 1 year after onset.

The Pupil

Close attention to pupil size and reactivity can provide valuable clues to many diagnoses of concern to the neurosurgeon. It is perhaps equally important for the clinician to recognize common pupil abnormalities that do not warrant further investigation. The value of observing for the presence of an RAPD is discussed earlier. This section addresses *anisocoria*, which is a difference in right and left pupillary size. Anisocoria is never caused by visual loss (i.e., afferent defects); pupillary equality is not affected even if one eye is normal and the other is blind. Anisocoria is an *efferent* problem that stems from abnormalities in ocular sympathetic or parasympathetic innervation of the iris musculature or the iris itself.

Pupillary size is determined by the net result of parasympathetic innervation to the strong pupillary sphincter (through the oculomotor nerve), sympathetic innervation of the much weaker pupillary dilator, and local iris factors that affect the "stiffness" of the iris stroma. Ptosis of the upper eyelid is an important accompanying clinical sign because the third cranial nerve and the sympathetic systems are involved in lid position. The oculomotor nerve innervates the powerful levator muscle, and the sympathetic nerves contribute a few millimeters of lid lift through Müller's muscle.[118]

Determining the Abnormal Pupil

The first and most important step in examining the pupils is to determine whether the larger or the smaller one is abnormal. If a problem exists in the parasympathetic system on one side, that pupil will be larger. In this setting, the difference in pupillary size is most apparent in bright light because that pupil does not constrict well. With a sympathetic outflow deficit, the difference in pupillary size is greatest in the dark, thereby implicating the smaller pupil. Simple, or physiologic, anisocoria is common, with a small difference in pupillary size (generally less than 0.5 mm) remaining constant in light and dark.

The Abnormally Large Pupil

When the larger pupil is abnormal, the most important concerns are oculomotor nerve compression, Adie's pupil, or pharmacologic mydriasis. Pupillary dilation in isolation, without any other sign of oculomotor nerve dysfunction, is unlikely to be caused by an oculomotor palsy. An *Adie "tonic" pupil* is generally manifested as unilateral mydriasis with the pupillary response to near focus being far better than the response to light; this *light-near dissociation* is also seen in "blind" eyes and bilaterally in patients with neurosyphilis or the dorsal midbrain syndrome. Redilation and relaxed accommodation occur very slowly after convergence and near focus, thus the designation as a *tonic* pupil. This condition is the result of an insult to the ciliary ganglion, with subsequent aberrant regeneration of pupillary and accommodative fibers.

Irregular reinnervation of the iris sphincter segments is seen as sector palsies or vermiform movements on slit-lamp examination. Supersensitivity of the pupillary sphincter can be identified with dilute pilocarpine testing (Fig. 13-22).[119]

Pharmacologic mydriasis can occur in many settings: contact with jimsonweed, contamination from a scopolamine patch (used for motion sickness) or other medications, or purposeful administration of mydriatic agents. Weak pilocarpine (0.1%) readily constricts the pupil as a result of neurogenic mydriasis but is ineffective if topical parasympathetic blocking drugs (e.g., atropine) or other causes are responsible for the mydriasis.

The Abnormally Small Pupil

When the smaller pupil is abnormal, an *oculosympathetic paresis* (e.g., Horner's syndrome) must be considered. Relative miosis and a slight ptosis (1 to 2 mm) may result from interruption of the oculosympathetic pathway anywhere along the three-neuron chain: from the hypothalamus to the ciliospinal center of Budge-Waller (C8-T1), across the lung apex to the superior cervical ganglion, or from the superior cervical ganglion by means of the carotid plexus sympathetic nerves to the pupillary dilator. Postganglionic interruption (at or distal to the superior cervical ganglion) is commonly benign or idiopathic, but preganglionic or central oculosympathetic pareses are associated with malignancy in about half the cases.[118] Pharmacologic testing with topical cocaine and apraclonidine is useful in confirming an

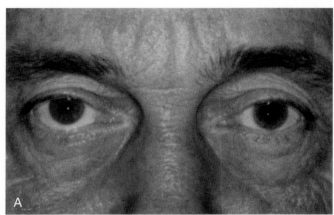
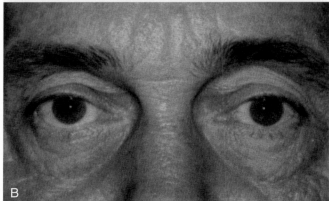

FIGURE 13-22 Adie's pupil. **A,** Anisocoria that was most noticeable in bright light developed in a 56-year-old asymptomatic individual. **B,** Clinical suspicion of a left Adie pupil was confirmed with 0.125% pilocarpine. Thirty minutes after drops were placed in both eyes, left pupillary sphincter supersensitivity was evident.

oculosympathetic paresis (Fig. 13-23).[120,121] Hydroxyamphetamine, previously used to aid in localizing the level of an oculosympathetic paresis, is no longer available.

Other Disorders

Dorsal Midbrain Syndrome

Lesions in the region of the pretectum and posterior commissure frequently produce characteristic signs. Dorsal midbrain syndrome (also known as *Parinaud's syndrome* or *mesencephalic syndrome*) consists of vertical gaze deficiencies, convergence spasm or paresis, bilateral mid-dilated pupils with light-near dissociation (poor reaction to light and good reaction to near), and convergence-retraction nystagmus. The nystagmus is unique to this syndrome and consists of rapid convergence with retraction of the globes on attempted upgaze. This result is most evident with an optokinetic stimulus moving downward because the fast upward component induces this finding (Video 13-4). Common causes include pinealomas, aneurysms of the vein of Galen, and noncommunicating hydrocephalus with distention of the third ventricle and the anterior aqueduct of Sylvius. This syndrome may also occur with stroke as one of the "top of the basilar" syndromes.[122]

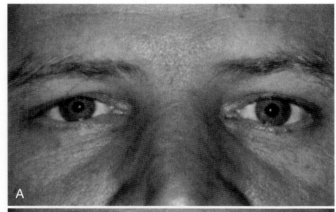
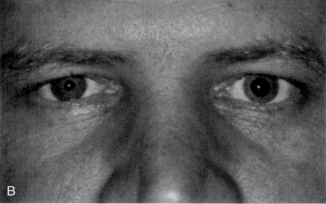

FIGURE 13-23 Horner's syndrome in a 37-year-old man with a history of right-sided cluster headaches being evaluated for right oculosympathetic paresis. **A,** Right ptosis and miosis. **B,** Forty minutes after bilateral instillation of 10% cocaine eyedrops, the left pupil dilates, but the right does not, thus confirming the diagnosis of oculosympathetic paresis. Paredrine (hydroxyamphetamine hydrobromide) testing (not shown) gave a similar result, which implicated the third-order neuron (postganglionic) lesion.

Ocular Myasthenia Gravis

Ocular myasthenia gravis can mimic a neuropathy of cranial nerves III (except pupil involvement), IV, or VI, alone or in any combination, but it is often manifested as elusive diplopia or ptosis that is not easily categorized.[123,124] Ocular symptoms are generally apparent before other systemic signs and symptoms, and in some patients, the disorder is confined to the ocular muscles.[124,125] Because this disorder of the neuromuscular junction causes apparent fatigue of muscular function, patients frequently report worsening symptoms (i.e., increasing ptosis or diplopia) as the day progresses and relief after a nap or rest. The orbicularis oculi is often involved and weak. This weakness may be demonstrated by having patients forcefully close their eyes against resistance. The diagnosis is sometimes difficult to make because the results of edrophonium chloride (Tensilon) testing, serum acetylcholine receptor antibody assay, repetitive electromyographic nerve stimulation, or trials of pyridostigmine bromide (Mestinon) may be unremarkable or equivocal. Single-fiber electromyography has the greatest sensitivity and specificity but is technically difficult. Correctly diagnosing this disease early in its course saves the patient a long and often expensive evaluation.

Orbital Graves' Disease

Because the signs and symptoms of orbital Graves' disease frequently occur in patients with normal thyroid function, normal results of thyroid function tests do not rule out the disease. Although associated with thyroid malfunction, the orbital disorder seems to run its own course, independent of success in treating the endocrine manifestations. Orbital Graves' disease is manifested in three ways: restrictive strabismus, proptosis with external eye disease, and compressive optic neuropathy. The disturbed motility pattern can be manifested as diplopia without an evident cause. Because the inferior and medial rectus muscles are generally involved first, the eyes are usually turned in (i.e., esodeviation) and down (i.e., hypodeviation).[111] Contrary to popular belief, significant muscle involvement can occur without any external manifestations. Strabismus surgery is contraindicated during the active phases of the disease, but prism correction in the spectacles is occasionally helpful.

Compressive optic neuropathy can also occur without fanfare and should always be included in the differential diagnosis of optic nerve pallor (or disc edema), despite a lack of obvious external signs. Optic nerve compression results from crowding of the orbital apex by enlarged extraocular muscles. Treatment usually consists of a trial of steroids for a defined period, followed by surgical decompression of the orbit or irradiation if the signs and symptoms persist.[126]

Enlargement and inflammation of the extraocular muscles can push the globe forward and cause exophthalmos. Orbital Graves' disease is the most common cause of unilateral or bilateral exophthalmos in adults. True upper eyelid retraction also occurs and exaggerates the exophthalmic appearance by exposing white sclera above the superior limbus. For these and other reasons, exposure and dry eye problems can become serious, both functionally and cosmetically. Occasionally, eyelid relaxation surgery is indicated to protect the cornea.

CONCLUSION

Because many neurosurgical disorders affect the afferent or efferent visual systems, the field of neuroophthalmology is of vital importance to the neurosurgeon. Many neuro-ophthalmic disorders require a multidisciplinary approach with contributions from neurosurgeons, ophthalmologists, neurologists, and others.

lesions in patients with sensorineural hearing loss. Such information is available from more formal measures of auditory system function.

Pure-Tone Audiometry

Air Conduction

Pure-tone threshold hearing sensitivity has developed to be the subjective procedure by which auditory sensitivity is determined. In the United States, the American National Standards Institute (ANSI) has established standards for the calibration of clinical audiometers. The output sound pressure level for standard circumaural or inserted earphones, or both, is specified when measured in a standard coupler, referred to as an artificial ear. The artificial ear simulates the impedance characteristics of the average human ear at the plane of the tympanic membrane. The decibel levels used in audiometers for the normal threshold for air conduction can be found elsewhere.[5]

Hearing loss (by air conduction) is assessed by determining the magnitude (in decibels) by which the patient deviates from the 0-dB hearing level (HL) (i.e., normal hearing). To determine hearing loss, hearing sensitivity is assessed at octave frequencies between 250 and 8000 Hz. There is increasing interest in assessing hearing between 8000 and 16,000 Hz, but testing in the ultra-audiometric range (10 to 20 kHz) is not routine.

In summary, pure-tone air conduction testing is the initial and critical measurement for subjective hearing loss. The measure provides an indication of the magnitude and configuration of the hearing loss as a function of frequency. However, little differential diagnostic information can be obtained from this description of audiometric configuration because auditory system dysfunction at various anatomic sites may result in similar patterns of loss of sensitivity. Other hearing tests have been developed for the purpose of distinguishing among the various sites of auditory dysfunction.

Bone Conduction

The primary audiologic tests used to distinguish conductive from sensorineural hearing loss are the comparative measures of air and bone conduction thresholds. The procedure for measuring bone conduction thresholds is similar to that for measuring air conduction thresholds, except that a vibrotactile stimulator transduces the signal, usually coupled to the mastoid of the ear under test. The diagnostic utility of the difference between air and bone conduction sensitivity is based primarily on two assumptions: that the air conduction threshold measures the function of the total auditory system, both conductive and sensorineural components, and that the threshold for bone conduction is primarily a measure of the integrity of the sensorineural auditory system and is not significantly influenced by the functional status of the external or middle ear. It has been demonstrated, however, that the external ear and middle ear do provide minor, but important contributions to the bone conduction threshold in the normal auditory system.[6] Consequently, some conductive disorders do cause minor, but significant alterations in bone conduction sensitivity because of changes in the contribution of the middle ear to the bone-conducted signal reaching the cochlea. Despite this limitation, the difference between air and bone conduction pure-tone thresholds provides the most definitive indication of the effect of disorders in the external and middle ear on threshold sensitivity. A thorough review of the clinical principles of bone conduction testing is provided by Dirks.[7] Examples of conductive and sensorineural hearing loss can be seen in Figures 14-5 and 14-6, respectively. Notice that in conductive hearing loss (see Fig. 14-5), hearing sensitivity by air conduction deviates from normal

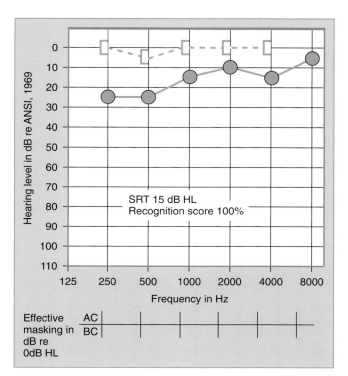

FIGURE 14-5 Air conduction (AC, *circles*) and bone conduction (BC, *square open brackets*) pure-tone threshold sensitivities are shown as a function of frequency in conductive hearing loss caused by otitis media. The speech reception threshold (SRT) is expressed as hearing level (HL) and the speech recognition score is given as the percentage of correct responses. ANSI, American National Standards Institute. *(Published with permission, copyright © 2009, P. A. Wackym, MD.)*

hearing (0-dB HL) but bone conduction sensitivity is within the normal limits. In sensorineural hearing loss (see Fig. 14-6), hearing sensitivity by both air conduction and bone conduction deviates equally from normal hearing (0-dB HL). Combinations of sensorineural and conductive hearing loss are called *mixed hearing loss*.

Masking

When a patient has a substantial difference in hearing sensitivity between the two ears, it is necessary to rule out the potential participation of the better hearing ear when testing the poorer hearing ear. Masking is defined by ANSI as the amount by which the threshold of audibility of a sound is raised by the presence of another (masking) sound.[8] As early as 1940, Fletcher observed that a restricted bandwidth of frequencies contained within a broadband noise was sufficient to effectively mask a pure-tone threshold.[9] Most clinical audiometers contain narrow bands of noise that encompass the critical band of frequencies necessary to mask frequency-specific stimuli.

The process of clinical masking can be rather complex, especially in patients with bilateral conductive hearing loss. The problem arises because the masking stimulus is presented by air conduction but must be intense enough to reach and raise the elevated threshold by air conduction. Overmasking occurs when the masking stimulus from the nontest ear crosses intracranially to the test ear to raise the threshold of that ear. The procedures developed for masking must take into consideration the air and bone conduction thresholds of both ears of the patient.

In some circumstances of severe bilateral conductive hearing loss, it may be impossible to obtain a threshold for bone

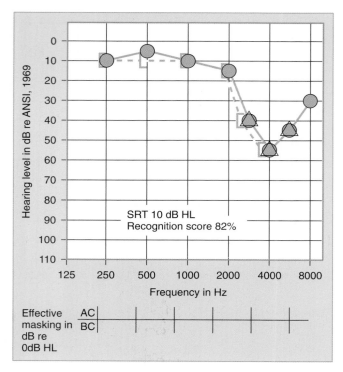

FIGURE 14-6 Air conduction (AC, *circles*) and bone conduction (BC, *square open brackets*) pure-tone threshold sensitivities are shown as a function of frequency in sensorineural hearing loss caused by exposure to industrial noise. Thresholds with masking are also indicated (*triangles*). The speech reception threshold (SRT) is expressed as hearing level (HL) and the speech recognition score is given as the percentage of correct responses. ANSI, American National Standards Institute. (*Published with permission, copyright © 2009, P. A. Wackym, MD.*)

conduction (or possibly air conduction) without overmasking. Fortunately, as described later in this section, acoustic immittance studies can be performed without regard to "masking dilemmas" and can give additional diagnostic information on the functional status of the middle ear. Studebaker has described the rules for clinical masking in detail.[10]

Speech Audiometry

Reduced speech recognition is among the most difficult problems faced by persons with hearing loss. Reduced speech recognition also provides differential diagnostic information on the probable site of the auditory lesion. Speech audiometry is therefore used to assess the receptive communicative ability of the patient and to predict the site of an auditory lesion. Two tests are performed in a standard auditory battery: a measurement of the sensitivity for speech, referred to as the speech recognition threshold (SRT), and a measurement of the recognition (discrimination) ability at suprathreshold levels.

Speech Recognition Threshold

Traditionally, the SRT is measured with the use of spondaic words, that is, two-syllable words in which equal stress is placed on each syllable, such as hot-dog, baseball, cowboy, and sidewalk. No standardized method for presentation of the words has been accepted, although practical means for standardization have been suggested.[11] The SRT is reported as the decibel HL below which the patient cannot successfully recognize the two-syllable words. It is expected that the SRT will

approximately equal the average hearing loss for pure tones in the midfrequency region (500 to 2000 Hz), regardless of the type of hearing loss (i.e., conductive or sensorineural). The SRT has little differential diagnostic significance, except in cases of pseudohypacusis, but it is used to provide a descriptive measure of hearing loss for speech and to confirm the pure-tone air conduction sensitivity measures.

Speech Recognition Measures

Measurement of speech recognition at suprathreshold levels is conducted with standardized lists of words or sentences. Standardized material has been chosen to meet specific criteria that enable comparison with everyday speech. The material available for use includes monosyllabic word lists, nonsense syllables, and sentences. The results are reported as the percent correct scores at a specified level above the SRT.

Persons with conductive hearing loss typically score high with these materials, whereas those with sensorineural hearing loss show decreased discrimination, depending on the magnitude and configuration of the sensorineural hearing loss and the site of the auditory lesion (i.e., cochlear or retrocochlear). Recognition of isolated speech segments is unaffected by conductive hearing loss (if the materials are presented at suprathreshold levels) because the encoding mechanisms of the cochlea and cranial nerve VIII are normal. When the presentation level overcomes the threshold sensitivity loss, the ability to understand speech segments is excellent; however, when the conductive mechanism is normal but lesions of the auditory system affect the cochlear or retrocochlear structures, the ability to understand the consonant elements of speech is affected. When the cochlear structures are normal but cranial nerve VIII or low-brainstem structures are affected by a space-occupying lesion, speech recognition can be severely affected. One of the early diagnostic signs of lesions of cranial nerve VIII or the low brainstem is severely reduced speech recognition scores in the presence of mild or moderate pure-tone hearing loss.

Figures 14-7 and 14-8 provide examples of the effects of conductive and sensorineural hearing loss on the SRT and speech recognition scores of two patients. Figure 14-7 is an example of conductive hearing loss secondary to otosclerosis. Notice the elevated pure-tone air conduction threshold and SRT, together with normal bone conduction sensitivity and excellent speech recognition score. Figure 14-8 is an example of sensorineural hearing loss secondary to Meniere's disease, which is discussed later. Notice the low-frequency sensorineural hearing loss, the mildly elevated SRT, and the diminished speech recognition score (64%). This example reveals the potential effect of a cochlear lesion site on speech recognition ability. Early in the course of Meniere's disease, it is unusual for speech discrimination ability to be abnormal. Review of Figures 14-5 and 14-6 reveals other examples in which conductive hearing loss from chronic otitis media (see Fig. 14-5) and sensorineural hearing loss from industrial noise trauma (see Fig. 14-6) affect speech and pure-tone results.

Objective Measures of Auditory System Function

Immittance Studies

Among the most significant advancements in the differential diagnosis of middle ear impairments and one that provides definitive information on cranial nerve VIII and low-brainstem function is measurement of acoustic immittance.[12] This procedure requires no active participation by the patient but provides objective evidence of middle ear function and a means of testing the

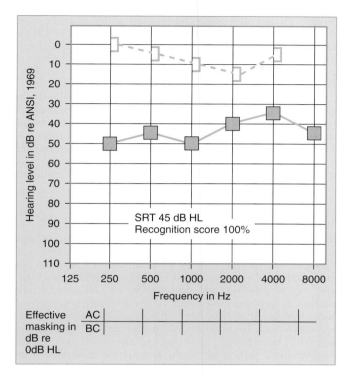

FIGURE 14-7 Air conduction (AC, *squares*) and bone conduction (BC, *square open brackets*) pure-tone threshold sensitivities are given as a function of frequency in conductive hearing loss caused by oto-sclerosis. The speech reception threshold (SRT) is expressed in hearing level (HL) and the speech recognition score is given as the percentage of correct responses. ANSI, American National Standards Institute. (*Published with permission, copyright © 2009, P. A. Wackym, MD.*)

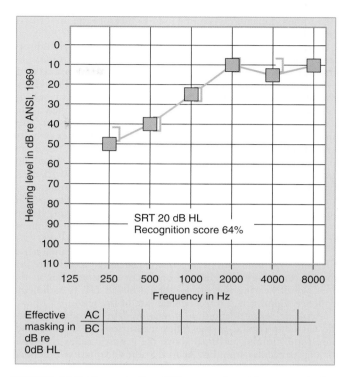

FIGURE 14-8 Air conduction (AC, *squares*) and bone conduction (BC, *square open brackets*) pure-tone threshold sensitivities as a function of frequency in sensorineural hearing loss caused by Meniere's disease. The speech reception threshold (SRT) is expressed as hearing level (HL) and the speech recognition score is given as the percentage of correct responses. ANSI, American National Standards Institute. (*Published with permission, copyright © 2009, P. A. Wackym, MD.*)

integrity of the acoustic reflex arc. The two procedures included in immittance studies are tympanometry and acoustic reflex measures.

Tympanometry

Tympanometry provides evidence of the relative change in impedance (or its reciprocal, admittance) with a change in ear canal air pressure at the plane of the tympanic membrane. The tympanogram provides indirect evidence of the mechanical integrity of middle ear structures when changes in ear canal air pressure are introduced. When pathologic conditions such as middle ear effusion, ossicular chain fixation, or ossicular chain discontinuity occur, concomitant changes in admittance at the plane of the tympanic membrane take place. Such changes in admittance affect the efficient transmission of acoustic energy across the middle ear space to the cochlea and introduce hearing loss. The changes in transmission characteristics can also be measured objectively by direct measures of changes in relative admittance. Clinical instruments are available by which changes in ear canal air pressure can be introduced while simultaneously measuring the effects of the changes in air pressure on transmission of energy through the middle ear to the cochlea. In a normal middle ear system, negative and positive (relative to atmospheric pressure) changes in air pressure produce predictable decreases in the relative transmission of energy through the middle ear space. When pathologic conditions such as middle ear fluid and ossicular chain fixation occur, the relative changes in admittance decrease, a finding indicative of a high-impedance (low-admittance) middle ear. When ossicular chain discontinuity and some

disorders of the tympanic membrane occur, the effect is decreased impedance (increased admittance) of the middle ear system. These measures of relative change in impedance with alterations in ear canal air pressure can also provide evidence of tympanic membrane perforations and the functional integrity of pressure equalization tubes that might have been placed in the tympanic membrane. The tympanogram provides objective evidence of the integrity of the middle ear system and differential diagnostic information on the underlying middle ear source of any resulting conductive hearing loss that might have been demonstrated on the pure-tone audiogram.

Acoustic Reflex

The acoustic reflex refers to the reflexive contraction of the stapedius muscle on delivery of an acoustic stimulus. The stapedius muscle contracts reflexively and bilaterally on presentation of an acoustic stimulus.[13] The muscle contraction results in a concomitant increase in impedance in the middle ear when measured at the plane of the tympanic membrane. Unfortunately, when middle ear pathologies introduce changes in middle ear impedance, it is not possible to measure evidence of further changes in impedance that might be introduced by contraction of the stapedius muscle. Only when tympanometry reveals the middle ear system to be functioning normally is it possible to test the integrity of the acoustic reflex arc.

When tympanometry has revealed the middle ear system to be functionally normal, two types of acoustic reflex measurements can be made: acoustic reflex threshold measures and acoustic reflex adaptation measures. The same equipment used to obtain the tympanogram can be used to measure the integrity of the acoustic reflex.

Constant air pressure is maintained in the external auditory canal, and impedance or admittance is monitored over time. The intensity of a reflex-inducing acoustic stimulus is increased until a change in impedance or admittance is observed. The lowest intensity at which the reflex-inducing acoustic stimulus results in a change in acoustic impedance or admittance is specified as the acoustic reflex threshold. Typically, lesions in cochlear sites produce a change in the threshold of the acoustic reflex only for wide-band noise stimuli, not for pure-tone stimuli, until the hearing loss exceeds approximately the 60-dB HL. When the hearing loss is of cochlear origin and the loss exceeds 60 dB, there may be an increase in the threshold of the acoustic reflex even for pure-tone stimuli. The acoustic reflex threshold measure can be used in cases of sensorineural hearing loss to provide differential diagnostic information on the site of the sensorineural hearing loss.[14]

In patients with a retrocochlear site of the lesion (cranial nerve VIII and low brainstem), the acoustic reflex may be elevated or absent. An abnormally elevated or absent acoustic reflex in the presence of hearing loss at less than a 60-dB HL is audiologic evidence supporting a retrocochlear site of the lesion.[15,16]

Acoustic reflex adaptation is measured by introducing (into the ear contralateral to the reflex-measuring tip) a 10-second, pure-tone stimulus at 10 dB above the acoustic reflex threshold for that particular stimulus. Acoustic reflex adaptation is defined as a decrease in impedance or admittance that exceeds 50% of the nominal impedance or admittance observed at the onset of the 10-second stimulus. This adaptation is not a function of the inability of the stapedius muscle to maintain contraction throughout a 10-second period, but rather an adaptation to the 10-second, continuous pure tone presented to the contralateral (test) ear. The test ear in acoustic reflex adaptation is the ear receiving the acoustic stimulation, not the ear in which the acoustic impedance or admittance is being measured. Acoustic reflex adaptation is typically observed only in ears in which there is a retrocochlear (cranial nerve VIII or low brainstem) disorder.

Figure 14-9 is an example of audiometric data from a patient with a left acoustic neuroma within the cerebellopontine angle. The pure-tone results reveal mild, left ear sensorineural hearing loss with a very poor speech recognition score (24%). The tympanograms were normal bilaterally, but there was no acoustic reflex identifiable with acoustic stimulation of the left ear. When the measuring tip was in the right ear, evidence of stapedius muscle contraction was observed only with ipsilateral stimulation. When the measuring tip was in the left ear, the stapedius muscle contracted only when the acoustic stimulus was presented contralaterally. As evidenced by acoustic reflex measures, this is the classic audiometric result seen in a patient with a left acoustic neuroma.

Auditory Brainstem Evoked Response Measures

Possibly the most powerful audiologic test available today in differentiating between cochlear and retrocochlear lesions is measurement of the auditory brainstem evoked response (ABR). The ABR is one of several clinically useful evoked auditory potentials and the one most often applied in site-of-lesion testing.[17] The ABR is typically evoked with a short-duration pulse delivered to the ear at a predetermined intensity. At high-intensity levels, the acoustic stimulus evokes as many as five amplitude peaks. The peaks were first identified and categorized by Jewett and Williston.[18] Three of these peaks (waves I, III, and V) are the major peaks and are generally accepted as corresponding to firing of the first-order neurons of cranial nerve VIII (wave I), the superior olivary complex (wave III), and the inferior colliculus (wave V). These three major waves are present at approximately 2-msec

intervals (in normal-hearing children and adults) after the onset of the acoustic stimulus at high-intensity levels (Fig. 14-10). As revealed in Figure 14-10, as the intensity of the stimulus is decreased, the amplitude of all peaks decreases, the latency of each peak increases, and the replicability of the early waves (I and III) decreases. Only wave V is identifiable at threshold levels.

Starr and Achor were among the earliest to use ABR results to describe a diverse set of patients with neurological disorders.[19] Patients with cortical problems had normal ABR values, whereas patients with acoustic nerve and low-brainstem disorders had abnormal ABR results. This early evidence has been corroborated by numerous other reports in which ABR values were abnormal in patients with cranial nerve VIII and low-brainstem disorders.[20,21]

Auditory Neuropathy

Results from auditory evoked potential recordings combined with otoacoustic emission (OAE) testing provide objective measures that can identify patients with auditory neuropathy. The term *auditory neuropathy*, coined by Starr and colleagues,[22] has been used to describe a group of patients with abnormal neural function demonstrated by absent or abnormal ABR results and absent middle ear reflexes but with normal outer hair cell function determined by normal OAE testing and cochlear microphonics. These patients also show evidence of poor speech discrimination, particularly in the presence of noise. Pure-tone thresholds vary widely in severity from normal to severe to profound and may be asymmetric or have a variety of configurations. Doyle and coworkers described the audiometric and electrophysiologic findings associated with auditory neuropathy.[23] The results obtained after performing ABR and OAE testing suggest an abnormality of the auditory system at the level of the inner hair cells, at the synapse between hair cells and the cochlear nerve, at the level of the cochlear nerve itself, or a combination of these sites.

The ABR results in patients with cochlear hearing loss typically reveal normal ABR replicability and latencies at high-intensity levels, but with an elevated ABR "threshold" (a function of the elevated hearing thresholds secondary to cochlear pathology). In patients with a retrocochlear site of a lesion, the site of the auditory lesion affects the results. If a space-occupying lesion is present in the brainstem but after the first-order neurons of cranial nerve VIII, wave I may be normal, but all subsequent waves may be absent or significantly delayed in latency. If the lesion affects function of the first-order neurons of cranial nerve VIII, there may be no replicable waveforms evoked by the acoustic stimulus. Figure 14-9 presents the ABR results in a patient with an acoustic neuroma within the left cerebellopontine angle. The ABR result at a 75-dB normalized HL in the right ear reveals a replicable waveform with normal absolute and interwave latencies. The response from the left ear reveals poor replicability of waves III and V, increased latency of waves III and V, and consequently, abnormal I-III and I-V interwave latencies.

The ABR is often used in the preoperative evaluation of patients suspected of having cranial nerve VIII and low-brainstem disorders. An additional application is use of the procedure for monitoring changes in auditory system function intraoperatively. Specifically, under conditions in which a replicable ABR can be evoked preoperatively, it is common to use the procedure intraoperatively to monitor the integrity of the cochlea and cranial nerve VIII (wave I) and evaluate more central auditory structures (waves III and V) as surgery progresses. Intraoperative changes in ABR wave latencies can be used to quantify the effects of surgical procedures on transmission characteristics within the auditory system, but these are not real-time measurements. Immediate postoperative ABR monitoring also provides objective

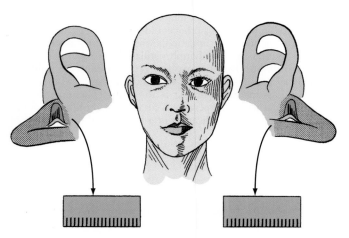

FIGURE 14-17 The left and right horizontal (lateral) semicircular canals are shown with the head in the anatomic position and stationary. The spontaneous resting afferent discharge rate is relatively constant and symmetrical between the two sides (approximately 80 spikes per second). *(Published with permission, copyright © 2009, P. A. Wackym, MD.)*

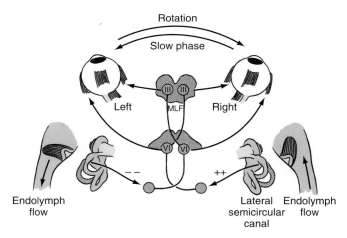

FIGURE 14-18 Normal horizontal (lateral) semicircular canals and the vestibulo-ocular reflex are demonstrated. With angular acceleration in the clockwise direction, there is ampullipetal deflection of the right cupula, which results in an increased afferent discharge firing rate (++). Flow of endolymph in the left horizontal canal causes ampullifugal deflection of the left cupula, which results in a decreased afferent discharge firing rate (– –). The increased firing rate on the right side causes a slow deviation of the eyes to the left. The fast phase of the nystagmus beats to the right. *(Published with permission, copyright © 2009, P. A. Wackym, MD.)*

ducts are able to signal angular acceleration or deceleration. Constant motion (acceleration) cannot be detected by the vestibular system.

The peripheral vestibular system represents a unique neurosensory system. At rest, the type I and type II vestibular hair cells and their primary afferent neurons have a relatively constant and symmetrical resting discharge rate of approximately 80 spikes per second (Fig. 14-17). This discharge rate increases if the stereocilia are deflected toward the kinocilium of each type I or type II vestibular hair cell, and it decreases if they are deflected away from the kinocilium (see Fig. 14-16). Transduction of accelerated motion is brought about by movement of the endolymph, which is coupled to the stereocilia and kinocilia of the neuroepithelium. All the kinocilia are oriented in the same direction relative to the long axis of each crista, and flow of endolymph in one direction results in the same discharge characteristics for all the hair cells in each individual end-organ. A further level of redundancy exists in the push-pull organization between both sets of vestibular apparatus (see Fig. 14-11). For example, with rotation to the right in the horizontal plane, there is relative flow of endolymph to the left (Fig. 14-18). The resting discharge rate from the right horizontal crista ampullaris is greatly increased as the cupula is deflected toward the vestibule (i.e., ampullipetal displacement), whereas the discharge rate from the left side decreases an equal amount as the cupula of the left horizontal crista ampullaris is deflected away from the vestibule (i.e., ampullifugal displacement) (Fig. 14-18). The vestibulo-ocular reflex (VOR) arc results in compensatory eye movements by stimulation of the medial and lateral recti muscles to maintain gaze (Fig. 14-18). The relationship between the vestibular receptors and eye movement is exploited in our objective testing of vestibular function, as described later in this chapter. Normally, this bilateral system is constantly at work, receiving signals and passing them on to regulate posture and movement of the body, limbs, and eyes. Under normal circumstances, the vestibular signals produced by each side are equal and opposite in magnitude bilaterally (Fig. 14-18). The paired otolithic organs function by similar mechanisms, except that type I and type II vestibular hair cells are coupled to gravitational force through the otolithic membrane and their overlying otoconia (see Figs. 14-13 to 14-15) and the kinocilia are polarized relative to a region called the *striola* (see Fig. 14-14). Consequently, conscious perception of this normal

vestibular activity does not occur. However, if there is an imbalance in the relative increase and decrease in afferent firing between sides, patients experience vertigo or impairment of gravitational perception (Fig. 14-19).

Vertigo is a hallucination of movement in any plane or direction. The senses of patients are deceived so that they feel themselves move or see abnormal movement of their surroundings. This abnormal perception of vestibular function may occur when one side is stimulated or impaired by an active intrinsic inner ear

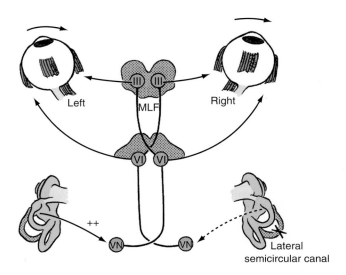

FIGURE 14-19 The horizontal (lateral) semicircular canals and the vestibulo-ocular reflex after unilateral ablation of the right horizontal canal are demonstrated. With absence of resting discharge afferent firing on the right, the normal left spontaneous firing rate appears to be increased (+ +) at the level of the vestibular nuclei. The relatively increased firing rate on the left side causes slow deviation of the eyes to the right (*top arrows*). The fast phase of the nystagmus beats to the left. *(Published with permission, copyright © 2009, P. A. Wackym, MD.)*

disease process (e.g., Meniere's disease), when it is unilaterally ablated (e.g., vestibular neurectomy, vestibular neuronitis), or when one ear is being subjected to caloric irrigation.

Nystagmus, the only sign of a vestibular disorder, may be spontaneous or induced. Spontaneous nystagmus is usually associated with some acute disturbance of the vestibular system, although it may be found in 5% to 10% of normal subjects. Nystagmus may be induced as a test of vestibular function, as described later.

When there is unilateral loss of vestibular function, as illustrated by ablation of the right horizontal semicircular canal shown in Figure 14-19, a relative increase in afferent discharge firing from the left horizontal crista is transmitted to the vestibular nuclei. There will be a slow tonic deviation of the eyes to the right and a rapid compensatory movement of the eyes to the left. The vestibular stimulus produces a relatively slow movement of the eyes, and the central stimulus produces a rapid return. This is the basis for vestibular nystagmus, which may be defined as an abnormal spontaneous or an induced involuntary, sustained-rhythmic, coupled movement of the eyes consisting of a slow (vestibular) phase in one direction followed by a fast (central) return in the opposite direction. Unfortunately, the direction of the nystagmus has erroneously been established according to the fast component, which may lead to some confusion when interpreting eye movements.

Nystagmus may also be defined in terms of its degree. First-degree nystagmus occurs only when gaze is in the direction of the fast component. Second-degree nystagmus occurs with gaze straight ahead; it is accentuated when looking in the direction of the fast component and absent when looking in the opposite direction. Third-degree nystagmus occurs in all directions of gaze, but it is progressively more accentuated as gaze turns toward the direction of the fast component.

Spontaneous vestibular nystagmus may also be classified as irritative and destructive. An irritating lesion produces nystagmus with the fast component to the same side, which is indicative of stimulation of a functional vestibular organ. After the irritating process has ablated vestibular function, the nystagmus is reversed so that the fast component is now toward the intact labyrinth, indicative of lack of function in the diseased vestibule.

TESTS OF VESTIBULAR FUNCTION

Spontaneous Nystagmus

Observation of spontaneous eye movements is facilitated by the use of Frenzel lenses. These glasses have 14- to 20-diopter lenses that eliminate visual fixation and magnify the patient's eyes, thereby resulting in easier visualization of the eyes. Small bulbs that further facilitate objective assessment of eye movements illuminate these goggle-like glasses. The pattern and character of the spontaneous nystagmus have both diagnostic and localizing value, but these issues are beyond the scope of this chapter. More information may be obtained in books by Baloh and Honrubia[36] and by Leigh and Zee.[37]

Labyrinthine Fistula Test

The fistula test is performed by compressing the air in the external auditory canal with a pneumatic otoscope. A positive result leads to transient conjugate deviation of the eyes toward the opposite side. Negative pressure causes deviation to the side of the affected ear. In the case of a perforated tympanic membrane in a patient with vertigo, the labyrinthine fistula test should always be performed. A positive fistula test result in a patient with chronic suppurative otitis media implies the presence of otic capsule erosion down to the endosteum of the labyrinthine cavity.

A positive fistula test with an intact tympanic membrane may be encountered in patients who have undergone fenestration or stapedectomy operations or in patients with Meniere's disease, traumatic or spontaneous perilymph fistulas, or otosyphilis.[38,39] For the test to be positive, the involved vestibule must be viable. A rare clinical manifestation of a labyrinthine fistula (also seen in severe endolymphatic hydrops) is the Tullio phenomenon. In such cases, the patient experiences rotatory or otolithic dysfunction with the sudden application of a loud sound to the affected ear.

Positional Tests

Positional tests should be done with the eyes open while wearing Frenzel lenses so that the eyes may be observed for nystagmus, or they may be performed with electro-oculography for objective measurement of eye movement. In the Hallpike maneuver (Fig. 14-20), the patient's head is placed in the following positions. The subject is seated with the feet on an examining table so that if supine, the head would hang over the edge of the table. The head is turned toward the examiner, who holds it between both hands. The subject is then suddenly placed in the supine position so that the head hangs slightly over the edge of the table and remains rotated toward the examiner. The examiner bends down with the subject and watches the eyes for positional nystagmus (Fig. 14-20) for at least 20 seconds. After the nystagmus has ceased, the patient is suddenly repositioned to sit upright, and the eyes are again observed for nystagmus. The test is repeated with the head turned in the opposite lateral direction.

Two types of abnormal responses may be seen. Static positional nystagmus is a type of positional nystagmus that remains as long as the position is held, although it may fluctuate in frequency and amplitude. It may be in the same direction in all positions or change directions in different positions. Direction-changing or direction-fixed static positional nystagmus can be associated with peripheral or central disorders.[36] In testing for benign paroxysmal positional nystagmus, after the head is placed in the head-hanging left, center, or right position, there is a latent period of 5 to 10 seconds. The characteristic nystagmus is rotary (i.e., torsional) in the ipsilateral eye (i.e., the side turned toward the examiner) and vertical in the contralateral eye (i.e., the side opposite the examiner). The neurology of these eye movements has been well characterized and is illustrated in Figure 14-21. The vertigo and nystagmus usually have an intense onset and attenuate in approximately 20 to 30 seconds. The nystagmus is always accompanied by vertigo, and its direction does not change. On repeating the test, the subsequent responses progressively fatigue, and they may not appear at all after two or three repetitions of the Hallpike maneuver. The pathophysiology is discussed later in the differential diagnosis of vertigo.

Objective Measurement of Vestibular Function

The two most widely applied methods for objectively studying vestibular function are electronystagmography (ENG) and rotatory testing.[1,36] Investigational methods such as posturography, stimulation of the vestibular nerve with a galvanic current, otolith function tests, and high-frequency vestibular autorotation tests are beyond the scope of this chapter but are considered in reviews by Baloh and Honrubia.[36]

Electronystagmography

ENG is an objective method of monitoring eye movements. It has been used widely for the diagnostic evaluation of patients with vertigo, dizziness, or unsteadiness. ENG depends on the fact that there are steady direct current potentials (i.e., corneal-retinal potentials) between the cornea and pigmented retina of each eye.

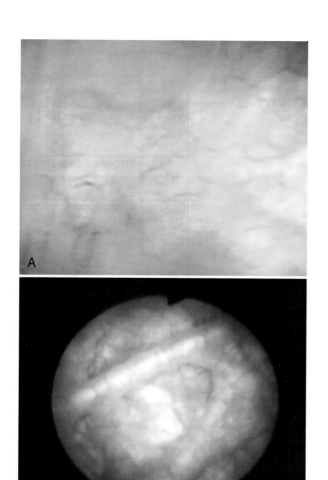

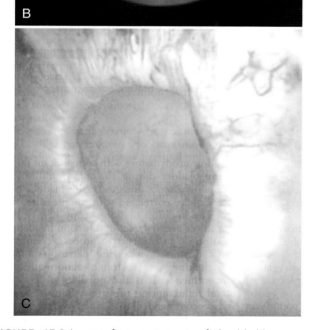

FIGURE 15-9 Images from cystoscopy of the bladder mucosa. **A,** Normal urothelium. **B,** Bladder wall trabeculation. **C,** Bladder wall diverticulum.

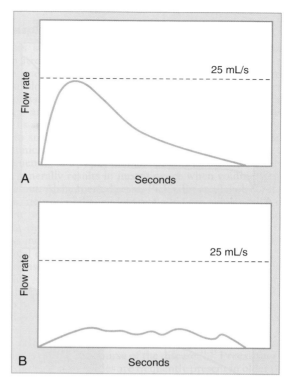

FIGURE 15-10 Uroflowmetry tracings. **A,** Normal uroflow pattern with a maximal flow rate of 25 mL/sec. **B,** Obstructed uroflow pattern with a maximal flow rate of less than 5 mL/sec.

accommodation during filling or bladder compliance, and the presence of involuntary bladder contraction (detrusor overactivity). Ideally, the study reproduces the symptomatology and will provide a physiologic correlation for a patient's complaints.

Bladder compliance, or the change in pressure divided by the change in volume, is determined to evaluate the ability of the bladder to fill with urine at low pressure. Decreased bladder compliance can be secondary to multiple conditions, including neurological disease affecting the spine or peripheral nerves. Low compliance can be a significant risk factor for the development of upper urinary tract complications (Fig. 15-11).[31] The presence of involuntary bladder contractions, or detrusor overactivity, can be either idiopathic or secondary to a neurological condition.

Pressure-Flow Studies and Uroflowmetry

The pressure-flow component of urodynamics assesses the voiding phase of the micturition cycle. Bladder pressure, intra-abdominal pressure, and urinary flow rates are simultaneously recorded during voiding. Specifically, readings can indicate the presence of bladder outlet obstruction, poor detrusor contractility (detrusor underactivity), or inadequate coordination of detrusor and sphincter function, such as in patients with detrusor sphincter dyssynergia.[32] Total voiding time, the use of abdominal muscles or pressure to void, and the ability to appropriately initiate and terminate micturition are also observed.

Electromyography

Sphincter EMG is used to record bioelectric potentials generated by the striated sphincter complex during bladder filling, storage, and micturition. EMG provides information on voluntary control

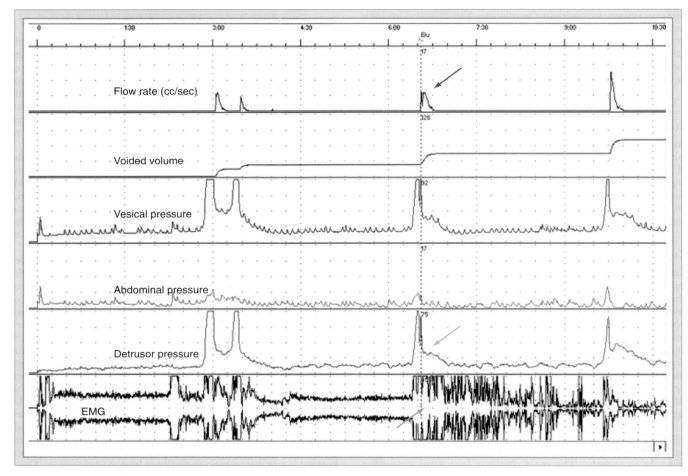

FIGURE 15-13 Full urodynamics tracing demonstrating detrusor-sphincter dyssynergia in a patient with a cervical spinal cord injury. The *dotted line* indicates the start of urine flow. Note the increased electromyographic (EMG) activity (*green arrow*) at the time of detrusor contraction (*red arrow*). Flow (*blue arrow*) is decreased because of increased outlet resistance.

loss of voluntary control.[48] Because of the preservation of external sphincter tone, urinary incontinence is usually secondary to poor emptying and overflow incontinence. Patients will have urinary retention during the period of spinal shock and require either intermittent or continuous catheterization to empty the bladder. Involuntary voiding between intermittent catheterizations indicates the return of reflex bladder activity. Spinal shock generally lasts 6 to 12 weeks but may continue as long as 1 to 2 years.[39]

Suprasacral Cord Injury

A complete lesion above the sacral portion of the spinal cord characteristically causes detrusor overactivity, smooth sphincter synergy (if below the T6 spinal column level), and striated sphincter dysynergy.[47,49] The dyssynergic striated sphincter causes a functional obstruction with poor bladder emptying and high detrusor pressure.[39] Smooth sphincter dyssynergy is present with lesions above T6. Functionally, the most common problem in patients with suprasacral SCI is failure of both filling/storage (because of detrusor overactivity) and emptying (because of striated or smooth sphincter dyssynergia, or both). Careful evaluation must be performed to identify risk factors for upper tract injury, including bladder overdistention, high storage pressure, vesicoureteral reflux, and complicated infection. The goal of treatment of suprasacral SCI is to maintain low storage and filling pressure with either medical or surgical therapy and to provide

suitable bladder emptying with intermittent or continuous drainage procedures (Fig. 15-13).

Autonomic dysreflexia is an extremely serious condition for patients with SCI. In patients with lesions of the spinal cord above the T6 sympathetic outflow tract, response to specific stimuli can cause a massive disordered autonomic discharge. The symptoms are pounding headache, hypertension, bradycardia, and flushing with sweating above the zone of the lesion. This is more common in patients with cervical injury.[50] The stimulus for autonomic dysreflexia is most often distention or manipulation of the bladder or rectum. However, any significant trauma (long-bone fracture, decubitus ulcer, and so on) or distention of hollow organs below the SCI may result in autonomic dysreflexia. Preventive medications, such as oral nifedipine or terazosin, have been used as prophylaxis against these events, but patients require careful monitoring during any provocative procedure.[51,52] The most important immediate treatment of autonomic dysreflexia is removal of the offending stimulus.

Spinal Stenosis

Spinal stenosis is narrowing of the spinal canal, nerve root canals, or intervertebral foramina. Compression of the nerve roots or cord may lead to neuronal damage, ischemia, or edema. Symptoms from compression are variable and based on the cord segment involved. Urodynamic findings will usually correlate with the area of the injury and the degree of damage.[53] Urodynamic studies are essential for determination of the appropriate urologic intervention. Treatment with decompression via laminectomy results in subjective improvement in 50% of patients with associated voiding symptoms.[54]

Neurospinal Dysraphism

Neurospinal dysraphism includes disorders of neural tube and vertebral arch development and is associated with a 90% incidence of lower urinary tract dysfunction.[55] Neurological examination and the level of spinal abnormality correlate poorly with findings on urodynamics and lower urinary tract dysfunction. The typical myelodysplastic patient has an areflexic bladder with an open bladder neck. This classic description is inconsistent, however, because many patients have detrusor overactivity or poorly compliant bladders.[56] There is a fixed external urethral sphincter, with 10% to 15% of patients having detrusor–striated sphincter dyssynergia. Patients usually suffer from incontinence as a result of filling pressures overcoming the low fixed sphincter pressures and transient increases in intra-abdominal pressure (stress incontinence).[57] At puberty, most patients with myelodysplasia report an improvement in continence but begin to suffer from the social implications of urinary leakage. Improved continence can be achieved with urethral bulking agents, urethral slings, and artificial urethral sphincters, If no incontinence is present but bladder emptying is incomplete, clean intermittent catheterization (CIC) is necessary for bladder drainage. With procedures that increase outlet resistance or detrusor-sphincter dyssynergia, careful monitoring of storage pressure is needed to prevent upper tract deterioration.

Tethered cord syndrome can be a primary or secondary result of spinal dysraphism, sacral agenesis, or scarring from initial release of a tethered cord. Preoperative urodynamic findings are abnormal in more than 50% of patients and should be checked before surgical intervention. Detethering for primary and secondary abnormalities may result in improvement in urodynamic parameters and rarely results in worsened lower urinary tract symptoms or bladder function.[58,59]

Disease at or Distal to the Sacral Spinal Cord

Sacral Spinal Cord Injury

Detrusor areflexia with normal compliance is the initial urodynamic finding after a sacral cord injury. Over time, decreased bladder compliance and elevated storage pressure may develop. The bladder outlet is classically described as a competent, but nonrelaxing smooth sphincter with a fixed external urethral sphincter not responsive to voluntary control.[39] Frequently, patients attempt to void by using Valsalva or Credé maneuvers to empty the areflexic bladder and overcome the functional obstruction at the fixed external sphincter and possible closed bladder neck.[48,49] Risk factors and goals for patients with sacral SCI are similar to those for patients with suprasacral SCI.

Disk Disease

Intervertebral disk protrusions most commonly involve the spinal roots at the L4-5 and L5-S1 interspaces. In 1% to 18% of patients, voiding dysfunction may occur as a result of nerve root compression.[41] Patients with voiding symptoms generally have difficulty voiding, exhibit straining or urinary retention, but are usually continent. Neurological examination will show reflex and sensory loss below the area of nerve root compression, as well as low back pain in a "girdle" distribution. The most common finding on urodynamics is an areflexic bladder with normal compliance and normal or incomplete denervation of the striated sphincter.[60] Irritative lesions of the nerve roots can occasionally cause detrusor overactivity.[61] Laminectomy may not improve bladder function, and it is important to obtain a preintervention urodynamic evaluation, which will allow the surgeon to discriminate between preoperative voiding dysfunction and changes resulting from surgical intervention.

Radical Pelvic Surgery

Voiding dysfunction after radical pelvic surgery is most common with abdominal perineal resection and radical hysterectomy. Voiding dysfunction may occur as a result of direct bladder or urethral injury, devascularization of the pelvic organs, or most commonly, tethering, encasement, or destruction of the innervations of the lower urinary tract. Lower urinary tract dysfunction after these procedures is reported in 10% to 60% of patients and is permanent in 15% to 20%.[62,63] The initial symptoms and neurourologic changes after radical pelvic surgery are similar to those after sacral cord injury. Commonly, these patients have urinary retention as a result of poor detrusor contractility and incontinence with coughing or a Valsalva maneuver because of fixed external sphincter tone. Urodynamic studies show decreased compliance and an open bladder neck with fixed striated sphincter tone.[39] Fortunately, some of the lower urinary tract dysfunction can be transient, but affected patients usually require CIC initially (Fig. 15-14).

TREATMENT OF NEUROUROLOGIC DISEASES

Once a diagnosis of the neurological or neurosurgical disease has been established and the neurourologic disturbance identified, attention should be given to the short- and long-term treatment of symptoms and prevention of long-term complications. Management of lower urinary tract symptoms is often complicated and must take into account a patient's overall level of function and neurological comorbidities, body habitus, family support system, and willingness to comply with intensive bladder management programs. There are four general goals in bladder management: (1) protecting renal function and the upper urinary tracts, (2) minimizing lower urinary tract complications, (3) treating the bothersome symptoms of neurourologic disease, and (4) choosing a management program compatible with individual patient goals and abilities.[64] To achieve these goals, treatment should focus on maintenance of low storage pressure, prevention of incontinence, promotion of efficient bladder emptying, and avoidance of infection. Because of the complicated and variable symptomatology of neurourologic disorders, management can be more easily divided into categories of lower urinary tract dysfunction rather than treatment of specific disease entities.

Failure to Store Urine (Incontinence)

Management of Detrusor Overactivity or Impaired Compliance

Timed Voiding, Pelvic Floor Exercises

Lifestyle and behavioral modification techniques are occasionally used in patients with mild detrusor overactivity and associated frequency, urgency, and urge incontinence. Lifestyle interventions include decreased fluid intake, avoidance of dietary irritants such as caffeine, bowel regulation and avoidance of constipation, and timed voiding. Bladder retraining and pelvic floor muscle exercises are behavioral modifications that allow a patient to use

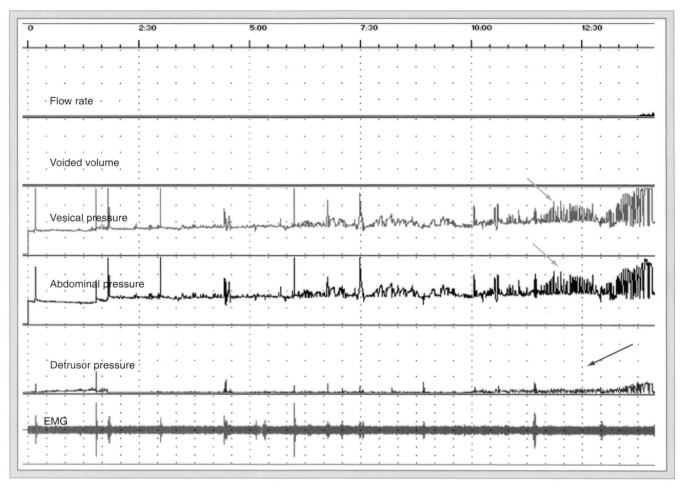

FIGURE 15-14 Full urodynamics tracing demonstrating detrusor areflexia in a patient after sacral spinal cord injury. Despite considerable straining (*red arrows*), there is no demonstrable detrusor contraction (*blue arrow*). Flow is minimal. EMG, electromyographic activity.

contraction of the pelvic striated muscles to inhibit detrusor contractions and urgency sensations through an inhibitory reflex pathway.

Medications

In the treatment of neurogenic detrusor overactivity and poor bladder compliance, the first-line therapy is usually anticholinergic medication. By inhibiting postganglionic parasympathetic stimulation of the detrusor muscle, anticholinergic medications can decrease bladder storage pressure, inhibit involuntary bladder contraction, improve compliance, increase functional bladder capacity, and reduce the symptoms of urgency, frequency, and urge incontinence.[65] There are many formulations of anticholinergic medications, ranging from nonselective to highly selective muscarinic receptor antagonists with various pharmacokinetic profiles. The side effect profiles among the agents also vary considerably. Extended-release and once-daily formulations and transdermal patches are available. Physiologic response can be manipulated through upward dose titration but is accompanied by increased side effects. The classic antimuscarinic side effects of dry mouth, constipation, confusion, and blurred vision necessitate a balance between efficacy and tolerability.[66] Intravesical therapies using dissolved anticholinergics in conjunction with oral therapy have been shown to enhance efficacy with reduction of side effects.[67] Although anticholinergic medications can treat

neurogenic detrusor overactivity and may improve compliance, it is important to remember to treat associated outlet abnormalities such as detrusor-sphincter dyssynergia if present or urinary retention may result.

Tricyclic antidepressants such as imipramine have both anticholinergic and sympathetic action, as well as a central nervous system effect, and decrease bladder contractility and increase sphincter resistance. Although the exact mechanism is not entirely clear, these agents have been used successfully for the management of urgency symptoms and urgency incontinence. The vanilloid receptor antagonists capsaicin and resiniferatoxin are currently being studied and have been shown to increase bladder capacity and decrease urge incontinence in patients with neurogenic and non-neurogenic detrusor overactivity after intravesical administration.[68]

Botulinum toxin A injections into the bladder are used to treat idiopathic or neurogenic detrusor overactivity and decreased bladder compliance. Usually, 100 to 300 units of the toxin is administered by endoscopic injection under local anesthesia. Although not yet approved by the U.S. Food and Drug Administration, botulinum toxin A injection is safe and successful in increasing functional bladder capacity, reducing intravesical pressure, and improving continence and quality of life.[69] A 50% reduction in incontinence episodes has been achieved in patients with neurogenic detrusor overactivity.[70] Optimal administration techniques and dosages have not been defined, and the benefits from injection last 6 to 9 months.[71] The risk for urinary retention is significant after injection, and patients may require CIC for bladder drainage. Side effects of botulinum toxin A injection are infrequently reported but include the development of resistance and systemic absorption with blurred vision, weakness, respiratory failure, and paresis.[72]

Sacral Neuromodulation

Patients refractory to medical treatment may benefit from sacral neuromodulation techniques, which use percutaneously placed electrodes in the S3 or S4 foramen to stimulate the afferent nerve fibers involved in sensory processing and micturition reflexes.[73] The exact mechanism of action is unknown. Success rates in patients with refractory urgency, frequency, and urge incontinence are approximately 60% at 5 years.[74] Experience in patients with neurogenic detrusor overactivity is limited, but preliminary results from smaller studies are promising.[75]

Augmentation Cystoplasty

Patients with intractable neurogenic detrusor overactivity may be candidates for physical enlargement of the bladder by augmentation cystoplasty. A vascularized segment of small bowel, colon, or stomach is placed as a patch after bivalving the bladder. This method prevents coordinated detrusor contractions and enlarges the functional bladder volume. Although it is highly effective in preventing high-pressure storage of urine and protects the upper urinary tracts, intermittent catheterization may be necessary because of impairment of bladder emptying. Risk factors postoperatively include metabolic disturbances, perforation, and malignancy.

Management of Outlet Deficiency

Deficiencies in the bladder outlet and sphincter mechanism can cause significant incontinence in neurogenic patients. The deficiencies can be related to intrinsic sphincter deficiency (open bladder neck), a poorly functioning external urethral sphincter, or bladder outlet injury from indwelling catheters or previous surgical procedures. Methods to prevent incontinence episodes focus on improving intrinsic sphincter function and urethral closure forces or restoring the anatomy of the bladder outlet and urethra. The increase in outlet resistance may cause dangerous elevations in intravesical pressure in some patients with poor detrusor compliance, thereby increasing the risk for upper tract injury.

Injectable Bulking Agents

Injection of urethral bulking agents is used to increase resistance within the urethra or at the bladder neck. Periurethral, transurethral, and transvesical injection techniques have been developed. A variety of agents have been studied, and collagen has been used most commonly. Collagen injections result in success (improved incontinence) rates of up to 85% for stress incontinence and long-term improvement rates of 65% at 3 years.[76] Results in children with neurogenic voiding disorders, specifically myelomeningocele, are less favorable, with only 15% improved with collagen injection.[77]

Sling Procedures

Management of outlet failure secondary to low bladder neck and urethral pressure can be overcome with increased resistance from sling procedures. Transvaginal (female) and perineal (male) slings composed of fascia can be placed to compress and obstruct the outlet. In neurogenic patients, reported continence rates are high for male and female patients after fascial slings.[78,79] Because of the tension necessary to promote continence, CIC is necessary, and there may be difficulty in intermittently passing a catheter. More recently, midurethral slings composed of polypropylene mesh at the midurethra have also demonstrated good continence rates with no erosion complications, although their use in the neurogenic population is limited.[80]

Artificial Urinary Sphincters

Implantation of an artificial urinary sphincter can be performed at the level of the bladder neck or bulbar urethra to establish continence. Artificial urinary sphincters are considered to have the highest continence rates and maintain the ability to spontaneously void. There are conflicting data regarding increased complication rates in neurogenic patients and whether concomitant bladder augmentation increases infection.[64] Long-term revision rates because of infection and mechanical failure are also significant.

Bladder Neck Closure

Failures of more conservative therapy or devastation of the bladder outlet can be managed by closure of the bladder outlet and supravesical urinary diversion. Bladder neck closure is performed through vaginal, abdominal, or combined surgical approaches.

Urinary Diversion

Urinary diversion is useful to establish independence from caregivers for patients who are unable to catheterize per urethra. The variety of diversion techniques will not be addressed but they can either exclude the native bladder or incorporate the bladder with the reconstruction. Diversions can be incontinent or continent and are chosen in accordance with a patient's functional and cognitive abilities. In the setting of bladder outlet failure, diversion is used as a last resort for patients with refractory incontinence from either end-stage bladder dysfunction or complete outlet devastation.

Failure to Empty Urine (Retention)

Urinary stasis can predispose to urinary tract infection, overflow incontinence, and elevated bladder pressure. The goals of treatment include either increasing bladder contractility, reducing outlet closure force, or otherwise emptying the bladder intermittently or continuously.

Management of Detrusor Acontractility (Underactivity)

Clean Intermittent Catheterization

The technique of intermittent catheterization is frequently the first line of treatment for patients with incomplete bladder emptying as a result of detrusor underactivity or urethral overactivity. Adequate manual dexterity is required. By serially emptying the bladder at regular fixed intervals, usually between 4 and 6 hours, patients may maintain freedom from the nuisance and complications of indwelling catheters. If leakage occurs between catheterizations, the frequency can be increased and anticholinergics can be added. The clean technique, popularized by Lapides, involves washing the catheter and hands with soap and water rather than sterility.[81] Although bacteriuria is common, symptomatic urinary infection is much less likely in neurogenic patients undergoing

CIC than in those with indwelling catheters, and there is a lower overall rate of complication when using CIC.[82] CIC decreases the risk for upper tract infection, bladder calculi, cystitis, and bladder compliance.[82,83] There is conflicting evidence comparing clean with sterile techniques, and patients who have recurrent symptomatic urinary tract infections with CIC may benefit from sterile or low-friction catheters.[64]

Indwelling Catheters

The Foley catheter and suprapubic cystostomy tube are useful in the management of detrusor areflexia and are often helpful in the management of acute neurological injury. The suprapubic tube can avoid the complications of urethral erosion, epididymitis, orchitis, prostatitis, and urethral stricture and is often more comfortable and manageable for the patient. However, indwelling catheters have been shown to be inferior to intermittent catheterization techniques in terms of rates of bacteriuria and urethral complications.[84] The irritation related to indwelling catheters can predispose to squamous metaplasia, which is a statistically significant risk factor for the development of squamous cell carcinoma of the bladder, a particularly aggressive form of cancer. Patients should undergo surveillance after placement of an indwelling catheter. It has been suggested that after 8 years of an indwelling catheter, the risk for malignancy is such that annual endoscopic surveillance of the bladder should be performed.[85]

Voiding with the Credé and Valsalva Maneuvers

Some patients with detrusor areflexia do not require intermittent catheterization and can empty their bladder by transmission of increased intra-abdominal pressure. To be successful, the abdominal pressure generated must overcome outlet closure forces. Patients should be checked for hydronephrosis because the increased voiding pressure may be transmitted to the upper tracts, especially in patients with already impaired compliance.[86]

Cholinergic Agonists

Bethanechol is a cholinergic agonist that might be expected to improve bladder contractility. Unfortunately, there is little evidence to support the use of cholinergic agonists alone for detrusor areflexia.[87]

Sacral Neuromodulation

The use of sacral neuromodulation, mentioned previously for refractory detrusor overactivity, has shown benefit in stimulating detrusor contraction in the setting of chronic nonobstructive urinary retention. In a randomized prospective trial, 83% of patients who received a permanent implant had improvement of their symptoms, with 69% of treated patients able to discontinue intermittent catheterization.[88] Its utility in the neurogenic patient population has not been extensively investigated.

Urinary Diversion

Patients who are unable to empty their bladder are at increased risk for infection, upper tract injury, overflow incontinence, and urolithiasis. Frequently, intermittent catheterization or other bladder management options are not feasible because of physical, cognitive, or situational limitations. An alternative to continuous bladder drainage with urethral or suprapubic catheters is urinary diversion, which can provide a low-pressure conduit for urine flow and thereby prevent urinary stasis. Surgery poses a significant risk, but the long-term results are favorable.[89,90]

Management of Detrusor–External Sphincter Dyssynergia

Patients with suprasacral SCI may have bladder outlet obstruction as a result of external or internal sphincter dyssynergia. Management of these patients is dependent on a variety of factors, most notably the ability to catheterize, the presence of autonomic dysreflexia, elevated bladder storage pressure, and incontinence. If left untreated, patients with detrusor–external sphincter dyssynergia will have reflux, upper tract injury, worsening bladder compliance, and eventually, renal failure.

External Sphincterotomy

Surgical transurethral endoscopic incision of the external urethral sphincter can be used to manage patients with detrusor–external sphincter dyssynergia and insufficient dexterity or functional status to perform CIC. Destruction of the sphincter mechanism produces complete urinary incontinence that can be managed with external condom catheters. Although the result will be low bladder pressure and low outlet resistance, the procedure is associated with the complications of hemorrhage and stricture and has a high rate of failure to relieve outlet obstruction.[91] Women are not candidates for this procedure because of the lack of an appropriate collection device and the severe skin breakdown associated with total incontinence.

Urethral Stenting

Prosthetic stent placement across the external sphincter can produce a similar effect as sphincterotomy by eliminating outlet obstruction. In the immediate postoperative period, surgical complications such as bleeding and failure are less common. However, the long-term complications of stent migration, encrustation, and stenosis can produce unsatisfactory results.

Botulinum Toxin A Injection

Direct injection of botulinum toxin A into the external sphincter can provide a minimally invasive and safe alternative to surgical ablation. Similar to other outlet reduction procedures, botulinum toxin A injection decreases intravesical pressure, improves urinary retention, and decreases autonomic dysreflexia.[92] The procedure is not approved by the Food and Drug Administration, is associated with significant expense for the patient, and requires reinjection every 3 to 9 months.

Management of Detrusor–Internal Sphincter Dyssynergia

Internal sphincter dyssynergia at the level of the bladder neck is found mostly in patients with spinal lesions above T6 and can lead to outlet obstruction. α-Adrenergic blocker medications can promote bladder smooth muscle relaxation at the level of the bladder neck. Cystoscopic incision of the bladder neck with electrocautery can also defunctionalize the internal sphincter.

SUGGESTED READINGS

Andersson KE, Arner A. Urinary bladder contraction and relaxation: physiology and pathophysiology. *Physiol Rev.* 2004;84:935-986.

Arunabh M, Badlani G. Urologic problems in cerebrovascular accidents. *Probl Urol.* 1993;1:41-53.

Bhatia N, Bradley W. Neuroanatomy and physiology: innervation of the lower urinary tract. In: *Female Urology.* Philadelphia: WB Saunders; 1983:12-32.

Blaivas JG. The neurophysiology of micturition: a clinical study of 550 patients. *J Urol.* 1982;127:958-963.

Blaivas JG, Chancellor MB. Neuro-urologic examination. In: Chancellor MB, Blaivas JG, eds. *Practical Neuro-urology: Genitourinary Complications in Neurologic Disease.* Boston: Butterworth-Heinemann; 1995:55-62.

Chancellor MB, Anderson RU, Boone TB. Pharmacotherapy for neurogenic detrusor overactivity. *Am J Phys Med Rehabil.* 2006;85:536-545.

Chancellor MB, Blaivas JG. Urologic symptoms of neurologic diseases. In: Chancellor MB, Blaivas JG, eds. *Practical Neuro-urology : Genitourinary Complications in Neurologic Disease.* Boston: Butterworth-Heinemann; 1995:49-54.

Deen HG Jr, Zimmerman RS, Swanson SK, et al. Assessment of bladder function after lumbar decompressive laminectomy for spinal stenosis: a prospective study. *J Neurosurg.* 1994;80:971-974.

de Groat WC. Integrative control of the lower urinary tract: preclinical perspective. *Br J Pharmacol.* 2006;147:S25-S40.

Dmochowski R, Sand PK. Botulinum toxin A in the overactive bladder: current status and future directions. *BJU Int.* 2007;99:247-262.

Elbadawi A. *Neuromuscular Mechanisms of Micturition: Neurourology and Urodynamics.* New York: Macmillan; 1988:3-35.

Esclarin De Ruz A, Garcia Leoni E, Herruzo Cabrera R. Epidemiology and risk factors for urinary tract infection in patients with spinal cord injury. *J Urol.* 2000;164:1285-1289.

Hsieh MH, Perry V, Gupta N, et al. The effects of detethering on the urodynamics profile in children with a tethered cord. *J Neurosurg.* 2006;105:391-395.

Karsenty G, Denys P, Amarenco G, et al. Botulinum toxin A (Botox) intradetrusor injections in adults with neurogenic detrusor overactivity/neurogenic overactive bladder: a systematic literature review. *Eur Urol.* 2008;53:275-287.

Lapides J, Diokno AC, Silber SJ, et al. Clean, intermittent self-catheterization in the treatment of urinary tract disease. *J Urol.* 1972;107:458-461.

Leng WW, Chancellor MB. How sacral nerve stimulation neuromodulation works. *Urol Clin North Am.* 2005;32:11-18.

Lue T. Physiology of penile erection and pathophysiology of erectile dysfunction. In: Wein AJ, Kavoussi LR, Partin AW, et al, eds. *Campbell-Walsh Urology.* Philadelphia: WB Saunders; 2007:718-749.

McGuire EJ, Woodside JR, Borden TA, et al. Prognostic value of urodynamic testing in myelodysplastic patients. *J Urol.* 1981;126:205-209.

O'Flynn KJ, Murphy R, Thomas DG. Neurogenic bladder dysfunction in lumbar intervertebral disc prolapse. *Br J Urol.* 1992;69:38-40.

Peterson A, Webster G. Urodynamic and videourodynamic evaluation of voiding dysfunction. In: Wein AJ, Kavoussi LR, Partin AW, et al, eds. *Campbell-Walsh Urology.* Philadelphia: WB Saunders; 2007:1986-2010.

Razdan S, Leboeuf L, Meinbach DS, et al. Current practice patterns in the urologic surveillance and management of patients with spinal cord injury. *Urology.* 2003;61:893-896.

Rovner E, Wein AJ. *Adult Voiding Dysfunction Secondary to Neurologic Disease or Injury, Lesson 6: AUA Update Series, vol. XVIII.* Houston: American Urological Association Office of Education; 1999:42-47.

Trop CS, Bennett CJ. Autonomic dysreflexia and its urological implications: a review. *J Urol.* 1991;146:1461-1469.

Wahle GR, Young GPH, Raz S, et al. Neurourology. In: Winn HR, ed. *Youmans Neurological Surgery.* 5th ed. Philadelphia: WB Saunders; 2004:357-384.

Weld KJ, Dmochowski RR. Effect of bladder management on urological complications in spinal cord injured patients. *J Urol.* 2000;163:768-772.

Yoshimura N, Chancellor MB. Current and future pharmacological treatment for overactive bladder. *J Urol.* 2002;168:1897-1913.

Full references can be found on Expert Consult @ www.expertconsult.com

now by using handheld computers)? What about interweaving artificial neuronal arrays with real neurons in the cortex or other brain regions to repair them after injury? Ideally, this could all be done with a genetic or epigenetic set of instructions, but this method might be so complicated that it prohibits all but the most general types of instructions, which would be insufficient to promote specific functions or abilities. The neuropsychologist and neurosurgeon have important roles to play in these future efforts.

The human brain is a lovely and complicated organ. Simply navigating through it for the purposes of surgical precision and efficacy has proved a challenge. Identifying the function of its various regions has proved as much of a challenge. For clinical neuropsychologists and cognitive neuroscientists, the past few decades have brought dramatic improvements in the ability to precisely evaluate patients, identify the functions of various brain regions, measure their change over time, and predict outcome. Clinical neuropsychologists and cognitive neuroscientists provide an essential service to the neurosurgeon and can be intellectual companions in the effort to resolve the remaining mysteries of the human brain.

SUGGESTED READINGS

Birbaumer N, Murguialday AR, Cohen L. Brain-computer interface in paralysis. *Curr Opin Neurol.* 2008;21:634.

Boller F, Grafman J, eds. *Handbook of Neuropsychology*, 2nd ed. Amsterdam: Elsevier Science; 2003.

Cicerone K, Levin H, Malec J, et al. Cognitive rehabilitation interventions for executive function: moving from bench to bedside in patients with traumatic brain injury. *J Cogn Neurosci.* 2006;18:1212.

Dubois B, Slachevsky A, Litvan I, et al. The FAB: a Frontal Assessment Battery at bedside. *Neurology.* 2000;55:1621.

Farace E. Role of Neuropsychological assessment in cancer patients. In: Meyers A, Perry JR, eds. *Cognition and Cancer.* New York: Cambridge University Press; 2008:33.

Frank MJ, Samanta J, Moustafa AA, et al. Hold your horses: impulsivity, deep brain stimulation, and medication in parkinsonism. *Science.* 2007;318:1309.

Gazzaniga MS, ed. *The Cognitive Neurosciences III.* 3rd ed. Cambridge, MA: MIT Press; 2004:1399.

Gelbard-Sagiv H, Mukamel R, Harel M, et al. Internally generated reactivation of single neurons in human hippocampus during free recall. *Science.* 2008;322:96.

Grafman J, Christen Y, eds. *Neuronal Plasticity: Building a Bridge from the Laboratory to the Clinic.* Berlin: Springer; 1999:190.

Jurado MA, Junque C, Vendrell P, et al. Overestimation and unreliability in "feeling of doing" judgments about temporal ordering performance: impaired self-awareness following frontal lobe damage. *J Clin Exp Neuropsychol.* 1998;20:353.

Kane RL. Standardized and flexible batteries in neuropsychology: an assessment update. *Neuropsychol Rev.* 1991;2:281.

Khuntia D, Mathew BS, Meyers CA, et al. Brain metastases. In: Meyers CA, Perry JR, eds. *Cognition and Cancer.* New York: Cambridge University Press; 2008:170.

Levin HS, Grafman, J, eds. *Cerebral Organization of Function after Brain Damage.* New York: Oxford University Press; 2000:392.

Lezak MD, Howieson DB, Loring DW, eds. *Neuropsychological Assessment.* 4th ed. Oxford, U.K.: Oxford University Press; 2004:1016.

Locke DEC, Cerhan JH, Malec JF. Behavioral strategies and rehabilitation. In: Meyers CA, Perry JR, eds. *Cognition and Cancer.* New York: Cambridge University Press; 2008:281.

McDonald BC, Saykin AJ, Ahles TA. Brain imaging investigation of chemotherapy-induced neurocognitive changes. In: Meyers CA, Perry JR, eds. *Cognition and Cancer.* New York: Cambridge University Press; 2008:19.

Meyers CA, Boake C, Levin VA, et al. Symptom management, rehabilitation strategies, and improved quality of life for patients with brain tumors. In: Levin VA, ed. *Cancer in the Nervous System.* New York: Churchill Livingstone; 1996:4492.

Ojemann G, Ojemann J, Lettich E, et al. Cortical language localization in left, dominant hemisphere. An electrical stimulation mapping investigation in 117 patients. *J Neurosurg.* 2008;108:411.

Owen AM, Coleman MR. Functional MRI in disorders of consciousness: advantages and limitations. *Curr Opin Neurol.* 2007;20:632.

Salazar AM, Warden DL, Schwab K, et al. Cognitive rehabilitation for traumatic brain injury: a randomized trial. Defense and Veterans Head Injury Program (DVHIP) Study Group. *JAMA.* 2000;283:3075.

Schiff ND, Fins JJ. Deep brain stimulation and cognition: moving from animal to patient. *Curr Opin Neurol.* 2007;20:638.

Schiff ND, Giacino JT, Kalmar K, et al. Behavioural improvements with thalamic stimulation after severe traumatic brain injury. *Nature.* 2007;448:600.

Schwab K, Grafman J, Salazar AM, et al. Residual impairments and work status 15 years after penetrating head injury: report from the Vietnam Head Injury Study. *Neurology.* 1993;43:95.

Shaw EG, Butler J, Case LD, et al. Pharmacological interventions for the treatment of radiation-induced brain injury. In: Meyers CA, Perry JR, eds. *Cognition and Cancer.* New York: Cambridge University Press; 2008:312.

Smith JA, Wefel JS. Neurocognitive testing in clinical trials. In: Meyers CA, Perry JR, eds. *Cognition and Cancer.* New York: Cambridge University Press; 2008:320.

Squire LR. The legacy of patient H.M. for neuroscience. *Neuron.* 2009;61:6.

Velliste M, Perel S, Spalding MC, et al. Cortical control of a prosthetic arm for self-feeding. *Nature.* 2008;453:1098.

Wefel JS, Collins R, Kayl AE. Cognitive dysfunction related to chemotherapy and biological response modifiers. In: Meyers CA, Perry JR, eds. *Cognition and Cancer.* New York: Cambridge University Press; 2008:97.

Wood JN, Grafman J. Human prefrontal cortex: processing and representational perspectives. *Nat Rev Neurosci.* 2003;4:139.

Full references can be found on Expert Consult @ www.expertconsult.com

Radiologic Fundamentals

CHAPTER 17

Computed Tomography and Magnetic Resonance Imaging of the Brain

Thomas Aquinas Kim ■ Aleksandrs Uldis Kalnins ■
Robert W. Prost

COMPUTED TOMOGRAPHY OF THE BRAIN

History and Fundamentals

Computed tomography (CT), also called computed axial tomography (CAT), was developed in the early 1970s by Sir Geoffrey Hounsfield and his colleagues in England.[1] It was possibly the single most important advance in medical imaging since the discovery of x-rays by Professor Wilhelm Roentgen. It represented the first commercially available imaging equipment that used the emerging technologic advances in computing to generate digital images displayed in gray scale. Its development revolutionized the evaluation of patients with neurological diseases and allowed noninvasive visualization of the inner body, which led to important diagnoses of diseases and abnormalities and played a key role in the diagnosis, management, and treatment of patients on a daily basis in the practice of medicine all over the world.[2] Although its place in imaging of the brain and spine have been somewhat supplanted by another revolutionary technology known as magnetic resonance imaging (MRI), CT remains a workhorse and important first study of choice in many aspects of neurosurgery. Furthermore, important advances in CT technology during the past decade, such as multidetector configurations in newer CT scanners and ever increasing speed of computer technology that now allow very fast CT scanning of a patient in seconds rather than minutes, have resulted in a strong resurgence in its use. Such advances have led to the development of CT angiography (CTA) and perfusion CT (pCT), which have become important in noninvasive evaluation of cerebrovascular diseases. In addition, portable CT scanners can now provide high-quality images for point-of-care imaging in an intensive care unit setting and thereby avoid potential risks associated with transport of critically patients.

CT can be performed in various planes that depend on patient position and the CT gantry angle within its limited arc. For example, direct coronal-plane CT imaging of the paranasal sinuses or brain can be performed with the patient in a supine, "hanging-head" position with the head of the patient literally hanging over the edge of the CT scanner table or with the patient in the prone position and the neck hyperextended. However, most commonly, CT imaging of the brain and spine is performed in the axial plane with the patient in a supine position on the scanner table and the head and neck in a neutral position. The need for a direct coronal patient position is less important since the advent of high-resolution multiplanar reconstruction capabilities on newer generation CT scanners. These reconstruction capabilities can generate axial images in 0.5- to 0.6-mm increments, which can then be reformatted into the sagittal, coronal, and oblique planes with image quality nearly identical to that obtained from direct scanning.[3,4]

A typical routine brain CT scan consists of 5-mm contiguous axial images through the entire brain from the skull base to the vertex without the intravenous injection of iodinated contrast material. This can be followed by another set of 5-mm axial images through the brain after the intravenous administration of a contrast agent, typically 100 mL of iodinated contrast material injected through an 18- or 20-gauge intravenous catheter. Scanning intervals can and do get adjusted for clinical need and indications such as patient age and size, need for higher resolution images of specific anatomy such as the orbits, temporal bone, and skull base, or CTA. With the newer multidetector CT scanners, these images can be reconstructed into submillimeter axial images that can be used to generate two-dimensional (2D) and three-dimensional (3D) reformatted sagittal and coronal images and thus better delineate parenchymal, vascular, and osseous anatomy.

CT is most often the first study of choice for evaluation of a patient with suspected acute intracranial pathology because of its ready availability, ease of use, short acquisition time, and high sensitivity for detection of acute hemorrhage and fractures. It can provide a wealth of information about the brain, including ventricular size, presence of brain edema, mass effect, presence and location of hemorrhage or masses, midline shift, evolving ischemic injuries, fractures, benign and malignant osseous pathology, and the paranasal sinuses. Its availability and short acquisition time also allow frequent repeat scanning of the brain, which can contribute to the management and follow-up of patients in the acute, subacute, and chronic phases in both inpatient and outpatient settings.[5-7]

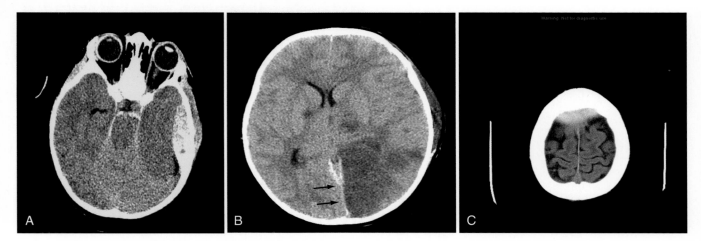

FIGURE 17-1 A, Non–contrast-enhanced head CT demonstrating an acute epidural hematoma over the left cerebral hemisphere. Note the biconvex contours of the hematoma. **B,** Postoperative CT shows multiple infarctions, including a large left posterior cerebral artery (PCA) distribution infarction (*arrows*) from compression of left PCA by the epidural hematoma. **C,** Epidural hematoma at the vertex (*arrows*) (different patient) extending across the interhemispheric fissure.

In neurosurgery, CT of the head is used for preoperative and postoperative evaluation of patients for hemorrhage, infarction, hydrocephalus, mass effect, fracture, and postsurgical assessment.[8-12] CT is the study of choice to evaluate for acute hemorrhage because it has higher sensitivity and specificity for this indication than MRI does. Intracranial hemorrhage is typically described in terms of its location within the head, such as epidural, subdural, subarachnoid, intraventricular, and parenchymal, with each of these different types of hemorrhages having sufficiently distinct appearances and locations. Epidural hemorrhage has a biconvex contour of its borders (Fig. 17-1A) in relation to the cranial vault and adjacent brain parenchyma and is usually the result of acute trauma associated with an acute fracture across branches of meningeal arteries that hemorrhage into the epidural space. Less commonly, rapid venous hemorrhage into the epidural space may occur and cause an epidural hematoma. The extent of an epidural hematoma is usually limited by periosteal dural insertions at the major sutures. However, an epidural hematoma can extend across the midline in the frontal region anterior to the coronal suture because it is not limited by the dural reflections within the anterior interhemispheric fissure (Fig. 17-1C).

A subdural hematoma (SDH) is more common than an epidural hematoma, particularly in older patients, and is generally associated with acute head trauma with or without an associated fracture. Its shape is different from an epidural hematoma because its deeper border against the brain parenchyma is concave and approximates the contour of the adjacent cerebral hemisphere convexity. An acute SDH is typically a result of venous hemorrhage and is not limited by the periosteal dural insertions at the major sutures. However, it is limited by the midline dural reflections within the interhemispheric fissure. The density of the blood in acute, subacute, and chronic SDH changes over time from hyperdense, to isodense, to hypodense (Fig. 17-2). However, a hyperacute SDH or an acute subarachnoid hemorrhage (SAH) in the presence of coagulopathy may sometimes appear isodense or hypodense.

Trauma is the most common cause of SAH, whereas rupture of an intracranial aneurysm is the most common nontraumatic cause of SAH. SAH extends freely within the subarachnoid spaces around the cerebral hemispheres, brainstem, and cerebellum and frequently, by reflux of cerebrospinal fluid (CSF), extends into the intraventricular spaces. It often leads to acute, subacute, or

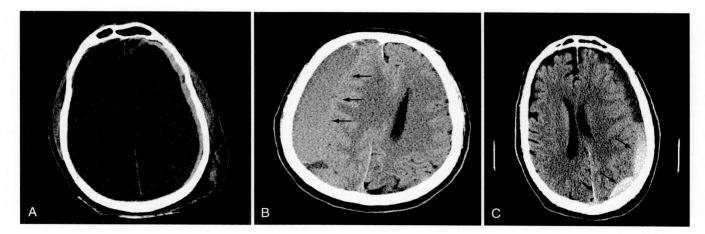

FIGURE 17-2 A, Non–contrast-enhanced head CT showing a thin left acute subdural hematoma (SDH). **B,** Right subacute, nearly isodense SDH (*arrows*). **C,** Acute-on-chronic SDH over the left frontal and parietal lobes.

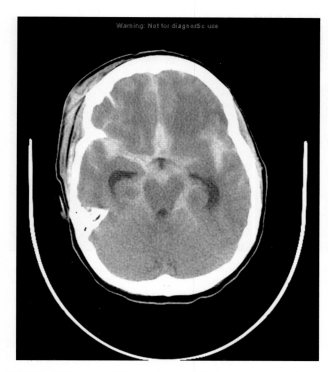

FIGURE 17-3 Acute diffuse subarachnoid hemorrhages within the suprasellar cistern, ambient cistern, and frontal and temporal sulci. There is dilation of both temporal horns of the lateral ventricles associated with communicating hydrocephalus.

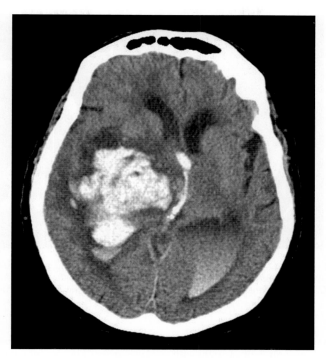

FIGURE 17-4 Non–contrast-enhanced head CT demonstrating an acute right thalamic hypertensive hemorrhage, midline shift to the left, intraventricular hemorrhage, and hydrocephalus.

chronic hydrocephalus because the blood products disrupt and obstruct the normal CSF drainage pathways (Fig. 17-3).

Parenchymal hemorrhages have many causes, including trauma, hypertension, vascular anomalies such as arteriovenous malformation (AVM) or cavernoma, infarction, neoplasm, infection, or vasculitis. They can be small or large and single or multiple, and patient prognosis depends on the cause, number, size, and associated mass effect of the hemorrhage, among other variables (Fig. 17-4).

Computed Tomographic Angiography

Advances in CT scanner technology have allowed an ever improving capacity for higher resolution images in the submillimeter range with shorter acquisition times. Such technologic improvements have led to imaging techniques such as CTA, which permits relatively noninvasive imaging of the major arteries and veins of the neck and brain after an intravenous injection of iodinated contrast material rather than the traditional catheter-based intra-arterial angiogram technique. This venous injection helps avoid the small risk for complications such as vascular dissection, renal injury, allergic reaction, and iatrogenic embolic strokes associated with traditional catheter angiography. CTA of the neck or brain is performed with a multidetector CT scanner, which allows rapid dynamic imaging of the anatomy of interest after a bolus intravenous injection of iodinated contrast material through a large-bore intravenous catheter (i.e., 18 gauge). Typically, submillimeter axial images are obtained and then reformatted into 2D sagittal and coronal image data sets at 1- to 2-mm intervals. 3D reconstruction images are usually obtained, but interpretation of the study is based primarily on the original axial data set and the 2D sagittal and coronal reformatted images. The diagnostic sensitivity and specificity of CTA approach that of catheter angiography for both the extracranial

and intracranial vasculature.[13,14] Although CTA cannot entirely replace traditional catheter angiograms, it is a very useful noninvasive screening study for the evaluation, management, and follow-up of patients with definite or possible aneurysms, as well as the evaluation of vasospasm, AVMs, traumatic dissection, stroke, and carotid or vertebral artery atherosclerotic stenosis (Figs. 17-5 and 17-6).[15]

Perfusion Computed Tomography

pCT is an example of new advances in imaging that provides physiologic information in addition to anatomic information. pCT is performed with the latest-generation multidetector CT scanners, which allow very rapid CT imaging of a particular anatomy, such as the cerebral hemispheres. During a bolus intravenous injection of iodinated contrast material at a rate of 4 to 5 mL/sec, rapid serial CT images of a chosen volume are obtained in multiple phases over an approximately 1-minute period. At the end of this acquisition, multiphase time-density curves corresponding to each voxel are generated within a 2D image of a multilevel image data set. The data from these images are further postprocessed with a mathematical algorithm that allows displays of the data in color maps representing such physiologic cerebral perfusion parameters as cerebral blood flow (CBF), cerebral blood volume (CBV), and mean transit time (MTT). The CBF, CBV, and MTT maps generated from this CT technique are, in part, quantitative; that is, the numerical values obtained from these images may be expressed in mL/100 g per minute for CBF, mL/100 g for CBV, and seconds for MTT.[16] pCT technology has been validated against other proven in vivo techniques such as xenon-enhanced CT and positron emission tomography (PET).[17,18]

pCT has been used to evaluate acute stroke, central nervous system (CNS) neoplasms, and ischemic sequelae of SAH-related

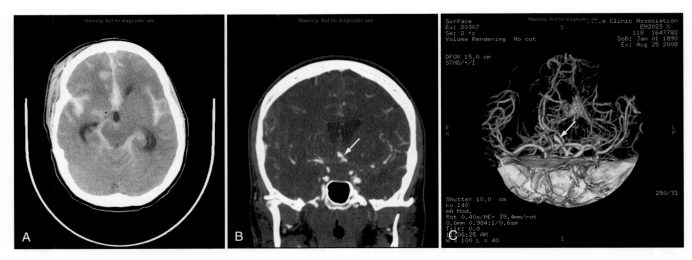

FIGURE 17-5 A, Non–contrast-enhanced head CT illustrating subarachnoid hemorrhage from a ruptured anterior communicating artery (ACOM) aneurysm. **B,** Coronal two-dimensional reformatted image from a brain CTA demonstrating an irregular ACOM artery aneurysm (*arrow*). **C,** Three-dimensional CTA reconstruction image of the ACOM aneurysm (*arrow*).

vasospasm. The most common use of the pCT technique is for the evaluation of a patient with an acute stroke. The various color maps of cerebral perfusion help determine the presence of salvageable ischemic penumbra during the first few hours after stroke, which may lead to more aggressive therapy such as an intra-arterial thrombolysis or thrombus extraction to permit rapid recanalization of occluded large intracranial arteries such as the supraclinoid segment of the internal carotid artery (ICA) or M1 segment of the middle cerebral artery (MCA) (Fig. 17-7).

The availability of physiologic data also helps in the diagnosis, management, and treatment of patients with a ruptured aneurysm and subsequent vasospasm, which may contribute to acute or subacute ischemic injury. Evaluation of these patients has typically relied on serial clinical assessment, non–contrast-enhanced head CT, and transcranial Doppler (TCD) ultrasound. There are recognized limitations with this evaluation protocol; in particular, non–contrast-enhanced CT and TCD may not accurately reflect the state of cerebral perfusion at an early enough stage to allow successful intervention for reversal of oligemia and ischemia. Baseline pCT and follow-up pCT can demonstrate the size and extent of brain areas at risk for stroke in patients in a neuro-

logical intensive care unit often before symptoms develop and permanent infarction occurs (Fig. 17-8). This early detection of at-risk areas may in some patients permit earlier medical and catheter-based intervention for vasospasm and thus prevent delayed ischemic injury.[19-21]

MAGNETIC RESONANCE IMAGING OF THE BRAIN

Physics and Techniques of Magnetic Resonance Imaging

History

The interaction of the intrinsic magnetic moment of the nucleus with an externally imposed magnetic field results in the phenomenon known as nuclear magnetic resonance (NMR). Two independent groups, Felix Bloch working with liquid water[22] and Edwin Purcell working with solid paraffin,[23] detected the hydrogen nucleus resonance in 1946 in bulk matter. Bloch further

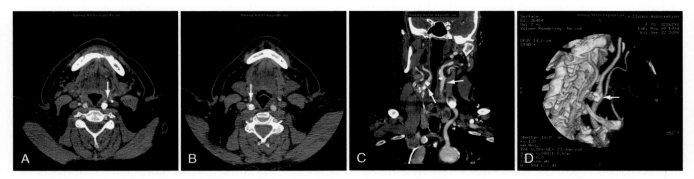

FIGURE 17-6 A and **B,** Source images from a neck CTA illustrating calcified atherosclerotic stenoses of the left internal carotid artery (ICA) and right ICA origins, respectively (*arrows*). **C,** Coronal 2D reformatted image showing calcified atherosclerotic disease of both common carotid artery bifurcations (*arrows*). **D,** Oblique three-dimensional reconstruction image from neck CTA showing calcified plaque in the left common carotid artery bifurcation (*arrow*).

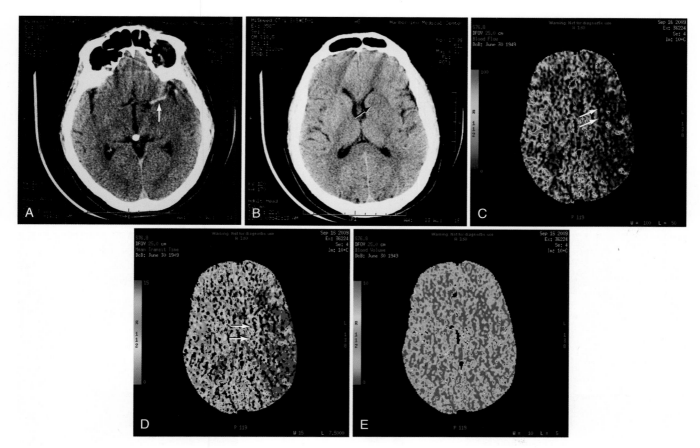

FIGURE 17-7 **A,** Non–contrast-enhanced head CT illustrating increased density of the M1 segment of the left middle cerebral artery (MCA; *arrow*)—the "dense MCA sign"—in a patient with an acute left hemispheric stroke. **B,** There are early ischemic changes with hypodensity within left lenticular nuclei (*arrow*). **C,** Perfusion CT showing a perfusion defect in the left MCA distribution on a cerebral blood flow (CBF) map (*arrows*). **D,** Perfusion CT mean transit time (MTT) map at the same level illustrating delayed MTT in the left MCA distribution (*arrows*). **E,** Perfusion CT cerebral blood volume (CBV) map at the same level illustrating a normal perfusion pattern that is symmetrical with the contralateral MCA territory. This pattern of CBF and MTT map perfusion defects and mismatched normal perfusion on the CBV map represents salvageable ischemic penumbra within the left MCA territory.

described the processes and time constants (T1 and T2) by which the resonance would dissipate.[24] This set the stage for the eventual development of MRI 30 years later. Between 1946 and 1976, NMR became a useful laboratory tool for probing molecular structure. Laboratory NMR instruments had small spaces for the sample, usually a small test tube. Use of NMR for larger objects, such as humans, required the development of larger magnets with larger sample spaces. The term *magnetic resonance imaging* is now used rather than NMR to allay patient anxiety about a test that has the word "nuclear" in it.

Basic Physics of Magnetic Resonance Imaging

Why Hydrogen?

Many nuclei bear a magnetic moment. Those relevant to biology include phosphorus 31, carbon 13, and sodium 23. However, all MRI systems use the resonance of the hydrogen nucleus for three reasons. First is the ease of detection of the MR signal. The hydrogen nucleus has the largest magnetic moment of any nucleus and is therefore the most detectable. Second is the natural abundance of hydrogen—99.99% for ^{1}H. By contrast, the abundance of ^{13}C is 1.1% (98% of carbon is ^{12}C, which has no magnetic moment). Third, hydrogen is contained in water, which

is in high concentration in the body; in the brain, the concentration of water is approximately 67% by weight.

Creating the Signal

To begin, the sample is immersed in a strong, constant magnetic field. A magnet that may be one of three designs creates the field. First is the electromagnet, similar in principle to a washing machine solenoid. Bloch and Purcell used these magnets in their original experiments. However, the maximal field strength that can be achieved is limited in practical applications to around 0.4 T (1 T = 10,000 G). An electromagnet consumes large amounts of electricity, and its use in MRI has therefore declined.

The second magnet type is a permanent magnet assembled from ferromagnetic material. The field strength of this type of magnet is limited to 0.3 T. Permanent magnets are generally used for small, low-cost open designs. MRI systems that accommodate large (>300 lb) or claustrophobic patients tend to use this technology.

The third and most widely used magnet type is the superconducting magnet. This design is also similar to a washing machine solenoid. However, unlike the solenoid, the wire is an alloy that conducts electricity without resistance when kept at temperatures within 15 degrees of absolute zero. An electric current is slowly driven into the magnet. Once the current reaches the desired

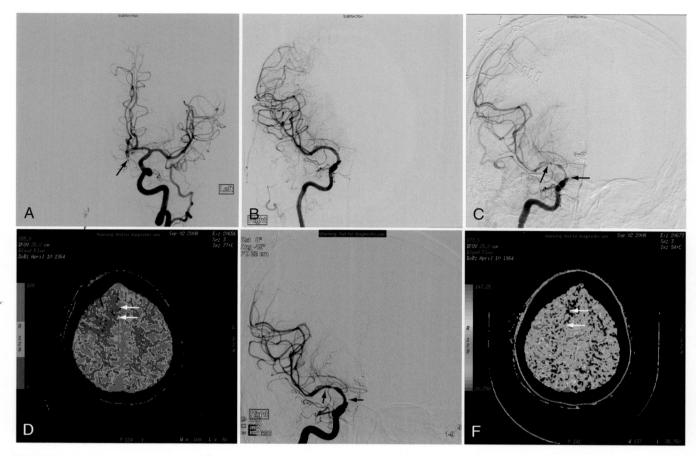

FIGURE 17-8 **A,** Anteroposterior (AP) left internal carotid (ICA) angiogram demonstrating a ruptured anterior communicating artery aneurysm (*arrow*). **B,** AP right ICA angiogram illustrating an absent A1 segment of the right anterior cerebral artery and no vasospasm. **C,** AP right ICA angiogram 7 days after admission showing severe vasospasm of the M1 segment of right middle cerebral artery (MCA) (*up arrow*) and supraclinoid right ICA (*left arrow*). **D,** Perfusion computed tomographic cerebral blood flow (CBF) map demonstrating vasospasm-induced decreased CBF (*blue* areas) within the right frontal lobe (*arrows*). **E,** AP angiogram (right ICA) after intra-arterial administration of verapamil showing improved MCA (*up arrow*) and ICA (*left arrow*) vessel caliber. **F,** Follow-up perfusion CT at the same level as in **D** illustrating restored CBF in the right anterior frontal lobe on a CBF color map (*arrows*).

level, the ends of the magnet wire are connected, which forces the current to circulate continuously without loss. Magnets of this type can remain at field strength for many years without the addition of electric current. Field strengths of up to 8 T can be achieved in these magnets, which can accommodate human subjects. Most MRI systems now use superconducting magnets, usually 1.0 to 1.5 T, although an increasing number of hospitals and imaging centers are now using 3-T clinical MRI systems.

When immersed in the strong, constant magnetic field, the spins in the sample experience a slight polarization. This polarization, known as M0, increases with increasing magnetic field. At 1.5 T, this polarization is very slight, about 1×10^{-5}. This translates to just 10 in 1 million nuclei being polarized.[25] The polarization competes with the randomizing effect of the thermal vibration (Fig. 17-9). It is only the polarized nuclei that contribute to the MR signal; hence, MRI systems with higher field strength produce better images.

We will use the classic model created by Bloch to describe the motion of the spins. Spins that align with the main field precess around the direction of the main field in a manner similar to the spinning of a toy top (Fig. 17-10). The rate of this precession is a product of the intrinsic magnetic moment (the gyromagnetic ratio) of the spin and the strength of the main magnetic field. The rate of precession is known as the Larmor or resonant frequency.[26] The spins aligned along B0 are rotated into a plane

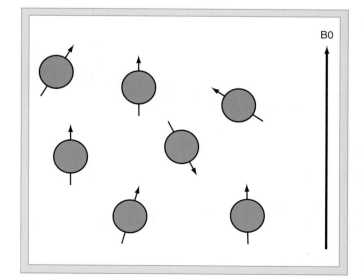

FIGURE 17-9 Illustration of nuclear spins in the magnetic field B0. The net alignment of spins is along B0. This is the source of M0, or longitudinal magnetization. In reality, the net aligned versus unaligned fraction is about 1 in 100,000 in a 1.5-T field at body temperature.

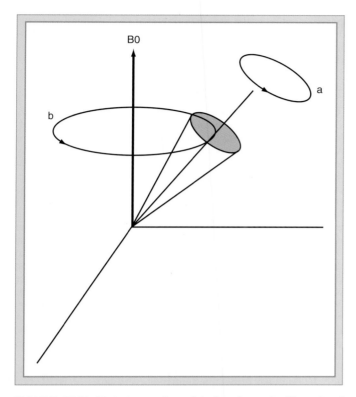

FIGURE 17-10 "Spinning top" model of nuclear spin. The spin of nucleus "a" creates the magnetic moment of the nucleus, which causes the spin to precess along circle "b" around magnetic field B0. The rate of this precession around B0 is called the *Larmor frequency.*

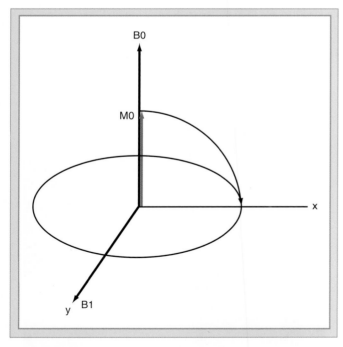

FIGURE 17-11 The applied (transmitted) radiofrequency magnetic field B1 causes the spin to experience a torque, which twists (nutates) the M0 magnetization into the transverse plane x-y, where it is referred to as Mxy.

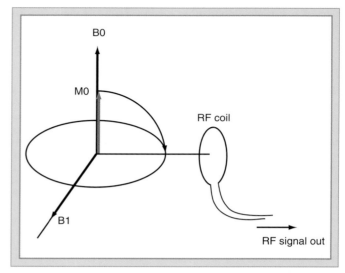

FIGURE 17-12 The radiofrequency (RF) coil both transmits and receives the signal from the spins in the transverse plane.

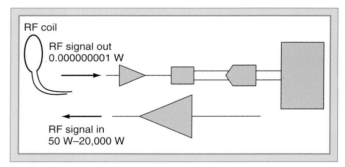

FIGURE 17-13 Bloch diagram of the transmit and receive scheme used in magnetic resonance imaging that illustrates the large disparity between the high radiofrequency (RF) power transmitted into the patient and the tiny RF signal received from the patient.

transverse to the direction of the main magnetic field by the action of a time-varying magnetic field called *B1* (Fig. 17-11). The B1 field is created by the radiofrequency (RF) transmitter and the antenna, known as the RF coil. The frequency of the B1 field matches the Larmor frequency of the spins. The B1 field is of brief duration, typically 1 to 10 msec, and is thus referred to as an RF pulse. The angle through which the spin is rotated is called the *flip angle*. The flip angle depends on the duration and amplitude of the RF pulse.

Detecting the Signal

To detect the MR signal, an RF coil is placed as shown in Figure 17-12. This may be the same coil used to transmit the B1 pulse. A time-varying magnetic field will be created at the coil by the magnetic field of the precessing spins (rotated in the transverse plane) as they pass by the RF coil. Magnetic induction (Faraday's law) causes the RF coil to produce an electric current, which can then be amplified and detected (Fig. 17-13). An interesting and important disparity should be noted. The amount of power used to produce the RF pulse is in the range of 100 to 20,000 W. The signal that is received from the object is on the order of 10^{-12} W. This received signal is no greater than the signals from radio or television stations, among other sources. To prevent interference from these external sources, MRI systems are enclosed in electrically shielded rooms, which are six-sided copper boxes.

Physics: Localizing the Signal

To this point, the sample has been polarized and excited and a signal detected, but the location of the spins that created the signal remains unknown. Suppose that two objects are in the magnetic field, both of which create a signal. To force each object to give off a unique signal, the magnetic field can be modified to vary as a function of position along the x-axis (Fig. 17-14). The resonant frequency of the spins is a function only of the magnetic field at that point in space. Thus, the spatial origin of the signal can be determined by the frequency of the received signal. In practice, this is done by creating a linear gradient that adds or subtracts to the main field as a linear function of offset from the origin. An MRI system has three gradients: x, y, and z. The gradient system serves two purposes in the MRI system. The first is to limit the excitation to a plane or slab (Fig. 17-15). If an RF pulse is transmitted during the time that a gradient is applied, only a slice or slab will be excited, the thickness of which depends on the amplitude of the gradient and the bandwidth of the RF pulse. The second purpose is to encode the spatial location of spins to form the MR image. In a slice, the two directions of encoding required are frequency and phase. Location along the frequency-encoding axis is accomplished by applying a gradient during the signal readout time. The orthogonal axis is encoded by applying a gradient somewhere between the time of excitation and reception and is called *phase encoding*. One unique value of

phase encoding is applied every time that the readout gradient is applied. Thus, the excitation and readout must be repeated to make an image. The rate at which the excitation is repeated is the TR time.

The Origin of Image Contrast

The intensity of a voxel in an image arises from the three principal factors. The first is the number of protons in the voxel, known as proton density. If this were the only image mechanism, MRI would be little more than a CT scanner. However, intensity in the voxel also depends on the relaxation rates of the spins. The first is T1, or the longitudinal relaxation rate (Fig. 17-16A). After excitation, the magnetization in the slice returns along the axis of the main magnetic field by interaction with other nonmoving hydrogen spins, typically those attached to large molecules. The magnetization returns along B0 as an exponential function of the ratio of T1 and the rate at which the excitation is repeated, or TR. The second relaxation rate is T2 (Fig. 17-16B). This rate describes the rates at which spins that have been excited into the transverse plane lose coherence. Each spin precesses at a rate that is determined by the magnetic field at the location of that spin. Macroscopic and microscopic field gradients, created by differences in the magnetic susceptibility of tissue, cause some of the excited spins to precess faster and some slower. Eventually, the spins are spread out uniformly, which produces no signal in the RF coil used to detect the spins.

Three principal image intensity factors—proton density, T1, and T2—influence the appearance of every voxel on MRI. For example, cortical bone is hypointense on MRI because the proton density (of mobile spins) is quite low. Lung parenchyma is usually hypointense because the T2 of lung tissue is so low that the signal is gone before it can be sampled. The long T1 of liquid water causes CSF to be dark on sequences that use short TR times.

An MRI scan user has a choice of pulse sequence parameters such as echo time (TE) and repetition time (TR). Maximal contrast between structures of interest may be achieved by the appropriate choice of sequence parameters. Conversely, inappropriate choices may result in failure to detect a lesion. Other endogenous sources of contrast include blood flow (magnetic resonance angiography [MRA]) and water-macromolecular T1-based interactions (magnetization transfer).

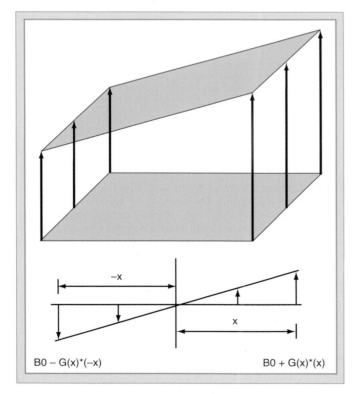

FIGURE 17-14 Magnetic field gradients alter the strength of the main magnetic field. A single gradient is designed to change the magnetic field along only one direction (x, y, or z). Three such gradients are required to localize signals in three dimensions.

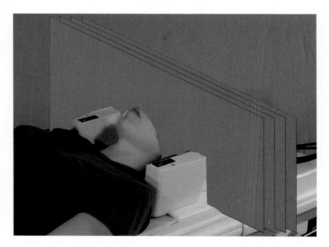

FIGURE 17-15 Slice selection illustrating a group of four excited axial slices relative to a patient. *(Radiofrequency head coil courtesy of Midwest RF LLC.)*

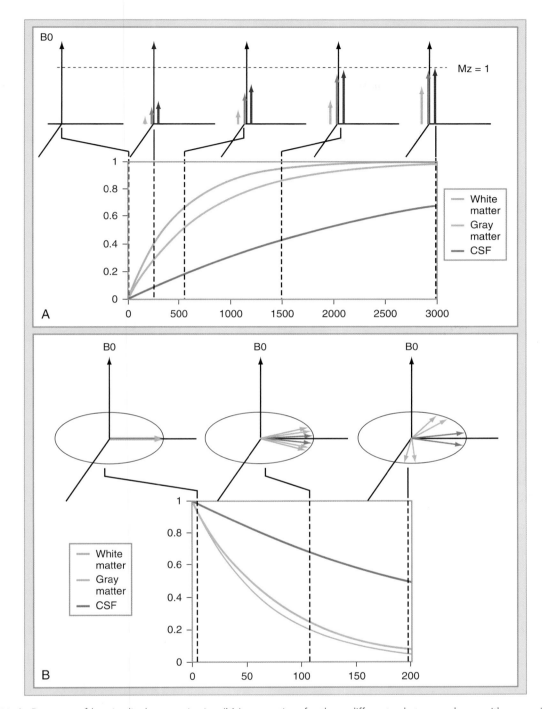

FIGURE 17-16 A, Recovery of longitudinal magnetization (Mz) versus time for three different substances shown with regrowing vectors and plotted. **B,** Decay of Mx versus time for three different substances. CSF, cerebrospinal fluid.

Spin Echo

After the spins have been rotated into the transverse plane by the initial 90-degree RF pulse (Fig. 17-17A), they begin to lose coherence because of the effects of local inhomogeneities (contributed by changes in tissue), inhomogeneities secondary to imperfections in the B0 field, and diffusion of water molecules (Fig. 17-17B). If a second RF pulse is transmitted at twice the amplitude of the first pulse, the relative direction of the spins can be reversed (Fig. 17-17C). Then, at the echo time, the spins will have nearly regained coherence (Fig. 17-17D). The effects of

magnetic field inhomogeneities are thus cancelled out. One loss, that caused by diffusion, cannot be reversed but is usually negligible in routine imaging. The resulting coherence produces the spin echo as described by Erwin Hahn in 1950.[27] If the 180-degree pulse is not used, the signal decreases with increasing echo time as T2*. With the 180-degree pulse included, the decrease is T2, with T2 always being greater than T2*.

The spin echo sequence is the mainstay of routine clinical imaging. By adjusting TE and TR times, proton density–, T1-, or T2-weighted images can be selected (Table 17-1).

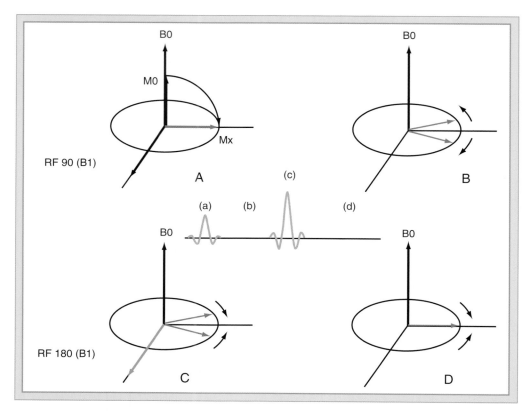

FIGURE 17-17 The spin echo starts with nutation of longitudinal magnetization (Mz) into the transverse plane (**A**). The magnetization decays over time (**B**) until the radiofrequency (RF) 180-degree pulse (**C**) reverses the direction of the spins, which then reform Mx at the echo time (**D**).

Gadolinium Contrast

Exogenous contrast enhancement is now a routine part of MRI. The most widely used is a gadolinium chelate. The gadolinium atom is strongly paramagnetic and acts to shorten the T1 relaxation time of nearby water protons in blood.[28] The agent does not pass the blood-brain barrier and thus becomes a marker for abruptions in the blood-brain barrier caused by neoplasm, infection, trauma, and infarction. The T1-shortening effect is also used for rapid MRA, which is performed by using a fast scanning protocol after the bolus injection of a contrast agent. In the brain, bolus injection of gadolinium with repeated echo planar imaging (EPI) has been used to image perfusion[29] and the blood volume of tumors.[30]

Fast Spin Echo

Fast spin echo (FSE) sequences decrease scan time by increasing the efficiency of data collection.[31] The increased efficiency can be used to either decrease scan time or increase the signal-to-noise ratio of the resulting images. Improved scan efficiency has resulted in the frequent application of FSE sequences in radiology, particularly in imaging of the CNS.

TABLE 17-1 Weighting of Magnetic Resonance Images

	SHORT TE	LONG TE
Short TR	T1 weighted	Mixed contrast—do not use
Long TR	Proton density weighted	T2 weighted

TE, echo time; TR, repetition time.

To understand this improved efficiency, it is necessary to understand how the data are collected. In a conventional spin echo sequence (Fig. 17-18A), a single line of k-space samples (called a *view*) is collected. For images that are not fractional excitation, the number of views is equal to the matrix size in the phase that encodes image direction. The next view is collected at TR time later, when the sequence is repeated. The entire k-space matrix must be collected before the images can be reconstructed. The TR time is set in accordance with the desired contrast (Table 17-1). The FSE sequence collects multiple views in each TR time (Fig. 17-18B). The number of views collected per TR time is known as the echo train length (ETL). An FSE sequence with an ETL of 4 has a total scan time a fourth that of a conventional spin echo sequence with equivalent TR. The ETL can be equal to the number of views in the sequence. This allows the entire image to be collected in a single TR time.

The improved efficiency of FSE sequences comes at the expense of image contrast purity because each view is collected at a different echo time (Fig. 17-18B). The effect is to create image blurring that worsens with increasing ETL or decreasing tissue T2. The relatively long T2 times of tissues in the neuraxis allow ETL values of 16 to be used routinely. To image uncooperative patients, single-shot FSE sequences can be used, but with some increase in image blurring.

Inversion Recovery

Image contrast can be further manipulated by transmitting a 180-degree RF pulse before the pulse sequence. The effect of using this pulse is to rotate the spins from their orientation along +z to −z (Fig. 17-19A). The longitudinal magnetization (Mz) signal regrows from −z to +z at a rate determined by the T1 of

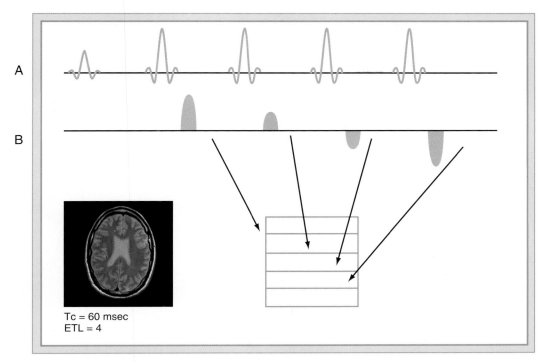

FIGURE 17-18 A, Multiple-echo spin echo sequence in which a single phase encoding is applied for all four echoes and each echo fills in the same sample line in four separate k-space matrices. The sequence must be repeated a number of times equal to the resolution in the phase-encoding direction of the image. **B,** A fast spin echo sequence applies a different phase encoding for each echo of the same sequence as in **A**. In this way, a single k-space matrix is filled four times faster. This yields one image in a quarter of the time required to complete the sequence in **A**. ETL, echo train length.

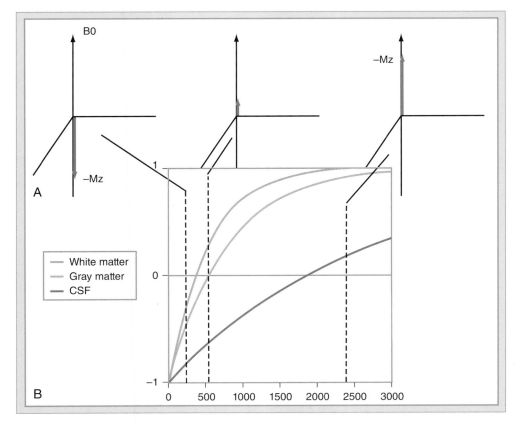

FIGURE 17-19 Inversion recovery sequence showing both the motion of the spins (**A**) and a plot of longitudinal magnetization (Mz) versus time (**B**). CSF, cerebrospinal fluid.

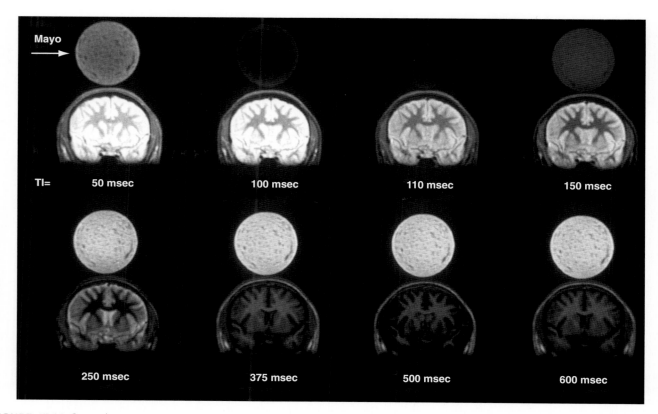

FIGURE 17-20 Coronal inversion recovery magnetic resonance images of a volunteer and a jar of mayonnaise. The nulling effect of certain T1 times on various substances is illustrated: T1 of 110 msec nulls mayonnaise, T1 of 150 msec nulls white matter, and T1 of 375 msec nulls gray matter.

the spins. The regrowth is plotted in Figure 17-19B for several tissues. If the 90-degree RF pulse is transmitted at the time at which Mz is 0, the tissue will produce no signal. Inversion recovery can be used to increase contrast between structures, such as gray and white matter, or to null signals that arise from protons of a known T1. A coronal image of a volunteer imaged at multiple T1 times is shown in Figure 17-20. The round object above the volunteer's head is a jar of mayonnaise. Fluid-attenuated inversion recovery (FLAIR) imaging[32] uses this method to null CSF while preserving signal from edematous tissue. The inversion pulse may be applied to a spin echo or gradient echo sequence.

Gradient Echo

The pulse that rotates Mz into the transverse plane, nominally a 90-degree pulse, does not have to be followed by an 180-degree pulse to produce an echo. In this case the sequence is referred to as a gradient echo because a readout gradient is used to form the echo. By eliminating the 180-degree pulse, sequence time is saved and TR time may be made very short—as little as 6 msec. In so doing, k-space can be filled very quickly and the scan can be completed in a matter of seconds rather than minutes as is the case with conventional spin echo. At the TR times used in conventional spin echo sequences, 500 to 2000 msec, the MR signal is strongest when the first RF pulse is 90 degrees. When the TR time is very short, the peak signal is obtained at a flip angle of less than 90 degrees. The flip angle becomes an important determinant of image contrast in gradient echo. Low flip angles,

typically 5 to 20 degrees, result in images that are more T2* weighted, whereas higher flip angles, 40 to 90 degrees, create more T1-weighted images. It is important to remember that gradient echo sequences do not yield the purity of contrast of a conventional spin echo sequence and that the T2 weighting in a conventional spin echo is replaced by T2* in gradient echo. The advantages of gradient echo are short scan times, utility for MRA, and the ability to visualize hemosiderin and ferritin. MRA does not use spin echo because flow is dephased and becomes invisible.

Echo Planar Imaging

The readout gradient used to form the echo in a gradient echo sequence can be repeated to collect additional k-space views in a manner similar to FSE.[33] Between repetitions of the readout gradient, a small phase-encoding gradient is applied that allows a different view to be collected during the subsequent readout gradient (Fig. 17-21). Only a single excitation is used to collect all the views in k-space. The entire image can be collected in approximately 40 msec. Applications that are highly sensitive to even minor patient motions use this sequence. Like FSE, EPI suffers from blurring caused by acquiring views at different echo times, but without rephasing of the RF 180-degree pulses. This effect limits the resolution obtainable. Although an FSE image may use a matrix of 256 × 256, EPI is limited to 128 × 128 or more typically 64 × 64 over the same field of view. Despite these limitations, EPI is essential for diffusion, perfusion, and functional MRI (fMRI).

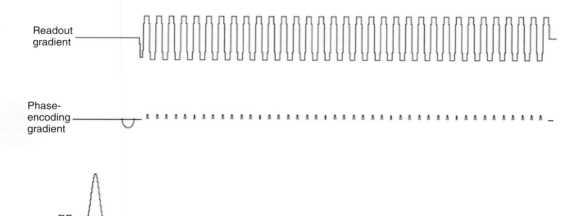

Readout gradient

Phase-encoding gradient

RF

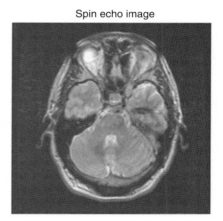

EPI image

Spin echo image

FIGURE 17-21 Sequence diagram and image from echo planar imaging (EPI). The readout gradient repeatedly reverses, which fills the k-space matrix in a single excitation. EPI is similar in concept to fast spin echo imaging, except for the repeated 180-degree radiofrequency pulses. In the absence of these pulses in EPI, susceptibility artifacts are present in areas adjacent to bone and air.

Diffusion-Weighted Imaging

Diffusion of water in the brain depends on the integrity of the cellular membrane and the osmotic balance of the neurons and astrocytes.[34] In ischemic processes, the diffusion of water first decreases because of cellular swelling and thus decreases the extracellular space. During recovery and into the chronic stage, the loss of cell wall integrity causes the diffusion to increase.

In the section on the spin echo, it was noted that the 180-degree pulse could not recover signal lost because of diffusion. If the water molecule moves between the time of the gradient that is applied before the 180-degree pulse and the gradient after the 180-degree pulse, the spin will experience a different B0 field. The different B0 field is due to the applied gradient and the total motion of the spin in that direction. The spin precesses at a different rate before and after the 180-degree pulse, thereby resulting in an accumulated phase error at the time of readout and a loss of signal. The farther that the spin wanders (*wander* is the correct term here because the motion is brownian) between gradient lobes, the greater the signal loss. Hence, a chronic infarct is hypointense. Conversely, when the cells swell and the spin motion is reduced to less than that of normal tissue, the diffusion loss is reduced to less than that of normal tissue and the region becomes hyperintense.

Perfusion-Weighted Imaging

Two main approaches are taken to measure tissue perfusion. Both methods use EPI sequences because like diffusion, the effect can be easily degraded by minor patient motion. The first method for imaging tissue perfusion is to create an endogenous contrast. This is done by presaturating the blood flowing into the organ with an RF pulse. EPI of the organ is performed with the presaturation on and off. By subtracting the two images, a tissue perfusion image is created.[35] The second method is by bolus injection of contrast material while repeatedly performing EPI. Time course images from EPI are then fitted to a model of the response of the tissue to the presence of the contrast agent, and an image of perfusion is made. This method is also known as a dynamic susceptibility contrast technique and requires a rapid intravenous bolus injection of gadolinium contrast material at a rate of 4 to 5 mL/sec, usually through an 18-gauge intravenous catheter, followed by normal saline injection. Manual or automatic postprocessing is required to generate color maps of various parameters of cerebral perfusion, such as CBV, CBF, mean time to enhance, and MTT.

Perfusion MRI is used clinically to evaluate patients with chronic ischemic disease, acute stroke, vasospasm after SAH, or intracranial neoplasms. It can also be used to distinguish recurrent neoplasm from radiation necrosis in patients who underwent radiation therapy for primary brain tumors.

Spectroscopy

The resonant frequency of a spin is determined not only by the B0 magnetic field and its associated imperfections but also by the molecule of which the nucleus is a part. The effect is slight, but not negligible. This phenomenon is known as chemical shift; that is, the chemical microenvironment of a given nucleus results in a slight change in the resonance frequency of the nucleus from that expected in its pure state. The difference between the resonant frequencies of the protons in water and the hydrogen atoms in the methylene groups in lipid are about 3.5 ppm. This translates to a difference of about 220 Hz for operation at 1.5 T. Between the water proton and fat proton resonances lie resonances of other moieties of interest in the brain. These include myoinositol, a sugar phosphate; choline, a key indicator of membrane turnover; creatine and phosphocreatine, part of the energy pool; glutamate and glutamine, the primary excitatory neurotransmitter and its astrocyte-recycled counterpart; N-acetyl aspartate (NAA), a key indicator of neuronal health; and lactate, an indicator of a shift to anaerobic metabolism. A spectrum of the resonances of the protons in these compounds is shown in Figure 17-22A. These resonances are included in every MR image of the brain. However, the concentration of each is lower than that of water by a factor of 5000 to 10000. To detect the resonances of the metabolites thus requires much larger voxels than imaging does: 2 cm³ versus 1 mm³ in imaging.

Two principal methods are used to collect spectroscopic data. The first, single-voxel spectroscopy, selects a voxel by using three successive RF pulses and then reads out the signal from the entire voxel. The second, chemical shift imaging, selects a larger volume or slice with one or more RF pulses. Phase-encoding gradients are then applied in one to three directions to yield 2D or 3D spectroscopy data sets. Reconstruction allows the selected region to be subdivided into separate voxels. An individual spectrum can then be extracted from a voxel, or a resonance may be selected and an image made of that resonance. Such 2D and 3D data sets can be postprocessed to generate color maps of metabolite distributions within the volume of brain evaluated with spectroscopy (Fig. 17-22B).

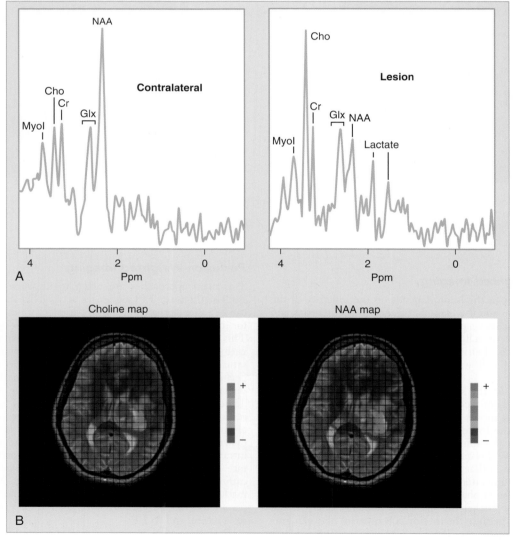

FIGURE 17-22 Magnetic resonance spectroscopy. **A,** Spectra extracted from a (¹H) chemical shift imaging data set. There is increased choline (Cho) resonance and decreased N-acetyl aspartate (NAA) resonance in the spectrum labeled "lesion." The spectra from the contralateral hemisphere show a normal pattern. Cr, creatine; Glx, glutamate and glutamine; Myo, myoinositol. **B,** Metabolite images made from the same data set used in **A**. The increased concentration of choline is seen in the lesion as the *red* area.

Spectroscopic data can be collected for several different nuclei present in the body, including phosphorus, carbon, and sodium. Exogenous substances that can be detected in the body include fluorine and lithium, both of which are found in psychoactive drugs. However, proton (hydrogen) spectroscopy is the most readily commercially available because of the high abundance of hydrogen, in the form of water and other hydrogen-containing molecules, in comparison to other nuclei. To perform spectroscopy using nuclei other than hydrogen also requires additional hardware and software to allow what is known as multinuclear spectroscopy. In the MRI literature that describes human imaging, the greatest literature volume exists for proton spectroscopy.

Clinical proton MR spectroscopy (MRS) has been commercially available for more than a decade. Nevertheless, MRS remains somewhat limited in use and is found in select academic medical centers and some large community hospitals because of the level of complexity in acquisition and postprocessing of data. However, in centers with active spectroscopy programs, clinical MRS can add value in the diagnosis, follow-up, and thus management of patients with various neurological diseases, including epilepsy, neoplasms, demyelinating disorders, metabolic diseases, and ischemic diseases.[36,37] The clinical applications of proton spectroscopy to neoplasms, stroke, and epilepsy are discussed later in this chapter.

Functional Magnetic Resonance Imaging

fMRI is used to image the change in the ratio of oxyhemoglobin to deoxyhemoglobin in cerebral blood in response to a stimulus.[38] Changes in the ratio within activated cortical structures are taken to be indicative of changes in the oxygen extraction fraction.[39] These changes are thought to occur in response to cortical function and the resulting upregulation of local metabolism. The change in the oxyhemoglobin-to-deoxyhemoglobin ratio alters the magnetic susceptibility of the blood because deoxyhemoglobin is less paramagnetic than oxyhemoglobin. This difference is manifested as a change in T2* in activated tissue.

The effect is slight; at 1.5 T the change in image intensity is less than 6%. To preclude interference from patient motion, the data are collected with EPI techniques. Images are repeatedly acquired at the same location over the course of the application of a stimulus pattern. By using the a priori knowledge of the stimulus pattern and cross-correlating it with the time course intensity data, a functional image may be made (Fig. 17-23).

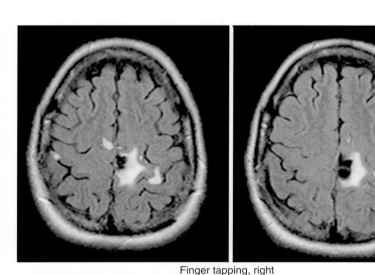

Finger tapping, right

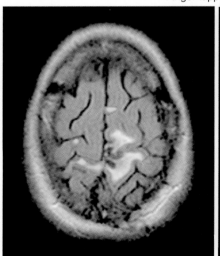
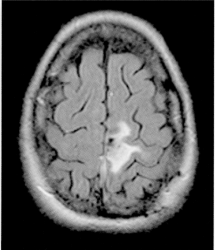

Lower extremity movement, right

FIGURE 17-23 Functional magnetic resonance imaging of a patient with a lesion near the left motor cortex. The functional data overlie a fluid-attenuated inversion recovery image.

Clinical Magnetic Resonance Imaging

Screening

The usual screening MRI of the brain begins with a sagittal localizer of the brain, which is then used to prescribe the remainder of the study. Typically, this includes T1- and T2-weighted axial images and, more recently, a FLAIR sequence, which results in increased lesion conspicuity, especially in the areas adjacent to CSF spaces (i.e., cortex, subcortical white matter, and periventricular deep white matter). At some centers, a gadolinium intravenous contrast agent is given routinely as a part of a screening examination. At other centers, gadolinium is administered at the neuroradiologist's discretion. The contrast-enhanced sequence usually includes an axial or coronal T1-weighted image, or both. Sagittal contrast-enhanced images can also be added as needed.

Generally, screening MRI of the brain includes the entire brain, orbits, and maxillofacial and skull base regions, including the craniocervical junction. Variable slice thickness, planes, and slice intervals are used. Usually, axial and coronal images are obtained as 5-mm-thick slices, with or without an interslice gap of 1 to 2 mm. Sagittal images are generally 4 to 5 mm in thickness with a 1- to 2-mm interslice gap. Contrast-enhanced images are almost always T1 weighted because the gadolinium contrast material's enhancement characteristics (T1-shortening effect) are best observed on T1-weighted images, although its effects may also be observed and quantified on T2-weighted images.

Tailored Magnetic Resonance Imaging

There are many different ways to perform a brain MRI examination. For patients in whom clinical suspicion of pathology is high, a more tailored examination instead of a screening study should be done to increase the likelihood of detecting relevant and clinically significant abnormalities. For example, in a patient with a suspected meningioma that involves the cavernous sinus, a more tailored study that includes thin 3-mm contiguous T1-weighted coronal images before and after contrast administration may better define extension of the tumor in relation to the optic chiasm, pituitary infundibulum, Meckel's cave, and orbital apex. Such a tailored study requires close communication between the neuroradiologist and the neurosurgeon before the study.

Neoplasms

Gliomas

Gliomas are the most common primary brain neoplasms in both adults and children and represent approximately half to two thirds of all brain tumors, respectively, encountered in these populations. Gliomas are usually categorized into four distinct histologic subgroups—astrocytomas, oligodendrogliomas, ependymomas, and choroid plexus tumors, which include the more common papillomas and rare carcinomas and xanthogranulomas.[40,41]

The MRI appearances of gliomas are quite varied, but in some cases these neoplasms can have a set of very distinct appearances and location that permit a correct preoperative radiologic diagnosis. In other cases, the MRI appearance is not specific and several differential diagnoses have to be entertained preoperatively. MRI appearances can also vary according to the neoplasm's histologic grade: lower grade tumors usually exhibit little or no peritumoral vasogenic edema, whereas higher grade tumors demonstrate prominent vasogenic edema associated with a local/regional mass effect or herniation, or both.[42,43] However, the sensitivity and specificity of MRI in assessing the degree of histologic anaplasia of a given neoplasm are limited.

Astrocytomas represent the largest subgroup of gliomas (about 20% to 30% of all gliomas). The histologic subtypes of astrocytomas (e.g., fibrillary, protoplasmic, or gemistocytic) cannot be distinguished by MRI. However, certain subtypes, such as the cystic pilocytic astrocytomas typically found in the cerebellum in children and subependymal giant cell astrocytomas in patients with tuberous sclerosis, may be diagnosed preoperatively by MRI because of their typical appearance, location, and clinical features. Astrocytomas are usually hypointense to normal brain tissue (cortex and white matter) on T1-weighted images and mildly to significantly hyperintense to normal brain on T2-weighted and FLAIR images. Although not completely reliable, in general, low-grade astrocytomas are usually well circumscribed and exhibit no or minimal peritumoral edema, whereas the higher grade anaplastic or glioblastoma multiforme varieties are usually more infiltrative in appearance with less well defined borders and are associated with significant surrounding edema. Low-grade tumors are generally homogeneous in signal characteristics on both T1- and T2-weighted images, whereas higher grade tumors are more likely to be heterogeneous; this reflects the heterogeneity observed by histology associated with the cystic and necrotic changes typically found in these tumors (Figs. 17-24 and 17-25). Rarely, certain astrocytomas demonstrate signal intensity characteristics that are similar or identical to those of CSF on T1- and T2-weighted images.[42,43] Some of these tumors are in fact predominantly cystic in composition, which explains their signal characteristics, but some are solid neoplasms whose parenchymal composition and organization (e.g., microcysts) mimic CSF signals on MRI. Therefore, with MRI, unlike CT, lesions that appear to have the same signal as that of CSF may not be cystic.

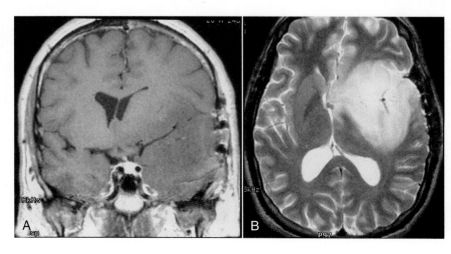

FIGURE 17-24 **A,** Spin echo T1-weighted coronal image with contrast enhancement demonstrating a low-grade astrocytoma as a hypointense mass in the left temporal lobe and inferior frontal lobe that is causing superior displacement of the M1 segment of the left middle cerebral artery. **B,** Fast spin echo T2-weighted axial image demonstrating that the lesion involves the left basal ganglia and insula, with a mild midline shift to the right. It is homogeneously hyperintense.

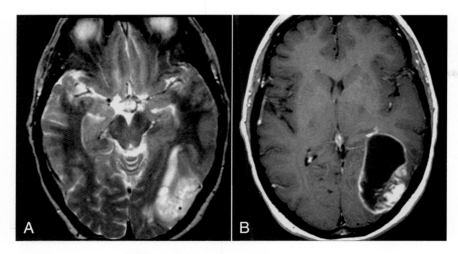

FIGURE 17-25 **A,** Fast spin echo T2-weighted axial image demonstrating a heterogeneously hyperintense mass in the left temporal and occipital lobes. **B,** Spin echo T1-weighted contrast-enhanced image demonstrating a large cystic anterior component with thin peripheral enhancement and a heterogeneously enhancing solid component along the posterolateral aspect of this glioblastoma multiforme.

Brainstem gliomas, which are usually of a fibrillary histologic type and more common in children, appear as a poorly defined mass within the brainstem with diffuse enlargement. They frequently demonstrate exophytic growth with partial or complete circumferential encasement of the basilar artery (Fig. 17-26).[44,45] Gliomatosis cerebri, in which the neoplasm is diffusely infiltrating without a discrete mass, is another astrocytoma subtype. The patient may often have nonfocal neurological findings such as headache, decline in mental status, or changes in personality; on MRI, extensive involvement of one or both cerebral hemispheres is observed, with diffusely abnormal T2 hyperintensity involving the subcortical and deep white matter.

Enhancement of astrocytomas on gadolinium-enhanced T1-weighted images can be quite variable. In general, higher grade tumors demonstrate more prominent enhancement than do lower grade tumors; however, exceptions do occur.[46] Therefore, the presence or absence of significant enhancement in a neoplasm, by itself, should not be used to suggest the degree of anaplasia. Interlobar, interhemispheric, or transtentorial macroscopic extension of astrocytomas (or any combination of such extension) and associated vasogenic edema can readily be seen on MRI, especially on T2-weighted and FLAIR images. However, MRI is more limited in the assessment of microscopic tumor infiltration at the tumor margins and in defining the border between the neoplasm and its non-neoplastic vasogenic edema. Contrast-enhanced T1-weighted images can improve the sensitivity of MRI both preoperatively and postoperatively when looking for recurrence. This might be further improved by MRS either in single-voxel or in 2D multivoxel (chemical shift imaging) forms. On MRS, a significantly elevated amplitude of the choline peak relative to that of creatine or NAA suggests a recurrent neoplasm, whereas absence of elevated choline on the background of mobile lipids and lactate would favor radiation necrosis or postsurgical changes, or both (Fig. 17-27).[47-49] Additional new MRI techniques such as perfusion MRI and activation fMRI are now being used for preoperative evaluation of tumor and for surgical planning (Fig. 17-28).[50-53]

Oligodendrogliomas, which arise from oligodendrocytes, are tumors of adults and have a peak incidence in the fourth to sixth decades. When made up predominantly or purely of oligodendrocytes, they behave in a benign manner. However, when the tumors are of mixed cell origin and contain both astrocytic and oligodendrocytic components, the astrocytic component often degenerates into a more anaplastic astrocytoma at recurrence. This occurs in about half of oligodendrogliomas. Calcifications are common in oligodendrogliomas, and histologically about 70% contain calcification.[40] On CT, about 30% to 40% of these tumors contain visible calcification. On MRI, calcifications are usually hypointense on T1- and T2-weighted images, but microcalcifications can demonstrate hyperintensity on T1-weighted images (Fig. 17-29). However, oligodendrogliomas, mixed oligoastrocytomas, and astrocytomas cannot be reliably differentiated by their MRI appearances.[54]

Ependymomas have protean MRI appearances with variable signal intensities on T1- and T2-weighted images, consistent with the variable cellularity and histologic composition found in these tumors. They are typically hypointense on T1- and hyperintense on T2-weighted images, but calcification or cystic

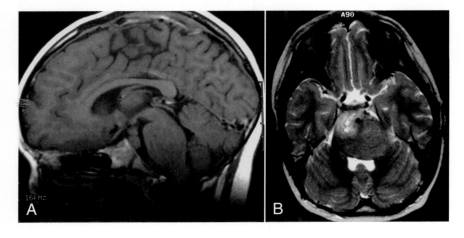

FIGURE 17-26 **A,** Spin echo T1-weighted sagittal image with contrast enhancement showing a diffusely enlarged pons and upper medulla. **B,** Fast spin echo T2-weighted axial image demonstrating heterogeneous signal characteristics in this brainstem glioma consisting of a mixture of hyperintense and isointense areas.

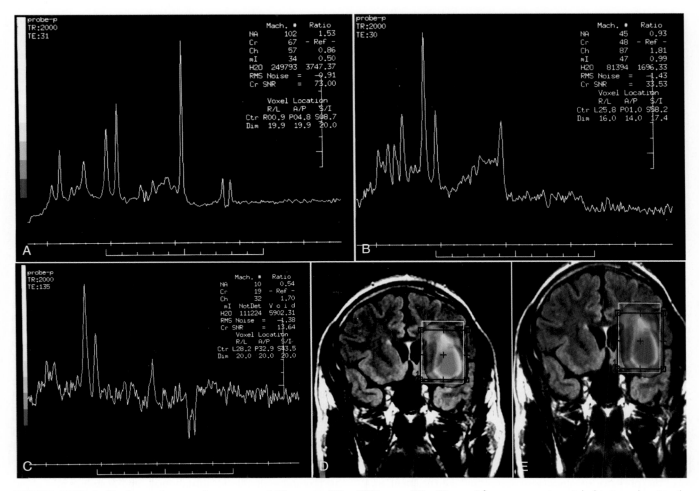

FIGURE 17-27 **A,** Single-voxel magnetic resonance (MR) spectra (TR = 2000 msec, TE = 35 msec) from an experimental phantom showing the expected normal appearance of proton (¹H) MR spectroscopy, except for the double lactate peaks. The dominant peak is for *N*-acetyl aspartate (NAA). Peaks for creatine, choline, and myoinositol are also seen. Refer to the labeled normal spectra from the contralateral hemisphere in Figure 18-22A. **B,** Abnormal single-voxel MR spectra (TR = 2000 msec, TE = 35 msec) from a patient with a frontal lobe mass showing reduced NAA amplitude and an increased amplitude of choline, consistent with a neoplasm. **C,** Single-voxel MR spectra (TR = 2000 msec, TE = 135 msec) from a different patient with a neoplasm showing a similar abnormal pattern and double lactate peaks, indicative of the presence of anaerobic metabolism and production of lactate by the neoplasm. **D,** Color metabolite map for choline from multivoxel MR spectroscopy (TR = 2000 msec, TE = 144 msec) in a patient with a progressive high-grade astrocytoma demonstrating an abnormally increased concentration of choline (displayed in *red*) in the left inferior frontal lobe.

FIGURE 17-28 **A,** Fast spin echo T2-weighted axial image at the level of the roof of the lateral ventricle shows a slightly hyperintense mass (*arrow*) surrounded by prominently hyperintense vasogenic edema (*arrowheads*). **B,** Axial cerebral blood volume image from a perfusion magnetic resonance imaging study demonstrating increased blood volume (*arrow*) within the mass lesion and a halo of decreased perfusion in the surrounding area of edema in a patient with a central nervous system lymphoma.

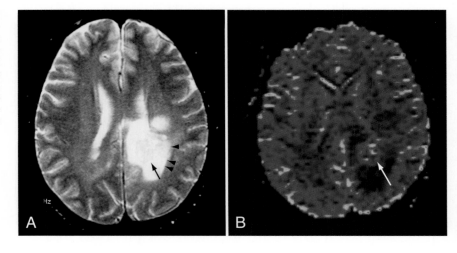

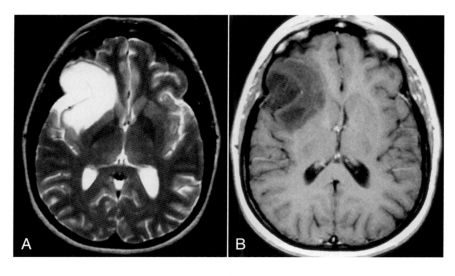

FIGURE 17-29 **A,** Fast spin echo T2-weighted axial image showing a well-circumscribed, homogeneously hyperintense mass involving the right frontal lobe, insula, and basal ganglia, without significant surrounding vasogenic edema. **B,** Spin echo T1-weighted contrast-enhanced axial image showing a heterogeneously hypointense mass with no significant enhancement within this oligodendroglioma.

or hemorrhagic components will often result in a variable heterogeneous MR signal and enhancement (Fig. 17-30).[55] Ependymomas can be found both in a supratentorial location typically within the lateral ventricles and in an infratentorial location within the fourth ventricle. They can demonstrate intraventricular or predominantly extraventricular appearances. A subtype called a *subependymoma* is typically manifested as a periventricular parenchymal mass.

Choroid plexus papillomas and carcinomas can develop within the ventricular system. In children, they typically occur in the atrium of the lateral ventricles, whereas in adults, they are more common within the fourth ventricle. They are generally T1 hypointense and T2 isointense to hyperintense with prominent enhancement (Fig. 17-31). Papillomas are well circumscribed and lobulated in contour, which corresponds to the classic "cauliflower"-like appearance in gross pathology.[56] Choroid plexus papillomas are frequently associated with communicating hydrocephalus. There is debate about the etiology of the hydrocephalus in these patients, but it probably represents some combination of overproduction of CSF by the tumor and obstruction to normal CSF absorption by arachnoid granulations as a result of cellular debris shred from the papilloma.

Meningiomas

Meningiomas are the second most common primary brain neoplasm. They occur at any age and in either sex but are usually found in middle-aged to older women. Meningiomas arise from arachnoid cap cells and are commonly found over the parasagittal cerebral convexity, sphenoid wing, parasellar region, tuberculum sella, olfactory groove, and cerebellopontine angle region. On MRI, meningiomas are usually isointense to gray matter on both T1- and T2-weighted images and can therefore be overlooked on a screening MRI study obtained without contrast enhancement.[57] Certain histologic subtypes such as syncytial and angioblastic meningiomas demonstrate hyperintensity on T2-weighted images.[58] When gadolinium contrast is administered, meningiomas are remarkably easy to detect because they exhibit reliably prominent and generally homogeneous enhancement (Fig. 17-32).[59] They are often associated with an enhanced thickened dura along the lateral margins of the tumor that is known as a "dural tail."[60] In some cases these dural tails represent the margins of tumor extension, whereas in most cases they represent reactive dural enhancement without tumor infiltration.[61] A dural tail is not unique to meningiomas and can be observed in other neoplastic and non-neoplastic processes, including exophytic gliomas, dural metastases, lymphoma, and granulomatous infections. Meningiomas sometimes have areas of necrosis, macroscopic calcification, hemorrhage, or cystic changes. Such findings lead to some heterogeneity of signal and enhancement (Fig. 17-33). Most meningiomas have relatively small amounts of vasogenic edema and are frequently found with no significant edema despite their large size. In some cases, however, they are associated with a large amount of vasogenic edema that resembles the edema observed with high-grade gliomas.[58]

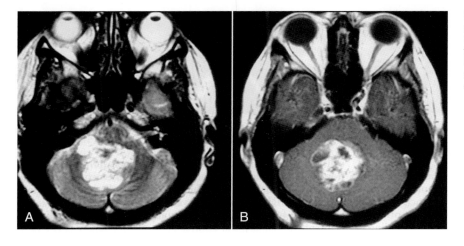

FIGURE 17-30 **A,** Fast spin echo T2-weighted axial image showing a lobulated hyperintense mass in the fourth ventricle with extension into the region of the right foramen of Luschka. **B,** Spin echo T1-weighted contrast-enhanced axial image demonstrating heterogeneous enhancement of this ependymoma.

FIGURE 17-36 A, Fast spin echo T2-weighted axial image showing a cystic mass in the left cerebellar hemisphere with distortion of the adjacent medulla. **B,** Spin-echo T1-weighted contrast-enhanced sagittal image showing peripheral enhancement of this cystic metastasis from breast carcinoma.

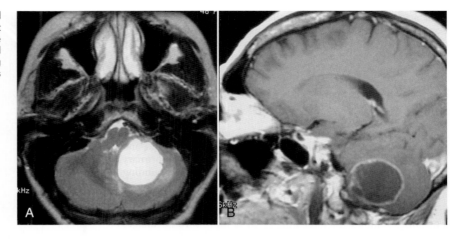

the porus acusticus. Vestibular schwannomas are usually isointense to hypointense to brain tissue on T1-weighted images and hyperintense to brain on T2-weighted images with prominent enhancement after intravenous gadolinium injection. When they are small (e.g., intracanalicular tumor), vestibular schwannomas typically enhance homogeneously (Fig. 17-38). However, with an increase in tumor size, cystic and necrotic foci can develop, which then contribute to more heterogeneous MRI signal characteristics and enhancement patterns (Fig. 17-39).

Vestibular schwannomas are the most common mass lesions in the cerebellopontine angle and represent about 75% of all masses in this location. The next most common mass in the cerebellopontine angle is a meningioma. Meningiomas tend to exhibit more intermediate T2 signal characteristics than do vestibular schwannomas and infrequently extend into the porus acusticus. Although the epicenter of a vestibular schwannoma is at the porus acusticus, a meningioma in this location is located eccentric to the porus acousticus.[68]

Other intracranial schwannomas include those from the trigeminal (cranial nerve V), facial (VII), glossopharyngeal (IX), vagus (X), spinal accessory (XI), and hypoglossal (XII) nerves. Of these, trigeminal nerve schwannomas are the most common.

Facial nerve schwannomas often appear as a lytic, enhancing mass in the petrous temporal bone in the region of the geniculate ganglion (Fig. 17-40).[69] The origin of a schwannoma that arises from cranial nerve IX, X, XI, or XII in the caudal aspect of the posterior fossa is difficult to ascertain on preoperative MRI and may be obvious only at the time of surgery.

Primitive Neuroectodermal Tumors

Primitive neuroectodermal tumors (PNETs) were first defined to describe large, solid hemispheric neoplasms made up of undifferentiated cells, often found in infants and young children, that could not be designated, because of their locations, as a retinoblastoma, medulloblastoma, pineoblastoma, or ependymoblastoma. However, most pathologists are of the opinion that these various neoplasms are similar in their histopathology. Therefore, the designation PNET is used to describe all these undifferentiated, primitive neoplasms found in children and young adults.[40] In the posterior fossa, PNETs arise from the germinal matrices surrounding the fourth ventricle in children and along the anterolateral cerebellar hemisphere in young adults. They can also occur in the supratentorial compartment as intraventricular

FIGURE 17-37 A, Fluid-attenuated inversion recovery axial image at the level of the centrum semiovale revealing multiple areas of abnormal hyperintensity within the sulci of both cerebral hemispheres. **B,** Spin-echo T1-weighted contrast-enhanced fat saturation image showing abnormal enhancement within these sulci in a patient with meningeal carcinomatosis from breast carcinoma.

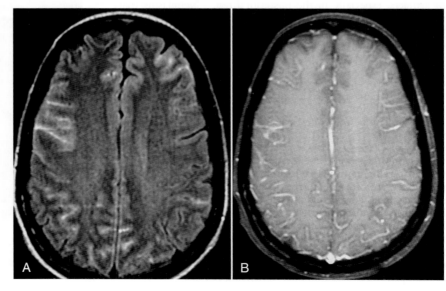

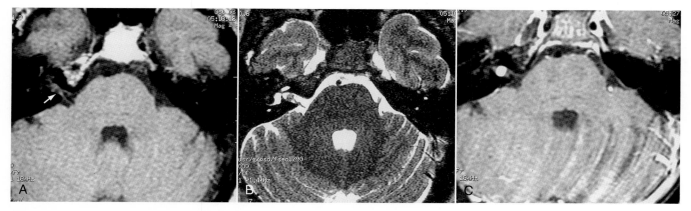

FIGURE 17-38 **A,** Spin echo T1-weighted non–contrast-enhanced axial image showing a small isointense mass with ill-defined borders in the right internal auditory canal (*arrow*). **B,** This high-resolution, fast spin echo T2-weighted image better delineates a small isointense intracanalicular mass. **C,** Spin echo T1-weighted contrast-enhanced axial image demonstrating prominent homogeneous enhancement of this small intracanalicular vestibular schwannoma.

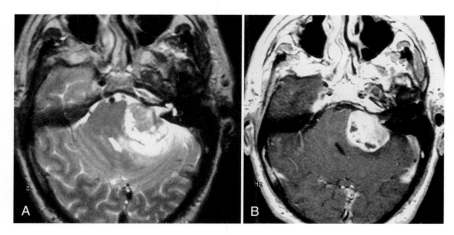

FIGURE 17-39 **A,** Fast spin echo T2-weighted axial image showing heterogeneous signal from a mass in the left cerebellopontine angle at the level of the left internal auditory canal (IAC). There is a significant mass effect on the brainstem, left cerebellar hemisphere, and fourth ventricle. **B,** Spin echo T1-weighted contrast-enhanced axial image showing the heterogeneous enhancement pattern of this large vestibular schwannoma, with minimal enhancement in the left IAC.

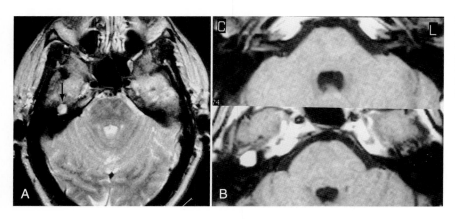

FIGURE 17-40 **A,** Fast spin echo T2-weighted axial image showing a hyperintense mass in the right petrous apex. **B,** Spin echo T1-weighted contrast-enhanced axial image demonstrating a homogeneously enhancing right facial nerve schwannoma at the level of the geniculate ganglion.

FIGURE 17-41 A, Fast spin echo T2-weighted axial image showing a heterogeneous posterior fossa mass with a cystic hyperintense anterior component and a solid isointense posterior component. There is nearly complete effacement of the fourth ventricle by this mass. **B,** Spin echo T1-weighted contrast-enhanced axial image showing a central focus of prominent enhancement with variable enhancement in the remainder of this primitive neuroectodermal tumor.

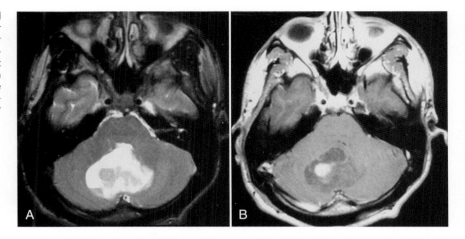

or intra-axial masses. PNETs are made up of small round cells and are hypercellular with a high nuclear-to-cytoplasm ratio. These characteristics contribute to their MRI signal characteristics, which are slightly hypointense to isointense to brain tissue on T1- and isointense on T2-weighted images. They demonstrate moderate to prominent enhancement on contrast-enhanced T1-weighted images. PNETs are typically homogeneous solid masses but can have cystic or necrotic components that result in more heterogeneous signal and enhancement characteristics (Fig. 17-41).[70]

Infections

MRI evaluation for meningitis is limited by its marginal sensitivity. With the advent of the FLAIR pulse sequence and especially with gadolinium-enhanced FLAIR studies, increased sensitivity for meningeal diseases is reported, but further large-scale prospective studies are required. A normal brain MRI study does not exclude meningitis. Therefore, the diagnosis of meningitis should still be made by chemical and bacteriologic examination of CSF. However, in a patient with high suspicion or a proven meningeal infection, MRI is valuable and can help ascertain the degree of involvement and the presence of any parenchymal involvement (i.e., encephalitis, infarction, or abscess formation). MRI also can help monitor a patient's response to therapy if an objective parameter, in addition to the clinical findings, is required.[71]

Viral meningitis, when visible on MRI, is typically manifested as diffuse meningeal enhancement on gadolinium-enhanced T1-weighted images (Fig. 17-42). When encephalitis is present (e.g., herpes encephalitis), the involved parenchyma reflects the presence of cytotoxic and vasogenic edema with hypointense T1 and hyperintense T2 signal characteristics involving both gray and white matter (Fig. 17-43). Effacement of local cortical sulci, hemorrhage, and prominent leptomeningeal enhancement may also be present.[72]

Bacterial meningitis is often associated with prominent diffuse meningeal enhancement. It is typically hematogenous, but it also results from direct extension of infections in the adjacent paranasal sinuses or mastoid air cells. Complications of bacterial meningitis include subdural empyema, infarction, and parenchymal abscess. An abscess is seen on T1-weighted images as a mass with a central nonenhancing or slightly enhancing T1 hypointense cavity with an enhancing wall of variable and irregular thickness that is surrounded by T1 hypointense and T2 hyperintense edema. The central cavity is typically hyperintense on T2-weighted images, but it can be isointense or hypointense, depending on its contents.[73] However, these MRI appearances are similar to those observed with a necrotic neoplasm. MRI findings can be crucial in distinguishing an abscess from a necrotic

neoplasm when other clinical or laboratory data are lacking. The enhancing wall of an abscess cavity is typically thinner along its medial/deeper aspect and thicker along its lateral/superficial aspect. The extent of associated edema may be smaller with an abscess, whereas a necrotic brain neoplasm such as glioblastoma multiforme usually has a large area of surrounding vasogenic edema.[74] Newer MRI techniques such as MRS and diffusion-weighted imaging (DWI) can help differentiate abscesses from necrotic neoplasm. In MRS, spectroscopic evaluation of an abscess reveals several amino acid signatures and abundant lactate and mobile lipids. These, however, are also observed in necrotic neoplasms. On DWI, an abscess cavity typically has a restricted diffusion pattern with a low apparent diffusion coefficient (ADC) and hyperintense signal on diffusion-weighted images (Fig. 17-44).[75,76] By contrast, a cystic/necrotic neoplasm has a relatively increased ADC with hypointense signal on diffusion-weighted images.

MRI can be used to image other infections such as tuberculosis, fungal infections, and cysticercosis. Tubercular meningitis usually involves the basal meninges and typically extends into the Virchow-Robin perivascular spaces of the basal ganglia, which may cause lacunar infarctions (Fig. 17-45).[77-79] Fungal infections involve the brain by direct extension from contiguous structures

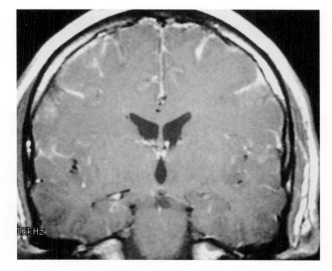

FIGURE 17-42 Spin echo T1-weighted contrast-enhanced coronal image demonstrating abnormal, thick meningeal enhancement in this patient with viral meningitis.

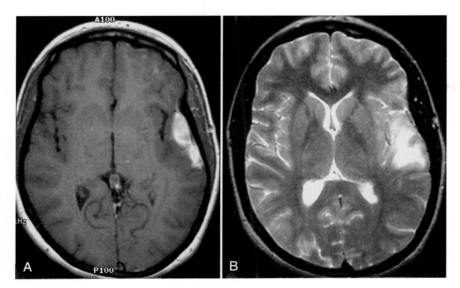

FIGURE 17-43 **A,** Spin echo T1-weighted non–contrast-enhanced axial image illustrating a lesion in the left anterior temporal lobe with a hypointense medial component and a hyperintense lateral component. **B,** Fast spin echo T2-weighted axial image showing the abnormal hyperintensity of this lesion, which represents a focus of encephalitis from herpes infection. The T1 hyperintense area represents subacute parenchymal hemorrhage.

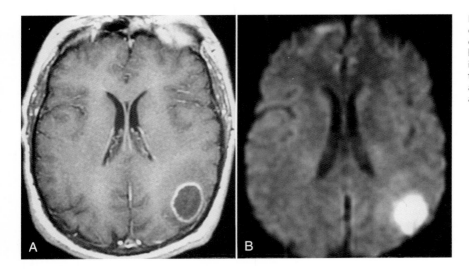

FIGURE 17-44 **A,** Spin echo T1-weighted contrast-enhanced axial image showing a ring-enhancing left parietal mass with surrounding hypointense edema. **B,** Axial diffusion-weighted image revealing abnormal hyperintensity within the nonenhancing central cavity, which indicates a marked restriction of water diffusion in this abscess cavity.

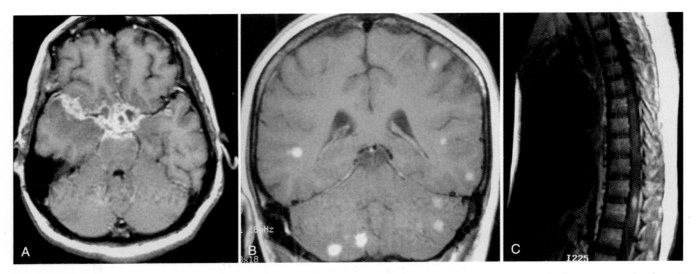

FIGURE 17-45 **A,** Spin echo T1-weighted contrast-enhanced axial image demonstrating diffuse basal meningeal enhancement with edema in the right temporal lobe in this patient with tubercular meningitis. **B,** Spin echo T1-weighted contrast-enhanced images showing multiple enhancing parenchymal nodules within the brain and thoracic spinal cord (**C**). They represent multiple tuberculomas associated with miliary tuberculosis infection.

FIGURE 17-46 Fast spin echo T2-weighted axial image (**A**) and spin echo T1-weighted contrast-enhanced axial image (**B**) revealing multiple cystic parenchymal lesions that are T2 hyperintense and T1 hypointense at the gray matter–white matter junction and in the periventricular region. These lesions are associated with central nervous system cysticercosis.

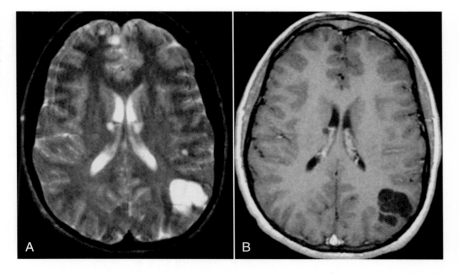

such as the paranasal sinuses, orbits, and mastoid or by a hematogenous route. These infections are usually found in diabetic patients or immunocompromised individuals. Meningitis and encephalitis with parenchymal abscesses are possible. In *Aspergillus* infection, the fungus has a propensity for vascular invasion, which results in hemorrhagic transformation of encephalitic foci.[80,81] Cysticercosis is an infection that results from infestation with a pork tapeworm. When these parasites die within the brain, parenchymal reaction to the dying parasites contributes to the edema, enhancement, and calcification seen on imaging. Cysticercosis appears as small, parenchymal lesions with punctate calcifications, intraventricular masses, or multiple lobulated T1 hypointense masses that expand the subarachnoid spaces (racemose form) (Fig. 17-46).[82,83]

Stroke and Vascular Diseases

Visualization of an acute infarction on MRI depends on several factors, including time after the ictus, stroke size, and location. Of these, time is the single most important factor. The high tissue contrast of MRI has decreased the time between the ictus and when an acute infarction can first be identified on imaging. Acute infarction appears as a hyperintense T2 lesion involving the cortical, white matter, or deep gray matter structures (or any combination). Larger cortical infarctions have associated effacement of adjacent sulci from cytotoxic edema. Abnormal hyperintensity in

cortical vessels within these sulci may be the first signs of an acute infarction, even before any significant changes in T2-weighted images are apparent. Slow vascular transit time within an infarction results in loss of the normal flow void and increased signal within these vessels. Absence of a normal flow void is occasionally observed in the setting of a large infarction involving the internal carotid or anterior, middle, or posterior cerebral artery territory. Acute infarction changes on MRI are usually present within 24 hours of the ictus and are often evident between 6 and 12 hours after the ictus. Cytotoxic edema increases during the first 1 to 2 weeks and resolves within 1 month. The infarcted area, in the chronic stage, exhibits local volume loss with compensatory enlargement of adjacent sulci, cisterns, and ventricles along with a hyperintense signal on T2-weighted images. If hemorrhage was present during the acute or subacute stages, T1 and T2 hypointensity, representing hemosiderin and ferritin, are present in the chronic stages.

Echo planar DWI has even further decreased the time required for MRI visualization of an acute stroke.[84] In animal models, DWI can demonstrate large vascular territory infarctions (e.g., ICA or MCA) within minutes after vessel occlusion.[85] In humans, acute infarctions can be demonstrated on DWI within 30 minutes to 1 hour. This implies that most acute infarctions should be visible on DWI by the time that a patient arrives at the hospital after the onset of stroke (Fig. 17-47).[86] Once present on MRI, the hyperintense infarction on DWI persists

FIGURE   17-47 Fluid-attenuated   inversion recovery axial image (**A**) showing abnormal hyperintensity in the left frontal lobe, temporal lobe, and insula, with corresponding abnormal hyperintensity on the diffusion-weighted image (**B**), in this patient with an acute middle cerebral artery infarction.

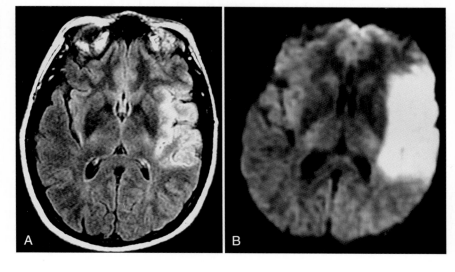

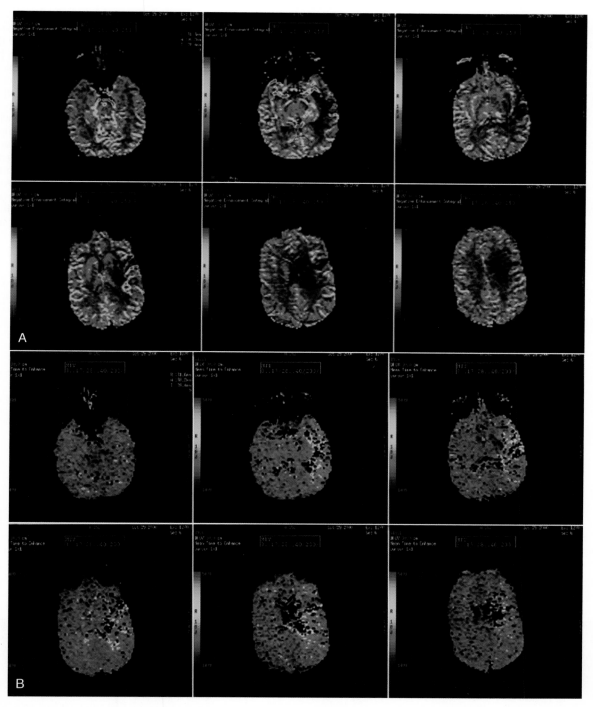

FIGURE 17-48 A, Images from a multiple-level relative cerebral blood volume (rCBV) map in a patient with left middle cerebral artery ischemic symptoms demonstrate decreased perfusion (*dark blue*) in the left basal ganglia and superior temporal lobe and within the deep white matter (*black*) of the left frontal and parietal lobes. **B,** Mean transit time (MTT) maps at the same levels demonstrate increased MTT (*yellow* and *green*) in the same areas.

for approximately 2 weeks, depending on size and location and the diffusion sensitivity factor (i.e., b value) that is used to obtain the diffusion-weighted images. After this period, subtle hyperintensity may remain and corresponds to the areas of abnormal hyperintensity on T2-weighted and FLAIR images. The degree of such hyperintensity on DWI is much less than that observed with an acute infarction. This phenomenon is known as the "T2 shine-through" effect and should not be confused with an acute infarction.[87]

Perfusion MRI, in the form of dynamic susceptibility imaging, shows promise in evaluation of cerebral perfusion, expressed as relative CBV or MTT. Again, using an echo planar technique, several hundred images of the brain can be obtained in less than 2 minutes. These raw images are then postprocessed to obtain a "map" of relative CBV or MTT, which is then used to qualitatively and quantitatively assess cerebral perfusion (Figs. 17-48 and 17-49). Along with diffusion-weighted images, these perfusion images can be used to determine the extent of ischemic brain that is at risk for infarction. The difference between the area of abnormally low perfusion and the area of abnormally low diffusion coefficients represents the ischemic penumbra that is at risk for infarction but still may be salvageable if treated.[88,89]

MRS can also play a role in acute stroke evaluation. Evidence of anaerobic metabolism (lactate production and decreased NAA) can be detected with ^{1}H-MRS when ischemia and infarction are present. Single-voxel or 2D chemical shift imaging (multivoxel) spectroscopy can therefore define the extent of ischemic tissue that is producing significant amounts of lactate. When 2D spectroscopy is performed, a map of areas with lactate production or areas with decreased NAA can be displayed and compared with maps of abnormal diffusion or perfusion to further delineate the cerebral tissue at risk for infarction.[90] MRS may also help predict clinical outcomes in young children with hypoxic ischemic CNS injury.[91]

Nonemergency MR evaluation of patients with symptoms of intracranial or extracranial ischemic vascular disease usually begins with a routine brain MRI study that includes T2-weighted and FLAIR images for maximal sensitivity to detect subacute and chronic evidence of cerebral ischemic disease. MRA of the brain to evaluate the major intracranial arteries and their proximal branches is now a well-established technique. MRA typically uses a 3D TOF technique with added magnetization transfer pulse to improve the visualization of distal branches (Fig. 17-50). An MR venogram to exclude major venous thrombosis can be performed with either 3D TOF or phase-contrast techniques, which can easily identify the major superficial and deep venous sinuses and veins (Fig. 17-51). MRA has acceptable accuracy in evaluation of the intracranial internal carotid, vertebral, and basilar arteries, as well as the proximal branches of the anterior, middle, and posterior cerebral arteries in the setting of significant atherosclerotic stenoses, vasospasm, or vasculitis (Fig. 17-52).[92] However, MRA is limited in its evaluation of medium-sized and small arteries. When such a disease process is clinically suspected and suggested

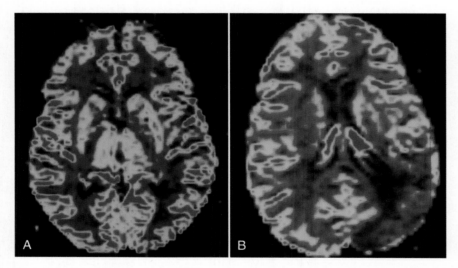

FIGURE 17-49 A, Normal relative cerebral blood volume (rCBV) map from a perfusion magnetic resonance imaging study at the level of the basal ganglia. **B,** rCBV map from a patient with an infarction in the left parietal and occipital lobes demonstrating reduced perfusion (*dark blue*) within the left parietal and occipital lobes.

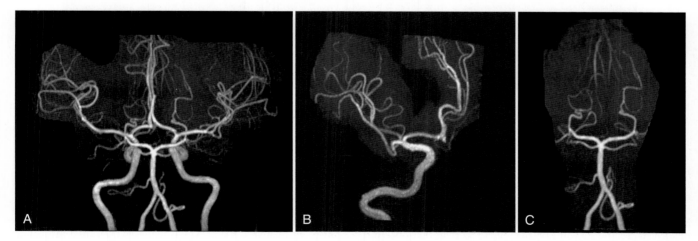

FIGURE 17-50 A, Postprocessed image from three-dimensional time-of-flight magnetic resonance angiography of the brain demonstrating major intracranial arteries, including the A2, M2, and P2 branches of the anterior, middle, and posterior cerebral arteries. **B,** Isolated "cutout" view of the right internal carotid artery and its intracranial branches. **C,** Isolated view of the posterior circulation.

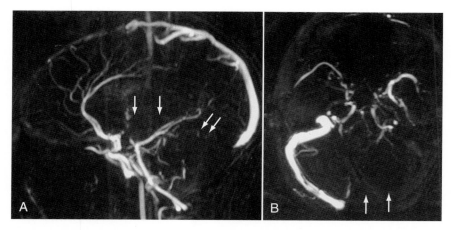

FIGURE 17-51 A, Postprocessed sagittal image from a two-dimensional time-of-flight magnetic resonance venogram (MRV) showing a normal appearance of the sagittal sinus but absence of signal from the deep internal cerebral veins, vein of Galen, and straight sinus, indicative of thrombosis of these venous structures. **B,** Postprocessed axial image from the same MRV showing thrombosis of the left transverse and sigmoid sinuses.

by a routine MRI study (i.e., abnormal lesions on T2-weighted or FLAIR images), conventional angiography is often warranted. Evaluation of the carotid and vertebral arteries in the neck can be performed with 2D or 3D TOF or phase-contrast MR techniques without the use of intravenous gadolinium contrast. The accuracy of these techniques in comparison to conventional contrast-enhanced angiography is well described.[93,94] A newer technique using a 3D spoiled gradient recalled (SPGR) pulse sequence obtained after rapid bolus intravenous injection of gadolinium can improve the accuracy of noninvasive MR vascular evaluation (Fig. 17-53).[95] Similar to brain CTA, MRA is increasingly being used as an initial noninvasive imaging study for intracranial aneurysms or as a follow-up imaging study for untreated or treated intracranial aneurysms.[95,96] MRA or CTA of a previously coiled or clipped aneurysm can be challenging because of inherent MR or CT artifacts generated by coils or clips. It is difficult to exclude a small recanalization or residual aneurysm on CTA because of a large amount of artifact from an aneurysm clip or coils. However, gadolinium bolus MRA of the brain may demonstrate recanalization of an intracranial aneurysm previously treated by endovascular coil embolization better than conventional TOF MRA without contrast enhancement (Fig. 17-54).[97,98]

Trauma

In acute CNS trauma, evaluation for a fracture or hemorrhage is still best done with a non–contrast-enhanced CT scan. However, because of its superior tissue contrast, MRI may better define small parenchymal abnormalities on T2-weighed, FLAIR, and gradient-recalled echo (GRE) images that may not be visible on CT. GRE is the most sensitive pulse sequence for acute/subacute blood breakdown products.[99] MRI also appears to be superior to CT in evaluating posterior fossa pathology because the usual posterior fossa beam-hardening artifacts typically observed on CT are absent. MRI is also useful in the evaluation of small cortical contusions and subdural and epidural hematomas because of its higher tissue contrast and the ease of multiplanar acquisition with MRI. Small subacute SDHs, which are often isodense and therefore subtle on CT, are typically T1 and T2 hyperintense on MRI and thus more conspicuous. The MRI appearances of subdural and epidural hematomas and hygromas are variable and depend on the age and history (i.e., repeat hemorrhages). In the acute and subacute stages, T1 and T2 signal characteristics are similar to those observed with parenchymal hematomas. They are T1 isointense to hypointense and T2 hypointense in the acute stage because of intracellular deoxyhemoglobin and methemoglobin and become T1 hyperintense and T2 hyperintense in the subacute stage from extracellular methemoglobin. In the chronic stage, parenchymal hemorrhages are hypointense on T1- and markedly hypointense on T2-weighted images as a result of susceptibility effects from intracellular ferritin and hemosiderin, which are mostly present in the interstitium and within macrophages. However, chronic SDHs (hygromas) are T1 hypointense and T2 hyperintense in signal, similar to those of CSF. This reflects the low-density fluid collection that is typically observed on CT. Some authors suggest that MRI with a FLAIR pulse sequence has high sensitivity for acute SAH, but significant debate remains about its accuracy in the presence of frequently observed CSF flow–related artifacts associated with this pulse sequence, especially in the basal cisterns.[100-102]

MRI is especially helpful in the evaluation of patients with diffuse axonal injury (DAI), which usually results from a high-speed acceleration and deceleration injury that causes mechanical stress on the brain and thus results in "shear" injuries.[103] The multiple, small and subtle shear injuries at the gray-white matter border, along the corpus callosum, and within the brainstem, typical of DAI, are much better evaluated with MRI than CT. The GRE pulse sequence, which is highly sensitive to areas of changes in susceptibility, is valuable when diffuse small parenchymal hemorrhages in the setting of trauma are evaluated. On T2-weighted and FLAIR images, these small superficial gray-white matter border lesions and deep pericallosal, deep gray matter, and upper brainstem lesions are hyperintense. If hemorrhagic, these lesions are also hypointense on GRE images because of changes in susceptibility associated with acute blood breakdown products such as deoxyhemoglobin and intracellular methemoglobin.[104] In the chronic stage, hemosiderin and ferritin result in hypointensity on T2-weighted and GRE images.[105]

Brain MRI can be useful when a patient with an acute head injury has minimal CT abnormalities but has profound neurological deficits. In addition, MRI may be helpful when an objective measure of extensive brain injury, particularly brainstem injury, is required before a patient's prognosis is discussed with the family. Newer MRI techniques such as DWI, perfusion MRI, and MRS may play additional roles in trauma patients to detect areas of ischemia and infarction.[106]

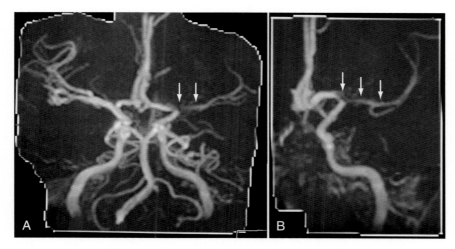

FIGURE 17-52 A, Three-dimensional time-of-flight brain magnetic resonance angiogram (MRA) demonstrating reduced flow signal within the distal intracranial segment of the left internal carotid artery (ICA) and proximal left middle cerebral artery (MCA) (compare with the right side). **B,** Magnified MRA view of the left ICA and MCA demonstrating thrombus within the terminal left supraclinoid ICA, proximal A1 segment of the anterior cerebral artery, and M1 segment of the MCA, with significantly diminished flow in the left MCA distribution distal to the thrombus.

Acute traumatic vascular injury at the skull base that involves the ICA or vertebral artery can be quickly and noninvasively evaluated with MRI. MRI is highly sensitive to high-grade vessel stenosis or occlusion from traumatic dissection, with demonstration of the absence of normal flow void in these vessels. Additional T1-weighted images with fat saturation in the neck and at the skull base readily identify the false lumen containing thrombus with subacute methemoglobin. 2D/3D MRA of the neck and the skull base can add additional information and display the relevant arterial tree from the aortic arch to the brain. Although conventional catheter angiography still remains the "gold standard," MRA in a posttraumatic, possibly unstable patient can help guide clinical management and direct further conventional angiographic evaluation once the patient is stable.

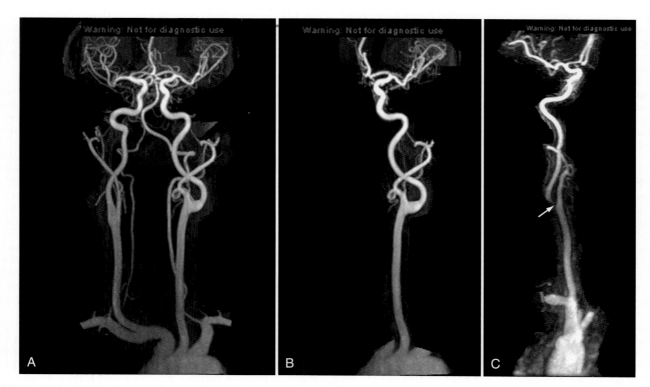

FIGURE 17-53 A, Three-dimensional gadolinium bolus neck magnetic resonance angiogram (MRA) demonstrating the major craniocervical arteries from the aortic arch to the proximal intracranial circulation. **B,** Isolated view of the left extracranial and intracranial carotid artery system. **C,** In a different patient, a gadolinium bolus neck MRA demonstrates a focal stenosis at the origin of the right internal carotid artery.

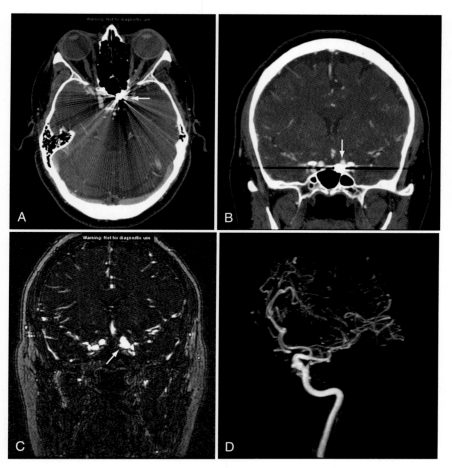

FIGURE 17-54 A, Axial image from a brain CTA at the level of the anterior clinoid process demonstrating prominent streak artifacts from previous endovascular coil embolization of a left parophthalmic internal carotid artery (ICA) aneurysm (*arrow*). **B,** A two-dimensional coronal reformatted image from the CTA data set is compromised by the artifacts, with poor visualization of the region of the aneurysm neck (*arrow*). **C,** Coronal image from a gadolinium bolus brain magnetic resonance angiogram (MRA) demonstrating small recurrent filling of the left ICA aneurysm (*arrow*). **D,** Three-dimensional reconstruction image from the MRA data set with a cutout view of the left ICA revealing definite small recanalization of the previously coiled aneurysm (*arrow*).

Vascular Malformations

Intracerebral vascular malformations include four distinct types: AVM, cavernous malformation (cavernous angioma or hemangioma), developmental venous anomaly (DVA, previously known as venous malformation or venous angioma), and capillary telangiectasia. All except capillary telangiectasia are typically visible on MRI. An AVM is a vascular malformation that consists of a nidus that lacks the normal capillary network with ensuing direct communication between abnormally enlarged thick-walled feeding arterial channels and thin-walled draining venous channels. The vessels often lack normal smooth muscle and elastic lamina layers. AVMs may often be associated with aneurysms of feeding arteries or the draining veins (venous varix). There is no normal parenchyma intermixed with an AVM, although some gliosis may be observed. On MRI, an AVM appears as a complex tangle of abnormally enlarged vessels that demonstrate flow voids because of a high-flow state. Secondary findings such as subacute and chronic blood breakdown products (methemoglobin, ferritin, and hemosiderin) can be found with corresponding areas of T2 and GRE hypointensity.[107] Similar small T2 hypointensity is also observed in the setting of calcifications associated with an AVM. Surrounding areas of edema, ischemia, or encephalomalacia may also be present.[108] These areas are visible on T2-weighted and FLAIR images as hyperintensity with or without loss of volume in the case of chronic atrophy. Thin, linear cortical T1 hyperintensity may also be observed if cortical laminar necrosis from chronic ischemia as a result of a physiologic steal phenomenon occurs in the parenchyma adjacent to the AVM. AVMs can also be further visualized with 2D or 3D MRA using either phase-contrast or TOF techniques (Fig. 17-55).[109] These MRI techniques can be used to diagnose AVMs and help in preoperative localization with 3D intraoperative guidance software. MRI is also useful in monitoring smaller AVMs treated by stereotactic radiosurgery (linear accelerator or Gamma Knife techniques).[110,111]

Cavernous malformations are slow-flow vascular malformations made up of abnormally large venous channels without associated abnormally enlarged feeding arteries or draining veins. They become symptomatic and also visible on MRI because they frequently bleed.[112] Typically, cavernous malformations are discrete parenchymal masses with heterogeneous hypointensity and hyperintensity on T1- and T2-weighted images as a result of blood breakdown products of various ages. When recent hemorrhage is present, reactive T2 hyperintense surrounding edema may be seen with associated local mass effect.[113] Multiple cavernous malformations are found in patients with vascular malformation syndromes. Because MRI, among all the imaging techniques, including conventional angiography, best visualizes these cavernous malformations, it is the study of choice in the initial evaluation and follow-up of patients with cavernomas (Fig. 17-56).

A DVA (as mentioned before, previously known as venous malformation or venous angioma) is not a pathologic vascular malformation. Instead, a DVA is a normal variant in which several prominent deep parenchymal veins drain a normal part of the brain and then drain into an unusually large superficial or deep draining vein. The angiographic and MRI appearance of these malformations has been described in the literature as resembling the "head of Medusa," a Greek mythologic figure with a head of "hair" made of multiple live serpents. Because this

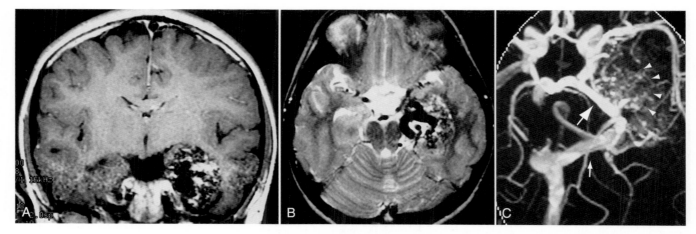

FIGURE 17-55 Spin echo T1-weighted contrast-enhanced coronal image (**A**), fast spin echo T2-weighted axial image (**B**), and postprocessed axial image from three-dimensional time-of-flight magnetic resonance angiography (**C**) illustrate a large left temporal lobe arteriovenous malformation with multiple flow voids within a large nidus (*arrowheads*) and prominently dilated feeding arteries (*large arrow*) and draining veins (*small arrow*).

is a benign entity and requires no intervention, its recognition on imaging studies is essential. DVAs have a typical imaging appearance on MRI that consists of several slightly prominent vessels with flow voids on T2-weighted images that drain into a larger draining vein.[114] They are best visualized on contrast-enhanced T1-weighted images (Fig. 17-57). DVAs may sometimes coexist with cavernous malformations. If a hemorrhage is present in the vicinity of a DVA, the cause of hemorrhage is most likely an occult cavernous malformation neighboring the DVA.

Capillary telangiectasia is a histopathologic diagnosis rather than a radiologic one. It is rarely diagnosed preoperatively. If capillary telangiectasia is visible on MRI, it appears as a nonspecific focus of T2 hyperintensity, which may be associated with subtle enhancement on contrast-enhanced T1-weighted images. Multiple capillary telangiectases are found in patients with ataxia-

telangiectasia syndrome, which affects both the CNS and other viscera.[115]

Seizure and Epilepsy

Imaging of a patient with a first-time seizure usually begins with a head CT without contrast, followed by a contrast-enhanced study if necessary. Causes of seizures such as stroke, hemorrhage, neoplasm, abscess, or benign cysts can often be adequately evaluated with CT. Routine brain MRI has higher sensitivity than CT for subtle parenchymal lesions and meningeal diseases. However, in epilepsy, where a recurrent seizure disorder is present, a more tailored MRI study is required to exclude a structural substrate for epilepsy, including mesial temporal sclerosis, subtle cortical

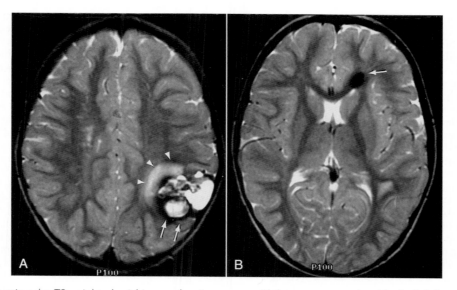

FIGURE 17-56 A, Fast spin echo T2-weighted axial image showing a mass with heterogeneous signal in the left frontoparietal lobes, central hyperintensity, and a peripheral rim of hypointensity with associated surrounding hyperintensity. This is a large cavernous malformation (*arrows*) with evidence of recurrent hemorrhages—blood breakdown products of different age surrounded by mild edema (*arrowheads*), suggestive of a recent episode of hemorrhage. **B,** Fast spin echo T2-weighted axial image at the level of the basal ganglia in the same patient illustrating a focus of abnormal hypointensity, representing hemosiderin, adjacent to the left frontal horn (*arrow*). This represents a focus of old hemorrhage from a smaller cavernous malformation.

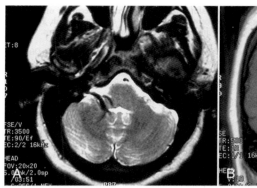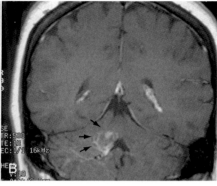

FIGURE 17-57 A, Fast spin echo T2-weighted axial image illustrating branching flow voids in the right brachium pontis region with extension into the adjacent cisternal space. **B,** Spin echo T1-weighted contrast-enhanced coronal image demonstrating a typical branching pattern of dilated veins in a venous malformation next to the fourth ventricle (*arrows*).

and subcortical neoplasms, or migration anomalies (heterotopias). These lesions may not be apparent on routine brain MRI examination because they are often quite small and have signal characteristics similar to adjacent normal brain tissue on both T1- and T2-weighted images.

Several different MRI protocols have been developed over the years to evaluate epilepsy patients. These protocols usually include a type of high-resolution, 3D, and heavily T1-weighted acquisition of the whole brain. An SPGR sequence is one such pulse sequence that can be obtained at 1-mm intervals in the axial, coronal, and sagittal planes. Small slice thickness along with its heavily T1-weighted parameters accentuates the signal difference between gray and white matter and thus improves the detection of small focal heterotopias and migration anomalies.[116,117] MRI acquisition with the use of phased-array surface coils over a part of the head instead of the usual head coil used for brain MRI may also improve resolution and sensitivity. These surface coils have an improved signal-to-noise ratio that is usually severalfold greater than that obtained with a routine head coil and have the flexibility to be placed directly over the part of the brain that is suspected of containing the epileptic focus. They are useful in the evaluation of small cortical or subcortical lesions, which may not otherwise be visible on routine brain MRI. The advantages of surface coils diminish for deeper structures because the signal decreases as the distance between the coil and the structure increases. Nonetheless, phased-array surface coils have been used successfully to evaluate the mesial temporal lobes in patients with complex partial seizures referable to the temporal lobes. In many of these patients, MRI correlates of mesial temporal sclerosis, such as hippocampal atrophy, abnormal T2 hippocampal hyperintensity, and disruption of the hippocampal internal architecture, are observed.[118-120] Such imaging of the mesial temporal lobes is best done in a coronal or modified coronal plane perpendicular to the anteroposterior axis

of the hippocampus at 1- to 20-mm intervals using T1, T2, and FLAIR images (Fig. 17-58).

Tailored MRI techniques are valuable in the preoperative imaging evaluation of epileptic patients. In particular, these techniques are useful in the preoperative evaluation and lateralization of the seizure focus in patients with temporal lobe epilepsy. Various MRI parameters can be used to diagnose the presence of mesial temporal sclerosis in patients with temporal lobe epilepsy, including qualitative techniques such as visual evaluation for asymmetrically and abnormally increased signal on T2 and FLAIR coronal images, decreased hippocampal volume, and larger than normal size of the temporal horn of the lateral ventricle within the ipsilateral temporal lobe. Quantitative measurements of these changes can be studied with 3D hippocampal volumetry to quantify the hippocampal atrophy and T2 relaxometry to quantify the change in T2 signal. Such MRI lateralization, when possible, has significant prognostic value for patients who undergo surgery to treat medically intractable temporal lobe epilepsy. Patients with a lateralizing MRI abnormality have a significantly greater seizure-free rate after hippocampal resection and partial temporal lobectomy than do those who do not demonstrate such a lateralizing abnormality on preoperative MRI.[121,122] MRS can also be used to study the mesial temporal lobes, including the hippocampus, in temporal lobe epilepsy. Single-voxel and 2D chemical shift imaging techniques are used to obtain proton MR spectra from the hippocampi and surrounding mesial temporal lobe structures. In MRS, neuronal concentration and integrity are ascertained by measuring the concentration of the neuronal marker metabolite NAA with an absolute quantitative technique or, more commonly, by a ratio that compares NAA with a reference metabolite such as creatine. A high accuracy rate in lateralization of the diseased hippocampus in patients with temporal lobe epilepsy is reported with the use of single-voxel or chemical shift imaging proton MRS.[47,123-125]

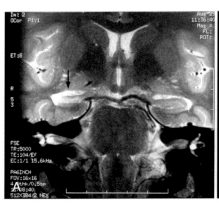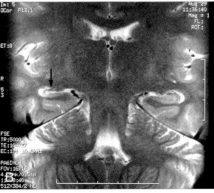

FIGURE 17-58 A, This high-resolution, fast spin echo T2-weighted coronal image obtained with phased-array surface coils demonstrates subtle abnormal hyperintensity in the right hippocampus (*arrow*) in a patient with temporal lobe epilepsy. **B,** A coronal image through the body of the right hippocampus demonstrates prominent asymmetric atrophy of the right hippocampus (*arrow*) in comparison to the contralateral left hippocampus.

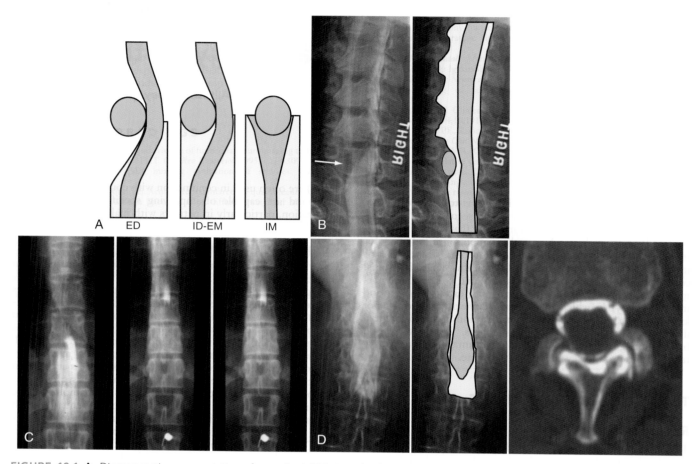

FIGURE 18-1 A, Diagrammatic representation of extradural (ED), intradural extramedullary (ED-EM), and intramedullary (IM) lesions of the spine. *Purple,* spinal cord; *orange,* mass; *tan,* subarachnoid space. **B,** Oblique view from a cervical myelogram demonstrating an extradural defect *(arrow)* from a herniated disk at the C6-7 level with cutoff of the nerve root. The diagram demonstrates the typical concave inward appearance of an extradural defect. **C,** Anteroposterior (AP) radiographs from a thoracic myelogram demonstrating an intradural extramedullary lesion. Contrast agent was introduced into the subarachnoid material below the lesion on the left and at C1-2 to outline the superior extent of the lesion on the right. One can see displacement of the cord silhouette to the left. **D,** AP views from a thoracic myelogram demonstrating an intramedullary mass at the conus. The contrast column in the subarachnoid space is splayed around the intramedullary mass. CT myelography demonstrates the enlarged conus.

and pathologic abnormalities with myelographic-like images. More recently, various forms of dual-energy multidetector CT have been introduced that can subtract out bone in both single slices and 3D multiplanar reformatted images (Fig. 18-3).

The disadvantages of myelography/CT myelography relate primarily to the introduction of contrast media into the subarachnoid space, use of ionizing radiation, and limited soft tissue discrimination. Myelography is an invasive procedure associated with postprocedural headaches (10% to 15%) and rare but possible complications such as nerve damage, formation of an iatrogenic epidermoid, infection, and arachnoiditis. The incidence of headaches severe enough to require treatment (e.g., epidural blood patch) is approximately 1%.

Magnetic Resonance Imaging

MRI has become the initial imaging technique for most patients with significant signs and symptoms of spinal disorders. It provides excellent contrast among different types of soft tissue. MRI without exogenous contrast material is capable of evaluating the extradural, intradural extramedullary, and intramedullary spaces. MRI is noninvasive and without the risks associated with ionizing radiation. Anatomic imaging can be performed in different planes, as well as used for volume acquisitions. It is the most sensitive modality and most specific technique for identifying abnormalities of the spinal cord, nerve roots, cerebrospinal fluid (CSF) space, soft tissues, and bone. When used with gadolinium complexed with diethylenetriaminepentaacetic acid (DTPA), MRI has even greater sensitivity for intramedullary disease, inflammatory changes, and reparative processes such as may be seen with postoperative changes and trauma. MRI is particularly efficacious for the evaluation of so-called red flag diagnoses such as osteomyelitis, neoplasia, and trauma.

Traditional clinical imaging has emphasized orthogonal T1- and T2-weighted imaging for morphologic assessment of the diskovertebral complex. These sequences also provide an evaluation of the changes in signal intensity associated with degenerative disk disease. Fast spin echo (SE) T2-weighted images have replaced conventional T2-weighted images because of their shorter acquisition times, but they provide no increased diagnostic advantage. Short tau inversion recovery (STIR) or fat-suppressed T2-weighted images have been added because they are more sensitive to marrow and soft tissue changes (Fig. 18-4). Although these standard sequences remain the mainstay of diagnostic MRI of the spine, new techniques continue to be evaluated in the hope of providing stronger correlation between imaging

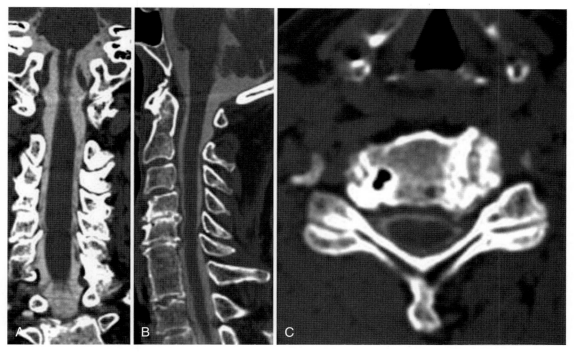

FIGURE 18-2 Coronal and sagittal multiplanar reformatted CT myelographic images obtained from the axial data set. Hypertrophic degenerative changes of the vertebral body margins and uncinate processes are producing extradural indentations on the subarachnoid space.

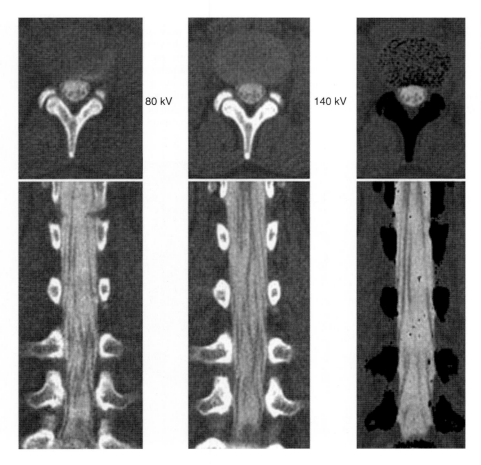

80 kV   140 kV

FIGURE 18-3 Dual-energy subtraction CT myelography. Primarily acquired axial and multiplanar reformatted coronal images through the lumbar region from a CT myelographic study were obtained with a CT scanner that uses two x-ray tubes. Different exposure factors using 80 and 140 kV produce data sets on which subtraction can be performed on the basis of attenuation differences related to the exposure factors.

FIGURE 18-4 MRI sequences. Sagittal T1-weighted spin echo, T2-weighted spin echo, and short tau inversion recovery (STIR) images through the lumbar spine demonstrate the different contrast obtained with different techniques. On the T1-weighted image, the vertebral body marrow has higher signal intensity than the intervertebral disk, primarily because of the fat content of the marrow space. On the T2-weighted spin echo image, the intervertebral disk has higher signal intensity than the vertebral body because of prolonged relaxation time related to both bound and unbound water species. This change in signal is probably a reflection of the health of the proteoglycans more than the total water content. The STIR sequence demonstrates decreased signal intensity of the marrow space and is the sequence that is most sensitive to marrow involvement. Note the degenerative changes at L4-5 and L5-S1. The decreased signal intensity of a degenerative disk is better noted on the T2-weighted and STIR sequences. Note the loss of the internuclear cleft as the degree of degeneration increases, as at the L5-S1 level.

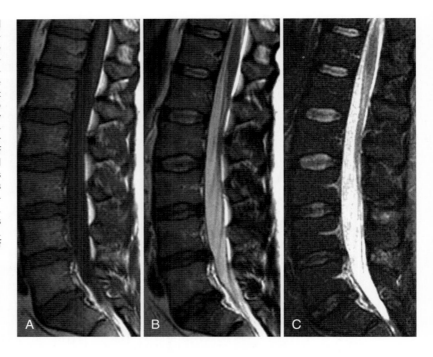

findings and patient symptoms. The utility of many of these techniques for the routine evaluation of degenerative disk disease remains unknown, and the number of patients in whom they have been evaluated remains small. Nevertheless, these approaches may be important for redefining the direction of spinal imaging from strictly anatomic imaging to imaging that combines more physiologic and functional information.[3] Techniques that have been evaluated include assessment of spinal motion (dynamic imaging, kinetic assessment, or axial loading), diffusion imaging (water or contrast agents), MR neurography, spectroscopy, functional MRI of the spinal cord, and ultrashort–echo time imaging. Of the variety of techniques available, only MR neurography and dynamic imaging have expanded beyond the experimental phase to demonstrate specific clinical utility (albeit in niche populations).

Dynamic Imaging

The utility of dynamic spine MRI remains unclear, in part because of the varied methods used. Methods used to date include axial loading in the supine position by means of a harness attached to a nonmagnetic compression footplate with nylon straps that can be tightened or the use of an upright open MRI system that allows flexion-extension imaging (Fig. 18-5).[4,5] Dynamic MRI has been used to evaluate for the presence of occult herniations, which may not be visible or be less visible when the patient is supine, to measure motion between spinal segments, and to measure canal or foraminal diameter when subjected to axial loading.[3,5-8] Hiwatashi and colleagues evaluated 200 patients with clinical symptoms of spinal stenosis and found 20 with detectable differences in caliber of the dural sac on routine and axial-loaded studies.[7] In 5 of these selected patients, all three neurosurgeons

FIGURE 18-5 Sagittal T2-weighted spin echo images through the cervical spine in flexion (**A**) and extension (**B**). Note the decreased anterior-posterior canal diameter on the extension image (7 versus 4 mm) at C3-4.

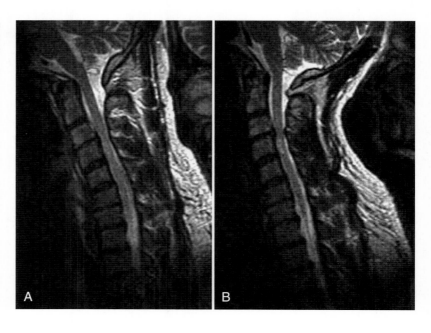

involved in the clinical evaluation changed their treatment recommendation from conservative management to decompressive surgery. Although a subset of patients may benefit from this type of evaluation, the benefit appears to be small for the added machine time and patient discomfort.

Neurography

A large and varied literature exists concerning the use of MR neurography for the evaluation of peripheral nerves, including the brachial and lumbar plexuses. Thin-section MR neurography uses high-resolution T1-weighted imaging for anatomic detail and fat-suppressed T2-weighted or STIR imaging to show abnormal nerve hyperintensity. Several reviews exist on this subject.[9-11] The technique is capable of depicting a wide variety of pathologic conditions involving the sciatic nerve, such as compression, trauma, hypertrophy, neuroma, and tumor infiltration.[12,13] MR neurography has 93% specificity and 64% sensitivity for diagnosis of the piriformis syndrome (piriformis muscle asymmetry and sciatic nerve hyperintensity).[14]

Ultrashort–Echo Time Imaging

Routine clinical MRI does not allow evaluation of tissues with very short relaxation times because echo times are on the order of 8 to 15 msec. Ultrashort–echo time sequences have been preliminarily evaluated for a number of tissues, including the spine. These sequences have echo times as short as 0.08 msec. The images show normal contrast enhancement, with high signal intensity from the longitudinal ligaments, end plates, and interspinous ligaments.[15-17]

Diffusion

Several authors have evaluated the apparent diffusion coefficient (ADC) in normal and degenerated intervertebral disks. Antoniou and associates evaluated the ADC in cadaveric human disks in relation to matrix composition and matrix integrity by using a stimulated echo sequence.[18] They found that the ADC in healthy subjects was significantly greater in the nucleus pulposus than in the annulus fibrosus. The ADC in the nucleus was noted to generally decrease with degeneration grade and age. A similar correlation of ADC measurements and annular degeneration was not found. The most notable correlations were observed between the ADC of the nucleus pulposus and the water and glycosaminoglycan content. Kealey and coworkers evaluated 39 patients with a multishot SE echo planar technique.[19] They found a significant decrease in the ADC of degenerated disks in comparison to normal disks. Kurunlahti and colleagues evaluated the ADC of disk and lumbar magnetic resonance angiograms in 37 asymptomatic volunteers.[20] Lumbar artery status correlated with diffusion values within the disks, thus suggesting that impaired blood flow may play an important role in disk degeneration.

Kerttula and collaborators compared disk ADC values in normal controls with those in patients with prior compression fractures (at least 1 year previously) and found that ADC values in the x and y directions decreased in degenerated disks and in disks of normal signal intensity in the area of trauma.[21] Diffusion tensor imaging has been evaluated for imaging of the annulus fibrosus[22] and for imaging defects or disruptions within the annulus.[3] Differences in diffusion have been demonstrated for the intervertebral disk in compressed versus uncompressed states.[23] Intravenous contrast enhancement may also be used to assess diffusion into the intervertebral disk. Normal disks enhance slowly after the injection of contrast material, which may be as much as 36% in animal models. This enhancement is modified by the type of contrast agent (ionic versus nonionic and molecular weight).[24,25] Ionic material diffuses less rapidly than nonionic

media into the disk. Degenerated disks with decreased glycosaminoglycan exhibit more intense and rapid enhancement.[26] Disk enhancement has been documented in normal and degenerated human lumbar disks.[27]

Cerebrospinal Fluid

CSF flow studies with cine MRI provide cardiac-gated gradient phase-contrast images that are displayed qualitatively as CSF flow images in a closed loop kinematic format. This same data set can be displayed quantitatively on a graph or in numerical format as analysis of values of flow velocity and volume flow rate. These images demonstrate the pulsatile motion of CSF, not the bulk flow. Pulsatile flow is a result of expansion of the brain during systole and relaxation during diastole and is therefore bidirectional, with CSF flowing caudally during systole and cranially during diastole. Typically, the signal intensity of normal CSF flow in these studies is demonstrated as hyperintense during systole, where there is caudal (downward) flow, and hypointense during diastole, where there is cranial (upward) flow. These images are usually displayed in the sagittal and axial planes. In general, the degree of pulsatile flow diminishes as it proceeds caudally. Clinically, these studies are most often used for the evaluation of CSF flow in patients with Chiari I and II malformations and for the assessment of syrinx cavities (Fig. 18-6).

Artifacts and Contraindications

Instrumentation, metal used as part of surgical procedures, and implanted electronic devices represent challenges for both CT and MRI. In the case of CT, metal can create beam-hardening artifacts that obscure adjacent soft tissue and osseous structures (Fig. 18-7). Multidetector studies with isotropic voxels and software used to decrease beam-hardening artifact can often decrease the image degradation caused by implanted metal.[28] Different types of metal produce different types of artifacts on MRI that may make the examination uninterpretable. The term *magnetic susceptibility* describes the manner and amount by which a material becomes magnetized in a magnetic field. Nonferrous magnetic metals may produce local electrical currents induced by the changing field, which causes distortion of the field and artifacts. These artifacts take two main forms: geometric distortion and signal loss secondary to dephasing (Fig. 18-8). Different techniques are more susceptible to these artifacts, and gradient echo images in particular are especially sensitive to differences in magnetic susceptibility and field homogeneity. Although metals can cause artifacts that render the examination uninterpretable, certain indwelling devices may be a contraindication to the entire examination. Certain types of aneurysm clips, cardiac valves, and vascular devices can result in harm to patients during an MRI examination. Some implantable devices may cease to function properly after an MRI study, and others may be a source of heating with deleterious biologic effects and burns. Readers are referred to publications and websites that track information related to contraindications.[28]

The primary disadvantages of MRI are related to its cost and safety concerns with respect to electronic devices or implants. The safety issues include heating, dislodgment, and malfunction, as well as image distortion in the presence of metal. Claustrophobia remains a significant problem that sometimes requires machines with a larger bore and sedation or general anesthesia.

Intravenous contrast agents are commonly used with both CT and MRI examinations. Both iodinated (CT) and paramagnetic substances (MRI) are cleared by the kidney and should be used with caution or not at all in patients with impaired renal function. Although this has been common knowledge with the iodinated contrast media used for CT, recent evidence has also documented various complications related to the use of paramagnetic contrast

further identify disk herniation and provide better morphologic characterization of various types of stenosis. MRI provides the greatest spectrum of morphologic findings. With MRI, degenerative changes are manifested as disk space narrowing; loss of T2-weighted signal intensity from the intervertebral disk; the presence of fissures, fluid, vacuum changes, and calcification within the vertebral disk; ligamentous signal changes; marrow signal changes; osteophytosis; disk herniation; malalignment; and stenosis.

Degenerative Disk Changes

The major cartilaginous joint (amphiarthrosis) of the vertebral column is the intervertebral disk. Each disk consists of an inner portion, the nucleus pulposus, surrounded by a peripheral portion, the annulus fibrosus. The nucleus pulposus is eccentrically located and is closer to the posterior surface of the intervertebral disk. With degeneration and aging, type II collagen increases outwardly in the annulus, and there is greater loss of water from the nucleus pulposus than from the annulus. This results in a loss of the hydrostatic properties of the disk, with an overall reduction in hydration in both areas to about 70%. In addition to water and collagen, the other important biochemical constituents of the intervertebral disk are the proteoglycans. The individual chemical structures of the proteoglycans are not changed with degeneration, but their relative composition is. The ratio of keratin sulfate to chondroitin sulfate increases, and there is a diminished association with collagen, which may reduce the tensile strength of the disk. The decrease in water-binding capacity of the nucleus pulposus is thought to be related to the decreased molecular weight of its nuclear proteoglycan complexes (aggregates). The disk becomes progressively more fibrous and disorganized, with the end stage represented by amorphous fibrocartilage and no clear distinction between the nucleus and annulus.[31-33] On T2-weighted images, central disk signal intensity is usually markedly decreased and at distinct variance to that seen in unaffected disks of the same individual. Work with T2-weighed SE sequences[34] suggests that MRI is capable of depicting changes in the nucleus pulposus and annulus fibrosus associated with degeneration and aging based on the loss of signal intensity (Fig. 18-9). In work with cadaver spines of various ages, absolute T2 measurements correlated more closely with the glycosaminoglycan concentration than with the absolute water content. Thus,

the signal intensity may not be related to the total amount of water but rather the state of the water. At present, the role that specific biochemical changes (proteoglycan ratios, aggregation of complexes) plays in the altered signal intensity is not well understood. Given that the T2 signal intensity in the disk appears to track the concentration and regions with a high percentage of glycosaminoglycan more than the absolute water content, it seems likely that the health and status of the proteoglycans are major determinants of signal intensity.[35] It has been proposed that annular disruption is the critical factor in degeneration and that when a radial tear develops in the annulus, there is shrinkage with disorganization of the fibrous cartilage of the nucleus pulposus and replacement of the disk by dense fibrous tissue with cystic spaces (Fig. 18-10).[36-40] Annular tears, also properly called *annular fissures*, are separations between annular fibers, avulsion of fibers from their insertions on the vertebral body, or breaks through fibers that extend radially, transversely, or concentrically and involve one or many layers of the annular lamellae. The term *tear* or *fissure* describes the spectrum of such lesions and does not imply that the lesion was caused by trauma (see Fig. 18-1). Although it is established that annular disruption is a sequela of degeneration and is often associated with it, its role as the causal agent of disk degeneration has not been proved. MRI is the most accurate anatomic method for assessing intervertebral disk disease. The signal intensity characteristics of the disk on T2-weighted images reflect changes caused by aging or degeneration. A classification scheme for lumbar intervertebral disk degeneration has been proposed that has reasonable intraobserver and interobserver agreement.[41] To date, however, there has been no correlation between disk changes on MRI and a patient's symptoms. With loss of water and proteoglycans, the nucleus pulposus is desiccated and friable with yellow-brown discoloration. Its onion skin appearance begins to unravel, and cracks, clefts, or crevices appear within the nucleus and extend into the annulus fibrosus. Fissuring, chondrocyte generation, and formation of granulation tissue may be noted within the end plate, annulus fibrosus, and nucleus pulposus of degenerative disks and are indicative of attempts at healing.[40] Radiolucent collections (vacuum disk phenomena) representing gas, principally nitrogen, occur at sites of negative pressure produced by the abnormal spaces.[42] The vacuum phenomenon within a degenerated disk is represented on SE images as areas of signal void (Fig. 18-11).[43] Although the presence of gas within the disk is usually

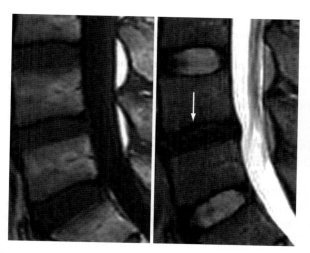

FIGURE 18-9 Degenerative disk. There is mild disk space narrowing (*arrow*) and loss of signal intensity on T2-weighted images of the L4-5 disk.

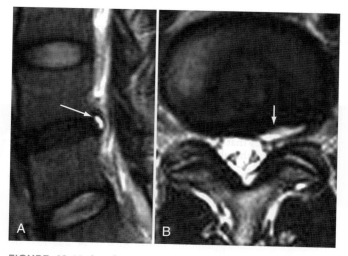

FIGURE 18-10 Annular tear seen on parasagittal (**A**) and axial (**B**) T2-weighted images through the L4-5 disk. Note the high signal intensity in the outer annulus/longitudinal ligament complex, which represents the area of annular disruption (*arrows*).

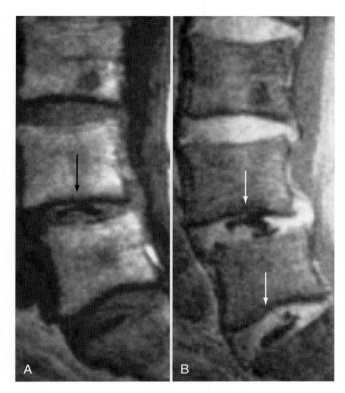

FIGURE 18-11 A and **B,** Vacuum phenomenon. Note the decreased signal intensity within the L4-5 disk, which is better seen on the gradient echo image (*white arrow*) than on the spin echo image (*black arrow*).

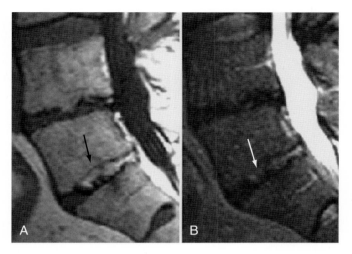

FIGURE 18-12 Intervertebral disk calcification (*arrows*). Note the high signal intensity on T1-weighted (**A**) and T2-weighted (**B**) images at the L5-S1 level.

suggestive of degenerative disease, spinal infection may (rarely) be accompanied by intradiscal or intraosseous gas.[44] As intervertebral osteochondrosis progresses, there may be calcification of the disk. Calcification has usually been described on MRI as a region of decreased or absent signal intensity. The loss of signal is attributed to a low mobile proton density, as well as, in the case of gradient echo imaging, to its sensitivity to the heterogeneous magnetic susceptibility found in calcified tissue. There is, however, variability in the signal intensity of calcium with various sequences, and the type and concentration of calcification are important factors. Hyperintense disks on T1-weighted MRI may be secondary to calcification (Fig. 18-12).[45] For concentrations of calcium particulates of up to 30% by weight, the signal intensity on standard T1-weighted images increases but then subsequently decreases.[46,47] These data probably reflect particulate calcium reducing T1 relaxation times by a surface relaxation mechanism. Hyperintensities that are affected by fat suppression techniques have also been noted within intervertebral disks and are thought to be related to ossification with lipid marrow formation in severely degenerated or fused disks.

Degenerative Marrow Changes

Changes in signal intensity of the vertebral body marrow adjacent to the end plates of degenerated disks are a long recognized and common observation on MRI of the lumbar spine.[48,49] However, despite a growing body of literature on this subject, their clinical importance and relationship to symptoms remain unclear.[50]

These marrow changes appear to take three main forms. Type I changes consist of decreased signal intensity on T1-weighted images and increased signal intensity on T2-weighted images

(Fig. 18-13). They have been identified in approximately 4% of patients scanned for lumbar disease,[49] in approximately 8% of patients after diskectomy,[51] and in 40% to 50% of chymopapain-treated disks, which may be viewed as a model of acute disk degeneration.[52] Histopathologic sections of disks with type I changes show disruption and fissuring of the end plate and vascularized fibrous tissue within the adjacent marrow that prolongs T1 and T2 times. Enhancement of type I vertebral body marrow changes is seen with the administration of gadolinium, and at times the changes extend to involve the disk itself and are presumably related to the vascularized fibrous tissue within the adjacent marrow. Type II changes are represented by increased signal intensity on T1-weighted images and isointense or slightly hyperintense signal on T2-weighted images (Fig. 18-14). They have been identified in approximately 16% of patients on MRI. Disks with type II changes also show evidence of end plate

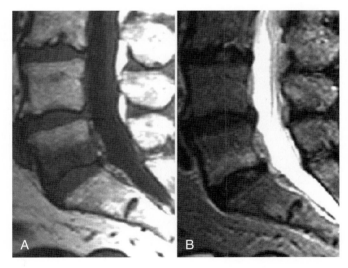

FIGURE 18-13 Type I degenerative marrow changes. Sagittal T1-weighted (**A**) and T2-weighted (**B**) images demonstrate decreased signal intensity of the L5 vertebral body adjacent to the degenerated disk space on T1 and increased signal intensity on T2.

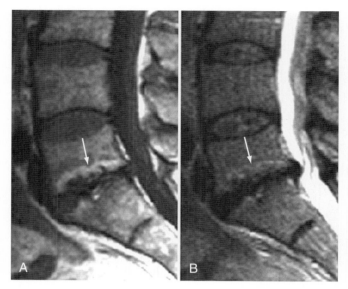

FIGURE 18-14 Type II degenerative marrow change (*arrows*). There is increased signal intensity along the opposing margins of L5 and S1 on both T1-weighted (**A**) and T2-weighted (**B**) images.

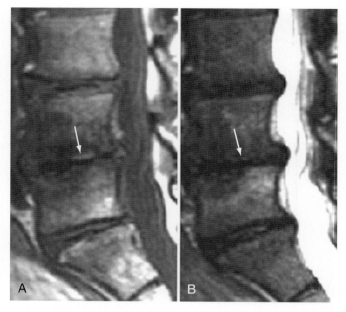

FIGURE 18-15 Type III degenerative marrow change (*arrows*). There is decreased signal intensity of the opposing vertebral body margins at L4-5 on both T1-weighted (**A**) and T2-weighted (**B**) images.

disruption, with yellow (lipid) marrow replacement in the adjacent vertebral body resulting in a shorter T1 time. Type III changes are represented by decreased signal intensity on both T1- and T2-weighted images and correlate with extensive bony sclerosis on plain radiographs. The lack of signal in type III changes no doubt reflects the relative absence of marrow in areas of advanced sclerosis (Fig. 18-15). Unlike types III, types I and II changes show no definite correlation with sclerosis on radiography.[53] This is not surprising when one considers the histology; the sclerosis seen on plain radiographs is a reflection of dense woven bone within the vertebral body, whereas the MRI changes are more a reflection of the intervening marrow elements.

Similar marrow changes have also been noted in the pedicles (Fig. 18-16). Although originally described as being associated with spondylolysis, they have also been noted in patients with degenerative facet disease and pedicle fractures.[54,55] The exact mechanism by which these marrow changes occur is not known. The association of these marrow changes with degenerative disk disease, facet changes, and pars and pedicle fractures suggest that they are a response to biomechanical stress.

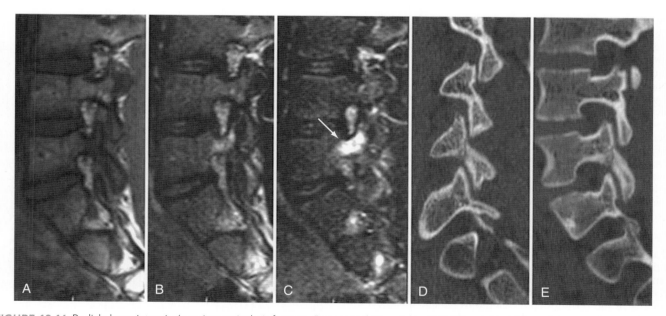

FIGURE 18-16 Pedicle hyperintensity/pars interarticularis fracture. Parasagittal T1-weighted (**A**), T2-weighted (**B**), and short tau inversion recovery (STIR) (**C**) images demonstrate high signal intensity within the pedicle of L4, which is best appreciated on the STIR sequence (*arrow*). Parasagittal (**D**) and sagittal (**E**) CT multiplanar reformatted images demonstrate a subacute fracture through the pars at L4-5.

Of these three types, type I changes appear to be more fluid and variable, a reflection of ongoing underlying pathologic processes such as continuing degeneration with associated changing biomechanical stresses. Of the three types, type I is most often associated with ongoing low back symptoms.[56-60] In a longitudinal study, the incidence of new degenerative marrow changes was 6% over a 3-year period, with most being type I.[58] In a study of nonoperated patients with low back pain, Mitra and associates found that 92% of type I changes converted either wholly or partially to type II (52%), became more extensive (40%), or remained unchanged (8%).[57] There was an improvement in symptoms in patients in whom type I changes converted to type II.

Some diskography studies in patients with degenerative marrow changes have suggested that type I marrow changes are invariably associated with painful disks.[61,62] Others have failed to reproduce this association,[63,64] and thus the relationship between degenerative marrow changes and diskogenic pain remains unproved.

Multiple authors have observed a variety of inflammatory mediators in association with degenerative marrow changes. Burke and colleagues observed an increase in proinflammatory mediators such as interleukin-6, interleukin-8, and prostaglandin E_2 in the disks of patients with type I marrow changes who were undergoing fusion for low back pain.[64] Ohtori and coworkers found that the cartilaginous end plates of patients with type I marrow changes had more protein gene product (PGP) 9.5 immunoreactive nerve fibers and cells immunoreactive for tumor necrosis factor (TNF) than did patients with normal end plates.[65] PGP 9.5 immunoreactivity was seen exclusively in patients with diskogenic low back pain. TNF immunoreactivity in end plates with type I marrow changes was higher than in those with type II marrow changes. The authors concluded that type I marrow changes represent a more active inflammation mediated by proinflammatory cytokines whereas type II and type III changes are more quiescent.[50] In a study of infliximab, a monoclonal antibody against TNF-α, Korhonen and associates found that it was most effective when there were degenerative type I marrow changes at the symptomatic level.[66] Nevertheless, the relationship of degenerative marrow changes to immunobiologic and cellular response mechanisms, although probably important, remains unclear.

In a study by Toyone and colleagues, 70% of patients with type I marrow changes had segmental hypermobility versus 16% with type II changes.[56] Probably the greatest indication that these marrow changes, particularly type I, are related to biomechanical instability is based on observations after fusion. Chataigner and collaborators suggested that patients with type I marrow changes have much better outcomes with surgery than do those with isolated degenerative disk disease and normal or type II marrow changes.[67] In addition, conversion of type I marrow changes to either normal or type II was associated with higher fusion rates and better outcomes. Other studies support the contention that persistence of type I changes after fusion suggests pseudarthrosis and is associated with persistent symptoms. Conversely, conversion of type I marrow changes to either normal or type II is associated with higher fusion rates and better outcomes (Fig. 18-17).[68-70] The conclusion is that fusion produces greater stability, reduces biomechanical stress, and accelerates the course of type I marrow changes toward improvement.

As further support that these fluid marrow changes reflect biomechanical stress, we have seen similar marrow conversion in the pedicles of vertebral bodies associated with symptomatic pars and pedicle fractures, as well as in those with severe degenerative facet joint disease. Pedicle marrow change to a normal or type II appearance is associated with improvement in symptoms.[71]

Degenerative Facet and Ligamentous Changes

The superior articulating process of one vertebra is separated from the inferior articulating process of the vertebra above by a synovium-lined articulation, the zygapophyseal joint. Like all diarthrodial synovium-lined joints, the lumbar facet joints are predisposed to arthropathy with alterations of the articular cartilage (Fig. 18-18). With disk degeneration and loss of disk space

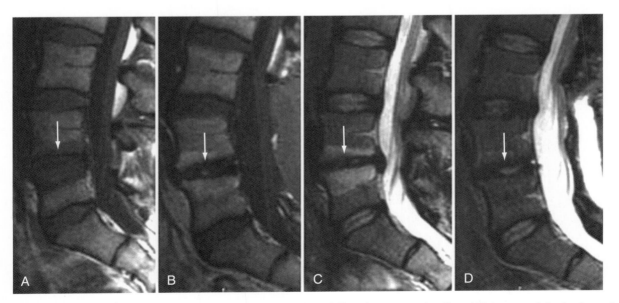

FIGURE 18-17 Conversion of type I marrow changes. Preoperative (**A** and **C**) and postoperative (**B** and **D**) images of the lumbar spine in a patient after lumbar fusion demonstrate typical type I marrow changes at the L4-5 level preoperatively (*arrows*). Postoperatively, the type I changes have converted to type II changes. The decreased signal on T1 is converted to an increased signal representing lipid marrow conversion. The increased signal intensity on T2 has resolved.

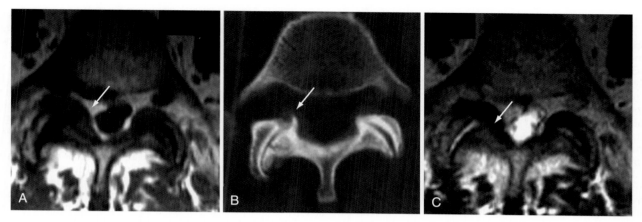

FIGURE 18-18 Degenerative facet changes (*arrows*) seen on T1-weighted (**A**), high-resolution CT (**B**), and T2-weighted spin echo (**C**) axial images through the L4-5 facets. Note the bony osteophyte along the anterior margin of the inferior facet at L4 on the right and the degenerative facet narrowing bilaterally. The bony changes are not as obvious on the T1- and T2-weighted images, but the findings of narrowing and asymmetrical soft tissue are clearly identifiable on MRI.

height, the increased stress on the facet joints with craniocaudal subluxation results in arthrosis and osteophytosis. The superior articular facet is usually more substantially involved. Facet arthrosis can result in narrowing of the central canal, lateral recesses, and foramina and is an important component of lumbar stenosis. However, it has been proposed that facet arthrosis may occur independently and be a source of symptoms on its own.[72,73] Synovial villi may become entrapped within the joint with resulting joint effusions. The mechanism of pain may be related to nerve root compression from degenerative changes of the facets or direct irritation of pain fibers from the innervated synovial linings and joint capsule.[73] Osteophytosis and herniation of synovium through the facet joint capsule may result in synovial cysts, although the cause of these facet joint cysts is unclear. There is a more straightforward relationship of synovial cysts with osteoarthritis and instability of the facet joints than with degeneration of the intervertebral disk alone. In a review of patients with degenerative facet disease, synovial cysts occurred at anterior or intraspinal locations in 2.3% of patients and at posterior or extraspinal locations in 7.3% (Fig. 18-19).[74] The important ligaments of the spine include the anterior longitudinal ligament, the posterior longitudinal ligament, the paired sets of ligamenta flava (connecting the laminae of adjacent vertebrae), the intertransverse ligaments (extending between transverse processes), and the unpaired supraspinous ligament (along the tips of the spinous processes). Because these ligaments normally

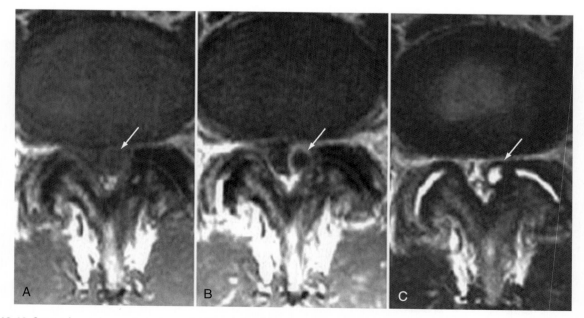

FIGURE 18-19 Synovial cyst demonstrated on axial T1-weighted (**A**), contrast-enhanced T1-weighted (**B**), and T2-weighted (**C**) images through the facets at L4-5. There are severe bilateral degenerative facet changes with distraction and fluid. On the T1-weighted image, there is an ill-defined soft tissue mass projecting medially off the left facet (*arrow*). On the contrast-enhanced T1-weighted image, this soft tissue mass (*arrow*) is now clearly outlined by peripheral enhancement. On the T2-weighted image this mass (*arrow*) is demonstrated to have high signal intensity suggestive of fluid.

provide stability, any alteration in the vertebral articulations can lead to ligamentous laxity with subsequent deterioration. Loss of elastic tissue, calcification and ossification, and bone proliferation at sites of ligamentous attachment to bone are recognized manifestations of such degeneration. Excessive lordosis or extensive disk space loss in the lumbar spine leads to close approximation and contact of the spinous processes and to degeneration of intervening ligaments.[75,76] Histologically, granulomatous reaction and perivascular cellular infiltration characterize the condition.

MORPHOLOGIC AND FUNCTIONAL SEQUELAE

Common potential complications of degenerative disk disease include alignment abnormalities, intervertebral disk displacement, and spinal stenosis. Various types of alignment abnormalities can exist alone or in combination, but the two most frequent are segmental instability and spondylolisthesis.

Instability

Segmental instability can result from degenerative changes involving the intervertebral disk, vertebral bodies, and facet joints that impair the usual pattern of spinal movement and produce motion that is irregular, excessive, or restricted. It can be translational or angular. Spondylolisthesis results when one vertebral body becomes displaced relative to the next most inferior vertebral body. The most common types are classified as degenerative, isthmic, iatrogenic, and traumatic. Degenerative spondylolisthesis is seen usually with an intact pars interarticularis, is related primarily to degenerative changes of the apophyseal joints, and is most common at the L4-5 vertebral level (Fig. 18-20). The predilection for degenerative spondylolisthesis at that level is thought to be related to the more sagittal orientation of the facet joints, which makes them increasingly prone to anterior displacement. Degenerative disk disease may predispose to or exacerbate this condition secondary to narrowing of the disk space, which can produce subsequent malalignment of the articular processes and lead to rostrocaudal subluxation.

Herniation

Herniation refers to localized displacement of nucleus, cartilage, fragmented apophyseal bone, or fragmented annular tissue beyond the intervertebral disk space. The disk space is defined rostrally and caudally by the vertebral body end plates and peripherally by the outer edges of the vertebral ring apophyses, exclusive of osteophytic formations. The term *localized* contrasts with the term *generalized*, the latter being arbitrarily defined as greater than 50% (180 degrees) of the periphery of the disk.[77]

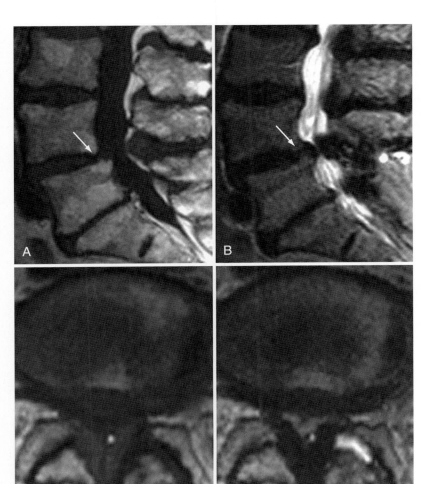

FIGURE 18-20 Degenerative spondylolisthesis. Sagittal T1- and T2-weighted spin echo images (**A** and **B**) of the lumbar spine. Grade I spondylolisthesis of L4 on L5 (*arrows*) is present, as well as severe central canal stenosis and thickening of the posterior ligaments. Axial T1- and T2-weighted images (**C** and **D**) through the L4-5 level. Note the severe central canal stenosis, thickened posterior ligaments, and severe bilateral degenerative facet changes.

Displacement, therefore, can occur only in association with disruption of the normal annulus or, as in the case of intravertebral herniation (Schmorl's node), a break in the vertebral body end plate. Because details of the integrity of the annulus are often unknown, the diagnosis of herniation is usually made by observation of localized displacement of disk material beyond the edges of the ring apophyses—that is, less than 50% (180 degrees) of the circumference of the disk (Fig. 18-21). Localized displacement in the axial (horizontal) plane can be focal, or less than 25% of the disk circumference, or broad based, between 25% and 50% of the disk circumference. The presence of disk tissue circumferentially (50% to 100%) beyond the edges of the ring apophyses may be called *bulging* and is not considered a form of herniation. A disk may have more than one herniation. The term *herniated disk* does not imply any knowledge of etiology, relationship to symptoms, prognosis, or need for treatment. When data are sufficient to make the distinction, a herniated disk may be more specifically characterized as protruded or extruded. These distinctions are based on the shape of the displaced material. Protrusion is present if the greatest distance, in any plane, between the edges of the disk material beyond the disk space is less than the distance between the edges of the base in the same plane (Fig. 18-22). Extrusion is present when, in at least one plane, any one distance between the edges of the disk material beyond the disk space is greater than the distance between the edges of the base in the same plane or when no continuity exists between the disk material beyond the disk space and that within the disk space (Fig. 18-23). Extrusion may be further specified as sequestration if the displaced disk material has completely lost any continuity with the parent disk. The term *migration* may be used to signify displacement of disk material away from the site of extrusion, regardless of whether it is sequestrated (Fig. 18-24). Herniated disks in the craniocaudal (vertical) direction through a break in the vertebral body end plate are referred to as intravertebral herniations. Nonacute Schmorl's node intrabody herniations are common spinal abnormalities regarded as incidental observations. They have been reported in 38% to 75% of the population.[78,79] Although intrabody herniations may occur as a result of end plate weakness secondary to bone dysplasia, neoplasms, infections, or any process that weakens the end plate or the underlying bone, most intrabody herniations probably form after axial-loading trauma, with preferential extrusion of nuclear material through the vertebral end plate rather than an intact and normal annulus fibrosus. It has been suggested that asymptomatic intrabody herniations may be traceable to a specific occurrence of acute nonradiating low back pain in the patient's history, which supports the concept that intrabody herniations (Schmorl's nodes) occur through sites of end plate fracture. Type I vertebral body marrow changes have been described surrounding acute interbody herniations.[80]

Stenosis

Spinal stenosis was defined in 1975 as any type of narrowing of the spinal canal, nerve root canals, or intervertebral foramina.[81] Two broad groups have been defined: acquired (usually related to degenerative changes) and congenital or developmental. Developmental stenosis can be exacerbated by superimposed acquired degenerative changes (Fig. 18-25). In the acquired type, there has been no association between the severity of pain and the degree of stenosis. The most common symptoms are sensory disturbances in the legs, low back pain, neurogenic claudication, weakness, and relief of pain by bending forward. The imaging changes are in general more extensive than expected from the clinical findings.[82] Patients with symptoms referable to spinal stenosis tend to have narrower spines than asymptomatic patients do. Although there appears to be a correlation between cross-sectional area and midsagittal measurements in patients with symptomatic spinal stenosis, absolute values and correlation between measurements and symptoms are lacking. The degree of stenosis is not static; extension worsens the degree of central and foraminal stenosis by 11%, whereas flexion appears to improve it by an average of 11%. Segmental instability, which can cause static and dynamic stenosis, is considered a cause of low back pain but is poorly defined.[83] Some evidence suggests that disk degeneration, narrowing of the spinal canal, and degenerative changes in the facets and spinal ligaments contribute to stenosis and that instability increases with age. Unfortunately,

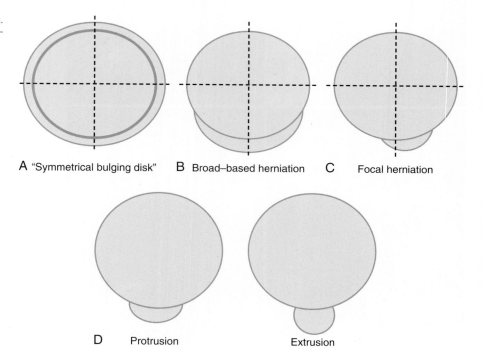

FIGURE 18-21 **A,** Symmetrical bulging disk. **B,** Broad-based herniation. **C,** Focal herniation. **D,** Protrusion and extrusion.

A "Symmetrical bulging disk"   B Broad–based herniation   C Focal herniation

D Protrusion   Extrusion

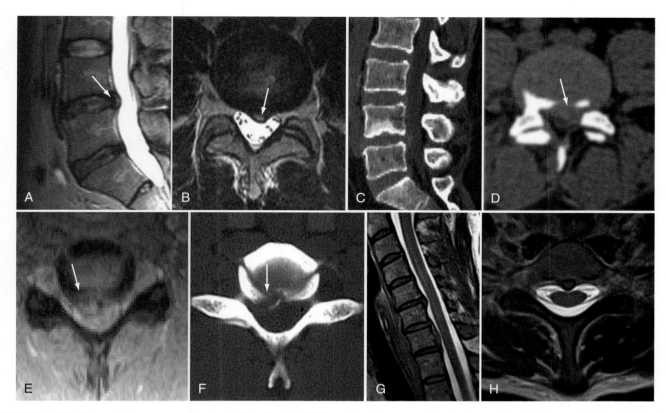

FIGURE 18-22 Disk protrusion seen on sagittal (**A**) and axial (**B**) T2-weighted images of the lumbar spine. On the sagittal image, the disk extends beyond the vertebral body margins, which on the axial image shows the base to be broader than the posterior extent (*arrows*). Sagittal multiplanar reformatted (MPR) (**C**) and axial (**D**) CT images through the lumbar spine. The sagittal MPR image demonstrates an ill-defined soft tissue mass projecting posteriorly at the L4-5 disk level. The broad-based disk protrusion is better depicted on the axial image (*white arrow*). Axial gradient echo MRI (**E**) and CT (**F**) at the C5-6 level. Note the broad-based right-sided disk protrusion (*arrow*). Sagittal (**G**) and axial (**H**) T2-weighted images of the cervical spine demonstrating disk protrusion at C5-6 and disk extrusion with an inferior fragment at C6-7. The axial image through the body of C7 demonstrates the rounded soft tissue mass centrally in the anterior epidural space.

there do not appear to be reliable prognostic imaging findings that correlate with surgical success or even predict whether patients will benefit from surgery.[84]

SIGNIFICANCE OF IMAGING FINDINGS

Given the high prevalence of degenerative morphologic alterations, the role of an imaging test is to provide accurate morpho-

logic information and influence therapeutic decision making.[85] A necessary component that connects these two purposes is accurate natural history data. Any study looking at the natural history of degenerative disk disease is confounded by the high prevalence of morphologic changes in the asymptomatic population.[86-88] Twenty percent to 28% of asymptomatic patients demonstrate disk herniations, and the majority have evidence of additional degenerative disk disease.[86-88] In a study of symptomatic patients

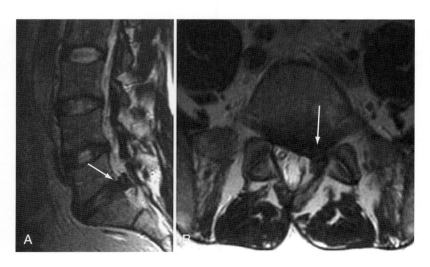

FIGURE 18-23 Extruded disk. Sagittal (**A**) and axial (**B**) T2-weighted images of the lumbar spine demonstrate disk extrusion (*arrow*) on the sagittal image with a narrow base. The axial image demonstrates posterior displacement of the S1 nerve root on the left as a result of this disk extrusion.

FIGURE 18-24 Disk extrusion and a free fragment seen on sagittal T1-weighted (**A**) and T2-weighted (**B**) images of the lumbar spine. There is disk extrusion and an inferior fragment (*white* and *black arrows*, respectively).

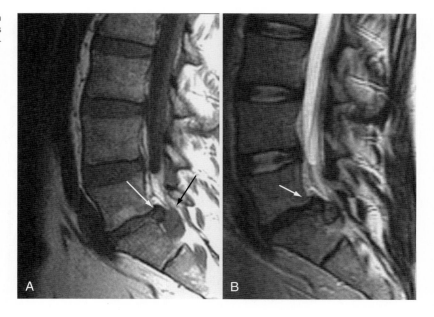

with low back pain or sciatica, the prevalence of disk herniation in those with low back pain and in those with radiculopathy at initial evaluation was similar.[89] There was a higher prevalence of herniation, 57% in patients with low back pain and 65% in patients with radiculopathy, than the 20% to 28% prevalence reported in asymptomatic series.[87,88] In studies of the natural history of disk herniation, many show regression of the disk fragment over time. In general, a third of patients with disk herniation at initial examination exhibit significant resolution or disappearance by 6 weeks and two thirds by 6 months.[89,90] The type, size, and location of herniation at diagnosis and changes in herniation size and type over time did not correlate with outcome. In fact, the presence of herniation on MRI was a positive prognostic finding.[89] Interestingly, not only do disk herniations have a tendency to regress, but new or larger ones may also appear after the onset of symptoms. In this study, new or larger disk herniations developed in 13% of patients in this symptomatic series over a 6-week period. The lack of prognostic value of imaging studies also applies to the conservative management of spinal stenosis. There do not appear to be reliable prognostic imaging findings that correlate with surgical success or even with whether patients will benefit from surgery.[84,91] Demographic and clinical features appear to predict the outcome of nonsurgical treatment, whereas the morphometric features of disk herniation and spinal stenosis in conjunction with clinical features are more powerful predictors of surgical outcome.[92]

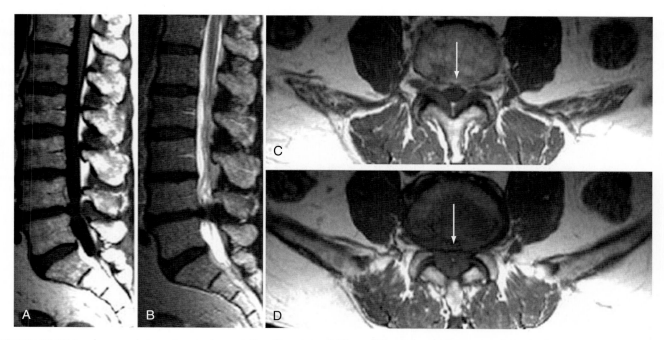

FIGURE 18-25 Lumbar canal stenosis noted on midline T1-weighted (**A**) and T2-weighted (**B**) images of the lumbar spine. There is diffuse central canal narrowing, evidence of a broad-based disk protrusion, and severe canal stenosis at L4-5. Contiguous axial T1-weighted images (**C** and **D**) of the L4-5 level demonstrate severe central canal stenosis (*arrows*).

Osteomyelitis

In general, the early findings of disk space infection on plain films consist of minimal disk space narrowing and erosion or indistinctness of the end plates. There may be adjacent paraspinal soft tissue swelling, which in the lumbar region may be detectable as enlargement of a paravertebral soft tissue shadow, in the thoracic region as a paraspinal mass, and in the cervical region as prevertebral soft tissue swelling. As the disease progresses, the disk space narrowing worsens, and destruction of the end plates becomes more obvious (Fig. 18-26). In healing, the disk space remains markedly narrowed or fuses.

Intense uptake in two adjacent vertebral bodies with loss of the disk space is seen on bone scans in patients with vertebral osteomyelitis. In the spine, it can be problematic to differentiate increased radionuclide uptake as a result of vertebral osteomyelitis from degenerative disk disease, benign compression fracture, or metastatic disease. The combination of gallium scanning or indium 111–labeled white blood cells and three-phase bone scanning may increase the specificity. Although highly specific, indium 111–labeled white blood cells demonstrate poor sensitivity for the diagnosis of vertebral osteomyelitis. Fluorodeoxyglucose (FDG)-PET imaging is capable of demonstrating the increased glucose metabolism in the inflammatory cells associated with osteomyelitis. The FDG-PET scan is not affected by metallic implants and may be useful in evaluating patients with hardware for infections. FDG-PET has better resolution than the more traditional nuclear medicine imaging and may be useful for differentiating bone from soft tissue infection. Low FDG uptake on PET has been shown in fractures and in pseudarthrosis, which may make it useful in differentiating these entities from vertebral osteomyelitis. Malignancies, however, often appear similar to osteomyelitis on nuclear medicine studies because both exhibit increased uptake.

CT is most useful for the detection of bony destruction and paraspinal soft tissue changes. The addition of intrathecal contrast material improves the delineation of epidural masses. CT demonstrates a decrease in attenuation of the affected vertebral body and disk. CT criteria for the diagnosis of pyogenic vertebral osteomyelitis include diffuse moth-eaten or permeative bone destruction, gas within the bone or adjacent soft tissues, involvement of the intervertebral disk primarily, and prevertebral soft tissue involvement.[77,81,93]

MRI has a sensitivity of 96%, a specificity of 92%, and an accuracy of 94% in the diagnosis of vertebral osteomyelitis.[55,93] The classic MRI appearance of vertebral osteomyelitis is as follows: a confluent decreased signal intensity of the intervertebral disk and adjacent vertebral bodies with an inability to discern a margin between the two on T1-weighted images, increased signal intensity of the vertebral bodies adjacent to the involved disk on T2-weighted images, and an abnormal configuration and increased signal intensity of the intervertebral disk and the presence of paravertebral soft tissue swelling.[93] The addition of gadolinium has been found to increase the accuracy of the diagnosis of vertebral osteomyelitis in equivocal cases.[82,93] The involved portions of the adjacent vertebral body and disk will typically enhance after the administration of gadolinium (Fig. 18-27).

The presence of abnormal soft tissue in a paraspinal epidural location raises the differential consideration of inflammatory phlegmon versus abscess. These soft tissue masses can produce various degrees of encroachment on the central canal and foramina. The typical phlegmon is a homogeneously enhancing soft tissue mass on T1-weighted images and is usually hyperintense on T2 and STIR images. An epidural abscess characteristically demonstrates a peripherally enhancing fluid or soft tissue collection (Fig. 18-28). Epidural metastases may look like phlegmon, and large migrated extruded disks may demonstrate peripheral enhancement and require differentiation from an abscess. Other differential considerations include epidural lipomatosis, which has a more characteristic fat signal on T1, and epidural hematomas, which are more variable on T1 and T2 and usually demonstrate loss of signal on gradient echo images as a result of the presence of blood by-products. More recently, it has been suggested that restricted diffusion is characteristic of an abscess.[94,95]

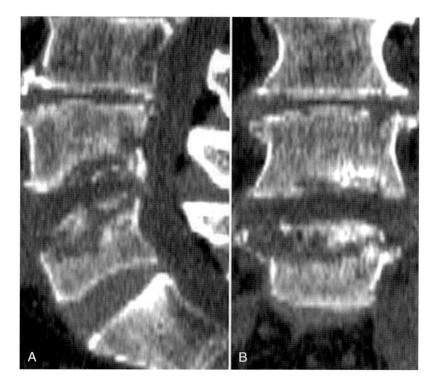

A   B

FIGURE 18-26 Vertebral osteomyelitis shown on sagittal (**A**) and coronal (**B**) multiplanar reformatted images from a CT data set of the lumbar spine. There are destructive changes of the adjacent vertebral body margins of L4 and L5 with an irregular contour and ill-defined soft tissue mass.

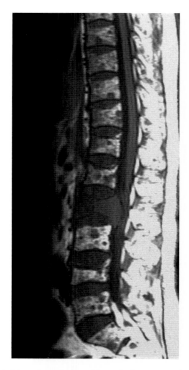

FIGURE 18-29 Metastases demonstrated on a sagittal T1-weighted spin echo image of the lumbar spine. Patchy as well as focal replacement of the marrow space is seen at all visualized levels. There is complete marrow replacement of the L2 vertebral body with loss of height and a convex posterior extension of the vertebral body into the spinal canal.

the typical appearance of an intraosseous hemangioma, variable signal intensity on T1- and T2-weighted images is not uncommon. Incidental intraosseous hemangiomas are a common finding on MRI of the spine. The primary differential consideration is another normal incidental finding, a lipid marrow rest. Vertebral body hemangiomas can extend extraosseously and, particularly in the thoracic region, can produce severe cord compression (Fig. 18-34).

Other primary tumors of bone such as osteomas, osteoblastomas, aneurysmal bone cysts, giant cell tumors, osteochondromas, chondrosarcomas, and osteosarcomas are much less common than metastatic disease and occur as solitary lesions that involve both bone and soft tissue. Unlike plain-film radiography, myelography, and CT, which focus primarily on the bony architecture of the spinal canal and its adjacent soft tissues, MRI focuses on the vertebral marrow space and nearby soft tissues. The characteristics used for differential considerations are different between the two approaches. The designations osteolytic and osteoblastic have no meaning with MRI. However, certain primary lesions involving the vertebrae have been noted to present a unique appearance on MRI. For instance, aneurysmal bone cysts have a somewhat unique MRI appearance consisting of numerous well-defined cystic cavities surrounded by a rim of low signal intensity and multiple fluid levels. These changes, however, are not specific in that other bony lesions such as osteosarcoma, chondroblastoma, and giant cell tumor of bone may mimic aneurysmal bone cysts.

Chordomas are typically seen on conventional radiographs as radiolucent lesions or heterogeneous destructive masses, usually of the sacrum or vertebral body. On CT, chordomas also appear destructive and may have a large paraspinal soft tissue mass.

FIGURE 18-30 Diffuse marrow replacement from metastatic disease visualized on sagittal T1-weighted (**A**) and T2-weighted (**B**) images and a posterior view from a whole-body technetium 99 bone scan (**C**). On the T1-weighted image there is diffuse decreased signal intensity of the visualized osseous structures. Note the higher signal intensity of the intervertebral disk than the vertebral body on this T1-weighted spin echo image. On the T2-weighted image there is diffuse decreased signal intensity of the marrow space. On the radionuclide study, diffuse increased activity is seen throughout the spinal column.

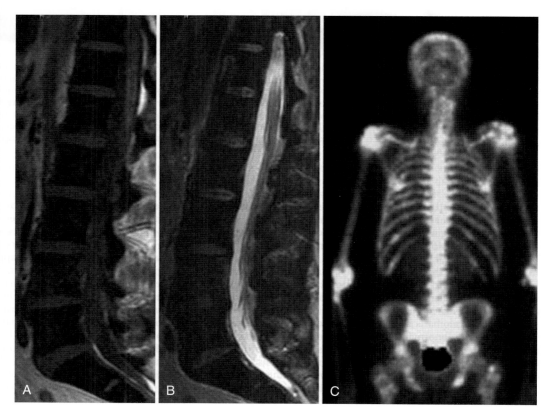

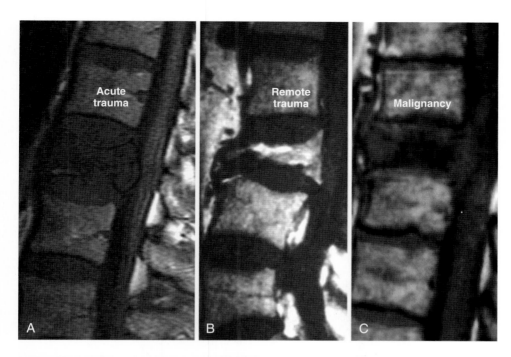

FIGURE 18-31 Vertebral body compression fractures from acute trauma (**A**), remote trauma (**B**), and malignant disease (**C**). The compression fracture caused by remote trauma demonstrates hyperintense signal within the vertebral body from increased lipid marrow content and is easy to distinguish from subacute or acute changes. Acute trauma and malignancy may be difficult to differentiate.

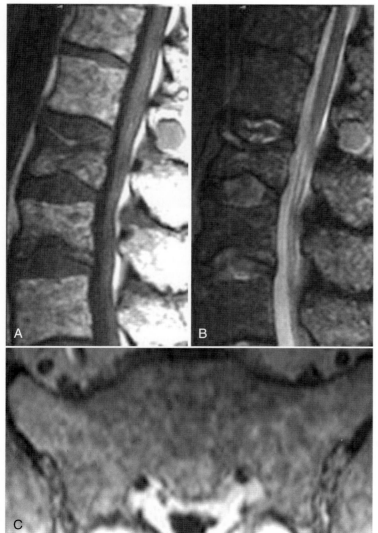

FIGURE 18-32 Multiple myeloma. Diffuse patchy heterogeneous marrow signal intensity of the visualized osseous structures is seen on both T1- (**A**) and T2-weighted (**B**) images. A more focal area of marrow replacement is noted in the spinous process of L1. There is loss of vertebral body height at L2 and L3.

FIGURE 18-33 Benign intraosseous hemangioma demonstrated on sagittal T1-weighted (**A**) and T2-weighted (**B**) images of the mid lumbar spine. On T1, there is an ovoid heterogeneous but predominantly increased signal intensity replacement of the normal marrow signal. On the T2-weighted image there is heterogeneous increased signal intensity in the same location. Axial T1-weighted (**C**) and T2-weighted (**D**) images through the hemangioma within the L2 vertebral body. The T1-weighted changes are a reflection of the fat within the hemangioma, and the T2-weighted changes are a reflection of the more vascular elements. Note the somewhat speculated core, which is characteristic of a hemangioma.

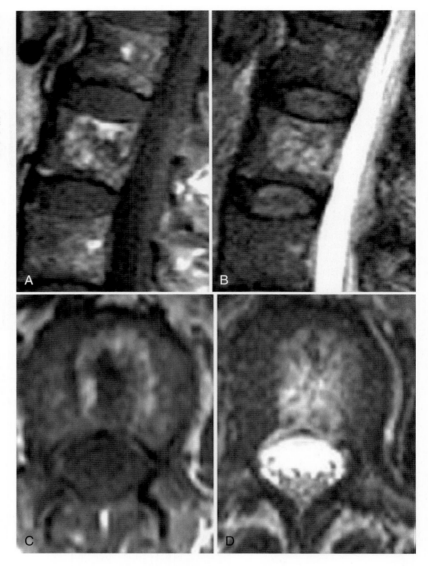

Sclerosis is seen in almost half the cases. The sacral coccygeal region is the most common location (50%), followed by the spheno-occipital (35%) and vertebral bodies elsewhere (15%). On MRI, chordomas typically appear as heterogeneous hypointense to isointense lesions on T1 and hyperintense lesions on T2 with low-signal septations indicative of fibrous stroma (Fig. 18-35).

Intradural Extramedullary Tumors

Intradural extramedullary tumors include meningiomas, nerve sheath tumors, embryonal tumors, paragangliomas, leptomeningeal metastases, and meningeal cysts (arachnoid cysts). Fifty percent of intradural extramedullary lesions are meningiomas or nerve sheath tumors. They are typically isolated and well circumscribed with marked homogeneous enhancement.

Meningiomas are most commonly located in the thoracic region in a lateral or posterolateral location. On conventional radiographs the only finding may be focal intraspinal calcification. On CT, an isointense to hyperintense mass, relative to muscle, is the usual appearance on a nonenhanced study. After intravenous contrast administration there may be homogeneous enhancement. Adjacent bone may be hyperostotic. The MRI findings of an intraspinal meningioma are similar to those seen intracranially. On T1-weighted images the mass is isointense with spinal cord. On T2 the mass remains isointense or slightly hypointense in comparison to adjacent spinal cord. Rarely, it may be hyperintense. There is usually prominent homogeneous enhancement after contrast administration (Fig. 18-36). An enhancing dural tail, commonly seen intracranially, is less common intraspinally.[101] The common differential consideration is a schwannoma or nerve sheath tumor, which often has higher signal intensity on T2-weighted images, may be cystic, and may be more commonly associated with hemorrhage. Other differential considerations are paraganglioma, epidermoid, arachnoid cyst, intradural metastasis, or lymphoma.

Schwannomas are characterized by a well-circumscribed intraspinal masses; they are most commonly located in an intradural extramedullary location. Fifteen percent may have an extradural component. An enlarged intravertebral foramen and thin pedicle are conventional radiographic signs of a long-standing mass. Schwannomas tend to be more hyperintense on T2-weighted images and have cystic changes or hemorrhage more often than meningiomas do. They are indistinguishable from solitary

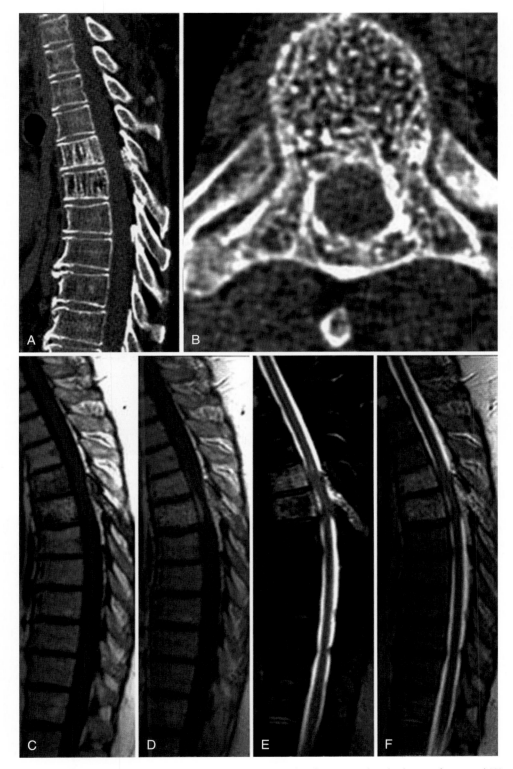

FIGURE 18-34 Extraosseous extension of a vertebral body hemangioma visualized on sagittal multiplanar reformatted (**A**) and axial source (**B**) images through the midthoracic spine. The striated osseous appearance on the sagittal image and the spiculated appearance on the axial image are characteristic of an intraosseous hemangioma. Note the extension into the pedicles and posterior elements on the axial image. Sagittal T1-weighted (**C**), contrast-enhanced T1-weighted (**D**), T2-weighted (**E**), and short tau inversion recovery (**F**) images through the thoracic spine. Striated hyperintense changes within the vertebral body are noted on T1 and T2. There is contiguous vertebral body involvement, as well as extension into the posterior elements. On the contrast-enhanced T1-weighted and T2-weighted images, there is evidence of extraosseous extension and soft tissue enhancement in the anterior epidural space.

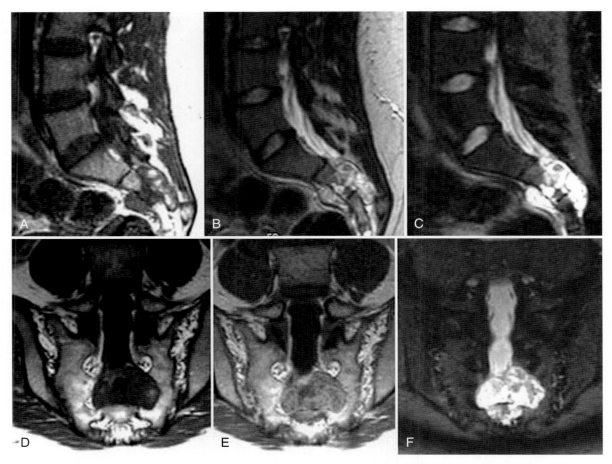

FIGURE 18-35 Chordoma demonstrated on sagittal T1-weighted (**A**), sagittal T2-weighted (**B**), and short tau inversion recovery (**C**) images of the sacral region. Coronal T1-weighted (**D**), contrast-enhanced T1-weighted (**E**), and fat-suppressed T2-weighted (**F**) images. There is a destructive mass involving the S2 body with an extraosseous soft tissue component involving the sacral canal and presacral soft tissues.

FIGURE 18-36 Meningioma seen on sagittal T1-weighted contrast-enhanced (**A**) and T2-weighted (**B**) images of the thoracic spine. An anterior extra-axial mass at the T10-11 level demonstrates homogeneous enhancement and is posteriorly displacing and markedly compressing the thoracic cord. There is a small superior dural tail noted (*arrow*). On the T2-weighted image, the mass is isointense with spinal cord. The hyperintense intramedullary signal within the thoracic cord presumably represents cord edema secondary to compression.

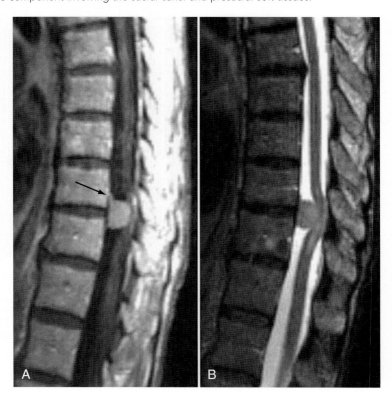

neurofibromas by imaging (Fig. 18-37).[102,103] Spinal involvement in neurofibromatosis is most common in type 2. Schwannomas in this condition may be solitary or multiple and can appear solid or cystic (Fig. 18-38).

Dermoid and epidermoid tumors are usually either intradural extramedullary (60%) or intramedullary (40%). The lower thoracic and lumbar regions are the most common locations. Conventional radiographs are generally normal but may demonstrate benign spinal canal widening with flattening of the pedicles and laminae. On CT these tumors are usually seen as well-demarcated masses with attenuation similar to that of CSF. The presence of calcification is more suggestive of a dermoid than an epidermoid tumor. Again, there may be focal osseous erosion or spinal canal widening. On MRI, dermoids are typically hypointense to hyperintense on T1 with variable signal intensities that reflect fat (hyperintense on T1) or calcium (decreased signal intensity on T1) (Fig. 18-39). Epidermoids are usually isointense on T1. Both tumors demonstrate increased signal intensity on T2-weighted images. Typically, these tumors do not enhance after contrast administration and may demonstrate restricted diffusion.

Myxopapillary ependymomas represent 90% of filum tumors. They occur exclusively in the conus and filum terminale, are slow growing, and may fill the entire spinal canal. Conventional radiographs and CT may demonstrate vertebral body scalloping and canal enlargement (Fig. 18-40).

Leptomeningeal disease is silent on conventional radiographs and on myelography is manifested by filling defects of variable size within the subarachnoid space. Non–contrast-enhanced CT is usually normal unless there is coexisting extradural disease, as in the case of metastatic breast or lung carcinoma. On MRI, leptomeningeal disease is generally isointense with the spinal cord and nerve roots and, when extensive, may be manifested as a diffuse increase in the signal intensity of the CSF space on T1-weighted images with a so-called ground-glass appearance. Nerve roots may appear blurred or less distinct. On T2-weighted images, leptomeningeal disease is usually isointense with neuroelements or may be manifested as thickened nerve roots within the subarachnoid space. On contrast-enhanced T1-weighted images, there is obvious enhancement that may be diffuse, nodular, or linear. The most common cause is hematogenous dissemination from extracranial neoplasms such as adenocarcinoma (Fig. 18-41) of the lung or breast, melanoma, lymphoma, and metastases. In children and young adults, primitive neuroectodermal tumors are most commonly manifested as leptomeningeal disease. Differential considerations include inflammatory

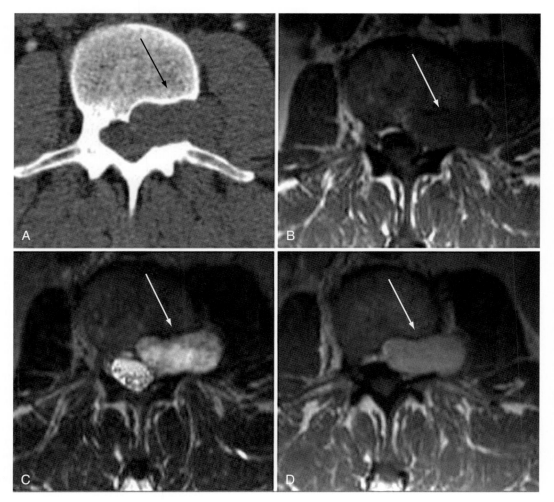

FIGURE 18-37 Schwannoma visualized on axial CT (**A**), T1-weighted (**B**), T2-weighted (**C**), and T1-weighted contrast-enhanced (**D**) images through the L2 vertebral body. A large lobulated dumbbell mass (*arrows*) is expanding the neuroforamina and remodeling the adjacent vertebral body. The T1 signal is isointense with neural structures. There is a somewhat heterogeneous increased signal on T2 and homogeneous enhancement after contrast enhancement.

FIGURE 18-38 Sagittal cervicothoracic (**A**) and thoracolumbar (**B**) T1-weighted contrast-enhanced images demonstrate multiple intradural extramedullary enhancing masses that represent schwannomas in this patient with neurofibromatosis type 2.

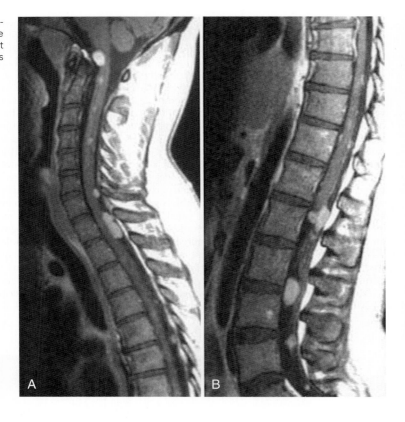

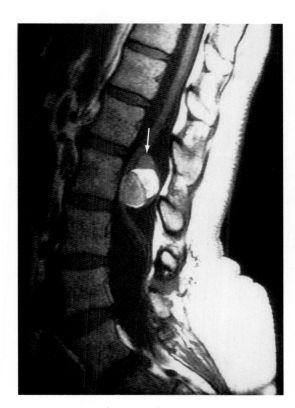

FIGURE 18-39 Dermoid. An intradural extramedullary mass (*arrow*) is displacing the conus anteriorly. This mass has variable signal intensity, with soft tissue, lipid, and heterogeneous regions noted. These lesions typically do not enhance.

conditions such as hemangic meningitis, granulomatous meningitis (tuberculosis and sarcoidosis), congenital hypertrophic polyradiculoneuropathy, thickened nerve roots secondary to inflammatory conditions such as Guillain-Barré syndrome, polyneuropathy associated with acquired immunodeficiency syndrome, and chronic interstitial demyelinating polyneuropathy and arachnoiditis (see Fig. 18-41).[104]

Arachnoid cysts are typically intradural extramedullary loculated CSF collections that can be manifested as space-occupying lesions. Type I is an extradural meningeal cyst that contains no neural tissue (Fig. 18-42). Type II includes extradural meningeal cysts that contain neural tissue, and type III includes intradural meningeal cysts. Type II, or perineural cysts/Tarlov's cysts, is more commonly encountered and contains nerve roots, often adherent to the cyst's wall. Type III consists of spinal intradural meningeal cysts (arachnoid cysts), which are thought to arise from the diverticulum of the arachnoid. When long-standing, they may produce posterior vertebral body scalloping and thinning of the pedicles with a widened intrapedicular distance on conventional radiographs. On myelography, intradural cysts produce an intrathecal filling defect and extradural effacement of the subarachnoid space. Depending on their size, they may result in spinal cord compression. On CT, non–contrast-enhanced studies show isoattenuation with adjacent CSF, and there may be evidence of cord displacement. After intrathecal contrast administration an intradural arachnoid cyst may be difficult to visualize if it is opacified, but it otherwise appears as a filling defect with a mass effect. Delayed imaging with postmyelographic CT often results in opacification of the cyst with decreased attenuation in the generalized subarachnoid space. On MRI, CSF signal intensity is that of CSF that does not usually share the same degree of pulsations as the general subarachnoid space. T2-weighted images are equivalent to CSF but again may lack CSF flow signal

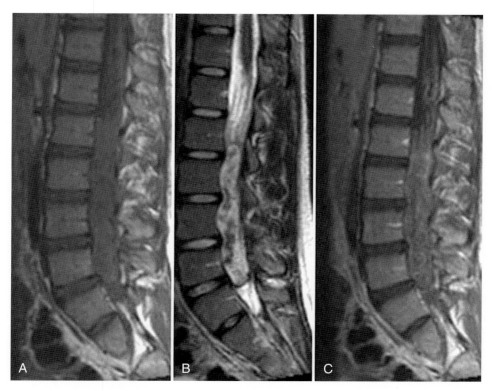

FIGURE 18-40 Myxopapillary ependymoma seen on sagittal T1-weighted (**A**), T2-weighted (**B**), and T1-weighted contrast-enhanced (**C**) images of the lumbar spine. The T1-weighted image shows a subtle mass filling the lumbar canal of L2 through L5. On the T2-weighted image this mass is noted to be heterogeneous with areas of both increased and decreased signal intensity. There is diffuse subtle enhancement after contrast administration, as well as evidence of enhancement more proximally in the region of the conus.

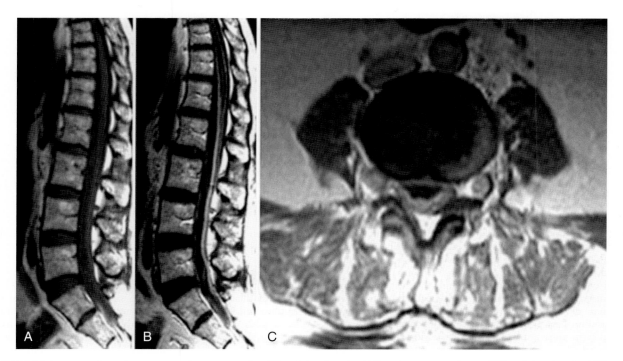

FIGURE 18-41 Leptomeningeal metastases demonstrated on T1-weighted sagittal (**A**) and contrast-enhanced T1-weighted sagittal (**B**) and axial (**C**) images. On the precontrast study, diffuse increased signal intensity of the cerebrospinal fluid space is seen in the distal lumbar region. After contrast administration there is enhancement of the surfaces of the distal thoracic cord and the traversing nerve roots in the lumbar region. An axial image through the region of the conus demonstrates enhancement of the surface of the distal cord and subarachnoid space.

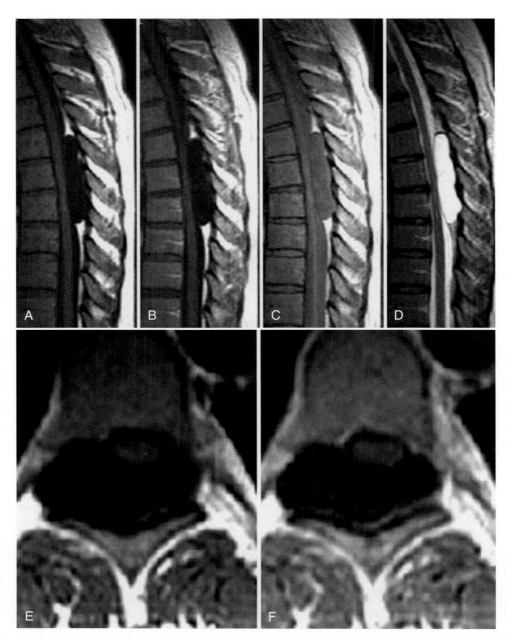

FIGURE 18-42 Type I arachnoid cyst visualized on sagittal T1-weighted (**A**), T1-weighted contrast-enhanced (**B**), short tau inversion recovery (**C**), and T2-weighted (**D**) images through the midthoracic region. There is a large cerebrospinal fluid (CSF)-like intradural extramedullary mass that is displacing the cord anteriorly and does not enhance. Axial T1-weighted images before (**E**) and after (**F**) contrast administration demonstrate the large posterior located intradural extramedullary CSF-like collection.

changes. There is no enhancement after contrast administration, and the walls of the cyst may be impossible to resolve. Differential considerations include large degenerative cysts, dural ectasia, and spinal cord herniation.

Spinal cord herniation occurs through a defect in the dura, which is usually ventral. Clinically, these patients usually have unexplained chronic progressive leg pain and myelopathy. Imaging findings are those of anterior displacement of the thoracic cord with apparent expansion of the dorsal subarachnoid space. It is usually located in the midthoracic region. On myelography, there is either displacement of the cord or a focal deformity anteriorly. CT myelography is helpful in defining the deformity. MRI demonstrates cord displacement anteriorly, which is usually focal. The increased dorsal subarachnoid

space can mimic the appearance of a type I arachnoid cyst (Fig. 18-43).[105,106]

Intramedullary Disease and Tumors

Intramedullary abnormalities are silent on conventional radiographic and CT imaging unless nonspecific cord expansion has developed. MRI is clearly the study of choice and is able to characterize abnormalities on the basis of morphology, changes in signal intensity, the presence or absence of contrast enhancement, and anatomic location and extent. In general, the location, length, cord morphology, signal intensity characteristics, contrast character or absence of contrast enhancement, and blood by-products are important morphologic considerations for the

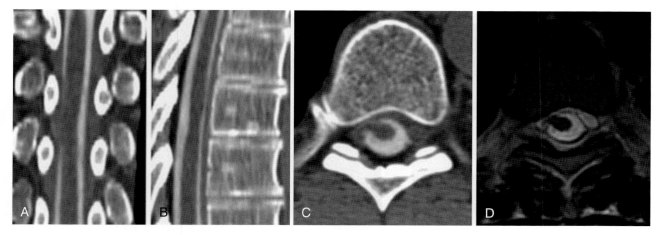

FIGURE 18-43 Thoracic cord herniation seen on coronal (**A**) and sagittal (**B**) multiplanar reformatted images from a CT myelogram. There is apparent displacement of the thoracic cord to the right and an increased cerebrospinal fluid dorsally. Axial CT myelography (**C**) and axial T2-weighted MRI (**D**) demonstrate herniation of the thoracic cord anteriorly and laterally on the right.

differential diagnosis. Differential considerations of intramedullary disease are demyelinating disease, tumor, hydrosyringomyelia, infection, ischemia, vascular malformation, acute disseminated encephalomyelitis, sarcoid, and changes related to trauma.

In patients with acute transverse myelitis and the onset of acute motor, sensory, and autonomic dysfunction in the absence of preexisting neurological disease and spinal cord compression, the main differential considerations are multiple sclerosis, postinfectious myelitis, metabolic changes, paraneoplastic syndromes, and infection.

Ten percent to 20% of patients with multiple sclerosis have isolated spinal cord disease, most commonly affecting the cervical region in the dorsal lateral aspect of the cord (Fig. 18-44). These usually appear as well-circumscribed hyperintense lesions on T2

with homogeneous, nodular, or ring enhancement after contrast administration. Long-standing disease is often manifested as cord atrophy. Top differential considerations are other intramedullary diseases, neoplasms, or other causes of acute transverse myelitis.

The most common primary neoplasms of the spinal cord are ependymomas and astrocytomas. In general, it is usually impossible to differentiate between the two with imaging. Typically, primary cord tumors demonstrate expansion of the cord, low signal intensity on T1, and high signal intensity on T2 with variable contrast enhancement. Ependymomas are more likely to have associated blood by-products and large satellite cysts (Fig. 18-45). When long-standing, ependymomas may have the conventional radiographic findings of canal widening and posterior

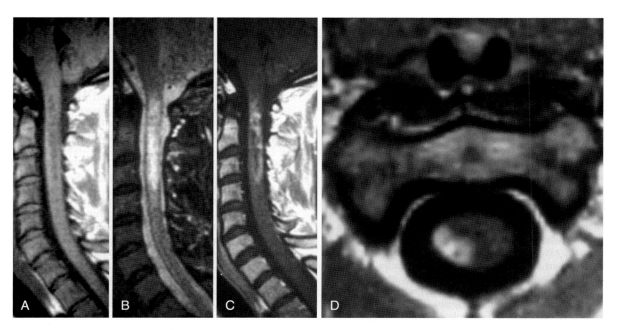

FIGURE 18-44 Multiple sclerosis demonstrated on T1-weighted (**A**), T2-weighted (**B**), contrast-enhanced sagittal T1-weighted (**C**), and axial contrast-enhanced T1-weighted (**D**) images. The T1-weighted image demonstrates patchy decreased signal intensity. There is increased signal in this region on the T2-weighted study. Patchy enhancement of the upper cervical cord is seen after contrast enhancement. The axial image after contrast administration demonstrates posterior lateral enhancement of the cord.

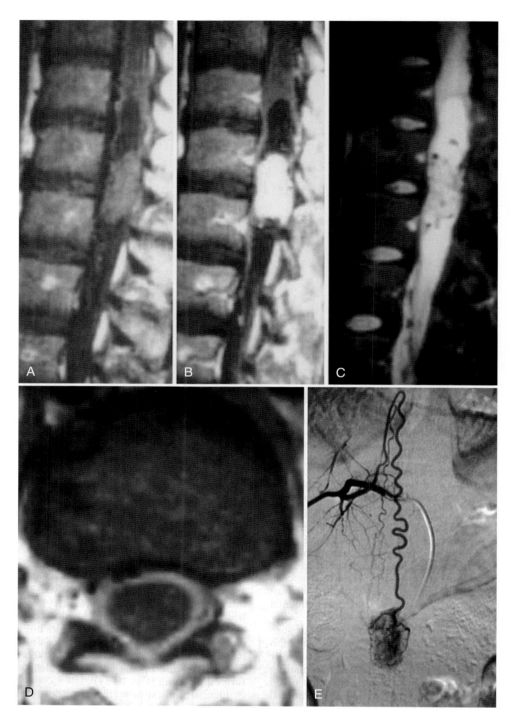

FIGURE 18-47 Hemangioblastoma visualized on sagittal T1-weighted (**A**), T1-weighted contrast-enhanced (**B**), and T2-weighted (**C**) images of the thoracolumbar junction. There is an intramedullary mass associated with adjacent cord edema or a syrinx. Homogeneous enhancement of this intramedullary mass is seen after contrast administration. The T2-weighted image demonstrates multiple areas of focal decreased signal intensity representing flow voids from the increased vascularity of the lesion. An axial T1-weighted image (**D**) demonstrates the associated cyst within the adjacent thoracic cord. An anteroposterior view from a spinal arteriogram (**E**) demonstrates an enlarged artery of Adamkiewicz feeding the hypervascular mass at the thoracolumbar junction.

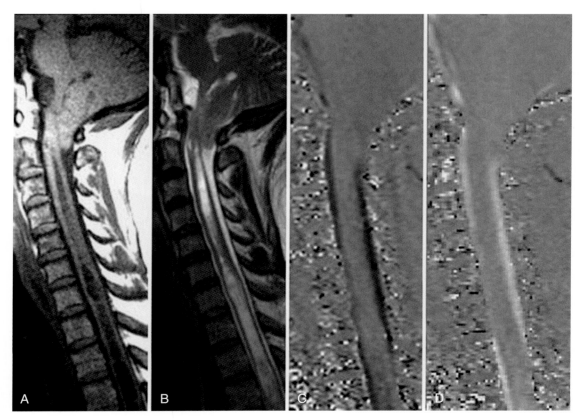

FIGURE 18-48 Syringomyelia seen on sagittal T1-weighted (**A**), T2-weighted (**B**), and cerebrospinal fluid (CSF) flow studies (**C** and **D**) of the cranial vertebral junction. There is a syrinx cavity within the cervical cord and a Chiari malformation with downward herniation of the tonsils. The CSF flow studies demonstrate an absence of flow dorsal to the upper cervical cord. There is absence of flow in the region of the cisterna magna as well.

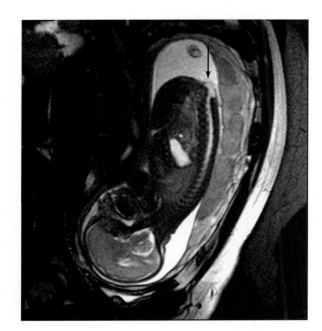

FIGURE 18-49 Sagittal T2-weighted image through a fetus demonstrating spinal dysraphism with herniation of the thecal sac (*arrow*). Resolution is not adequate for determining whether neural elements are present.

Diastematomyelia, the most common neurenteric or split notochord entity, may require several imaging modalities for full anatomic delineation (Fig. 18-53). Plain films may show spina bifida, intersegmental laminar fusion, anomalies of the vertebral bodies, and kyphoscoliosis. For septal definition, axial SE T2-weighted MRI, axial gradient echo T2-weighted MRI, CT, or CT myelography may be necessary. Other commonly associated abnormalities, including a thickened filum, developmental tumors (lipomas, dermoid/epidermoid), and hydromyelia, can be depicted.

There may be a bone or cartilaginous spur within the cleft in the cord. For accurate definition, a combination of sagittal, coronal, and axial MRI, CT, or CT myelography may be necessary. The conus is located below the L2 level in more than 75% of patients, and there is often an associated thickened filum. Hydromyelia is present in approximately 50% of patients, and the spinal column is almost always abnormal.

IMAGING OF VASCULAR DISORDERS OF THE SPINE

Vascular disorders of the spine can be divided into two groups: vascular malformations of the spine and spinal cord and parenchymal injury as a result of hemorrhage or stroke. Evaluation of patients with potential vascular disease of the spine is frequently challenging. MRI is the screening procedure of choice for detection of vascular abnormalities of the spine. It is capable of identifying cord enlargement, cord enhancement, and changes in

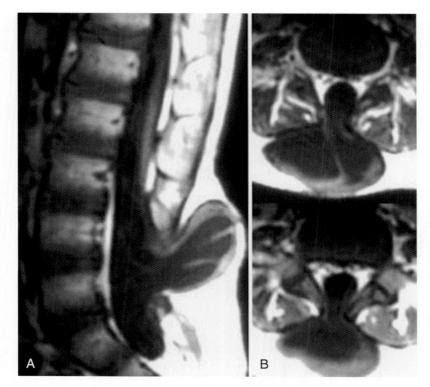

FIGURE 18-50 Myelomeningocele demonstrated on sagittal (**A**) and axial (**B**) T1-weighted images through a dysraphic defect in the distal region through which both neural elements and cerebrospinal fluid have herniated. The placode is adherent dorsally, and the nerve roots are splayed more ventrally.

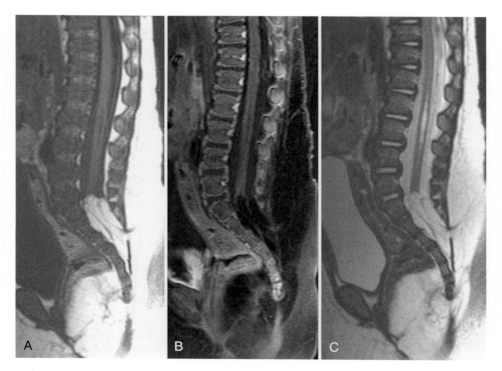

FIGURE 18-51 Lipomyelomeningocele seen on sagittal T1-weighted (**A**), fat-suppressed T1-weighted (**B**), and T2-weighted (**C**) images of the lumbosacral region. A tethered spinal cord terminates in a lipomeningocele in the lumbosacral region that is communicating with a presacral lipoma. A syrinx cavity is present in the tethered cord in the upper lumbar region.

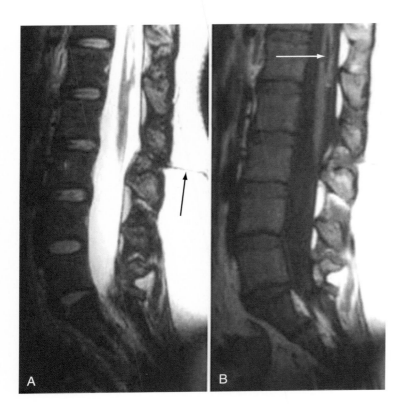

FIGURE 18-52 Dermal sinus visualized on sagittal T2-weighted (**A**) and T1-weighted (**B**) images of the lumbar region. A sinus track (*black arrow*) passing intraspinally is associated with a tethered cord at the L3 level. There is a syrinx cavity within the cord at the L1 level (*white arrow*).

signal intensity related to flowing blood within arterial or venous structures. The presence of blood products that may be more remote can also be identified, especially on gradient echo imaging. In addition to static imaging, both contrast-enhanced and time-of-flight techniques are available for MRA examination. MRI can reliably detect or exclude spinal vascular abnormalities and provide important localization information, but it lacks the capacity to accurately classify the subtypes. Even when there is good depiction of the arterial and venous anatomy with MRA techniques, catheter-based angiography is required for further therapeutic management. Once a diagnosis is made or suspected, the patient my warrant further evaluation with either conventional spinal angiography or CTA.

Vascular Malformations of the Spine and Spinal Cord

Spinal vascular malformations are a heterogeneous group of non-neoplastic vascular abnormalities that account for 3% to 16% of spinal mass lesions. The current classification system is based on the angioarchitecture and hemodynamics of the lesion as defined by spinal angiography. The major groups of spinal vascular malformations include spinal-dural arteriovenous fistulas (SDAVFs) (Fig. 18-54), spinal cord arteriovenous malformations (SCAVMs) (Fig. 18-55), perimedullary spinal cord arteriovenous fistulas (SCAVFs) (Fig. 18-56), and cavernous malformations (Fig. 18-57).[111]

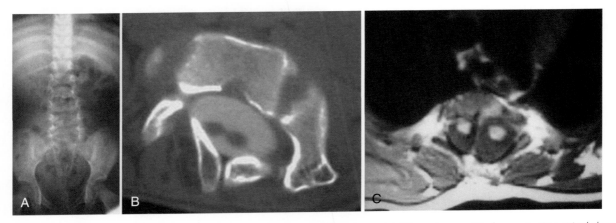

FIGURE 18-53 Anteroposterior radiograph of the thoracolumbar region (**A**) and an axial CT myelogram (**B**) demonstrating spinal dysraphism with widening of the interpedicular distance in the lumbar region and anomalies of the vertebral bodies and posterior elements. Axial T1-weighted MRI at a slightly higher level (**C**) demonstrates a septum separating two spinal cords. There appears to be two separate dural coverings.

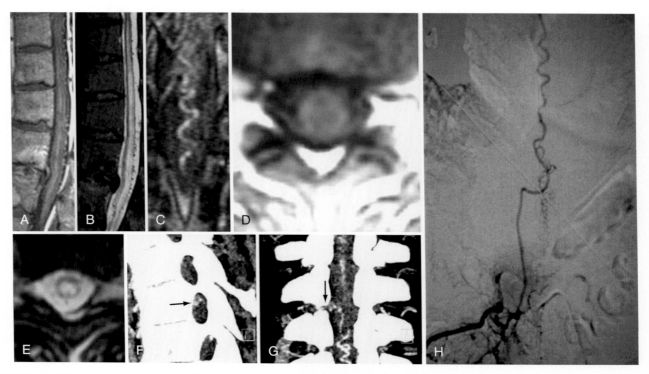

FIGURE 18-54 Type I dural arterial venous fistula seen on T1-weighted contrast-enhanced (**A**), T2-weighted (**B**), and magnetic resonance angiographic (MRA) (**C**) images of the distal thoracic region. Multiple enhancing vessels are noted along the surface of the thoracic cord on the T1 contrast-enhanced image. Diffuse increased hyperintensity is apparent within the cord on the T2-weighted image, as well as multiple small focal flow voids along the surface. MRA demonstrates an enlarged draining venous plexus. Axial T1-weighted (**D**) and T2-weighted (**E**) images of the thoracic cord demonstrate the decreased signal intensity on T1 and increased signal intensity on T2 within the spinal cord centrally secondary to the cord edema. Sagittal (**F**) and coronal (**G**) multiplanar reformatted images from a CT angiogram of the thoracic cord. Note the prominent radicular vessel leading to the dural fistula, which then shunts into the venous plexus on the surface of the thoracic cord (*arrow*). A spinal arteriogram (**H**) demonstrates a dural fistula fed from an intercostal artery that shunts into the venous plexus along the surface of the cord.

FIGURE 18-55 Type II arteriovenous malformation (AVM) shown on sagittal T2-weighted images (**A** and **B**) and a spinal arteriogram (**C**) of the cervical cord. The sagittal T2-weighted images demonstrate an intramedullary mass with heterogeneous signal at the C2 level and flow voids along the surface of the cervical cord. A lateral view from the spinal arteriogram demonstrates opacification of the AVM nidus fed from the anterior spinal artery.

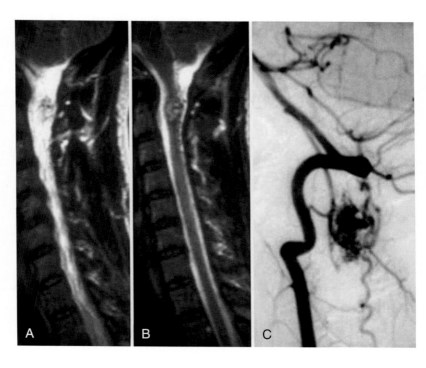

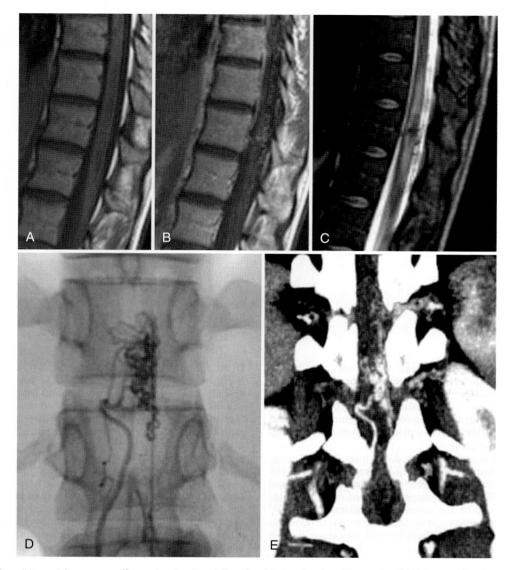

FIGURE 18-56 Type IV arterial venous malformation (perimedullary fistula) visualized on T1-weighted (**A**), T1-weighted contrast-enhanced (**B**), and T2-weighted (**C**) images at the level of the distal thoracic cord. On the T1-weighted image there is subtle decreased signal intensity within the thoracic cord suggestive of edema. On the contrast-enhanced T1-weighted image, multiple enhancing vessels are seen along the surface of the thoracic cord. On the T2-weighted image there is increased signal within the cord secondary to edema and a focal low signal that presumably reflects compressed perimedullary vessels. An anteroposterior spinal arteriogram (**D**) and CT angiogram (**E**) demonstrate filling of the vascular malformation on the surface of the cord by a radicular artery. In contradistinction to type I, shunting in this pathology is at the cord level and not at the dura.

SDAVFs are the most common spinal vascular malformation and represent up to 80% of all spinal malformations. Males are affected in 80% to 90% of cases, and they are usually seen initially in the fourth or fifth decade of life. Anatomically, SDAVFs are arteriovenous shunts in the dura, most commonly adjacent to the intervertebral foramen or in the nerve root sleeve. The arterial supply usually arises from a dural branch of the radicular artery and drains directly into the pial veins of the cord via an intradural vein. This abnormal drainage pattern results in venous hypertension and spinal cord edema. Hemorrhage with SDAVFs is rare. There are four basic types of arterial vascular malformations of the spinal cord: I, AV fistulas between dural branches of the spinal ramus of the radicular artery and an intradural medullary vein; II, intramedullary glomus malformation; III, extensive juvenile malformation; and IV, intradural perimedullary AV fistulas.

Type I: Dural arteriovenous malformations (AVMs). These AVMs have a male preponderance with the usual manifestation in the fifth to eighth decades. Patients usually exhibit progressive radiculomyelopathy secondary to venous hypertensive myelopathy.[112] Subarachnoid hemorrhage and venous infarction are uncommon. MRI is the screening procedure of choice. There is usually cord enlargement, cord enhancement, and central increased high signal on T2-weighted imaging with sparing of the cord peripherally. Low T2 signal on the cord periphery is highly suggestive of venous hypertensive myelopathy (SDAVF). Flow voids are encountered on the surface in 45% of patients.[113,114]

Type II: Intramedullary glomus AVMs. Nineteen percent to 45% of spinal AVMs are initially evaluated because of subarachnoid intraspinal hemorrhage. Arterial aneurysms are identified in more than 40% of patients.[115]

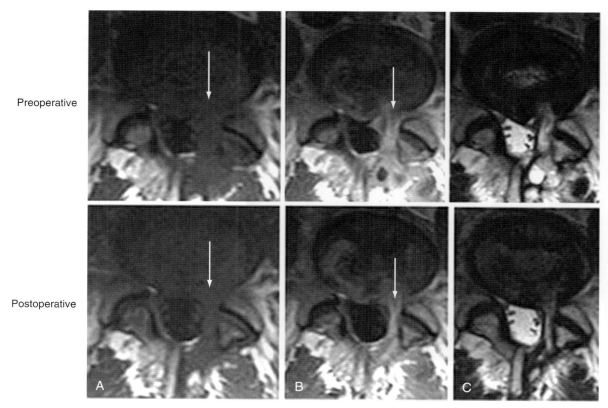

Preoperative

Postoperative

FIGURE 18-59 Axial T1-weighted (**A**), contrast-enhanced T1-weighted (**B**), and T2-weighted (**C**) images through the L4-5 disk in a patient after left-sided laminectomy and diskectomy. The immediate preoperative study demonstrates aberrant soft tissue (*arrows*) in the anterior and left lateral epidural space. This enhances in a relatively homogeneous fashion after administration of contrast material. There is mild deformity of the thecal sack. Eight weeks postoperatively, there has been reexpansion of the thecal sack and some retraction of the aberrant soft tissue, which still continues to demonstrate homogeneous enhancement. This is epidural fibrosis.

considerations include crowding of nerve roots with stenosis, leptomeningeal seeding of neoplasms, or meningitis[119,120] (Fig. 18-65).

In patients with metallic implants, screw artifact can make visualization of the foramina and nerve roots very difficult, although the central canal can still be seen adequately in most cases. Metal artifact can be minimized by using a variety of techniques, including fast SE sequences, smaller voxel size, enlargement of the field of view, or the use of higher readout bandwidth.

Moreover, geometric distortion occurs along the frequency in the coded direction. Frequency in coding directed parallel to the axis of an implant improves image quality except at the tip.

Computed Tomography

CT and CT myelography are essential tools for imaging postoperative patients. Screw artifact can be minimized to allow greater visualization of the foramina and lateral recesses. The presence

FIGURE 18-60 Scar tissue seen on axial T1-weighted images before (**A**) and after (**B**) contrast enhancement in a patient after a left-sided laminectomy. On the precontrast T1-weighted axial image there is aberrant soft tissue (*arrow*) in the left anterior epidural space. After contrast administration there is relative homogeneous enhancement of this aberrant soft tissue (*arrow*) without evidence of a mass effect. This is scar tissue.

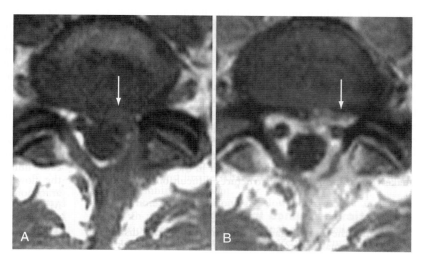

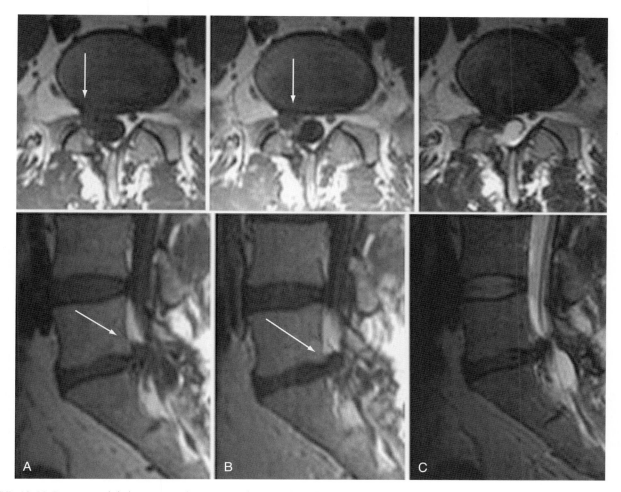

FIGURE 18-61 Recurrent disk herniation demonstrated on axial and sagittal T1-weighted (**A**), contrast-enhanced T1-weighted (**B**), and T2-weighted (**C**) images through the lumbar spine in a patient after a right-sided laminectomy at the L5-S1 level. On the pre–contrast-enhanced T1-weighted axial and sagittal images there is aberrant soft tissue (*arrows*) in the right anterior and lateral epidural space. After the administration of contrast material, there is mild peripheral enhancement of aberrant soft tissue (*arrows*) surrounding a nonenhancing core.

of pseudarthrosis in spinal fusion patients is best assessed with fine-cut CT. Postprocessing of the images with sagittal and coronal reconstructions can aid in the assessment of fusion. Hardware placement and integrity can also be assessed in this manner. Myelography can enhance the ability to visualize compressive and intrinsic lesions of the neural elements.

Plain Films

Although largely supplanted by CT for the assessment of spinal fusion, plain radiographs can be very useful in postoperative patients. They are a cheap, fast, effective way to assess the position and competence of spinal hardware. Moreover, 3-ft antero-posterior and lateral films are essential in the evaluation of deformity and correction of deformity. Dynamic imaging with flexion and extension images is also helpful in the assessment of spinal stability and the presence of pseudarthrosis.

EVALUATION OF SPINE TRAUMA

Plain radiography, MRI, and CT are all used in evaluation of the posttraumatic spinal column and are often complementary. Appropriate indications for imaging the spine in trauma include pain, neurological deficit, altered consciousness, and the presence of a high-risk mechanism of injury. The Canadian C-spine Rule Study confirmed that "low-risk" patients (ambulatory, no midline tenderness, no immediate onset of pain, able to sit, or victims of simple rear-end motor vehicle collisions) who could actively rotate their heads 45 degrees in both directions do not require imaging.[121]

Computed Tomography

CT scanning has been shown to be significantly more sensitive and more time efficient than plain films for detection of cervical fractures in the setting of acute spinal trauma. The widespread availability of high-quality CT scanners, the ability to rapidly acquire images, and the ability to construct multiplanar and 3D images make CT the ideal screening test for cervical fracture. The sensitivity of CT scanning for acute cervical fractures ranges from 90% to 99% with specificities of 72% to 89%. The sensitivity of plain films in the acute setting ranges from 39% to 94%.[122-124] Moreover, a number of studies have demonstrated limitations in the ability of plain films to detect injuries to the upper cervical spine and occipital condyles.[125,126] Because of its greater sensitivity and wide availability, CT is quickly becoming the initial screening modality for bony injury in the cervical spine.

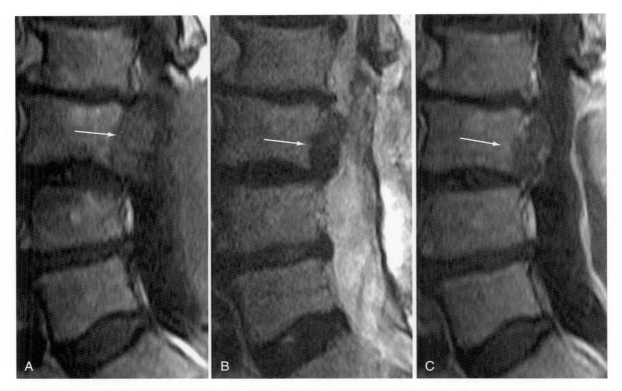

FIGURE 18-62 Postoperative epidural hematoma (*arrows*) visualized on sagittal T1-weighted (**A**), T2-weighted (**B**), and contrast-enhanced T1-weighted (**C**) images of the lumbar spine in a patient after laminectomy. A large soft tissue mass (*arrows*) is situated in the anterior epidural space behind the body of L3. It has soft tissue signal intensity on T1 but markedly decreased signal intensity on T2. After administration of contrast agent there is minimal peripheral enhancement. Note the posterior laminectomy defect. This was found to be an epidural hematoma at surgery.

CT has been shown to be superior to plain radiography in assessing fractures of the thoracic and lumbar spine as well. Campbell and coauthors[127] reported that 20% of burst fractures diagnosed by CT were misdiagnosed as stable wedge compression fractures on plain films. CT is better at detecting fractures of the dorsal elements, malalignment, and intracanalicular fragments.

Plain Films

CT has largely supplanted plain-film imaging as the modality of choice for the evaluation of osseous injury to the spine. However, plain films can be very useful in the evaluation of trauma patients, particularly when CT is unavailable.

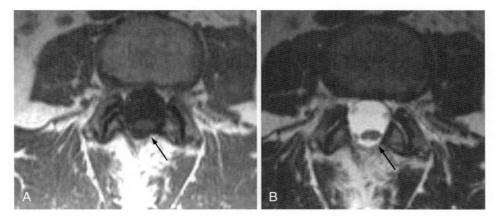

FIGURE 18-63 Group I arachnoiditis. Axial T1-weighted (**A**) and T2-weighted (**B**) images of the lumbar spine show evidence of a laminectomy defect. Portions of the traversing nerve roots are clumped posteriorly (*arrows*).

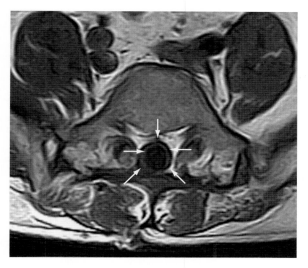

FIGURE 18-64 Group II arachnoiditis demonstrated on an axial T1-weighted spin echo image through the lumbar spine. There is a laminectomy defect and a thin rim of soft tissue signal intensity on the thecal sac that appears adherent peripherally. No individual traversing nerves are identified centrally (*arrows*).

Plain films are also critical in the evaluation of instability in the absence of bony injury. Stability of the cervical spine is best assessed with dynamic imaging that includes flexion and extension views. An increase in the atlantodental interval or greater than 3.5-mm horizontal displacement of the vertebral body between flexion and extension can be indicative of spinal instability. This examination should be performed only on alert, cooperative patients without neurological injury or radiographic evidence of unstable spinal injuries. Frequently, cervical mobility is limited by pain and muscle spasm at the time of the initial injury. Flexion and extension views may be more helpful when performed in a delayed fashion 7 to 10 days after the injury.[128]

Magnetic Resonance Imaging

MRI provides the best evaluation of soft tissue pathology and is the only means of directly evaluating the spinal cord. The information obtained is often complementary to evaluation of the bony structures by CT. Information about disk herniations, hematoma formation, and ligamentous and muscular injury can be instrumental in determining the appropriate treatment for the patient. MRI is indicated in a trauma patient with a neurological deficit or when there is suspicion of a soft tissue or vascular injury. STIR sequences can detect bone edema and aid in differentiating the acuity of fractures. Heavily T2-weighted sequences can be used to evaluate for nerve root avulsions and pseudomeningocele development. MRA and fat-saturated T2 sequences can be used to screen for vascular injuries. Ligamentous and soft tissue injuries are best visualized on fat-saturated T2 images. The normal anterior and posterior longitudinal ligaments are seen as continuous hypointense lines along the ventral and dorsal aspects of the vertebral bodies. In the presence of soft tissue injury, areas of increased T2 signal or discontinuity of the ligament may be seen. MRI is the modality of choice for the evaluation of a variety of posttraumatic conditions, including myelomalacia, cord tethering, syrinx formation, and the presence of dural AV fistulas.[128]

Although MRI can be very useful in the setting of acute trauma, it has not gained widespread use because of a variety of factors. The requirement for special ventilators and monitors can often make it difficult or even impossible to image critically ill trauma patients. MRI in patients with bullet fragments within the spine remains controversial. Most bullets are nonferrous; however, the composition of the embedded projectile is rarely known in the acute setting. There is a theoretical risk that a ferrous fragment may become mobile in the magnetic field and result in greater damage to surrounding structures, although this

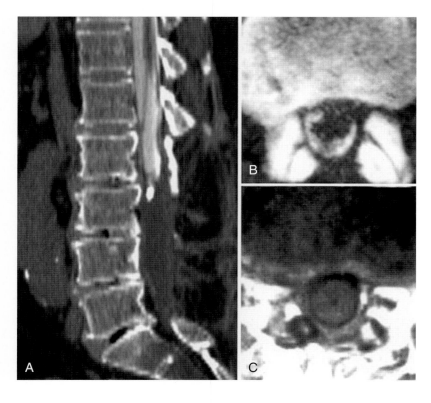

FIGURE 18-65 Group III arachnoiditis. Sagittal multiplanar reformatted CT myelogram (**A**), axial CT-myelogram (**B**), and a T1-weighted spin echo image (**C**) show complete blockage of the flow of contrast material at the L2-3 level. A laminectomy defect is seen together with evidence of calcification along the posterior margin of the thecal sac. The axial CT myelogram demonstrates a soft tissue mass within the thecal sac, as evidenced by soft tissue signal intensity on the axial T1-weighted image.

has never been reported. Finally, limited access to MRI scanners and qualified technicians decreases the usefulness of MRI in the acute setting at many centers.

SUGGESTED READINGS

Anson J, Spetzler R. Classification of spinal arterovenous malformations and implications for treatment. *BNI Q*. 1992;8:2-8.

Boden SD, Davis DO, Dina TS, et al. Abnormal magnetic-resonance scans of the lumbar spine in asymptomatic subjects: a prospective investigation. *J Bone Joint Surg Am*. 1990;72:403-408.

Bradley WG Jr. ACR appropriateness criteria. Low back pain. *AJNR Am J Neuroradiol*. 2007;28:990-992.

Carragee EJ, Kim DH. A prospective analysis of magnetic resonance imaging findings in patients with sciatica and lumbar disc herniation: correlation of outcomes with disc fragment and canal morphology. *Spine*. 1997;22:1650-1660.

Cook AM, Lau TN, Tomlinson MJ, et al. Magnetic resonance imaging of the whole spine in suspected malignant spinal cord compression: impact on management. *Clin Oncol*. 1998;10:39-43.

Dagirmanjian A, Schils J, McHenry M, et al. MR imaging of vertebral osteomyelitis revisited. *AJR Am J Roentgenol*. 1996;167:1539-1543.

Egelhoff JC, Bates DJ, Ross JS, et al. Spinal MR findings in neurofibromatosis types 1 and 2. *AJNR Am J Neuroradiol*. 1992;13:1071-1077.

Gilbertson J, Miller G, Goldman M, et al. Spinal dural arteriovenous fistulas: MR and myelographic findings. *AJNR Am J Neuroradiol*. 1995;16:2049-2057.

Jensen MC, Brant-Zawadzki MN, Obuchowski N, et al. Magnetic resonance imaging of the lumbar spine in people without back pain. *N Engl J Med*. 1994;331:69-73.

Korhonen T, Karppinen J, Paimela L, et al. The treatment of disc-herniation induced sciatica with infliximab: one year follow-up results of FIRST II, a randomized controlled trial. *Spine*. 2006;31:2759-2766.

Maravilla KR, Bowen BC. Imaging of the peripheral nervous system: evaluation of peripheral neuropathy and plexopathy. *AJNR Am J Neuroradiol*. 1998;19:1011-1023.

Milette PC. Reporting lumbar disk abnormalities: at last, consensus! *AJNR Am J Neuroradiol*. 2001;22:428-429.

Modic MT, Obuchowski NA, Ross JS, et al Acute low back pain and radiculopathy. *Radiology*. 2005;237:597-604.

Modic MT, Steinbert PM, Ross JS, et al. Degenerative disc disease; assessment of changes in vertebral body marrow with MR imaging. *Radiology*. 1988;166:193-199.

Morrison JL, Kaplan PA, Dussault RG, et al. Pedicle marrow signal intensity changes in the lumbar spine: a manifestation of facet degenerative joint disease. *Skeletal Radiol*. 2000;29:703-707.

Ohtori S, Inoue G, Ito T, et al. Tumor necrosis factor–immunoreactive cells and PGP 9.5–immunoreactive nerve fibers in vertebral endplates of patients with discogenic low back pain and Modic type 1 or type 2 changes on MRI. *Spine*. 2006;31:1026-1031.

Rahme R, Moussa R. The Modic vertebral endplate and marrow changes: pathologic significance and relation to low back pain and segmental instability of the lumbar spine. *AJNR Am J Neuroradiol*. 2008;29:838-842.

Ross JS, Obuchowski N, Zepp R. The postoperative lumbar spine: evaluation of epidural scar over a 1-year period. *AJNR Am J Neuroradiol*. 1998;19:183-186.

Ross JS, Masaryk TJ, Modic MT, et al. MR imaging of lumbar arachnoditis. *AJR Am J Roentgenol*. 1987;149:1025-1032.

Schenarts PJ, Diaz J, Kaiser C, et al. Prospective comparison of admission computed tomographic scan and plain films of the upper cervical spine in trauma patients with altered mental status. *J Trauma*. 2001;51:663-668.

Shellock F. *Magnetic Resonance Procedures: Health Effects and Safety*. Philadelphia CRC Press; 2001.

Stiel IG, Wells GA, Vandemheen KL, et al. The Canadian C-spine rule for radiography in alert and stable trauma patients. *JAMA*. 2001;286:1841-1848.

Thomsen H. Nephrogenic systemic fibrosis: a serious late adverse reaction. *Eur Radiol*. 2006;12:2619-2621.

Ulmer JL, Elster AD, Mathews VP, et al. Lumbar spondylolysis: reactive marrow changes seen in adjacent pedicles on MR images. *AJR Am J Roentgenol*. 1995;164:429-433.

Widder S, Doig C, Burrowes P, et al. Prospective evaluation of computed tomographic scanning for spinal clearance of obtunded trauma patients: preliminary results. *J Trauma*. 2004;56:1179-1184.

Full references can be found on Expert Consult @ www.expertconsult.com

CHAPTER 19

Physiologic Evaluation of the Brain with Magnetic Resonance Imaging

Amish H. Doshi ■ Pascal Bou-Haidar ■ Bradley N. Delman

Although the first magnetic resonance imaging (MRI) sequences provided largely anatomic information, over the past 20 years there have been considerable advances in the development of physiologic sequences that better illustrate disease processes. With MRI, radiologists are increasingly able to suggest more specific disease processes with greater accuracy. Perfusion and diffusion imaging allow rapid diagnosis of ischemia and infarction and can identify the so-called ischemic penumbra that may be rescued with aggressive therapy. The integrity of white matter tracts can be established with diffusion tensor imaging (DTI), and the more recent development of tractography allows graphic visualization of these tracts. Cerebrospinal fluid (CSF) flow patterns are demonstrated by performing cardiac-gated scanning to characterize bulk shifts in water. Blood oxygen level–dependent (BOLD) imaging characterizes changes in flow and oxygenation to specific areas of the brain during specific tasks to characterize the site and degree of brain activation. Spectroscopy offers a more specific understanding of metabolites in different areas of the brain and can therefore indicate areas of necrosis, anaerobic metabolism, and regions of accelerated cell membrane turnover or identify specific metabolites characteristic of specific disease processes.

DIFFUSION-WEIGHTED IMAGING

Diffusion-weighted imaging (DWI) has become an important tool in routine evaluation of the brain on MRI. On modern scanners a diffusion sequence may take 30 seconds or less, so many sites have added this technique to a standard brain-imaging protocol. Although DWI had initially been used predominantly to identify areas of acute ischemia, the appearances of other specific disease entities have been well characterized with this imaging method.

DWI characterizes differences in the brownian motion of water molecules, depending on their local environment. In bulk, water molecules can move freely in any direction. Biologic systems typically impede the free motion of water in one or more directions. Thus, cellular structure, permeability barriers, and various macromolecules within the brain parenchyma may all restrict the free diffusion of water molecules. Normally, restriction tends to be greater within the intracellular space than within the extracellular space[1]; thus, extracellular water molecules can diffuse more freely than intracellular molecules.

Physics

The imaging technique most often used for DWI is an echo planar imaging (EPI) sequence. In EPI, two separate and equal magnetic gradients are applied to opposite sides of the radiofrequency (RF) pulse during image acquisition. Use of these bipolar pulsed gradients allows detection of diffusional motion by changes in the magnitude of the moving spins from phase dispersion. Water molecules that do not travel significantly between excitation pulse and read pulse will not dephase significantly and will therefore retain much of their initial signal. Thus, in pathologic

states, the increased signal on DWI reflects an abnormal decrease in water diffusivity, typically caused by either loss of normal extracellular space (as seen in cytotoxic edema) or the presence of a highly viscous, proteinaceous, or cellular environment.[1,2] It is worth noting that loss of signal is not due to travel of water from one imaging voxel to another, but rather motion within the voxels themselves. Indeed, the average motion of a water molecule at 40°C is 2.5×10^{-3} mm^2/sec, which translates into motion of 22 μm in 100 msec; this is considerably smaller than the typical 1- to 2-mm voxel dimension.[3]

The magnitude of diffusion sensitization of DWI is determined by the "b-value," which in turn is related to the duration, strength, and time interval between the magnetic gradients. Therefore, higher b-values confer more sensitive DWI and thus yield improved contrast and ability to identify areas of water restriction; however, higher b-values also result in loss of signal, as well as noisier images, which may then have reduced utility. The b-value that is typically used in clinical assessment is approximately 800 to 1000 sec/mm^2,[4] but with certain applications, such as vertebral imaging or characterization of intracranial tumors, b-values may range from 500 to 2000 sec/mm^2 or greater.

The rate of diffusional motion is characterized by the apparent diffusion coefficient (ADC). This quantitative estimate of diffusivity can be achieved by acquiring two sets of images with different b-values, which can eliminate the effects of spin density and T1 and T2 relaxation. In clinical practice, one of the b-values would measure approximately 1000 sec/mm^2, as indicated earlier. The other b-value is typically 0 sec/mm^2, which reflects an image that does not have any motion-probing gradient applied (yielding so-called B0 images). ADC maps quantify differences between B0 and B1000 images and therefore nullify "T2 shine-through," a condition in which high B1000 signal is primarily due to high T2 signal rather than water restriction (Fig. 19-1). Thus, true restricted diffusion, as seen with acute ischemia, will demonstrate high signal on DWI and corresponding low signal on ADC maps.[1]

Clinical Uses and Applications

In clinical use, diffusion images are acquired in at least three directions, with the resulting images mathematically averaged to generate the *trace image* in which regions of normal white matter and gray matter appear fairly uniform. The normal brain shows slight variation in diffusion signal based on cellular structure. Gray matter has marginally higher signal on DWI, probably reflecting differing T2 properties rather than true differences in the ADC. Areas that are essentially water (most notably CSF) are dark on DWI sequences because of the free motion of water molecules in bulk water.[5]

The most completely characterized application of DWI is for the diagnosis and management of patients with acute cerebral ischemia. When perfusion does not meet the metabolic demand of territorial parenchyma, energy-dependent sodium-potassium adenosine triphosphatase ion pumps may fail. The resulting ion flux leads to the accumulation of water within the intracellular

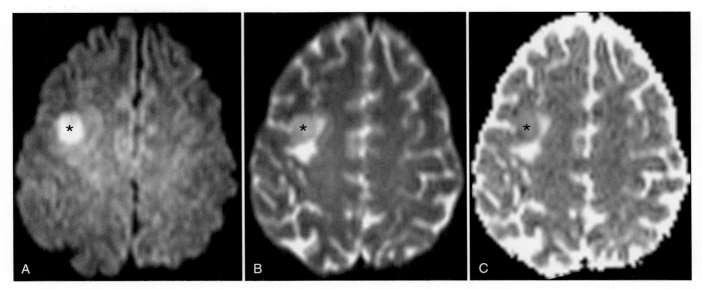

FIGURE 19-1 Breast carcinoma metastasis producing a T2 shine-through artifact. **A,** Axial diffusion trace image demonstrating a rounded focus of increased diffusion signal in the right posterior frontal lobe (*asterisk*). **B,** Corresponding T2 image (B0 image) showing increased signal in the same distribution (*asterisk*), thus suggesting that the diffusion signal may not reflect true restriction. **C,** Apparent diffusion coefficient map confirming that this area is not dark, so the lesion does not truly restrict diffusion.

compartment (cytotoxic edema). Neuronal swelling crowds the extracellular space, with resulting restricted motion of extracellular water molecules that is manifest as high DWI signal; these changes may be seen within minutes of tissue infarction. Normal brain ADC values range from approximately 740 to 840×10^{-6} mm^2/sec, with considerable overlap between white matter and gray matter values.[6] Parenchyma with ADC values of less than 500 to 550×10^{-6} mm^2/sec is almost certainly in the process of irreversible infarction. Intermediate ADC values (550 to 700×10^{-6} mm^2/sec) may reflect parenchyma that is ischemic yet still viable; it is this tissue that may be potentially salvageable with appropriate intervention. Although DWI is frequently identified as the most sensitive sequence for detecting infarction, other complementary sequences (such as the perfusion sequences described later) can help define an apparent impending infarction and define tissue at risk for infarction, the so-called *ischemic penumbra*.[7,8]

As infarcts age, the ADC and DWI patterns mature at differing rates. Although both become abnormal within minutes, the ADC increases from low signal to isointensity more rapidly, in most instances within 5 to 14 days. The ADC then continues to rise over the ensuing weeks to remain positive for the life of the patient, corresponding with encephalomalacia. DWI normalizes more slowly. It may reach isointensity with surrounding brain as long as 4 to 5 weeks after the infarction, and it will take even longer for signal to decline further in the setting of encephalomalacia (Fig. 19-2).

Certain intracranial neoplasms demonstrate restricted diffusion. Many of these neoplasms are tumors that are high in cellularity, with resulting high signal on DWI and low signal on the ADC map (i.e., true diffusion restriction). Examples include lymphoma, medulloblastoma, and portions of high-grade gliomas. Some tumors demonstrate restriction without high cellularity. Hence, although both epidermoid cysts and arachnoid cysts closely follow fluid intensity on T1, T2, and fluid-attenuated inversion recovery (FLAIR) sequences, the high DWI signal and heterogeneous low signal on the ADC map conferred by desquamated debris allow confident diagnosis of an epidermoid. Arach-

noid cysts, which instead contain simple fluid, demonstrate facilitated diffusion and therefore have the opposite diffusion pattern (low DWI signal and high ADC signal).[9]

Brain abscesses are typically peripherally enhancing lesions that are usually surrounded by significant vasogenic edema. Occasionally, these lesions can be difficult to differentiate from other peripherally enhancing masses such as necrotic tumors. The central cavity of an abscess demonstrates high signal on DWI and low signal on ADC maps. The restricted diffusion is most likely attributed to the high viscosity of proteinaceous fluid and the hypercellularity of inflammatory cells.[10-12]

Seizure activity can induce changes in water diffusivity because of cellular swelling and fluctuation in extracellular fluid. Cortical restricted diffusion has been seen with prolonged seizure activity, presumably caused by an imbalance between oxygen delivery and consumption.[13] Focal parenchymal changes in the postictal state can be seen as hyperintense signal changes on T2-weighted sequences with variability in DWI signal. In the setting of ischemia related to seizure activity, DWI may initially demonstrate restricted diffusion as a result of cytotoxic edema, but the restricted diffusion can later progress to decreased diffusion signal, which may represent gliosis of the involved tissue.[14]

DWI also aids in the diagnosis and further characterization of other disease processes. Restricted diffusion can be seen in zones of active demyelination in such disease processes as multiple sclerosis and progressive multifocal leukoencephalopathy (Fig. 19-3), in areas of active inflammation typically seen in the medial temporal lobes in herpes simplex encephalitis, in the anterior deep gray nuclei of the basal ganglia and along a discontinuous cortical ribbon in Creutzfeldt-Jacob disease, in some phases of hemorrhage, and in some encephalopathies and leukodystrophies.[1,9]

As indicated earlier, facilitated diffusion can be seen in patients with encephalomalacia and arachnoid cysts, with resulting low signal on DWI and high signal on ADC maps. Other entities with a similar pattern include cystic lesions, vasogenic edema, transependymal spread of CSF in hydrocephalus, tumor necrosis, and radiation necrosis.

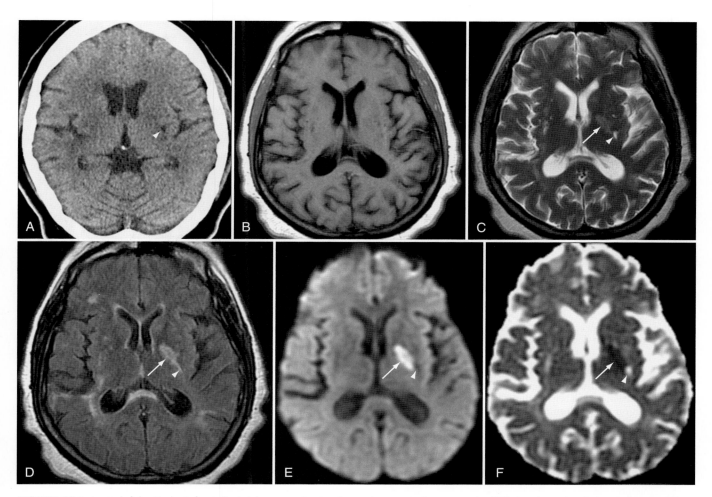

FIGURE 19-2 Acute left lenticular infarct. **A,** Axial non–contrast-enhanced computed tomography (CT) showing a focal chronic lacunar infarct (*arrowhead*), but no area suspicious for acute infarction. **B,** Axial T1-weighted image obtained 3 hours after CT showing no definite infarction. **C,** T2-weighted image showing an area of vague lenticular edema (*arrow*) distinct from the chronic lacunar infarct (*arrowhead*). **D,** A fluid-attenuated inversion recovery (FLAIR) T2-weighted image also shows the lenticular edema (*arrow*). The chronic lacunar infarct (*arrowhead*) is less conspicuous on FLAIR than on T2 imaging, probably related to the canceling effect of volume loss and gliosis on this sequence. **E,** Diffusion-weighted imaging showing increased signal corresponding with the infarct (*arrow*) in **C** and **D**, whereas the chronic focus (*arrowhead*) has no restriction. **F,** The apparent diffusion coefficient map is dark in the area of edema, thus confirming true restriction of diffusion (*arrow*). The lacunar infarction is mostly bright, which suggests facilitated diffusion, as is seen with volume loss (*arrowhead*).

Pitfalls and Limitations

EPI techniques allow ultrafast acquisition times, thereby almost eliminating motion artifact. However, the long echo train lengths needed to obtain the data render these sequences sensitive to both chemical shifts and magnetic susceptibility. Lipid suppression can be used to resolve some effects of chemical shift. Eddy currents result from the use of rapidly alternating gradients; these currents may result in significant distortion or misregistration between directional acquisition, which translates into blurring and loss of soft tissue contrast in the resulting trace image. Traditional DWI is prone to areas of susceptibility, most notably about the skull base, paranasal sinuses, and petrous bone, where air-bone-tissue interfaces are present.[5,15,16] In addition, the presence of paramagnetic and ferromagnetic material such as blood products or metal from surgery, trauma, or dental hardware can produce significant artifact, seen as ghosting, image distortion, and susceptibility artifact (Fig. 19-4). Newer techniques (periodically rotated overlapping parrallel lines with enhanced reconstruction [PROPELLER], BLADE, and others) use a rotating acquisition frame to minimize the effect of such artifacts and increase the sensitivity for abnormalities in previously challeng-

ing areas; however, these sequences may be associated with a significant increase in scanning time.

DIFFUSION TENSOR IMAGING AND TRACTOGRAPHY

Physics

DTI, a refinement of DWI, characterizes the dominant vector of water motion within voxels. In contrast to DWI, where typically only 3 directions (motion-probing gradients) are obtained, DTI requires at least 6 directions to resolve the mathematical ambiguities related to oblique fiber trajectories. Some centers increase signal either by acquiring multiple acquisitions in these 6 directions or by acquiring 25 or more directions; however, with both techniques, the additional scan time increases the risk for patient motion during the sequence and subsequent misregistration of the data.

As mentioned in the discussion on DWI, the water motion illustrated on diffusion sequences is predominantly extracellular,

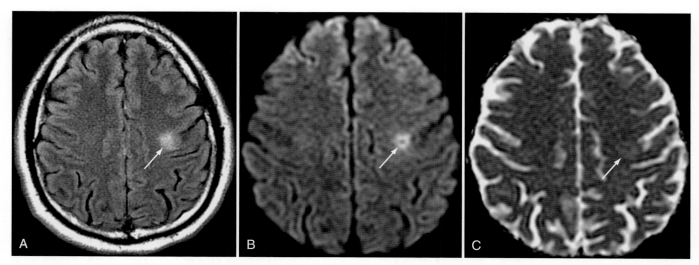

FIGURE 19-3 Forty-two-year-old man infected with human immunodeficiency virus and progressive multifocal leukoencephalopathy. **A,** Axial fluid-attenuated inversion recovery T2-weighted image showing a nonspecific area of high signal, possibly edema, near the vertex (*arrow*). **B,** Diffusion-weighted imaging showing a small area of corresponding signal abnormality, with restricted diffusion noted preferentially at the periphery (*arrow*). **C,** A slight increase in signal on the apparent diffusion coefficient map suggests T2 shine-through (*arrow*). Ordinarily, progressive multifocal leukoencephalopathy does not enhance, but with the polydrug regimen and immune reconstitution, one may see more distinctive restriction of diffusion and enhancement, both of which are absent in more indolent cases.

and the vector of motion tends to parallel the white matter tracts. In DTI, the acquisition of at least six directions allows mathematical construction of a tensor ellipsoid whose major axis points in the direction of the dominant fiber tract within a voxel.[17] In voxels in which white matter tracts are homogeneous and nearly

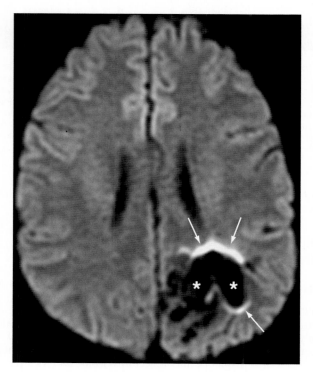

FIGURE 19-4 Axial trace diffusion image showing susceptibility around an arteriovenous malformation. This lesion had been embolized previously. There is significant signal loss within the embolized bed (*asterisks*) and a halo of high signal distortion around the margin of the embolized nidus (*arrows*). Note that posteromedially, where a small amount of patent nidus remains, one sees low signal flow voids but considerably less susceptibility and distortion.

colinear, this ellipsoid is thin and elongated in a so-called *prolate* or cigar-shaped configuration, with the dominant axis (major *eigenvector*) being significantly greater than the two perpendicular axes (minor *eigenvectors*). Such ellipsoids are *anisotropic*; that is, they represent voxels whose fibers have a strong directional bias. When white matter tracts are not as colinear (i.e., when there are many crossing or divergent fibers) or in areas of gray matter or CSF, the tensor ellipsoid is nearly spherical. These ellipsoids are further characterized as *isotropic*; that is, they lack significant directional bias.

Once tensors have been calculated, they may be presented for interpretation in numerous ways. A mean diffusivity map portrays average molecular motion that is independent of tissue directionality, so voxels with high motion such as water will be bright and voxels with low motion such as gray matter will be dark. A fractional anisotropy (FA) map represents the colinearity and integrity of fibers, and therefore large tracts with parallel white matter bundles, as seen in the callosum fibers and descending corticospinal tract, appear white (FA approaches 1). CSF, gray matter, and crossing white matter tracts all lack parallel axonal configuration and thus appear dark or black (FA approaches 0). Color-encoded directional maps overlay fiber directional data on an FA image, with typical color assignments of red representing transverse fibers, green representing anteroposterior fibers, and blue representing superoinferior fibers; brighter or more saturated fibers indicate greater colinearity and hence greater anisotropy (Fig. 19-5).

Tractography is a mathematical method of tracking theoretical fiber trajectories by using vector data to incrementally advance to adjacent voxels. Tracking is typically initiated by placing a source "seed" over an area of interest. A second "target" seed can be placed to determine a destination focus to which the trajectory must run, or the second seed may be omitted to allow tracking software to course spontaneously to determine all potential tracts leading from the source seed.

Clinical Uses and Applications

DTI can be a very useful tool for demonstrating the integrity or compromise of tracts running between different areas of the brain. Four classic patterns of abnormal fiber orientation have

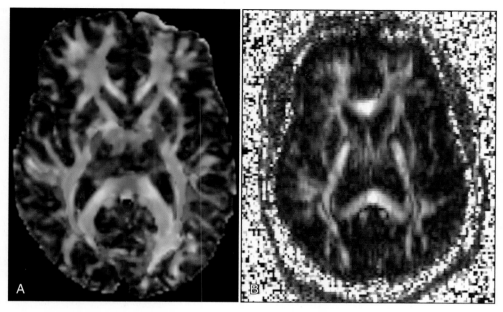

FIGURE 19-5 Normal diffusion tensor maps. **A,** Color-encoded diffusion tensor map showing primary tract orientations. By convention, *red* indicates right-left fibers, *green* indicates anterior-posterior fibers, and *blue* indicates superior-inferior fibers. Oblique directions are represented by intermediate colors, so for example, as splenial fibers leave the midline and angle toward the occipital lobe, they change from *red* to *orange* to *yellow* to *lime-green* to *green*. **B,** Fractional anisotropy map indicating the degree of anisotropy within given voxels. The voxels containing nearly colinear fibers (e.g., genu, splenium, posterior limb of the internal capsule) appear bright, with fractional anisotropy approaching 1. The gray matter has proportionately fewer fibers that are more arbitrarily oriented; they appear dark and have fractional anisotropy approaching 0. Note that when fiber tracts cross, for example, lateral to the posterior margins of the ventricles, signal drops completely because conventional acquisition and processing techniques are unable to resolve discordant orientation data.

been described: (1) deviated but otherwise preserved fiber tracts, (2) edematous tracts with diminished FA but preserved fiber tract orientation, (3) infiltrated tracts with diminished FA and abnormal fiber tract orientation, and (4) frank destruction of fiber tracts with negligible anisotropy.[18] Figures 19-6 and 19-7 illustrate varieties of tract disruption.

Such assessment of tracts can aid in planning treatment and determining prognosis, thereby allowing surgeons and radiation oncologists to protect tracts that are preserved while more aggressively addressing tracts that have already been destroyed. This has tremendous surgical importance because with these data a surgeon can maximize resection while minimizing risk to adjacent structures. A study by Kikuta and colleagues involving patients who had undergone resection for arteriovenous malformations (AVMs) found that incomplete tractography of the optic radiation was associated with visual field loss postoperatively.[19] Such information not only assists in surgical planning but also helps prepare patients for potential outcomes of surgery. In addition, for patients undergoing surgery to treat brain tumors near the motor pathways, tractography may be used to identify initial sites for electrocortical stimulation, thus facilitating faster localization of eloquent cortex during surgery.

Applications of DTI extend beyond tumor evaluation. Preliminary studies suggest that DTI may be sufficiently sensitive to detect early changes in vulnerable regions in individuals with certain cognitive disorders, even at the presymptomatic or preclinical stages.[20] Additional uses for tractography include assessment of patients with multiple sclerosis, and early studies in stroke patients suggest that DTI can aid in prognosis and may detect corticocortical rewiring.

DTI and tractography have recently been applied to the spinal cord, an area previously too degraded by artifact to image successfully. Some authors now suggest that FA data from DTI may be useful in distinguishing surrounding cord edema from tumor.[21] In spinal cord AVMs, FA values in surrounding cord may improve after embolization and correlate with enhanced patient outcome.

Pitfalls and Limitations

A major limitation of conventional DTI is its poor distinction of crossing fiber tracts. When a voxel contains a homogeneous population of similarly oriented fibers, calculation of the dominant vector or water motion is straightforward. However, when a voxel contains crossing fibers, a simple tensor calculation is unable to reflect the more complex fiber configuration. In this instance, the major eigenvector may be calculated as the average of all voxel fibers, and as a result the eigenvector may not represent any of the dominant tracts.[22] Newer techniques such as high–angular resolution diffusion imaging (HARDI) and Q-ball imaging may use 100 or more directions along with complex mathematical techniques to better characterize intravoxel tract ambiguity.[23]

The DTI sequence is also prone to artifacts that result in local field distortion and sometimes signal dropout. Thus, the diffusion signal may be compromised in regions adjacent to postoperative air, blood products, and surgical clips or embolic material. As in DWI, eddy currents can also distort images in DTI and result in image misregistration and computational errors; in these instances, correction software can compensate for at least some of the distortion to yield more accurate maps.

Tractography depends on user input to define tracts of interest. Incorrect or suboptimal region-of-interest placement will result in misrepresented tracts. Mathematical assumptions will also influence tractography generation, with tract validity being dependent on appropriate definition of the maximal angulation within a voxel, the minimum FA value to tolerate while generating the tract, and the total path length. Because signal in the cord is more variable than signal in the brain and because the cord moves with CSF pulsation, spinal tractography proves considerably more

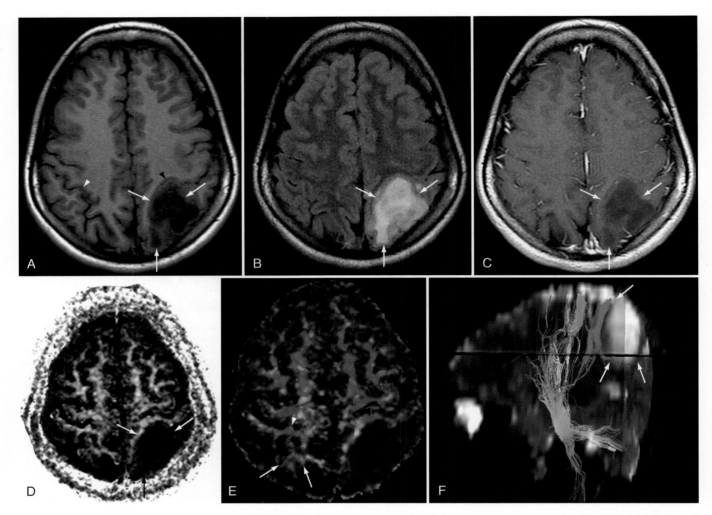

FIGURE 19-6 Infiltrating parietal glioma. **A,** Axial T1-weighted image showing a slightly heterogeneous low-signal mass within the left parietal white matter (*arrows*), with the mass causing effacement of the overlying sulci. The intraparietal sulcus is compressed and displaced anteriorly (*black arrowhead*). The normal right intraparietal sulcus is shown for reference (*white arrowhead*). **B,** Fluid-attenuated inversion recovery T2-weighted image showing high signal corresponding with low intensity on T1 (*arrows*), and there is little enhancement after gadolinium (**C**) (*arrows*). **D,** Fractional anisotropy map showing loss of anisotropy corresponding to tumor (*arrows*). **E,** Tensor color map demonstrating anterior displacement and more strongly inferior (more *blue*) orientation of fibers within postcentral gyral white matter (*black arrowhead*) than in the normal position on the contralateral side (*white arrowhead*). Note that the normal white matter anatomy seen posteriorly on the right (*hatched arrows*) is obliterated on the left. **F,** Diffusion tractography showing displacement of fibers around the tumor (*arrows*).

challenging. In general, tractography in the cervical cord is easier to generate than in the thoracic cord, at least in part because of the greater pulsation effects in the mid and lower cord.[21]

MAGNETIC RESONANCE ANGIOGRAPHY

Evaluation of the intracranial vascular system is important in the diagnosis and planning of treatment of many vascular-related disease processes such as aneurysms, AVMs, infarction, and sinus venous thrombosis. Although the "gold standard" for evaluation of many vascular entities is currently digital subtraction angiography (DSA), magnetic resonance angiography (MRA) offers an alternative for the assessment of intracranial vessels that is both noninvasive and does not require the use of ionizing radiation. The three main varieties of MRA used clinically are time-of-flight (TOF), phase-contrast (PC), and contrast-enhanced (CE) techniques. Each MRA is typically postprocessed by a technologist before interpretation to yield maximum intensity projections that can be rotated in space for a three-dimensional (3D) effect (Fig. 19-8).

Physics

TOF MRA is performed by applying repetitive pulses to stationary tissues in a discrete volume of the brain, which results in saturation or suppression of signal in these tissues. Blood flowing into the volume has not been saturated and is therefore fully magnetized; this in-flowing blood therefore provides the only significant signal within the imaging slab. The intrinsic contrast that is derived from flowing blood eliminates the need for injection of contrast material to visualize the intracranial vessels. The pulse sequence used typically consists of a gradient recalled echo (GRE) sequence, which is acquired with either a two-dimensional (2D) or 3D technique. 2D TOF images are obtained as contiguous or slightly overlapped sections, whereas 3D TOF images are derived from one or more overlapping 3D volumes. Of these two methods, 3D TOF is more commonly used than 2D TOF because of its superior spatial resolution.[24]

In PC MRA, the vascular contrast is obtained by applying a bipolar phase-encoding gradient and a velocity-encoding (VEnc) factor.[25,26] Phase shifts in moving spins or flowing blood are

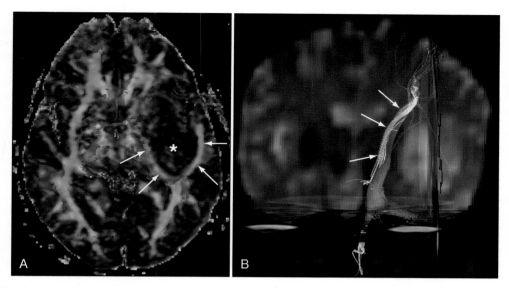

FIGURE 19-7 Diffusion tensor characterization of white matter integrity around a glioma centered near the sylvian point. **A,** The lesion itself has low anisotropy (*asterisk*) because of its high cellular nature and lack of organized white matter tracts. The surrounding white matter is splayed and compressed (*arrows*). As the compressed arcuate fasciculus extends posteriorly around the mass, the color orientation changes from *green* (anteroposterior) to *yellow* (anteroposterior oblique) to *orange* (transverse oblique) to *red* (transverse); as these fibers project anteriorly again, the colors repeat in reverse. **B,** Tractography demonstrates that the corticospinal tracts are deviated medially (*arrows*) but appear grossly intact.

obtained when gradients with opposing polarities are applied twice during a single RF excitation. This method results in nulling of signal from stationary tissue while exploiting signal from flowing blood. Visualization of blood flow depends on the velocity of the flow. In specific encoding orientations, middle-gray usually represents no flow, whereas progressively increasing shades of white or black indicate directionally encoded higher

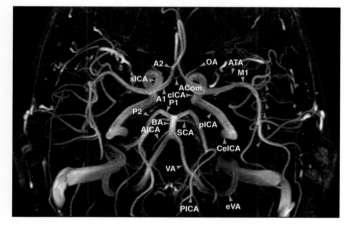

FIGURE 19-8 Collapsed maximum intensity projection of a three-dimensional time-of-flight magnetic resonance angiogram. Although the technique is optimized to evaluate for visualization of arteries, veins with high flow are also seen, including the sigmoid/jugular systems and sphenoparietal drainage. A1, first segment of the anterior cerebral artery; A2, second segment of the anterior cerebral artery; ACom, anterior communicating artery; AICA, anterior inferior cerebellar artery; ATA, anterior temporal artery; BA, basilar artery; CeICA, cervical internal carotid artery; cICA, cavernous internal carotid artery; eVA, extracranial vertebral artery; M1, first segment of the middle cerebral artery; OA, ophthalmic artery; P1, first segment of the posterior cerebral artery; P2, second segment of the posterior cerebral artery; pICA, petrous internal carotid artery; PICA, posterior inferior cerebellar artery; *purple arrowheads,* sylvian middle cerebral artery branches; SCA, superior cerebellar artery; sICA, supraclinoid internal carotid artery; VA, intracranial vertebral artery.

velocities up to the predefined VEnc factor. Blood that flows at velocities higher than the VEnc factor will demonstrate aliasing, a situation in which signal intensity "wraps around" and will therefore be opposite that expected. In other words, if flow in a certain direction matches the VEnc factor, it will be encoded as white, but any greater velocity in that direction will actually appear as black. Because arterial flow is more rapid than venous flow, the typical arterial VEnc factor intracranially measures greater than 60 to 80 cm/sec, whereas slow flow within veins and venous sinuses is best imaged with a VEnc factor of 20 cm/sec or less.[26] Images generated from this technique provide not only direction of flow but also magnitude of flow.

CE MRA uses a high-resolution T1-weighted technique in which the vessels are accentuated by a bolus of gadolinium chelate. The 2% to 3% concentration of gadolinium contrast agent in blood (by volume) causes a marked T1-shortening effect in vessels with a resultant increase in vessel signal. CE MRA provides anatomic information related to lumen diameter and the concentration of contrast material in vessels rather than physiologic information reflecting the flow rate, as calculated with TOF and PC techniques. Advantages of CE MRA over non-CE techniques include higher signal-to-noise ratios, decreased susceptibility to artifacts caused by pulsatility and flow, shorter image acquisition times, and temporal resolution that illustrates patterns of flow over time. Older CE MRA paradigms (e.g., elliptic-centric techniques) had collected full RF spectral data during the bolus, so only about three full-volume MRA repetitions could be acquired per minute. However, with that technique, the intended arterial-phase imaging was frequently obscured by venous enhancement. The need for improved temporal resolution led to the development of time-resolved CE MRA, such as TRICKS (time-resolved imaging of contrast kinetics) and TREAT (time-resolved echo-shared angiography technique).[24] These sequences improve temporal resolution by repetitively acquiring the center of the RF spectrum along with varying peripheral portions during each acquisition; data missing from unsampled regions are interpolated by using data obtained at other points in time. This development enables more rapid 3D acquisitions before, during, and after transit of a contrast bolus, thereby allowing identification of the arterial, capillary, and venous phases.[27,28]

Clinical Uses and Applications

The angiographic modality with unparalleled spatial and temporal resolution is DSA. However, manipulation of catheters in the aorta or in the carotid or vertebral arteries, even by an experienced operator, is associated with a 1.3% risk for a cerebral event.[29] Therefore, in clinical practice most institutions still use noninvasive techniques such as computed tomographic angiography (CTA) or MRA for preliminary evaluation of the vascular tree in the clinical setting of infarction, aneurysm, AVM, dural arteriovenous fistula (AVF), and veno-occlusive disease.

Stroke

A cerebrovascular accident, or stroke, is major cause of morbidity and mortality. It is the third most common cause of death in the United States, with approximately 795,000 cases occurring annually. The majority of these cases are caused by atherosclerotic disease, which results in stenosis and progressive occlusion of an arterial vessel. This can lead to ischemia and potential infarction of the brain tissue involved. MRA has been used to study the major arterial intracranial vessels to evaluate the effect of atherosclerotic disease. Specifically, 3D TOF MRA has been used as a screening method in stroke patients because it is minimally invasive and provides a reasonable assessment of the degree of vessel occlusion. Studies have shown 100% detection of vessel occlusion on 3D TOF MRA when correlated with DSA; however, grading of stenosis is less accurate (61%) when using MRA.[30] Additionally, visualization of vessels that demonstrate slow or turbulent flow can be improved with the use of contrast material injected intravenously. For example, CE MRA has been shown to offer better visualization of the internal cerebral and middle cerebral arteries that exhibit artifactual narrowing on 3D TOF MRA because of slow or turbulent flow.[31] Although such limitations exist, TOF MRA remains an important sequence for evaluation of the intracranial arterial circulation in patients with acute neurological symptoms.

Intracranial Aneurysms

Detection of intracranial aneurysm can be done with noninvasive techniques such as MRA and CTA. 3D TOF MRA has been shown to have an overall sensitivity of 87% and specificity of 95% for the detection of intracranial aneurysms (Fig. 19-9). The sensitivity for detection of aneurysms larger than 3 mm is greater than that for aneurysms 3 mm or smaller (94% versus 38%) on older 1.5T scanners.[32] At a magnetic field strength of 3T, aneurysms as small as 1 mm can be detected.[33] Both TOF MRA and

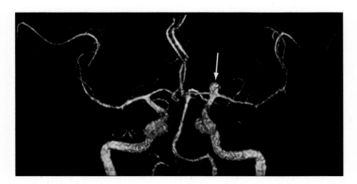

FIGURE 19-9 Surface rendering of a three-dimensional time-of-flight magnetic resonance angiogram reveals an aneurysm at the left internal carotid artery bifurcation (*arrow*).

CE MRA are optimized to show vessel lumens; apical thrombus may remain undetected unless MRA is correlated with conventional sequences that are more sensitive for nonflowing blood.

Studies have shown similarities and differences between 3D TOF MRA and CE MRA in the detection of aneurysms. One study demonstrated no significant difference in the quality of the images and equal detection rates for both techniques.[34] Another study showed that 3D TOF MRA detected more aneurysms than CE MRA did,[35] whereas a third study indicated a sensitivity of 100% and a specificity of 94% for CE MRA, hence suggesting that CE MRA may be superior to the 3D TOF technique.[36] Thus, there remains no clear consensus regarding which modality is superior, but both provide relatively accurate noninvasive methods for the detection of aneurysms.

MRA has also been studied for the follow-up of intracranial aneurysms treated by coil embolization. Serial studies have been performed with the use of both 3D TOF and CE MRA after treatment to evaluate for delayed aneurysm configuration because recanalization is estimated to occur in 10% to 40% of patients.[37] Studies evaluating residual flow in coil-treated aneurysms have shown a sensitivity and specificity of 81% and 90.6%, respectively, for 3D TOF MRA and 86.8% and 91.9%, respectively, for CE MRA.[38] It has been suggested that CE MRA may be slightly more sensitive in evaluating residual slow flow.[24] DSA does remain the gold standard for evaluation of residual filling in treated aneurysm, but studies have shown 86% to 94% agreement between 3D TOF MRA evaluation and DSA.[39-41]

Vascular Malformations

AVMs and AVFs are typically evaluated with DSA because of its excellent spatial and temporal resolution. However, MRA techniques may also provide an accurate noninvasive method for preoperative planning and evaluation of AVMs.[42,43] 3D TOF MRA and PC MRA allow characterization of flow in abnormal vessels, but they do not provide information on the hemodynamics of vascular malformations.[44] Because definition of the architecture in and around malformations (e.g., arterial feeders, nidus size, and draining veins) is crucial in the evaluation of AVMs, advances in temporal resolution have had a large impact on noninvasive evaluation of these abnormalities. Indeed, ultrafast CE MRA and time-resolved CE MRA techniques have been shown to define relationships between lesions and the vasculature better than TOF and routine CE MRA techniques.[45,46] Specific types of time-resolved CE MRA such as TRICKS MRA have been developed to provide hemodynamic information that gives one the ability to detect processes previously undetectable on noninvasive imaging, such as early venous drainage (Fig. 19-10).[24] For example, in a small series of 40 patients, time-resolved MRA at 3 T was shown to be a reliable technique for the evaluation and surveillance of dural AVFs.[47]

Intracranial Venous System and Sinus Venous Thrombosis

MRA techniques can be applied to study the intracranial venous system. Although arterial flow provides robust signal on 3D TOF sequences, the slower flow in veins provides more limited signal with 3D techniques. 2D TOF techniques are used instead because they offer excellent sensitivity for slow flow and less saturation effects than with 3D TOF techniques (Fig. 19-11).[48] 2D TOF best depicts flow perpendicular to the scanning plane, so areas of turbulent or tortuous flow (e.g., from the straight sinus through the transverse sinus through the sigmoid sinus) may require imaging in more than one acquisition plane to adequately represent flow patterns. In addition to TOF magnetic resonance venography (MRV), 2D or 3D PC MRV may be used because

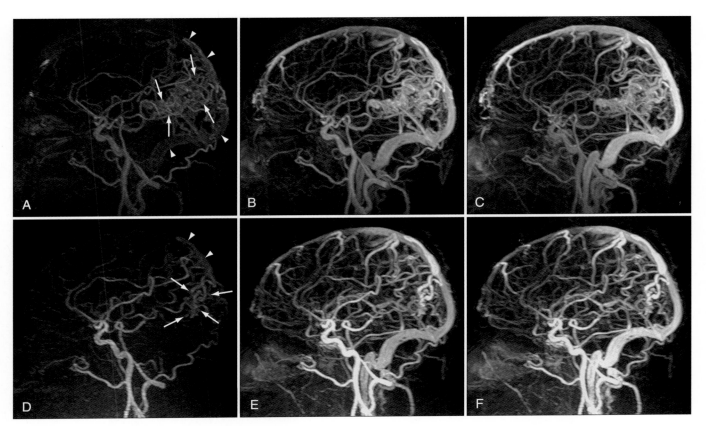

FIGURE 19-10 Time-resolved contrast-enhanced magnetic resonance angiography showing embolization of an arteriovenous malformation. All images are thick-section maximum intensity projections at progressively later points in time during the bolus transit. **A-C,** Pre-embolization scans at early arterial (**A**), slightly later (**B**), and discrete venous (**C**) phases. The corresponding postembolization images **D** to **F** parallel **A** to **C**. In the pre-embolization arterial scan (**A**), a large posterior cerebral artery feeder supplies an abnormal large wedge-shaped parietal-occipital area (*arrows*). The presence of venous enhancement in this early arterial phase (*arrowheads*) confirms abnormal shunting. The arterial phase in the postembolization image (**D**) shows a considerable reduction in the volume of the perfusing nidus, with a small focus remaining posteriorly (*arrows*). Note that even with the small residual nidus there is still early venous enhancement (*arrowheads*).

these techniques can indicate not only the rate of flow but also the directionality of flow. However, the dependence of PC MRV on operator-defined VEnc parameters may complicate its use,[49] with incorrect assumptions at the time of scanning potentially leading to artifacts on the final images.

MRV can be enhanced by exploiting the paramagnetic effects of intravenous gadolinium. CE MRV has been shown to provide significantly better visibility of venous structures, including deep cerebral veins, than possible with the TOF technique. Selected venous structures studied in a small group of patients demonstrated visibility of 99% with CE MRV and 72% with TOF MRV. CE MRV can also be helpful in reducing the effects of turbulent flow on visualization of the venous sinuses.[50]

Pitfalls and Limitations

Various MRA techniques can serve as an alternative to DSA imaging, although limitations in both spatial and temporal resolution still render DSA the gold standard in evaluating most neurovascular pathologies. However, MRA is used widely because it is noninvasive (or minimally invasive if gadolinium is injected). Therefore, it is important to be familiar with limitations of the various vascular MR techniques.

Spin dephasing can occur when blood flow is complex or turbulent and when vessels are in close proximity to tissues with short T1 properties, such as fat and subacute hemorrhage (met-

hemoglobin). This configuration may result in loss of signal on TOF and PC MRA. Slow flow can also result in similar loss of signal on these imaging sequences because of spin saturation.[51,52] Flow saturation effects can be diminished by using the "multiple overlapping thin slab acquisition" (MOTSA) technique for 3D TOF MRA (Fig. 19-12). Most institutions use three or four such slabs in an MRA acquisition through the head; this technique improves flow signal in vessels but lengthens imaging times.

Velocity aliasing can be seen with PC MRA when true velocities exceed the VEnc parameter of the imaging sequence.[53] This may result in the perception of motion opposite the actual direction of blood flow; however, experienced radiologists will recognize the abrupt transition from black to white (or vice versa) as artifactual. In addition, factors such as lengthier acquisition times, lower spatial resolution, and artifacts related to pulsatile flow have limited the use of PC MRA in comparison to TOF and CE MRA.[54] Thus, many sites reserve PC MRA to answer specific questions about flow directionality rather than including it as a standard imaging sequence.

Studies have reported high sensitivity and specificity ranging from 94% to 96% for 3D TOF MRA in the evaluation of intracranial stenosis. However, the MRA technique has a tendency to overestimate the degree of stenosis. A small study demonstrated overestimation of stenosis in 37% of diseased intracranial arterial segments with 3D TOF MRA when compared with DSA.[55] Even though such measurement errors do limit the positive predictive

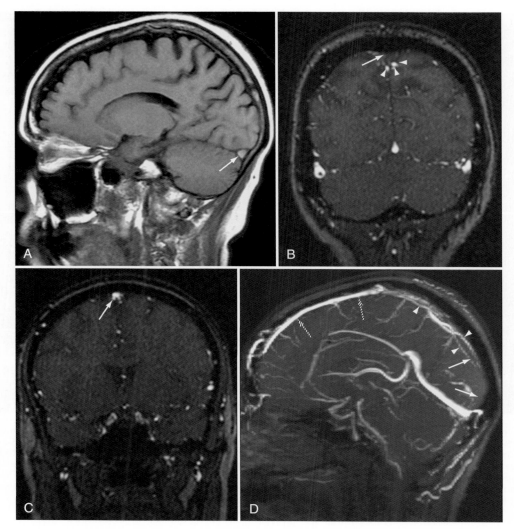

FIGURE 19-11 Dural venous thrombosis. **A,** Sagittal paramidline non–contrast-enhanced T1-weighted image demonstrating increased signal in the transverse sinus (*arrow*), suggestive of thrombosis rather than flowing blood. **B,** Coronal source data from two-dimensional time-of-flight magnetic resonance venography posteriorly shows low signal where the superior sagittal sinus is expected (*arrow*), but flow within adjacent cortical veins is well seen (*arrowheads*). **C,** More anteriorly, flow is confirmed in the superior sagittal sinus (*arrow*), which drains anteriorly. **D,** A sagittal maximum intensity projection of time-of-flight venography data better defines the flowing superior sagittal sinus anteriorly (*hatched arrows*) but not posteriorly (*arrows*). Flow within cortical veins (*arrowheads*) should not be mistaken for patency of the superior sagittal sinus.

value of TOF MRA in evaluating intracranial stenosis, this technique is still frequently used because of its high negative predictive value and its noninvasive technique.[44]

Failure to visualize appropriate signal in a normally flowing sinus may relate to MRV acquisition in a plane parallel to that of venous flow. This is a common limitation in the interpretation of these images and often mandates closer assessment of the source images. In instances in which true thrombosis is suspected, the acquisition plane may be modified, or CE MRV may be performed to improve sinus visualization.[49]

PHASE-CONTRAST MAGNETIC RESONANCE IMAGING OF CEREBROSPINAL FLUID FLOW

CSF flow studies have been used to evaluate a variety of conditions related to defined or suspected hydrocephalus. In particular, PC MRI provides a method for both qualitative and quantitative assessment of intracerebral and cervical CSF flow. The technique

is a reliable and rapid tool available for characterization of CSF flow dynamics. In most instances, gating can be achieved with a pulse oximeter.

Physics

As in PC MRA, a PC acquisition can be used to quantify the rate and directionality of CSF flow. A similar bipolar gradient is applied to stationary tissue to cancel the magnetization from stationary spins and null the signal from these tissues. CSF that moves through the plane of acquisition between two separate gradient pulses will experience a net phase shift that is proportional to its velocity along a selected axis.[56,57] The VEnc factors used in PC CSF studies are typically lower than those used for PC MRA, averaging 10 to 15 cm/sec. Imaging is usually acquired in the midline sagittal plane, although other orthogonal or oblique planes can be prescribed as well if needed.

PC CSF study differs from PC MRA in its use of cardiac gating. Hence, with this technique, magnitude and direction of

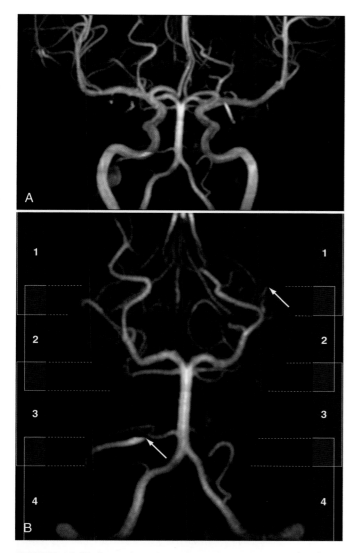

FIGURE 19-12 Coronal maximum intensity projections of a three-dimensional time-of-flight magnetic resonance angiogram (**A**) and segmented projection of the vertebrobasilar system only (**B**). The sequences are ordinarily acquired by using multiple overlapping slabs to increase the conspicuity of vessels. Where slabs overlap (indicated schematically by bright *green* reflecting slabs 1 plus 2, or 2 plus 3, or 3 plus 4), one sees better signal but also abrupt increase in venous signal (*arrows* in **B**).

flow can be segregated by phase in the cardiac cycle. Sixteen phases are typically acquired through the cardiac cycle, with triggering generally based on detection of each electrocardiographic R wave.[58] In patients with normal sinus rhythm, adequate data are acquired through the cardiac cycle. Certain arrhythmias may compromise gating, however, and limit signal, particularly in the later phases.

Clinical Uses and Applications

PC MRI has been used to evaluate CSF flow in a wide range of cerebral disorders, including communicating hydrocephalus, normal-pressure hydrocephalus, and aqueductal stenosis. Recently, analysis of CSF pulsation in the axial plane at the foramen magnum has improved our understanding of the role of CSF flow disturbances in patients with symptomatic Chiari I malformations. PC MRI has been used to demonstrate elevated

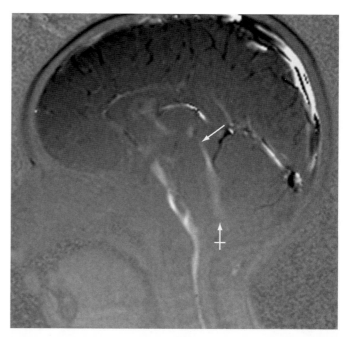

FIGURE 19-13 Normal cerebrospinal fluid (CSF) flow pattern. A superior-inferior sensitized image from a phase-contrast CSF flow study shows flow through the aqueduct (*arrow*), through the fourth ventricle, and past the outlet foramina (*hatched arrow*).

peak systolic velocities through the subarachnoid space and foramen magnum in these patients in comparison to normal subjects.[59]

Normal Cerebrospinal Fluid Flow

PC MRI sequences are usually analyzed in both static and cine formats. Typically, CSF flow sequences will generate magnitude, phase, and three orthogonal PC flow-encoded sets. Of greatest utility are the directional series that characterize flow within a structure. In the case of midline CSF flow from the third ventricle through the fourth ventricle outlet foramina, the most useful direction would conform most closely to the z-axis (Fig. 19-13). Shades representing one direction versus another may vary by scanner vendor; in practice, radiologists typically refer to the structures with known flow patterns (e.g., the deep venous system) to determine which shades represent which directions of flow.

During a normal cardiac cycle, there is rhythmic movement of not only CSF but also brain parenchyma. Cardiac pulsations are transmitted through the intracranial arteries and capillaries and result in motion within the CSF. The relationship between the cardiac cycle and CSF is perceived as normal oscillatory CSF flow. During systole, expansion of the cerebral arterial vessels creates a pressure wave within the subarachnoid CSF. This pressure wave is transmitted through the intracranial subarachnoid space and results in outflow of CSF through the foramen magnum into the compliant spinal CSF space. In diastole, the arterial relaxation and resulting change in intracranial pressure cause CSF to flow back into the cranium through the foramen magnum.[57,60] PC MRI techniques can be used to demonstrate the pulsatile flow within the CSF compartments and have been used to demonstrate the mechanical coupling between blood flow and CSF flow.[61-64] Cine CSF flow studies have shown that normal CSF pulsations exhibit a timed sequence of oscillatory flow at specific sites in the ventricular system and subarachnoid spaces.[58] The full length of the aqueduct can often be outlined by upward

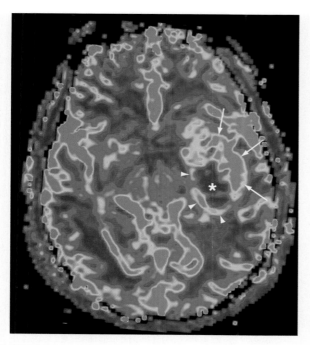

FIGURE 19-17 Relative cerebral blood volume map of a patient with a large necrotic glioma. The area of suspected viable tumor has variable blood patterns. Centrally, where necrosis was identified on anatomic imaging, there is little or no blood volume (*asterisk*). A thin band of increased blood volume is seen along the medial aspect of the cavity (*arrowheads*), but it is the lateral aspect of the cavity (*arrows*) that shows the most prominent perfusion pattern. Characterization of such blood flow patterns may aid surgeons by identifying the most metabolically active areas for biopsy planning so that the pathologist can grade the most aggressive portion of the tumor.

parameters are related by the equation CBF = CBV/MTT.[77] It is worth noting that unlike CT perfusion, in which image density is linearly dependent on contrast concentration, in MR perfusion the relationship of signal to contrast concentration is curvilinear. As a result, most contrast MR perfusion studies in the brain will refer to *relative CBV* and *relative CBF*, and therefore comparison of suspected pathologic perfusion with normal contralateral perfusion is necessary.

A less prevalent variety of dynamic scanning is *permeability* imaging (Fig. 19-18). Although gadolinium does not normally pass through the blood-brain barrier (BBB), when the BBB is disrupted there is slow extravasation of contrast material into surrounding tissue. The pattern and rate of extravasation can be documented by dynamic repetitive acquisition of rapid T1-weighted MR images. This technique enables calculation of the microvascular permeability of the BBB. Permeability may be followed by perfusion imaging in one study session, with the added advantage that the permeability scan pre-enhances pathologic tissue and thus results in more normal return of the perfusion curve to baseline during PWI.

Arterial spin labeling (ASL) does not use intravenous gadolinium but instead assesses perfusion by labeling protons in the large arteries of the neck.[78,79] These labeled protons then course intracranially within the blood pool and result in diminished signal. A second acquisition is generated without water labeling to serve as a baseline volume. Hemodynamic parameters and maps are generated on the basis of differences between the two acquisitions (Fig. 19-19).[80]

Another technique used for obtaining perfusion images without gadolinium enhancement depends on the BOLD technique, which is discussed further in the section "Functional Magnetic Resonance Imaging."

Clinical Uses and Applications

The combination of PWI and DWI in patients with brain ischemia can help distinguish viable tissue that is at risk for infarction (i.e., the penumbra) from the nonviable infarcted tissue core, which would have DWI restriction and markedly reduced CBV (Fig. 19-20).[77] In addition to its application in cerebral ischemia from large-artery stenosis, as well as small-vessel disease, PWI can be used to characterize changes in perfusion in such entities as vasculitis, moyamoya, and vasospasm (Fig. 19-21). This holds particular promise in the assessment of peripheral ischemia in the setting of vasospasm (as from subarachnoid hemorrhage), which is difficult to quantify with catheter angiography.

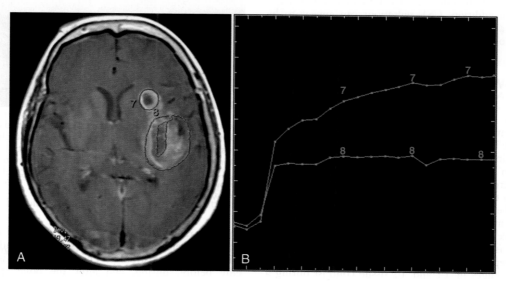

FIGURE 19-18 Permeability map in the same patient as in Figure 19-17. **A,** Axial T1-weighted gadolinium-enhanced image showing region-of-interest placement and (**B**) corresponding time-dependent enhancement curves. Curve 7 from the more anterior cavity shows a rapid first-phase rise and continued rise in the second phase at a lower rate. This is suggestive of radiation necrosis. Curve 8 from the necrotic cavity more posteriorly shows a rapid rise in the first phase but leveling out in the second phase. This is suggestive of viable tumor.

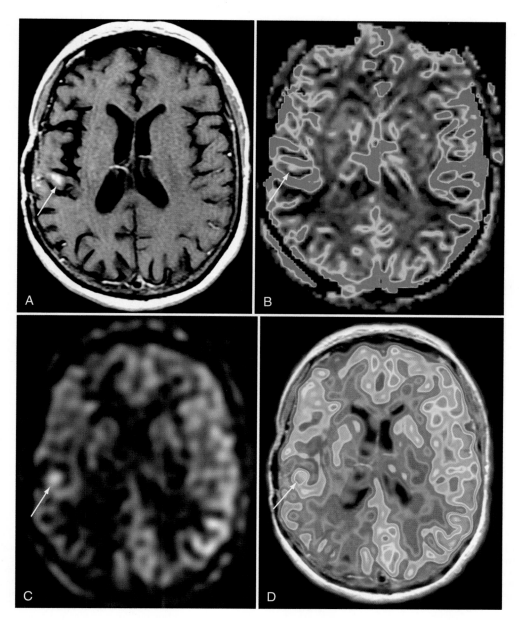

FIGURE 19-19 Tumor recurrence. **A,** Axial T1-weighted contrast-enhanced image revealing a nodular area of enhancement in the right superior temporal lobe (*arrow*). **B,** Relative cerebral blood volume map showing a very subtle nodule of increased perfusion (*arrow*) that could escape detection among the many sylvian vessels. **C,** Continuous arterial spin labeling map showing the focus of increased perfusion (*arrow*) more clearly than possible with the gadolinium bolus technique. In both **B** and **C** there is generalized diminished perfusion to the right hemisphere, particularly posteriorly, from previous radiation therapy. **D,** A colorized spin labeling image from **C** superimposed on the anatomic image from **A** confirms that both abnormalities (*arrow*) represent the same process.

Perfusion examinations are also frequently performed to estimate the hemodynamics of brain tumors. Perfusion data can aid in the differential diagnosis, with increased perfusion seen in gliomas as a result of angiogenesis related to aggressiveness and tumor viability.[81] PWI has also become useful after treatment in distinguishing radiation necrosis from tumor recurrence.[82] Both tumor growth and radiation necrosis will exhibit contrast enhancement related to disruption of the BBB, but the enhanced perfusion of neoplastic tissue (similar to or greater than adjacent "normal" tissue) contrasts with the diminished perfusion in radiation necrosis. Identification of zones of hyperperfusion may also help the surgeon target the most metabolically active area if the patient requires subsequent biopsy.[83]

Pitfalls and Limitations

As a technique optimized to image susceptibility, dynamic susceptibility contrast imaging is also exquisitely sensitive to static structures in and around the brain that induce a strong magnetic field inhomogeneity. Thus, chronic blood products (hemosiderin), calcification, metal, or air (postoperative or in a paranasal sinus/mastoid cell) can cause artifacts and distortion of the perfusion data set. At standard slice thicknesses and gaps, small regions of hypoperfusion may escape detection, and attempts to increase resolution will reduce signal and prolong the scan time with a resulting reduction in temporal resolution.

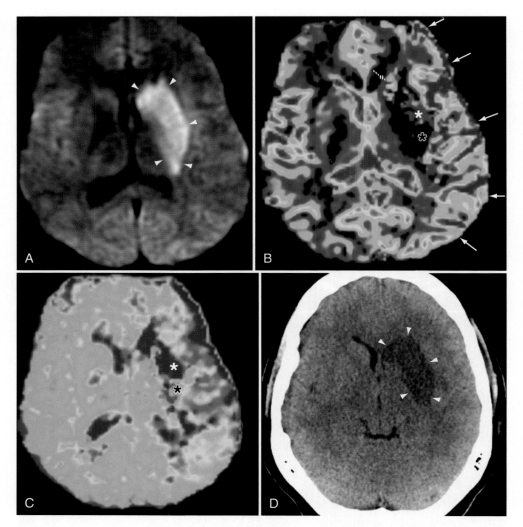

FIGURE 19-20 Diffusion-perfusion mismatch. **A,** An axial diffusion-weighted image obtained within 8 hours of the onset of symptoms reveals a large focus of restricted diffusion primarily conforming to the left lenticular nucleus, with additional involvement of the caudate head antero-medially and the anterior and posterior limbs of the internal capsule (*arrowheads*). This was dark on the apparent diffusion coefficient map and corresponded with acute infarction. **B,** A dynamic susceptibility perfusion imaging cerebral blood volume map shows variable patterns within the infarct bed; the spectrum ranges from very low blood volume in the posterior lenticular nucleus (*black asterisk*), to slightly higher volume in the mid and anterior lenticular nucleus (*white asterisk*), to an increased vascular pool (greater than the contralateral side) in the left caudate head (*hatched arrow*). There is a generalized increased volume in the more superficial left middle cerebral artery territory (*arrows*). **C,** The mean transit time map parallels the blood volume map, with prolonged transit time through the penumbra, but the posterior lenticular infarct (*black asterisk*) and internal capsule have slightly more rapid transit than does much of the remaining infarct bed (*white asterisk*). **D,** Delayed axial nonenhanced computed tomography shows that the final infarct territory (*arrowheads*) correlates well with the diffusion abnormality; the more superficial penumbra did not ultimately infarct.

With regard to tumors, distinction between tumor growth/recurrence and radiation necrosis can still be confusing and problematic, especially since both processes may coexist in similar areas.[84] In addition, calculation of relative CBV can be grossly inaccurate in lesions such as glioblastoma multiforme, in which there is severe breakdown of the BBB.[78] Furthermore, the extent of tumor infiltration into adjacent tissue is suboptimally characterized, particularly in areas where there is early infiltration but not yet neovascularity. Finally, tumor histology cannot reliably be inferred from perfusion data because some of the lower grade cerebral tumors such as oligodendrogliomas can have markedly increased perfusion that would otherwise be more suggestive of higher grade tumors.

FUNCTIONAL MAGNETIC RESONANCE IMAGING

Physics

Functional MRI (fMRI) characterizes brain hemodynamic activity by indirectly revealing areas of neuronal activation after various stimulation by motor, visual, auditory, and tactile sensory input, most commonly in the form of "block paradigms." Shortly after presentation of stimuli (or the onset of motor activity), the increase in cortical activity leads to increase in local CBF. The oxygen delivered by this increased blood flow is greater than the demand of tissue for oxygen, and as a result there is a net

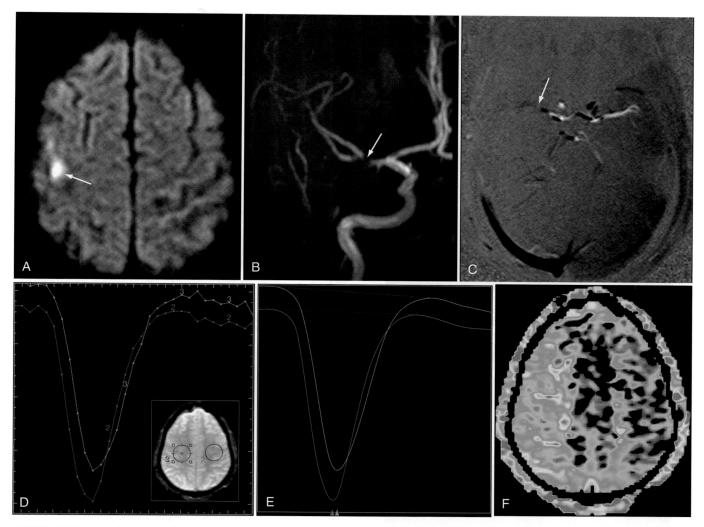

FIGURE 19-21 Sixty-five-year-old patient with a history of coronary heart disease evaluated for acute left upper extremity weakness. **A,** Focus of restricted diffusion in the right precentral gyrus (*arrow*) was confirmed on an apparent diffusion coefficient map. **B,** A frontal maximum intensity projection of a 3D TOF MRA through the right internal carotid artery and tributaries confirms the stenosis (*arrow*), with irregular calibers of the more distal branches. **C,** Phase-contrast magnetic resonance angiography, with left flow indicated in *white* and right flow indicated in *black*, demonstrates a focal narrowing in the luminal profile (*arrow*) and poor flow more distally. **D,** Region-of-interest intensity curves over the central white matter in each hemisphere (right, *green*; left, *purple*). The more gadolinium that perfuses a vessel, the greater the drop in signal. **E,** Smoothed curves showing the slight delay in perfusion to the right (the *green arrowhead* indicates the later peak). The area under the curve, bounded by the curve itself and a line drawn between the shoulders of the curve, is proportional to blood volume. **F,** The resulting blood volume map shows increased volume to essentially the entire right middle cerebral artery territory. Vasodilation is an early autoregulatory responses to diminished pressure.

increase in oxyhemoglobin in the capillary bed. This increase in oxyhemoglobin is associated with a relative decrease in deoxyhemoglobin, whose paramagnetic properties ordinarily cause a reduction in local signal. Hence, with the reduction in deoxyhemoglobin comes a transient net increase in local signal.[85] Because this technique depends on variation in oxygenation levels in blood, it is frequently referred to as BOLD imaging (Fig. 19-22).

BOLD EPI therefore identifies areas of increased MR signal from activated brain cortex. In practice, typical paradigms consist of three or four sets of alternating "on" periods, where sensory stimulation, cognitive tasks, or motor activity is present, and "off" periods, which are free of such stimulation. Differences between "on" and "off" measurements help determine where blood flow is affected by the stimulus or activity. Activation maps are generated by determining the statistical threshold above which true activity is likely. This activation pattern is then typically color-coded and superimposed on a high-resolution T1-weighted MRI

sequence of the same section or on a 3D model for anatomic recognition.[86]

Clinical Uses and Applications

Mapping of cognitive functions has clear implications for surgical planning (Fig. 19-23). Preoperative identification may limit intraoperative awake testing if certain functions are localized away from the surgical bed. Functional data can be further exploited by processing in conjunction with DTI data; a site of activation can serve as a seed for DTI tractography to identify the trajectory of fibers (such as pyramidal tracts) that emanate from certain cortical areas so that they may be avoided during surgery.[87]

fMRI may also be used to demonstrate the eloquent regions of the brain and to determine right/left dominance. Most studies are sufficient to demonstrate the location of sensorimotor, speech, and auditory areas of the cerebral cortex.[88]

When interpreting the MRS data it is crucial to consider what metabolites are found in normal spectra and at what concentrations. Conspicuity of metabolites is affected by the echo time (TE) used, which ranges from very short (25 msec or less) to intermediate (144 msec) to long (288 msec).

N-Acetylaspartate (NAA, 2.0 ppm) is the highest peak in normal spectra and is classically described as a marker for neuronal integrity and density. Malignant tumors and neuronal death are associated with a decline in NAA.

Choline (3.2 ppm) is a metabolic marker of membrane density and integrity. Malignant tumors show an increase in the choline peak because of increased cell membrane turnover; however, elevated choline can also be seen in inflammatory processes as well.

Creatine (3.0 and 3.94 ppm) is a marker of energy metabolism. Because creatine values are relatively stable, the ratio of another metabolite to creatine helps normalize the concentration of that metabolite.

Glutamate and glutamine represent the Glx complex (2.1 to 2.5 ppm). Glutamate is the most abundant excitatory neurotransmitter, but the Glx complex is typically best seen with very short echo times and may not be well resolved on intermediate or long echo clinical scans.

Lactate (1.33 pm) is not seen under normal conditions but is present in scenarios of anaerobic glycolysis, such as in brain ischemia and seizures. At intermediate echo times (TE = 144 msec), it is an inverted doublet, seen below the baseline, whereas at TE = 288 msec it has a positive peak.

Myoinositol (3.56 ppm) is a glial marker that is found almost exclusively in astrocytes and is believed to reflect the degree of glial proliferation.

Alanine (1.48 ppm) has a role in the citric acid cycle and can be increased in meningiomas.

Lipid (0.8 to 1.2 ppm) may be seen as a broad peak or two peaks at longer echo times, but it may be better visualized on MRS with short echo times. Lipid can be seen in areas of increased cell turnover, but its presence may also indicate voxel contamination by fat in the diploic space, the scalp, and subcutaneous tissues when the voxel is placed near one of these structures.[94]

A quick assessment is frequently used to characterize the three most prominent metabolites in normal brain parenchyma: NAA, creatine, and choline. The imaginary line that connects the peaks of these metabolites normally slopes up from the left to the right at approximately 45 to 50 degrees, a so-called normal *Hunter's angle*. A reduction in this angle is seen with neuronal destruction. Reversal of this angle (with the choline peak higher than the NAA peak) is strongly suggestive of tumor but can be seen with ischemic processes, inflammatory conditions, and even neurodegenerative disease.

Clinical Uses and Applications

MRS is now perhaps most widely used for the characterization of brain neoplasms (Fig. 19-26). In general, with increasing grade of glioma, one sees a reduction in the NAA peak and elevation of the choline peak (Fig. 19-27). The ultimate diagnosis is made by pathologic evaluation, but MRS can aid in determining the prognosis in some patients; for example, the percent change in the choline-NAA ratio has been shown to be useful for predicting progression of brain tumor in children. Overall, spectroscopy should be considered as a supplement to other imaging data in tumor analysis. Integration of spectroscopy data with perfusion data, enhancement pattern, and the remaining conventional MRI sequences increases the accuracy of predicting tumor grade and differentiating radiation necrosis from tumor recurrence.

In addition to tumors, recent work has shown the utility of MRS in other conditions. In seizure disorders, spectroscopy may be used to lateralize the side of hippocampal sclerosis by demon-

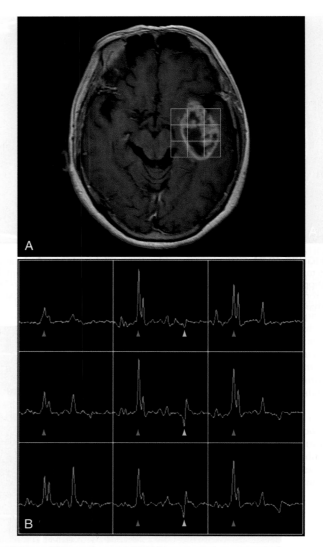

FIGURE 19-26 Infiltrating medial temporal glioma. **A,** Axial contrast-enhanced image showing the predominant peripheral enhancement with central stippling and necrosis. The overlying grid shows voxel locations. **B,** A magnetic resonance spectroscopy grid as defined in **A** shows the greatest lipid-lactate (*yellow arrowheads*) concentration in the central column, whose voxels contain the greatest apparent degree of necrosis. There is also a prominent choline signal (*purple arrowheads*) in virtually every voxel.

strating decreased NAA and elevated Glx and myoinositol. It can also demonstrate bilateral temporal sclerosis, but correlation and confirmation with electroencephalography are advised.[95] MRS may detect early changes in Alzheimer's dementia before gross findings on MRI, with decreasing NAA and increasing myoinositol observed in the occipital, temporal, parietal, and frontal regions. In imaging of patients with traumatic brain injury, reductions in the NAA-creatine and NAA-choline ratios have been shown to be a reliable index for an unfavorable outcome and may help to identify which patients have a greater likelihood of regaining consciousness.[96,97] Certain metabolic conditions have characteristic metabolite aberrations, such as the markedly elevated NAA in Canavan's disease, which reflects a deficiency in the myelin synthesis pathway. In practice, MRS and DWI can be considered complementary methods for evaluating neurometabolic disease to give detailed information about the neurochemistry of affected brain areas.[98]

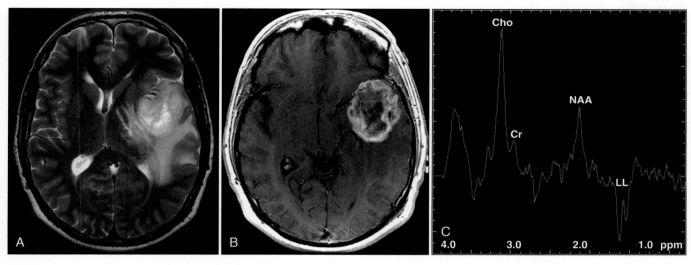

FIGURE 19-27 Infiltrating glioma. **A,** Axial T2-weighted image demonstrating a necrotic mass centered in the medial left temporal lobe, with significant edema extending through much of the temporal lobe and into the gangliocapsular structures. **B,** Contrast-enhanced T1-weighted image showing heterogeneous enhancement predominantly about the periphery with finer strands of enhancement central amid necrosis. The *purple box* defined placement of the single spectroscopy voxel. **C,** Spectroscopy performed at intermediate echo time (TE = 144 msec) demonstrates an inverted lactate doublet at 1.3 to 1.4 ppm (LL), a dramatically elevated choline peak at 3.2 ppm (Cho), and a small residual *N*-acetylaspartate (NAA) peak at 2.0 ppm. Other metabolites, including the glial cell marker myoinositol, as well creatine (Cr) and glutamine derivatives, are also seen between 3.5 and 4.0 ppm.

Pitfalls and Limitations

The concentrations of normal metabolites in the brain vary in different age groups. Metabolites in normal subjects younger than 2 years differ from the spectral patterns seen in subjects 2 years and older (through adulthood). In these young children there is a reversal of the NAA-creatine and choline-creatine ratios. Changes are also seen in the elderly, who exhibit a normal decline in the level of NAA.

As stated earlier, the grade of an astrocytic tumor as a guide is thought to be proportional to the choline concentration. In evaluating the spectra of brain tumors, some highly malignant tumors such as glioblastoma multiforme may artifactually show low choline because of extensive necrosis. Furthermore, it is not uncommon to find some low-grade gliomas with very high choline-creatine and choline-NAA ratios. It is widely appreciated, however, that because of the heterogeneity of tumor, there is a significant overlap in the spectroscopy indices used to grade gliomas.[99]

SUGGESTED READINGS

Barnett A. Theory of Q-ball imaging redux: implications for fiber tracking. *Magn Reson Med.* 2009;62:910-923.

Barrett T, Brechbiel M, Bernardo M, et al. MRI of tumor angiogenesis. *J Magn Reson Imaging.* 2007;26:235-249.

Brandes AA, Tosoni A, Spagnolli F, et al. Disease progression or pseudoprogression after concomitant radiochemotherapy treatment: pitfalls in neurooncology. *Neuro Oncol.* 2008;10:361-367.

Cha S. Neuroimaging in neuro-oncology. *Neurotherapeutics.* 2009;6:465-477.

Detre JA. Clinical applicability of functional MRI. *J Magn Reson Imaging.* 2006; 23:808-815.

Hattingen E, Blasel S, Dettmann E, et al. Perfusion-weighted MRI to evaluate cerebral autoregulation in aneurysmal subarachnoid haemorrhage. *Neuroradiology.* 2008;50:929-938.

Heiss WD, Sorensen AG. Advances in imaging. *Stroke.* 2009;40:e313-314.

Holdsworth SJ, Bammer R. Magnetic resonance imaging techniques: fMRI, DWI, and PWI. *Semin Neurol.* 2008;28:395-406.

Lacerda S, Law M. Magnetic resonance perfusion and permeability imaging in brain tumors. *Neuroimaging Clin N Am.* 2009;19:527-557.

Olivot JM, Marks MP. Magnetic resonance imaging in the evaluation of acute stroke. *Top Magn Reson Imaging.* 2008;19:225-230.

Ozsarlak O, Van Goethem JW, Maes M, et al. MR angiography of the intracranial vessels: technical aspects and clinical applications. *Neuroradiology.* 2004; 46:955-972.

Paldino MJ, Barboriak DP. Fundamentals of quantitative dynamic contrast-enhanced MR imaging. *Magn Reson Imaging Clin N Am.* 2009;17:277-289.

Roberts TP, Mikulis D. Neuro MR: principles. *J Magn Reson Imaging.* 2007; 26:823-837.

Soares DP, Law M. Magnetic resonance spectroscopy of the brain: review of metabolites and clinical applications. *Clin Radiol.* 2009;64:12-21.

Sunaert S. Presurgical planning for tumor resectioning. *J Magn Reson Imaging.* 2006;23:887-905.

Thurnher MM, Law M. Diffusion-weighted imaging, diffusion-tensor imaging, and fiber tractography of the spinal cord. *Magn Reson Imaging Clin N Am.* 2009;17:225-244.

Tieleman A, Deblaere K, Van Roost D, et al. Preoperative fMRI in tumour surgery. *Eur Radiol.* 2009;19:2523-2534.

Wallace RC, Karis JP, Partovi S, et al. Noninvasive imaging of treated cerebral aneurysms, part I: MR angiographic follow-up of coiled aneurysms. *AJNR Am J Neuroradiol.* 2007;28:1001-1008.

Wolf RL, Detre JA. Clinical neuroimaging using arterial spin-labeled perfusion magnetic resonance imaging. *Neurotherapeutics.* 2007;4:346-359.

Zou Z, Ma L, Cheng L, et al. Time-resolved contrast-enhanced MR angiography of intracranial lesions. *J Magn Reson Imaging.* 2008;27:692-699.

Full references can be found on Expert Consult @ www.expertconsult.com

CHAPTER 20

Molecular Imaging of the Brain with Positron Emission Tomography

William P. Melega ■ Antonio A. F. De Salles

Advances in our understanding of the molecular mechanisms of diseases are providing the clinician with new targets for therapeutic intervention. Long-term evaluation of these therapies will be necessary to provide critical information about efficacy, and an essential assessment modality will be the noninvasive molecular imaging technology of positron emission tomography (PET). PET is used to assess rates of biologic processes in vivo throughout the brain and body by using subnanomolar concentrations of radioactively labeled biologic probes. As such, PET provides quantitative radioassays of biochemical activity without producing significant disturbances in the biologic system being assessed. The types of data obtained with PET extend across different levels of biologic function. For example, PET can be used to assess glucose metabolic rates, blood flow, blood-brain barrier permeability, enzyme activity, synthesis and release of neurotransmitters, neuroreceptor densities, mood states, substance abuse, and most recently, gene expression.[1,2] In the brain, PET has been used to image alterations in neurochemical activities related to normal development, aging, and disease states. For both the basic researcher and clinician, assessment of central nervous system function with PET has been extended to studies of quantitative features of motor, visual, somatosensory, behavioral, and cognitive function. In pharmacology studies, novel approaches have been developed to measure the in vivo pharmacokinetic and pharmacodynamic actions of therapeutic drugs in human subjects with tracer doses.[3] For clinical applications, PET is used for the detection of tumor and planning of surgical procedures. Multiple PET studies over time can also be used to provide a chronologic record of the subject's disease status and treatment efficacy.

This chapter presents the major principles of PET and an overview of the PET imaging modality. Selected examples are used to illustrate the positive impact of PET on the differential diagnosis of brain dysfunction.

BASIC PRINCIPLES OF POSITRON EMISSION TOMOGRAPHY

The essential components of PET are as follows:

1. Production of the positron-emitting radionuclide in a cyclotron
2. Radiopharmaceutical synthesis procedures to attach the positron-emitting radionuclide to a molecule of interest, which is called a *tracer* or *probe*
3. Positron tomograph camera (PET scanner) to measure the photons resulting from positron-electron annihilation and computer algorithms to construct images based on localization of the positron-emitting radionuclides
4. Tracer kinetic model for the interpretation of temporal changes in the regional distribution, accumulation, and clearance of the positron-emitting radionuclides

Each of these topics is described here in sufficient detail to enable the reader to interpret PET data from human studies.

References to comprehensive reviews on each topic are included for further study.[4,5]

The Cyclotron and Radiochemical Procedures

Positron-emitting radionuclides are generated in a cyclotron. In this machine, charged particles (protons, deuterons, or negative hydrogen ions) are accelerated in a circular path to achieve sufficient kinetic energy. The particles are then directed to bombard a stable isotope and the resultant interaction creates a new, unstable, proton-rich isotope. This isotope becomes a more stable atom by a nuclear process in which a proton is converted to a neutron, a positron (the antiparticle of the electron with the same mass but positively charged), and a neutrino. The positron and neutrino are emitted from the nucleus of the radioactive species at a characteristic decay rate, depending on the particular isotope. The positron-emitting isotopes most often produced for PET studies are radioactive forms of oxygen (^{15}O), nitrogen (^{13}N), carbon (^{11}C), and fluorine (^{18}F). These isotopes have decay rates in the range of minutes to hours (e.g., half-lives of 2 minutes for ^{15}O and 109 minutes for ^{18}F) and are ideally suited for biologic imaging because there is sufficient time to image their presence in the body without producing long-term radiation exposure (see Table 20-1 for the physical characteristics of radioisotopes). These radioisotopes can be readily incorporated into a wide variety of molecules, including the labeling of physiologic substrates (e.g., glucose, amino acids), neuroreceptor ligands, and substrates and inhibitors of enzymes. The injectable end product is then introduced into the body, usually by intravenous injection. Because these compounds are injected in minute quantities (subnanomolar concentrations) and do not produce pharmacologic effects, they are referred to as biologic tracers or probes. The tracer is then distributed throughout the body in accordance with its delivery, uptake, and metabolism characteristics. Throughout this time, the tracer continues to decay and emit positrons and neutrinos. The neutrinos pass through the body and are not detected. Wherever the tracer is trapped in tissues, the positrons travel only a short distance (≈ 1 mm) and lose energy in collisions with electrons in the tissue, until they collide with nearby electrons, which results in annihilation of the two particles and conversion of their masses into two gamma-ray photons, referred to as annihilation photons. These photons each have an energy of 511 keV and are projected linearly at approximately 180 degrees to each other. They have a high probability of escaping the body without attenuation, which allows their detection. A pair of detectors set at 180 degrees to each other can register the arrival of these photons and localize the positron emitter along that line of travel, referred to as a coincidence line, or line of response. For a given localized concentration of positron emitters, the resultant photon pairs are emitted in all directions and can be detected by a circumferential ring of scintillation detectors (Fig. 20-1). On combining the lines of response from many different angles, the data are reconstructed with a mathematical algorithm (special coincidence technique called a *reconstruction algorithm*) to establish their distribution pattern, a pattern that corresponds to

TABLE 20-1 Physical Properties of Selected Positron-Emitting Radionuclides

RADIONUCLIDE	HALF-LIFE	MAXIMAL POSITRON ENERGY (MeV)
^{18}F	109.7 min	0.64
^{11}C	20.4 min	0.96
^{13}N	9.96 min	1.19
^{15}O	2.07 min	1.72
^{22}Na	2.6 yr	0.55
^{64}Cu	9.7 min	0.65
^{68}Ga	67.6 min	1.89

regional concentrations of the radionuclide. These profiles are then used to produce tomographic brain images, which can then be coregistered with computed tomography (CT) or magnetic resonance imaging (MRI) to obtain precise anatomic localization.[6]

For a PET brain study, the tracer, on injection, is distributed and accumulated in tissues as a function of time. Accordingly, different time intervals of data acquisition (frames) are used to discriminate these time-dependent changes in regional concentrations of activity. Immediately after injection of the tracer, short time frames of 1 minute or less are acquired to image the rapid changes in radioactivity, whereas at later times, longer time frames of 5 to 10 minutes suffice. These temporal and spatial distributions of radioactivity are then fitted to a kinetic model that has been designed to quantify the biologic process being investigated.

Camera and Brain Imaging

The PET camera is a sophisticated imaging instrument that is used to measure the photons generated from positron-electron annihilation. The PET camera can acquire data in intervals that range from seconds to minutes, thereby allowing monitoring of many biologic processes. The quality and quantity of the acquired data from a particular PET camera are a function of technical parameters, some of which are described later. These parameters are often listed in the methods sections of PET studies because they provide critical information on the quality of the data acquisition.

Sensitivity refers to the fraction of positron emission events within a field of view that is detected by the camera. As the relative sensitivity of a camera increases, more counts from the same amount of radioactivity are detected, which results in an increase in the signal-to-noise ratio and therefore better image quality.

Spatial resolution, or the ability to accurately locate events, refers to the smallest distance between two points that can be distinguished by the PET scanner. This parameter defines the ability of the camera to differentiate spatial activity and is based primarily on the camera detector elements, with smaller elements providing better detail. A typical clinical PET camera has a spatial resolution of 5 to 8 mm; small animal scanners have a resolution as low as 2 mm.[7] With recent advances in detector and scanner design technology, the sensitivity and spatial resolution of PET have dramatically improved, especially as data collection has evolved from a two- to a three-dimensional mode of acquisition (which increases the number of gamma rays being collected). State-of-the-art PET cameras can now image subregional cortical and subcortical structures throughout the brain (Fig. 20-2).

Full width at half-maximum (FWHM) is a technical term that refers to the width of a gaussian-shaped curve at half its maximal peak value. When activity is acquired from a single point source, the PET camera has a limited ability to accurately locate that

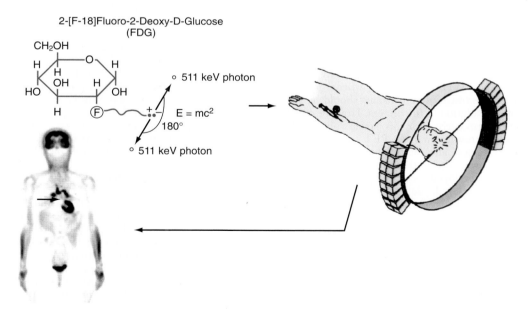

FIGURE 20-1 The positron-electron interaction results in their annihilation and the coincident emission of two 511-keV photons at 180 degrees to each other. Detection of the essentially simultaneous arrival of these annihilation photons at the positron emission tomography camera detectors establishes a coincidence line (line of response). In an actual tomogram that registers the photons emitted from regions of accumulated radioactivity, there are about 1 to 2 million detector pair combinations that can record these events simultaneously. For a subject injected with [^{18}F]fluoro-2-deoxy-D-glucose (FDG), the distribution and accumulation of radioactivity throughout the entire body can be imaged by sequentially moving the subject through the ring of detectors. The *darker areas* represent regions of higher glucose metabolic rates. *(Adapted from Phelps ME. PET: The merging of biology and imaging into molecular imaging. J Nucl Med. 2000;41:661-681.)*

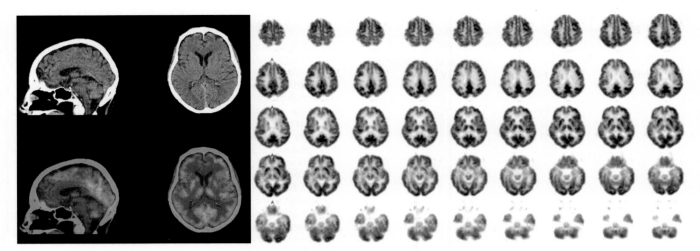

FIGURE 20-2 [^{18}F]Fluoro-2-deoxy-D-glucose (FDG) and positron emission tomography (PET)–computed tomography (CT) imaging. **Left,** The two columns show the tomographic planes of sagittal (*column 1*) and transaxial (*column 2*) CT data (*top row*) and the PET data overlaid on the CT images (*bottom*). **Right,** Transaxial planes of FDG-PET images covering the superior to inferior extent of the brain. The *darker areas* represent regions of higher glucose metabolic rates and clearly delineate cortical and subcortical structures. (*Courtesy of D. H. Silverman, M.D., Ph.D., Department of Molecular and Medical Pharmacology, David Geffen School of Medicine, University of California, Los Angeles.*)

activity, which results in a spatial distribution of that activity that resembles a bell-shaped curve. The corresponding FWHM for that distribution is used to define the spatial resolution of the PET camera (i.e., objects that are closer together than one FWHM cannot be distinguished).

Partial volume correction describes methods for removing errors in the regional quantification of activity caused by analysis of regions that are smaller in width than twice the spatial resolution of the camera (i.e., regions with a diameter less than two times the FWHM). For example, if the FWHM is expressed as 4 to 5 mm, any structure less than 10 mm will be affected by concentrations of radioactivity in the surrounding areas. If the structure of interest has a higher concentration than adjacent structures, its concentration of radioactivity will be underestimated. In contrast, if the structure of interest has a lower concentration than adjacent structures, its radioactivity will be overestimated. In general, a region of interest should be quantified only when its size is twice that of the FWHM. Therefore, whenever a small region of interest is quantified, its dimensions should be stated relative to the spatial resolution of the camera. However, further processing of the data can correct for this partial volume effect, provided that the spatial resolution of the PET camera, the exact size and shape of the region, and the relative concentrations of radioactivity are all known. The methods of partial volume correction that have been developed require an MRI scan or other anatomic brain image of the individual.[8]

Image reconstruction refers to the mathematical process of creating an image from a series of detection events obtained from the PET camera. Radioactive decay events are detected as lines of response, and a reconstruction algorithm is used to determine the distribution of radioactivity from the summation of all observed lines of response. The most commonly used reconstruction algorithm initially was called *filtered backprojection (FBP)*. With FBP, the counts from all detector pairs are projected back along the lines of response where they originated, which results in overlapping of backprojections and a corresponding two-dimensional distribution of emission origins. Before projection, these data are processed with a mathematical filter algorithm, relatively graded from sharp to smooth, to improve the signal characteristics. Sharp filters result in better spatial resolution and more statistical noise, whereas smooth filters result in less resolution and a reduction in statistical noise.[9] The FBP method is increasingly being replaced by iterative reconstruction methods (e.g., maximal likelihood estimation) that essentially begin with an estimated image based on the intersection of lines of response followed by comparison of its calculated projection data with the actual projection data. With subsequent iterations, the image is revised until convergence is achieved, with limiting factors being the technical features of the detector system.

Tracer Kinetic Models

Hundreds of PET tracers have been synthesized for research in animal and human imaging studies. A representative list of positron-labeled compounds is presented in Table 20-2 to illustrate the wide range of imaging applications. It should be emphasized that the initial PET data acquisition reflects the total radioactivity in a region over the time that the data were acquired. Because only radioactivity is measured in the brain and not the relative concentrations of the tracer and its metabolites, optimal use of a particular PET tracer requires an appropriate tracer kinetic model to interpret the observed changes in radioactivity levels. Tracer kinetic models provide a mathematical framework by which the time course of tracer distribution and changes in regional concentrations of accumulated radioactivity are used to derive rates of biologic processes.

To construct kinetic models, the biologic process is categorized into compartments (e.g., plasma and a tissue region would represent a two-compartment model) and then formulated by differential equations that describe exchange of the isotope between compartments.[10] In general, models contain parameters that are used to determine transport rates of the tracer into and out of the region of interest, the extent of tracer-receptor binding, and enzymatic activities. The images that are constructed from these parameters and subsequent model fitting are referred to as parametric images.

A typical three-compartment tracer kinetic model is presented in Figure 20-3. After intravenous injection of the tracer, the time course of the tracer concentration in plasma (obtained from arterial blood samples) is determined. This plasma-time activity curve is referred to as the input function and is used to provide a quantitative parameter on tracer availability to the brain as a function of time.

Additionally, FDG has been used in conjunction with FDOPA to provide a complementary assessment of compensatory regional alterations in glucose metabolism.[22] These PET assessments have been used to differentiate idiopathic Parkinson's disease from related movement disorders.

An alternative to FDOPA assessment of striatal dopamine system integrity is obtained with PET tracers that bind selectively to the presynaptic DAT and thereby may provide an index of its terminal density.[23] For example, the cocaine congener N-(3-^{18}F-fluoropropyl)-2β-carbomethoxy-3β-(4-iodophenyl)nortropane ([18]FPCIT), which has high binding affinity for the DAT (Fig. 20-5), has been used to show how the pathology in Parkinson's disease progresses from unilateral to bilateral striatal dopamine deficits and that their magnitude correlates with the severity of behavioral symptoms.[24] Other [18]FPCIT-PET studies have

revealed 50% decreases in mean striatal DAT binding in patients with early-stage Parkinson's disease who were imaged within 2 years of diagnosis, thus suggesting that significant nigrostriatal degeneration had occurred by the time that the first symptom appeared.[25]

For the postsynaptic striatal dopamine system, PET tracers have been synthesized for the dopamine D_1 and D_2 receptors.[26] These receptors subserve different functions based on their signal transduction mechanisms of stimulation and inhibition of adenylyl cyclase, respectively.[27] At present, PET studies of dopamine receptors have been limited to the assessment of receptor density and, in some instances, receptor affinity.

Nonetheless, changes in apparent ligand-receptor binding are indicative of dysfunctional neurotransmission at the synapse. For example, changes in D_2 receptor density in patients with

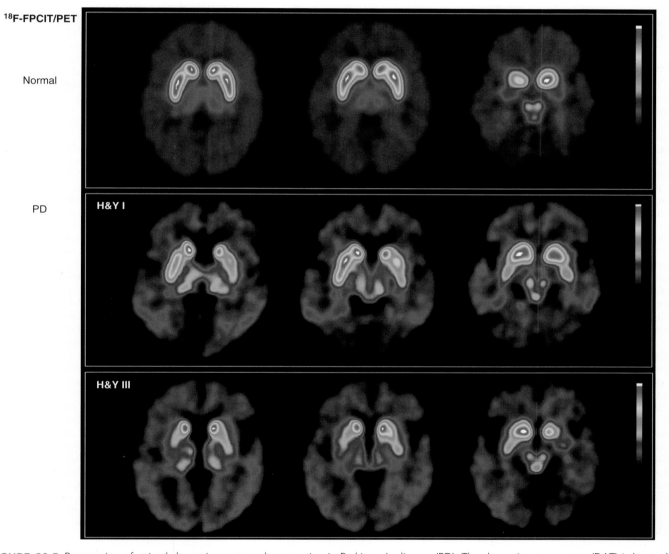

FIGURE 20-5 Progression of striatal dopamine system degeneration in Parkinson's disease (PD). The dopamine transporter (DAT) is located at the presynaptic terminal, and its density in the striatum can be used as an index of dopamine system integrity. The positron emission tomographic images show the striatal uptake of N-(3-^{18}F-fluoropropyl)-2β-carbomethoxy-3β-(4-iodophenyl)nortropane ([18]FPCIT), a ligand with high binding affinity for DAT, for a normal volunteer (*top row*) and two patients with PD (*middle row*: Hoehn & Yahr (H&Y) stage I; *bottom row*: H&Y stage III). [18]FPCIT uptake is reduced predominantly in the putamen, unilaterally in early-stage PD (*middle row*) and more pronounced bilaterally (*bottom row*) with disease progression. *(From Kazumata K, Dhawan V, Chaly T, et al. Dopamine transporter imaging with fluorine-18-FPCIT and PET. J Nucl Med. 1998;39:1521-1530.)*

Parkinson's disease as a result of compensatory reactions to the ongoing disease process have been measured with PET.[28] Subregional striatal alterations that show larger increases in D_2 receptor binding in the putamen than in the caudate have also been detected (see Fig. 20-4). These relative differences in receptor density are paralleled by a similar pattern of increases in FDG metabolism; that is, metabolic rates in the putamen are greater than those in the caudate.

PET can also provide in vivo assessments of the efficacy of neurosurgical interventions. In the United States, two National Institutes of Health–sponsored double-blind trials were conducted in which fetal mesencephalon cells were transplanted into the striatum of patients with Parkinson's disease.[29,30] Although clinical improvements appeared only marginal and the primary end points were not met, the integrity of the grafts to survive in the host striatum was unequivocally demonstrated with FDOPA–PET studies (Fig. 20-6). At present, novel neurorepair and neurorestoration strategies are being developed that include stereotactic delivery into the brain of neuronal growth factors (e.g., glial cell line–derived neurotrophic factor, genetically engineered viral vectors that deliver genes of interest, and stem cells). The long-term efficacy of these interventions will be assessed by PET.

Huntington's Disease

The neurodegeneration associated with this autosomal dominantly inherited disease results in a significant loss of the medium spiny GABAergic (secreting γ-aminobutyric acid [GABA]) neurons of the striatum. Because these cells contain the majority of dopamine receptors in the striatum, a decrease in dopamine receptor binding accompanies their loss.[31] Accordingly, changes in dopamine receptor binding were targeted for assessment with PET. Because striatal GABAergic neurons express D_1 and D_2 receptors, PET studies initially focused on alterations in these receptor densities by using the D_1 receptor ligand [^{11}C]SCH 23390 and the D_2 receptor ligand [^{11}C]raclopride. PET studies have shown that progression of Huntington's disease is accompanied by significant reductions in both striatal D_1 and D_2 receptor binding.[31]

Additionally, FDG studies have shown that the striatum of carriers with asymptomatic Huntington's disease mutations has reductions in FDG activity characteristic of the disease. These results are in contrast to the normal appearance of the same structures on MRI, thus illustrating that significant biochemical alterations are not necessarily paralleled by a similar degree of morphologic change.

Hence, detection by PET of asymptomatic disease and progression of Parkinson's and Huntington's disease demonstrates that biochemical reserves, redundancies, and compensatory responses can mask altered function up to a certain limit. Longitudinal assessment of these processes with PET now presents the opportunity to determine subsets of individuals who are likely to benefit from neuroprotective and neurorestorative therapies. As access to PET expands to the broader clinical community, medical evaluation will shift to such early detection—when, as these studies show, there is significant residual function that can become the target of intervention. In the future, neurosurgeons will increasingly rely on PET for planning of intervention treatments and assessment of outcomes.

Dementias and Mental Illness

Clinically, early dementia is difficult to differentiate from related pathologies associated with aging processes. Here, as with movement disorders, the goal of present and future research is to develop PET tracers that can be used for early diagnosis and assessment of the efficacy of therapy.

At present, FDG-PET can diagnose Alzheimer's disease and distinguish it from patterns of normal aging.[16] Specifically, hypo-

metabolism can be detected in cortical neuronal pathways, which represents the summative effect of decreases in regional synaptic activity. These deficits are most prominent in the parietal and temporal lobes rather than the motor and visual cortex and become more marked and widespread with increasing disease severity.[32,33] Additionally, the hypometabolism is not generalized to subcortical structures such as the basal ganglia and thalamus.

It is now apparent that the major histopathologic aspects of Alzheimer's disease, namely, amyloid plaques and neurofibrillary tangles, are present in brain before the onset of cognitive decline.[34-36] The predominant role hypothesized for β-amyloid in producing neuronal dysfunction has made it an attractive target for in vivo PET imaging, whereby disease progression and the efficacy of interventions designed to reduce the amyloid burden could be assessed. Recent advances in imaging amyloid in the brain have been achieved by using novel PET ligands that are modifications of histologic dyes with high binding affinity for amyloid. The most promising compound currently used for imaging amyloid is N-methyl-[^{11}C]2-(4′-methylaminophenyl)-6-hydroxybenzothiazole, also referred to as the Pittsburg-B Compound ([^{11}C]-PIB).[37] Patients with Alzheimer's disease imaged with [^{11}C]-PIB show greater retention of [^{11}C]-PIB in cortical regions associated with accumulation of amyloid than in the pons or cerebellum, where there is little or no amyloid (Fig. 20-7). Multiple studies of Alzheimer's disease patients with [^{11}C]-PIB and FDG imaging have now shown that the apparent amyloid burden remains relatively high and stable over a 2-year period while cerebral glucose metabolism continues to decline, thus suggesting that amyloid accumulation precedes the associated loss of cognitive function.[38]

PET has also contributed to refinement of the diagnosis and surgical treatment of mental illnesses such as severe major depression[39] and obsessive-compulsive disorders.[40] A clinical response to antidepressants is associated with decreases in rates of glucose metabolism in the limbic (subgenual cingulate cortex, hippocampus, insula, and pallidum) and striatal regions, with increases in the dorsal cortical (prefrontal, parietal, anterior, and posterior cingulate) regions.[41] Mayberg and colleagues used the findings of increased blood flow in the subgenual cingulate cortex to identify a target for deep brain stimulation to abate the symptoms of medically refractory major depression. Their early work demonstrated the integral role played by the subgenual cingulate cortex in both normal and pathologic shifts in mood.[42] Increases in limbic and paralimbic blood flow, as measured with PET, occur in the subgenual cingulate cortex and anterior insula during sadness. Furthermore, there is a significant inverse correlation between blood flow in the subgenual cingulate cortex and the right dorsolateral prefrontal cortex.[43] In 2005, Mayberg and associates implanted deep brain stimulation electrodes into the bilateral subgenual cingulate cortex in six patients with medically refractory major depression. With stimulation, patients reported positive emotional phenomena.[44] In the acute postoperative period, the patients experienced reproducible increases in activity and mood scores that were not seen during sham stimulation. Chronic stimulation at high frequency probably resulted in reduced functional stimulation in the site. Subsequently, significant improvement in behavioral responses and remission of depression were observed in four of the six patients at 6 months. These well-conducted studies showed the effectiveness of PET in enhancing our knowledge of brain function and leading to effective diagnosis and therapeutic interventions.

Changes in FDG-PET patterns of cortical uptake in the frontal areas have also been demonstrated in patients with internal capsule lesions,[45] as well as with deep brain stimulation for the management of obsessive-compulsive disorder.[46] Thus, evidence is accumulating to support the use of PET for determination of targets and follow-up of patients undergoing neurosurgical interventions for mental illness.

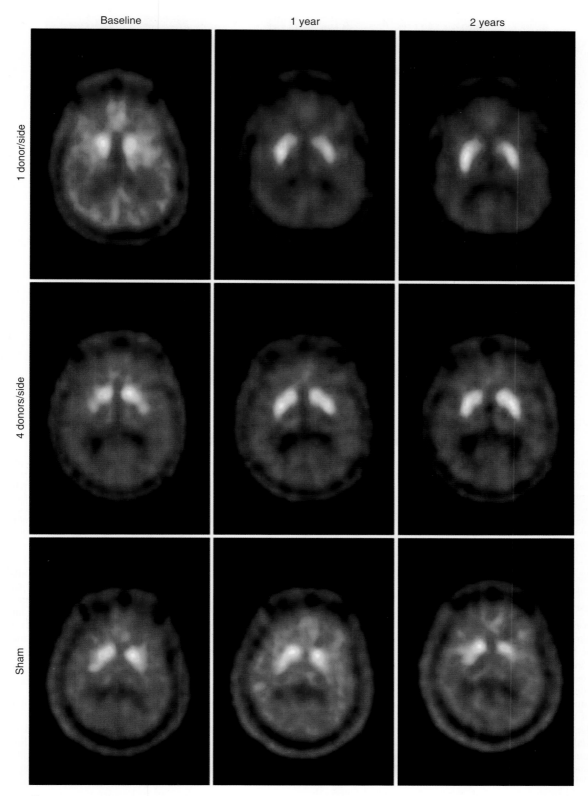

FIGURE 20-6 [^{18}F]6-Fluoro-L-dopa (FDOPA) imaging of fetal nigral cell transplantation into the striatum of patients with Parkinson's disease. Longitudinal positron emission tomography studies show baseline putaminal deficits in FDOPA uptake in patients with Parkinson's disease and subsequent striatal FDOPA increases at 1 and 2 years after fetal cell transplantation (*top row*: patient with one donor per side; *middle row*: patient with four donors per side). The sham/placebo patient (*bottom row*) shows further reductions in FDOPA uptake over the same time period, a finding suggesting disease progression. *(From Olanow CW, Goetz CG, Kordower JH, et al. A double-blind controlled trial of bilateral fetal nigral transplantation in Parkinson's disease. Ann Neurol. 2003;54:403-414.)*

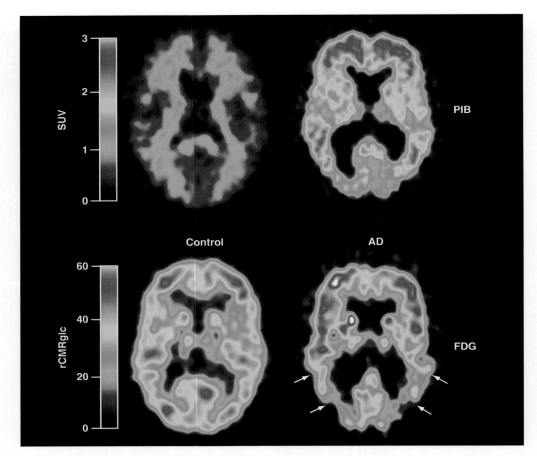

FIGURE 20-7 Imaging brain amyloid burden in patients with Alzheimer's disease (AD). The positron emission tomography (PET) tracer N-methyl-[11C]2-(4′-methylaminophenyl)-6-hydroxybenzothiazole, also referred to as [11C]PIB, has high binding affinity for amyloid in vivo. [11C]PIB-PET studies show that in frontal and temporoparietal brain regions known to contain amyloid there is significantly greater [11C] retention in a patient with AD (*right column*) relative to a healthy control subject (*left column*); the standardized uptake value (SUV) represents the tissue concentration of tracer as measured by the PET scanner divided by the injected dose per kilogram of patient body weight. 2-[18F]Fluoro-2-deoxy-D-glucose (FDG) studies obtained within 3 days in a patient with AD show hypometabolism in the temporoparietal cortex (*arrows; bottom right*) and apparent preserved metabolic rate in the frontal cortex. (*From Klunk WE, Engler H, Nordberg A, et al. Imaging brain amyloid in Alzheimer's disease with Pittsburgh Compound-B. Ann Neurol. 2004;55:306-319.*)

CLINICAL APPLICATIONS

Epilepsy

The outcome of epilepsy surgery is directly linked to accurate localization of the focus of the seizures. Improvements in techniques for localization of the seizure focus have resulted from advances in brain imaging. Currently, electroencephalography (EEG) is used to localize the focus, and imaging studies are used to corroborate the EEG findings. In the future, imaging studies will be incorporated into standard protocols for localization because of the high degree of accuracy of PET and volumetric MRI studies. This trend evolved from earlier findings with pneumoencephalography that demonstrated hippocampal atrophy, but modern imaging techniques can decrease the use of invasive EEG methods such as implantation of grids and depth electrodes.[47]

FDG-PET scanning first demonstrated focal seizure abnormalities in the absence of structural changes.[48] Currently, single-photon emission computed tomography (SPECT), magnetoencephalography (MEG), and magnetic resonance spectroscopy (MRS) are also capable of showing abnormalities consistent with seizure foci in the absence of structural changes.[49] It is likely that these imaging modalities will provide complementary data for specific clinical situations. PET imaging with [11C]flumazenil is also used to detect focal abnormalities. [11C]Flumazenil is an antagonist with high binding affinity for the benzodiazepine site on $GABA_A$ postsynaptic receptors. The region of the epileptogenic focus is localized by detecting a reduced area of [11C]flumazenil binding, which can be overestimated as a larger area of hypometabolism when imaged with interictal FDG-PET.[50] The merits of PET are discussed in this section; other modalities are evaluated elsewhere in this volume.

Temporal Lobe Epilepsy

Temporal lobe epilepsy has been extensively studied with PET because of the prevalence of its surgical treatment.[51,52] At present, the process of resecting the seizure focus is divided into three phases. Phase I consists of noninvasive studies for localization of the seizure focus as defined by the semiology of the seizure, by scalp EEG findings, including needle electrodes (e.g., sphenoidal electrodes), and by imaging studies. Phase II is undertaken only if the phase I studies fail to localize the seizure focus. Phase II consists of invasive EEG studies, including electrocorticography with strips, grids, and depth electrodes implanted stereotactically. Because phase II studies substantially increase the morbidity of the surgical process, it is desirable to minimize their use.[53] Phase III is resection of the seizure focus.[54] Ideally, all the information necessary for characterization of the resection is obtained before the surgical procedure.

The need for accurate noninvasive localization becomes even more pressing for minimally invasive neurosurgery such as radio-surgery, which is now available for the treatment of focal epilepsy.[55] FDG-PET has been the most reliable imaging technique for lateralization of the seizure focus in temporal lobe epilepsy and for identification of cortical dysplasias, even when findings on MRI are unremarkable.[56,57] FDG-PET has provided detailed information on cell firing in minute foci, such as the origin of electrical discharges resulting in gelastic seizures in patients with hypothalamic hamartoma.[58] Radiosurgery directed to such hypermetabolic foci can lead to significant decreases in and even complete resolution of seizures.[59]

The University of California, Los Angeles, group showed in a retrospective study of patients undergoing temporal lobe resection that the use of FDG-PET resulted in 86% sensitivity and 100% specificity for lateralization of the seizure focus.[53] This study demonstrated that localization was correct in all patients with glucose hypometabolism. Of the patients studied, only 14% of those undergoing resection did not have glucose hypometabolism in the resected lobe.[51,52] These results were reproduced in a study in which all patients with unilateral temporal lobe hypometabolism as assessed by FDG-PET had congruent results with invasive EEG studies.[57] Additionally, FDG-PET correlated with the semiology of the seizure. Patients with only aura and staring spells showed regional hypometabolism that was confined to the mesial temporal lobe structures, whereas patients with posturing as a component of their complex partial seizures had hypometabolism extending to the frontolateral cortex and motor cortex regions. Patients with complex automatism had hypometabolism in widespread areas, including the ipsilateral and contralateral limbic structures.[47] At present, neuronal loss in the seizure focus is the most plausible hypothesis for the interictal hypometabolism detected by FDG-PET. Although hypometabolic regions distant from the focus are also observed, these decreases may arise secondarily from diaschisis (see Fig. 20-10) as a result of primary loss of neurons in the region of the seizure focus.[60]

MRI volumetric measurements of the hippocampus and amygdala also have high sensitivity and specificity in determining the seizure focus.[61] T2 relaxometry denoting gliosis in the hippocampus offers additional information when MRI is used.[62] When hippocampal atrophy is present, neuronal loss is highly predictable, especially in the CA1 subfield. Such characterization corresponds to FDG-PET–defined hypometabolism, and the PET results are more reliable than those obtained with T2 relaxometry.[63] The results of visual inspection, including volume and T2 relaxometry, reached a concordance of 90% with EEG lateralization; the addition of volumetric calculations generated with computer workstations brought this concordance to 97%. The congruency of EEG, MRI volumetric, and T2 relaxometric findings with FDG-PET hypometabolism is now considered sufficient for lateralization of the focus.

Further information on lateralization can be obtained with MRS.[64] MRS offers quantitative tissue spectra of *N*-acetylaspartate (NAA), choline, creatine, phosphocreatine, and lactate in the epileptic zone. NAA is found in neurons, whereas choline and creatine are found predominantly in glia. Therefore, relative decreases in NAA may represent neuronal loss, and increases in choline and creatine may denote gliosis.

In one study of 16 patients with unilateral temporal lobe epilepsy as determined by EEG, concordance of these results with the NAA/choline + creatine ratio was observed for all subjects.[65] Similar studies reported by others show that determination of the seizure focus based on MRI, MRS, and FDG-PET may be sufficient for surgical resection without invasive recordings.[66,67] Algorithms based on imaging and recording studies can be used for decisions on resection (Table 20-3). It remains to be demonstrated whether only one of these techniques can provide sufficient accuracy for such determination.

TABLE 20-3 Algorithm for Defining the Seizure Focus in Temporal Lobe Epilepsy

Electroencephalography	+	+	+	+	+
Magnetic resonance imaging	+	−	+	−	−
Positron emission tomography	+	+	−	−	−
Invasive electroencephalography	0	0	0	+	−
Resection*	Yes	Yes	Yes	Yes	No

*Resection can be performed with certainty of localization of the seizure focus.

Additional information can be obtained with SPECT. Although interictal SPECT offers inferior imaging results relative to FDG-PET, SPECT may be adequate for ictal studies because of its availability and the longer half-life of the imaging agents (6 hours) compared with FDG (110 minutes).[49] Immediate postictal injection of technetium 99m hexamethyl-propylene-amine oxine followed by scanning can show cerebral hyperperfusion in the focus and surrounding areas of the epileptogenic zone.

MEG is likely to provide localization similar to EEG. As MEG becomes more available, the combination of MEG and FDG-PET or MRI and MRS may suffice for complete determination of the locus of the seizure focus without the need for ictal EEG or invasive recordings.

Extratemporal Lobe Epilepsy

Similar to localization of temporal lobe epilepsy foci, extratemporal foci are also identified on FDG-PET in interictal studies as areas of glucose hypometabolism. EEG recordings and MRI detection of abnormalities on T1-weighted images or T2 relaxometry also provide localization, but volumetric studies do not reveal extratemporal seizure areas. For example, in patients with infantile spasms and normal findings on MRI, cortical dysplastic areas are identified by hypometabolic changes seen on FDG-PET. Based on such PET characterization, successful surgical results were achieved in the early 1990s.[48,56] Advanced MRI techniques can now detect abnormalities in a substantial number of patients with normal conventional MRI findings.[68] Additionally, the improved resolution of MRS in combination with FDG-PET can be used in the surgical treatment of extratemporal lobe epilepsy. The use of PET fusion techniques and functional MRI data will assist in localization of the focus and facilitate the stereotactic surgical approach by providing functional mapping of the surrounding brain regions.[69-73]

Brain Tumors

Applications of PET studies of brain tumors range from diagnosis and grading of gliomas to postsurgical assessment of gliomas and metastatic tumors. The consequences of therapy, including hemodynamic changes and alterations in tumor metabolism in relation to normal brain, have been used to interpret clinical observations during the evolution of these diseases. Changes in blood-brain barrier permeability and protein synthesis rates within the tumor region have provided insight into the limitations and effects of treatment on the tumor. At present, PET is used in clinical practice to determine the efficacy of treatment and to differentiate tumor recurrence from tissue necrosis.

Tumor Metabolism

Regional cerebral blood flow (CBF), cerebral blood volume (CBV), oxygen extraction fraction (OEF), and cerebral oxygen

FIGURE 20-8 [^{18}F]Fluoro-2-deoxy-D-glucose–positron emission tomography (PET) (**A**) and gadolinium-enhanced T1-weighted magnetic resonance imaging (**B**) show a metastatic melanoma in the corpus callosum at the time of stereotactic radiosurgical treatment. The *arrow* points to the tumor in the PET image. Notice the ring of hypermetabolism surrounding a center of hypometabolism representing the lesion.

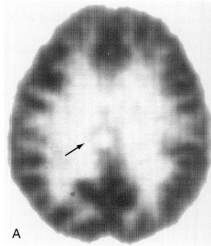
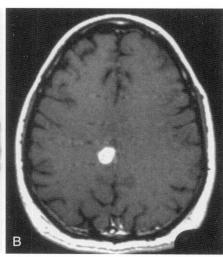

utilization (CMRO$_2$) have been evaluated by [^{15}O]CO$_2$, [^{11}C]CO, and [^{15}O]CO as tracers and constant infusion of [^{15}O]H$_2$O.[74] Surprisingly, it has been shown that oxygen extraction and utilization are decreased in primary brain tumors in comparison to normal brain tissue.[75] Moreover, there appears to be an uncoupling of regional CBF and regional CBV. CBF in gliomas is rather variable, particularly in high-grade gliomas. For example, edematous areas surrounding the tumor have decreased blood flow and oxygen utilization but normal oxygen extraction and are therefore not considered ischemic. These metabolic characteristics are altered by dexamethasone administration or radiotherapy.[76] Dexamethasone causes a decrease in CBF and CBV in both hemispheres of patients with brain tumors, and radiotherapy effects a decrease in CMRO$_2$ and CBF in the tumor, with an increase in these parameters in the opposite hemisphere.[68] These findings are in accord with the rapid clinical improvement of patients with brain tumors undergoing steroid therapy. Similarly, the effects of radiotherapy on CBF and metabolism explain the clinical improvement of patients undergoing this therapy.

Tumor characterization with FDG-PET has been correlated with the histologic grade of primary brain tumors.[77-80] Hypermetabolism is observed in high-grade gliomas because the rate of cell growth is directly related to tumor metabolism (Fig. 20-8).[79,81] Areas of hypermetabolism in low-grade gliomas may suggest histologic deterioration to a higher grade. Therefore, FDG-PET has prognostic value because the histologic grade of a primary brain tumor determines the prognosis and treatment options, as has been confirmed by several investigators.[82,83] For example, patients with MRI-detected low-grade gliomas can postpone undergoing biopsy if they are monitored carefully with serial FDG-PET and MRI. Then, when surgery is indicated, the FDG-PET profiles of tumor delimitation can be used to guide stereotactic biopsy to the areas most likely to yield the correct tumor grade.[84]

Hypometabolism, as measured by FDG-PET, has been the defining characteristic of low-grade gliomas. Areas of high glucose uptake in a low-grade glioma suggest malignant degeneration. However, differentiation of low-grade glioma histology based on FDG-PET imaging is problematic. Glucose metabolic rates are generally lower in low-grade astrocytomas and oligodendrogliomas than in normal brain tissue. Moreover, oligodendrogliomas have slightly higher metabolism than do low-grade astrocytomas. It has been suggested that histologic differentiation of these two tumors may be accomplished with [^{11}C]methionine-PET.[85] Oligodendrogliomas have significantly higher uptake of this tracer than do low-grade astrocytomas, and this observation may be related to cell density and turnover in each of these tumors. Higher cell turnover, presumably present in oligodendrogliomas,[86] may also account for this difference. During the follow-up period, FDG-PET studies have value in differentiating radiation necrosis from tumor recurrence; radiation necrosis has very low cell turnover, and consequently, that region does not accumulate FDG significantly (Figs. 20-9 to 20-11; see also Fig. 20-8). This differential diagnosis is important for patients with malignant gliomas and metastatic tumors undergoing multimodality therapy.[85,87]

Several other tracers have been used in brain tumor research, but most are related to breakdown of the blood-brain barrier and add little to the already exquisite imaging capabilities of MRI with gadolinium enhancement. They do add, however, to the study of alterations in various transport mechanisms across the blood-brain barrier.[88] For example, [^{11}C]methyl-glucose measures the facilitated diffusion rate of glucose, rubidium 82 uses the same active transport carrier as potassium,[89] and [^{11}C]albumin studies can be used to assess pinocytosis mechanisms related to the transport of much larger molecules and proteins.[89,90] This unique ability of PET to image specific aspects of blood-brain barrier permeability makes it attractive for follow-up studies of chemotherapy trials.

The rationale for the use of amino acid tracers for imaging tumors is based on the relatively higher amino acid uptake and protein synthesis rates in tumors than in normal tissue. The excellent tumor delineation, particularly at early imaging times (10 to 15 minutes after injection), obtained with both amino acid and amino acid analogue tracers that are not substrates for protein synthesis suggests that it is the increase in transport activity that underlies the relatively higher tracer uptake in tumors.

Studies using FDOPA as an amino acid analogue (Fig. 20-12) have now shown that this tracer is sensitive for the detection of primary brain tumors and is superior to FDG (Fig. 20-13). FDOPA imaging is also helpful in the detection of tumor recurrence in the presence of radiation necrosis, but it has no specificity for tumor grade. Recent studies of amino acid PET tracers suggest that they are also more sensitive than FDG for imaging some recurrent tumors, in particular, recurrent low-grade astrocytomas. For example, the finding of high uptake versus no uptake of the amino acid [^{18}F]fluoroethyltyrosine ([^{18}F]FET) was shown to strongly correlate with malignant progression of nonspecific findings on MRI.[91]

Other new applications of PET tracers that image important aspects of tumor biology include the use of 3′-deoxy-3′-[^{18}F]fluorothymidine, which can serve as an index of cell proliferation.[92]

Unfortunately, differentiation of tumor recurrence and radiation necrosis is still not definitive with these amino acid PET

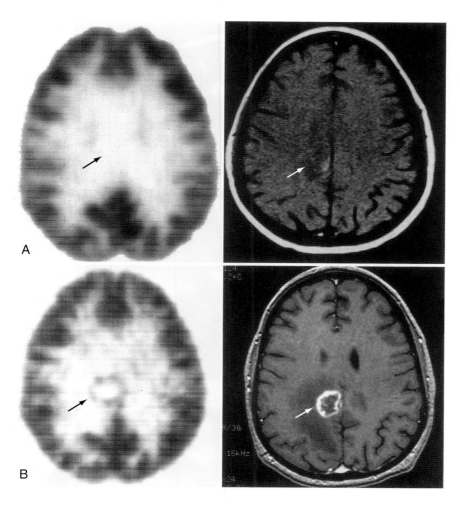

FIGURE 20-9 A, [^{18}F]Fluoro-2-deoxy-D-glucose (FDG)–positron emission tomography (PET) (*left*) and magnetic resonance imaging (MRI) (*right*) 3 months after stereotactic radiosurgery for a melanoma. *Arrows* show the location of the previous tumor (presented in Fig. 20-8). **B,** FDG-PET and gadolinium-enhanced T1-weighted MRI at the time of recurrence, 3 months later. PET is instrumental in differentiating tumor recurrence from radiation necrosis, a distinction that cannot be ascertained with MRI. *Arrows* point to the tumor recurrence.

tracers. Therefore, PET continues as a complementary imaging technique in the management of brain tumors.[93] Nonetheless, PET provides clinically relevant information for precisely targeting therapy (radiosurgery, gene therapy) by identifying the most biologically active areas within the tumor mass, as defined by breakdown of the blood-brain barrier seen on other imaging modalities such as MRI and CT.

Brain Injury

PET is unique in its ability to study brain energy metabolism because it is the only imaging modality that can provide all the parameters of energy metabolism (CBF, CBV, CMRO$_2$, OEF, and CMRGlu) in the human brain in vivo.[94] These parameters were briefly mentioned in the section on assessment of brain tumor metabolism. Their clinical relevance is exemplified by their use in assessing aspects of neurovascular disease. Alterations in these cerebrovascular factors are intimately related to areas of cerebral ischemia and provide both therapeutic and prognostic value when analyzed in situations of stressed cerebral tissue. For example, arterial obstruction or traumatic brain injury with a decrease in cerebral perfusion pressure (CPP) can be differentiated by different PET tracers. Patterns of cerebral vascular activity can be detected by PET with ^{15}O-, ^{11}C-, or ^{18}F-labeled tracers, depending on the viability of the stressed tissue.[95]

Brain Energy Metabolism Parameters

CBF is maintained within physiologic levels by blood pressure and by chemical autoregulation.[96] When CBF falls to critical levels, CMRO$_2$, OEF, and CMRGlu reflect the functional status of the tissue. Oxygen supply is continuously required in viable tissue, so OEF increases accordingly to maintain a normal CMRO$_2$. The uncoupling of glucose metabolic rates from CBF and oxygen extraction reflects tissue stress that may be due to ischemia, traumatic injury, or seizure disorder. These changes have been characterized in relation to CPP.[94] Briefly, a fall in CPP of up to 40% of baseline can be compensated if autoregulation is intact. A fall in CPP of 40% to 60% leads to levels of oligemia that are compensated by an increase in OEF to maintain CMRO$_2$ and CMRGlu within normal limits. A 60% to 80% fall in CPP reaches levels of the ischemic penumbra. In this situation, OEF cannot compensate for the fall in CBF, and CMRO$_2$ starts to decrease, with a consequent increase in glucose anaerobic metabolism (i.e., glycolysis). A fall of 80% or greater in CPP is accompanied by irreversible tissue damage. At this point, CBF is below critical levels, and as CBV decreases because of cerebral edema and stasis, OEF becomes variable as a result of large areas of tissue death. CMRO$_2$ is then further decreased because of lack of metabolism, as indicated by concomitant decreases in CMRGlu.

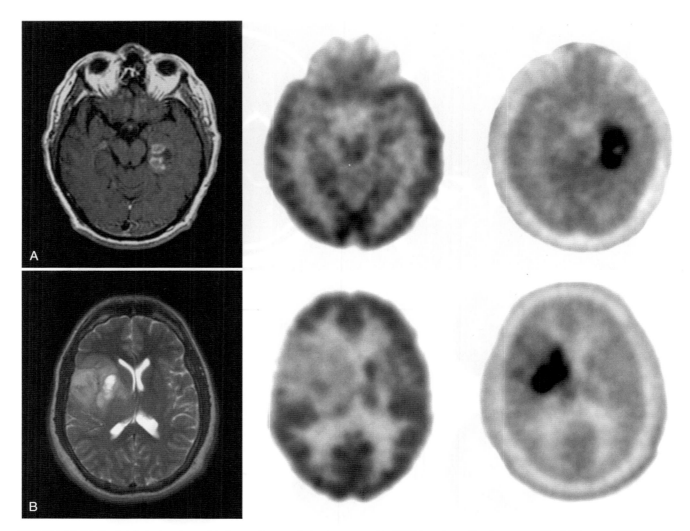

FIGURE 20-13 Radiolabeled amino acids for positron emission tomographic (PET) imaging of brain tumors. The PET tracer [18F]fluoro-L-dopa (FDOPA), which has been extensively used to assess striatal dopamine system integrity, is representative of the 18F-labeled aromatic amino acid analogues recently applied to tumor imaging. FDOPA imaging at early time periods of 10 to 15 minutes after injection shows higher [18F] uptake in tumor tissue than in normal brain tissue. **A** and **B,** Comparison of magnetic resonance imaging (*left*), [18F]fluorodeoxyglucose-PET (*middle*), and FDOPA–PET (*right*) images of newly diagnosed tumors. Glioblastoma (**A**) and grade II oligodendroglioma (**B**) show better contrast with FDOPA for differentiating tumor and normal tissue. *(From Chen W, Silverman DH, Delaloye S, et al. 18F-FDOPA PET imaging of brain tumors: comparison study with 18F-FDG PET and evaluation of diagnostic accuracy. J Nucl Med. 2006;47:904-911.)*

Clinical Implications

The diagnosis of "misery-perfusion syndrome" has implications in the clinical management of patients with stroke, head trauma, or subarachnoid hemorrhage secondary to bleeding from an aneurysm or arteriovenous malformation. Misery-perfusion syndrome is characterized by a decrease in CBF with normal $CMRO_2$ maintained by a compensatory increase in OEF (Table 20-4). Measures to increase CBF in this circumstance can result in progression from the phase of tapping into the perfusion reserve (also called *oligemia)* to true tissue stress, the ischemic penumbra, and irreversible tissue damage.[97] Such measures may include the simple use of rheologic agents and triple-H therapy (hypertension, hypervolemia, and hemodilution) or surgical procedures such as arterioplasty, extracranial-to-intracranial arterial bypass, or carotid endarterectomy. Advantage is taken of the perfusion reserve to achieve an increase in CBV. There is a consistent increase in CBF, which leads to an increase in intracranial pressure during the initial phase of exhaustion of "autoregulation,"

as well as in oligemia and the ischemic penumbra (see Table 20-4). This has particularly ominous repercussions not just for patients with severe head injury but for patients with borderline high intracranial pressure from cerebral infarction or subarachnoid hemorrhage as well. Maintenance of adequate CPP becomes the sine qua non, not only in these pathologic circumstances but also during general anesthesia, when patients with brain tumors have a risk for increased intracranial pressure.

Prolonged periods of inadequate CPP from any pathologic situation result in the accumulation of metabolites that have an important impact in the reperfusion phase.[98] Terms such as *luxury perfusion,*[99] *hyperperfusion, relative luxury perfusion,* and *true hyperemia* denote levels of vasodilation and paralysis secondary to metabolic influences in the cerebral vasculature. The degree of tissue damage depends on several factors, including the type and maturity of the tissue[98] and tissue activity at the time of the metabolic demand. Determining the extent of the oligemic state and the degree to which penumbral areas have evolved to a state of irreversible damage is important for certain clinical trials and for

TABLE 20-4 Fall in Cerebral Perfusion Pressure and Its Effects on Brain Energy Metabolism

CPP FALL	CBF	CBV	OEF	CMRO$_2$	CMRGlu
<40%	Normal	Increase	Normal	Normal	Normal
40%-60%*	Decrease	INCREASE	Increase	Normal	Normal
60%-80%†	Decrease	Increase	INCREASE	Decrease	Decrease
>80%‡	DECREASE	Decrease	Variable	Decrease	Decrease

The use of capital letters represents a greater change in brain energy metabolism.
*Oligemia.
†Penumbra.
‡Irreversible damage.
CBF, cerebral blood flow; CBV, cerebral blood volume; CMRGlu, cerebral metabolic rate of glucose consumption; CMRO$_2$, cerebral metabolic rate of oxygen consumption; CPP, cerebral perfusion pressure; OEF, oxygen extraction fraction.

the definition of inclusion criteria.[100] Only PET studies can offer the detailed regional analysis necessary for these important decisions.

Regional aberrations in cerebral metabolism also appear in unique situations such as seizures, intracranial hematomas, and head trauma.[101] In these situations, significant uncoupling of CBF and glucose metabolism can be detected by FDG-PET studies during the acute and subacute periods (Fig. 20-14). Hypermetabolism in the acute stage of traumatic brain injury has been well characterized.[102] However, its regional nature and relationship to posttraumatic events, such as areas of contusion, subclinical seizures, and relief of pressure by surgical intervention, have only recently been demonstrated by serial FDG-PET studies.[103] The pathophysiologic substrate of this hyperglycolysis has not been defined. Its presence and degree have been unequivocally related to prognosis after traumatic brain injury,[102] although the repercussions for tissue recovery are currently unknown. In addition to these acute changes in cerebral metabolism that have been confirmed by PET studies, other alterations during the rehabilitative period are suggestive of brain plasticity. For instance, it has been demonstrated that recruitment of motor areas in nondamaged parts of the brain can affect recovery of lost regional function.[104]

IN VIVO DRUG MONITORING

Molecular imaging with PET can also be applied to various types of pharmacokinetic and pharmacodynamic studies. For example, many drugs can be labeled with ^{11}C without altering their struc-ture. In PET studies, the distribution of these ^{11}C-labeled drugs throughout the brain can then be determined at tracer doses. With this methodology, the distribution and temporal profile of a drug can be imaged in humans, thereby obviating the need for animal studies, whose results are often difficult to extrapolate to the human condition because of species-dependent differences in drug metabolism.

An excellent example of a PET-based pharmacokinetic study in humans was conducted with deprenyl, an irreversible monoamine oxidase B (MAO-B) inhibitor used for Parkinson's disease.[105] To determine the regional MAO-B distribution in brain, ^{11}C]deprenyl was synthesized for use as a PET tracer. [11]C] Deprenyl-PET imaging studies then showed that the MAO-B content is 60% higher in the thalamus and basal ganglia than in cortical regions and the cerebellum. Subsequently, a series of ^{11}C]deprenyl-PET studies were used to estimate the half-time for MAO-B synthesis in vivo in individual subjects. First, a ^{11}C] deprenyl-PET scan was obtained for determining baseline values of brain MAO-B content. Before the next ^{11}C]deprenyl-PET scan, the individuals were administered deprenyl in pharmacologic doses (5 mg/day for 7 days) to achieve essentially total irreversible inhibition of MAO-B. Thereafter, a second ^{11}C] deprenyl-PET scan was obtained. Relative to the pretreatment scan values, ^{11}C]deprenyl binding after administration of deprenyl was reduced by 90%, thus indicating nearly complete inactivation of the enzyme. Multiple scans in the individuals during the next 2 months revealed a protracted recovery of MAO-B binding, which was attributed to the time course needed for synthesis of new enzyme. These data were used to calculate a

CT FDG-PET

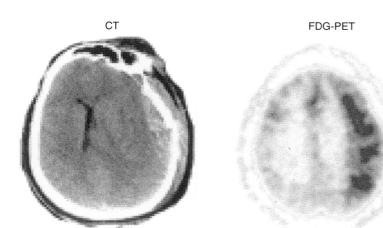

FIGURE 20-14 Computed tomography (CT) (*left*) shows a subdural hematoma after severe head trauma. [^{18}F]Fluoro-2-deoxy-D-glucose–positron emission tomography (FDG-PET) (*right*) shows significant regional hypermetabolism after drainage of the hematoma. The *darker areas* represent higher metabolic rates. The PET study was conducted 5 days after surgery. (*From Bergsneider M, Hovda D, Shalmos E, et al. Cerebral hyperglycolysis following severe traumatic brain injury in humans: a positron emission tomography study. J Neurosurg. 1997;86:241-251.*)

Perioperative Care

CHAPTER 21

Neuroanesthesia: Preoperative Evaluation

Deepak Sharma ■ Arthur M. Lam

The neuroanesthesiologist's goals can be divided into three periods—the *preoperative period*: (1) prepare the patient and family for the planned surgical procedure both physiologically and psychologically, (2) evaluate and optimize the patient's preoperative condition, (3) plan the anesthesia and elaborate the risks entailed to the patient and family; the *intraoperative period*: (4) render patients unconscious and insensitive to surgical and psychological trauma, (5) minimize the stress response to the surgical procedure, (6) maintain and optimize intraoperative physiologic function, (7) provide optimal operating conditions to facilitate surgery; and the *postoperative period*: (8) ameliorate pain after surgery without compromising patient safety, and (9) provide reassurance to the patient and family. The relative importance of these goals varies according to the patient and the nature of the surgical procedure. This chapter addresses general and neurosurgical procedure–specific considerations in the preoperative evaluation.

The preanesthetic evaluation is defined as the process of clinical assessment that precedes the delivery of anesthesia care for surgical and nonsurgical procedures. The primary aim of preanesthetic evaluation is to minimize the overall patient morbidity associated with surgery and anesthesia. This goal is achieved by assessing the patient's medical condition and the balance between anesthetic risk and surgical benefit, optimizing the medical condition within the limitations of the surgical circumstances, and formulating the best possible anesthesia plan. Other benefits may include improved safety of perioperative care, optimal resource utilization, improved outcomes, and patient satisfaction.[1] Hence, the objectives of preanesthetic evaluation include the following:

1. Establish rapport with the patient and immediate family members/significant others to minimize their anxiety and have a cooperative and relaxed patient
2. Provide information to the patient and family regarding anesthetic techniques and procedures and the associated risks and benefits and postoperative management issues, including pain control and possible need for postoperative mechanical ventilation in a major procedure
3. Evaluate the past medical, surgical, and anesthetic history and current medications to establish a baseline profile
4. Review the relevant personal, family, and social history and history of allergies
5. Perform a general physical examination, including recording of vital signs and examination of individual systems, particularly the nervous and cardiopulmonary systems

6. Interpret the relevant laboratory data and arrange for further investigations and consultations if deemed necessary to eliminate unnecessary preoperative standing "screening tests" and limit investigations to only appropriate ones, with obvious economic savings
7. Optimize the patient's physiologic condition
8. Stratify patient risk regarding morbidity and mortality based on the considerations just presented
9. Formulate an anesthesia plan and organize resources for perioperative care and postoperative recovery
10. Document informed consent for the proposed anesthetic technique and procedures

The preanesthetic evaluation may be performed well in advance of the planned surgery for most elective procedures during a visit to the preanesthetic evaluation clinic. Otherwise, it may be performed at the bedside in the hospital ward or intensive care unit the "night before" for inpatients or on the day of surgery for morning-admission patients. For urgent and emergency procedures, this evaluation may of necessity take place just before surgery. The consensus of the American Society of Anesthesiologists (ASA) Task Force on preanesthesia evaluation is that an initial record review, patient interview, and physical examination should be performed before the day of surgery for patients with high severity of disease.[1] Of patients with low severity of disease, those undergoing procedures with high surgical invasiveness should have the interview and physical examination performed before the day of surgery, whereas those undergoing procedures with medium or low surgical invasiveness may be interviewed and examined on or before the day of surgery.[1] Although the task force cautions that the timing of such assessments may not be practical with the limitation of resources, it recommends that at a minimum, a focused preanesthetic examination should include assessment of the airway, lungs, and heart and documentation of vital signs.[1]

Preanesthesia clinics are ideally run by anesthesiologists with or without the assistance of trained nurses. These clinics have been shown to improve operating room efficiency and minimize unexpected delays and cancellations because of poorly prepared patients.[2,3] To be able to run smoothly, however, good organization, concise guidelines and protocols, and adequate medical support are required. Additional staffing issues are also important considerations.

It has been shown that the patient's preoperative condition predicts postoperative mortality and morbidity.[4-8] In one study, preoperative evaluation of patients led to a change in the proposed anesthesia plan in up to 15% of healthy individuals and 20% of ill patients.[9] Although these changes in plan do not necessarily reduce patient morbidity, they can lead to delays caused by the need to obtain different drugs and equipment and further specialist consultations and result in increased operating room downtime and cost. Establishment of a preanesthesia assessment clinic streamlines the process and obviates this potential source of delay. In a study from Stanford University, implementation of a preanesthetic evaluation clinic produced an 87.9% reduction in day-of-surgery cancellations.[3] It is estimated that $30 to $40 billion is spent annually on preoperative testing and subsequent follow-up in North America alone, 50% of which could be saved by the appropriate and selective ordering of tests.[10] In one study, implementation of a preoperative clinic, in which tests were ordered at the anesthesiologist's request, resulted in a savings of $112.09 per patient. This equated to an annual potential saving of more than $1.01 million at one institution.[3]

To ensure smooth transition from patient referral to surgical intervention, preoperative communication among neurosurgeons, anesthesiologists, neurophysiologists, and the laboratory is essential. To the extent that the anesthesiologist must be acquainted with the surgical and neurophysiologic monitoring needs of the procedure, the neurosurgeon equally needs to be aware of the anesthetic concerns. Good communication between the surgical and anesthesia teams allows exchange of ideas and an opportunity to address concerns, to the benefits of the surgeon, the anesthesiologist, and most of all, the patient.

GENERAL PREANESTHETIC EVALUATION

Optimal preoperative status may not be the same as optimal daily living status, and thus when reviewing the patient, the effects of anesthesia, positioning, surgery, and postoperative pain must be considered in relation to the patient's surgical state and medications. The patient's preexisting medical condition, unrelated to the proposed surgical procedure, may require more intense scrutiny than the pathologic process being treated.

The ASA classification of physical status is a universally accepted system used for stratification of a patient's preexisting health status (Table 21-1). Although it does not take into account surgical risk and is not primarily designed for prediction of outcome, it has been found to correlate with perioperative morbidity and mortality.[11-13] In fact, ASA physical status 3 to 5 has been found to independently predict perioperative cardiovascular

TABLE 21-1 ASA Classification of Physical Status

ASA PHYSICAL STATUS	DISEASE STATE
1	A normal healthy patient
2	A patient with mild systemic disease
3	A patient with severe systemic disease
4	A patient with severe systemic disease that is a constant threat to life
5	A moribund patient who is not expected to survive without the operation
6	A patient declared brain-dead whose organs are being removed for donor purposes

ASA, American Society of Anesthesiologists.
Excerpted from the Relative Value Guide 2008 of the American Society of Anesthesiologists. A copy of the full text can be obtained from ASA, 520 N. Northwest Highway, Park Ridge, IL 60068-2573.

complications in intracranial surgical patients and is also a risk factor for perioperative mortality.[8]

History and Physical Examination

Careful evaluation of the patient will rate the severity of the medical problems and detect risks for asymptomatic disease. A good starting point is the primary disease process requiring surgical intervention, which may alert the anesthesiologist to potential problems such as trauma and a full stomach, head injury and the development of coagulopathy, or intracranial aneurysm and the need for blood pressure control. Thereafter, the evaluation should focus on each system. The specific neurosurgical aspects are discussed separately later in this chapter. The general approach is summarized here.

Medical History

1. Medical history related to the intended surgical procedure
2. Medical history related to other constitutional diseases that may or may not have a bearing on the intended procedure
3. History of previous surgery and anesthesia (insight into problems with airway management, intravenous access, postoperative pain, nausea/vomiting, and other problems)
4. Current medications (anticonvulsant therapy is associated with increased resistance to nondepolarizing muscle relaxants and hence an increased requirement for them; steroid administration might be associated with hyperglycemia and adrenal suppression) and allergies (e.g., allergy to latex, antibiotics, adhesive tape)
5. Personal history (smoking, alcohol, recreational drug use—all of which have bearing on anesthesia and intraoperative care)
6. Relevant family medical history and social/religious background (e.g., Jehovah's Witnesses, which would limit blood transfusion by adherence to faith)
7. Physical examination and assessment of organ system function
8. Ancillary laboratory investigations

General Physical Examination

Before proceeding to examination of individual systems, a general physical examination should be conducted and take into account the patient's level of consciousness, mental status, build, nutrition, and vital parameters. Patients with malignant tumors and those with high cervical lesions might be emaciated with significantly reduced muscle mass. Conversely, obesity might be coexistent in many patients. Obese individuals have an increased likelihood of associated diabetes, hypertension, coronary artery disease, restrictive lung disease, sleep apnea, and gastroesophageal reflux, which might warrant alteration of the anesthesia plan. Difficulty with tracheal intubation may be encountered more frequently in obese than in lean individuals,[14] and the pharmacologic profile of anesthetic agents may also be altered.[15] Some neurosurgical patients might be dehydrated because of reduced intake of fluids (as a result of impaired consciousness), vomiting, or the use of diuretics and contrast agents. Correction of significant dehydration before induction of anesthesia can prevent postinduction hypotension in such patients. Significant blood loss is a possibility with surgery for intracranial aneurysms, arteriovenous malformations (AVMs), vascular tumors, craniosynostoses, and extensive spine problems. Preanesthetic evaluation should look for preexisting anemia and attempt to correct it preoperatively or arrange for intraoperative transfusion on a case-by-case basis. Recording of preoperative vital parameters (heart rate, blood pressure) provides baseline values for intraoperative management, which is particularly important in surgeries requiring strict hemodynamic control (e.g., aneurysms and AVMs).

Perhaps the most crucial aspect of the general examination is assessment of the patient's airway. Although the primary neurosurgical problem may be responsible for potential difficulties in intubation and airway management, inadequate management of the airway may adversely affect the neurological outcome. Routine maneuvers used for airway management may worsen spinal instability in patients with cervical lesions and lead to increased intracranial pressure (ICP) with potentially devastating consequences in patients with decreased intracranial compliance. Hence, the patient's airway should be assessed carefully for ease of ventilation and difficulty of tracheal intubation, in conjunction with specific surgical needs such as hemodynamic stability and spine immobilization. Mallampati scoring[16] thyromental distance, presence of overbite or underbite, and the range of neck flexion-extension collectively provide an estimate of the risk for difficult intubation.[17] Some specific situations in which a difficult airway should be anticipated include patients who have recently undergone supratentorial craniotomy, in whom mouth opening might be significantly reduced secondary to ankylosis of the temporomandibular joint,[18] acromegalic patients undergoing pituitary surgery,[19] and patients with cervical spine lesions. Recognition of potential airway difficulty allows proper planning with the availability of accessory equipment and resources, as well as formulation of a back-up plan, and results in improved patient safety and efficient use of operating time.

Assessment of System Functions

Neurological System

The importance of complete assessment of the neurological system of a patient scheduled for a major neurosurgical procedure cannot be overemphasized. Although most patients would have received a complete assessment by the attending neurologist or neurosurgeon by the time that they are evaluated for anesthesia, careful documentation would nonetheless facilitate planning for anesthesia and anticipation of potential perioperative complications. Moreover, because the signs and symptoms may change in the interim as a result of progression of the pathologic process, the preanesthetic examination will provide a baseline for postoperative comparison.

Patients with a depressed level of consciousness preoperatively are likely to have a reduced anesthetic need for induction and more likely to have a slow or delayed emergence postoperatively and need for postoperative mechanical ventilation. Such patients should not receive any sedative or narcotic agents unless they are under continuous supervision, preferably in the operating room itself with vigilance for respiratory depression. Moreover, in patients with previous motor deficits, exacerbation of focal neurological signs may develop after sedative doses of benzodiazepines and narcotics.[20] The presence of brainstem lesions or lower cranial nerve dysfunction, or both, predisposes patients to an increased risk for aspiration postoperatively. Finally, life-threatening hyperkalemia secondary to succinylcholine administration may develop in patients with preexisting motor deficits.[21] Succinylcholine has also been reported to cause hyperkalemia in patients with ruptured cerebral aneurysms independent of the presence of motor nerve disturbances,[22] although this appears to be uncommon. Elevated ICP is often manifested as headache with nausea and vomiting, but it can also lead to olfactory nerve dysfunction with loss of the sense of smell. Unilateral uncal herniation would result in a dilated unresponsive ipsilateral pupil, which should be distinguished from incidental anisocoria, or a unilateral third nerve palsy resulting from compression by a space-occupying lesion. Field of vision might be significantly limited in patients with pituitary and other suprasellar tumors and should be documented for postoperative comparison. Dysfunction of the trigeminal and

facial nerves may interfere with mask ventilation and tracheal intubation. A patient with a damaged vagus nerve may have a hoarse voice secondary to vocal cord paralysis and may be at increased risk for airway obstruction.

Respiratory System

Risk for perioperative respiratory complications is increased in patients with preexisting obstructive or restrictive pulmonary disease. Perioperative hypoxemia or hypercapnia is more likely to occur and in turn can further aggravate an already compromised cardiorespiratory status. Patients with a history of pulmonary disease require an assessment of their baseline status, and any element of potential reversibility should be addressed.[23-25] Smoking is a common important risk factor for both cardiovascular and pulmonary disease and is associated with a threefold increase in perioperative morbidity. Cessation of smoking for 6 to 8 weeks is recommended for reactivation of mucociliary clearance, but as little cessation as 24 hours can reduce carboxyhemoglobin levels and improve oxygenation.[26] The presence of reactive airway disease indicates an increased risk for bronchospasm with airway manipulation and tracheal extubation and an increased risk for coughing and laryngospasm during emergence.

In patients with symptomatic obstructive pulmonary disease, preoperative pulmonary function testing, including flow-volume loops before and after the administration of bronchodilators, and arterial blood gas sampling allow assessment of reversibility and determination of preoperative optimization. An abnormally high $Paco_2$ or low Po_2 preoperatively is predictive of postoperative respiratory complications. In patients with significant impairment, elective postoperative mechanical ventilation after a major neurosurgical procedure may be indicated. Some patients with sleep apnea might be using continuous positive airway pressure devices at home, and it is important to ensure that the same device is available postoperatively.

Management of upper respiratory tract infection preoperatively in children is controversial because the effects on the airway last for 2 to 4 weeks after clinical resolution. The patient is at increased risk for perioperative respiratory morbidity during this period.[27] Postponement of elective surgery must be balanced against the risk for progressive neurological disability or the occurrence of a potentially catastrophic complication during the waiting period.

Patients with decreased levels of consciousness because of intracranial pathology and those with high spinal lesions or lower cranial nerve paralysis might have preexisting atelectasis preoperatively, which puts them at increased risk for postoperative mechanical ventilation. Aspiration pneumonitis or superimposed pneumonia, or both, can also develop. A restrictive pattern of lung disease often occurs in patients with craniovertebral junction anomalies preoperatively and persists in the postoperative period.[28] Some patients, such as those with head injury, spinal cord injury, or subarachnoid hemorrhage (SAH), might be intubated and mechanically ventilated preoperatively and usually remain intubated postoperatively as well.

In their systematic review of preoperative pulmonary risk stratification for noncardiothoracic surgery for the American College of Physicians, Smetana and colleagues found good evidence to support the following patient-related risk factors as being predictive of postoperative pulmonary complications: advanced age, ASA class 2 or greater, functional dependence, chronic obstructive pulmonary disease, and congestive heart failure.[29] They also found fair evidence indicating increased risk in patients with impaired sensorium, abnormal findings on chest examination, cigarette use, alcohol use, and weight loss.[29] Although asthma is not a risk factor if well controlled, perioperative risk may be increased if it is poorly controlled.[29] Important procedure-related risk factors include neurosurgery, emergency surgery, and prolonged surgery.[29] The value of preoperative testing in estimating pulmonary risk is controversial. Even though an abnormal chest radiograph does indicate increased risk for postoperative pulmonary complications and spirometry may provide some risk stratification, among potential laboratory tests for stratifying risk, a serum albumin level of less than 35 g/L is the most powerful predictor.[29]

Cardiovascular System

Anesthesia, surgical positioning, and surgery itself put additional demands on the cardiovascular system. Moreover, intraoperative maintenance of hemodynamic stability is important to avoid adverse neurological effects in neurosurgical patients. The presence of cardiovascular disease significantly increases the risk associated with anesthesia, and optimizing the patient's condition can significantly improve outcome. The overall risk of cardiac patients undergoing a noncardiac procedure has traditionally been assessed with the Goldman index.[4] However, it has now been superseded by the Revised Cardiac Risk Index.[5] According to this index,[5] the presence of three or more of the following factors is associated with a cardiac morbidity rate of 9%: (1) high-risk surgery, (2) history of ischemic heart disease, (3) history of congestive heart failure, (4) history of cerebrovascular disease, (5) preoperative treatment with insulin, and (6) preoperative serum creatinine level greater than 2.0 mg/dL. Because most patients undergoing intracranial procedures often have two or more of these risk factors, careful evaluation of the other organ systems is important to quantify risk for cardiac morbidity. Preanesthetic evaluation should also be focused on detecting and assessing the physiologic effects of cardiovascular conditions known to be associated with specific neurosurgical conditions, such as hypertension and coarctation of the aorta in patients with aneurysms.

Coronary artery disease is associated with diabetes mellitus, hypertension, smoking, hypercholesterolemia, and peripheral vascular disease. The presence of angina is a significant risk factor—although unstable or resting angina predicts the highest risk for postoperative cardiac complications, the risk with angina on exertion can be minimized with appropriate intraoperative management. Left ventricular dysfunction with symptoms of cardiac failure (dyspnea on mild exertion, orthopnea, peripheral edema) is indicative of significantly reduced cardiac output, which can worsen with general anesthesia. Mannitol must be used carefully and judiciously or not at all in patients with left ventricular failure. Hypertension is a common preexisting condition and is frequently inadequately controlled. These patients often have reduced plasma volume, thus making them more susceptible to the systemic vasodilatory effects of anesthetic agents, which can result in cardiovascular instability and labile blood pressure intraoperatively. Moreover, in patients with chronic hypertension, increased cerebrovascular resistance causes the lower and upper limits of cerebral blood flow (CBF) autoregulation to shift to higher pressure levels, and such patients consequently have poor tolerance of acute hypotension.[30,31] However, adaptive hypertensive changes in CBF autoregulation may be reversible with adequate control of blood pressure.[30,31] Patients with evidence of myocardial ischemia or myocardial infarction (MI) are at increased risk for postoperative MI, congestive heart failure, malignant arrhythmias, and death.

Preoperative cardiac evaluation must be carefully tailored to the circumstances and nature of the surgical illness. Given an acute surgical emergency, preoperative evaluation might have to be limited to simple and critical tests (such as rapid clinical assessment, hematocrit, electrolytes, renal function, and electrocardiography [ECG]), with a more extensive evaluation conducted after surgery. In patients in whom coronary revascularization is not an option, it is often not necessary to perform a noninvasive stress test. In general, preoperative tests are recommended only

if the information obtained will result in a change in the surgical procedure performed, a change in medical therapy or monitoring during or after surgery, or postponement of surgery until the cardiac condition can be corrected or stabilized. A cardiology consultation should be sought if deemed necessary and surgical circumstances allow. Preoperative evaluation by a cardiologist may involve changes in medications, additional preoperative tests or procedures, or recommendations for higher levels of postoperative care.

The American College of Cardiology/American Heart Association (ACC/AHA) 2007 guidelines on perioperative cardiovascular evaluation and care for noncardiac surgery grade clinical risk factors as major, intermediate, and minor.[32] The presence of one or more of the major risk factors (active cardiac conditions) mandates intensive management and may require delay or cancellation of surgery unless the surgery is being performed on an emergency basis. Major risk factors include

- Unstable coronary syndromes (e.g., unstable or severe angina)
- Decompensated heart failure
- Significant arrhythmias (e.g., high-grade atrioventricular block, supraventricular arrhythmias with an uncontrolled ventricular rate, symptomatic ventricular arrhythmias/bradycardia)
- Severe valvular disease (severe aortic stenosis or symptomatic mitral stenosis)

According to the guidelines,[32] intermediate-risk factors include

- History of ischemic heart disease
- History of compensated or previous heart failure
- History of cerebrovascular disease
- Diabetes mellitus
- Renal insufficiency

A history of MI or abnormal Q waves on ECG is listed as a clinical risk factor, whereas acute MI (defined as at least one documented MI 7 days or less before the examination) or recent MI (more than 7 days but 1 month or less before the examination) with evidence of important ischemic risk by clinical symptoms or noninvasive study is an active cardiac condition. This definition reflects the consensus of the ACC Cardiovascular Database Committee. If a recent stress test does not indicate residual myocardium at risk, the likelihood of reinfarction after noncardiac surgery is low. Despite the lack of adequate clinical trials on which to base firm recommendations, it appears reasonable to wait 4 to 6 weeks after an MI to perform elective surgery.[32]

Minor predictors are recognized markers for cardiovascular disease that have not been proved to increase perioperative risk independently, such as advanced age (>70 years), abnormal findings on ECG (left ventricular hypertrophy, left bundle branch block, ST-T abnormalities), rhythm other than sinus, and uncontrolled systemic hypertension.

The guidelines recommend the following stepwise approach to perioperative cardiac assessment for noncardiac surgery[32]:

Step 1 (Need for Emergency Noncardiac Surgery)

Further cardiac assessment or treatment is not warranted, and emergency surgery may proceed with perioperative surveillance, postoperative risk stratification, and risk factor management. The cardiologist may provide recommendations for perioperative medical management and surveillance.

Step 2 (Patients with Active Cardiac Conditions)

The presence of unstable coronary disease, decompensated heart failure, severe arrhythmia, or severe valvular heart disease warrants evaluation and treatment according to the ACC/AHA guidelines, with cancellation or delay of surgery until the cardiac problem has been clarified and treated appropriately. However, depending on the results of investigations and cardiac interventions and the risk associated with delaying surgery, it may be appropriate to proceed to the planned surgery with maximal medical therapy.

Step 3 (Patients Undergoing Low-Risk Surgery)

Interventions based on cardiovascular testing in stable patients rarely result in a change in management, and it is appropriate to proceed with the planned surgical procedure in such patients.

Step 4 (Patients with Good Functional Capacity and No Symptoms)

Functional status is a reliable predictor of perioperative and long-term cardiac events. In highly functional asymptomatic patients, management will rarely be changed by the results of any further cardiovascular testing. It is therefore appropriate to proceed with the planned surgery. In patients with known cardiovascular disease or at least one clinical risk factor (ischemic heart disease, compensated or previous heart failure, diabetes mellitus, renal insufficiency, and cerebrovascular disease), perioperative heart rate control with beta blockade is considered appropriate. However, results from the Perioperative Ischemic Evaluation Study (POISE) indicate that the reduced cardiac morbidity with perioperative beta-blocker therapy in patients not previously taking beta blockers is achieved at the expense of an increased stroke rate and an overall increase in mortality.[33]

Step 5 (Symptomatic Patients and Patients with Poor or Unknown Functional Capacity)

In this scenario, the presence of clinical risk factors determines the need for further evaluation. If the patient has one or two clinical risk factors, it is reasonable to either proceed with the planned surgery, with consideration of beta blockade for heart rate control, or perform cardiac testing if it will change management. In patients with three or more clinical risk factors, the surgery-specific cardiac risk is important, which in turn is related to the degree of hemodynamic cardiac stress (alterations in heart rate, blood pressure, vascular volume, pain, bleeding, clotting tendencies, oxygenation, neurohumoral activation, and other parameters) associated with the surgery. In patients undergoing intermediate-risk surgery (including head and neck surgery and carotid endarterectomy [CEA]), data are insufficient to determine the best strategy.

Gastrointestinal System

Patients at risk for aspiration include those with full stomachs, bowel obstruction, and gastroesophageal reflux. Patients with cranial nerve dysfunction involving the 9th and 10th cranial nerves, as well as those with decreased level of consciousness, are also at risk if they have not been fasting. In these patients, general anesthesia with rapid-sequence induction and cricoid pressure should be undertaken to minimize the risk for aspiration.

Renal System

Patients needing neurosurgical interventions sometimes have coexistent renal dysfunction that might be acute or chronic. Acute renal failure can be prerenal, renal, or postrenal, depending on its cause. In contrast, chronic renal failure is attributable most commonly to hypertensive nephrosclerosis, diabetic nephropa-thy, chronic glomerulonephritis, and polycystic renal disease. Patients with kidney disease represent an anesthetic challenge because they may have autonomic neuropathy, encephalopathy, fluid retention (congestive heart failure, pleural effusion, ascites) and yet intravascular volume depletion, hypertension, metabolic acidosis, electrolyte imbalance (hyperkalemia, hyponatremia, hypocalcemia), anemia, and delayed gastric emptying, among other manifestations. The generalized effects of azotemia mandate a thorough evaluation of patients in renal failure. Signs of fluid overload or hypovolemia should be sought. Hematocrit, serum electrolytes, coagulation studies, blood urea nitrogen, and creatinine measurements are advisable. A chest radiograph and arterial blood gas analysis might be required in patients with breathlessness, and the electrocardiogram should be examined for signs of hyperkalemia or hypocalcemia, as well as ischemia and conduction blocks. Severely anemic patients may require preoperative red blood cell transfusions. Preoperative drug therapy should be carefully reviewed for drugs with significant renal elimination. Dosage adjustments and measurement of blood levels are sometimes necessary to prevent drug toxicity.

Intravascular volume depletion, injection of contrast dye, and use of aminoglycoside antibiotics, angiotensin-converting enzyme inhibitors, and nonsteroidal anti-inflammatory drugs (NSAIDs) are risk factors for acute deterioration in renal function and must be avoided. Hypovolemia appears to be a particularly important factor in the development of acute postoperative renal failure. The emphasis in management of these patients is on prevention because of the high mortality associated with postoperative renal failure. Optimal management may require preoperative dialysis in certain situations, the usual indications being severe acidosis or volume overload, hyperkalemia, metabolic encephalopathy, and drug toxicity. Patients with nausea, vomiting, or gastrointestinal bleeding should undergo rapid-sequence induction with cricoid pressure. Volume status is often difficult to assess and may necessitate invasive monitoring, including placement of intra-arterial and central venous pressure catheters. Neuromuscular blocking agents not dependent on renal function for elimination should be selected. Mannitol is contraindicated in anuric patients. Postoperative mechanical ventilation is sometimes required in patients with renal failure because inadequate spontaneous ventilation with progressive hypercapnia can result in a respiratory acidosis that may exacerbate any preexisting acidosis, lead to potentially severe circulatory depression, and dangerously increase the serum potassium concentration.

Hematologic System

Postoperative intracranial hemorrhage is a potentially lethal catastrophe. Thus, any bleeding tendency should be investigated thoroughly and corrected preoperatively. If deemed necessary, appropriate clotting factors and platelets should be made available at the time of surgery.[34] Patients taking NSAIDs such as aspirin should have their medications stopped for a week before intracranial surgery.[35] This decision may have to be modified in patients suffering from transient ischemic attacks, in whom the risk associated with discontinuation may exceed the benefits.

Endocrine System

Patients with diabetes mellitus who are about to undergo surgery require special attention because hyperglycemia is associated with hyperosmolarity, infection, and poor wound healing. More importantly, it may worsen neurological outcome after an episode of cerebral ischemia. Nonetheless, hypoglycemia is also detrimental because the brain depends on glucose for its energy supply. Close monitoring of glucose perioperatively is therefore essential, and treatment with insulin is often required to maintain euglycemia, but sulfonylureas and metformin should not be used

TABLE 21-2 Mayo Clinic Preoperative Classification of Risk*

GRADE	NEUROLOGICAL FINDINGS	MEDICAL FINDINGS	ANGIOGRAPHIC FINDINGS	RISK FOR MI/STROKE
1	Stable	No defined risk	No major risk	1%
2	Stable	No defined risk	Significant risk	2%
3	Stable	Major risk	With or without risk	7%
4	Unstable	With or without risk	With or without risk	10%

*Medical risk: angina, MI (<6 months), congestive heart failure, severe hypertension (blood pressure of 180/110 mm Hg), chronic obstructive lung disease, age 70 years or older, severe obesity. Neurological risk: progressing deficit, new deficit (<24 hours), frequent daily transient ischemic attacks, multiple cerebral infarcts. Angiographic risk: contralateral carotid artery occlusion, internal carotid artery siphon stenosis, proximal or distal extension of plaque, high carotid bifurcation, presence of soft thrombus.
MI, myocardial infarction.

anticipate blood loss with a need for transfusion and sometimes long, technically difficult surgery requiring maximal brain relaxation.

Although most commonly used anesthetic regimens have been shown to be acceptable in patients undergoing elective supratentorial surgery because short-term outcomes are not affected,[57] lower subdural ICP and better brain relaxation have been observed during anesthesia maintained with propofol than with isoflurane or sevoflurane.[58] Hence, intravenous anesthetics may be preferable over inhaled agents in patients thought to be disposed to intraoperative brain swelling. In contrast, a recent multicenter trial did not find the anesthetic regimen to affect brain bulk assessment or ICP, whereas hyperventilation was found to decrease the risk for increased brain bulk.[59]

Vascular Diseases

Ischemic Cerebrovascular Disease

Patients with arteriosclerotic carotid disease are often scheduled for CEA and, less frequently, for extracranial/intracranial revascularization. The cerebral vascular disease is but one manifestation of the underlying disorder of generalized atherosclerosis. Patients who undergo CEA commonly have significant coronary artery disease, arterial hypertension, peripheral vascular disease, chronic obstructive pulmonary disease, diabetes mellitus, or renal insufficiency.[60] The predominant symptoms and any neurological deficits should be recorded because neurologically unstable patients are more likely to suffer perioperative stroke. The Mayo Clinic classification of preoperative risk is used widely (Table 21-2).[61]

Data from the North American Symptomatic Carotid Endarterectomy Trial (NASCET) suggest that increased surgical risk is associated with five baseline variables: (1) hemispheric versus retinal transient ischemic attack as a qualifying event, (2) a left-sided procedure, (3) contralateral carotid occlusion, (4) an ipsilateral ischemic lesion on CT, and (5) irregular or ulcerated ipsilateral plaque.[62] A review of medical, non–stroke-related complications in patients enrolled in NASCET reported cardiac complications to be the most common cause of postoperative medical morbidity and responsible for all fatalities.[63] The NASCET results indicated that a history of MI or unstable angina and hypertension are independent risk factors for medical complications. Conversely, aggressive blood pressure control in patients undergoing CEA, including preoperative treatment of hypertension, has been associated with improved outcome, thus emphasizing preoperative treatment of high blood pressure.[64] Despite the fact that routine coronary angiography before CEA has been suggested by some, there is no evidence to suggest

improved cardiac outcome attributable to preoperative coronary angiography. Hence, a prudent approach is to assume that all patients scheduled for CEA have associated atherosclerotic heart disease and base perioperative risk and the need for further investigation and intervention on patients' functional status. Although diabetes mellitus was not an independent risk factor for medical complications in NASCET patients,[63] it does increase the risk for perioperative stroke or death.[65] Because hyperglycemia adversely affects outcome after temporary focal or global ischemia, it is best to optimize the blood glucose level preoperatively and manage it carefully in the perioperative period to avoid both hyperglycemia and hypoglycemia.

Aneurysmal Subarachnoid Hemorrhage

The most important aspect of the preoperative evaluation of patients with intracranial aneurysms is assessment of the patient's neurological status and grading of SAH. Classically, SAH is graded with the Hunt and Hess scale (Table 21-3).[66] This grading system has prognostic importance because patients with higher grades of SAH have higher morbidity and mortality. However, higher grades are also more likely to be associated with vasospasm, elevated ICP,[67] impaired cerebral autoregulation,[68,69] and

TABLE 21-3 Modified Hunt and Hess Clinical Scale*

GRADE	CRITERIA
0	Unruptured aneurysm
I	Asymptomatic or minimal headache and slight nuchal rigidity
II	Moderate to severe headache, nuchal rigidity, but no neurologic deficit other than cranial nerve palsy
III	Drowsiness, confusion, or mild focal deficit
IV	Stupor, mild or severe hemiparesis, possible early decerebrate rigidity, vegetative disturbance
V	Deep coma, decerebrate rigidity, moribund appearance

*Serious systemic diseases such as hypertension, diabetes, severe arteriosclerosis, chronic pulmonary disease, and severe vasospasm seen on arteriography result in placement of the patient in the next less favorable (higher) category.
Modified from Hunt WE, Hess RM. Surgical risk as related to time of intervention in the repair of intracranial aneurysm. *J Neurosurg.* 1968;28:14-20.

TABLE 21-4 World Federation of Neurological Surgeons Grading Scale

WFNS GRADE	GCS SCORE	MOTOR DEFICIT
I	15	Absent
II	14-13	Absent
III	14-13	Present
IV	12-7	Absent or present
V	6-3	Absent or present

GCS, Glasgow Coma Scale; WFNS, World Federation of Neurological Surgeons.
From Drake C. Report of World Federation of Neurological Surgeons Committee on a universal subarachnoid hemorrhage grading scale. *J Neurosurg.* 1988;68:985-986.

impaired cerebrovascular reactivity to CO_2.[69] A worse clinical grade is also associated with a higher incidence of cardiac arrhythmia and myocardial dysfunction,[70] hypovolemia, and hyponatremia.[71,72] All these observations are crucial for anesthetic management of these patients.

An alternative scale for grading the severity of SAH is that of the World Federation of Neurological Surgeons, which is based on the Glasgow Coma Scale and the presence or absence of a motor deficit (Table 21-4).[73] The Fisher scale is based on the amount of subarachnoid blood seen on CT, which correlates with risk for the development of vasospasm (Table 21-5).[74] While examining the CT scan, the anesthesiologist can also assess the degree of mass effect, midline shift, cerebral edema, and hydrocephalus, which can help anticipate intraoperative brain swelling.

A variety of medical conditions are known to be associated with the development of cerebral aneurysms and SAH. The preoperative evaluation should look for any of these associated conditions, which include hypertension, coarctation of the aorta, polycystic kidney disease, and fibromuscular dysplasia, as well as a history of smoking, and take into consideration the specific anesthetic concerns with any of these conditions if they exist in a given patient.[75]

Patients with SAH frequently have a contracted intravascular volume that may be multifactorial: altered sensorium associated with reduced fluid intake, use of diuretics and radiographic contrast agents (for diagnostic imaging), bed rest, supine diuresis, negative nitrogen balance, decreased erythropoiesis, and iatrogenic blood loss. In some patients, hypovolemia may be

paradoxically associated with hyponatremia secondary to increased release of atrial natriuretic peptide (cerebral salt wasting syndrome)[76] and may be related to the subsequent development of vasospasm.[77] Erroneous attribution of hyponatremia to the syndrome of inappropriate secretion of antidiuretic hormone may lead to treatment by fluid restriction, thereby increasing the risk for delayed cerebral ischemia and MI.[78] Hypertonic or isotonic saline should be used judiciously to correct the hyponatremia associated with SAH.[79] Other significant electrolyte abnormalities include hypokalemia and hypocalcemia. Preoperative treatment should be aimed at correcting the electrolyte abnormalities while maintaining normal intravascular status.

ECG changes, primarily involving ST-segment changes or T-wave inversion, are common and occur in 40% to 60% of patients suffering from SAH.[80] Three causes could account for the ECG abnormalities in these patients: coincidental MI, SAH-induced MI, or ECG changes without infarction. The ECG changes, however, usually correlate with the neurological dysfunction in that they are more prevalent in patients with poor-grade SAH,[81,82] but they do not affect surgical morbidity or mortality.[83] They do not necessarily correlate with ventricular dysfunction, although the presence of symmetrical inverted T waves and severe QTc-segment prolongation on serial ECG has been shown to be indicative of ventricular dysfunction.[84] Echocardiographic ventricular dysfunction can occur in 10% to 20% of patients and is also more prevalent in patients with high-grade SAH.[26,85] Acute ST-segment elevation is rare with SAH and should be viewed with suspicion for MI. Cardiac enzymes and echocardiography are required to rule out MI and to ascertain the degree of ventricular dysfunction in these patients,[81] and elevated levels of troponin and brain natriuretic protein are associated with a poor prognosis.[86] Although anesthetic risk is increased if MI has occurred, this must be balanced against the risk of rebleeding from postponing surgery. Unless the patient is hemodynamically unstable, has poor ventricular function (ejection fraction <30%), or is clinically in heart failure, surgery should proceed with appropriate hemodynamic monitoring.[87] In contrast, in patients with poor ventricular function refractory to medical management, it would be prudent to defer surgery until the patient is hemodynamically stable; alternatively, endovascular

TABLE 21-5 Fisher Grading of CT Scans in Patients with Subarachnoid Hemorrhage

GRADE	CT SCAN FINDING
1	No blood detected
2	Diffuse thin layer of subarachnoid blood (vertical layers <1 mm thick)
3	Localized clot or thick layer of subarachnoid blood (vertical layers ≥1 mm thick)
4	Intracerebral or intraventricular blood with diffuse or no subarachnoid blood

CT, computed tomography.
From Fisher C, Kistler J, Davis J. Relation of cerebral vasospasm to subarachnoid hemorrhage visualized by computerized tomographic scanning. *Neurosurgery.* 1980;6:1-9.

TABLE 21-6 Electrocardiographic and Myocardial Dysfunction Seen in Patients with Subarachnoid Hemorrhage

BENIGN CHANGES

Sinus bradycardia
Sinus tachycardia
Atrioventricular dissociation
Premature ventricular contractions
Nonspecific ST depression
T-wave inversion
U wave

POSSIBLE WALL MOTION ABNORMALITY

Symmetrical T-wave inversion
Prolonged QT interval (>500 msec)
ST-segment elevation

POSSIBLE MYOCARDIAL INJURY

Q wave
ST-segment elevation
Elevated myocardial enzymes
Elevated troponin I

is reduced and right ventricular hypertrophy may develop secondary to pulmonary hypertension. Lung function should be carefully assessed, as should any increased risk for difficult tracheal intubation and airway control.

Acquired lesions include herniated disks, spinal stenosis, tumor, infection, and trauma. Those afflicted may have neurological symptoms, the severity of which needs to be carefully evaluated preoperatively. Their presence indicates that the spinal cord is at risk, either directly from pressure (slipped disk, tumor) or indirectly from hypoperfusion. Effort is made to prevent further cord damage, maintain adequate blood flow, and avoid secondary insults. Patients seen on an emergency basis after spinal injury usually have actual cord compromise from trauma or instability. Up to 20% of these patients may have concurrent injury to other organ systems.

Certain procedures may require intraoperative "wake-up" tests, and hence the use of a rapid-offset anesthetic technique is required. Informing the patient and reassurance are important aspects of the preoperative visit. In other patients, somatosensory and motor evoked potentials may be monitored, and the anesthetic technique has to be planned accordingly so that it does not interfere with such monitoring. Preoperatively, the neurological assessment should note both the present symptoms and their response to movement. Patients who report worsening of symptoms with motion and who are lucid and cooperative may be candidates for awake fiberoptic intubation of the trachea. Patients with cervical spine pathology may require awake fiberoptic intubation even in the absence of symptoms. In patients who are intoxicated or otherwise uncooperative, rapid-sequence anesthetic induction followed by direct laryngoscopy with manual in-line stabilization is indicated. Succinylcholine is a quick-onset short-acting neuromuscular blocking agent that is ideally suited for urgent tracheal intubation. However, in patients with denervation injury, it can cause an acute elevation in the serum potassium level and lead to cardiac standstill. Because proliferation and development of the extrajunctional receptors responsible for this potentially lethal complication develop over time, it is safe to use succinylcholine in first 48 hours after the injury. Beyond this period, it is best to avoid succinylcholine in patients with significant denervation injury and use alternative quick-onset nondepolarizing muscle relaxants such as rocuronium.

Methylprednisolone therapy is usually started in patients with spinal cord injury and should be continued through the intraoperative period.[96] The prone position is most commonly used and necessitates a firmly secured airway and placement of adequate intravenous and arterial lines before turning the patient. The preoperative interview should include providing the patient information about possible complications of the prone position, including orbital edema, facial swelling, and airway swelling, which may warrant elective postoperative ventilation, as well as the potential for postoperative visual loss.[97] Patients with a history of coronary artery bypass may have an increased risk for myocardial ischemia because of compression of the graft against the chest wall.

Adequate ventilatory effort depends on the integrity of the phrenic nerve (C3-5) and the innervation of the intercostal muscles. A spinal cord injury above C3 will result in a ventilator-dependent patient.[98] An inability to cough and clear secretions increases the risk for respiratory insufficiency and occurs with loss of intercostal muscle action and chest wall excursion. Elective tracheal intubation and ventilation may be required preoperatively, as indicated by the parameters listed in Table 21-10.

Cardiovascular collapse is common after acute cervical cord trauma. Immediately at the time of trauma, activation of the sympathetic nervous system leads to a slight increase in cardiac contractility, as well as mean arterial pressure and systemic vascular resistance. In some patients this intense sympathetic discharge can result in neurogenic pulmonary edema, followed

TABLE 21-10 Indications for Tracheal Intubation in Spinal Cord–Injured Patients

Maximal expiratory force less than +20 cm H_2O
Maximal inspiratory force less than −20 cm H_2O
Vital capacity less than 15 mL/kg or 1 L
PaO_2/FiO_2 less than 250
Severe atelectasis on chest radiographs

by the onset of spinal shock characterized by bradycardia and hypotension with reduced contractility.[99] The spinal shock can last from 1 to 4 weeks. During this period there is complete vasoparalysis. Vasoconstriction for maintenance of cardiac filling pressure cannot take place, and fluid resuscitation is required to correct the relative hypovolemia and restore cardiac output. Because contractility is also reduced, inotropic support may be required. Invasive hemodynamic monitoring with placement of a central venous or pulmonary artery catheter will facilitate management of these patients during the acute period.[100]

Epilepsy Disorders

Epileptic patients can be encountered by the anesthesiologist for a number of reasons, including resection of the epileptic focus, electrocorticographic recording, diagnostic radiologic procedures, nonepilepsy surgery, and management of status epilepticus. Surgery for epilepsy can be performed with the patient under general anesthesia or under local anesthesia with minimal intravenous sedation. A sleep-awake-sleep technique is frequently used, with or without an artificial airway.[101,102] Awake craniotomy allows the surgeon to communicate with a sedated, yet cooperative patient and precisely map the location and extent of resection. An important part of the preanesthetic evaluation is counseling of patients regarding the procedure to allay their fear and anxiety. With the introduction of propofol, it is now possible to induce short periods of "deep anesthesia" during the painful period to maximize patient comfort without sacrificing the subsequent need for a lucid and cooperative patient.[102] Intraoperative electrocorticography has shown that high-dose propofol does not cause seizures[103] and that it does not interfere with mapping, provided that the infusion is suspended for 15 minutes before recording.[104] Good preoperative rapport with the patient nevertheless facilitates this process. In some centers, patient-controlled sedation has been used with some success.[105]

The newer anesthetic drugs have minimal effects on the electrocorticogram and do not interfere with mapping—hence patients with increased ICP or impaired cerebral autoregulation can safely undergo general anesthesia with controlled ventilation to prevent intraoperative brain swelling from retention of carbon dioxide—and provide spontaneous breathing under sedation alone. For all epileptic patients, it is important to note that the use of phenytoin makes them more resistant to nondepolarizing neuromuscular blocking drugs,[106] and these patients may also have an increased requirement for opioids.[107] Placement of a stereotactic frame is a potential airway concern for the anesthesiologist. Ventilation by mask can be difficult, and direct laryngoscopy could be impossible. If tracheal intubation is required, fiberoptic laryngoscopy or intubation with a laryngeal mask airway may be required and must be readily available. Laryngeal mask airways are useful under these conditions and should always be considered.[108] Any sedation technique carries a potential risk for overmedication with the associated loss of protective airway reflexes or the onset of severe respiratory depression. Thus, during the preoperative evaluation, special attention should be paid to airway assessment and the need for airway adjuncts.

Neuroradiology

With the exception of very young children, most neuroradiologic procedures are performed on sedated patients under local anesthesia. Anesthetic assistance is usually requested for children, uncooperative adults, and debilitated patients at high risk. Monitored sedation may be adequate even in children.[109] The aim is to provide a calm, comfortable, and cooperative patient. The technique of patient-controlled sedation with propofol has also been used successfully for interventional radiologic procedures.[110] However, patients with mass lesions and intracranial hypertension who would benefit from avoidance of sedation-induced hypercapnia need general anesthesia with controlled ventilation. General anesthesia and complete immobility are also desirable for embolization of AVMs, endovascular coiling of aneurysms in many centers, and intraluminal balloon angioplasty for cerebral vasospasm.

The preoperative assessment must therefore take into consideration both the nature of the neuroradiologic procedure and the medical and psychological condition of the patient. Added to the anesthetic challenge is the fact that the procedure is performed in an area remote from the familiar operating room environment, where technical and expert assistance are more readily available. For this reason, preoperative evaluation must include anticipation of complications and formulation of back-up plans. All necessary drugs and equipment must be immediately available. For procedures in the MRI suite, anesthetic and monitoring equipment must be MRI compatible.

CONCLUSION

Although the general principles governing intracranial hemodynamics and function are the same, patients undergoing different surgical procedures for different pathologic conditions can have vastly different anesthetic and monitoring requirements. Successful intraoperative management of these challenging patients requires a basic understanding of the pathophysiology and surgical demands of the procedure, all of which start with a thorough preoperative evaluation and preparation of the patient.

SUGGESTED READINGS

American College of Cardiology/American Heart Association Task Force on Practice Guidelines (Writing Committee to Revise the 2002 Guidelines on Perioperative Cardiovascular Evaluation for Noncardiac Surgery); American Society of Echocardiography; American Society of Nuclear Cardiology; Heart Rhythm Society; Society of Cardiovascular Anesthesiologists; Society for Cardiovascular Angiography and Interventions; Society for Vascular Medicine and Biology; Society for Vascular Surgery, Fleisher LA, Beckman JA, Brown KA, et al. ACC/AHA 2007 guidelines on perioperative cardiovascular evaluation and care for noncardiac surgery: executive summary: a report of the American College of Cardiology/American Heart Association Task Force on Practice Guidelines (Writing Committee to Revise the 2002 Guidelines on Perioperative Cardiovascular Evaluation for Noncardiac Surgery). *Anesth Analg.* 2008;106:685-712.

American Society of Anesthesiologists Task Force on Preanesthesia Evaluation. Practice advisory for preanesthesia evaluation: a report by the American Society of Anesthesiologists Task Force on Preanesthesia Evaluation. *Anesthesiology.* 2002;96:485-496.

Dernbach PD, Little JR, Jones SC, et al. Altered cerebral autoregulation and CO_2 reactivity after aneurysmal subarachnoid hemorrhage. *Neurosurgery.* 1988;22:822-826.

Diringer MN, Lim JS, Kirsch JR, et al. Suprasellar and intraventricular blood predict elevated plasma atrial natriuretic factor in subarachnoid hemorrhage. *Stroke.* 1991;22:577-581.

Drummond JC, Dao AV, Roth DM, et al. Effect of dexmedetomidine on cerebral blood flow velocity, cerebral metabolic rate, and carbon dioxide response in normal humans. *Anesthesiology.* 2008;108:225-232.

Fisher CM, Kistler JP, Davis JM. Relation of cerebral vasospasm to subarachnoid hemorrhage visualized by computerized tomographic scanning. *Neurosurgery.* 1980;6:1-9.

Gelb AW, Craen RA, Rao GS, et al. Does hyperventilation improve operating condition during supratentorial craniotomy? A multicenter randomized crossover trial. *Anesth Analg.* 2008;106:585-594.

Goldman L, Caldera DL, Nussbaum SR, et al. Multifactorial index of cardiac risk in noncardiac surgical procedures. *N Engl J Med.* 1977;297:845-850.

Gronert GA, Theye RA. Pathophysiology of hyperkalemia induced by succinylcholine. *Anesthesiology.* 1975;43:89-99.

Hunt WE, Hess RM. Surgical risk as related to time of intervention in the repair of intracranial aneurysms. *J Neurosurg.* 1968;28:14-20.

Lee LA, Roth S, Posner KL, et al. The American Society of Anesthesiologists Postoperative Visual Loss Registry: analysis of 93 spine surgery cases with postoperative visual loss. *Anesthesiology.* 2006;105:652-659.

Lee TH, Marcantonio ER, Mangione CM, et al. Derivation and prospective validation of a simple index for prediction of cardiac risk of major noncardiac surgery. *Circulation.* 1999;100:1043-1049.

Mallampati SR, Gatt SP, Gugino LD, et al. A clinical sign to predict difficult tracheal intubation: a prospective study. *Can Anaesth Soc J.* 1985;32:429-434.

North American Symptomatic Carotid Endarterectomy Trial Steering Committee: North American Symptomatic Carotid Endarterectomy Trial: Methods, patient characteristics, and progress. *Stroke.* 1991;22:711-720.

Paciaroni M, Eliasziw M, Kappelle LJ, et al. Medical complications associated with carotid endarterectomy. *North American Symptomatic Carotid Endarterectomy Trial (NASCET).* 1999;30:1759-1763.

Petersen KD, Landsfeldt U, Cold GE, et al. Intracranial pressure and cerebral hemodynamic in patients with cerebral tumors: a randomized prospective study of patients subjected to craniotomy in propofol-fentanyl, isoflurane-fentanyl, or sevoflurane-fentanyl anesthesia. *Anesthesiology.* 2003;98:329-336.

POISE Study Group; Devereaux PJ, Yang H, Ysusf S, et al. Effects of extended-release metoprolol succinate in patients undergoing non-cardiac surgery (POISE trial): a randomised controlled trial. *Lancet.* 2008;371:1839-1847.

Rasmussen M, Bundgaard H, Cold GE. Craniotomy for supratentorial brain tumors: risk factors for brain swelling after opening the dura mater. *J Neurosurg.* 2004;101:621-626.

Report of World Federation of Neurological Surgeons Committee on a universal subarachnoid hemorrhage grading scale. *J Neurosurg.* 1988;68:985-986.

Rozet I, Vavilala MS, Lindley AM, et al. Cerebral autoregulation and CO_2 reactivity in anterior and posterior cerebral circulation during sevoflurane anesthesia. *Anesth Analg.* 2006;102:560-564.

Skucas AP, Artru AA. Anesthetic complications of awake craniotomies for epilepsy surgery. *Anesth Analg.* 2006;102:882-887.

Smetana GW, Lawrence VA, Cornell JE; American College of Physicians. Preoperative pulmonary risk stratification for noncardiothoracic surgery: systematic review for the American College of Physicians. *Ann Intern Med.* 2006;144:581-595.

Thal GD, Szabo MD, Lopez-Bresnahan M, et al. Exacerbation or unmasking of focal neurologic deficits by sedatives. *Anesthesiology.* 1996;85:21-25.

Van der Bilt IA, Hasan D, Vandertop WP, et al. Impact of cardiac complications on outcome after aneurysmal subarachnoid hemorrhage: a meta-analysis. *Neurology* 2009;72:635-642.

Wolters U, Wolf T, Stützer H, et al. ASA classification and perioperative variables as predictors of postoperative outcome. *Br J Anaesth.* 1996;77:217-222.

Full references can be found on Expert Consult @ www.expertconsult.com

CHAPTER 22

Avoidance of Complications in Neurosurgery

Nirit Weiss ■ Kalmon D. Post

As with all neurosurgical procedures, avoidance of complications is as important as treatment of disease. In general, avoidance of surgical complications requires attention to making the correct diagnosis, choosing the appropriate surgery, and correctly selecting patients. This chapter is intended to review how to prevent complications of neurosurgical procedures in general, with additional emphasis placed on the specific complications that might be encountered in particular approaches to the spine and brain.

Avoidance of complications in neurosurgery begins with the correct selection of patients who are likely to benefit from the surgical intervention planned. When possible, patients with nonmedical issues that have a known association with poor outcomes, such as workers' compensation claims or pending lawsuits, should be investigated further to determine the patient's motivation for recovery.[1-7] Taking the time to explain the probable risks and benefits of the procedure allows the patient to make an informed decision and protects the surgeon in the event of an adverse outcome from claims of inadequate consent. The remainder of this chapter focuses on prevention of complications once the patient has arrived in the operating room. Intraoperative complications may be related to anesthetic issues, positioning of the patient, or technical or anatomic aspects of the specific surgery selected.

Before induction of anesthesia, the surgeon and anesthesiologist must discuss the case in detail and review what is likely to happen and the possible risks. Ideally, an experienced neuroanesthesiologist should be available for neurosurgical procedures. Adequate venous access, placement of a single- or double-lumen tube as required by the surgical approach, and insertion of an intracardiac central venous pressure line to potentially remove air emboli must be planned in advance. The presence of blood products in proximity to the operating room and notification of the blood bank that more may be required depend on the scope of the surgical procedure. Antibiotics should be administered within 1 hour before incisions to ensure therapeutic blood levels.[8]

COMPLICATIONS RELATED TO PATIENT POSITIONING

After the anesthesiologist has determined that the airway has been adequately secured and that all lines and monitoring equipment are in place, the patient is ready to be positioned. Several common positioning errors can lead to complications,[9-21] but most can be prevented with meticulous positioning protocols.

Supine Positioning

Exposure, bleeding, and complications such as air embolism depend on the angle of the head relative to the operative site and the patient's heart. Overflexing the neck may lead to kinking of the endotracheal tube in the pharynx or obstruction of the jugular vein, which may increase venous pressure in the head and cause increased bleeding or decreased perfusion. The heels, gluteal area, shoulders, and head need to be sufficiently padded. Prefer-

ably, rolls are placed under both knees so that they are slightly flexed, and the feet should be suspended by padding under the calves. This position prevents heel pressure ulcers and compression on the Achilles tendon. If the arms are to be secured at the patient's side, adequate padding of the elbow and wrist and any points of contact with monitoring devices need to be verified before the procedure starts.

Prone Positioning

Nerve palsies and compression injuries are the most frequent complications seen and the most easily preventable. Radial and ulnar neuropathies can occur as a result of positioning the patient in the prone position with the arms extended if padding is inadequate or an inappropriate position is used. Keeping the arms in a mildly flexed position prevents excessive traction in either direction. Padding may be in the form of sheets or blankets placed under the elbows and forearms, or egg-crate foam padding can be used. Brachial plexus injuries can occur with rostral or caudal traction on the shoulders[22] and is frequently seen in the prone position when the arms are extended in the cruciate position or too far above the head. Downward traction, such as when the shoulders need to be pulled down for x-ray localization in the low cervical or cervicothoracic junction, can also cause brachial plexus injury. If possible, any tension placed on the patient's shoulders during radiography should be removed after the x-ray film has been obtained. Neurophysiologic monitoring of the ulnar nerve with somatosensory evoked potentials during spinal procedures has been shown to be effective in correcting and preventing position-related stretch injuries to the brachial plexus.[23,24] Another common peripheral neuropathy associated with the prone position is inadequate padding of the anterior superior iliac crest, which can lead to pain or numbness in the distribution of the lateral femoral cutaneous nerve.[25] A rare complication is obstruction of the external iliac artery or femoral artery from prolonged compression in the inguinal region.[26,27]

Starting at the top, the face and head should be gently suspended without any compression on any one area (discussed later in the chapter in further detail). If the patient is being placed on chest rolls or chest bolsters, the ideal position is to have the shoulders slightly overhanging the chest rolls. Breasts should be tucked between the two rolls to prevent excessive pressure. Prone positioning on a spinal table (e.g., Jackson table, Orthopedic Systems, Inc., Union City, CA) requires placement of the hip pads (of a size appropriate for the patient) so that the top of the pad is at the anterior superior iliac crest. The thigh pads are placed just below the hip pads. The ankles should be allowed to dangle off the edge of the leg supports, if possible. Inadequate padding of the anterior superior iliac crest can cause pressure necrosis of the overlying skin. Male genitalia should be examined to verify that they are not being compressed between the thighs or gluteal folds and that a Foley catheter, if present, is not causing undue traction on the penis. The knees need to be padded, and a padded roll should be placed underneath the ankles so that the feet hang suspended.

The abdomen should be hanging suspended to prevent venous compression and improve venous return to the heart. This point is critical because excessive venous compression can lead to significant intraoperative bleeding secondary to epidural venous hypertension. If the abdomen cannot be adequately suspended, the three-quarter prone position can be used instead (discussed later), particularly in morbidly obese patients, who may not fit on any chest bolstering system, such as the Kamden frame, the four-post Relton frame, or chest rolls. This position allows the abdomen to remain free while the surgeon works from behind, but the position also makes intraoperative radiography very difficult.

Another difficulty with positioning for spine surgery is the difference between the ideal position for a decompressive procedure, with the spine and hips flexed, and that for spinal fusion, with the spine in a more lordotic position and the hips and spine in neutral positions. Many patients have been subjected to iatrogenic flat-back syndrome because of improper position during a fusion procedure.[28]

Surgeons must be aware of the potential for unilateral or bilateral blindness after prolonged prone surgery. Causes have been hypothesized to be occlusion of the retinal artery or vein, direct trauma, orbital compartment syndrome, and ischemic optic neuropathy. Although rare, devastating complications have been described even when no direct trauma occurred, and therefore patients' eyes should be checked frequently during the procedure. Minimizing blood loss and hypotensive episodes and maintaining a slightly elevated head of the bed may reduce the chance for this complication. If orbital compartment syndrome is suspected, emergency orbital decompression is the best chance for recovery.[29-33]

Lateral Positioning

The lateral or three-quarters lateral decubitus position carries with it specific risks for peripheral nerve injuries. Stretch on the brachial plexus can be prevented by placement of an axillary roll slightly thicker than the diameter of the upper part of the arm. This roll should be placed approximately four fingerbreadths below the armpit to prevent compression of the long thoracic nerve. Failure to place an adequately sized roll may lead to excessive stretch of the brachial plexus, with the greatest effects on the C5 and C6 nerve roots. The upper extremities need to be supported in relatively neutral positions to prevent ulnar neuropathies. Horner's syndrome can occur when the head is inadequately padded and allowed to hang laterally in such a manner that excessive tension is placed on the superior cervical ganglion.[34] Excessive traction on the lateral femoral cutaneous nerve can be caused by undue extension of the upper part of the leg at the hip while bending the dependent leg. Compression of the common peroneal nerve can occur as a result of inadequate padding laterally under the knee.

Intraoperative Monitoring

Various electrophysiologic modalities can be used to detect subtle signs of neurological compromise before they become fixed deficits. The use of intraoperative monitoring can reduce the likelihood of significant neurological deficits in the appropriate circumstances. Some positioning complications can be avoided with the concomitant use of intraoperative monitoring.[9,35-39] At our institution, we use motor evoked potentials or somatosensory evoked potentials before and after positioning that may result in injury to the cervical cord. We have found excellent correlation between the lack of changes in evoked potentials and patient outcome. Monitoring is not necessary or indicated in all cases because it is time-consuming, can cause inappropriate movement of the patient, results in bleeding, and has the potential for needlestick injury to the operating room staff. However, in procedures with a potential for significant risk to the cord or neural structures, neurological monitoring is a helpful adjunct to the surgeon. Electrophysiologic neurological monitoring can consist of somatosensory evoked potentials, motor evoked potentials, intraoperative electromyographic responses, nerve action potential monitoring, direct spinal cord stimulation, and other methods.[36,37,40-44] The information gleaned from these modalities can be used to determine whether manipulation of the neural elements is compromising conduction. Numerous authors have published series in which the surgeon has changed some portion of the procedure as a reaction to changes in electrophysiologic monitoring.[9,35-39,43-48] Changes in ulnar nerve somatosensory evoked potentials can also indicate traction injury to the brachial plexus and is increasingly being used to monitor positioning, even with lumbar and thoracic procedures.[23,24]

Although not appropriate to monitor for position-related changes, direct epidural electrode motor evoked potential monitoring provides real-time evaluation of the spinal motor tracts and allows quantification of the measured output. This technique may be used during intramedullary spinal cord tumor resection and has been suggested to be helpful in minimizing injury during intramedullary resection.[49]

Cranial Fixation Complications

Positioning of the head for cranial fixation is a frequent source of complications. In sacral, lumbar, and midthoracic surgery performed in the prone position, the head does not need to remain immobile, nor does the cervical spine need to be kept straight. In these circumstances, the head is positioned on loose foam padding (with a cutout for the airway and no compression on the eyes), or the head is turned to the side on loose padding. The objective is to prevent compression on the eyes, face, and forehead. However, for many types of cranial, craniocervical, cervical, or cervicothoracic surgery, it is necessary to firmly immobilize the head and prevent unwanted motion of the neck. Several devices can be used to immobilize the head, the most effective of which is the Mayfield head clamp. This clamp involves three-point pin fixation into the skull so that the skull and neck are rigid relative to the table and, assuming that the body is adequately secured to the table, rigid relative to the body. Because it is more difficult to correct spine deformities after the head is secured in this manner, if part of the goal is to reconstitute cervical lordosis, this issue needs to be considered when positioning.

Pin site complications include lacerations,[50] skull fractures, associated intracranial hemorrhage (i.e., epidural, subdural, or subarachnoid hemorrhages), and infections that can lead to osteomyelitis.[51-56] Lacerations can be prevented by making sure that the two-pin arm swivels freely so that the force is evenly distributed between the two pins without one pin being shielded from tension, which can potentially result in pivoting on the other pin. If the pins are placed into muscle, it is wise to recheck tension on the single pin to make sure that the muscle has not settled and reduced the pressure. The three pins should be placed slightly below the center of gravity of the head when it is in final position to prevent gravity or personnel from pulling the head down and out of the pins. Ideally, the pins should not be placed directly into the coronal suture or temporal squamosal bone because these bones are most prone to fracture.[57-59] Pins should be tightened to 60 to 80 lb in adults and 40 to 60 lb in children younger than 15 years. Pins are generally avoided in children younger than 2 years; however, some skull clamp systems do exist for these patients for procedures in which they are required.[60]

Pivoting within the pins by one of these methods or by inadequately locking the clamp before positioning the patient can result in changes in neck position (which can cause cervical spinal cord injury), lacerations, or compression on the eyes and subsequent blindness. These complications can also occur with Gardner-Wells–type tong traction.

Other forms of head support include the horseshoe headrest and the four-cup headrest. Because the horseshoe headrest is not a rigid form of fixation, the head may shift during the procedure, and thus it is imperative that the anesthesiologist continuously observe for any signs of movement. The four-cup headrest is an excellent alternative to the horseshoe, although blindness, skin and scalp compression, and abnormal cervical motion are possible with either support. Alopecia has been reported as a result of scalp compression.[61-67]

Dependent Edema

One complication associated with the prone position is the development of orofacial edema when the head is dependent. This complication occurs more frequently with longer procedures and when the spine is more flexed for facilitation of the surgical approach. Such edema can be prevented by minimizing the amount of fluid given by the anesthesiologist and by placing the patient slightly more in a reverse-Trendelenburg position to elevate the head relative to the heart. Facial edema can result in lingual or laryngeal edema and resultant airway obstruction. If obstruction occurs, the patient should be kept intubated until the edema has improved or resolved. Premature attempts at extubation can result in hypoxia and may necessitate emergency tracheotomy.

CATASTROPHIC MEDICAL COMPLICATIONS

Venous Air Embolism

In positioning patients for neurosurgical procedures, the anesthesia team and the surgeons must be aware of the gradient between the patient's head and the right atrium. Venous air embolism (VAE) is most often encountered with the patient in the seated position for posterior fossa surgery or cervical spine surgery.[68-73] It has also been described in patients who have undergone procedures in the prone, supine, and lateral positions.[68,71-77] Dehydration or blood loss leading to decreased central venous pressure may potentiate the risk for VAE. Patients with a patent foramen ovale or a known right-to-left shunt should be given special consideration before the seated position is used because the risk for paradoxical air embolism after VAE appears to be higher.

Most VAEs are thought to be caused by air entering noncollapsible veins, dural sinuses, or diploic veins. They also have arisen from central venous lines and pulmonary artery catheters. Air travels from the head down the venous system to the heart and eventually to the lungs, where pulmonary constriction and pulmonary hypertension ensue, or in patients with a right-left heart shunt, paradoxical air embolism may occur. Peripheral resistance decreases, and cardiac output initially increases to compensate and maintain blood pressure. Later, as the volume of air infused increases, cardiac output drops, as does blood pressure. Without intervention, cardiac arrest may occur.

Given the dangers of VAE, early detection of the embolus is paramount in reducing the severity of this complication. Monitors used to detect emboli include precordial Doppler ultrasonography, capnography or mass spectrometry, transesophageal echocardiography, transcutaneous oxygen, esophageal stethoscope, and right heart catheter.[68,69,71-74,77] The most sensitive are transesophageal echocardiography and Doppler, followed by expired nitrogen and end-tidal carbon dioxide. Electrocardiographic changes, hypotension, and heart murmurs are late signs. Because no single monitor is completely reliable, two or more should be used simultaneously. In awake patients, the presence

of a cough may be the earliest sign of VAE, and it can be treated before the VAE becomes hemodynamically significant.[78] Detection of VAE has increased over the past several decades, but serious morbidity and mortality have decreased. Its incidence varies from 1.2% to 60%, with morbidity and mortality rates of less than 3% in most series.

Treatment of VAE includes aspiration of air through a right atrial catheter, discontinuation of nitrous oxide because it may enlarge the air bubble, and administration of pure oxygen. Surgeons should immediately seal the portals of entry with bone wax, electrocautery, and full-field irrigation. Arrhythmias, hypotension, and hypoxemia should be corrected quickly. Repositioning the patient in the left lateral decubitus position may facilitate removal of air from the right atrium. Stabilization of the patient's hemodynamic status becomes the first priority, and the procedure may have to be prematurely terminated if hemodynamic stabilization cannot be achieved easily.

Deep Venous Thrombosis and Pulmonary Embolism

Deep venous thrombosis (DVT) and pulmonary embolism are major contributors to morbidity and mortality in postoperative neurosurgical patients. The incidence of DVT, as measured by the labeled fibrinogen technique, ranges from 29% to 43%.[79-91] Most DVTs are asymptomatic and never come to medical attention. Pulmonary embolism, however, is thought to subsequently occur in 15% of such patients.[80,84,89,92,93] Significant thrombi are thought to arise from the popliteal and iliofemoral veins. Risk factors include prolonged surgery and immobilization, previous DVT, malignancy, direct lower extremity trauma, limb weakness, use of oral contraceptives, gram-negative sepsis, advanced age, hypercoagulability, pregnancy, and congestive heart failure.[79,81,83-89,92-100]

A diagnosis of DVT made by clinical examination is generally unreliable. Ankle swelling, calf pain, calf tightness, and a positive Homans sign may all be absent, even in the presence of significant DVT. Doppler ultrasonography and impedance plethysmography are useful in detecting proximal venous thrombosis and are the mainstay of diagnosis, with sensitivities exceeding 90%. When Doppler results are equivocal, extremity venography can be used to diagnose distal and proximal DVTs.

Because of the often-fatal result of pulmonary embolism, prophylaxis against DVT is of major importance in neurosurgery. Many studies have confirmed the utility of sequential pneumatic leg compression devices in preventing DVT.[80,81,83,84,89,90,101,102] These devices are placed on the patient preoperatively and should be continued until the patient is ambulatory. Early mobilization of postoperative patients is important in preventing thrombus formation. The prophylactic use of low-dose (minidose) subcutaneous heparin (e.g., 5000 IU twice daily) has been well studied over the past 25 years and has been demonstrated to be efficacious in preventing DVT.[86,102-107] However, some studies have shown an increase in the rate of postoperative intracranial bleeding with minidose administration of heparin.[102,103] Low-molecular-weight heparin (LMWH) has more recently been used for DVT prophylaxis in surgical patients. Several meta-analyses have been conducted, but it remains unclear whether unfractioned heparin or LMWH is superior for DVT prophylaxis in neurosurgical patients or whether increased efficacy correlates with increased hemorrhagic complications.[108-111]

Despite the use of such prophylactic methods, thrombi inevitably develop in one or both lower extremities in some patients. Management options include full-dose heparinization or inferior vena cava interruption. In the immediate and early postoperative period, many neurosurgeons believe that neurosurgical patients with documented DVT should undergo transvenous Greenfield filter placement.[80,81,83,84,88,89,98,102] There appears to be a general consensus that full anticoagulation is acceptable 1 to 3 weeks after surgery; our institution uses the 1-week rule. Treatment with intravenous heparin (target partial thromboplastin time of 45 to 60 seconds) is followed by oral warfarin sulfate (target international normalized ratio of 2) when not contraindicated. Anticoagulation should be continued for 6 weeks to 3 months in uncomplicated cases. Gastrointestinal bleeding is the most common serious complication encountered.

Patients experiencing pulmonary embolism complain of pleuritic chest pain, hemoptysis, and dyspnea. Jugular venous distention, fever, rales, tachypnea, hypotension, and altered mental status may be found on physical examination. Arterial blood gas determination reveals a Po_2 of less than 80 mm Hg in 85% of patients, accompanied by a widened alveolar-arterial gradient. The level of fibrin degradation products is elevated in most cases. In patients with massive embolism, right axis deviation, right ventricular strain, or right bundle branch block may be identified on electrocardiography. Chest radiography demonstrates an effusion or infiltrate in 90% of cases. A nuclear medicine ventilation-perfusion scan is sensitive in detecting pulmonary embolism but is not specific. The entire clinical scenario, including patient examination, laboratory results, and radiographic evaluation, leads to the diagnosis.[80,84,89,93,112-116] Spiral computed tomography (CT) has become the preferred diagnostic study for pulmonary embolism.[117] However, pulmonary angiography is the "gold standard" and may be necessary to confirm the diagnosis in as many as half of patients.

Guidelines similar to those discussed for treatment of DVT should be used for the treatment of pulmonary embolism. Patients suffering from a massive, life-threatening embolus, however, should be fully anticoagulated despite the risk for intracranial hemorrhage. This subset of patients usually requires ventilatory support and vasopressor therapy to ensure adequate oxygenation and blood pressure. Because thrombolytic therapy with urokinase or streptokinase has a higher risk for complications than does treatment with heparin, with no significant improvement in outcome, these modes of therapy have largely been abandoned. When all else fails, pulmonary embolectomy may be performed as a lifesaving measure.

Hemorrhagic and Transfusion-Related Issues

Two significant and somewhat similar complications related to bleeding are diffuse intravascular coagulation and transfusion reactions. Both are a consequence of excessive bleeding and transfusions. The first results in a consumptive coagulopathy and further paradoxical bleeding. The other is a reaction to incompatible blood and can result in fever, rash, or shock. Both can be prevented by meticulous hemostasis. When bone is bleeding in an area where the need for fusion precludes the use of bone wax, thrombin-soaked Gelfoam can be rubbed on the bleeding bone surfaces and acts in much the same way as bone wax. When hemostasis alone is not enough to minimize transfusion requirements, as with some long spinal procedures, autologous blood salvage (e.g., Cell Saver) can be used to recycle the patient's own blood. Other modalities to minimize allogeneic transfusions include autologous blood donation (with or without the use of preoperative erythropoietin), hemodilution, or induced hypotension. Patients about to undergo neurosurgery should, when medically suitable, avoid the use of aspirin products in the week before surgery and other nonsteroidal anti-inflammatory agents on the day before surgery.

Wound Complications

Because of the vascularity of the scalp, most cranial wounds heal well. Postoperative pseudomeningocele formation from persis-

tent leakage of cerebrospinal fluid (CSF) is more common when the normal CSF reabsorption pathways are impaired, as with hydrocephalus, subarachnoid hemorrhage, and meningitis. CSF finds the path of exit of least resistance from the head.

Several potential problems related to the wound area and wound closure can be anticipated and prevented. The first category is postoperative blood collections, or hematomas. Ideally, postoperative hematomas can be prevented by meticulous hemostasis during the procedure, but such is not always the case. The use of postoperative drainage devices (e.g., Hemovac, Jackson-Pratt drain) in wounds for which hemostasis was difficult to achieve before closure can reduce the incidence of postoperative hematoma. Postoperative drainage may also be advantageous in patients in whom postoperative anticoagulation may be required because some of these patients have slightly delayed hematoma formation.[118] An obese patient undergoing spine surgery may have significant serous exudation that can continue for up to 5 days or longer postoperatively. It is best to keep a drain in the submuscular space during this time to prevent a postoperative seroma that can become infected.

Several factors can predispose to loss of wound integrity. Prolonged steroid use, irradiation or chemotherapy, reoperations, and malnutrition can predispose patients to poor wound healing. Patients who are likely to lie on their incisions because of an inability to move or the location of an incision are also likely to experience wound breakdown because of pressure-related ischemia and failure to heal adequately. Known or unknown intraoperative violations of sterility may lead to subcutaneous infection and resultant loss of wound integrity. Failure to use perioperative antibiotics can also lead to local infection and failure of the incision line. Maintenance of a dry, sterile wound area results in better wound healing, and if a dressing becomes significantly stained or wet, it must be changed immediately. One way to prevent wound breakdown in a compromised host is the use of an incision that avoids the impaired area. Craniotomies may require a larger incision, such as a bicoronal or larger curvilinear incision that avoids a focused radiation area. In spine surgery, this means use of a paramedian incision. By removing the incision from the avascular midline plane and creating a vascularized myocutaneous flap, patients with cancer or severe malnutrition can have the same or better wound-healing rates as healthy patients. By making the incision off the midline, the pressure is also not directly on the wound and the instrumentation.

Other modalities being investigated include the use of cultured keratinocytes or fibroblasts injected back into the wound area, supplemental or hyperbaric oxygen therapy for several days after surgery, and injection of various growth factors into the wounds.

RISK FACTORS RELATED TO ANATOMY OR TECHNIQUE IN SPECIFIC SURGERIES

Cranial Surgery

Postoperative Seizures

The risk for postoperative seizures within the first week after supratentorial procedures has been well described in the literature.[119-132] The underlying cause of these seizures may be metabolic derangements, cerebral hypoxia, preoperative structural defects, stroke and vascular abnormalities, or congenital seizure disorder. Manipulation of brain tissue, postoperative edema, and hematoma formation are common causes of surgically induced seizures. The overall incidence of immediate and early seizures after craniotomy is 4% to 19%.

It is important to identify any risk factors that may contribute to the development of seizures postoperatively. Lesions of the tumor size, approximately 43%, after high-dose Gamma Knife radiosurgery for vestibular schwannomas that correlates with deterioration of facial and trigeminal function. The effect is much smaller at lower doses.[244] Because tumor control is greater with larger doses of radiation, fractionated stereotactic radiosurgery is usually performed to allow increased control of growth while minimizing risk to the facial, cochlear, and trigeminal nerves.[245] Intracanalicular tumors may be associated with higher cranial nerve morbidity when treated with radiosurgery.[246] Improvements in target imaging and reduction in doses have led to lower cranial nerve morbidity.[241,243]

Radiosurgery has also been applied to cranial base meningiomas. The morbidity rate is about 5% to 8%.[238,239,247,248] Most complications involve transient cranial nerve palsies and occur 3 to 31 months after surgery. High radiation doses applied to Meckel's cave increase risk for the development of trigeminal neuropathy.[239] Radiosurgery is also used to treat gliomas and brain metastasis. Preliminary reports indicate a morbidity rate of about 10% and a mortality rate of 1%.[249] Early complications can involve increased ICP, which may lead to death.[250] Radiotherapy for brain parenchymal lesions can result in seizure complications. Patients with lesions in the motor cortex are especially susceptible to seizures after radiosurgery.[251] Gamma Knife radiosurgery for trigeminal neuralgia is generally well tolerated and associated with minimal morbidity. Loss of facial sensation has been reported infrequently.[252]

Spine Surgery

Cerebrospinal Fluid Leak or Pseudomeningocele Formation

Prevention of CSF leakage is critical for optimizing wound healing, for preventing neural elements from herniating through the defect in the dura and leading to pain syndromes or neurological deficits, and for eliminating positional headaches. It is generally accepted that reduction of intraspinal CSF pressure facilitates healing of a dural defect. This can be achieved by maintenance of strict bed rest or by placement of a CSF diversion drain, such as a lumbar drain. The use of spinal subarachnoid drains after a CSF leak is supported as an adjunct.[253-257] One treatment element that seems to be accepted almost uniformly as being beneficial is the use of fibrin glue sealants.[258-263] The sealant can be prepared autologously in the operating room, from cryoprecipitate obtained from the blood bank, or from commercial kits made from donated blood products. Regardless of the cause, fibrin glue sealants, when applied in the area of the dural repair, dramatically increase the rate of healing. The use of dural replacements is more controversial. Repair with fascia, AlloDerm, Duragen, or other techniques is more a matter of choice than evidence-based medicine.

Primary repair of a dural violation, when possible, is clearly indicated. Multiple surgeons have documented increased infection rates and decreased fusion rates associated with CSF leaks.[255,262-265] In addition to CSF leaking from the durotomy, nerve roots have been known to herniate into the durotomy and result in painful syndromes.[266]

A tight, multilayer closure is critical to prevent local CSF collections from leaking outward to the skin. If a CSF leak exists, organisms have a portal of entry and may cause meningitis. Any CSF leak should be treated immediately by oversewing of the wound and institution of some form of CSF pressure–reducing strategy. The decision to revise a wound rather than treat conservatively depends on several factors, including the tightness of the dural and fascial closure, the presence of and size of the subfascial collection, and the patient's underlying ability to heal a wound spontaneously. A CSF pseudomeningocele, even in the absence of an external leak, can increase the likelihood of local infection.

Instrumentation-Related Risks

Instrumentation has increased the incidence of complications in all series that have compared the results of instrumented with noninstrumented fusions.[267-270] This finding is not surprising in that instrumentation adds time, complexity, and an implanted foreign body to the operative procedure. Fusion rates are uniformly higher in instrumented cases, and most experienced spine surgeons believe that the risks are outweighed by the benefits of rigid segmental fixation. However, each surgeon must feel confident and comfortable with any technique because morbidity rates vary from surgeon to surgeon.[268,271-289]

Identification of the correct level is critical for most spine operations. Whether preoperative or intraoperative, the use of radiography or fluoroscopy to adequately identify the level in question is vital for medical and legal documentation. Surgical operations at the wrong level can be prevented by identifying landmarks with radiographs, but surface and deeper landmarks must be correlated. One common problem is failure to take into account the downward projection of the spinous process; for example, a needle placed on one spinous process but in front of the next lower body may lead to confusion about the level. Obvious bony landmarks (e.g., loss of a pedicle or a fracture seen on the localizing film) can facilitate identifying the surgical site. Subtle findings, such as the location of unique osteophytes or compression fractures, can assist in localization when obvious findings are absent. The use of a tangible marker, such as a bite from bone with a rongeur or placement of a stitch into a spinous process, reduces ambiguity later in the procedure.

The use of intraoperative imaging has grown dramatically. Ultrasonography as an intraoperative localizing device can help verify the correct level and locate hidden, deep lesions within the spinal cord.[290-293] More medical centers are using portable and dedicated MRI and CT scanners for determination of the adequacy of procedures for resection of tumor or osteophytes, placement of instrumentation, or other needs of the surgeon. Stand-alone MRI scanners have been developed that function in an operating room or even as an operating room.[294] Some of these modalities require specialized equipment that is compatible with the modality (e.g., nonmagnetic instruments for intraoperative MRI). Each has its advantages and limitations, and the use of these devices depends on the needs of the surgeon and the institution. Intraoperative CT scanners are available, as are fluouroscopy-based systems that create three-dimensional reconstructions resembling CT scans. These modalities can be useful in confirming the adequacy of decompression or screw placement before leaving the operating room.

Stereotactic navigational adjuncts have increasingly been used in spine surgery.[294-298] The accuracy of stereotaxis depends on the quality of the scan used, the position of the patient intraoperatively and in the scanner, performance of the stereotactic portion of the procedure before any resection or opening that would distort the landmarks used for calibration, and user-dependent variables. Currently, numerous intraoperative navigation techniques are available that rely on preoperative CT, intraoperative three-dimensional reconstruction from planar fluoroscopy, or three-dimensional reconstruction using intraoperative isocentric circumferential fluoroscopy. All appear to provide accuracy with respect to screw placement.[299-303] Although each system has its pros and cons, there is no evidence that one system is clearly superior to another.[301] Miniature robotic systems are also being developed to improve the accuracy of targeting and screw placement.[302,303] Navigational techniques are increasing being applied to spinal arthroplasty procedures, as well as fusion procedures.[304]

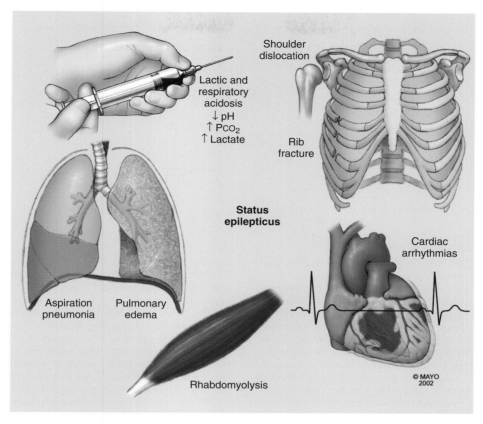

FIGURE 24-3 Systemic effects of status epilepticus. *(©Mayo, 2002.)*

Nonconvulsive status epilepticus is very difficult to diagnose and is probably less common. It frequently follows a clearly defined generalized tonic-clonic seizure or occurs in elderly patients with a major irreversible brain injury. Clinical hallmarks are a decrease in the level of consciousness or fluctuation in responsiveness. Patients may have fluttering of the eyelids or eye deviation as the only signs of nonconvulsive status epilepticus.

Management of seizures begins with aspiration precautions. Respiratory support with manual bagging is commonly sufficient, but progression to status epilepticus requires mechanical ventilation and placement of a central line.

Benzodiazepines—in particular, lorazepam—are the preferred first-line drugs for acute control of tonic-clonic seizures. Lorazepam terminates seizures in more than 80% of patients.[23]

Intravenous administration of phenytoin or fosphenytoin usually follows treatment with benzodiazepines. Newer alternative drugs such as levetiracetam have fewer side effects and are now available as intravenous and oral formulations. Data are insufficient to use levetiracetam for the treatment of status epilepticus, but it remains a preferable drug in patients with single seizures. The recent Food and Drug Administration acceptance of intravenous levetiracetam (15-minute intravenous infusion of 1000 mg) may increase its role in the treatment of refractory status epilepticus, but levetiracetam has been effective mostly in patients with nonconvulsive or focal status epilepticus.

Failure of lorazepam and fosphenytoin in adequate doses to control seizures indicates transition to refractory status epilepticus. The different approaches for refractory status epilepticus have seldom been compared in a prospective controlled study. At this point, either increasing doses of barbiturates or midazolam should be used for treatment.[24] Propofol is another alternative, but high doses are needed. Propofol infusion syndrome, or sudden cardiovascular collapse with metabolic acidosis, is a serious complication that limits the routine use of this otherwise very effective medication.[25] Drugs used for seizures and status epilepticus are presented in Table 24-3.

ASSESSMENT OF NUTRITIONAL NEEDS

Early feeding of the gut to ensure adequate nutrition is part of daily care. Outcome studies in patients with severe strokes and head injury suggest that early nutritional support reduces mortality and the incidence of nosocomial infections.[26-28] The main goal of nutrition should be to preserve muscle mass and provide adequate fluids, minerals, and fats.[29,30]

Malnutrition should be recognized during emergency admission of patients with severe head injury or fulminant meningitis, conditions that are more prevalent in alcoholics and illegal drug users. Vitamin B_1 (thiamine) deficiency might lead to the development of Wernicke-Korsakoff syndrome (confusional state, horizontal and vertical nystagmus, gaze palsy, and ataxia of gait). Intravenous administration of thiamine (100 mg intravenously initially and then 100 mg daily for 5 to 7 days) prevents the development of Wernicke-Korsakoff syndrome after carbohydrate loads.

Malnutrition causes significant lung malfunction by impairing the respiratory muscles, decreasing the respiratory drive, and diminishing lung defense mechanisms. At the same time, overfeeding with excessive carbohydrate calories may lead to hypercapnia, which reduces the success of weaning. Caloric needs can be estimated by weight and approximate 25 to 30 kcal/kg per day. The nutritional needs of patients with critical neurological illness should be calculated with the Harris-Benedict formula to obtain the basal energy expenditure (BEE) in calories. The Harris-Benedict equations are based on weight in kilograms, height in centimeters, and age in years. For men, BEE = 66.5 + (13.75 ×

TABLE 24-3 Intravenously Administered Drugs Typically Used for the Treatment of Status Epilepticus

DRUG	LOADING DOSE	RATE OF ADMINISTRATION	GOAL
Lorazepam	4-8 mg	Push	Not available
Phenytoin	18-20 mg/kg	50 mg/min	10-20 µg/mL
Fosphenytoin	18-20 mg PE/kg	150 mg PE/min	10-20 µg/mL
Phenobarbital	10-20 mg/kg	30-50 mg/min	10-40 µg/mL
Pentobarbital	10-15 mg/kg	1-3 mg/kg/hr	NS on EEG
Valproate	20-30 mg/kg	20 mg/min	NS on EEG
Lidocaine	2-3 mg/kg	50 mg/min	NS on EEG
Propofol	1-3 mg/kg	1-5 mg/kg/hr	NS on EEG
Midazolam	0.2 mg/kg	4 mg/min	NS on EEG

EEG, electroencephalogram; NS, no seizure activity; PE, phenytoin equivalent.

weight) + (5.003 × height) − (6.775 × age), and for women, BEE = 655.1 + (9.563 × kg) + (1.850 × cm) − (4.676 × age).

The integrity of the gut is maintained by enteral feeding and greatly challenged by parenteral nutrition. It is prudent to consider postpyloric feeding in patients with neurological catastrophes because gastric atony increases the risk for aspiration. However, drug absorption in the jejunum may be unreliable. Enteral feeding should preferably be carried out by continuous infusion with a volumetric pump. Current protocols recommend that feeding start at 25 mL/hr and the volume be increased by 25 mL/hr every 4 hours until the goal of nutrition is achieved.[31] In patients with a gastric residual volume of greater than 250 mL, feeding should be withheld for 4 hours and then restarted at the same rate but with a more gradual increase. Problems with enteral feeding are frequent and include diarrhea, nausea, and abdominal distention.

Gastrostomy placement should be considered in patients with a prolonged need for enteral nutrition because of impaired swallowing mechanisms. Gastrostomy should also be considered if recovery from dysphagia is not anticipated for 2 to 3 weeks.

Parenteral nutrition is rarely used in the NICU. It is much more complex, has the potential for more complications, and requires close monitoring of laboratory values. Energy requirements are again estimated with the Harris-Benedict equation. Mechanical or metabolic complications occur in about 50% of patients undergoing parenteral nutrition.

ASSESSMENT OF PROPHYLAXIS AND NEED FOR ANTICOAGULATION

Patients with acute brain injury and hemiparesis have a higher incidence of DVT because of lack of mobility of the affected limb. Clinically apparent DVT was reported in 2% to 5% of patients with ischemic stroke,[30,32] whereas subclinical DVT occurred in 28% to 73%, mostly in the paralyzed extremity.[33]

No observational studies are available to clarify the incidence of DVT in patients with intracerebral hemorrhage. One study demonstrated that DVT was detected at day 10 in 16% of patients wearing elastic stockings alone.[34] In another study, 5% of patients with intracranial hemorrhage died of PE within the first 30 days.[35]

Only general recommendations can be made for postoperative neurosurgical patients. The most recent consensus statement published by the American College of Chest Physicians in 2004 recommended mechanical methods (intermittent pneumatic compression with or without elastic stockings) as the standard of care.[36] The use of unfractionated heparin was left to the discretion of the physician, but the use of low-molecular-weight heparin was discouraged.[36] Only one randomized clinical trial compared low-dose unfractionated heparin with no prophylaxis in craniotomy patients and found an 85% reduction in DVT in heparinized patients.[37]

The use of DVT prophylaxis in patients with traumatic head injury is another challenging situation. Several studies have tried to address the safety of anticoagulation in patients with recent hemorrhagic contusions. One study demonstrated no increased risk for hemorrhage in patients treated with unfractionated heparin within 72 hours.[38] Another comprehensive study of 150 patients with hemorrhagic traumatic brain injury tested enoxaparin, 30 mg twice daily subcutaneously, starting 26.5 ± 11.5 hours after head injury. Overall, 23% of the patients demonstrated progression of the hemorrhagic lesion on CT. Nineteen percent had enlarging lesions before anticoagulation, but only 4% demonstrated an increase after initiation of anticoagulation. In 8% of patients who underwent craniotomy, hemorrhagic complications developed and required reoperation.[39] These studies emphasize the potential dangers with the use of unfractionated heparin, and no definitive recommendation can be made.

Full anticoagulation is indicated for patients with cardioembolic strokes, acute DVT, or PE. It might be considered in patients with critical stenosis or acute occlusion of the carotid artery.[40] Anticoagulation is used frequently in patients with high-grade basilar artery stenosis or recent basilar artery occlusion despite a virtual lack of any evidence of effectiveness. Anticoagulation is resumed in patients with a mechanical heart valve and recent cerebral hematoma, usually after a 10- to 14-day interval.

The weight-based nomogram for the use of intravenous heparin has been shown to be more effective than the standard-care nomogram.[41] Heparin boluses are not recommended in neurological patients because of the increased incidence of intracerebral hemorrhage. The activated partial thromboplastin time (aPTT) is used to monitor heparin therapy closely, with values ranging from 1.5 to 2.0 times the baseline aPTT (50 to 75 seconds) being recommended. Bleeding is possible at any location with heparin but frequently occurs in the gastrointestinal tract as a result of stress ulcers. Bilateral adrenal hemorrhage might be manifested as sudden shock without any evidence of overt blood loss.[42] Retroperitoneal hemorrhage should be considered in patients with a rapid decrease in hematocrit, in those with labile blood pressure, and especially when a recent cerebral angiogram or endovascular procedure has been performed. Thrombocytopenia secondary to the development of heparin-induced antibodies is another well-established complication. It is usually delayed by 5 to 10 days after the initiation of heparin therapy and might be associated with hemorrhagic and ischemic complications.[43,44]

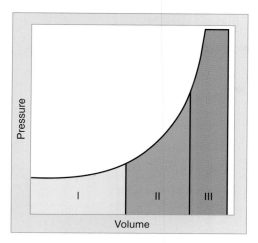

FIGURE 24-4 Pressure-volume curve. Zone 1, fully compensated for an increase in volume; zone 2, failing compensatory mechanisms with a slow rise in intracranial pressure (ICP); zone 3, exponential rise in ICP indicating absent compensation with shifting of brain tissue occurring.

ASSESSMENT OF INTRACRANIAL PRESSURE

Intracranial pressure (ICP) is tightly controlled. According to the Monro-Kellie model, overall intracranial volume is constant because of the rigidity of skull, which does not permit any expansion. An increase in the volume of any component leads to a compensatory decrease in other components or eventual displacement of brain tissue through the tentorial opening or foramen of Magnum and possibly brainstem displacement and loss of brainstem function. Several compensatory mechanisms may prevent this complication. First, CSF may shift from the ventricular or subarachnoid space into the spinal compartment. Second, reduction of intracranial blood volume is achieved by collapse of veins and dural sinuses and by changes in the diameter of cerebral vessels. If the limits of the compensatory mechanisms are exceeded, a minimal increase in intracranial volume will lead to a precipitous rise in ICP (Fig. 24-4).

Autoregulation is usually severely impaired in patients with acute neurological injury. Severe diffuse traumatic brain injury, aneurysmal subarachnoid hemorrhage, diffuse brain infection, or any type of bilateral global cerebral injury may virtually eliminate any autoregulation and thus compensatory mechanisms for control of ICP.

Monitoring of ICP is an integral function of the NICU. Indications for placement of ICP monitors include a coma from severe traumatic brain injury, and massive cerebral edema from infarction. ICP can be reduced by decreasing total intracranial volume, which is achieved by withdrawal of CSF via ventricular drainage, reduction of cerebral tissue volume (osmotic dehydration), or removal or decompression of an intracranial mass.[45]

Head position should be neutral to reduce any possible compression of the jugular veins. Head elevation of 30 degrees is considered standard.[46] Patients should be made comfortable, and pain, bladder distention, and agitation should be avoided because these factors might increase ICP.

The patient should be maintained in a euvolemic state. Hypovolemia caused by fluid restriction does not have an impact on ICP but may result in hypotension and unnecessary risk to already compromised brain tissue.

Hyperventilation is one method of reducing ICP. Hypocapnia causes cerebral vasoconstriction, which in turn reduces cerebral blood flow. This effect is maintained for several hours, after which it becomes ineffective because of compensatory rapid buffering of alkalotic CSF.[47] Moreover, monitoring of brain tissue oxygenation has demonstrated that even a small reduction in Pco_2 causes a decrease in cerebral oxygenation in comatose patients.[48] Aggressive hyperventilation might thus decrease cerebral blood flow to levels approaching ischemia. Consequently, hyperventilation should be used only as a bridging measure while other means of ICP control are being instituted.

Osmotic diuresis is the mainstay of medical therapy for elevated ICP. The most widely used diuretic agents for the treatment of increased ICP are mannitol and hypertonic saline. The basic mechanism of this intervention is transport of extracellular water to the intravascular space.[49] Mannitol not only facilitates the movement of extracellular water but also might increase CSF absorption. This osmotic gradient remains the overriding mechanism, but other mechanisms of action are increased cerebral blood flow from transient hypervolemia and hemodilution resulting in a decrease in blood viscosity.[50] Cerebral blood volume, however, remains much the same as the result of a compensatory reflex vasoconstriction of the cerebral arterioles. Mannitol is typically used in a 20% solution, and the agent is excreted through the kidneys. The initial dose is 1 g/kg, which is then tapered to 0.25 to 0.5 g/kg. Rarely, higher doses (up to 2 g/kg) are needed to reduce ICP. The effect is apparent within 15 minutes, and failure to respond to mannitol is a sign of poor compliance and failing compensatory mechanisms. Not infrequently, it is a reason for decompressive surgery to allow more volume expansion within the skull. The maximal effect lasts about 60 minutes. The adverse reactions of mannitol, including congestive heart failure and profound pulmonary edema, are a result of rapid intravascular expansion.

Failure of mannitol to control ICP should lead to a trial of hypertonic saline. In a recent retrospective study, hypertonic saline was effective in 75% of patients deteriorating from increased ICP.[51] Hypertonic saline can be administered only by central venous access, especially when given in more concentrated solutions. Brief hypotension, caused by a sudden reduction in peripheral vascular resistance in reaction to a sudden osmotic load, is the most common side effect of administration of hypertonic saline and can be avoided by slow administration lasting 10 to 15 minutes. No cases of central pontine myelinolysis were documented after treatment with a 23.4% solution.[51] Cardiac arrhythmia is another potential complication of this treatment.

Failure to respond to osmotic agents might lead to the use of barbiturates. Barbiturates are useful in reducing ICP even in patients resistant to standard medical and surgical therapies. This treatment is far from benign, however, and is associated with multiple complications, including myocardial depression, infections, hypotension, and skin breakdown. Vasopressors are commonly needed to maintain blood pressure and cerebral perfusion pressure. Suppression of the EEG to the level of burst suppression is often needed to achieve adequate ICP control, and this requires high doses. Therapy is usually maintained for several days until stabilization of the clinical situation. Barbiturate therapy can be withdrawn slowly by reducing the infusion rate by 50% each day, but because of a very prolonged half-life, improvement in consciousness may not occur for 7 to 10 days.

MONITORING OF DETERIORATION AFTER ACUTE BRAIN INJURY

One of the most distinctive tasks in the NICU is monitoring for neurological decline, and the burden is on the neurosciences nursing staff. Their assessment will lead to further evaluation and often initial measures to prevent further worsening.

TABLE 24-4 Causes of Clinical Deterioration in Selected Disorders

DISORDER	CAUSES OF CLINICAL DETERIORATION	CLINICAL SIGNS OF DETERIORATION
Aneurysmal subarachnoid hemorrhage	Acute hydrocephalus Delayed cerebral ischemia Rebleeding Expanding lobar hematoma Seizures	Decline in consciousness Upward gaze palsy Pinpoint pupils Sudden loss of upper brainstem reflexes and transient apnea
Ganglionic or lobar hemorrhage	Expanding volume	New aphasia or hemiparesis Eye deviation and eyelid twitching Decreased consciousness Worsening hemiparesis Acute anisocoria or wide fixed pupil and extensor posturing
Cerebellar hematoma	Rebleeding Compression of the 4th ventricle and acute hydrocephalus Displacement of the pons	New Cushing's signs Pinpoint pupils and downward gaze Comatose and need for intubation Sudden coma with extensor posturing and midposition pupils
Hemispheric infarct	Hemorrhagic conversion Brain swelling	Gradual decline in consciousness New-onset cerebral ptosis
Traumatic brain injury	New contusional lesions Malignant cerebral edema Extension of subdural or epidural hematoma	New fixed dilated pupil New decerebrate or decorticate responses

Brain function can currently be evaluated with the use of monitors for ICP, brain tissue oxygenation, and microdialysis, and each of these devices may signal neuronal distress. Video-EEG monitoring may be used in patients with a fluctuating level of consciousness after a single seizure and to titrate antiepileptic drugs. However, most NICUs will have to rely on repeated expert neurological examination and neuroimaging.

Deterioration in a patient with an acute brain injury is disease specific but predictable. Examples are shown in Table 24-4. In many instances, neurological deterioration is due to further displacement of brain tissue and, eventually, brainstem displacement. A lateral shift in brain tissue distorts the thalamus and mesencephalon. These patients have a decline in consciousness (thalamus-mesencephalon). A unilateral fixed dilated (varying from a difference of 2 to 5 mm) pupil is seen early and can be followed by bilateral fixed pupils. The pontine reflexes remain intact. This course, however, can be mimicked by acute lesions in the thalamus that suddenly extend asymmetrically to the mesencephalon (e.g., a thalamic hemorrhage). Lesions in the cerebellum may produce compression of the brainstem, but more often at the pontine level. Most notable is a predominance of pontine signs with possible bilateral miosis and loss of both corneal reflexes and the oculocephalic reflex. Frequent episodes of bradycardia with or without hypertension may occur (Cushing's sign). A mass located more centrally will distort the thalamus and mesencephalon in a vertical plane and cause fixed midposition (4 to 6 mm) pupils initially. Asymmetric compression of the mesencephalon with anisocoria and a larger pupil or an oval-shaped pupil on the side with the lesion may be seen. Motor responses vary from decorticate to extensor responses, sometimes even with variation throughout the day and no evidence of other signs of deterioration. In patients with a gaze preference toward the expanding mass, gaze may reverse as a result of thalamic compression. Brief episodes of periodic lateral gaze may

occur. Further vertical displacement of the entire thalamus-mesencephalon pontine structure may take place, but only after the upper brainstem has been destroyed directly from compression. It may occur with bilateral thalamic compression as a result of diffuse brain edema. Patients who lose all brainstem reflexes generally lose their pontomesencephalic reflexes at onset and medulla function later. A common progression is the appearance of flaccidity and no motor response with loss of the pontomesencephalic reflexes and, finally, failure to trigger the ventilator indicative of brain death.

Fluctuating consciousness with transient eye deviation and frequently eye fluttering may indicate seizures. There is evidence that seizures, when monitored 24 hours a day for several days after head injury, may be more common than appreciated, and in any such patient EEG monitoring is warranted. Patients with cortical ischemic and hemorrhagic lesions, encephalitis, and major tumor surgery are at high risk.

Serial CT remains the most useful method of monitoring structural CNS lesions. Portable CT may be even more helpful, but no comparative studies have yet been performed. CT is able to document enlargement of the ventricles, signs of a mass effect with further displacement of the pineal gland and septum pellucidum, obliteration of the basal cisterns and sulcal effacement, compression of the brainstem, and intraventricular extension of hemorrhage, among other signs of a changing lesion.

CONCLUSION

Care of critically ill neurological patients is not a simple combination of critical care and neurological assessment, but an amalgamated treatment plan that is specific for the cause of the injury. Surely, many of the intensive care principles apply to acutely ill neurological patients, but some specific interventions are available for this category of patients. There has been better understanding of medical and neurosurgical care of critically ill neurological patients. There has also been better understanding of the mechanisms of clinical deterioration and ways to recognize them. Our approach to critically ill neurological and neurosurgical patients is to avoid further injury, which might not only reduce recovery potential but also shift patients into a permanently disabled category.

SUGGESTED READINGS

Becker PS, Miller VT. Heparin-induced thrombocytopenia. *Stroke.* 1989;20: 1449-1459.

Carmona Suazo JA, Maas AI, van den Brink WA, et al. CO_2 reactivity and brain oxygen pressure monitoring in severe head injury. *Crit Care Med.* 2000;28:3268-3274.

Kirby DF. As the gut churns: feeding challenges in the head-injured patient. *JPEN J Parenter Enteral Nutr.* 1996;20:1-2.

Lacut K, Bressollette L, Le Gal G, et al. Prevention of venous thrombosis in patients with acute intracerebral hemorrhage. *Neurology.* 2005;65:865-869.

Norton B, Homer-Ward M, Donnelly MT, et al. A randomized prospective comparison of percutaneous endoscopic gastrostomy and nasogastric tube feeding after acute dysphagic stroke. *BMJ.* 1996;312:13-16.

Norwood SH, McAuley CE, Berne JD, et al. Prospective evaluation of the safety of enoxaparin prophylaxis for venous thromboembolism in patients with intracranial hemorrhagic injuries. *Arch Surg.* 2002;137:696-702.

Ropper A, Rockoff M. *Physiology and Clinical Aspects of Raised Intracranial Pressure.* New York: McGraw-Hill; 1993.

Wijdicks EFM. *The Comatose Patient.* Oxford University Press; 2008.

Wijdicks EFM. *The Clinical Practice of Critical Care Neurology*, 2nd ed. Oxford University Press; 2003.

Wijdicks EFM, Bamlet WR, Maramattom BV, et al. Validation of a new coma scale: the FOUR score. *Ann Neurol.* 2005;58:585-593.

Full references can be found on Expert Consult @ www.expertconsult.com

PART 2

General Principles and Surgical Techniques

CHAPTER 25

Surgical Planning: Overview

Martin Weiss ▪ Gabriel Zada ▪ Alexander A. Khalessi

Comprehensive planning represents an axiomatic prerequisite for any neurosurgical procedure. "Failing to prepare is preparing to fail" holds particularly true in neurosurgical cases given the unforgiving nature of the human nervous system. Thorough preoperative consideration of the technical goals and potential pitfalls ensures the safest and most efficacious outcome for the patient. Effective planning allows the surgeon critical flexibility and latitude in managing deviations from the intended operative course. Indeed, the experience and ability to detect and handle the most adverse intraoperative events should be a goal for any surgeon. By taking the necessary steps to ensure adequate preparation for a case, the surgeon may prevent or avoid many significant neurosurgical complications.

Any surgical procedure demands a working preoperative diagnosis. Effective intervention requires a theoretical understanding of the pathophysiology involved or a directed effort to acquire further information. The surgical plan should therefore not only be based on a working diagnosis but also designed to accommodate changes in the operative plan as the case proceeds. Admittedly, even sound planning generates an incomplete preoperative state of information. Intraoperative findings or surgical pathology results, if anticipated, allow the reasoned pursuit of alternative surgical goals. Due consideration of nonsurgical diagnoses (e.g., prolactinoma, lymphoma) and alternative modalities (e.g., medical therapy, radiation therapy, radiosurgery) represents a crucial component of preoperative planning. Surgical planning thereby seamlessly blends with a larger treatment plan to minimize morbidity and optimize timely diagnosis and treatment of disease.

This chapter outlines a generalized approach to preoperative neurosurgical planning, emphasizing key considerations and adjunctive measures essential to optimization of patient outcomes beyond the incision.

PREOPERATIVE EVALUATION

Before any neurosurgical procedure, the surgeon must complete a comprehensive evaluation of the patient. Detailed history, physical examination, and review of the patient's laboratory results and radiographic studies are paramount. Symptom time course and onset represent central features of the suspected disease and complement a focused neurological history. Pertinent negatives must be duly considered, and a strict accounting of preoperative deficits will be critical to establishment of a baseline

with which to compare the patient's postoperative examination findings. Moreover, inquiring about the side of hand dominance is significant in many cranial procedures. Further review of a patient's past medical and surgical history, medications, allergies, and any pertinent social or familial considerations should be undertaken.

A complete review of systems is routinely performed. The physical and neurological examination should be performed soon before the procedure and documented in the medical chart. The complete neurological examination includes an assessment of mental status and speech ability, cranial nerve function (including the first cranial nerve), motor and sensory function, reflexes, and cerebellar and gait testing. Formal visual field and acuity examination may be indicated before selected cases if sellar or suprasellar disease exists. Rectal examinations for tone, volition, sensation, and the bulbocavernosus reflex may be necessary in instances of spinal disease. Other aspects of the patient's overall medical status demand consideration in every case; many neurosurgical patients will have significant comorbidities requiring preoperative attention. The goals of surgery should always be considered as they relate to the patient's overall medical status and personal preferences.

Routine laboratory values are indicated before any nonemergent surgical procedure and should be obtained to screen for a number of underlying systemic conditions that may pose a risk to a patient undergoing general anesthesia and surgery. A qualitative β-human chorionic gonadotropin assessment should be performed for every woman of childbearing age before surgery. Baseline renal function and electrolyte levels are determined and evaluated further as necessary. Any suggestion of infection, such as an elevated white blood cell count, positive cultures, elevated erythrocyte sedimentation rate, or elevated C-reactive protein level, should be considered, especially in elective cases or if hardware implantation is planned.

Underlying anemia must be worked up and corrected accordingly. Any suggestion of bleeding diathesis or coagulopathy should be investigated further and corrected. Preoperative laboratory investigations geared toward these issues include platelet count, prothrombin time (international normalized ratio), partial thromboplastin time, and bleeding time (if necessary). Many patients currently take anticoagulant or antiplatelet agents for a number of underlying medical comorbidities. Plans for discontinuation or reversal of these agents (or perhaps initiation of these agents in select endovascular cases) should be addressed at least 1 week before surgery.

Blood typing and screening, or crossmatching for reserve units and additional blood products, should be requested from the blood bank and verified in advance. If sellar disease exists, a full or selective endocrine panel is drawn to assess for deficiencies in any number of hormonal axes. The thyroid and cortisol axes are of paramount importance, and deficiencies must be identified and repleted before any surgical procedure is performed. Ruling out nonsurgical lesions, such as prolactinomas, additionally necessitates judicious review of preoperative laboratory work.

Preexisting cardiac disease is commonly encountered in the neurosurgical patient population. Preoperatively, patients should undergo a detailed cardiovascular history to assess exercise tolerance and to screen for angina or congestive heart failure. Should there be preexisting disease or if a patient has significant risk factors, clearance or risk assessment from a cardiologist may be required before an elective case. A 12-lead electrocardiogram and plain chest film are obtained in the majority of adult patients before routine surgery. If further cardiac work-up is indicated, exercise treadmill testing, echocardiography, nuclear medicine study, or coronary angiography may be performed to further assess the degree of cardiac risk.

Hypertensive patients require adequate blood pressure control on multiple visits before undergoing general anesthesia for an elective case. In general, any cardiac condition that poses a risk to the patient's overall condition should be addressed before an elective neurosurgical procedure. The degree of cardiac risk, if present, must always be accounted for and weighed against the urgency of the neurosurgical procedure. Any perioperative measures that may improve cardiac monitoring or function should be planned in conjunction with the anesthesia team, and include invasive cardiac monitoring and perioperative medications. In the setting of baseline anemia or anticipated blood loss, large-bore intravenous access is critical to the timely delivery of blood products and prevention of a hypovolemic intraoperative insult.

Baseline pulmonary disease is also encountered frequently in the general neurosurgical population. Comorbidities such as asthma and chronic obstructive pulmonary disease may limit optimal provision of anesthesia during a neurosurgical case and should be addressed with a thorough preoperative evaluation. Historical details, including a smoking history, merit special attention by the physician. A plain chest radiograph, pulmonary function tests, and chest computed tomographic scans are within the battery of tests that may be indicated for preoperative work-up. Once again, perioperative medications, including steroids and beta agonists, may be indicated for patients with pulmonary disease and should be discussed with the anesthesia staff. Instances involving severe ventilatory compromises may limit positioning options (i.e., protracted prone positioning), and coincident structural lesions (i.e., lung masses) may dictate the laterality of the neurosurgical approach to midline structures.

Some neurosurgical patients will present with malnutrition or failure to thrive in relation to their disease process. Many afflictions prevalent in the population of neurosurgical patients render them unable to tolerate a normal diet. Because of their mental status, paralysis, or any number of airway or cranial nerve issues, some patients rely on alternative sources of nutritional intake. These may include nasogastric tubes, percutaneous gastric tubes, and parenteral routes of intake for nutritional supplementation. Before any neurosurgical case, a patient's nutritional status should be considered and optimized. A serum prealbumin level can be monitored to assess and observe a patient's nutritional status. A consultation with a nutritionist can be invaluable in optimizing a patient's status before major surgery. Patients who have undergone previous surgery or radiation therapy or those receiving chronic steroid treatment may present additional wound healing concerns that require additional preoperative planning to achieve adequate wound healing. Diabetes, especially in the setting of poor glycemic control, may further compromise

wound healing. Hemoglobin A_{1c} levels may be used to screen for this clinical scenario. In certain situations, specialized tissue transfer techniques, such as rotational pedicle-based vascular flaps or free flaps, are required, often in conjunction with a separate team of specialty surgeons.

Once a complete evaluation of a patient's neurologic and systemic disease has been thoroughly considered and a surgical plan formulated, a frank discussion with the patient and any other individuals involved in the patient's care should take place. The goals of surgery and potential barriers to the achievement of these goals should be clearly and honestly delineated. For nonemergent cases, the benefits and risks of the recommended procedure and its alternatives are reviewed, and any additional questions are answered by the surgeon. Informed consent should be obtained before the initiation of any nonemergent procedure. The consent process includes information about the placement of any permanent implants or hardware that may be used as well as the potential for the transfusion of blood products if necessary.

RADIOGRAPHIC IMAGING

Before the initiation of any surgical procedure, the correct array of radiographic imaging is obtained and reviewed thoroughly by the surgeon. Consultation with a neuroradiologist may be beneficial in select cases. Preoperative images frequently include plain films, computed tomographic imaging, magnetic resonance imaging, angiography, and a variety of additional modalities. The surgeon should ensure that the correct sequences have been performed and reviewed before the case. The images should be available to the surgeon for the duration of the procedure. In addition to static images, dynamic studies such as flexion-extension views may provide insight into the responsible pathologic process. Certain pathologic entities involve abnormalities of flow, which make dynamic studies (i.e., assessment of flow in an arteriovenous malformation) important in the preoperative evaluation.

Intraoperative imaging and image-guided neurosurgery are increasingly used surgical adjuncts that require additional preoperative planning steps. Image guidance navigation systems may be used for a variety of neurosurgical cases and require particular preoperative imaging sequences. The timing of image acquisition in relation to the operation should be considered, as some patients require early admission for these sequences to be obtained. Intraoperative fluoroscopy is commonly used during select spine or skull base cases and is set up before the case. Intraoperative magnetic resonance imaging has been used during the past decade or so in a variety of tumor cases and requires specific steps for preoperative setup and preparation of instrumentation. Intraoperative angiography and fluorescein angiography are commonly used during cerebrovascular cases and also require prior planning. Cannulation of the femoral artery and initial imaging for intraoperative angiography are frequently performed and set up before the operative portion of the case.

ANESTHESIA

Before the initiation of the surgical procedure, the surgeon should review the operative plan with the anesthesia team. Optimal physiologic parameters (blood pressure, volume, temperature) and any additional methods of monitoring required during the procedure should be reviewed. The proper use of ventriculostomy and lumbar drain catheters should be reviewed before surgery when these modalities are to be used. In pediatric cases or other cases in which the degree of bleeding is of paramount concern, a plan for monitoring and repletion of blood or any additional products should be in place. Planning for autologous blood recovery systems or normovolemic hemodilution may be undertaken when a significant degree of bleeding is anticipated.

Particular requirements for the administration of anesthetic medications for induction and the duration of the case should be reviewed with the anesthesiologists, including the selection of paralytic agents or total intravenous anesthesia. This is of key importance when neurophysiologic monitoring will be performed. Plans for electroencephalographic burst suppression must also be discussed with the anesthesia team before the surgery. In certain functional and tumor cases, neuroleptic anesthesia is desired to assess the patient during the procedure. Anesthesia for awake craniotomy or deep brain stimulator placement requires additional preparation on the part of the anesthesia team, and the timing and depth of anesthesia must be preplanned. The perioperative administration of medications such as antibiotics, steroids, hemostatic or anticoagulation agents, and antiepileptic drugs is frequently indicated and discussed with the anesthesia team, in addition to affirmation of the side or site of surgery in a formal "time-out" procedure. A review of a patient's allergies should be readily available and alternative medications selected for existing conflicts.

Any concerns about spinal stability should be noted before positioning and intubation. Fiberoptic intubation may be required in instances of cervical instability or spondylosis, in which the extension required for standard intubation places the neural elements at risk. Certain surgical positions require additional means of patient monitoring, which are planned before surgery. A typical example of this is the requirement for central venous Doppler monitoring for air emboli in the case of sitting craniotomies. Notably, the use of the Mayfield skull clamp in cranial cases and posterior cervical cases allows stable head fixation. Somatosensory and motor evoked potential baselines before and after final positioning further confirm safe preparation and manipulation of the patient before definitive surgical intervention.

SELECTION OF SURGICAL APPROACH

In general, the selected surgical approach allows the most direct and maximal access to the pathologic process, with minimal morbidity to surrounding structures. Any surgical instrumentation that may be required to perform the operation should be requested and tested before initiation of the procedure. Vascular lesions require detailed consideration of flow dynamics and proximal control in preparation for a bleeding event. Likewise, surgical manipulation generally minimizes traction or compression of nervous structures. For instance, resection of extra-axial tumors is thereby best accomplished by mobilization out and away from adjacent nervous structures.

Considerations for Cranial Procedures

For cranial procedures, the surgical approach and position should be planned and any equipment for positioning set up in advance. This may include devices for cranial fixation and for positioning the body or extremity support. If surgical navigation is to be used, it should be set up, registered, and verified before the procedure begins. Neurophysiologic monitoring, such as somatosensory, motor, or brainstem auditory evoked responses, must be anticipated and discussed with the anesthesia and neuromonitoring teams before surgery. The method of visualization to be used for the procedure, such as the operating microscope, surgical loupes, or an endoscopic system, should be selected and tested before surgery. Any adjunctive measures for brain relaxation, such as placement of a ventriculostomy catheter or lumbar drain, should be considered in advance. Drill equipment, including electric or pneumatic setup, and any additional drill bits or attachments should be selected and tested. Instruments or products required for hemostasis, such as monopolar and bipolar cautery, collagen sponge, Surgicel, and thrombin, should be discussed with the operating room staff before surgery so that they are ready for use at the onset of the case.

Tumor Cases

Before craniotomy procedures for neoplastic diseases, a surgeon should have a working diagnosis and a plan prepared. If a biopsy procedure is to be performed, the method of acquisition is planned in advance. This may be done by stereotactic frame-based procedures, image-guided neuronavigation through a bur hole or open craniotomy, or direct open biopsy. The surgical pathologist should be notified and on standby before the initiation of surgery. A plan is prepared in advance as to how the case should proceed after initial assessment of the frozen biopsy specimen. A surgeon should plan for a variety of scenarios, depending on the results of the biopsy. In certain cases, complete tumor resection is indicated. In other cases, partial resection, decompression, or palliation is attempted. Other biopsy results may suggest a medically treatable condition, and the decision to terminate surgery may be made at that time. Tumors that appear especially vascular on imaging studies may require preoperative neurointerventional embolization. Instruments required for tumor resection are anticipated and may include special transsphenoidal or skull base instrument sets, endoscopic equipment, and the Cavitron ultrasonic aspirator. If the potential for a cerebrospinal fluid leak near the skull base exists, the abdomen may be prepared for a fat or fascial graft harvest. Injection of fluorescein dye into the subarachnoid space may be warranted to improve detection of a cerebrospinal fluid leak and should be done before positioning.

Operative Planning for Cerebrovascular Cases

The surgical management of complex cerebrovascular disease can often be greatly facilitated by thorough preoperative planning. When possible, an approach is selected that offers exposure of the entire lesion and proximal vasculature. Preparation for a potential intraoperative aneurysm rupture is a requirement, and a plan must be established in relation to when in the procedure this event occurs. Additional steps to achieve proximal vascular control of cerebral aneurysms and arteriovenous malformations are frequently mandated. Methods of proximal control include temporary aneurysm clipping, intraoperative balloon occlusion, and exposure of proximal vessels in the neck. If necessary, a balloon test occlusion is performed in advance to ascertain whether a given vessel can be sacrificed. In cases of anticipated reconstruction or bypass procedures, preoperative studies are performed to ensure that feeder and recipient vessels are sufficient, and mapping of the vessel course with a Doppler instrument may be required. In cases in which no feeding vessel is accessible, a venous or arterial graft harvest site may be selected and prepared on the basis of the flow demand of the target distribution. Intraoperative angiography may be used for a variety of reasons during cerebrovascular cases, including proximal control, suction-decompression, and assessment of persistent filling of vascular lesions and parent vessels. Indocyanine green fluorescence angiography is an alternative measure that can be used intraoperatively to assess the distribution of cerebral blood flow. A wide variety of aneurysm clips should be available to the surgeon to treat complex aneurysms, including various sizes and configurations of straight and fenestrated clips. Temporary and permanent aneurysm clips should be readily available in the event of an intraoperative rupture. Verification of distal artery patency after aneurysm ligation can be performed with a micro-Doppler flow probe, fluorescence or intraoperative angiography, or an endoscope.

Planning of Spine Procedures

For spine cases, the surgical approach must also be selected, and equipment required for positioning should be ready. This may include a standard radiolucent surgical table or the Jackson surgical table. The Wilson frame may be desirable in a variety of cases to induce flexion to facilitate intralaminar access. Equipment to perform imaging for surgical localization, such as plain radiography, fluoroscopy, or image-guided navigation systems, should be available. Monitoring of somatosensory and motor evoked potentials, if desired, is set up before the case is started. Additional instrumentation for exposure, stabilization, and fusion should be sterilized and prepared for the case. This may include retractor sets, dilator sets, and any combination of grafts, plates, screws, and rods that may be required to complete the case. When a bone fusion is desired, the surgeon should have a plan for use of autograft, allograft, or any number of additional fusion products available. If iliac crest graft harvesting is required, this should be planned and the field prepared preoperatively.

CONCLUSION

The complexity of neurological surgery demands the employment of all means and methods available to the surgeon to maximize the safety of the patient and to enhance the surgical procedure. Surgical success therefore begins well before setting foot in the operating theater. In the patient's history, in the laboratory work-up, in review of the radiographic findings, and in an appraisal and discussion of the risks and a tempering of expectations, the foundation for the operative enterprise is built. The goal is to use a team familiar with the necessary operative equipment, with a reliance on other disciplines to enable a plan of care to facilitate the likelihood of a successful intervention. Neurosurgery will always remain among the most audacious of human endeavors; preoperative planning provides the footing to help patients and diminish the burden of neurological disease.

CHAPTER 26

Positioning for Cranial Surgery

R. Webster Crowley ■ Aaron S. Dumont ■ M. Sean McKisic ■ John A. Jane Sr

Although it is not always adequately emphasized, positioning of the patient for intracranial procedures remains a critical step in a successful surgery. Optimal positioning allows the surgical team to complete their objective in the most effective fashion in many ways; for example, ideal positioning may reduce or eliminate the need for brain retraction, help provide a clear and bloodless field, reduce intracranial pressure and avoid venous obstruction, present the anatomy and pathology in the ideal perspective for the surgeon, and minimize the chance of avoidable complications such as brachial plexus stretch injuries and pressure neuropathies. This chapter reviews fundamental principles of positioning for the most common approaches to cranial disease.

PTERIONAL (FRONTOTEMPORAL) CRANIOTOMY

The pterional craniotomy, otherwise known as the frontotemporal craniotomy, is considered to be the craniotomy most commonly performed by the neurosurgeon. Its versatility has made it a fundamental component of the neurosurgeon's repertoire, and it (or its derivatives, such as the cranio-orbito-zygomatic approach) has become the craniotomy of choice for a large number of procedures. These procedures include but are not limited to the vast majority of supratentorial intracerebral aneurysms and pathologic processes of the anterior and middle cranial fossae, the central skull base, and in select instances, the posterior cranial fossa.

Positioning for the pterional craniotomy begins with placement of the patient supine on the operative table. The patient is then placed in the Mayfield-Kees head fixation or similar cranial immobilization apparatus. When possible, we prefer to position the pins such that the single pin is placed in the frontal bone contralateral to the operative target, approximately 2 to 3 cm above the brow. The dual pins are then placed in the occipital bone on the ipsilateral side. It is usually preferable to place the pins along the axial plane; however, depending on the extent of the planned skin flap, it may be necessary to orient the pins along the sagittal plane. Others, however, advocate placing the single pin posteriorly, a decision that typically comes down to the surgeon's preference.[1] Regardless of this decision, careful attention should be paid to avoid the frontal sinus anteriorly and the mastoid air cells posteriorly. Once the patient is in pins, a shoulder roll is placed under the ipsilateral shoulder along the long axis of the patient. This allows adequate rotation without compromising venous return by obstructing the jugular veins in the neck. We also generally place the patient in some reverse Trendelenburg to promote brain relaxation and to allow the head to be fixed higher than the level of the heart.

Once the patient's body has been positioned correctly, the head can be adjusted. Appropriate positioning of the head requires a combination of head flexion, rotation, and neck extension that is designed to provide the ideal surgical trajectory while minimizing brain retraction. The head is first rotated toward the contralateral shoulder. The degree of rotation can vary greatly and is largely dependent on the desired surgical target. For example, internal carotid artery disease is often approached from 5 to 20 degrees of contralateral rotation; anterior communicating artery aneurysms may require up to 60 degrees of rotation to allow optimal visualization of the anterior communicating artery complex. In general, for approaches requiring wide opening of the sylvian fissure, avoidance of excessive rotation is preferred because the greater the contralateral rotation, the more the temporal lobe and its operculum obstruct the trajectory into the sylvian fissure. Once the desired degree of rotation is obtained, the head is laterally flexed slightly, followed by an extension of the neck. This last maneuver should present the malar eminence as the highest point on the patient and aids in retraction by allowing gravity to pull the frontal lobe from the skull base. Once it is in position, the head fixation device is secured to the table (Fig. 26-1). The patient's arm that is adjacent to the scrub nurse or technician is padded and tucked close to the body; the other arm is supported on an arm board to provide unfettered access for the anesthesiologists. Pillows and padding are placed under the patient's knees and feet, and the patient is secured to the table with a padded safety belt or padding and tape. In cases in which significant bed rotation is anticipated during the surgery, additional tape or belts are applied to secure the patient to the table.

TEMPORAL AND SUBTEMPORAL APPROACH

The temporal or subtemporal craniotomy (or derivatives such as a middle fossa, extended middle fossa approach) may be performed alone (such as for petrous apex disease, other disease of the middle fossa, or basilar apex aneurysms). It may also be performed in conjunction with another approach, such as the pterional or lateral suboccipital craniotomy.[2]

In preparation for the subtemporal craniotomy, the pins are placed for a lateral park bench position. This is accomplished by placing the single pin of the Mayfield-Kees head clamp into the frontal bone 2 to 3 cm above the ipsilateral brow and the dual pins in the occipital bone along the axial plane at midline and contralateral to the surgical site. Once in pins, the patient is placed on the side opposite the operative site on top of a vacuum-ready beanbag, with the inferior arm extended perpendicular to the patient's body on an arm board. In this position, it is critical to place a small axillary roll under the inferior axilla to avoid compression or other injury to the axillary artery or brachial plexus. Once the dependent arm is properly positioned and the beanbag is hardened, padding is placed between the superior arm and the patient's body. The arm is then placed in neutral position along the long axis of the torso, with slight flexion at the elbow before it is secured. For the subtemporal approach or middle fossa approach, correct head positioning is critical. The patient is placed in reverse Trendelenburg position to place the head above the level of the heart. In addition, the neck is laterally flexed, with the dependent ear being brought toward the ipsilateral shoulder. This also uses gravity to facilitate gentle retraction

CHAPTER 27

Patient Positioning for Spinal Surgery

Peter D. Angevine ■ Paul R. Gigante ■ Paul C. McCormick

To obtain optimal outcomes from spinal surgery, any operation must be performed effectively and safely. Achieving the surgical objectives depends, in part, on the surgical field being positioned in a way that facilitates the procedure. The surgeon must select the appropriate surgical approach and then position the patient properly to ensure a safe surgical corridor. At the same time, the surgeon must ensure the patient's safety during the procedure. Particularly during long procedures and operations performed with the patient prone or lateral, morbidity may occur as a result of the patient's position. Appropriate positioning and attention to detail will minimize the probability of complications and facilitate the surgical procedure.

EQUIPMENT

Table

A basic electric operating table may be used for many spinal procedures (Fig. 27-1). Operations in the supine position, such as anterior cervical procedures and anterior lumbar fusions in the distal lumbar spine (L3-S1), are easily performed with such a table. Reversing the table may improve clearance under the table for the fluoroscopic unit. A lateral approach for thoracic, thoracolumbar, and lumbar procedures may also be performed on an electric table. For thoracoabdominal and retroperitoneal flank approaches, it is often helpful to place the level of pathology at the table break and flex the patient laterally.

A posterior approach for thoracic and lumbar procedures may also be performed on a standard operating table with either a Wilson frame or padded bolsters. If an instrumented lumbosacral arthrodesis is planned, however, care must be taken to ensure adequate lumbar lordosis. We generally do not use a Wilson frame for posterior thoracolumbar procedures that include instrumentation and fusion because of the possibility of inadvertently causing an iatrogenic flat-back deformity.

There are many advantages to modular spine-specific operating tables such as the Jackson Spinal table (Mizuho OSI, Union City, CA) (Fig. 27-2). The carbon fiber frame is radiolucent and low profile to allow 360-degree fluoroscopy and the use of intraoperative CT scanners such as the O-arm (Medtronic Navigation, Louisville, CO). Modular components allow customization for each procedure and for a wide range of patient phenotypes. The head may be secured in a foam headrest, in a rigid fixator, or with traction. The legs may be supported in a sling to allow lumbar flexion or on a rigid tabletop to enhance lordosis (Fig. 27-3). Finally, intraoperative repositioning for anterior-posterior or posterior-anterior surgery is facilitated with a rotational capability that obviates the need for moving the patient from one table to another.

Head Holders

The simplest method for supporting the head of a patient in the prone position is a purpose-made foam head holder. Cutouts for

the eyes and endotracheal tube are the main safety features. An improvement over this system is the combination of a foam head holder and a rigid support. A mirrored base holds the support and allows the anesthesiologist to ensure that there is no pressure on the eyes.

Other head support options include a table-mounted three-pin skull clamp. This offers the greatest degree of control of the position of the head and cervical spine, but intraoperative repositioning is cumbersome. Craniocervical traction may also be used for spinal surgery in the prone position. Gardner-Wells tongs are the standard equipment for this; several weights totaling at least 15 lb should also be available.

Other Equipment

Although safe, effective patient positioning can be achieved without a large amount of specialized equipment, a few additional items are useful. A beanbag with a suction port effectively supports patients in a lateral position for a thoracotomy or retroperitoneal flank approach. Armrests for prone and supine cases should be available. A variety of foam pads such as doughnuts, kneepads, and arm supports are necessary. Disposable heating blankets such as those available for the Bair Hugger system (Arizant, Inc., Eden Prarie, MN) are used to prevent intraoperative hypothermia.

PRINCIPLES OF POSITIONING

Surgical Access

The primary goal of operative patient positioning is to allow the surgeon to achieve the surgical objectives. Selection of the surgical approach is based on the location and nature of the pathology and the specific planned procedure, and the patient's position is based on the chosen approach. Although a patient undergoing spinal surgery does not usually need to be positioned as exactingly as for intracranial procedures, surgical exposure is often facilitated by proper patient positioning. Operative considerations such as access for fluoroscopy or radiography and placement of table-mounted retractors should be anticipated by the surgeon and appropriate accommodations made.

In some circumstances, fluoroscopy or radiography is used before preparing and draping the patient, both to mark the incision and to confirm that surgical access is possible with the planned approach. For example, the trajectory for placing an odontoid screw is evaluated with the patient in the supine position to ensure that the patient's habitus and position will allow the proper angle for screw placement.

Patient Safety and Protection

Patient safety and avoidance of morbidity are important secondary considerations in operative positioning. Although the overall approach (posterior, anterior, lateral) is selected to allow

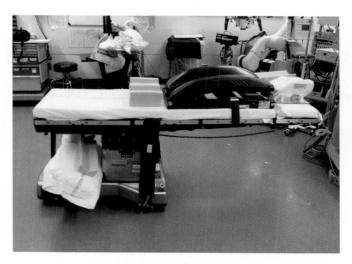

FIGURE 27-1 A standard electric operating room table may be used for many spinal operations. The bed is used in a reverse position to allow clearance underneath for the fluoroscopy unit. Either a Wilson frame (shown here) or padded bolsters may be used to support the patient.

achievement of the surgical objective, it is meticulous attention to the specific details of positioning that ensures that patients do not suffer adverse sequelae from their position during the procedure. Properly padding all areas that may be exposed to pressure and placing extremity joints in relaxed, natural positions are basic preventive measures. Other important considerations may include head positioning and facial pressure and the relationship of the operative field to the level of the heart.

Neuropathies and Prevention

Ulnar neuropathy, one of the most common postoperative neuropathies, accounts for a third of all nerve injury claims in the American Society of Anesthesiologists Closed Claims Study database.[1] Although the etiology of postoperative peripheral nerve injury is not entirely known, it is thought to be related to

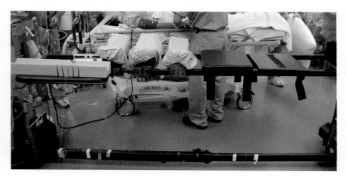

FIGURE 27-3 For lumbar and lumbosacral instrumented fusions, the spine table is set up with flat boards to support the legs. This maximizes hip extension and optimizes lumbar lordosis.

intraneural capillary ischemia resulting from nerve overstretch or compression, perhaps exacerbated by prolonged intraoperative hypotension. The ulnar nerve appears to be more vulnerable to ischemia than the median and radial nerves, with a reported incidence of 0.04% after noncardiac surgery to 37% in one series of cardiac patients who underwent detailed postoperative sensory testing. The time of onset of ulnar nerve symptoms varies from immediately after surgery to 3 days postoperatively. The duration of symptoms tends to vary across reports, with some completely resolving spontaneously in days and others persisting for years after the initial insult.[2] Risk factors for postoperative ulnar neuropathy include diabetes, increased age, and male gender.[3]

Anatomically, the ulnar nerve appears to be particularly susceptible to direct compression as it courses through the superficial condylar groove at the elbow. Elbow flexion, especially to greater than 110 degrees, can tighten the cubital tunnel retinaculum and directly compress the nerve,[4] and external compression in the absence of flexion may compromise the nerve. With the patient in the supine position, direct pressure on the ulnar nerve at the elbow is significantly higher if both forearms are pronated than if they are in a neutral and supinated position (Fig. 27-4).[5]

Brachial plexus neuropathy may have findings similar to ulnar neuropathy but may additionally be characterized by symptoms such as shoulder pain, scapular winging, and shoulder weakness.

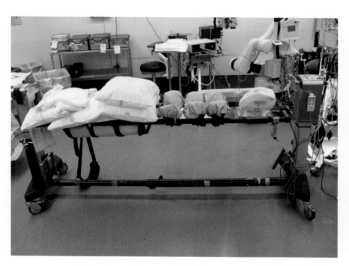

FIGURE 27-2 A dedicated spine table, here a Jackson Spinal Table, allows a greater range of height adjustment, full 360-degree clearance around the patient, and the use of multiple positioning pads and support devices. In addition, it is radiolucent.

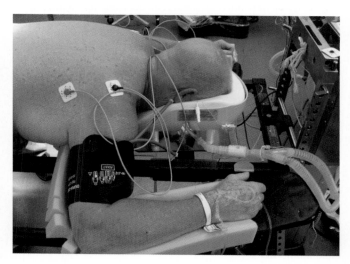

FIGURE 27-4 The arms are abducted to 90 degrees and the elbows flexed to 90 degrees or a bit less. The axillae and ulnar aspects of the arms are well padded. Note also the use of a helmet-type head holder with a reflective surface to ensure that no pressure is placed on the eyes. The neck is in relatively neutral alignment.

The incidence of brachial plexopathy during posterior spinal surgery has been estimated to be between 3.6% and 15%, as compared with 0.02% in a large study of 15,000 general surgical patients. Most patients achieve partial or full functional recovery, although some have persistent symptoms at late (1- to 3-year) follow-up.[6,7]

The majority of brachial plexus injuries are manifested as upper trunk injuries after surgery in the supine position and as lower trunk injuries after procedures in the prone position. The brachial plexus may be especially vulnerable to stretch in a prone-positioned patient with elbow flexion and shoulder abduction. Patients with congenital anomalies such as cervical ribs and shoulder contractures may have an increased susceptibility to stretch injury.

Some investigators have suggested intraoperative somatosensory evoked potential (SSEP) monitoring as a way to detect impending nerve injury. One retrospective study of 1000 spinal surgeries determined that the overall incidence of position-related upper extremity SSEP changes was 6.1%, with the lateral decubitus position (7.5%) and prone "superman" position (7.0%) having the highest incidence of position-related upper extremity SSEP changes. In this study, postoperative deficits did not develop in any patient who had positionally reversible SSEP changes.[8]

Lower extremity neuropathies have not been well studied in spinal surgery because they typically occur in patients undergoing surgery in the lithotomy position and after lower extremity orthopedic procedures. Injury to the common peroneal nerve has been reported more frequently than injury to any other lower extremity peripheral nerve, probably because of its vulnerable anatomic location. The common peroneal nerve is fixed in a superficial location as it traverses the head of the fibula, which leaves it susceptible to direct compression injury by devices that hold the legs in place. The legs should be padded and well protected at the level of the fibular head, particularly for procedures in the lateral decubitus position.[9]

In the event of a new postoperative neurological deficit, it is important to distinguish peroneal nerve injury from an acute L5 radiculopathy. A peroneal neuropathy is characterized by complete plegia of dorsiflexion and eversion without significant pain complaints, whereas an L5 radiculopathy usually results in dermatomal pain and sensory deficit accompanied by weakness of dorsiflexion, toe extension, and foot inversion.[10]

The lateral femoral cutaneous nerve (LFCN) originates from the L2-3 nerve roots and travels along the lateral border of the psoas major muscle and across the ilium toward the anterior superior iliac spine (ASIS). Because of its anatomic exit below the ASIS, compression neuropathy of the LFCN by posts or pads that support the pelvis may develop in patients who are placed in the prone position. In patients who sustain perioperative injury to the LFCN, hypoesthesia of the anterolateral aspect of the thigh usually develops, but some experience pain and dysesthesia as well. Few studies have been conducted to assess the incidence of positioning-related LFCN injury, although most estimates are around 20%. One study in particular estimated the incidence of LFCN injury to be 23.8% in patients who underwent prone spinal surgery with use of the Relton-Hall frame. All these patients experienced resolution of symptoms within 1 week to 2 months postoperatively.[11]

Soft Tissue Injuries

The patient's soft tissues must also be assiduously protected. Prolonged pressure leads to local ischemia and, in severe cases, tissue necrosis. The risk for injury may be minimized by, first, ensuring that sensitive structures do not bear significant pressure and, second, by distributing the pressure over a wide surface with careful padding. Materials that contact the skin should be permeable to prevent moisture buildup. Before placing the patient in the final position, an inspection should be performed to ensure that there are no electrocardiographic leads, intravenous line connectors, or other devices located in areas that will rest on the supporting pads.

With the patient in either the lateral or the prone position, the abdomen should be as free as possible. In the lateral position, the free abdomen will tend to fall anteriorly away from the spine, thereby facilitating a thoracoabdominal or retroperitoneal flank approach. With the patient positioned prone, having the abdomen free decreases intra-abdominal pressure. This both facilitates ventilation of the patient and decreases pressure in the valveless epidural venous plexus and thus reduces epidural bleeding.

Proper positioning of the breasts, particularly for relatively large women placed in the prone position, can be difficult. Adequate support of the upper thoracic region is necessary to achieve neutral cervical alignment and a stable operative platform. In general, the breasts are positioned so that they are medial and caudal to the supporting pads. Particular care is taken to ensure that direct pressure on the nipples is avoided, if possible.

Breast implants may pose a difficult positioning problem as well. The implants tend to be less compressible and less mobile than natural breast tissue, and it may be difficult to avoid direct pressure on the implants. It is important to discuss this potential problem with the patient beforehand and explain the risk for soft tissue injury from pressure and the rare possibility of implant rupture.

Head Positioning

Secure, neutral positioning of the cervical spine is a fundamental principle of patient positioning for all spinal operations, not just those directly involving the cervical region. Patients with degenerative disease in the thoracolumbar region frequently have concomitant cervical spondylosis and may therefore be at risk for postoperative cervical myeloradiculopathy if improperly positioned.

There are three main methods for providing head support and maintaining neutral cervical alignment. For lateral and supine cases, soft supports such as doughnut-shaped foam or gel pads or pillows may be used. Appropriately sized pads should be selected to avoid hyperextension, hyperflexion, or excessive lateral flexion. A specialized foam head holder with or without a custom rigid support may also be used to support the head for prone procedures. These are most appropriate for relatively short operations that do not involve the cervical or upper thoracic region.

Rigid head-holding devices may also be used. Three-point pin fixation devices with a table-mounted holder, such as the Mayfield system (Integra, Plainsboro, NJ), are familiar to most neurological surgeons, but perhaps less so to orthopedic surgeons. Proper positioning of the pins is necessary to prevent slippage of the head in the holder and to minimize the likelihood of perforating the skull. One benefit of rigid head fixation is that the occipitocervicothoracic region can be precisely aligned and the position maintained throughout the operation. A military prone position to reduce a malaligned dens fracture, for example, can be readily achieved, confirmed with fluoroscopy, and securely held during surgery. If a long instrumented fusion is planned, care must be taken during positioning to ensure proper alignment in all three planes and avoid creating an iatrogenic deformity.

Finally, traction systems can be used to secure the head. They allow some movement of the head and neck during surgery, which can have at least two benefits. First, by setting up dual vectors for traction, alignment of the spine can be altered during surgery by the surgeon while still scrubbed (Fig. 27-5). Second, the small amount of movement produced by the placement of upper thoracic pedicle screws might cause dislodgment of the head from a rigid fixator; a properly adjusted traction system

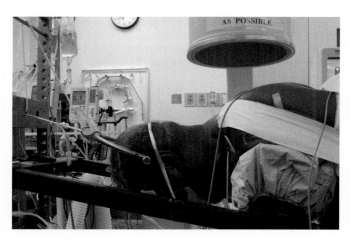

FIGURE 27-5 By using two ropes for the traction setup, one can change the alignment of the spine safely and effectively during surgery.

allows a safe amount of movement and eliminates this potential complication.

Visual Loss and Its Prevention

Postoperative visual loss (POVL) is an infrequently recognized but devastating complication of spinal surgery. Given that the estimated incidence of POVL has varied considerably across the surgical literature and was thought to be escalating in the mid-1990s, the American Society of Anesthesiologists created a POVL registry in 1999. Interim analyses of the POVL registry suggested a frequency of 0.0008% in noncardiac surgical patients undergoing procedures as disparate as hip arthroplasty, thoracotomy, and neck dissection. POVL in spinal surgery appears to be up to 100 times more frequent, with an incidence of roughly 0.08%.[12]

The most common cause of POVL in spinal surgery is ischemic optic neuropathy (ION) (89% of registry cases), which is more frequently unilateral than bilateral. POVL may also be attributed to central retinal artery occlusion (11% of registry cases). Although the precise etiology of ION in spinal surgery remains unclear, the leading hypothesis attributes ION to compromised blood flow in the optic nerve as a result of increased venous pressure and interstitial edema. Seventy-two percent of all ION cases were associated with prone spinal surgery; it occurred both in patients whose heads were maintained in facial supporters and in those for whom Mayfield pins alone were used for the entirety of the procedure. These data demonstrate that ION occurs independent of external pressure on the globe. Early data also suggested a relationship between POVL and prolonged anesthetic duration (94% of procedures had an anesthetic duration of 6 hours or longer), as well as between POVL and significant blood loss (82% of patients had estimated blood loss of 1 L or greater).[13]

Air Embolism

Air embolism is a concern that occurs almost exclusively when operating with a patient in the sitting position. This position is used by some surgeons for cervical foraminotomies and has been described for cervicothoracic osteotomies. With the operative field located significantly above the heart, air may be entrained into open, uncoagulated venous channels and result in air embolism. This may be more likely to occur with vascular channels in bone, which cannot collapse under atmospheric pressure. A precordial Doppler probe may help diagnose an air embolism early, and a long venous line with the tip in the right atrium may be

used in an attempt to aspirate air. If air embolism is suspected during surgery, the field should be flooded with sterile irrigation fluid and the position changed to bring the head close to the level of the heart, if possible.

Spinal Alignment

As increasing numbers of instrumented fusions are performed, spinal surgeons are recognizing the relationship between achieving and maintaining proper spinal alignment and good clinical outcome. For procedures in which no arthrodesis is performed, such as lumbar microdiskectomy or cervical foraminotomy from a posterior approach, the patient's intraoperative position may be optimized to facilitate safe, thorough neural decompression. This usually involves a moderate amount of regional flexion. If the spine is instrumented as an adjunct to fusion, however, care should be taken to place the spine in anatomic alignment to avoid creating an iatrogenic deformity such as lumbar hypolordosis ("flat back"). There are important considerations specific to each spinal region that the surgeon should address when checking the patient's position before surgery.

Proper alignment of the occipitocervical region is essential for good patient outcomes after instrumentation and arthrodesis of the region from the occiput to C2. Improper positioning can lead to an overly extended position and an inability of patients to see their body. Excessive flexion or retraction can make swallowing difficult. Finally, coronal or axial (rotational) malalignment will require patients to compensate for head tilt or rotation to maintain level, forward gaze.

One option to ensure proper occipitocervical alignment is to place the patient in a halo and vest preoperatively. Adjustments can then be made to the patient's position before surgery. This strategy may be appropriate for patients who will require halo-vest immobilization postoperatively. It is less useful for procedures in which repositioning during the procedure is necessary or advantageous, such as combined transoral decompression and posterior occipitocervical fixation and arthrodesis. There can also be practical issues in accommodating the halo and vest on the operating table.

Estimating the chin-brow angle from fluoroscopy or radiographs can be difficult. We generally use a combination of low-magnification fluoroscopy, which maximizes the field of view and the ability to judge the relationship between the occipitocervical region and the subaxial cervical spine, and direct inspection of the relationship between the head and the torso. In some cases this does require the surgeon to scrub out of the sterile field to look under the surgical drapes.

When performing instrumentation and arthrodesis of the subaxial cervical spine, the surgeon must attend to the restoration or preservation of normal cervical lordosis. Patients who are fixed in a straight alignment are likely to complain about their head and neck position or pain, or both. To facilitate laminectomies, foraminotomies, and placement of lateral mass fixation, we prefer an intraoperative position of relative neck flexion. By using the dual-vector traction system described earlier, we can easily place the patient into cervical lordosis before rod placement and grafting. Although well-placed lateral mass screws can tolerate modest amounts of corrective force during rod placement, their relatively low pullout strength and the lack of a good salvage fixation option in the event of pullout has led us to try to achieve the final alignment through patient positioning and to use the fixation to maintain rather than achieve the final lordotic alignment (see Fig. 27-5).

Alignment of the cervicothoracic region deserves special mention. Without careful attention, it is easy to position the patient so that there is relative cervicothoracic kyphosis and a straight subaxial cervical spine. This is a particularly debilitating position in that the patient's head juts forward from the upper thoracic region and forward gaze is maintained only through

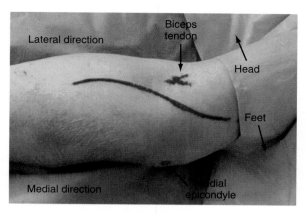

FIGURE 28-4 The incision for exposure of the anterior interosseous nerve.

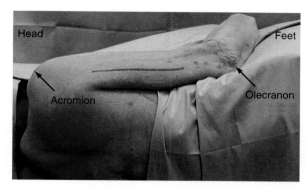

FIGURE 28-5 A patient in the lateral decubitus position for exposure of the radial nerve. Note that in this position, the surgeon may move from the posterior aspect of the patient to the anterior aspect of the patient to reach the radial nerve distal to the spiral groove.

median nerve lies lateral to the brachial artery. As there are no branches of the nerve in the arm, it is easily mobilized and traced both proximally and distally.

In Forearm

SURGICAL EXPOSURE

The incision begins 2 to 3 cm above the medial epicondyle over the medial intermuscular septum. Moving inferiorly, it crosses the elbow flexion crease obliquely and just medial to the biceps brachii tendon (Fig. 28-4). The incision continues distally over the bicipital aponeurosis in a gentle curve toward the midline of the forearm. The incision then moves distally down the forearm, following the interval between the flexor digitorum superficialis and brachioradialis. The incision is opened proximally, and the median nerve is located in the interval between the biceps brachii and the medial intermuscular septum. The nerve is traced into the forearm, and the lacertus fibrosus crosses its path obliquely. The nerve next passes deep to the pronator teres muscle. As the nerve is traced, it dives between the two heads of this muscle. The nerve then moves deep to the arch of the flexor digitorum superficialis, and this arch is divided. The median nerve may then be traced to the wrist, where it lies between the flexor carpi radialis and the flexor digitorum superficialis.

The anatomy and surgical exposure of the median nerve in the wrist are covered in other chapters.

Radial and Posterior Interosseous Nerve

In Arm

POSITIONING

If the radial nerve needs to be exposed only from the triangular interval, where it emerges into the posterior compartment of the arm, to the spiral groove, the patient may be placed in the lateral decubitus, the prone, or the supine position. I find that the lateral decubitus position offers the most comfortable positioning for this exposure. If the nerve must be exposed on both sides of the spiral groove, the posterior and anterior surfaces of the arm must be available for exposure. Once again, the patient may be positioned in the lateral decubitus, prone, or supine position. In the lateral position, the surgeon must be able to move freely from

the posterior aspect of the arm to the anterior aspect. In the supine position, the arm must be able to swing freely over the patient's body so that the posterior aspect of the arm is easily exposed.

SURGICAL EXPOSURE

The incision is made on the posterolateral aspect of the arm. An incision in a line connecting the acromion and olecranon, both of which are easily palpated, exposes the sulcus between the long and lateral heads of the triceps (Fig. 28-5). The fascia is incised along the lateral border of the long head of the triceps. The interval between the long and lateral heads is divided bluntly. Retraction of the superficial muscle exposes the radial nerve and profunda brachii artery. The radial nerve may then be traced distally as it passes from the posterior compartment into the anterior compartment of the arm.

In Forearm

POSITIONING

The patient is placed in the supine position with the arm on an arm board. The shoulder is abducted and externally rotated. The hand is fully supinated. The operator is most comfortable superior to the arm, just lateral to the neck and head of the patient.

SURGICAL EXPOSURE

The incision begins 3 to 4 cm proximal to the elbow flexion crease in the interval between the biceps brachii and brachioradialis muscles. It crosses the elbow flexion crease obliquely and then curves down onto the forearm lateral to the biceps brachii tendon. The incision should reach the midline of the forearm 4 to 5 cm distal to the elbow flexion crease and then continue distally in the forearm just radial to the midline. The nerve may be identified in the interval between the biceps and brachioradialis just proximal to the elbow flexion crease. The nerve is then traced down into the plane between the brachioradialis and extensor carpi radialis longus muscles. The posterior interosseous nerve should be traced distally as it passes under a vascular leash of vessels, inferior to the arcade of Frohse and into the supinator muscle.[5]

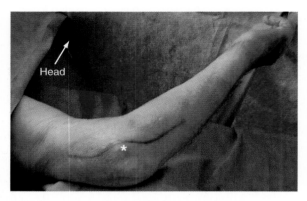

FIGURE 28-6 A patient positioned with an incision drawn for an ulnar nerve exposure. The *asterisk* marks the palpated olecranon.

Ulnar Nerve

In Elbow and Forearm

POSITIONING

The patient is placed in the supine position with the arm on an arm board. The shoulder is abducted and externally rotated. The hand and forearm are fully supinated, and the elbow is gently flexed. The surgeon works from a position between the abducted arm and the patient's body. A seated position is often the most comfortable for operating.

SURGICAL EXPOSURE

Exposure of the nerve within the cubital tunnel begins with a skin incision 5 cm proximal to the medial epicondyle that curves gently up and over the epicondyle (Fig. 28-6). The incision then continues down onto the forearm for another 4 to 5 cm. The posterior cutaneous nerve of the forearm may cross the operative field, and it should be identified and protected. Once the skin is retracted, the nerve may be found within the cubital tunnel and traced both proximally and distally as needed. Further details may be found in Chapter 28.

Lower Extremity

Sciatic Nerve

ANATOMY

The ventral rami of the fourth lumbar to third sacral nerve roots unite to form the sciatic nerve. In the lesser pelvis, the nerve lies anterior to the piriformis muscle. Just caudad to this muscle, the nerve enters the buttock through the sciatic foramen. The nerve then moves laterally in an oblique direction beneath the gluteus maximus muscle toward the midline of the posterior aspect of the leg. The nerve descends in the thigh close to the midline. In the majority of individuals, the nerve divides into tibial and common peroneal branches at the mid to distal third of the thigh.

Once divided, the common peroneal nerve then moves obliquely across the distal thigh to travel on the lateral aspect of the popliteal fossa. Close to its origin, one or more branches of the peroneal nerve leave to contribute to the formation of the sural nerve. The tibial nerve will also contribute to the formation of the sural nerve. Moving distally, the nerve then crosses the lateral head of the gastrocnemius muscle to reach the area just posterior to the fibular head. Once it curves over the posterior rim of the fibular head, it enters a tunnel formed by the two heads of the peroneus longus muscle and the fibular neck. The common peroneal nerve divides into superficial and deep branches. The superficial portion of the nerve takes a relatively straight course to innervate the peroneus longus muscle and continues descending distally to innervate the peroneus brevis muscle.

The deep peroneal nerve, once it is past the neck of the fibula and after it passes beneath the fibrous lateral edge of the peroneus longus, gives off geniculate branches and branches to the tibialis anterior. The nerve descends in the anterior compartment of the leg lateral to the tibialis anterior. In the very distal leg, the nerve divides into medial and lateral terminal branches.

The tibial nerve continues the line of the sciatic nerve after its bifurcation in the mid to distal third of the thigh. In the popliteal fossa, the tibial nerve becomes more superficial, first lying posterior and lateral to the popliteal vessels and then crossing obliquely to their medial side before moving into the leg. It travels distally in the leg between the gastrocnemius and the tibialis posterior muscles. Finally, the nerve curves anteroinferiorly into the sole of the foot behind the medial malleolus, deep to the flexor retinaculum and between the tendons of the flexor hallucis longus and the flexor digitorum longus. The nerve in the so-called tarsal tunnel ends at this level as it divides into medial and lateral plantar nerves. A calcaneal branch is also given off at this level. The sural nerve, a cutaneous branch of the tibial nerve, arises at the mid or lower aspect of the popliteal fossa. It gives off branches to the skin on the lower lateral leg and heel.[6] The terminal portion of the sural nerve is the lateral dorsal cutaneous nerve that supplies sensation to the lateral foot and small toe.

POSITIONING

After intubation and induction of general endotracheal anesthesia on a stretcher, the patient is placed on the operating table in the prone position on abdominal bolsters. The arms are brought forward on arm boards. The ipsilateral buttock and leg are draped.

SURGICAL EXPOSURE

A curvilinear incision in a reverse question mark shape is fashioned. The stem of the question mark will follow the midline of the posterior aspect of the thigh; the curve will follow the inferior margin of the gluteus muscle around the contour of the buttock and up onto the lateral aspect of the buttock (Fig. 28-7). After the skin is incised, the inferior margin of the gluteus maximus muscle is located. At the midline of the leg, just inferior to the edge of the gluteal muscle, a fat pad is found. The sciatic nerve is located within this fat. For more proximal exposure, the gluteus muscle must be divided. A cuff of muscle both medially and laterally must be left for reattachment at the completion of the case. Once the muscle is divided, it is reflected in a unit medially for exposure of the sciatic nerve in the buttock. Exposure of the sciatic nerve more proximal to the sciatic notch will require an abdominal extraperitoneal approach.[7]

In exposure of the nerve distally, the posterior femoral cutaneous nerve travels superficially and should not be confused with the sciatic nerve. For more distal exposure, the incision may be extended distally along the posterior midline of the thigh, tracing the nerve beneath the long head of the biceps femoris muscle and on to its division into the common peroneal and tibial nerves (Fig. 28-8).

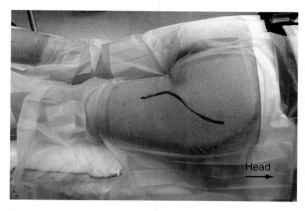

FIGURE 28-7 A patient positioned with an incision drawn for a sciatic nerve exposure. The patient is in the prone position on abdominal bolsters. The incision may be extended distally as needed.

Peroneal Nerve

POSITIONING

The patient is placed on the operating table in the prone position on abdominal bolsters. The arms may be either tucked to the side or brought forward on arm boards. The midline of the popliteal fossa and just superior to it should be marked. The biceps femoris tendon can usually be palpated at the lateral aspect of the popliteal fossa and should also be marked. Last, the fibular head should be palpated and marked.

SURGICAL EXPOSURE

The skin incision is laid out so that the proximal end is just superior to the popliteal fossa. In the medial-lateral direction, it lies midway between the biceps femoris tendon and the midline of the fossa. Care should be taken in making the skin incision, particularly around the fibular head, as the nerve is surprisingly superficial. As the nerve is followed distally beyond the popliteal fossa, a thick fascial covering is encountered that is contiguous

with the fibrous lateral edge of the peroneus longus muscle. This edge should be incised, revealing a portion of the muscle. This muscle may also be incised to expose the nerve further. Dissection should continue to fully expose and identify both the superficial and deep branches of the nerve. The deep branch must be traced around the neck of the fibula.

Tibial Nerve

In Leg

POSITIONING

The tibial nerve at the level of the popliteal fossa is explored in the prone position. After intubation and induction of general endotracheal anesthesia, usually on a stretcher, the patient is placed on the operating table on abdominal bolsters. The arms may be either tucked to the side or brought forward on arm boards. The midline of the popliteal fossa and just superior to it should be marked.

SURGICAL EXPOSURE

The patient is in the prone position with the midline marked. The incision begins at the midline and extends distally to run obliquely across the popliteal fossa. It then cuts laterally across the fossa and continues down the leg just medial to the midline. Once the skin and subcutaneous tissue are divided, the tibial nerve may be located in the midline in close approximation to the popliteal artery and vein. Much beyond the popliteal fossa, the nerve is difficult to expose and will require a medial leg incision.

At Tarsal Tunnel

POSITIONING

The patient is placed in the supine position with a bolster under the contralateral buttock.

SURGICAL EXPOSURE

The incision runs in a curvilinear fashion in a radius approximately 2 to 3 cm around the posterior aspect of the medial malleolus. The incision should also extend at least 5 cm proximal to the malleolus up into the leg and 5 cm distal to the malleolus out onto the foot, paralleling the medial border of the plantar foot pad. The skin is incised, and after a small amount of dissection, the tendons that course through the tunnel are immediately apparent. Just posterior to these tendons, the nerve, posterior tibial artery, and vein will be located. The artery and vein are often intertwined with the nerve at this level, making the dissection more difficult. As the nerve is traced distally, further sectioning of the flexor retinaculum reveals the nerve dividing into medial and lateral plantar nerves and a calcaneal branch. The proximal belly of the abductor hallucis muscle may overlie the area where the nerve divides. The belly of the muscle must be partially sectioned to visualize this last portion of the nerve.

Sural Nerve

POSITIONING AND SURGICAL EXPOSURE

Positioning for exposure of the sural nerve will most often depend on the reason for operation. If sural nerve exposure is required

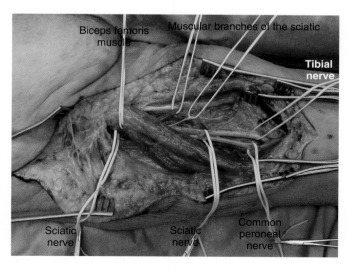

FIGURE 28-8 The sciatic nerve fully exposed.

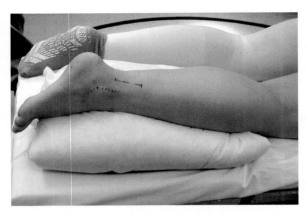

FIGURE 28-9 A patient positioned for exposure of the sural nerve. The lateral malleolus is marked.

for harvesting a cable graft and the primary nerves to be operated on require the body to be placed in a supine position (e.g., brachial plexus, femoral nerve), the sural nerve may be harvested from a supine position. It is somewhat awkward to perform in this position, particularly as the nerve is traced more proximally, but it can be accomplished. The knee should be bent and the leg tilted medially to facilitate exposure. An incision is laid out two fingerbreadths posterior and two fingerbreadths superior to the lateral malleolus. If sural nerve exposure is required for operations that are performed in the prone position (e.g., harvesting

of a cable graft for sciatic nerve), the sural nerve is easily exposed through the same incision as outlined for a supine position. This positioning is much less awkward for the operator, but the exposure and anatomy are identical to those encountered in supine positioning (Fig. 28-9).

The nerve and muscle tendon are fairly superficial, and care should be exercised accordingly in making the incision. The skin and subcutaneous tissue are exposed. If the nerve is not immediately visible, it will lie slightly anterior in the fat layer just beneath the subcutaneous tissue. Care should be taken not to disrupt the lesser saphenous vein that travels with the nerve. If it is traced proximally, the nerve may be followed, accompanied by the lesser saphenous vein, until its disappearance beneath the two heads of the gastrocnemius muscle.

SUGGESTED READINGS

DeMaura W, Gilliert A. Surgical anatomy of the sural nerve. *J Reconstr Microsurg.* 1984;1:31-39.

Hall HC, Mackinnon SE, Gilbert RW. An approach to the posterior interosseous nerve. *Plast Reconstr Surg.* 1984;74:435-437.

Henry AK. Exposures in the lower limb. Section IV. In: Henry AK, ed. *Extensile Exposure,* 2nd ed. New York: Churchill Livingstone; 1973:180-307.

Kerr AT. The brachial plexus of nerves in man, the variations in its formation and its branches. *Am J Anat.* 1918;23:285-395.

Kline DG, Kott J, Barnes G, Bryant L. Exploration of selected brachial plexus lesions by the posterior subscapular approach. *J Neurosurg.* 1978;49:872-880.

Maniker A. *Operative Exposures in Peripheral Nerve Surgery.* New York: Thieme; 2005.

Walsh JF. The anatomy of the brachial plexus. *Am J Med Sci.* 1877;74:387-399.

Full references can be found on Expert Consult @ www.expertconsult.com

The facial nerve lies within a small fat bed between the layers of the deep temporal fascia, posterior to the superficial temporal artery and vein, at the level of the zygomatic arch.[15] The facial nerve lies deep to the superficial temporal fascia in the temporoparietal region within the subgaleal tissue. It courses 2.5 cm anterior to the tragus and 1.5 cm lateral to the orbital rim within the deep temporal fascia and innervates the frontalis from its lateral aspect.[18] Therefore, when elevating a pericranial flap, care should be taken to preserve the frontal branch of the facial nerve as it runs along the undersurface of the subgaleal fascia on the lateral border of the frontalis muscle.

Cadaveric studies have revealed that the superficial temporal artery does contribute to the blood supply of the periosteum and skull in the frontoparietal region whereas the deep temporal artery supplies the calvaria in the temporal region. The outer table of the posterior cranial vault is supplied by the occipital artery.[20,21] The frontoparietal bone survives by its attachment to the middle meningeal artery, a branch of the maxillary artery; however, one study has depicted it perforating between the diploic spaces and the superficial temporal artery.[20]

Clinical Considerations

With this understanding of the pertinent regional anatomy, one can now choose the incision that affords the greatest exposure and reliable closure. In general, the most appropriate craniotomy approach for a particular lesion is often the one that provides the shortest traversal through brain tissue. The frontosphenotemporal or pterional craniotomy, commonly used for access to anterior aneurysms and parasellar, sphenoid, and anterior skull base tumors, was traditionally described as involving an incision from the root of the zygoma to the linea temporalis and anteriorly to the center of the forehead, as seen in Figure 29-8.[22] The forehead is the most aesthetic part of the calvaria; it is visible in its entirety

and forms the medial and lateral walls of the orbit.[10] It is described as containing five aesthetic units: two temporal, two brow, and one central component, as illustrated in Figure 29-9. Standard reconstructive principles advocate replacement of an entire aesthetic subunit when 50% or more of the subunit is altered to avoid the "patchwork" appearance that results when only a portion of an aesthetic unit is replaced.[10] Use of a coronal incision is oftentimes superior to a pterional incision in providing better exposure and cosmetic result because it preserves all the aesthetic units of the forehead (see Fig. 29-8). The coronal incision is longer, however, and necessitates additional operative time. When elevating the coronal flap, care should be taken to preserve the frontal branch of the facial nerve in the galeal or subgaleal plane (depending on the anatomic location). The skull is exposed either through elevation of periosteum with the flap or by incising the periosteum after a galeal flap is raised. In the temporoparietal region, however, the temporalis muscle overlies the skull. Numerous techniques have been described to decrease potential injury to the temporal branch of the facial nerve when dissecting in this region.[23] Elevation of the temporalis muscle with the scalp incision is a reliable means of protecting the facial nerve; however, detachment of the muscle from its superior insertion results in retraction of the muscle inferiorly and an unfavorable cosmetic outcome of temporal wasting. One study proposed leaving a cuff of temporalis muscle superiorly attached to the skull to provide an adequate scaffold for reapproximating the muscle fibers and consequently reducing resultant temporal wasting while protecting the facial nerve.[23]

A subtemporal craniotomy involves the use of a horseshoe-shaped flap to approach tentorial, clivus, and basilar artery lesions, as depicted in Figure 29-8.[22] It is based on the superficial temporal and posterior auricular pedicles, with the former providing the majority of the blood supply. Design and use of this flap imply persistence and flow through these arteries. Incisions in the periphery of the scalp are at risk of transecting vital neurovascular trunks and may result in hypoesthetic, poorly vascularized tissue. Landmarks described earlier should be used to predict where the superficial temporal and posterior auricular arteries, as well as the regional cutaneous nerves, are located to avoid complications.

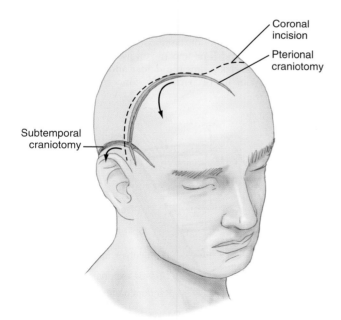

FIGURE 29-8 Craniotomy incisions. Pterional craniotomy violates the aesthetic units of the forehead and provides limited exposure when compared with a coronal incision. A subtemporal craniotomy incision places local vascular pedicles and cutaneous nerves at risk. The main vascular supply to the scalp originates at the periphery; it branches and establishes an extensive interconnected network as it runs medially.

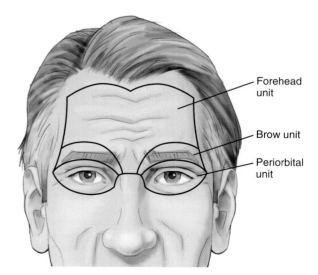

FIGURE 29-9 Forehead aesthetic units. Five aesthetic units of the forehead have been described: one central superior, two temporal, and two brow components. If 50% or more of one unit is involved in the resection, the entire aesthetic unit should be replaced. (*Adapted from Wells, M. Scalp reconstruction. In Mathes SJ:* Plastic Surgery. *Philadelphia: Saunders; 2006:607-610.*)

A midline suboccipital craniotomy imparts an inconspicuous scar and takes advantage of the avascular raphe between the two bellies of the occipitalis muscle to optimize wound healing and closure.[22] The region of the posterior scalp territory that lies inferior to the superior nuchal line is not supplied by the centripetal vascular network but rather by direct musculocutaneus perforators from the splenius and trapezius muscles.[16]

Reliable closure is complicated by many factors, including radiation, embolization, previous scalp surgery, and advanced age (>60 years). If, for example, the superficial temporal artery was embolized in a patient and one desired to use the subtemporal craniotomy approach, placement of the anterior incision to incorporate the blood supply of the supraorbital or supratrochlear vessels, branches of the internal carotid artery, would provide supplemental blood supply and ensure a more reliable closure. Similar principles apply when designing a flap based on a vessel that is either within or adjacent to irradiated scalp. Conservative flap length and avoidance of extension of the flap beyond the midline in tissues with poor vasculature, such as irradiated tissue or in patients older than 60 years, are recommended.

CLOSURE

With understanding of the considerations necessary for planning the most appropriate incision, discussion of the various factors that the surgeon can manipulate to optimize closure is warranted. Management of a simple, atraumatic, noncontaminated wound is best achieved with primary closure, with the goal being to obliterate potential dead space, distribute tension evenly along deep suture lines, and maintain suture tensile strength until tissue tensile strength is adequate.[24] Monofilament suture is a single-strand suture with proven resistance to the ingress of bacteria as compared with multifilament suture.[25] Monofilament suture also has decreased drag when passed through tissues, which may contribute to a decreased inflammatory response when compared with multifilament suture. Although infection is minimized, monofilament suture exhibits less tensile strength than multifilament suture does.[25] For purposes of galea and scalp closure, infection plays a larger role in surgical management and therefore supports the use of monofilament over multifilament suture in most circumstances. Absorbable suture provides temporary wound support, with final resorption being due to enzymatic or hydrolytic degradation of the suture material. Absorption is affected by the local environment, which must be taken into consideration when choosing the type of suture. As the wound heals, however, the absorption and relative loss of suture strength over time should be slower than the gain in tissue tensile strength.[25] Nonabsorbable suture provides constant tensile strength. One can select the optimal suture by choosing the smallest suture capable of achieving the desired "tension-free" closure.[25]

Tension-free closure is highly desirable for wound closure. In general, scalp defects of 2 cm or less can be closed primarily.[9] Simple primary closure of the scalp can be performed in two layers with approximation of the galea first, followed by epidermal closure. Deeper tissues bear the majority of the tension and therefore require suture material with appropriate tensile strength and minimal reactivity, such as longer lasting absorbable monofilament suture. An interrupted stitch is the preferred closure technique because it avoids compromising the vessels within the galea supplying the scalp. The detraction of this approach is that it requires longer operating time. Vertical mattress, continuous, and locking sutures are discouraged because they impair the blood supply to the flap. Well-vascularized skin is typically closed with continuous nonabsorbable monofilament suture to provide wound support with only slight tissue reaction. Metallic staples may be used in regions of compromised vascularity to improve the potential for uncomplicated wound healing.

Although some degree of undermining is often performed in most scalp closures, extensive undermining in the subgaleal plane predisposes to scar formation, hematoma, and vascular compromise with potential flap necrosis. Even though quantitative studies using tensiometric measurements have demonstrated no significant correlation between undermining and reduction in surface tension, clinically, the effect is more appreciated.[26] Deep-plane fixation is another surgical technique used to help disperse tension-vector forces away from the skin into deeper planes capable of sustaining such forces.[6] By placing a series of sutures several centimeters lateral to the wound edge, tension force on superficial tissue is minimized. In theory, deep-plane fixation augments wound healing; however, there is no statistically significant difference in the amount of resection afforded by these means.[6,26] Although surgeons continue to design techniques to limit tension in tissues, the most important determinant of optimal scalp closure is skin laxity, an inherent property of skin elastin.

When tension-free closure is not possible with primary closure, one should consider the options depicted in the reconstructive ladder presented in Figure 29-10.[4] The reconstructive ladder offers a systematic approach to wound closure with the goal of restoring form and function. Defect size, anatomy, and the quality of the surrounding tissue limit the options for reconstruction. The easiest form of skin replacement is an autogenous skin graft. The advantage of a split-thickness graft is the abundance of donor sites (thigh, buttock, abdomen); however, the disadvantage is that the graft is thin and usually hairless and requires a well-vascularized bed for survival and ingrowth. Full-thickness grafts have the advantage of being thicker, contain hair follicles, and often serve as more homogeneous color matches; however, they also require a well-vascularized bed and produce a more morbid donor site than split-thickness grafts do.

Small defects of the scalp can be reconstructed with "random-pattern" advancement flaps based on the subdermal plexus, with care taken to avoid transecting hair follicles, as previously depicted in Figure 29-7.[4] Larger defects may necessitate the use of a skin graft or local flaps, such as the bilobed flap used to cover defects less than 25 cm² or fasciocutaneous flaps such as the Orticochea three- and four-flap technique.[4,10] Local techniques require the area surrounding the defect and donor tissue to be healthy, which can be of particular concern in patients with

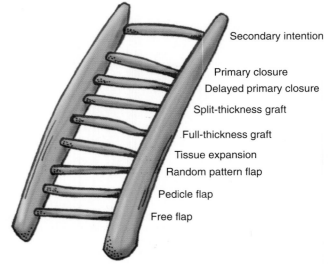

Secondary intention

Primary closure
Delayed primary closure

Split-thickness graft

Full-thickness graft

Tissue expansion

Random pattern flap

Pedicle flap

Free flap

FIGURE 29-10 Reconstructive ladder for a systematic approach to choosing the most appropriate reconstructive option.

resected cancer, infection, or radiation exposure. Pectoralis major, latissimus dorsi, and trapezius musculocutaneous flaps have been used for reconstruction of the temporal area.[4] The ideal free flap contributes well-vascularized tissue with a pedicle of sufficient length to allow the anastomoses to be distanced from the original zone of injury.[27] Free flap reconstruction requires advanced surgical skill but offers a viable, single-stage reconstruction of large cranial defects in wounds with vascular compromise, such as those with radiation exposure, previous surgery, or infection.

CONCLUSION

With thorough understanding of the basics of wound healing, pertinent surgical anatomy, and reconstructive options, reliable and reproducible closure can be obtained with an optimal cosmetic outcome.

SUGGESTED READINGS

Abul-Hassan HS, von Drasek Ascher G, Acland RD. Surgical anatomy and blood supply of the fascial layers of the temporal region. *Plast Reconstr Surg.* 1986;77:17-23.

Argenta LC, Friedman R, Dingman RO, et al. The versatility of pericranial flaps. *Plast Reconstr Surg.* 1985;76:695-702.

Browning J. Surgical pearl: the use of petroleum jelly in performing scalp surgery. *J Am Acad Dermatol.* 2006;55:515-516.

Buchfelder M, Ljunggren B. Part 2. The osteoplastic flap. *Surg Neurol.* 1988;30:428-433.

Easwer HV, Rajeev A. Cosmetic and radiological outcome following the use of synthetic hydroxyapatite porous-dense bilayer burr-hole buttons. *Acta Neurochir (Wien).* 2007;149:481-486.

Edlich RF, Kenney JG, Morgan RF, et al. Antimicrobial treatment of minor soft tissue lacerations: a critical review. *Emerg Med Clin North Am.* 1986;4:561-580.

Frechet P. Minimal scars for scalp surgery. *Dermatol Surg.* 2007;33:45-56.

Goel A. Tenting stitches for the scalp. *Br J Neurosurg.* 1992;6:357-358.

Horowitz JH, Persing JA, Nichter LS, et al. Galeal-pericranial flaps in head and neck reconstruction. *Am J Surg.* 1984;148:489-497.

Horowitz JH, Persing JA, et al. Galeal-pericranial flaps in head and neck reconstruction. *Am J Surg.* 1984;148:489-497.

Houseman ND, Taylor GI, Ran WR. The angiosomes of the head and neck: anatomic study and clinical applications. *Plast Reconstr Surg.* 2000;105:2287-2313.

Inaba Y, Inaba M. Prevention and treatment of linear scar formation in the scalp: basic principles of the mechanism of scar formation. *Aesthet Plast Surg.* 1995;19:369-370.

Kahn DS, Pritzker PH. The pathophysiology of bone infection. *Clin Orthop Relat Res.* 1973;96:12-19.

Kolt J. Use of adhesive surgical tape with the absorbable continuous subcuticular suture. *ANZ J Surg.* 2003;73:626-629.

Lorenz PH, Longaker MT. Wound healing: repair biology and wound and scar treatment. In: Mathes SJ, ed. *Plastic Surgery.* Philadelphia: Elsevier; 2006:209-234.

Marty F, Montandon D, Gumener R, et al. Subcutaneous tissue in the scalp: anatomical, physiological, and clinical study. *Ann Plast Surg.* 1986;16:368-376.

Mathes SJ, Hansen SL. Flap classification and applications. In: Mathes SJ, ed. Plastic Surgery. Philadelphia: Elsevier; 2006:365-482.

Mehrara BJ, McCarthy JG. Repair and grafting of bone. In: Mathes SJ, ed. Plastic Surgery. Philadelphia: Elsevier; 2006:639-718.

Orchard DC, McColl D. The subgaleal pulley suture. *Aust J Dermatol.* 1999;40:118-119.

Rodeheaver G, Edgerton MT. Antimicrobial prophylaxis of contaminated tissues containing suture implants. *Am J Surg.* 1977;133:609-611.

Seery G. Scalp surgery: anatomic and biomechanical considerations. *Dermatol Surg.* 2001;27:827-834.

Taylor GI, Ives A. Vascular territories. In: Mathes SJ, ed. Plastic Surgery. Philadelphia: Elsevier; 2006:317-364.

Tolhurst DE, Carstens MH, Greco RJ, et al. The surgical anatomy of the scalp. *Plast Reconstr Surg.* 1991;87:603-612; discussion 613-614.

Tremolada C, Candiani P, Signorini M, et al. The surgical anatomy of the subcutaneous fascial system of the scalp. *Ann Plast Surg.* 1994;32:8-14.

Tubbs RS, Salter EG, Wellons JC, et al. Landmarks for the identification of the cutaneous nerves of the occiput and nuchal regions. *Clin Anat.* 2007;20:235-238.

Wells MD. Scalp reconstruction. In: Mathes SJ, ed. *Plastic Surgery.* Philadelphia: Elsevier; 2006:607-632.

Whetzel TP, Mathes SJ. Arterial anatomy of the face: an analysis of vascular territories and perforating cutaneous vessels. *Plast Reconstr Surg.* 1992;89:590-603.

Winn HR, Jane JA, Rodeheaver G, et al. Influence of subcuticular sutures on scar formation. *Am J Surg.* 1977;133:257-259.

Wu T. Plastic surgery made easy: simple techniques for closing skin defects and improving cosmetic results. *Aust Fam Physician.* 2006;35:492-496.

Yaremchuk MJ. Acquired cranial bone deformities. In: Mathes SJ, ed. Plastic Surgery. Philadelphia: Elsevier; 2006:547-562.

Full references can be found on Expert Consult @ www.expertconsult.com

CHAPTER 30

Advantages and Limitations of Cranial Endoscopy

Jeroen R. Coppens ■ William T. Couldwell

Endoscopy was first used intracranially in the treatment of hydrocephalus at the beginning of the 20th century. Several eras of increased interest in cranial endoscopy during the past century have been linked to new technologic developments, and the endoscope's latest renaissance has expanded its potential applications by decreasing the risk of cerebrospinal fluid (CSF) leaks for skull base lesions. The endoscope has proved its utility in cranial surgery and has given the neurosurgeon more adaptability because it can be used alone or in combination with other open or microscopic techniques. Current indications for the use of intracranial endoscopy as well as the limitations still encountered with an endoscopic technique versus a microsurgical technique are reviewed.

HISTORY OF ENDOSCOPY

The earliest use of the endoscope intracranially was reported by Lespinasse in 1910 for the treatment of hydrocephalus.[1] Dandy[2] used the technique more extensively and became known as the "father of neuroendoscopy". Interest in cranial endoscopy was driven by the lack of alternative treatments of hydrocephalus in the first half of the 20th century. Endoscopic techniques evolved from fulguration or obliteration of the choroid plexus to fenestration techniques involving the ventricles and subarachnoid planes. The first endoscopic third ventriculostomy was reported by Mixter[3] in 1923. Limited development in the technology for endoscopes combined with the placement of the first valved shunt by Nulsen and Spitz[4] in 1949 decreased the interest in cranial endoscopy until the advent of rod lens endoscopes in 1960.[5] Better illumination and resolution of the image enabled the application of the endoscope in the context of cranial neurosurgery. In 1973, Fukushima and colleagues[6] introduced the modern endoscope, which could be used for the biopsy of intraventricular lesions, cyst fenestration, and treatment of hydrocephalus. The use of the endoscope in transsphenoidal approaches was introduced by Guiot, although he later abandoned the technique because it offered inadequate visualization.[7-9] Bushe and Halves[10] were the first to report the use of a modern endoscope in pituitary surgery in 1978. A few other reports emerged in the 1970s describing the use of an endoscope as an adjunct to the microscope in transsphenoidal approaches.[10-12] Application of the endoscope to the sella turcica did not grow in popularity until the mid-1990s, when endoscopic sinus surgery had virtually replaced open techniques in use by otolaryngologists.[9,13] Modern endoscopic cranial surgery developed from a combination of the growth in popularity of minimally invasive surgery through keyhole approaches[14,15] and the development of purely endoscopic approaches to the skull base leading to functional endoscopic pituitary surgery.[16]

ENDOSCOPIC INSTRUMENTATION AND GENERAL PRINCIPLES

Endoscopes are generally classified as either rod lens endoscopes or fiberoptic endoscopes (fiberscopes) on the basis of the technology used. Rod lens endoscopes transmit images through a series of lenses and are always rigid scopes. They provide a clearer image and better illumination than fiberscopes do. Fiberscopes transmit images through fiberoptic threads and can be maneuvered without image distortion. The resolution of fiberscopes is proportional to the number of fibers in the endoscope. Because of the nature of optic fibers, which may be flexed without breaking, fiberscopes can be fixed or flexible. However, rigid fiberscopes allow more pixel fibers than flexible or steerable fiberscopes do.

Flexible fiberscopes have the smallest diameter and can be used as a stylet within a ventricular catheter. They do not have a working channel but are appropriate for visualizing catheter placement and ensuring an intraventricular position. They have not been shown to improve the surgical outcome in hydrocephalus as no superiority of any specific location of catheter placement has been demonstrated.[17,18]

Steerable fiberscopes permit varying degrees of bending of the tip of the endoscope. A working channel is present, and its orientation is adjustable, enabling the instruments to reach all of the structures visualized. The diameter of the scope varies with the number of optic fibers; the larger scopes provide a better image quality.

Rigid fiberscopes exist in a variety of lengths and diameters. A working channel is present, but targets can be used only on a straight line from the bur hole. The quality of vision remains inferior to that of rod lens endoscopes.

Rod lens endoscopes are used overwhelmingly in cranial endoscopy because of the superior quality of the image obtained. They are heavier because of the mandatory attachment of the camera and fiberoptic cable for the light source. An assortment of viewing angles is available (e.g., 0-, 30-, 70-, 120-degree angled endoscopes; Fig. 30-1). Up to two working channels are available on certain types of rod lens endoscopes through which instrumentation can be used. These working channels can also be used in addition to a trocar sheath, enabling the surgeon to use different viewing-angle endoscopes without the need to reinsert them through brain tissue. Different sheaths are available with one to multiple channels for inserting instruments, providing irrigation, or supplying suction.[19] Instrumentation in the form of varying forceps, scissors, suction, or coagulation has been developed. The 0- and 30-degree endoscopes are the most widely used. The 0-degree scope minimizes the risk of disorientation, but the instruments inserted through the working channel remain in the periphery of the field of vision.[18] The 30-degree endoscope allows better control of the instruments and, with simple rotation, provides an angle of view with a surface area twice as large as that of a 0-degree endoscope.

The optimal use of the endoscope requires a light source combined with a camera and monitor. Halogen, mercury vapor, and xenon light sources are available. The light source is connected to the endoscope through a fiberoptic cable, and its intensity can be modulated. Xenon light sources provide the best illumination for neuroendoscopy.[18] The camera is connected to the endoscope by an adapter and transmits the image to a video monitor for viewing by the rest of the surgical team. Cameras are available as a single-chip or a three-chip charge-coupled device.

SUGGESTED READINGS

Cappabianca P, Alfieri A, de Divitiis E. Endoscopic endonasal transsphenoidal approach to the sella: towards functional endoscopic pituitary surgery (FEPS). *Minim Invasive Neurosurg.* 1998;41:66-73.

Couldwell WT, Weiss MH, Rabb C, et al. Variations on the standard transsphenoidal approach to the sellar region, with emphasis on the extended approaches and parasellar approaches: surgical experience in 105 cases. *Neurosurgery.* 2004; 55:539-547; discussion 547-550.

Dandy W. An operative approach for hydrocephalus. *Bull John Hopkins Hosp.* 1922;33:189-190.

Das K, Spencer W, Nwagwu CI, et al. Approaches to the sellar and parasellar region: anatomic comparison of endonasal-transsphenoidal, sublabial-transsphenoidal, and transethmoidal approaches. *Neurol Res.* 2001;23:51-54.

de Divitiis E, Cappabianca P. Microscopic and endoscopic transsphenoidal surgery. *Neurosurgery.* 2002;51:1527-1529; author reply 1529-1530.

Fries G, Perneczky A. Endoscope-assisted brain surgery: part 2—analysis of 380 procedures. *Neurosurgery.* 1998;42:226-231; discussion 231-232.

Guiot J, Rougerie J, Fourestier M, et al. [Intracranial endoscopic explorations.] *Presse Med.* 1963;71:1225-1228.

Iantosca MR, Hader WJ, Drake JM. Results of endoscopic third ventriculostomy. *Neurosurg Clin North Am.* 2004;15:67-75.

Kassam A, Snyderman CH, Mintz A, et al. Expanded endonasal approach: the rostrocaudal axis. Part I. Crista galli to the sella turcica. *Neurosurg Focus.* 2005; 19(1):E3.

Kassam A, Snyderman CH, Mintz A, et al. Expanded endonasal approach: the rostrocaudal axis. Part II. Posterior clinoids to the foramen magnum. *Neurosurg Focus.* 2005;19(1):E4.

Kehler U, Brunori A, Gliemroth J, et al. Twenty colloid cysts—comparison of endoscopic and microsurgical management. *Minim Invasive Neurosurg.* 2001;44: 121-127.

Liu JK, Das K, Weiss MH, et al. The history and evolution of transsphenoidal surgery. *J Neurosurg.* 2001;95:1083-1096.

Liu JK, Decker D, Schaefer SD, et al. Zones of approach for craniofacial resection: minimizing facial incisions for resection of anterior cranial base and paranasal sinus tumors. *Neurosurgery.* 2003;53:1126-1135; discussion 1135-1137.

Mixter W. Ventriculoscopy and puncture of the floor of the third ventricle: preliminary report of a case. *Boston Med Surg J.* 1923;188:277-278.

Nulsen FE, Spitz EB. Treatment of hydrocephalus by direct shunt from ventricle to jugular vein. *Surg Forum.* 1952;2:399-402.

Oi S, Abbott R. Loculated ventricles and isolated compartments in hydrocephalus: their pathophysiology and the efficacy of neuroendoscopic surgery. *Neurosurg Clin North Am.* 2004;15:77-87.

Perneczky A, Fries G. Endoscope-assisted brain surgery: part 1—evolution, basic concept, and current technique. *Neurosurgery.* 1998;42:219-224; discussion 224-225.

Rao G, Klimo P Jr, Jensen RL, et al. Surgical strategies for recurrent craniofacial meningiomas. *Neurosurgery.* 2006;58:874-879; discussion 879-880.

Spencer WR, Das K, Nwagu C, et al. Approaches to the sellar and parasellar region: anatomic comparison of the microscope versus endoscope. *Laryngoscope.* 1999; 109:791-794.

Zweig JL, Carrau RL, Celin SE, et al. Endoscopic repair of cerebrospinal fluid leaks to the sinonasal tract: predictors of success. *Otolaryngol Head Neck Surg.* 2000;123:195-201.

Full references can be found on Expert Consult @ www.expertconsult.com

CHAPTER 31

Thorascopic Spine Surgery

Rudolf Beisse

The applications of endoscopic spine surgery have been expanded since the first publications spanning nearly two decades.[1-6] Operating techniques have been standardized and unified and today are safe procedures with low complication rates that are comparable to those of open procedures, presuming the existence of adequate training and manual skills of the surgeon.[7] Thus, endoscopic operations on the spinal column no longer represent exceptional interventions but have become standard procedures in spine surgery. Thoracoscopic techniques can be used to approach the anterior column of the spine in the area between the third thoracic vertebra and the third lumbar vertebra because endoscopic splitting of the diaphragm also allows the exposure of the upper sections of the lumbar spine. The application potential includes anterior release procedures, with incision and resection of ligaments and intervertebral disks; removal of fragmented disks or sections of vertebrae, including anterior decompression of the spinal canal; replacement of vertebral bodies with biologic or alloplastic materials; and ventral stabilization procedures with implants designed for use in endoscopic spine surgery. In addition, percutaneous endoscopic techniques are used for minimally invasive treatment of degenerative disk disease of the thoracic and lumbar spine.

PRINCIPLES

The principle of thoracoscopic spine surgery includes the use of a rigid scope and long instruments that are inserted through small incisions between intercostal spaces. The thoracic cavity is used as a preformed operative corridor after the lung has been collapsed on one side by a double-lumen intubation. The image of the operation site is transmitted onto video screens. Because a two-dimensional image is provided by the system, new skills are required to assess the depth and angle of the instruments used.

INDICATIONS

Overall, the range of indications for the technique described here can be defined as follows:

- Anterior reconstruction of unstable fractures of the thoracic spine and thoracolumbar junction[8]
- Posttraumatic, degenerative, and tumor-related narrowing of the spinal canal[9]
- Disk-ligament instability
- Posttraumatic deformity of healed fractures with or without instability[10]
- Revision surgery (i.e., implant removal, infection, implant failure and loosening)[11]
- Preparation and release of the anterior column in tumor and metastasis
- Sympathectomy for hyperhidrosis[12]
- Protruded disk removal in degenerative disk disease of the thoracic spine[6]

TECHNICAL REQUIREMENTS

Trocars

Reusable, flexible, threaded trocars that are black with a diameter of 11 mm are used to reduce light reflections and the pressure on the intercostal nerves and vascular bundle. Air insufflation is not required, and thus valves within the trocars are not necessary.

Image Transmission

The key to any endoscopic technique is image recording and transmission. "You will do what you can see," and therefore true high-definition video technique has also revolutionized the endoscopic technique, which now provides an endoscopic view comparable to images that the microscope is able to provide. A high-intensity xenon light source is required to illuminate the thoracic cavity. A rigid, long, 30-degree scope enables positioning of the camera far away from the working portal, thus facilitating undisturbed working and variable adjustment of the angle of vision. The intraoperative view is transmitted onto two or three flat screens (Fig. 31-1).

Instruments

Complete sets of instruments for soft tissue and bone preparation are manufactured by contemporary instrument manufacturers (Fig. 31-2). Instruments should have a nonreflective surface and a depth scale on both sides and be ergonomically designed with big handles for safe control and handling. The technique by which they are used is called the three-point anchoring technique, which means that every sharp and potentially dangerous instrument is guided by both hands; one hand is based on the chest wall, always controlling and sometimes neutralizing unexpected forces and movements of the instrument (see Video 31-9).

 Video 31-9 can be found on Expert Consult @ www.expertconsult.com

Implants

Several implants for anterior instrumentation that can be used for endoscopic, mini-open, or open spine surgery are now available. Most of them are based on the principle of a cannulated screw and plate system, first allowing the implantation of K wires under fluoroscopic control to be used as landmarks, followed by the insertion of screws. Biomechanically tested four-point fixation implants provide adequate angular stability, which is necessary for single anterior instrumentation (Fig. 31-3).[13]

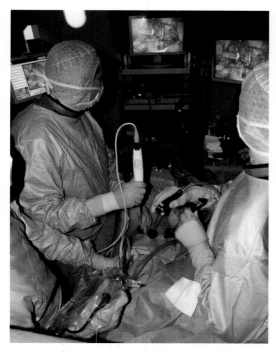

FIGURE 31-1 Thoracoscopic surgery at the spine: all portals, the 30-degree scope, and the instruments are inserted. The surgical team is looking at three high-definition flat screen monitors.

For vertebral body replacement, bone graft (autograft or allograft) or mechanical devices can be used and filled or surrounded with the autologous bone harvested from the corpectomy site. A wide variety of expandable titanium cages is currently available.[14]

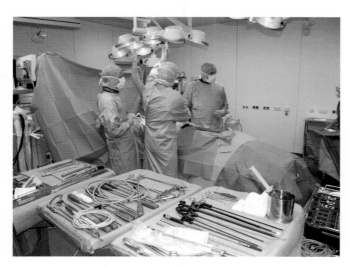

FIGURE 31-2 A whole set of long instruments for endoscopic soft tissue preparation and bone resection and devices for thoracoscopic implantation of a stabilizing implant are prepared to be used for the thoracoscopic procedure.

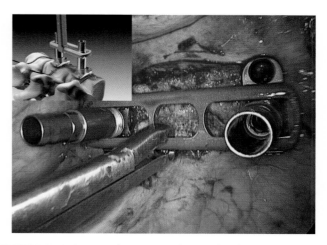

FIGURE 31-3 Screw and constraint plate implant for endoscopic and open instrumentation at the anterior column of the thoracic and lumbar spine (MACS TL, Aesculap, Tuttlingen, Germany).

PREOPERATIVE REQUIREMENTS

Education of the Patient

The patient should be informed about the following approach-specific risks and hazards:

- Injury to the spinal cord, spinal nerves, and sympathetic trunk (deafferentation syndrome), with neurological deficits
- Injury to the greater vessels, thoracic duct, and segmental vessels
- Possibility of conversion to a conventional thoracotomy
- Injury to spleen, diaphragm, and kidney
- Port and diaphragmatic hernia

Anesthesia

A pulmonary function test and breathing therapy are commonly performed preoperatively to assess the patient's vital parameters. Routine bowel preparation is commonly used to decrease intra-abdominal pressure and tension on the diaphragm. The thoracoscopic operation is performed under general anesthesia. Double-lumen tube intubation and single-lung ventilation are applied as routine. Proper placement of the endotracheal tube is confirmed by bronchoscopy. A Foley catheter, central venous line, and arterial line for continuous blood pressure assessment are placed. For postoperative pain relief, a peridural analgesic is inserted in the thoracic region.

Positioning of the Patient

All endoscopic operations at the anterior column of the thoracic spine and the thoracolumbar junction are performed with the patient lying on his or her side (Video 31-1). The approach side is determined by the preoperative computed tomographic (CT) scans and depends on the position of the major vessels shown in the scans and the surgery that is planned. Because of the great variability of the vascular anatomy, firm rules are no longer set for selection of the approach side by the height of the lesion.

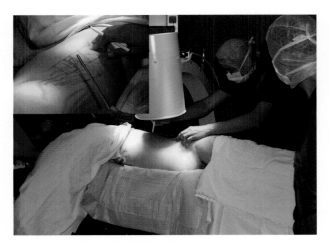

FIGURE 31-4 With the patient placed in a true lateral position, the affected section of the spine is accurately projected to the lateral thoracic and abdominal wall and marked with use of a C-arm amplifier.

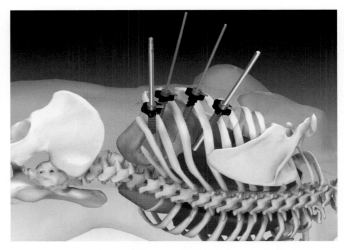

FIGURE 31-5 Placement of the trocars and instruments for an endoscopic intervention at the thoracolumbar spine.

The patient is stabilized in the side-lying position with four supports and a special U-shaped cushion for the legs. It is possible to use a vacuum mattress, but its construction height can make the manipulation of instruments under C-arm control and conversion to the open procedure more difficult.

Marking the Portals

As a routine, four portals are used: scope portal, working portal, suction-irrigation portal, and retractor portal (Video 31-2). Their location and, in particular, the position of the working portal are crucial for the endoscopic operation to proceed in the optimal fashion. For this reason, the lesion is first displayed in the lateral projection (with reference to the patient's body) under precise adjustment of the image intensifier, and a marker is used to draw the injured spinal section onto the lateral thoracic wall (Fig. 31-4). The working portal is drawn in directly above the lesion. The trocar for the endoscope is marked either caudal or cranial to the working portal, depending on the height of the lesion, and following the axis of the spine. The distance from the working portal is approximately two intercostal spaces. The entry points for suction and irrigation and for the retractor are then located ventral from these portals.

After skin disinfection and sterile draping, single-lung ventilation is begun in consultation with the anesthetist. As the first approach, the portal in the farthest cranial position is always selected because the risk of injury to the liver, spleen, and diaphragm is comparatively minor in this position. The approach is made by the mini-thoracotomy technique, providing the possibility of examining the immediate surroundings of the insertion site with the fingers before the trocar is introduced (Video 31-3). The rigid 30-degree endoscope is then carefully inserted, and the thoracic cavity is first inspected to rule out the existence of adhesions or parenchymal lesions. The other three trocars and then the instruments are subsequently introduced under endoscopic control.

OPERATIVE TECHNIQUES

Approach to the Thoracolumbar Junction

This operation is also performed using single-lung ventilation (Video 31-4).[8,11,15,16] Here, too, the approach side is decided by the location of the major vessels, which can be identified from the preoperative computed tomographic scan. In most cases, the best approach to the thoracolumbar junction is from the left. Placement of the trocars and instruments is illustrated in Figure 31-5.

As a first step, the affected section of the spine is drawn onto the skin of the lateral abdominal and thoracic wall under image intensifier control. Careful attention is paid to correct projection of the vertebrae, whose end plates and anterior and posterior margins should be displayed in the central beam, in sharp focus with no double contour. This marking is taken as the sole reference for subsequent placement of the portals.

The working portal is situated directly above the lesion; the portal for the endoscope is located over the spine two or three intercostal spaces away from the working portal in a cranial direction. The portals for the retractor and the suction-irrigation instrument are situated ventrally from this point.

The dome-like diaphragm is firmly connected at its margins with the sternum, ribs, and spine and arches up into the thoracic cavity. Topographically speaking, the attachment sites of the diaphragm to the spine are at the level of the first lumbar vertebra, whereas the lowest point of the thoracic cavity projects with the phrenicocostal sinus at the level of the baseplate of the second lumbar vertebra (Fig. 31-6). This makes it possible to place a trocar intrathoracically in the phrenicocostal sinus, which, after incision of the diaphragm attachment to the spine, provides access to the retroperitoneal section of the thoracolumbar junction down to the baseplate of the second lumbar vertebra. This requires a 4- to 5-cm–long incision following the attachment of the diaphragm; access to the L1-2 intervertebral disk can be obtained with a shorter incision of 2 to 3 cm (Fig. 31-7).[15-17]

To prevent a postoperative diaphragmatic hernia, an incision that runs parallel to the diaphragmatic attachment is preferred. Because of the dome-like architecture of the diaphragm, an increase in intra-abdominal pressure from a semicircular incision parallel to the attachment causes the resected margins to come together and to adhere spontaneously, whereas a radial incision in direct proximity to the orifices of the aorta and the esophagus weakens the diaphragm fixation and causes the resected margins to gape. In addition, it is recommended that every incision in the attachment longer than 2 cm be sutured endoscopically to prevent hernia formation.

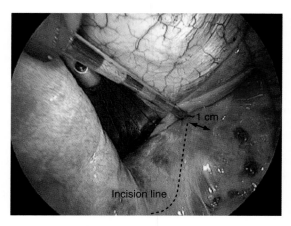

FIGURE 31-6 Typical operation site at the thoracolumbar section of the spine. The *interrupted line* runs parallel to the attachment of the diaphragm and indicates the line of incision for access to the subdiaphragmatic section of the thoracolumbar junction, L1, and L2.

Endoscopic Treatment of Spinal Trauma (Anterior Reconstruction)

Landmarks

As a first step, landmarks are set under image intensifier control to serve as orientation points for the surgeon and camera operator during the subsequent course of the operation (Video 31-5). For this, the K wires associated with the implant are used; these are then replaced by cannulated screws with integrated clamping elements. If no implant is used, marker points can be set onto the parietal pleura under fluoroscopic control by use of the cautery or ultrasonic knife. Thus, these K wires also define the later position of the screws, and they are placed near the end plates between the posterior and central thirds of the vertebra. To achieve this in the thoracolumbar junction region, the psoas muscle must be mobilized ventrad to dorsad, thus avoiding irritation of the fibers of the lumbar plexus. Through positioning of the K wires near the end plates, injury to the segment vessels is avoided, and the screws are anchored in a region of higher bone density.

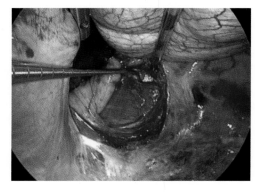

FIGURE 31-7 Partial detachment of the diaphragm reveals the retroperitoneal fat, the anterior border of the psoas muscle, and the spine. A fan-shaped retractor is inserted into the diaphragm gap.

Preparation of the Segment Vessels

Following the connecting line between the K wires, the pleura is opened, and the segment vessels are exposed with a Cobb raspatory. These vessels are mobilized subperiosteally from both sides, ligated twice with titanium clips ventrally and dorsally, and raised slightly with a nerve hook. The vessels are dissected with the endoscopic hook scissors. The lateral aspects of the vertebral body and the disks are exposed with the raspatory (Video 31-6).

Cannulated Screw Insertion

The K wires are now overdrilled with a cannulated broach, and the lateral cortex of the vertebral body is opened (Video 31-7). The working trocar is exchanged for a speculum through a switching stick, and the clamping element is tightened with a screw. The length of the screw has been previously measured against the preoperative computed tomographic scan and subsequently defines whether a monocortical or bicortical screw fixation is to be attempted. The direction of the screw can be altered after removal of the K wire and checked in both planes under C-arm monitoring. The connecting line between the screws and the anterior boundary of the clamping elements now defines an area of safety within which the partial removal of the vertebral body and the disks is performed. The ventral and dorsal extent of the partial corpectomy thus defined also then corresponds to the dimensions of the planned vertebral body replacement, which has a transverse diameter between 16 mm (thoracic) and 20 mm (lumbar).

The intervertebral disks are incised laterally with a knife, and the disk space is opened with a slightly offset osteotome (Video 31-8). The posterior osteotomy is then performed with a straight osteotome from disk space to disk space on the connecting line between the screws. The scale on the osteotome shows the corresponding depth, which in the anterior direction should be about two thirds of the diameter of the vertebra. The line of the anterior osteotomy runs along the anterior boundary of the clamping elements; to be sure of avoiding unintentional perforation of the anterior vertebral wall (and adjacent vessels), an osteotome that is slightly angled to the rear is used. The central section of the vertebral body is now removed with a rongeur, and the removed cancellous bone is preserved for later implantation adjacent to the vertebral body replacement (Video 31-9). Using a curet and rongeurs, the intervertebral disks are then resected and the end plates are freshened up. When titanium cages are implanted, any weakening of the load-bearing end plates must be avoided. In monosegmental fusion with a tricortical pelvic crest graft, the subchondral bone lamella on the cranial end plate is removed to assist healing of the bone graft.

Insertion of the Bone Graft

In monosegmental reconstructions and fusion, a tricortical bone graft taken from the iliac crest is used. After the corpectomy defect has been measured, the iliac crest is prepared and exposed. Using an oscillating saw and chisel, the bone graft is harvested and firmly connected to a graft holder. The graft is inserted in a centered position into the defect, which has to be fluoroscopically checked in both planes (Video 31-10).

For vertebral body replacement in a bisegmental reconstruction, I mostly use the hydraulically working Hydrolift (Aesculap, Center Valley, PA) with continuously variable distraction and adaptation of the end plates. Before the vertebra replacement is implanted, the extent and clean preparation of the implant site in the anterior sagittal direction and in its depth should be verified by palpation with a probe hook under image intensifier control.

Two Langenbeck hooks are inserted into the incision for the working portals, and the incision is widened slightly. The vertebral body replacement is then gradually introduced through the chest wall into the thoracic cavity and positioned over the defect in the vertebral body with a holder. Once again, it is determined that no soft tissue, in particular the ligated segment vessels, has slipped between the corpectomy defect and the vertebral body replacement. The vertebral body replacement device is then implanted into the planned central position in the vertebral body and distracted. The implant is surrounded with the cancellous bone harvested from the partial corpectomy. An antibiotic medium (e.g., gentamicin-collagen) can be added to the spongiosa. After the corpectomy defect zone has been filled with spongiosa, it is covered with a fibrin fleece.

Ventral Instrumentation with a Constraint Plate Implant

Because the screws and so-called clamping elements belonging to the implant were placed into position as a first step before the beginning of the partial corpectomy, now the plate just has to be fastened and the ventral screws of the four-point fixation inserted (Video 31-11). The distance between the screws is defined with a special measuring instrument to select a plate of the correct length. This is introduced lengthwise into the thoracic cavity through the incision for the working portal, laid onto the clamping elements with a holding forceps, and there definitively fixed with nuts with a starting torque of 15 Nm. The plate can be brought into direct bone contact with the lateral vertebral body wall by tightening the bone screws. The ventral screws are inserted after temporary fixation of a targeting device and opening of the cortex. Because of the heart shape of the vertebral body, the ventral screws are usually 5 mm shorter than the dorsal screws. The fixation of the angle-stable implant ends with the insertion of a locking screw that locks the polyaxial mechanism of the dorsal screws (Fig. 31-8).

Final Stages of the Endoscopic Operation

In every case, radiographs are taken in both planes with the C-arm to check the position of the implant before the operation is concluded (Video 31-12). For operations on the thoracolumbar junction that include incision of the diaphragmatic attachment, an incision longer than 2 cm should be closed with endoscopic suturing. Two or three adapting sutures are sufficient, depending on the extent of the incision. The suture does not need to be watertight.

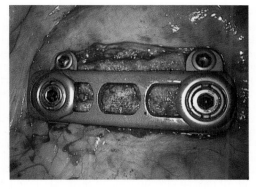

FIGURE 31-8 Thoracoscopic anterior instrumentation with a four-point stabilization constraint plate and screw system.

The entire thoracic cavity is again inspected endoscopically, and the site is irrigated and cleaned of blood residue.

A 20 Charrière thoracic drainage tube is inserted through the suction-irrigation portal. The instruments are removed under endoscopic monitoring. After consultation with the anesthetist, the lung is reinflated and ventilated. The complete reinflation of the lung is checked endoscopically before the endoscope is removed.

In the four incisions for the portals, adapting sutures are applied to the musculature, and the skin is closed by suturing. The thoracic drainage is connected to a water seal chamber, and a suction of 15 cm H_2O is applied. The patient is usually extubated while still on the operating table.

SPECIAL INDICATIONS

Removal of Posterior Wall Fragments: Endoscopic Anterior Decompression[9]

Depending on the level of stenosis, compression of the spinal canal can lead to a neurological deficit. The spectrum of injuries to the spinal canal, medullary cone, and cauda equina ranges from simple contusion to complete tearing of the neural structures. As long as the structures have not been severed, recovery of function and sensory deficits may be possible in principle. Thus, the indications for anterior decompression are present when significant narrowing and a neurological deficit remain after primary dorsal reduction and stabilization.

Operative Technique

Completion of the partial corpectomy and adjacent diskectomies is recommended before the canal decompression. The next step is to identify the pedicle of the fractured vertebral body. In traumatic burst fracture, the pedicles are nearly always preserved, and the retropulsed fragment usually is located medial to the pedicle. Thus, the retropulsed fragment is trapped between the two pedicles and is difficult to remove or reduce.

Therefore, resection of the ipsilateral pedicle with a punch is recommended before removal of the retropulsed fragment is attempted. For this reason, resection of the ipsilateral pedicle has a dual importance: it exposes the spinal canal, and it frees the retropulsed fragment from the pincer grip of the pedicles. A Cobb elevator is used to expose the ipsilateral pedicle subperiosteally and to push away the nerve root dorsally without having separated the root from the surrounding soft tissue. The inferior margin of the pedicle is identified with a nerve hook, and the pedicle is transected with a punch, which can be facilitated by thinning the pedicle with a high-speed bur beforehand. Removal of the dorsocranial section of the vertebral body together with the base of the pedicle exposes the posterior margin fragment and brings the dura into view. The compressing fragment can now be lifted off the dura under direct view, mobilized in the direction of the partial corpectomy, and resected. A nerve hook is used under image intensifier control to document the completeness of the posterior margin fragment resection in both planes. In cases with posterior wall resection, an expandable titanium cage is used as a vertebral body replacement because of its greater primary stability and the smaller risk for dislocation. The operation concludes with the ventral instrumentation and suturing of the diaphragm attachment.

Case Report

A 43-year-old man was referred to our hospital demonstrating severe back pain at the thoracolumbar junction, weakness of the lower extremities below T12, and moderate bowel and bladder

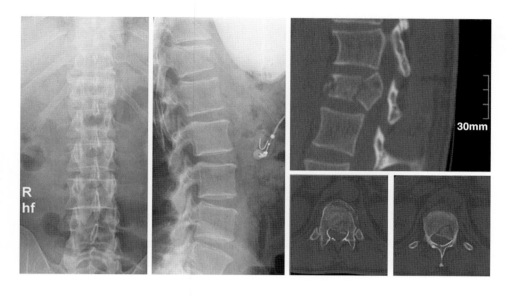

FIGURE 31-9 L1 complete burst fracture type A 3.3 with severe compromise of the spinal canal causing neurological deficit Frankel C.

dysfunction. After radiologic diagnostics and neurological examination, the patient was brought to the operating room for dorsal reduction and stabilization by internal fixator followed by thoracoscopic anterior decompression and reconstruction (Figs. 31-9 to 31-11).

Removal of Protruded Herniated Disk: Endoscopic Treatment of Degenerative Disk Disease

Only 0.15% to 1% of all operative procedures due to degenerative disk disease are done to treat thoracic disk protrusion.[18-20] As a specialty of the thoracic region, there is a "calcified disk" and an "intradural disk herniation" (Fig. 31-12). These removal procedures are technically demanding. Because of a smaller diameter of the thoracic spinal canal in conjunction with a spinal cord of bigger volume at these levels, there is little space to accommodate disk herniation. In consequence, small disk protrusions might cause significant symptoms. Depending on the localization and expansion of herniation—medial, mediolateral, intraforaminal, or extraforaminal—typical symptoms of thoracic disk herniation can be described.

Operative Treatment Options

The following procedures[21] are available, fitting the needed level and herniation site:

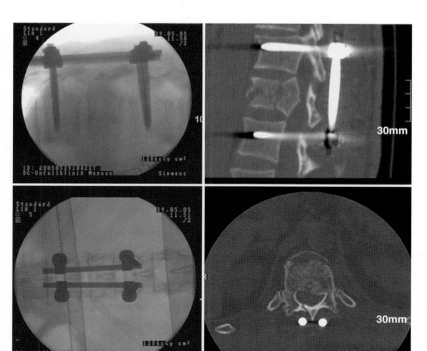

FIGURE 31-10 Immediate dorsal reduction and stabilization by internal fixator to achieve indirect decompression by ligamentotaxis.

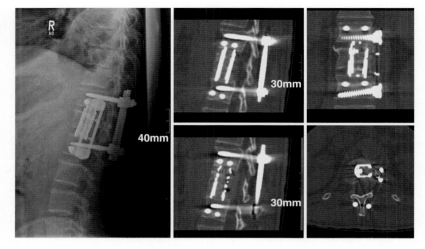

FIGURE 31-11 Thoracoscopic reconstruction of the anterior column with anterior decompression (i.e., posterior wall resection, vertebral body replacement, and anterior instrumentation).

- Transthoracic approach, open or endoscopic (T4-11, central disk herniation, with or without calcification)
- Lateral extracavitary approach (T6-12, centrolateral disk herniation)[22]
- Transfacet approach, pedicle preserving (all levels, centrolateral disk herniation)[21]
- Transpedicular approach (all levels, centrolateral disk herniation)[23]

Because of the high morbidity of the open transthoracic approach, indications were few. The advent of a tissue-preserving thoracoscopic approach[6,12,24] led to greater numbers of indications, centrolateral and lateral disk herniations remaining to be approached posterolaterally. The thoracoscopic approach and operative technique are described here (Video 31-13).

Special Anatomic Considerations

The difference between the thoracic spine on the one hand and the cervical and lumbar spine on the other is the presence of rib-attached vertebrae. Excluding the first thoracic vertebra, every rib articulates with the costovertebral joint through a cranial and a caudal part onto the neighboring vertebral bodies. Because of that anatomic situation, the rib head covers the dorsal disk space and the ipsilateral pedicle. Therefore, rib head removal is a key procedure for access to the disk space. The nerve root

and the outgoing segmental vessels form a bundle next to the rib head caudally, riding in a bony groove along the caudal rib ventrally. With the spinal canal opened, the dorsal borders of most vertebrae are concavely shaped; this is confirmed preoperatively on axial computed tomographic views. Therefore, the fluoroscopic visible back wall is created by summation effect; the anatomic concave back wall is ventral to that line.

Operating Room Setup

Positioning the Patient

The side for the approach has to be chosen primarily by the localization of the disk herniation and the adjacent great vessels. In cases of centromedial and right lateral herniation, the approach from the right side is preferred (Fig. 31-13).

Confirmation of the Operative Site

Verification of the level of disease can be demanding before the main procedure is started. Several methods are recommended to ensure that the right intervertebral disk space is addressed. Dickman and Rosenthal[12] recommend a preoperative radiograph of the chest to localize the level. Large osteophytes seen on computed tomographic scans or plain radiographs can be used as

FIGURE 31-12 Calcified herniated disk at the level of T9-10 with severe narrowing of the spinal canal and cord in a 54-year-old woman, causing myelopathy and belt-like back pain.

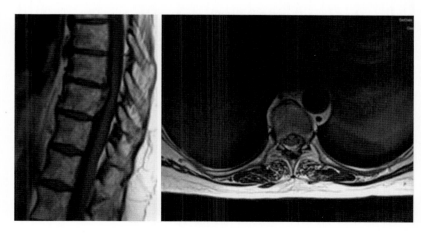

TABLE 34-1 Types of Communicating Hydrocephalus

DEFECTS OF FLOW IN THE SUBARACHNOID SPACE

Leptomeningeal inflammation

Infections

Hemorrhage

Meningitis

Carcinomatosis

Foreign matter

Tonsillar elongation/prolapse or basilar impression

Masses (neoplastic and non-neoplastic)

DEFECTS OF ABSORPTION OF CSF AT THE ARACHNOID GRANULATIONS

Congenital deficiency, i.e., absence of arachnoid granulations

Raised cerebral venous sinus pressure

ABNORMALITIES IN CSF

Excessive production of CSF or abnormally high CSF volumes

Raised intraventricular CSF pulse pressure, e.g., in the presence of a choroid plexus papilloma

Increased CSF viscosity secondary to high protein content, e.g., in the presence of spinal neurofibromas

IDIOPATHIC

CSF, cerebrospinal fluid.
From Pickard JD. Adult communicating hydrocephalus. *Br J Hosp Med.* 1982;27:35.

Isolated Fourth Ventricle Syndrome

The term "entrapped fourth ventricle" has also been used to describe the situation in which the fourth ventricle no longer communicates with the third ventricle, as well as the basal cisterns. Patients with prolonged infection or multiple shunt operations are particularly at risk for this syndrome. It is thought that secondary aqueduct stenosis from adhesions, obstruction of the foramina of Luschka or Magendie, or infective debris pooling in the basal cisterns may be responsible for this condition. Patients may have the typical symptoms and signs of hydrocephalus or more atypical symptoms such as lower cranial nerve dysfunction. Occasionally, an entrapped fourth ventricle is an incidental finding on imaging.

Slit Ventricle Syndrome

The lateral ventricles may collapse in some patients secondary to overshunting or remain at a fixed size because of subependymal gliosis. This may lead to intermittent or complete shunt malfunction. Patients may experience raised ICP without ventricular enlargement, and therefore imaging findings may be falsely reassuring in such cases (unresponsive ventricles). Symptomatic patients may respond to a change in valve setting if a programmable valve is in situ or to revision surgery (change of valve or incorporation of an antisiphon device to prevent overdrainage). Patients with progressive neurological deterioration secondary to raised ICP may require subtemporal decompression. When the ventricles are slit intermittently, endoscopic third ventriculostomy may be possible during periods of relative ventricular dilation. Please see Chapter 186 for a discussion of these issues in children, including shunt removal.

PATHOPHYSIOLOGY (see also Chapter 33)

Formation, Circulation, and Reabsorption

The total volume of CSF in the cranial-spinal axis is approximately 150 mL, distributed equally between the two compartments. However, net CSF production is about 0.35 mL/min (500 mL/day), which results in a CSF turnover rate of approximately three to four times per day. Intracranially, CSF is produced mainly by the choroid plexus of the ventricles (70% to 80%).[4] The remaining amount is produced by the ependymal lining of the ventricles, by the brain's capillary bed, and by metabolic water production. The proportion of CSF produced in the ventricular system is unequal; the vast majority of CSF produced by the choroid plexus is from the lateral ventricles, although small amounts are produced in the third and fourth ventricles. CSF is formed by filtration of plasma through fenestrated capillaries and active transport of water and solutes through the epithelial cells of the choroid plexus at the blood-CSF barrier.

CSF circulates through the ventricular system and exits through the foramina of Luschka and Magendie into the cerebellomedullary cistern and onward to the spinal cavity and the subarachnoid spaces of the cerebral convexities. Circulation of CSF is thought to be driven by hydrostatic pressure generated by cerebral arterial pulsation and changes in venous pressure secondary to respiration, change of posture, and other mechanisms.[5,6] CSF is resorbed by arachnoid villi that protrude from the subarachnoid space into the lumen of the dural sinuses. Solutes pass via one-way bulk flow into the venous circulation. The exact mechanism of this process has not been fully elucidated but may involve differential pressure between CSF and the venous system and one-way valves formed by overlapping endothelial cells lining the arachnoid villi.[5] Figure 34-1 illustrates the concepts just discussed.

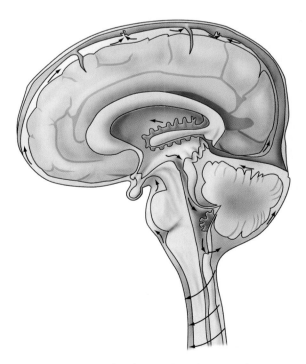

FIGURE 34-1 Circulation of cerebrospinal fluid.

Cerebrospinal Fluid Obstruction and Sequelae

Experimental models of acute ventricular obstruction have provided an understanding of the pathophysiologic processes occurring after disruption of the CSF circulation. Initial rapid ventricular dilation is followed by effacement of the cerebral sulci, fissures, and basal cisterns. Transependymal passage of CSF occurs through either an intact or disrupted ependymal lining and results in periventricular edema. Absorption of CSF occurs in the edematous white matter via alternative pathways, such as direct absorption into blood via the blood vessels.[7] Destruction of tracts secondary to edema and subsequent gliosis of damaged tissue are believed to occur within the periventricular white matter, with relative sparing of gray matter.[8] The resulting white matter damage and reduction in cerebral blood volume may progress to cerebral atrophy. This concept may explain the persistence of neurological deficits in some patients despite successful reduction of ventricular volume after shunt surgery. As a result of some or all of these processes, pathologic compensation for raised ICP may be reached. In a minority of cases, CSF production is reduced because of atrophy of the choroid plexus.[7]

Progressive Ventriculomegaly in the Context of Normal Pressure and the Concept of Combined Dementia

The confounding situation of progressive ventricular dilation in patients with NPH has led to many theories regarding the underlying pathophysiologic processes occurring in this condition. Hakim and Adams originally proposed that as ventricular enlargement progresses, the biomechanical forces required to maintain the ventricles in a dilated state are smaller.[9] Distortion of tissue, including white matter tracts and blood vessels, may lead to damage and ischemia. Loss of elasticity within the brain parenchyma may result in a pressure gradient between the ventricles and periventricular tissue. The resulting excess fluid in the interstitial space may lead to failure of drainage of toxic metabolites. There is also evidence of disruption of cerebral blood flow or distortion of blood vessels, which is believed to lead to watershed ischemia and deep lacunar infarcts. The pattern of disruption of cerebral blood flow in white matter has been demonstrated to take the form of a U-shaped relationship with distance from the ventricles, with the maximal reduction occurring adjacent to the ventricles and progressive normalization toward the subcortical white matter.[10]

NPH is also thought to be a CSF circulation disorder resulting from an imbalance between production and absorption. Abnormalities in the aging brain may make it uniquely susceptible to intermittent spikes of B waves and result in progressive ventriculomegaly. It has been demonstrated that resistance to CSF outflow increases in a nonlinear fashion with advancing age despite a decrease in the rate of CSF production, which also occurs with increasing age.[11] Failure of efficient CSF turnover may also result in an accumulation of potentially toxic metabolic products, such as β-amyloid peptides (Aβ) and tau protein. Such aggregates are thought to be neurotoxic and contribute to small-vessel damage and subsequent leakage of additional toxic metabolites into the interstitial space.[12] Moreover, it has been proposed that the two changes noted in aging, reduced CSF production and increased resistance to CSF outflow, may be implicated in a common pathway in the pathophysiology of Alzheimer's disease and NPH. A predominance of reduced CSF production and turnover may be manifested as Alzheimer's disease, and conversely, NPH may result from a predominant increase in CSF outflow resistance. A spectrum of disease may exist, including a subset of patients who either have both conditions or have risks for the development of both even if one process is predominant.[13]

TABLE 34-2 Common Initial Features of Acute versus Chronic Hydrocephalus

ACUTE—RAISED INTRACRANIAL PRESSURE

Headaches
Nausea and vomiting
Deterioration in gait or balance
Papilledema
Upgaze palsy—setting sun sign
Parinaud's syndrome—pressure on the suprapineal recess
Abducens palsy—long intracranial course

CHRONIC

Headaches
Deterioration in gait or balance
Urinary incontinence
Cognitive and attention deficits (subcortical dementia)
Personality changes (e.g., aggression, apathy)
Empty sella
Impingement or atrophy of the corpus callosum

INITIAL FEATURES OF HYDROCEPHALUS

Both communicating and obstructive hydrocephalus may give rise to the same symptoms and signs (i.e., those of hydrocephalus or raised ICP). Alternatively, both types may be associated with normal CSF pressure or spontaneously arrest. The initial features specific to NPH are discussed in the following section. Table 34-2 lists the common symptoms and signs in patients with acute versus chronic hydrocephalus.

NORMAL-PRESSURE HYDROCEPHALUS

Clinical Findings and Differential Diagnoses

The concept of a "symptomatic occult hydrocephalus with 'normal' CSF pressure" was described by Hakim and Adams in 1965 in their landmark paper of observations based on three cases, two secondary and one idiopathic.[9] Current guidelines deal primarily with idiopathic as opposed to secondary NPH, which occurs after trauma (such as the two patients in 1965), subarachnoid hemorrhage, intracranial surgery, or meningitis. The manifestations of secondary NPH may be delayed, sometimes many years after the incident in question. Most cases seen by clinicians are of the idiopathic variety. Despite advances in the diagnosis and management of this condition, the exact pathogenesis of NPH remains uncertain. The classic finding in patients with NPH is a clinical triad of symptoms—gait disturbance, dementia, and urinary incontinence. Patients may or may not have the complete triad of symptoms. In addition, many other symptoms have been reported, such as lethargy, apathy, impaired wakefulness, and visuospatial disturbances.

Gait Disturbance

Gait disturbance is the most common initial symptom and occurs in almost 90% of patients.[7] Ojemann and colleagues in 1969 noted that gait disturbance could be an initial manifestation of NPH,[14] thereby changing the emphasis from earlier descriptions of cognitive disturbance being the primary initial symptom. Fisher subsequently presented a series of 16 patients with shunt-responsive hydrocephalus in which gait disturbance was the initial manifestation in 12 of them.[15] In that series, dementia preceded gait disturbance in 1 patient and occurred at the same time in 3 patients. However, in 11 cases of shunt failure, dementia came first in 9 patients and gait disturbance was relatively less severe or was absent.

Common initial symptoms include unsteadiness, recurrent falls, shuffling, and reduced walking speed. More advanced symptoms include difficulty initiating gait and imbalance on turning. Gait in patients with NPH is described as being "magnetic" in nature, characterized by a broad base and slow, small steps with reduced height clearance as though the feet are "stuck to the floor." Patients may have difficulty rising from a chair or complain of their legs "giving way."[16] Patients may have disturbances in stance with a tendency to lean forward and imbalance exacerbated by eye closure.[14,17]

The gait disturbance may be difficult to distinguish from other types of frontotemporal pathology. The gait abnormality is often confused with Parkinson's disease because patients with NPH may appear to have features of lower limb parkinsonism such as rigidity, shortened stride length, and difficulties in balance and turning. This is particularly applicable in patients in whom other hallmarks of Parkinson's disease are not present, such as tremor, lead pipe rigidity, and a mask-like facies. However, unlike patients with Parkinson's disease, who are able to increase their stride length and walking cadence with the aid of external cueing such as counting, patients with NPH have a gait apraxia that does not respond to such aids. In addition, patients with NPH tend to mobilize with a relatively preserved arm swing.

Increased tone and brisk tendon reflexes in the legs are unusual in patients with shunt-responsive NPH, and there is absence of weakness or dysdiadochokinesis. The presence of upper motor neuron signs or lower limb weakness may be indicative of cervical myelopathy and lumbar canal stenosis, respectively. Other structural lesions of the brain and spine should be considered, such as tumors or cerebrovascular ischemic damage. Poor balance may reflect an underlying sensory neuropathy, and in such instances, diabetic neuropathy and autonomic dysfunction should be considered. However, these conditions are common in the age group of patients seen with NPH. The finding of comorbid pathologies might be significant but may not exclude patients from having a favorable outcome from shunt surgery if NPH accounts for a major proportion of the initial symptomatology.

The anatomic basis for gait disturbance in patients with NPH remains controversial. In 1947, Yakovlev proposed a theory that paraplegia in patients with hydrocephalus is caused by compression of the internal capsule fibers by the distended third ventricle. However, the general lack of upper motor neuron signs and upper limb involvement in NPH would suggest that such a theory may not account for the characteristic gait apraxia seen in this condition. Indeed, a study using motor evoked potentials and central motor conduction time in both the upper and lower limbs in patients with NPH did not demonstrate any evidence of major pyramidal tract dysfunction or subclinical upper limb involvement in patients who responded to shunt surgery. Prolonged central motor conduction time was seen in the lower limbs of patients who did not improve after surgery.[17] However, such methods may be insufficiently subtle to detect small lesions or reversible white matter damage occurring as a result of tissue distortion from hydrocephalus. Pyramidal tract damage may represent progression of these lesions to an end-stage phase of NPH that cannot be reversed by surgery.

Urinary Incontinence

Urinary incontinence may be a separate symptom or may be a consequence of gait disturbance or cognitive impairment. Some patients have urinary frequency rather than true incontinence. This symptom is thought to be due to involvement of the sacral fibers of the corticospinal tract.[18] Because urgency of micturition

and incontinence are both common problems in older age, the clinical finding may be that of a change or worsening of urinary symptoms rather than a new problem.

Cognitive Impairment

NPH is estimated to account for less than 5% of all cases of dementia. It is essential that patients undergo neuropsychological testing to distinguish the pattern of dementia in NPH from other conditions such as age-related cognitive decline as a result of neurodegenerative processes, including Alzheimer's disease. The pattern of NPH appears to be a subcortical frontal dysexecutive syndrome.[19,20] Cognitive deficits in patients with NPH typically include memory loss, reduced attention, difficulty planning, slowness in thought, and apathy. There may be speech disturbance because of dysexecutive or motivational problems.[16] This pattern differs from the cortical deficits of aphasia, apraxia, and agnosia seen in patients with Alzheimer's disease.[21]

The most difficult differential diagnosis to consider in the context of NPH is Binswanger's disease, a form of subcortical vascular encephalopathy. Patients with this condition exhibit a predominantly frontal cognitive deterioration and gait disturbance (ataxia or motor dysfunction, or both), although focal neurological signs may be present. The pathologic changes occurring in patients with Binswanger's disease are believed to be the result of small-vessel ischemia and subsequent extensive white matter damage. Neuropsychological testing demonstrates features consistent with a frontal subcortical type of dementia, which is similar to the pattern noted in NPH. Similar magnetic resonance imaging (MRI) features may be seen, including ventriculomegaly and the coexistence of MRI white matter changes, such as deep white matter hyperintensities and subcortical lacunar infarctions. Table 34-3 summarizes the list of differential diagnoses for the clinical triad in NPH, aside from other hydrocephalus disorders.

Neuroradiologic Features

Guidelines published by the Idiopathic NPH Study Group[16] include a set of imaging criteria required to justify the diagnosis of idiopathic NPH. Imaging in the form of computed tomography (CT) or MRI is required to establish the diagnosis of NPH. Important differential diagnoses to rule out include obstruction of CSF pathways as a result of tumor or similar pathology, significant cerebral atrophy, and evidence of cerebrovascular ischemia. Ventricular enlargement not entirely attributable to cerebral atrophy or congenital enlargement (Evans' index >0.3 or comparable measure) should be present. Evans' index is defined as the maximal width of the anterior ventricular horns divided by the maximal width of the calvaria at the level of the foramen of Monroe. An alternative measurement is the bicaudate ratio, which has been demonstrated to have excellent interobserver agreement and is more sensitive to changes in ventricular size.[22] This is the minimal intercaudate distance divided by the brain width along the same line. Significant ventriculomegaly is defined as a ratio of 0.25 or greater with this method.

There should also be one of the following supportive features: enlargement of the temporal horns of the lateral ventricles not entirely attributable to hippocampus atrophy; callosal angle of 40 degrees or greater; evidence of altered brain water content, including periventricular signal changes not attributable to microvascular ischemic changes or demyelination; or aqueductal or fourth ventricular flow void on MRI. Other imaging findings were acknowledged to be supportive of the diagnosis but not required, including a brain imaging study performed before the onset of symptoms demonstrating the absence of ventriculomegaly or smaller ventricles, a radionuclide cisternogram showing delayed clearance of the radiotracer over the cerebral convexities

TABLE 34-3 Differential Diagnoses for the Clinical Triad in Normal-Pressure Hydrocephalus, Aside from Other Hydrocephalus Disorders

GAIT DISTURBANCE

Vascular
Cerebrovascular disease
Stroke
Multi-infarct dementia
Binswanger's disease

Neurodegenerative
Parkinson's disease
Alzheimer's disease
Progressive supranuclear palsy
Frontotemporal dementia

Miscellaneous
Peripheral neuropathy
Cervical myelopathy
Lumbar canal stenosis
Diabetic neuropathy
Autonomic dysregulation
Spinal neoplasm

DEMENTIA

Vascular
Cerebrovascular disease
Stroke
Multi-infarct dementia
Binswanger's disease
Cerebral autosomal dominant arteriopathy, subcortical infarcts, and leukoencephalopathy

Neurodegenerative
Parkinson's disease
Alzheimer's disease
Progressive supranuclear palsy
Frontotemporal dementia
Corticobasal degeneration

URINARY INCONTINENCE

Structural
Bladder outflow obstruction
Benign prostatic hypertrophy

Bladder innervation
Autonomic dysregulation
Lumbar canal stenosis

Miscellaneous
Medications—anticholinergics, diuretics

Data from Idiopathic Normal-Pressure Hydrocephalus Guidelines; Relkin N, Marmarou A, Klinge P, et al. Diagnosing idiopathic normal-pressure hydrocephalus. *Neurosurgery.* 2005;57:S4; and expert opinion.

after 48 to 72 hours, cine MRI showing an increased ventricular flow rate, or a single-photon emission computed tomography (SPECT)-acetazolamide challenge showing decreased periventricular perfusion that is not altered by acetazolamide.[16]

The imaging finding of deep white matter hyperintensities in a patient with NPH has been shown to be inversely correlated with shunt responsiveness.[23] Such white matter hyperintensities are probably a marker of comorbidity, with patients being more prone to general complications of surgery when they are present.

However, other studies have demonstrated that the presence of these lesions may not be predictive of a poor outcome after shunt surgery. This was the subject of an MRI study by Tullberg and colleagues, who used conventional MRI sequences to examine these lesions and other MRI variables in a group of NPH patients undergoing surgery.[24] The authors found no correlation between the presence of these parameters and poor outcome after surgery. Akiguchi and associates further demonstrated that there was improvement in ventriculomegaly and mean total scores for white matter lesions in patients who clinically improved after surgery, thus implying that these white matter lesions may be reversible.[25] In this patient cohort the majority had parkinsonism (71%), but other coexisting comorbid conditions, such as small-vessel disease (29%), hypertension (41%), and diabetes (35%), were also found. Eighty-eight percent of patients had white matter lesions noted on CT or MRI. These contradictory findings illustrate the continuing debate regarding the presence of deep white matter hyperintensities and their correlation to small-vessel disease.

Supplementary Prognostic Testing

Guidelines on the value of supplementary tests conclude that a single standard for the prognostic evaluation of patients with idiopathic NPH is lacking. However, supplementary tests can increase the prognostic accuracy to greater than 90%.[26]

Three supplementary tests are currently recommended as options:

- Lumbar puncture "tap test"
- External lumbar drainage
- Measures of CSF outflow resistance

The method of choice depends on local experience and the availability of equipment. Direct ICP measurement may be useful to exclude other more acute causes of hydrocephalus but does not contribute to prognostic assessment. Radionuclide cisternography is no longer a favored option because this technique does not improve the diagnostic accuracy of combined clinical and CT criteria in patients with presumed NPH.[27]

A lumbar puncture "tap test" has been shown to produce a specificity of 100% with a sensitivity of 26%,[28] provided that it is performed at a high volume (i.e., withdrawal of 40 to 50 mL of CSF). Symptomatic improvement after removal of CSF has a high positive predictive value (73% to 100%) of a probably favorable outcome with shunt placement.[26] It has to be remembered that improvement after a shunt is often delayed in many patients, so a simple tap test would not be expected to reveal all patients who might benefit from a shunt. However, the low sensitivity of the "tap test" precludes using this method as a diagnostic tool for exclusion. Nonetheless, a lumbar puncture is often used as a first-line investigative tool to establish that CSF pressure is within the normal range (5 to 18 mm Hg/7 to 24 cm H_2O) and that no biochemical or microbiologic abnormalities are present. Prolonged external lumbar drainage in excess of 300 mL is associated with high sensitivity (50% to 80%), specificity (80%), and positive predictive value (80% to 100%).[26,28] However, this method requires inpatient stay and carries a risk for the complications of nerve root irritation, hemorrhage, and CSF infection.

Measurement of CSF outflow resistance, thought to reflect the CSF absorption pathways, is well established. Fluid is injected into a CSF space (e.g., ventricles or lumbar sac) either by bolus or infusion. CSF outflow resistance can then be calculated with a pressure-volume study and used to assess the CSF circulation for signs of disturbance.[29] The advantage of this technique is that it requires only day attendance and can also be performed through a preimplanted ventricular reservoir device. In the Dutch NPH study, outflow resistance greater than 18 mm Hg/mL per minute had a specificity of 87% and a sensitivity of 46%.[30]

Compliance of the cerebrospinal space is inversely proportional to the gradient of CSF pressure p and the reference pressure p_o [45,46]:

$$C = \frac{1}{E \times (p - p_o)}$$

The biologic significance of p_o remains a matter of debate. Through various mathematical manipulations, it is possible to derive equations that

1. Replicate a CSF infusion study.
2. Replicate the effects of a bolus injection of CSF.
3. Demonstrate the variation in compensatory parameters such as RAP* and the pressure-volume index, which is independent of resting CSF pressure. A full account of this point has been presented elsewhere.[47]

More sophisticated models have been formulated but have yet to become useful in clinical practice.[48-52]

Monitoring of Intracranial Pressure

ICP monitoring is relevant in patients with chronic forms of hydrocephalus and in some patients with possible shunt malfunction but confusing symptoms and signs. Although isolated measurements of CSF pressure in patients with communicating hydrocephalus and NPH may be in the normal range, overnight monitoring may reveal dynamic phenomena such as increased Lundberg "B waves."[53] B waves are slow waves of ICP lasting 20 seconds to 2 minutes. These waves are almost universally present in ICP recordings, probably even in healthy volunteers.[36,54,55] The presence of B waves for more than 80% of the period of ICP monitoring is thought to indicate that it is much more likely than not that shunting would be helpful. Various attempts at more precise quantification have yet to be generally accepted.

Monitoring of ICP can be performed safely with intraparenchymal probes. ICP monitoring via lumbar puncture or a needle inserted into a preimplanted reservoir is used less frequently. Connection of the pressure monitor to a computer performing

---

*RAP is the correlation coefficient between changes in mean CSF pressure and its pulse amplitude over the period of 3 to 5 minutes. RAP close to 0 signifies good compensatory reserve and RAP close to +1 indicates compensatory reserve exhausted.

real-time analysis is very helpful. The best results can be derived from overnight ICP monitoring. If this is impossible, a minimum of 30 minutes of ICP monitoring is required. Instant manometric lumbar CSF pressure measurements may be helpful but are known to be misleading[56] (Fig. 34-16). In patients with normal CSF dynamics, baseline pressure should be normal (i.e., <15 mm Hg) on overnight monitoring. Vasogenic waves of ICP, particularly intensive during the REM phase of sleep, are probably also present in normal conditions. The presence of vasogenic waves greater than 25 mm Hg for a period of around 10 minutes should be classified as intermittent intracranial hypertension. The average overnight RAP index should be less than 0.6 in patients with good compensatory reserve.[57,58] The overnight magnitude of slow waves is considered increased when their average value is greater than 1.5 mm Hg. The presence of plateau waves is always a bad prognostic sign. An example of pathologic overnight ICP recording is presented in Figure 34-17.

During the recording, detection of pulse amplitude proves that the ICP waveform is properly being transmitted to the transducer. Lack of amplitude implies an invalid pressure recording in most cases.[59] In our own material there is no evidence that pulse amplitude is a strong predictor of outcome after shunting as reported by other authors.[59] Analysis of a subgroup of idiopathic NPH patients with a stable follow-up assessment suggested that when the pulse amplitude is large (>3 mm Hg), improvement is very likely (>90% patients improve). When the pulse amplitude is less than 2 mm Hg, improvement is as equally probable as lack of improvement.

There is no difference in amplitude between males and females. Pulse amplitude increases slightly with age but does not show any correlation with the duration of symptoms of NPH or their severity. However, pulse amplitude is lower in patients with idiopathic NPH and no any evidence of coexisting cerebrovascular disease than in patients with clear evidence of vascular problems.[60] After shunting, pulse amplitude decreases. Differences are significant both at baseline and during infusion studies.[61] In shunted patients, pulse amplitude is lower in the context of normally functioning shunts than in patients with blocked shunts.

Clinical Tests of Cerebrospinal Fluid Dynamics

Measurement of the resistance to CSF outflow (R_{CSF} or R_{out}) is useful both in evaluating nonshunted patients with chronic forms

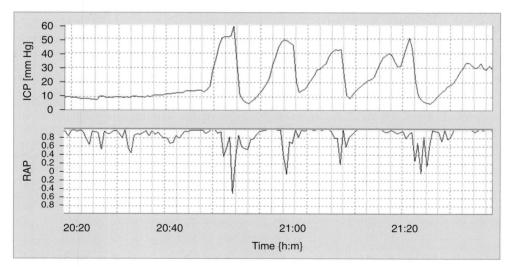

FIGURE 34-16 Example of recording of intracranial pressure (ICP) in a patient after subarachnoid hemorrhage with moderate ventricular dilation and normal baseline pressure (10 mm Hg). The computer recording indicated a regular pattern of plateau waves up to 60 mm Hg. The patient had previously undergone a series of manometric lumbar cerebrospinal fluid measurements with very mixed results: some measurements indicated normal pressure, and some indicated acutely elevated pressure.

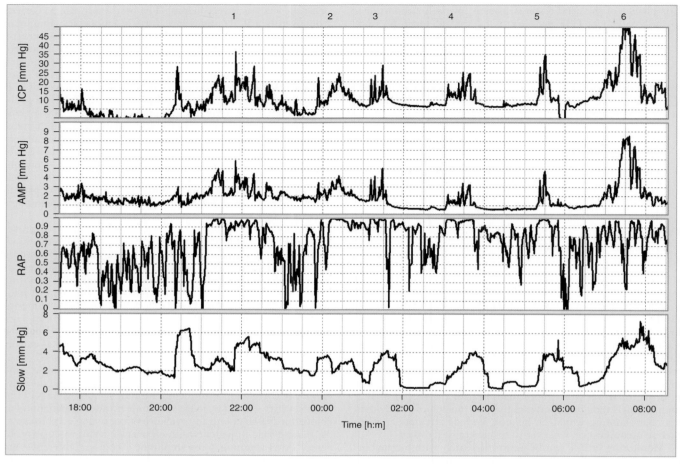

FIGURE 34-17 Example of overnight intracranial pressure (ICP) monitoring. Baseline pressure was normal (around 12 mm Hg) with periodic increases (probably during the random eye movement phase of sleep; they are indicated by numbers above the frame). Slow waves increased their power in these periods, and the compensatory reserve was worse (the RAP index increased to +1). During episodes 1 and 5, ICP increased above 25 mm Hg for only a short period (<5 minutes), but during episode 6 it increased to up to 50 mm Hg for 20 minutes. Overall cerebrospinal fluid dynamics was assessed as being disturbed. AMP, pulse amplitude.

of hydrocephalus and in assessing patients who are suspected of having shunt malfunction. Several methods of measuring resistance to CSF outflow have been described, from bolus injections into the CSF space (rapid but confounded by compliance and vasogenic phenomena), to servocontrolled constant-pressure tests, or controlled infusion studies (lumbar as in the original Katzman-Hussey test, lumboventricular, and ventricular).

The computerized infusion test[62,63] is a modification of the traditional constant-rate infusion as described by Katzman and Hussey.[64] The method requires infusion of fluid into any accessible CSF compartment proximal to any suspected block. The options are a lumbar tap or intraventricular infusion via a subcutaneously positioned reservoir connected to an intraventricular catheter or shunt antechamber. In such cases, two hypodermic needles (25 gauge) are used: one for the pressure measurement and the second for the infusion. There is an approximate 0.5% risk of introducing infection during CSF infusion studies, which has to be weighed against the risk of misdiagnosis or unnecessary shunt revisions.

During the infusion, the mean pressure and pulse amplitude readings over time are calculated (Fig. 34-18A and B). Resistance to CSF outflow can be calculated by simple arithmetic as the difference between the value of the plateau pressure during infusion and the resting pressure divided by the infusion rate. Precise measurement of the final pressure plateau is not possible when

strong vasogenic waves arise or excessive elevation of pressure above the safe limit of 40 mm Hg is recorded. However, computerized analysis produces results even in difficult cases when the infusion is terminated prematurely. The algorithm uses time series analysis for retrieval of volume-pressure curves (Fig. 34-18C), least-mean-square model fitting (Fig. 34-18A), and examination of the relationship between pulse amplitude and mean CSF pressure (Figure 34-18D).

Although not all patients with abnormal CSF circulation may improve after shunting, the computerized infusion test is important because it provides a baseline value of CSF dynamics, which is useful in further management of the disease. Such testing can be invaluable in cases of chronic hydrocephalus in which the architecture of the ventricles remains unchanged (i.e., striking ventriculomegaly is present after shunting). Examples include stiffening of the ventricular ependymal wall from prolonged subacute infection and NPH when there may be loss of periventricular parenchymal elasticity.

Differentiation between Brain Atrophy and Normal-Pressure Hydrocephalus

CSF dynamics in patients with NPH is characterized by a normal baseline pressure (ICP <18 mm Hg). Resistance to CSF outflow

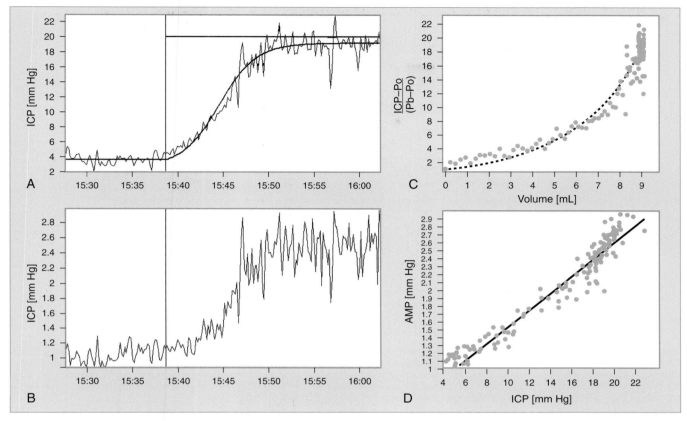

FIGURE 34-18 Methods of identification of the model of cerebrospinal fluid (CSF) circulation during infusion at a constant rate. **A,** Recording of real CSF pressure (intracranial pressure [ICP]) versus increasing time during infusion with an interpolated modeling curve.[7] Infusion at a constant rate of 1.5 mL/min starts from the *vertical line.* **B,** Recording of pulse amplitude (AMP) during infusion. It is customarily presented as different variables, in addition to mean ICP. The rise in AMP is usually well correlated with the rise in ICP. **C,** Pressure-volume curve. On the x-axis, an effective increase in volume is plotted (i.e., infusion and production minus reabsorption of CSF). On the y-axis is the increase in pressure measured as a gradient of the current pressure minus the reference pressure P_o relative to baseline pressure P_b. **D,** Linear relationship between pulse amplitude and mean ICP. The intercept of the line with the x-axis (ICP) theoretically indicates the reference pressure P_o.

(>13 mm Hg/mL per minute) is increased. The B waves recorded during infusion studies are regular. Pulse amplitude is well correlated with mean ICP. Compensatory reserve at baseline is usually good (RAP index <0.6), and the elastance coefficient is usually slightly increased (E >0.2 1/mL)—see Figure 34-19.

Patients suffering predominantly from brain atrophy have normal CSF circulation. Infusion studies in these patients typically demonstrate low opening pressure, resistance to CSF outflow, and low pulse amplitude (ICP <12 mm Hg, R_{CSF} <12 mm Hg/mL per minute, amplitude <2 mm Hg). Compensatory reserve at baseline is very good (RAP <0.5) as a result of the low elasticity of the atrophic brain (E <0.2 1/mL). Vasogenic waves are rather limited during the period of the recording. Mean ICP increases smoothly during the infusion and decreases in a similar fashion after infusion, similar to the inflation and deflation of a balloon (Fig. 34-20).

Noncommunicating and Acute Hydrocephalus

Lumbar infusion is not recommended in patients with noncommunicating hydrocephalus because of the risk for brain herniation in the event of uncontrolled CSF leakage. However, this type of hydrocephalus may not always be easy to detect by imaging. In the few cases in which lumbar infusion is performed, resistance to CSF outflow may be normal (noncommunicating hydrocephalus) because the lumbar infusion is not able to detect the proximal narrowing in CSF circulatory pathways. In acute hydrocephalus,

resistance to CSF outflow, resting pressure, and pulse amplitude are elevated, whereas paradoxically, elasticity is relatively low (ICP >15 mm Hg, pulse amplitude >4 mm Hg, E <0.20 1/mL).

Obstructive hydrocephalus can be safely assessed by ventricular infusion (via a reservoir). Typically, high intracranial resting pressure and high resistance to CSF outflow are demonstrated (ICP >15 mm Hg, R_{CSF} >13 mm Hg/mL per minute). Elasticity is high (>0.20 1/mL), RAP is elevated above 0.6, and the pulse amplitude is high (>4 mm Hg), findings indicative of poor compensatory reserve. Acute communicating hydrocephalus has a similar pattern of parameters, with frequent deep vasogenic waves (including plateau waves[53]).

Testing of Cerebrospinal Fluid Dynamics in Shunted Patients

Evaluation of CSF dynamics in shunted patients may prove very helpful in those with suspected shunt malfunction. The 0.5% risk of introducing infection has to be weighed against the avoidance of unnecessary revisions. In the event of proven shunt malfunction requiring revision surgery, CSF infusion studies may allow certain components to be targeted, such as a suspicion of valve malfunction or distal blockage. Infusion studies may be performed as previously described. Many shunts have accessible antechambers or have had reservoirs inserted within the shunt circuit. However, bur hole valves are generally unsuitable for

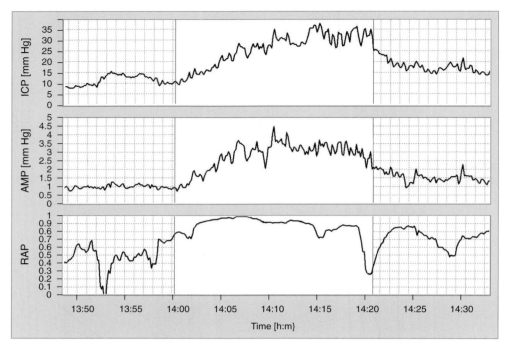

FIGURE 34-19 Example of an infusion study in a patient suffering from normal-pressure hydrocephalus with a normal baseline pressure (9 mm Hg), normal baseline pulse amplitude (AMP), and good compensatory reserve (RAP index at baseline <0.6). During infusion at a rate of 1.5 mL/min (between the *vertical bars*), pressure increased to 35 mm Hg (resistance to CSF outflow was 17.8 mm Hg/mL per minute), pulse amplitude increased proportionally to mean intracranial pressure (ICP), the RAP coefficient increased to +1 (indicating a decrease in compensatory reserve during the infusion), and slow vasogenic waves appeared in the ICP and AMP recordings.

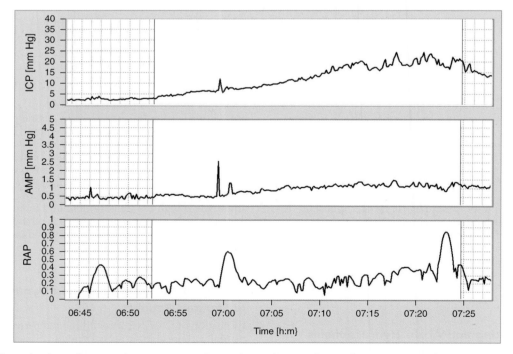

FIGURE 34-20 Example of an infusion study in a patient with atrophy predominantly. Baseline pressure was low (3 mm Hg) and increased only slightly to 18 mm Hg during infusion at a rate of 1.5 mL/min, which resulted in a normal value of resistance to CSF outflow (10 mm Hg/mL per minute). Compensatory reserve was good, even during infusion (RAP did not increase), pulse amplitude (AMP) increased very modestly in response to rising ICP, and there were very few slow waves in the recording.

infusion study access. With pressure measurement via the shunt antechamber, the presence of a CSF pressure pulse wave and an increase in pressure in response to coughing should indicate transmission of pressure between the needle and the CSF space. This is used to confirm patency of the ventricular catheter.

When a shunt drains properly, resting pressure remains at or below the shunt's operating pressure. Infusion studies or overnight ICP monitoring repeated with a shunt in situ should always be considered and the results compared with the tests performed before surgery. Abnormal cerebrospinal compensatory parameters, such as high resting pressure, increased resistance to CSF outflow, low compensatory reserve, increased activity of slow waves, or a high amplitude of the pulse waveform, should return to normal after successful shunting.[61,65] In valves with low hydrodynamic resistance and a well-defined opening pressure, a sharp plateau of the pressure trend is seen about 1 to 5 mm Hg above the level of the shunt's operating pressure.[66] The magnitude of this plateau should not exceed a value as derived from the following equation:

$$\text{Critical pressure} = \text{Shunt operating pressure} + \\ + R_{shunt} \times \text{Infusion rate} + 5 \text{ mm H}$$

where R_{shunt} is the hydrodynamic resistance of the opened shunt and 5 mm Hg is a "safety margin" and a credit for possible nonzero abdominal pressure (in patients with possible increased abdominal pressure, this value should be increased to 10 to 15 mm Hg). When shunt operating pressures and R_{shunt} are measured in the laboratory, these parameters provide invaluable guidelines for shunt testing in vivo[67]; see Figure 34-21 for examples of a working (A) and blocked (B) shunt.

When a shunted patient has low-pressure headaches, small or slit ventricles, subdural collections, or chronic hematomas, CSF overdrainage should be considered. Overdrainage related to body posture may be assessed with a tilting test. When the baseline pressure measured in the horizontal body position is low (usually negative), overdrainage is possible. A change in posture to sitting generally produces a further decrease in pressure. If the pressure decreases to a value lower than −10 mm Hg (the 95% confidence limit for ICP in the upright position in nonshunted patients is around −8 mm Hg), overdrainage is likely (Fig. 34-22).

The majority of contemporary valves usually have low hydrodynamic resistance,[68] a feature that may result in overdrainage from periodic oscillations in cerebrovascular volume. The expanding cerebrovascular bed acts like the membrane of a water pump with a distal low-resistance valve.[69] Early morning headache should not be always assumed to be "high pressure." It may be a consequence of the low pressure caused by nocturnal overdrainage.

In shunted patients with slit ventricles, baseline pressure recorded from the shunt antechamber may not demonstrate a pulse waveform. In this situation, collapse of the ventricular walls around the proximal catheter results in the lack of pressure transmission. A pulse waveform often appears after infusion starts as the buildup of pressure opens up the ventricular cavity (Fig. 34-23).

MANAGEMENT

Surgical management is required for patients with symptomatic acute or chronic hydrocephalus. Surgery is recommended for patients with idiopathic NPH and a favorable risk-to-benefit ratio.[70] Medical therapies, such as acetazolamide and repeated lumbar puncture, do not have a role in longer term management but may be used as temporizing measures before definitive treatment. Surgical management of any obstructive lesion, such as a tumor, may be required in addition to CSF diversion. The two main forms of surgical management for hydrocephalus are shunt insertion and endoscopic third ventriculostomy. Endoscopic

choroid plexus coagulation is favored in some units, but the results of a randomized controlled trial are awaited. Relief from symptomatic hydrocephalus and prevention of neurological deterioration may be achieved with or without a significant reduction in ventricular size, particularly in patients with chronic hydrocephalus.

Shunt Insertion

The most commonly used shunt in modern neurosurgery is a ventriculoperitoneal shunt. A ventricular catheter is placed into the lateral ventricles, usually from a frontal or occipital approach, and connected to the remainder of the shunt system. The ideal trajectory of the ventricular catheter would avoid areas of functional neuroanatomy and the choroid plexus while being at sufficient depth for CSF drainage to occur through all distal drainage openings despite changes in ventricular size. Stereotactic or image-guided placement of ventricular catheters is increasingly being used with normal or small ventricles to reduce the incidence of misplaced ventricular catheters. When raised ICP is associated with small ventricular size, such as benign intracranial hypertension, placement of a lumboperitoneal or lumbopleural shunt may be the preferred option. Ventriculoatrial shunts were previously in common use and may still be the treatment of choice in patients with significant truncal obesity, extensive abdominal abnormalities, or a history of multiple abdominal procedures. Indeed, it is possible to place the distal end of a shunt into any visceral cavity, such as the pleural cavity. Other more unusual shunt options that have been described include the Torkildsen shunt (ventricle to the cisternal space) and the Sinushunt (ventricle to the venous sinus). In addition to shunts placed within the ventricle, treatment of hydrocephalus may involve drainage of one or more cystic or subdural cavities, such as an arachnoid cyst or subdural hygroma.[71]

It is usual practice to incorporate a valve mechanism into the shunt circuit at the time of insertion. CSF drainage can be regulated either by pressure or by flow. Antisiphon devices to prevent overdrainage can be attached to the shunt circuit if required. Some valves incorporate such devices. Reservoir devices can also be fitted to allow access for subsequent CSF analysis or interrogation of CSF hydrodynamics. Some valves have separate reservoir chambers within their design. Many modern valves are programmable and allow subsequent adjustments in differential pressure after implantation. This permits changes to be made in the valve setting after insertion, often on an outpatient basis. The type of valves selected for patients with acute hydrocephalus is based on local experience, published data, and available supplementary information, such as drainage requirements assessed by external ventricular or lumbar drainage. In patients with NPH, no series has demonstrated a significant benefit with a particular type of shunt or valve, although there is a trend favoring low-pressure valves.[72] Patients with low-pressure hydrocephalus may require a valveless shunt system. Shunt devices are discussed in greater depth later.

Endoscopic Third Ventriculostomy

Patients with obstructive hydrocephalus may benefit from endoscopic third ventriculostomy rather than shunt insertion (see Chapter 36). This technique involves passing an endoscope (rigid or flexible) through the lateral ventricles (usually via one of the frontal horns) directly into the third ventricle. If the floor of the third ventricle can safely be visualized, a stoma can be created within it to allow fluid to drain directly into the basal cisterns. The advantage of this procedure over a shunt is that it avoids the potential morbidity of shunt infection and lifelong risk for revision. This procedure has little role in the management of true communicating hydrocephalus. However, some patients with NPH have a late-onset form of relative aqueduct stenosis. In

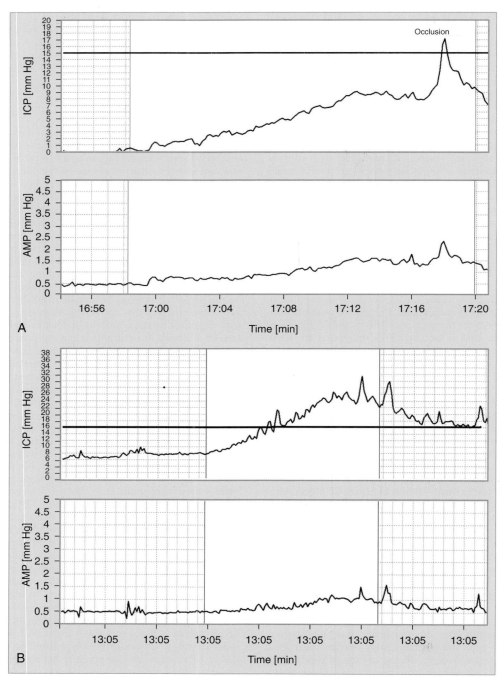

FIGURE 34-21 Examples of infusion studies performed in shunted patients through a shunt prechamber with a working and blocked shunt. **A,** Patient with a Strata Valve set for 1.5 in situ. Pulse amplitude (AMP) was low but clearly recordable, thus confirming the patency of the ventricular drain. Opening pressure was low, and during infusion the pressure increased to a value below the "critical threshold" for this valve (*thick horizontal line*). During infusion, transcutaneous occlusion (external compression of the siphon control device) was performed. Such a compression stops drainage through the valve. Pressure started to rise immediately, thus confirming that shunt system was patent. **B,** Patient with a Hakim Programmable Valve set at 100 mm H_2O. Pressure increased well above the "critical threshold" (*horizontal line*). Spontaneous vasogenic waves were recorded during the test. A pulse waveform was present on the recording. Distal obstruction of the shunt system was confirmed during revision of the shunt. ICP, intracranial pressure.

these patients, there is a mismatch between the degree of ventriculomegaly in the lateral ventricles and third ventricle and between the aqueduct of Sylvius and the fourth ventricle. This implies that the hydrocephalus has an obstructive element (although the hydrocephalus is still "communicating" in terms of the chronic signs and symptoms). In this situation, endoscopic third ventriculostomy may be considered. Gangemi and coauthors reported improvement in 72% of NPH patients with this technique and a relatively low complication rate (intracerebral hemorrhage in 4%).[73]

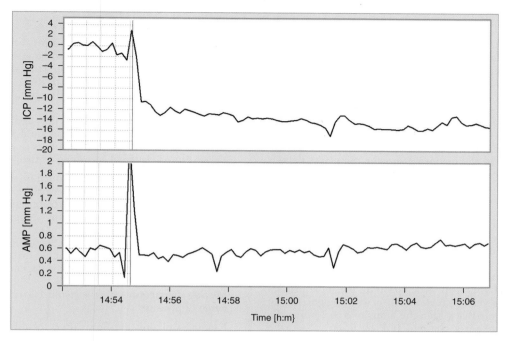

FIGURE 34-22 Overdrainage test showing an excessive decrease in intracranial pressure (ICP) during sitting up at the time point indicated by the *vertical line* (below −14 mm Hg). During sitting up, pulse amplitude (AMP) may not change.

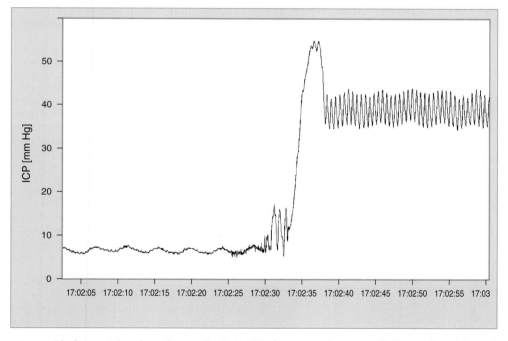

FIGURE 34-23 In patients with slit ventricles, the pulse amplitude (AMP) of intracranial pressure (ICP) is rarely visible on the recording. During infusion into the shunt prechamber, all fluid is drained distally—recorded pressure is equivalent to shunt operating pressure plus the pressure gradient along the distal tube plus abdominal pressure. A respiratory wave may be visible; it is commonly transmitted from the abdominal space. In patients with a membrane siphon–preventing device, occlusion of the device can be performed during infusion (17:02). Pressure increases quickly to very high values (in this case >50 mm Hg), collapsed ventricles open within a relatively short time, and pressure stabilizes at a lower level with a pulse wave clearly visible. The "stabilization pressure" is elevated, because in slit ventricles syndrome an intraparenchymal ICP is usually high. Ventricles may stay open for a longer time, but more frequently they collapse again after the end of the infusion.

SHUNTS

The ability of a shunt system to drain CSF continuously in a repetitive manner over a long-term period is crucial in the management of hydrocephalus. Contrary to popular opinion, a shunt constitutes a complex hydrodynamic system of highly nonlinear flow characteristics. A wide variety of shunt products (more than a hundred generic types, with numerous subtypes and performance levels—not including some homemade devices in use in developing countries) are manufactured. There is little systematic knowledge available with which their comparative cost-effectiveness can be judged by the practicing surgeon. Similarly, there is very little knowledge of whether a specific type of shunt can be matched to an individual pattern of disturbed CSF circulation.

An operating flow pressure of around 0.3 mL/min marks the range of ICP that can be measured in a patient with a properly functioning shunt in a horizontal body position. In ball-on-spring valves, this pressure is very stable over time but is sensitive to dynamic changes in ICP. This type is in contrast to silicone membrane valves, in which the operating pressure may vary within a range of 4 to 6 mm Hg in low, medium, or high ranges. Randomized trials have failed to demonstrate the superiority of different types of valve construction.[74] It is well recognized that physiologic ICP is variable within the limits of 0 to 15 mm Hg. Artificial attempts to set a constant ICP by using valves with minutely determined opening pressure and very low hydrodynamic resistance may not be useful.

Generally, a shunt consists of three parts: inlet tubing (ventricular or lumbar drain), which is a thin short tube with an inner diameter of 0.9 to 1.2 mm; a valve; and a distal drain, a longish silicone rubber tube—see Figure 34-24.

Contemporary CSF drainage devices may be divided into different groups according to the mechanism of CSF drainage control:

1. Fixed differential pressure valves, in which the inlet-outlet pressure gradient opens the valve and then controls the flow of fluid through tubing connecting the proximal (ventricles or lumbar subarachnoid space in most cases) and distal (e.g., peritoneal or atrial) spaces.
2. Adjustable differential pressure valves, which work similarly but allow the opening pressure to be externally adjusted via magnetic programming. Differential pressure (fixed or adjustable) valves are aimed at control of ICP.
3. Flow-regulating valves, in which flow is stabilized, irrespective of the differential pressure.
4. Accessory devices, which control flow and prevent overdrainage in the upright position (antisiphon devices).

Valves can be classified according to their construction:

1. Silicon membrane—flow is controlled by an elastic membrane that changes the area of the outlet orifice.
2. Ball-on-spring—flow depends on compression of a spring (flat or helical) supporting a ball moving along the cone that constitutes the outlet orifice.
3. Miter valve—flow depends on deflection of the silicon miter controlling the diameter of the outlet orifice.
4. Proximal or distal slit valves—flow depends on the area of a slit in soft silicone rubber.
5. Moving diaphragm—flow is stabilized within a certain fixed range of pressure.

Examples of pressure-flow curves of differential and flow-regulating valves are shown in Figure 34-25. Differential pressure valves are characterized by opening/closing pressure (pressure above/below the point at which flow starts/ceases) and an inverse of the slope of the curve within the range of full drainage (≥0.3 mL/min), which is termed the *resistance of the valve*. In flow-regulating valves, the resistance of the valve (within the range of regulation) is infinitely high. In most differential pressure valves, the resistance is very low (lower than physiologic resistance to CSF outflow).[68]

Opening and closing pressure may be programmed externally in some models. Magnetic programming was used for the first time in a French model—the Sophy Programmable Valve. The next generation of programmable valves was designed by S. and C. Hakim. Much more precise programming (18 steps) was achieved. The programmable Strata valve followed, a programmable equivalent of the popular fixed-pressure Delta Valve, integrated with a membrane siphon controlling device.[75] Patients should be counselled regarding the possibility that some magnetic fields may modify the setting of these valves under some circumstances, such as in an MRI scanner. Some valves are more prone to this problem than others.[76] In pediatric patients with programmable valves, parents should be made aware that strong magnetic toys could potentially result in a change in the setting of the valve. Newer adjustable valves (Pro-GAV [B. Braun, Melsungen, Germany] and Polaris [Sophysa, Orsay, France]) offer mechanisms that are able to prevent accidental readjustment, even in a 3-T MRI scanner.

Because the majority of contemporary valves have low hydrodynamic resistance, the net resistance of a shunt depends to a great extent on the diameter and length of the distal drain. In patients in whom clinical complications related to overdrainage are likely to develop, implantation of an antisiphon device should be considered. However, the risk for overdrainage related to vasomotor nocturnal waves may still be high.[29] A standard peritoneal open-end catheter (usually around 90 cm long, 1.1 to 1.2 mm in diameter) provides a resistance of 2.5 to 3.5 mm Hg/mL per minute. This may amount to 100% to 200% of the overall resistance of the valve itself. It must be recognized that shortening of a drain decreases overall shunt resistance, thus making it potentially more susceptible to overdrainage.

The hydrodynamic resistance of the drain is inversely proportional to the fourth power of its diameter. Therefore, many thin lumboperitoneal shunts with a small internal diameter (0.9 mm)

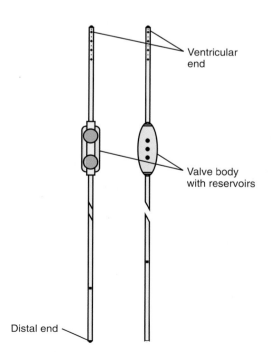

Ventricular end

Valve body with reservoirs

Distal end

FIGURE 34-24 Components of a shunt system: proximal drain, valve, and distal drain.

PART 3

MANAGEMENT OF ADULT HYDROCEPHALUS 3b

CHAPTER 35

Shunting*

Marvin Bergsneider ■ Eric Stiner

Hydrocephalus is a commonly encountered disorder that occurs either as a primary condition or as the sequela to an intracranial hemorrhage, a space-occupying lesion, or meningitis. For more than a half-century, a cerebrospinal fluid (CSF) shunt has been the mainstay for treatment of hydrocephalus. Although many consider shunting a relatively simple procedure, problems with CSF shunts are common, costly, and sometimes debilitating. Within the first year, shunts fail at extraordinary rates of up to 40% and show nearly a 10% infection rate.[1-4] Thus, the shunt operation has one of the highest associated complication rates in neurosurgery. Furthermore, cases of hydrocephalus can be some of the most complex and challenging clinical scenarios facing a neurosurgeon.[5,6]

The aim of this chapter is to help neurosurgeons choose the type of shunt, valve setting, and shunt location that will offer the highest probability of a good outcome while avoiding complications and revisions. Unfortunately, there are scant class I and class II evidentiary data on which to base guidelines pertaining to shunting methods and materials for adult hydrocephalus patients. Our recommendations are therefore derived from personal experience (more than 6000 outpatient encounters and 700 surgical procedures on adult hydrocephalus patients during a 14-year-period), insight drawn from our clinical studies,[7-9] and information gleaned from the literature.

Although this chapter is entitled *Shunting*, neurosurgeons should reflexively consider endoscopic third ventriculostomy an alternative when appropriate.[7,10] The "knee-jerk" response to proceed automatically with a shunt operation, particularly in patients presenting with shunt failure, robs the patient of an opportunity to live shunt free. Clinicians should investigate the etiology and ventricular anatomy in every case of hydrocephalus. In some cases, even patients whose physicians previously said that they had "communicating" hydrocephalus in fact have a ventricular obstruction that clinicians can readily visualize by modern high-resolution magnetic resonance imaging (MRI) technology (such as the CISS [constructive interference in steady state] or FIESTA [fast imaging employing steady-state acquisition] sagittal sequences[7,11,12]). Adult patients shunted in early childhood have a particularly high incidence of noncommunicating (intra-ventricular) hydrocephalus in our experience.

KEY POINT

In the initial evaluation of a newly diagnosed hydrocephalus patient or a previously shunted one, an essential component of the evaluation is to determine whether an endoscopic third ventriculostomy (or related procedure) is appropriate.

VALVE DESIGN AND TERMINOLOGY

Probably the most important component of a shunt system is the valve. Neurosurgeons can choose from more than 125 commercially available valves.[13] During the past 50 years, the predominant theme in the evolution of valve design has been the goal of preventing CSF overdrainage. This includes the introduction of anti-siphon devices, flow-restricting elements, multistage valves, and adjustable valves. It is important to understand that manufacturers have little or no direct in vivo intracranial pressure or CSF flow data to back up advertised claims, such as "preventing excessive flow while allowing constant physiological drainage" or "regulates flow through the valve at a rate close to that of CSF secretion, therefore minimizing the risks of underdrainage or overdrainage." Our studies[8] demonstrate that the in vivo behavior of even the simplest shunt, the ventriculoperitoneal shunt with a standard differential pressure valve, is poorly predicted by the first-order, steady-flow equations that are the basis of the many valve designs.

In our opinion, there is no single valve mechanism, design, or arrangement that is clearly the "best," nor one that will be adequate for every hydrocephalus patient. There are some valves and valve settings, however, that are poorly suited for adult hydrocephalus and will likely result in a higher complication rate. Hydrocephalus is a heterogeneous disorder, with a wide range of intracranial pressures, ventricular compliance, and CSF profiles across patients. It is somewhat fortunate that many valve designs work satisfactorily, at least in the short term, in the majority of patients. The main challenges arise from problematic patients, such as those suffering from headaches, subdural hematomas, repeated shunt obstructions, slit ventricle syndrome caused by chronic overdrainage, and so on. Shunt management is often a trial-and-error process, one in which knowledge of valve design and function can greatly help in the selection of a better choice should a revision be necessary.

The following is a primer on shunt valve design and characteristics with which every neurosurgeon placing shunts should be familiar.

*The senior author (M. B.) has received travel stipends from Codman & Shurtleff, Medtronic, and Sophysa. The senior author has served on Advisory Boards for Codman & Shurtleff and Medtronic. Clinically, the UCLA Adult Hydrocephalus Center uses Codman, Medtronic, Sophysa, Aesculap, and Integra products.

Differential Pressure Valve

The basic building block of most shunt valves is a differential pressure "check valve" mechanism. The basic design of John Holter continues in some form more than half a century after its development.[14] In most current valve designs, it consists of a tiny ball situated on a ring, with a spring pushing the ball downward on the ring. CSF passes through the ring, elevating the ball if the pressure exceeds the pressure exerted by the spring. This creates a one-way flow mechanism because reverse flow will not occur as the ball sits down onto the ring.

Opening of this valve mechanism depends on the *differential pressure* across the ring. For example, if the spring is exerting downward pressure of 100 mm H_2O, CSF will flow if the difference between the inlet and outlet pressures is greater than 100 mm H_2O, regardless of whether the inlet pressure is positive or negative.

A common misconception is that the valve opening pressure must be lower than the ventricular pressure (as measured at the time of surgery) for CSF to flow down the shunt. Our studies demonstrate that this is clearly an invalid assumption. In a study of patients with normal-pressure hydrocephalus (NPH), intracranial pressure was statistically lower at all head-of-bed elevations compared with preoperative values, even with the valve set at 200 mm H_2O opening pressure. For example, despite a mean preoperative intracranial pressure of 164 ± 64 mm H_2O, the mean postoperative intracranial pressure was 125 ± 69 mm H_2O ($P = .04$).[8]

The finding that an intracranial pressure reduction occurs even with a very high valve opening pressure might appear counterintuitive and physiologically untenable, but this misconception arises from a perpetuated oversimplification of intracranial pressure and CSF flow hydrodynamics. The concepts of CSF opening pressure (which, by default, is a mean pressure) and bulk CSF flow have been the standards of hydrocephalus pathophysiology teaching for decades. In reality, the intracranial pressure waveform is pulsatile, with significant elevations of intracranial pressure occurring because of coughing and Valsalva maneuvers as well as intrinsic vasomotor changes. The interaction between pulsatile intracranial pressure and the one-way valve mechanism (inherent to differential pressure valves) is poorly studied. Our continuous intracranial pressure recordings demonstrate that peak intracranial pressures often exceed 200 mm H_2O among patients with a mean intracranial pressure of 164 mm H_2O.[7] Even taking into account distal intra-abdominal pressure, one-way CSF egress occurs during these peaks, thereby lowering the mean intracranial pressure. The one-way flow check-valve phenomenon results in the shunt's draining CSF even with opening pressures exceeding the mean intracranial pressure. This demonstrates that use of a low-pressure valve setting is not necessary and results in excessive CSF drainage in many patients.

Most commercially available CSF shunt valves contain a differential pressure valve mechanism in one form or another. For some, it is the sole valve mechanism, whereas in others, it is the first in-series component of the valve assembly. Examples of ball-spring valves are the Medtronic Strata valve, the Codman Hakim programmable and Precision valves, and the Aesculap proGAV valve. A simpler, less accurate mechanism consists of a valve mechanism derived from two apposing semirigid membranes. These valves, which include the Medtronic, Pudenz, and Codman distal slit valves, are manufactured and then individually tested to determine the approximate opening pressure. They are then segregated into different bins covering a range of pressures. For example, the "medium-pressure valve" bin would contain valves ranging from 50 to 90 mm H_2O opening pressure.

Adjustable ("Programmable") Valves

A "programmable" or adjustable valve is created by adding a mechanism that enables precise changes of the spring tension of a differential pressure valve. There are several competing designs enabling this—all incorporating a magnetic actuation of a rotor. Strictly speaking, these valves are not truly programmable and are better considered as merely *adjustable* valves. Adjustable valves arose from the realization that fixed-pressure differential pressure valves result in either overdrainage or underdrainage in a significant number of adult patients. The overdrainage side of this argument is supported by data from the Dutch Normal-Pressure Hydrocephalus Study,[15] one of the few prospective, randomized studies performed in adult hydrocephalus. This study demonstrated that subdural hygromas occurred in 71% of patients with low-pressure valve shunts versus 34% of patients randomized to medium-pressure shunts. Given the likelihood that expanding or large subdural hygromas are a risk for subdural hematoma, this is one example that there is clearly a risk of selecting too low of an opening pressure. The analysis of our series of 114 consecutive idiopathic NPH patients, each treated with an initial valve opening pressure of 200 mm H_2O, revealed a subdural hygroma incidence of 4%.[7] As shown in Figure 35-1, combining the results of the Dutch Normal-Pressure Hydrocephalus Study with our experience suggests a direct relationship between subdural hygromas and valve opening pressure.

Another justification for the routine use of adjustable valves is based on the range of "final" valve opening pressures when these valves are used. In our retrospective evaluation of 114 consecutive NPH patients surgically treated with a CSF shunt,

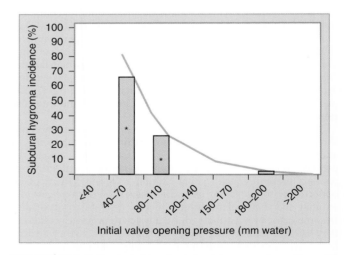

FIGURE 35-1 Estimated risk of subdural hygroma formation with idiopathic NPH. The Dutch Normal-Pressure Hydrocephalus Study[15] documented a subdural hygroma (effusion) incidence of approximately 70% and approximately 30% with low- and medium-pressure differential pressure valves, respectively (data signified with an *asterisk*). We encountered a 4% incidence among patients with an initial valve setting of 200 mm H_2O. Combining these data sets results in a direct relationship between valve opening pressure and subdural hygroma incidence. The hygroma incidence for other valve designs and arrangements has not been well documented. (*From Bergsneider M, Miller C, Vespa PM, Hu X. Surgical management of adult hydrocephalus. Neurosurgery. 2008;62:SHC643-660.*)

the histogram distribution of the final valve opening pressure revealed a roughly gaussian distribution, with most patients in the range of 120 to 140 mm H_2O (Fig. 35-2).[7] This finding closely agrees with that of other large NPH studies.[16] With the wide distribution of final valve pressures shown in Figure 35-2 (from <40 to >200 mm H_2O), it is difficult to fathom how a fixed-pressure valve could adequately serve this population unless there is a way of selecting the appropriate valve pressure preoperatively. Although some have suggested algorithms to do so,[16,17] none has been independently evaluated or validated.

Some neurosurgeons remain reluctant to use adjustable valves on a routine basis (or at all). On their side are the results of a prospective, randomized trial comparing the Codman Hakim adjustable valve and a standard differential pressure valve that failed to demonstrate a difference in shunt failure rates.[4] This study, however, was primarily a pediatric study and, in our opinion, not conclusive with regard to adult hydrocephalus. Arguments that these valves are unreliable, or malfunction more frequently than fixed valves do, are not supported by any clinical study (or our clinical experience with the implantation of more than 400 of these devices). There is a fear that in certain patients, particularly in patients with chronic headache or with particular psychosocial issues, the clinician will be plagued with continued requests for valve adjustments. In our experience, this has not materialized to any significant degree. Perhaps the biggest drawback is cost. Currently, adjustable valves are two to three times more costly compared with fixed-pressure valves, and there is no clinical study comparing cost-effectiveness. A direct comparison of cost utilization would have to factor in the morbidity associated with repeated operations and associated operative risks when fixed-pressure valves are used.

Another drawback of adjustable valves has been MRI compatibility. Because the rotors harbor permanent magnets, there is an inherent susceptibility to large magnetic fields, especially MRI scanners. To date, two manufacturers (Sophysa Polaris and Aesculap proGAV) have designed a locking mechanism that in theory prevents resetting of the valve when the patient is brought in and out of the MRI scanner. The first-generation adjustable valves (Sophysa Sophy, Codman Hakim, and Medtronic Strata valves) are all susceptible to high magnetic fields, and therefore the valve setting must be verified after an MRI scan. In our practice, we specifically use valves with locking mechanisms in patients in whom it is anticipated that future MRI studies are required (such as any patient with a brain tumor).

Commercially available adjustable valves have different opening pressure ranges. Because of physical limitations and spring properties, the maximum and minimum valve opening pressures are constrained. The best example is the Sophysa Polaris valves, which come in the following ranges: 10-140, 30-200, 50-300, and 80-400 mm H_2O (SPVA-140, SPVA, SPVA-300, and SPVA-400, respectively). The Codman Hakim and Medtronic Strata valves are available in only one range of pressure settings. There are no evidence-based guidelines for selection of the most appropriate valve pressure range for any given patient. In our practice, we have some adult patients who require a pressure setting of 10 mm H_2O and others who do best at 400 mm H_2O. See our recommendations on valve pressure selection later.

Both the Aesculap proGAV and Codman Hakim adjustable valve have multiple, smaller discrete settings (from 0 to 200 mm H_2O or 30 to 200 mm H_2O, respectively). Both the Medtronic Strata and Sophysa Polaris valves have only five settings, thereby necessitating a larger jump between steps. We are not aware of any clinical study demonstrating an advantage of smaller steps, although changes as small as 10 mm H_2O can result in clinical responses.[16] Our current management algorithm typically involves making valve adjustments of 30 mm H_2O; only in uncommon scenarios are smaller adjustments apparently beneficial.

Siphon-Control and Anti-Siphon Devices

We refer to these collectively as anti-siphon devices (ASDs), although there are mechanical and marketing differences between them. ASDs are add-on devices, meaning that they are used in conjunction with (immediately distal to) a differential pressure valve mechanism. These devices have been used clinically for more than 30 years.[18]

In general, the device is based on a membrane that is mechanically coupled to the subcutaneous tissue overlying it.[18] The pressure differential between the internal valve lumen and the atmosphere, transmitted across the skin and ASD membrane, determines the flow-pressure characteristics of the ASD device. When the intraluminal pressure becomes significantly negative (relative to atmospheric pressure), the membrane is drawn inward—interacting with other fixed components of the ASD and thereby creating an increased pressure gradient. The original ASD was a separate component (Heyer-Schulte) that had to be inserted into the shunt. The Heyer-Schulte ASD fell into disfavor because of a variety of reasons, typically underdrainage, and has been largely supplanted by a more advanced design marketed by Medtronic.[19] The Medtronic Delta chamber is found in the Delta valve (fixed-pressure apposing membrane differential pressure valve with integral Delta chamber) and Strata valve (adjustable ball-ring differential pressure valve with integral Delta chamber).

ASDs were developed on the basis of the premise that "siphoning" is the etiology of shunt-related CSF overdrainage. Shunt overdrainage has existed since the inception of the shunt.[13,20-22] This phenomenon, better termed gravity-dependent drainage, occurs as the result of gravity-driven CSF flow down the distal catheter when the patient is in the upright position. Early studies[20] documented significantly negative intracranial pressures in shunted patients in the upright position. At the time, it was natural to assume that overdrainage complications (such as subdural hematomas) were due to this gravity-dependent drainage.

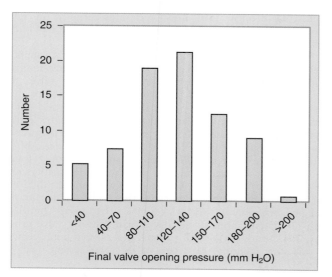

FIGURE 35-2 Range of valve opening pressures in the treatment of idiopathic NPH. Histogram of final differential valve opening pressure values shows a gaussian distribution centered at approximately 140 mm H_2O. The wide range of valve opening pressures required indicates that no single valve opening pressure is appropriate for the treatment of idiopathic NPH. *(From Bergsneider M, Miller C, Vespa PM, Hu X. Surgical management of adult hydrocephalus. Neurosurgery. 2008;62:SHC643-660.)*

Our intracranial pressure studies in idiopathic NPH patients,[8] as well as those of others,[15] suggest that gravity-dependent drainage is likely to play a lesser role in the etiology of overdrainage complications. As any person assumes an upright position, intracranial pressure decreases whether they have a shunt or not. As a matter of fact, in the standing position, most people have a slightly subatmospheric intracranial pressure. When you place a shunt with a differential pressure valve, the curve of intracranial pressure versus head-of-bed elevation in shunted patients nearly parallels that of the pre-shunt state (Fig. 35-3).[8] In other words, a shunt with a differential pressure valve essentially lowers the intracranial pressure nearly equally across the head-of-bed angulation range. The degree of intracranial pressure reduction is largely a function of the valve opening pressure.

KEY POINT

In vivo intracranial pressure data suggest that the etiology of shunt "overdrainage" with differential pressure valves is in many cases, if not most, a result of too low of a valve opening pressure selection, rather than so-called siphoning.

There is little clinical evidence to support the contention that ASDs prevent overdrainage. A large, prospective, randomized study comparing a standard differential pressure valve, the Medtronic Delta valve, and the Orbis-Sigma valve found no statistical difference in the rate of ventricular reduction, the final ventricle size, or the incidence of clinical shunt failure.[1,23] A follow-up single-armed prospective study[3] to the prospective, randomized trial comparing the Codman Hakim adjustable valve with a standard differential pressure valve[4] similarly revealed that the programmable Strata valve also failed to show any benefit in pediatric patients.

For some hydrocephalus patients, the presence of an ASD is detrimental.[24-29] This so-called low-pressure hydrocephalus syndrome, of which the incidence has not been quantified but is presumed to be less than 5%, occurs both in childhood and in adults. Given the low incidence of low-pressure hydrocephalus, we do not think that this "risk" constitutes a contraindication to the general use of products with ASDs. For clinicians who routinely use ASD devices, however, it is important that they become familiar with the signs and symptoms of low-pressure hydrocephalus.[7,24] In our experience as well as that of others,[30] the addition of an ASD can be effective in patients with clinically symptomatic overdrainage.

KEY POINT

A patient who fails to improve clinically (or deteriorates), a patient who remains with significant ventriculomegaly that did not change, a patient who has low measured intracranial pressure, or a patient with an ASD should not be written off as a nonresponder. The diagnosis of low-pressure hydrocephalus should be considered.[24]

Flow Restriction Devices

Another approach taken to counteract shunt overdrainage is the incorporation of a CSF flow restriction mechanism. The premise is that shunt overdrainage occurs as a result of an excessive rate of CSF drainage. It follows that by limiting the maximum CSF flow rate, overdrainage should be averted.

There are several different design approaches to achieve flow restriction. The Integra Orbis-Sigma II valve was designed to directly address flow restriction by use of a multistage needle-valve design. Depending on the differential pressure, a needle is raised or lowered through a small orifice. The diameter of the needle at any given point will determine the cross-sectional area through which the CSF can flow. The manufacturer claims that in stage I, it functions as a low-pressure differential pressure valve to minimize underdrainage complications. When conditions "favor postural or vasogenic overdrainage," the needle moves to stage II, and the valve functions as a flow regulator to maintain flow within "physiologic limits." Last, the manufacturer claims that if intracranial pressure elevates abruptly, the valve opens widely to function as a "safety valve," allowing rapid CSF flow.

There is scarce in vivo clinical evidence, however, to support these manufacturer claims. A large, prospective, randomized study comparing a standard differential pressure valve, the Medtronic Delta valve, and the Orbis-Sigma valve (the original design, predating the Orbis-Sigma II) found no statistical difference in the rate of ventricular reduction, the final ventricle size, or the incidence of clinical shunt failure.[1,23] In a retrospective study comparing the Orbis-Sigma valve with a standard differential pressure valve in NPH, Weiner and colleagues[31] found no significant difference in the time to initial malfunction (shunt survival) between the Orbis-Sigma valve and the differential pressure valve shunts. There were three subdural hematomas and one infection in the Orbis-Sigma valve group compared with no complications in the differential pressure valve group ($P = .11$). Nearly 90% of all patients experienced improvement in gait after shunting, regardless of the valve system that was used.

Remarkably, there exist some in vivo data of measured CSF flow rate through shunts. Miyake and associates[17] created an externalized loop connected to an indwelling ventriculoperitoneal shunt and measured CSF flow rates in patients with NPH. They assessed the Codman adjustable (differential pressure valve) and Orbis-Sigma valves. They demonstrated that shunt flow differed across patients, but in general, flow increased as the adjustable valve setting was lowered regardless of whether the patient was

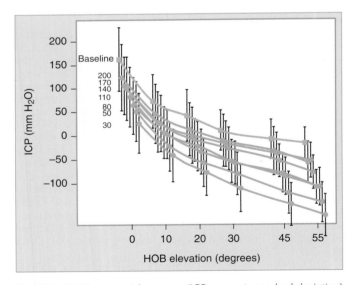

FIGURE 35-3 Intracranial pressure (ICP, mean ± standard deviation) versus head-of-bed (HOB) elevation curves through the full range of differential pressure opening pressures (200, 170, 140, and so on) measured in idiopathic NPH patients treated with a ventriculoperitoneal shunt.[8] The pre-shunt baseline curve (*gray line, filled gray square*) was obtained from the same group of patients. Note that the preoperative and postoperative curves roughly parallel one another, demonstrating the limited role of "siphoning" as the cause of overdrainage in idiopathic NPH patients.

recumbent or sitting. At higher opening pressures of the adjustable valve (140 to 200 mm H_2O) in the recumbent position, the flow was intermittent, whereas at the lowest setting of 30 mm H_2O, the flow rate was 100 to 200 μL/min. In the sitting position, the shunt flow rates were higher, ranging from 200 and 600 μL/min. For the Orbis-Sigma valve, the flow rates were very similar to the adjustable valve set at 200 mm H_2O in both the recumbent and sitting positions. This actual in vivo flow data would appear to contradict the Orbis-Sigma manufacturer's concept that in stage I, it functions as a low-pressure differential pressure valve. There are no in vivo data available either to confirm or to refute the manufacturer's claims regarding stage II and stage III activity.

The Orbis-Sigma II valve was studied in a single-armed, prospective, multicenter clinical study that included 270 adult hydrocephalic patients.[32] Shunt obstruction occurred in 14% of patients. The probability of having experienced a shunt failure–free interval was 71% at 1 year and 67% at 2 years; no difference was observed in shunt survival in pediatric versus adult groups. According to the authors, "overdrainage" occurred in only 2% of patients, although their definition of overdrainage was very narrowly defined. Clinical underdrainage was not assessed.

Another approach to flow restriction is the incorporation of a high-resistance element. The Codman Siphonguard is a coiled helical device that is placed immediately distal to a differential pressure valve (adjustable or fixed pressure). Unlike some ASDs, the Siphonguard device is unaffected by scar tissue encapsulation or external pressure. According to the manufacturer, the mechanical design "detects the difference between the normal and excessive flow and closes the primary pathway only when excessive flow occurs. The secondary pathway is always open and allows for the slow release of CSF when the primary pathway is closed." To our knowledge, to date, there are no published clinical studies evaluating the Siphonguard device. In vitro bench-top testing from an independent laboratory[33] demonstrates that switching between the primary and secondary pathways was initiated at a fluid flow rate between 700 and 1800 μL/min. On the basis of the data of Miyake and associates[17] presented earlier, in which measured flow rates did not exceed 600 μL/min, it is unclear whether the flow-restricting circuit would be activated at all in NPH. Similar flow data do not exist for younger hydrocephalus patients to our knowledge, although presumably the flow rates may be higher than in patients with NPH. Unlike gravity-dependent devices, both the Orbis-Sigma and Siphonguard designs potentially mitigate overdrainage that may occur in the recumbent position.

In our anecdotal experience, we have found that the Siphonguard appears to alleviate or to prevent the transient headaches that shunted patients complain of after sneezing, coughing, or bending over. These headaches, which are common in shunted patients, are rarely problematic and therefore typically do not require surgical intervention.

Medtronic manufactures a peritoneal catheter with a smaller internal diameter, which also achieves a fixed added flow resistance. This catheter is intended to be used in conjunction with a valve. To date, there have been no published clinical studies addressing the clinical efficacy or pitfalls of this approach. Interestingly, Sotelo and coworkers[34] reported the use of a valveless shunt that instead incorporated a peritoneal catheter with a highly precise cross-sectional internal diameter of 0.51 mm. At the end of the observation period of 44 ± 17 months, the failure rate of the shunting device was 14% for the high-resistance valveless shunt compared with 46% for controls (P < .0002). Shunt endurance was 88% for patients with the valveless shunt and 60% for patients with conventional valve shunts. Signs of overdrainage developed in 40% of patients treated with valved shunts but apparently were not observed in patients with the high-resistance valveless shunt.

Gravitational Devices

As discussed earlier, gravity-induced CSF flow (commonly referred to as siphoning) is considered by many to be the primary cause of overdrainage. To offset the negative pressures generated by the long hydrostatic column, the gravitational (also termed hydrostatic) device interposes a very high differential pressure valve while the patient is in the upright position. This is accomplished by a mechanical mechanism that diverts the CSF into one of two parallel differential pressure valves. When the patient is in the recumbent position, a low (lower) opening pressure is operational. CSF is diverted to the high-pressure valve in the upright position.

This approach is not new (the Integra horizontal-vertical valve has been marketed for more than two decades), but recent improved designs have offered a graded transition (Aesculap proGav and shunt-assist valves) as well as a wider selection of the low- and high-pressure (fixed) valve settings. If used alone without a series adjustable differential pressure valve, gravitational devices do not prevent overdrainage or underdrainage clinical conditions.[35] It was subsequently recommended that these gravitational devices be used in series distal to an adjustable differential pressure valve, although this too has been beset with technical problems.[36] Our preliminary experience with the add-on Aesculap shunt-assist valve is that like the Delta ASD device, it is effective in alleviating overdrainage headaches.

Other Valve Characteristics

There are other practical considerations to valve selection. One is the physical profile of the valve—particularly with adjustable valves. A high-profile (prominent) valve housing can have significantly negative cosmetic consequences, especially in alopecic patients. Moreover, prominent housings are more likely to cause overlying skin breakdown in susceptible patients (chronic steroid use, elderly patients, incisions overlying the valve). Another consideration is length of the valve assembly. For occipitally placed ventricular catheters, multiple series devices (such as adjustable valve plus gravitational device) may result in the latter situated in the neck region rather than overlying the skull.

Most valve assemblies have an integrated reservoir (also known as a tapping chamber), although some require a separate component to be added on proximally. It is our opinion that every shunt system should have a tapping chamber for access to CSF (for either CSF sampling or shunt patency assessment).

SHUNT OVERDRAINAGE AND UNDERDRAINAGE DEFINED

Overdrainage

This term means different things to different people. In our view, it is a condition that is (1) caused by excessive CSF drainage or intracranial hypotension and (2) of clinical significance. Overdrainage typically is manifested as either postural headaches (with or without nausea or other ill feelings) or imaging evidence of pathological subdural fluid collections.

Overdrainage symptoms are equivalent to a post–lumbar puncture or "spinal" headache. We know from the lumbar puncture literature that depending on needle size and design, the incidence of post–dural puncture headaches is 1% to 30%.[37] Presumably, most subjects after lumbar puncture experience some period of intracranial hypotension, but only a minority are sensitive to the state. This means that the mere presence of negative intracranial pressure is not pathognomonic of overdrainage. In fact, our studies and those of others[8,20] document that some degree of intracranial hypotension is the norm in shunted patients (data exist primarily for differential pressure valve shunts), but only a small percentage complain of postural headaches.

KEY POINT

In shunted patients undergoing continuous intracranial pressure monitoring, the finding of negative intracranial pressures in the upright position is not diagnostic of shunt overdrainage—there must be accompanying symptoms to establish this diagnosis.

The determination of postural headaches is straightforward in most cases. The patient will have clearly recognized that the headache or other symptoms occur within minutes of assuming an upright position and are alleviated immediately with recumbency. Intracranial pressure monitoring is not needed in such cases. Furthermore, postural headaches can occur in the setting of unchanged ventricle size, with a reduction in ventricle size, or with the presence of subdural fluid collections. Increasing the valve opening pressure (by at least 30 mm H_2O) usually alleviates postural headache symptoms within 1 hour of the intervention. The use of adjustable valves obviates the need for a shunt revision in most of these cases. In the situation in which the patient is already at the maximum valve opening pressure of an adjustable valve (or has a fixed pressure or other valve), a shunt revision is typically required either to add an ASD or gravitational device or, with the latter scenario, to change the valve to an adjustable valve with a higher range of pressures. If postural headaches are mild, conservative measures such as hydration can often bide the patient over until the body re-equilibrates and the symptoms abate spontaneously.

Less commonly, headache may not be the main symptom of shunt overdrainage. Some patients complain of only nausea, whereas others have difficulty concentrating. For patients who have new-onset headaches not present before the shunt operation, there should be a clinical suspicion of overdrainage even if there is no clear postural relationship.

In general, overdrainage headaches do not occur in a delayed manner. In other words, a patient who has been doing fine for months will not spontaneously present with overdrainage symptoms. Exceptions to this rule might include new subdural fluid collection and inadvertent shunt adjustment (such as with an MRI).

The development of subdural fluid collections is a second possible manifestation of shunt overdrainage. Subdural hygroma (also known as effusion) formation is relatively common in the shunted NPH population. Small subdural hygromas (<5 mm) are usually asymptomatic[15] and are often associated with improvement in NPH symptoms because they occur only in conjunction with reduction of the ventricular system. As a result, the presence of a subdural hygroma is not by itself diagnostic of shunt overdrainage. Expanding or large subdural hygromas are more worrisome and, many would agree, are risk factors for the development of acute hemorrhage (subdural hematoma). A non–trauma-related subdural hematoma in a shunted patient is obviously an overdrainage presentation.

It is our observation that shunted patients undergoing a contrast-enhanced MRI study sometimes show diffuse pachymeningeal enhancement—the same finding that is used to diagnose spontaneous intracranial hypotension. Given that most shunts generate some degree of intracranial hypotension, this enhancement pattern is not necessarily indicative of clinical overdrainage. If postural symptoms are present, however, the finding may support an overdrainage diagnosis.

"Slit" or collapsed ventricles are typically a manifestation of chronic overdrainage. Clearly, not all patients with slit (or unilateral slit) ventricles are symptomatic, but it is generally agreed that this state increases the risk of ventricular shunt obstruction. The apposition of the ventricular catheter to the ventricular wall

increases the chance of ingrowth of ependymal cells or choroid plexus. The adult slit ventricle syndrome is an ill-defined disorder, but the key components are "slit" or "collapsed" ventricles seen on computed tomography or MRI in a symptomatic, shunted patient. The incidence is unknown but represents about 5% of the non-NPH evaluations in our clinic.[7] Although relatively few in number, these patients represent a disproportionate amount of clinical effort expended with frequent emergency department visits and requests for office visits. The syndrome occurs more commonly in patients who have been shunted for many years, either as an adult or in childhood. In addition, it is our observation that a significant proportion of patients with adult slit ventricle syndrome have previously unrecognized noncommunicating hydrocephalus.

Common symptoms of adult slit ventricle syndrome include intermittent headaches that become more frequent and intense over time. The etiology of these intermittent headaches has been unclear but may be related to periods of insufficient CSF drainage. In addition, collapse of the ventricular system lowers intracranial compliance, further amplifying elevations in intracranial pressure during shunt underdrainage. At shunt revision, the typical intraoperative finding is nearly total but not complete obstruction of the ventricular catheter (typically only one or two holes are patent). Left untreated, the symptoms may progress to more continuous headaches, presumably due to completed mechanical obstruction of the shunt system. Therefore, the slit ventricle syndrome is actually an underdrainage syndrome created by a preceding period of overdrainage.

Underdrainage

In many cases, shunt underdrainage is easy to recognize. This includes patients who were obviously symptomatic from hydrocephalus and then fail to improve after shunt surgery or see a return of their symptoms with clinical deterioration. Similarly, interval enlargement of the ventricles is diagnostic of underdrainage.

It is the patient in whom the association between clinical findings and ventriculomegaly is uncertain and fails to improve after shunt surgery (or only minimally improves) who represents a clinical challenge. This is especially problematic in NPH patients because there always exists some doubt in the diagnosis. As a result, the failure to improve might be attributed to an incorrect diagnosis (an underrecognized weakness of many NPH clinical studies).

For example, what if there is no clinical improvement in a patient with suspected NPH despite the valve's being brought down to its lowest setting? After confirming shunt patency, many might consider such a patient a "nonresponder" and therefore by inference misdiagnosed. For patients in this scenario who remain with significant ventriculomegaly, the low-pressure hydrocephalus state should be considered.[25,29] For these patients, clinical improvement strongly coincides with reduction in the ventricular size, and only with significant negative intracranial pressure does reduction in the ventricular size occur. Not surprisingly, this state occurs with higher incidence in patients with ASDs.[24-29]

In NPH, if imaging reveals a reduction in ventricular size, a patient should be considered a nonresponder if no clinical improvement occurred. Downward adjustments in valve opening pressure are unlikely to benefit the patient and instead increase the risk of subdural hematoma.

If underdrainage is suspected, shunt obstruction is always a consideration. Based largely on the experience with pediatric hydrocephalus, many neurosurgeons use nuclear medicine isotope studies to determine shunt patency.[38-41] At our center, however, we have found fewer indications for this study, and it is now rarely ordered. The primary reason is that the results of the study seldom alter the clinical decision tree. As noted before, many cases of shunt malfunction are readily identified on the basis of the history or imaging findings, and a "confirmatory" patency study is not needed and perhaps is relatively contraindicated. In more clinically challenging cases, the question of shunt patency arises in association with the possible nonresponder. If the patient remains with unchanged (large) ventricle size and has not improved clinically (with a reasonable suspicion of clinical hydrocephalus), the results of a nuclear medicine study will unlikely alter the management plan. If no flow is found (which could be a false-positive finding because CSF drainage may occur only if the patient is allowed to assume the upright position for some time), the patient needs a shunt revision. Even if shunt flow is documented, one should pursue other interventions. For example, if there is an ASD, remove it. If the patient has a fixed-pressure valve or a flow-restricting valve, change it to an adjustable differential pressure valve (no ASD). It is our observation that ventriculoatrial shunts provide more drainage than ventriculoperitoneal shunts do, and therefore we offer a shunt revision to a ventriculoatrial shunt as well. It is only the case in which the patient has a ventriculoatrial shunt with a differential pressure valve set to 30 mm H_2O or less that an operative intervention is not recommended. Therefore, the results of a nuclear medicine study (positive or negative) likely would not obviate a shunt revision (for these selected patients).

KEY POINT

In NPH, documentation of shunt patency with a nuclear medicine isotope study is not diagnostic of a shunt nonresponder. Functional underdrainage must be considered.

VALVE SELECTION

There are no evidenced-based guidelines to support any recommendations. If the prospective pediatric hydrocephalus valve studies[1,3,4,23,42] are extrapolated to the adult population, no one valve design would appear to hold an advantage. Most would agree that NPH is clearly a distinct entity from pediatric hydrocephalus forms, and therefore the relevance of these studies can be challenged. On the basis of peer-reviewed published clinical studies and our large experience, we see no reasonable justification for not using an adjustable valve for NPH. Although adjustable valves are not the panacea, the use of a nonadjustable valve for the treatment of NPH exposes the patient to an unacceptable underdrainage or overdrainage risk.

In our view, the more difficult question pertains to the younger adult age group (18 to 65 years). Our routine practice includes the use of an adjustable valve for all adult patients, although admittedly, there are fewer published data to support this practice. What is not known is whether the added cost can be justified relative to the selective benefit in this cohort. Because we have no way of differentiating which patients might or might not benefit from the use of an adjustable valve, we do not think that the cost of the device should dictate the decision because an adjustable valve will be equivalent to or better than a standard fixed differential pressure valve for any given adult patient.

The next concern is whether an adjustable valve should be used alone or in conjunction with another device. There is no evidence demonstrating that valve designs incorporating an ASD, a flow-restricting device, or a gravitational device lower the incidence of overdrainage complications. In our opinion, what is important is that the clinician understand the potential pitfalls and risks of each valve type (including the stand-alone differential pressure valve) and be able to recognize possible shunt overdrainage or underdrainage states.

The second decision in valve selection is choosing the initial opening pressure. Our experience during the past decade is largely limited to the use of an adjustable, stand-alone differential pressure valve. For NPH, it is our experience that approximately 96% of patients are aptly treated with a valve pressure range between 30 and 200 mm H_2O. About 2% will have clinical overdrainage despite a valve pressure setting of 200 mm H_2O, and the other 2% will have underdrainage at a setting of 30 mm H_2O. An adjustable valve with a range from 10 to 240 mm H_2O would meet the needs of more than 99% of NPH patients on the basis of our experience. In our practice,[7,24] the valve pressure for all NPH patients is initially set at 200 mm H_2O, and the opening pressure is then sequentially lowered to effect.

We recommend that younger, non-NPH patients receive even higher opening pressure settings (upper opening pressures of 300 or 400 mm H_2O) or, alternatively, that an ASD, flow-limiting device, or gravitational device be incorporated in series with the "standard" adjustable valve (30 to 200 mm H_2O).

SHUNT CONFIGURATION

Cerebrospinal Fluid Access

For routine shunt placement, we prefer a frontal (precoronal) ventricular puncture shunt rather than a posterior or occipital shunt. A retrospective analysis of shunt operations from the U.K. Registry study demonstrated that frontal catheters were adequately placed in 67% of cases, whereas occipital catheters were adequate in 52%.[43] Moreover, we typically use frameless stereotaxis for the shunt ventricular catheter placement in patients with a bifrontal distance (maximum distance of lateral frontal horns) of less than 40 mm to increase the chances of optimal catheter placement. The tip of the catheter should reside just anterior to the ipsilateral foramen of Monro to keep it away from the choroid plexus. If the ventricles are large, the catheter is first positioned orthogonal to the skull, then angled slightly about 5 degrees anteriorly before the freehand insertion. The ideal depth is typically 6 cm of catheter at the dura.

As a general rule, every shunt incision should be carefully planned so that it does not directly overlie a shunt component. Failure to do so increases the risk of skin breakdown. We routinely place a modified titanium bur hole cover (one sector removed) over the frontal bur hole site after the catheter is situated. This prevents dimpling of the skin into the bur hole, which can result in poor cosmesis and sometimes discomfort.

Some neurosurgeons routinely use ventricular endoscopy to assist ventricular shunt placement. A multicenter trial demonstrated no benefit from this strategy.[44] In our opinion, endoscopy is not a substitute for stereotaxis. A poor initial trajectory may not be remediable by attempted endoscopic catheter placement.

Distal Site

During the past decade, our center has performed a similar number of ventriculoperitoneal and ventriculoatrial shunts. We have found a nearly identical complication rate between the two techniques.[7] We use a pragmatic decision-making process. If the patient is not obese and has no history (or probability) of peritoneal adhesions, a ventriculoperitoneal shunt is offered. Otherwise, a ventriculoatrial shunt is recommended. There is a growing literature on laparoscopy-assisted peritoneal catheter placement for obese patients and patients with peritoneal adhesions.[45-49] For the very cases in which laparoscopy is indicated, a ventriculoatrial shunt can usually be performed instead. As a result, we have used laparoscopic assistance in only two cases during a 14-year period.

Ventriculoatrial Shunt Technique

We routinely use a modified percutaneous technique.[50-52] With use of a sterile intraoperative ultrasound unit[53] to visualize the needle cannulation of the internal jugular vein (Fig. 35-4), only a 5-mm incision is needed. We use an 8 French peel-away vascular access kit and fluoroscopic visualization to place the tip of the catheter at the distal superior vena cava (we still use the term *ventriculoatrial shunt* for simplicity). We avoid placement of the catheter in the atrium to minimize the risk of sinus arrhythmias.

There continues to be reluctance for ventriculoatrial shunt placement. The perception that the infection rate is higher with ventriculoatrial shunts in comparison to ventriculoperitoneal shunts is not supported by the literature.[7,54] One concern is shunt nephritis, an immune complex–mediated glomerulonephritis that results from long-term, subacute bacteremia (typically an indolent species, such as *Staphylococcus epidermidis*).[55] During the last 15 years, with placement of more than 250 ventriculoatrial shunts, we have seen one case of documented shunt nephritis. This condition is not unique to ventriculoatrial shunts, having been reported in ventriculoperitoneal shunts as well.[56,57] Patients present with fever of unknown origin and microscopic hematuria. It underscores the importance of a shunt tap in shunted patients in whom another obvious source of infection cannot be identified. Shunt cultures should be kept in the incubator for at least 5 days to identify indolent bacterial forms.

The percutaneous ventriculoatrial shunt approach is performed in a specific order. Once the components are tunneled and situated, the patient is placed in Trendelenburg position for the ultrasound-guided placement of the distal ("atrial") catheter. Once this has been accomplished and the table returned to the neutral position, the dura is incised and the ventricular catheter is inserted. This order eliminates CSF loss while the patient is in the Trendelenburg position. The final assembly of the ventriculoatrial shunt is at the retroauricular incision site, where the distal valve is connected to the proximal portion of the atrial catheter. This has to be done last because the atrial catheter has to be cut to the correct length based on the localization of the distal tip.

Ventriculoperitoneal Shunt Technique

For most cases, we mark an incision about 4 to 5 cm below the costal margin and centered at the lateral border of the rectus musculature (Video 35-1). Typically, the mini-laparotomy can be accomplished easily with a horizontal incision of 3 cm or less. The (appendectomy) retractor is used for exposure in the pre–

rectus fascia space only. After the superficial rectus fascia is opened transversely, the rectus muscle separated vertically in a muscle-sparing fashion, an open Cushing forceps is all that is needed to provide exposure of the deep rectus fascia. This fascia is picked up with two Crile hemostats, and a 3- to 4-mm incision is made with Metzenbaum scissors. Pulling up on these hemostats brings this deep fascial plane superficial to the rectus muscle, thereby allowing the approach by such a small skin incision. In about half the cases, the peritoneum is adherent to this fascial layer, and the peritoneal cavity will be encountered. In the other cases, the peritoneum can be picked up with two mosquito hemostats and incised with the Metzenbaum scissors; the peritoneum cavity can then be confirmed by gently probing with the Penfield 4 instrument. Closure is performed in layers, with a single 3-0 absorbable suture reapproximating the deep fascia (we do not use a purse-string suture) and interrupted 3-0 absorbable sutures in the superficial fascia and dermis layers. We do not use skin sutures, staples, or subcuticular sutures, but instead only use Steri-Strips and Mastisol for maximal cosmesis.

Video 35-1 can be found on Expert Consult @ www.expertconsult.com

Challenges occur when a thick preperitoneal fat layer is encountered or if the omentum is large and it is difficult to confirm entrance into the peritoneal cavity. More troublesome is encountering peritoneal adhesions. If this occurs, a larger exposure may be required to be able to digitally explore the peritoneal space. As noted before, a ventriculoatrial shunt is a better choice in patients suspected of having peritoneal adhesions.

As noted before, our center has extremely limited experience with laparoscopy-assisted placement of peritoneal catheters. It is our experience that with the approach described, the incision is small and not a cosmetic issue. Therefore, the rationale of using laparoscopy for cosmetic purposes is difficult to justify in our opinion. One of the known complications of ventriculoperitoneal shunts is retraction of the peritoneal catheter into the subcutaneous pocket underlying the wound. In this case, a laparoscopic technique proposed by Nfonsam and coworkers[58] is appealing in that the shunt tunneler penetrates the peritoneum under laparoscopic visualization away from the open incision sites.

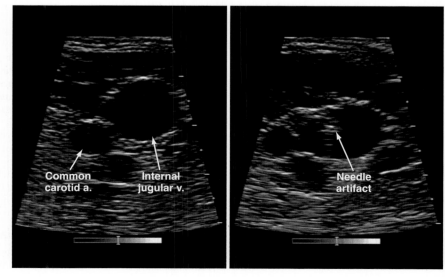

FIGURE 35-4 Image captures taken from an intraoperative 7.5-MHz portable ultrasound unit (Site-Rite, Bard Access Systems, Salt Lake City, Utah). *Left,* Normal tranverse plane anatomy, clearly demonstrating the common carotid artery and internal jugular vein. *Right,* Real-time ultrasonography allows visualization of the needle insertion into the vein (usually about 1.5 cm below skin surface), avoiding the artery and inadvertent puncture of the lung.

Common carotid a.   Internal jugular v.   Needle artifact

Third Ventriculostomy

The fenestration through the floor of the ventricle is made bluntly with a blunt trocar, closed forceps, or a laser wire. Sharp fenestration and cautery are not recommended because both these techniques increase risk to the basilar artery complex, a disastrous scenario. Some authors maintain that fenestrations may create tension along the walls of the third ventricle and increase the risk for postoperative hypothalamic dysfunction,[32] but we have not found this to be problematic. Others use a small Doppler probe to locate the basilar complex definitively before fenestration, especially in patients with opaque third ventricular floors.[39]

The fenestration is then dilated to 4 to 6 mm in diameter by using a double-balloon catheter, Fogarty balloon, spreaders, or forceps. Next, the endoscope is perched atop the ostomy to inspect the subarachnoid spaces for membranes such as the membrane of Liliequist. These, too, must be carefully fenestrated or the operation will be at risk for failure. A rule of thumb is that if the endoscope can fit within the fenestration, it is large enough. After the fenestration, the floor of the third ventricle should pulsate and flap with the respiration and heart rates. These pulsations have been shown to be a strong predictor of ETV success.[40]

Closure and Postoperative Issues

Once the procedure is completed, the endoscope should be withdrawn slowly to inspect for hemorrhage and contusions before final removal. Some authors use fibrin glue or Gelfoam sponge to occlude the tract through the cortex. This can potentially prevent subdural hygromas and leakage of CSF. We do not routinely occlude the tract but rather close the dura mater in a single close watertight fashion.

The use of external ventricular drains postoperatively is a controversial topic. Many surgeons will use them to measure intracranial pressure postoperatively or as an emergency safety valve in the event of patient deterioration or ETV failure. However, detractors of the use of drains point out that the presence of an external drain can promote leakage and wound pseudomeningocele and, if open, may not permit the necessary pressure head to encourage flow through the ventriculostomy and thereby cause false-negative failures. Our goal is to limit the use of external drains except in select cases in which the patient is in a morbid state, is at a high risk for failure, or is at high risk for hemorrhage during and after the procedure.

Many centers encourage the use of subcutaneous bur hole reservoirs after ETV. These can be tapped in emergency or potentially infectious scenarios and can also be used postoperatively to measure intracranial pressure.[39,41] However, ventricular reservoirs may encourage patency of the cortical tract and thus promote CSF leakage; their use may also disallow the possibility of rendering the patient hardware free.

As stated previously, ventriculomegaly in patients who have undergone ETV decreases at a much slower rate and to a much less extent than in patients with implanted shunts.[38] Therefore, we perform postoperative imaging (CT) at 6 to 8 weeks rather than on postoperative day 1 as is our practice in patients with shunts. Typical in-hospital stays for patients after ETV vary between 1 and 3 days, with most patients going home on postoperative day 2; this is longer than their counterparts with shunts.

COMPLICATIONS

Preoperative informed consent and postoperative patient monitoring require a detailed understanding of both the types and frequencies of complications associated with ETV. Despite allowing the patient to be hardware free and therefore invulnerable to shunt infection, ETV is certainly not without risk, espe-cially in the short term. The risk for ETV failure was described earlier and ranges from 10% to 50% in most studies. This variation is a result of the wide range of causes of hydrocephalus. The overall complication rates for this procedure vary from 5.8% to 16% (Table 36-1). These rates vary primarily based on indications for or cause of the hydrocephalus, patient comorbidity, surgeon experience, and vigilance in reporting.

Major complications that should be disclosed to the patient before surgery include CSF leakage (1% to 6%), meningitis (1% to 5%), cranial neuropathies (1% to 2%), seizures (1%), and medical complications (2% to 9%). Overall hemorrhage rates vary from 1% to 3.6% and include intraventricular bleeding requiring either abandonment of the procedure or reoperation (hemorrhage blocking the ostomy), postoperative hematoma, or rare catastrophic basilar injury. Hypothalamic injuries are generally underreported, especially pathologic weight gain, and include diabetes insipidus, amenorrhea, and precocious puberty.[32]

Hydrocephalic patients treated with ETV must be considered treated and not cured; therefore, they require follow-up just like their counterparts with shunts. This is especially important because rapid delayed deterioration has been reported in upward of 1 in 200 ETV patients.[7] Sixteen such cases have been reported, with a staggering mortality rate of 81%. All the survivors except 1 have been disabled as a result of the rapid deterioration.[42]

REPEATED ENDOSCOPIC THIRD VENTRICULOSTOMY AFTER PRIMARY FAILURE

When hydrocephalic patients who have previously undergone ETV fail the treatment, they generally have the usual signs and symptoms of raised intracranial pressure and increased ventricular size on CT from their postoperative baseline. Persistent wound pseudomeningocele and delayed CSF leaks are also highly suspicious symptoms suggestive of ETV failure.

Such patients with ETV failure should undergo MRI with high-resolution T2-weighted sagittal sequencing. This sequence will allow the clinician to evaluate ventricle size, the presence or absence of an interruption in the floor of the third ventricle (ostomy), and whether a flow void exists through the opening. If the opening is present with or without a flow void, serial lumbar punctures to encourage flow through the ostomy can be considered.[43] If there is no resolution after two or three attempts, CSF shunting is mandated. In a patient in whom neither an opening nor a flow void is seen on MRI, re-exploration or repeated ETV is warranted. During re-exploration, if an opening is visualized and is of adequate size, conversion to a CSF shunt is suggested. In the event that the ostomy is occluded either by debris or by scar tissue, refenestration is warranted. Gangemi and coauthors reported that in 10 of 110 patients who worsened clinically after primary ETV, 4 were found to have occluded ostomies on MRI and agreed to undergo a repeat ETV procedure.[27] All 4 improved clinically.

CONCLUSION

ETV is a useful technique for treating adult hydrocephalus, with success rates varying from 50% to 90%. Patient selection is key to achieving clinical success. Causes of hydrocephalus most favorable for consideration of ETV in the adult population are LIAS, secondary (lesional) obstructive hydrocephalus, NPH, and secondary ETV revisions of patients with pediatric-onset hydrocephalus who have a shunt. Detailed knowledge of the intricacies of each of these causes and their success rates, awareness of the potential risks and complications, and expertise in normal and anomalous ventricular anatomy will allow successful performance of ETV.

TABLE 36-1 Reported Rates of Complications in Patients after Endoscopic Third Ventriculostomy

PAPER	PATIENT POPULATION (AGE IN YEARS)	SAMPLE SIZE	CSF LEAK (%)	MENINGITIS (%)	HEMORRHAGE (%)	HYPOTHALAMIC INJURY (%)	CRANIAL NEUROPATHY (%)	SEIZURE (%)	RAPID DELAYED DETERIORATION OR DEATH (%)	WOUND INFECTION (%)	MEDICAL COMPLICATIONS (%)	OVERALL COMPLICATION RATE (%)
Drake[7]	Pediatric (0-20)	368	3.6	2.8	1.4	1.4	1.4	3.75	0.5	—	—	13.6
Jenkinson et al.[15]	Adult (16-79)	190	1.0	0	2	—	1	—	0	—	—	5.8
Hader et al.[32]	Pediatric and adult	131	6.1	5.3	2.3	6.1	2.3	1	—	1.5	—	16*
Gangemi et al.[27]	Adult NPH only	110	1.8	—	3.6	—	—	—	0	1	—	6.4
Dusick et al.[22]	Adult (17-88)	108	—	1	1.9	—	—	1	1.9	—	8.3	14.8

*Eight percent for primary endoscopic third ventriculostomy and 31% for endoscopic third ventriculostomy in lieu of shunt revisions.
Zeros indicate that the authors clearly stated that they had no such complications; dashes indicate that such complications were not discussed or reported.
CSF, cerebrospinal fluid; NPH, normal-pressure hydrocephalus.

SUGGESTED READINGS

Amini A, Schmidt RH. Endoscopic third ventriculostomy in a series of 36 adult patients. *Neurosurg Focus*. 2005;19(6):E9.

Bergsneider M, Miller C, Vespa PM, et al. Surgical management of adult hydrocephalus. *Neurosurgery*. 2008;62(suppl 2):643-659; discussion 659-660.

Bondurant CP, Jimenez DF. Epidemiology of cerebrospinal fluid shunting. *Pediatr Neurosurg*. 1995;23:254-258; discussion 259.

Del Bigio MR. Cellular damage and prevention in childhood hydrocephalus. *Brain Pathol*. 2004;14:317-324.

Drake JM. Endoscopic third ventriculostomy in pediatric patients: the Canadian experience. *Neurosurgery*. 2007;60:881-886; discussion 886.

Drake J, Chumas P, Kestle J, et al. Late rapid deterioration after endoscopic third ventriculostomy: additional cases and review of the literature. *J Neurosurg*. 2006;105:118-126.

Enchev Y, Oi S. Historical trends of neuroendoscopic surgical techniques in the treatment of hydrocephalus. *Neurosurg Rev*. 2008;31:249-262.

Fukuhara T, Luciano MG. Clinical features of late-onset idiopathic aqueductal stenosis. *Surg Neurol*. 2001;55:132-136; discussion 136-137.

Gangemi M, Maiuri F, Naddeo M, et al. Endoscopic third ventriculostomy in idiopathic normal pressure hydrocephalus: an Italian multicenter study. *Neurosurgery*. 2008;63:62-67; discussion 67-69.

Hader WJ, Drake J, Cochrane D, et al. Death after late failure of third ventriculostomy in children. Report of three cases. *J Neurosurg*. 2002;97:211-215.

Hader WJ, Walker RL, Myles ST, et al. Complications of endoscopic third ventriculostomy in previously shunted patients. *Neurosurgery*. 2008;63:ONS168-174; discussion ONS174-175.

Hellwig D, Grotenhuis JA, Tirakotai W, et al. Endoscopic third ventriculostomy for obstructive hydrocephalus. *Neurosurg Rev*. 2005;28:1-34; discussion 35-38.

Jenkinson MD, Hayhurst C, Al-Jumaily M, et al. The role of endoscopic third ventriculostomy in adult patients with hydrocephalus. *J Neurosurg*. 2009; 110:861-866.

Longatti PL, Fiorindi A, Martinuzzi A. Failure of endoscopic third ventriculostomy in the treatment of idiopathic normal pressure hydrocephalus. *Minim Invasive Neurosurg*. 2004;47:342-345.

Patwardhan RV, Nanda A. Implanted ventricular shunts in the United States: the billion-dollar-a-year cost of hydrocephalus treatment. *Neurosurgery*. 2005;56:139-144; discussion 144-145.

Simon TD, Riva-Cambrin J, Srivastava R, et al. Hospital care for children with hydrocephalus in the United States: utilization, charges, comorbidities, and deaths. *J Neurosurg Pediatr*. 2008;1:131-137.

St. George E, Natarajan K, Sgouros S. Changes in ventricular volume in hydrocephalic children following successful endoscopic third ventriculostomy. *Childs Nerv Syst*. 2004;20:834-838.

Tisell M, Hoglund M, Wikkelso C. National and regional incidence of surgery for adult hydrocephalus in Sweden. *Acta Neurol Scand*. 2005;112:72-75.

Warf BC. Hydrocephalus in Uganda: the predominance of infectious origin and primary management with endoscopic third ventriculostomy. *J Neurosurg*. 2005;102:1-15.

Full references can be found on Expert Consult @ www.expertconsult.com

CHAPTER 37

Pathophysiology of Subdural Hematomas

Brent O'Neill ■ Jack Wilberger ■ Adam Wilberger

Chronic subdural hematoma (CSDH) is frequently encountered in neurosurgical practice and occurs at a rate of 1 to 2 per 100,000 per year. Nonetheless, there has been ongoing debate over the fundamental pathophysiologic mechanisms of the development, evolution, and recurrence of CSDH. Virchow[1] in 1857 first described pachymeningitis haemorrhagica and ascribed the condition to dural inflammation; however, by the early 20th century, the traumatic nature of CSDH was established and widely accepted. During the subsequent century, through ultrastructural analysis of subdural membranes and various components of CSDH fluid, a complex pathophysiology has evolved.

PATHOPHYSIOLOGY OF THE DEVELOPMENT OF CHRONIC SUBDURAL HEMATOMAS

Grossly, CSDHs may vary in color from clear yellow to dark purple and in consistency from thin liquid to semisolid. A thin, often translucent inner membrane and a thicker outer membrane often encapsulate the hematoma.[2,3] The contents of the hematoma and the histology of the outer membrane have been the focus of investigation on the mechanisms by which CSDHs develop and expand.[2-6]

In 1932, Gardner first proposed the osmotic gradient theory as the predominant pathophysiology of CSDH. He postulated that the increased protein content in CSDH fluid causes ingress of fluid as a result of increased oncotic pressure.[7] Although CSDH fluid contains high levels of protein and lipid, Weir showed CSDH fluid to be isosmotic to both blood and cerebrospinal fluid.[8] Instead of an osmotic force pulling plain water into the CSDH, microscopic examination of fluid from CSDHs of any age reveals fresh erythrocytes, thus indicating that clinically silent rehemorrhage or progressive leakage of fresh blood into the CSDH is ongoing.[9,10]

The probable source of rebleeding is the CSDH membranes. These membranes consist of blood vessels, eosinophils, smooth muscle cells, fibroblasts, and myofibroblasts supported by a matrix of collagen and elastin.[4,5,11] The membranes arise from cleavage of the dural border layer, which results in dural border cells on both sides of the hematoma cavity. Some elements of both the inner and outer membranes resemble this dural border layer; however, the presence of blood vessels and eosinophils and attenuation of the remaining cells set a CSDH membrane apart.[4]

Blood vessels are absent in the normal dura-arachnoid interface. Neovasculature is abundant, but just in the outer CSDH membrane. Abnormal dilated sinusoids measuring as large as 1000 μm, with an incomplete basement membrane and attenuated endothelial cells, share the outer membrane with rapidly growing microcapillaries. Both vessel types are composed of endothelial cells with irregular surface because of numerous pseudopod-like structures extending into the vascular lumen.[6] Erythrocytes and platelets in various stages of degeneration are frequently found deposited in the perivascular space.[4,6] These sinusoids contain gap junctions as large as 8 μm, sufficient to allow leakage of plasma and even red blood cells into the hematoma cavity.[12]

Inflammatory mediators present in CSDH fluid may potentiate chronic rebleeding of the fragile neovasculature. Kallikrein, bradykinin, and platelet-activating factor (PAF) have all been identified at significant levels in CSDH fluid. These inflammatory mediators stimulate vasodilation, increase vascular permeability, prolong the clotting time, and release tissue plasminogen activator (t-PA) from endothelial cells.[13-15] Other work has focused on disturbances of the prostaglandin system (local and potentially systemic) as possible components in the pathophysiology.[16]

Eosinophil degranulation in the outer membrane may be the source of the fibrinolytic factors and inflammatory mediators causing local coagulopathy and cell destruction in the CSDH. An abundance of eosinophils in the outer membrane has been noted for decades.[17,18]

EVOLUTION OF CHRONIC SUBDURAL HEMATOMAS

As early as 1826, Bayle proposed that repeated bleeding episodes cause the ongoing expansion of CSDHs.[1] Decades of clinical experience and modern technologies—including computed tomography, magnetic resonance imaging, advanced microscopy, molecular biology techniques, and other innovations—have further supported his theory. In an early computed tomographic study, Bergström and colleagues[19] showed that acute subdural hematomas undergo a predictable loss of attenuation over time, but that some CSDHs return to high attenuation. They postulated that this change reflects an instance of sudden or chronic rebleeding as predicted by Bayle.[19]

As discussed previously, the presence of defective neovasculature certainly potentiates the process of rebleeding and absorption of plasma proteins into the subdural space, but this does not fully explain the growth of CSDHs. Normal hemostatic mechanisms should halt the process long before the CSDH reaches a clinically significant size.[15,19,20] Instead, considerable evidence supports the presence of a localized coagulopathy within the CSDH.

Labadie and Glover[21] analyzed fluid from two recurrent CSDHs. They found accelerated clot formation by the partial thromboplastin time and normal formation by the prothrombin time; however, the clots formed were structurally defective in comparison with controls. They postulated that the clots within CSDHs degrade rapidly, a supposition supported by high levels of fibrin degradation products (FDPs) and low mean plasminogen in their fluid samples.[21] FDPs inhibit coagulation, platelet aggregation, and fibrin polymerization and promote the activity of t-PA.[22]

Subsequent studies have identified lower levels of all coagulation factors in CSDH fluid than in plasma. Factors II, V, VII, VIII, and X are disproportionately depleted.[23] These findings reflect a phase of accelerated fibrinolytic activity after the rapid

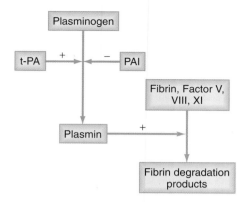

FIGURE 37-1 Mechanisms involved in the pathogenesis of chronic subdural hematoma. PAI, plasminogen activator inhibitor; t-PA, tissue plasminogen activator.

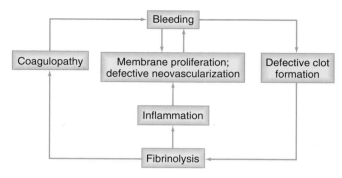

FIGURE 37-2 Defective clot formation and increased fibrinolysis contribute to rebleeding into the chronic subdural hematoma.

and defective clot formation. The end result is a milieu of anticoagulant proteins (chiefly FDPs) and depleted coagulation factors.[2,21-24]

The source of this accelerated fibrinolysis may be t-PA. t-PA transforms plasminogen into plasmin, which, in turn, degrades fibrin to fibrin split products (Fig. 37-1). Investigations by Ito and associates[25] found a threefold increase in t-PA in the outer membranes of CSDHs as opposed to the dura. Weir and Gordon[24] corroborated Ito and colleagues' work by showing increased t-PA and decreased α_2-antiplasmin (an inhibitor of plasminogen activation) in CSDH fluid.

Other authors have suggested that the PAF derived from lysis of red blood cells may stimulate the synthesis and release of t-PA, as well as induce chemotaxis of inflammatory cells to the CSDH membranes. They found increased levels of PAF in CSDH fluid and elevated plasma levels of PAF in patients with CSDH versus healthy volunteers. The latter observation may suggest a systemic predilection to the development of CSDH.[15]

In measurements of CSDH fluid from 23 patients, Lim and coworkers[22] found a correlation between the ratio of t-PA–to–plasminogen activator inhibitor (PAI) and hematoma size. These authors postulated that PAI may interrupt the hyperfibrinolysis to slow the growth of CSDHs or promote gradual spontaneous resorption.[22]

Localized coagulopathy and defective clot formation within the CSDH completes the cycle of bleeding, membrane formation, defective vascularization, fibrinolysis, coagulopathy, and rebleeding (Fig. 37-2).[3,22]

TREATMENT OF CHRONIC SUBDURAL HEMATOMAS

Surgical Therapy

Effective treatment of CSDH does not seem to require treating the underlying pathophysiology. In 1925, Putnam and Cushing[26] published an extensive work on CSDHs and advocated craniotomy with complete removal of the outer membrane and hematoma contents as the procedure of choice.[26] As noted earlier, the pathophysiology of CSDH development and evolution would appear to support such an approach; however, clinical experience has been to the contrary.

Svien and Gelety[27] reported in 1964 that CSDH patients treated by bur hole drainage had better outcomes and lower reoperation rates than did those undergoing craniotomy.[27] Tabaddor and Shulmon[28] corroborated this finding with a 1977 study comparing twist drill craniostomy, bur holes, and crani-

otomy. The craniotomy group had the highest mortality rate and poorest outcomes.[28]

More recent debate has focused on the value of irrigating the CSDH cavity. It has been proposed that washing out the coagulopathic and hyperfibrinolytic milieu of the CSDH fluid would minimize recurrence; however, at least two recent studies failed to corroborate a benefit of irrigation. Suzuki and associates[29] found closed system drainage without irrigation to be as effective as closed system drainage with irrigation.[29] Smely and coauthors[30] reported that twist drill drainage without irrigation was superior to bur hole drainage with irrigation, although other studies have shown contrary results. Thus, clinical experience would suggest that many aspects of the pathophysiology of CSDH are self-limited and need not be addressed at surgery.[3]

Medical Therapy

Medical therapy, including corticosteroids, osmotic agents, and angiotensin-converting enzyme (ACE) inhibitors, may interrupt the pathophysiology of CSDH. Eosinophils (present in the outer membranes of many CSDH specimens) have been invoked as driving the hyperfibrinolysis, vasodilation, and vascular permeability of CSDH. Corticosteroid therapy decreases leukocyte chemotaxis, inhibits degranulation, and has been shown to inhibit neomembrane formation and prevent clot enlargement in one experimental model of CSDH.[31] The membranes of patients undergoing osmotic therapy have been demonstrated on ultrastructural analysis to lack new capillary growth and have decreased vascular permeability, thus suggesting potential clinical therapeutic use of these agents.[32] In this regard, some clinical evidence supports the potential efficacy of these treatments. Bender and Christoff[33] reported a series of 97 CSDH patients with symptoms ranging from headache to stupor managed primarily with bed rest, mannitol and, later in the study, corticosteroids. In 75 cases the CSDH resolved, and only 2 of these patients had residual deficits. Twenty-two of the original 97 patients failed medical management and required surgery. The authors noted more rapid neurologic improvement after introducing corticosteroids to the treatment regimen, thereby allowing shorter hospitalization.[33]

Neovascularization is a key component of membrane formation and probably the primary source of renewed hemorrhage. Recent evidence suggests that ACE inhibitor therapy may interrupt this pathophysiology by systemically inhibiting vascular endothelial growth factor. A recent retrospective review of 438 CSDH patients found a lower percentage of hematomas in patients regularly taking ACE inhibitors than in age-matched controls, thus suggesting that ACE inhibitor therapy prevents the evolution of CSDH. They also found a statistically significant decrease in the postoperative recurrence rate (5% with ACE inhibition versus 18% without).[34] It remains to be seen whether ACE inhibitor use initiated at the time of diagnosis of CSDH has similar clinical benefit.

RECURRENCE

Reported recurrence rates of CSDH range from 2% to 37%, largely because the pathophysiologic mechanisms have not been fully elucidated. Theories range from recurrent outer membrane bleeding, to brain stiffness preventing reexpansion, to altered cerebral blood flow and its effects on reexpansion. These theories remain the subject of debate because, as noted, removal of the outer membrane is not necessary to achieve lasting CSDH resolution, and the patient population most subject to the development of CSDH tend to have atrophic, stiff brains with preexisting derangements in blood flow.[35-39]

CONCLUSION

CSDHs are prone to progressive expansion by way of episodic rebleeding and leakage of blood from fragile vessels within the membranes. The contents of a CSDH possess both coagulopathic and inflammatory properties that potentiate this expansion. Fresh blood leaked into the CSDH forms defective clot that is prone to hyperfibrinolysis, which, in turn, drives the inflammation, coagulopathy, and membrane formation. Understanding this multifactorial pathophysiology is important for optimizing treatment and minimizing recurrence.

SUGGESTED READINGS

Bender MB, Christoff N. Nonsurgical treatment of subdural hematomas. *Arch Neurol*. 1974;31:73-79.

Glover D, Labadie EL. Physiopathogenesis of subdural hematomas. Part 2: Inhibition of growth of experimental hematomas with dexamethasone. *J Neurosurg*. 1976;45:393-397.

Hirashima Y, Endo S, Kato R, et al. Platelet-activating factor (PAF) and the development of chronic subdural haematoma. *Acta Neurochir*. 1994;129:20-25.

Hirashima Y, Nagahori T, Nishijima M, et al. [Analysis of plasma and hematoma lipids related to choline glycerophospholipid in patients with chronic subdural hematoma.] *Neurol Med Chir (Tokyo)*. 1994;34:131-135.

Ito H, Komai T, Yamamoto S. Fibrinolytic enzyme in the lining walls of chronic subdural hematoma. *J Neurosurg*. 1978;48:197-200.

Ito H, Yamamoto S, Komai T, et al. Role of local hyper-fibrinolysis in the etiology of chronic subdural hematoma. *J Neurosurg*. 1976;45:26-31.

Killeffer JA, Killeffer FA, Schochet SS. The outer neomembrane of chronic subdural hematoma. *Neurosurg Clin N Am*. 2000;11:407-412.

Labadie EL, Glover D. Local alterations of hemostatic-fibrinolytic mechanisms in reforming subdural hematomas. *Neurology*. 1975;25:669-675.

Müller W, Firsching R. Significance of eosinophilic granulocytes in chronic subdural hematomas. *Neurosurg Rev*. 1990;13:305-308.

Putnam TJ, Cushing H. Chronic subdural hematoma: its pathology, its relation to pachymeningitis hemorrhagica and its surgical treatment. *Arch Surg*. 1925;11:329-393.

Stoodley M, Weir B. Contents of chronic subdural hematoma. *Neurosurg Clin N Am*. 2000;11:425-434.

Svien HJ, Gelety JE. On the surgical management of encapsulated subdural hematoma: a comparison of the results of membranectomy and simple evacuation. *J Neurosurg*. 1964;21:172-177.

Weigel R, Hohenstein A, Schlickum L, et al. Angiotensin converting enzyme inhibition for arterial hypertension reduces the risk of recurrence in patients with chronic subdural hematoma possibly by an antiangiogenic mechanism. *Neurosurgery*. 2007;61:788-793.

Weir B. The osmolality of subdural hematoma fluid. *J Neurosurg*. 1971;34:528-533.

Weir BK, Gordon P. Factors affecting coagulation, fibrinolysis in chronic subdural fluid collections. *J Neurosurg*. 1983;58:242-245.

Wilberger J. Pathophysiology of evolution and recurrence of chronic subdural hematoma. *Neurosurg Clin N Am*. 2000;11:435-438.

Yamashima T, Shimoji T, Komai T, et al. [Growing mechanism of chronic subdural hematoma: light and electron microscopic study on outer membranes of chronic subdural hematoma (authors' transl).] *Neurol Med Chir (Tokyo)*. 1978;18:734-752.

Yamashima T, Yamamoto S. How do vessels proliferate in the capsule of a chronic subdural hematoma? *Neurosurgery*. 1984;15:672-678.

Full references can be found on Expert Consult @ www.expertconsult.com

TABLE 38-3 CT Classification According to Nomura and Colleagues[111]

1 Hyperdensity
2 Isodensity
3 Hypodensity
4 Mixed density
5 Layering type

first widely available imaging modality that allowed visualization of CSDH, and neurosurgeons may be more familiar with interpretation of blood and its degradation products on CT than on MRI. Furthermore, MRI is a time-consuming and more expensive method, and it depends on a cooperative patient. In that regard, it should be considered that 18% of patients with CSDH have neuropsychiatric deficits when CSDH is diagnosed. Up to 15% of patients are comatose and need intensive care equipment,[62] which often is not compatible with the high magnetic fields of MRI scanners.

In the majority of cases, CSDH appears hyperintense on T2-weighted (Fig. 38-6A) or proton-weighted images because blood degradation products, especially methemoglobin, give a hyperintense signal on such images. The variability in signal intensity is greater on T1-weighted images. Although nearly 50% of CSDH images appear hyperintense (Fig. 38-6B), hypointense, isointense, and mixed intensities are also seen in CSDH. Hypointense or isointense signals were interpreted as fresh rebleeding into the cavity.[123] Therefore, it is not surprising that the recurrence rate is higher with the latter than with high-intensity hematomas on T1-weighted images. The inner architecture of CSDH noted on MRI suggests similarities with the findings on CT, but no correlation was found between the appearance in the two different techniques.[109] Hematomas with low density, isodensity, and mixed density on CT may all appear as homogeneous hyperintense lesions on MRI.

CSF is characterized by a hypointense signal on proton-weighted images. Subdural fluid collections with low intensity on proton-weighted images may therefore be lesions other than CSDH.[109] Because subdural hygroma is an important differential diagnosis, MRI can provide elementary information to differentiate both entities.

Other Imaging Modalities

The use of positron emission tomography,[125] single-photon emission computed tomography,[126] and xenon-enhanced CT[95] is reserved for scientific purposes. To date, these methods have limited influence in individual decision making.

CONTEMPORARY TREATMENT

The approach to management of patients with CSDH ranges from a simple "watch and wait" strategy to large craniotomies with marsupialization of hematoma membranes.[5] Pharmaceutical treatment was suggested in the past.[103,127,128] Spontaneous

TABLE 38-4 CT Classification According to Naganuma and Colleagues[112]

1 Homogeneous density
2 Laminar type
3 Layering or separated type
4 Trabecular density type

resolution of CSDH occurs only rarely.[112] Scientific reports on successful nonsurgical treatment of CSDH are also rare and date back to the 1960s and 1970s. The results are controversial and in reality cannot be construed as providing an alternative to surgical treatment. Conservative treatment has thus far included corticosteroids and bed rest. Glover and Labadie demonstrated a reduced rate of membrane formation in an animal model with corticosteroid treatment.[129] The effect of dexamethasone was thought to be anti-inflammatory[129] or antiangiogenic.[130] Another approach included long-term application of mannitol and bed rest.[131] The promising results of a pilot study, however, could not be reproduced in a randomized investigation because the side effects of long-term immobilization became more prominent in elderly patients.[132] No parameters were defined in the past that might help decide in favor of a nonsurgical approach. It is common sense to carefully monitor asymptomatic patients in whom the presence of CSDH was proved by CT or MRI. Once clinical symptoms develop, however, surgical management is mandatory in the majority of cases.

New pathophysiologic aspects might have an impact on conservative treatment in the future. In particular, detection of the angiogenic cytokines responsible for development of the well-known leaky vessels within the outer membrane of a hematoma might offer new and promising targets to be blocked by pharmacologic agents. Recently, it was shown that the antiangiogenic properties of angiotensin-converting enzyme inhibitors could reduce the rate of recurrences in CSDH, as well as levels of vascular endothelial growth factor within the hematoma.[133] Prospective trials with other antiangiogenic substances are under way.

An important issue in the perioperative and postoperative management of patients with CSDH is the question of whether anticonvulsive prophylaxis should be administered. The literature on this topic does not provide any guidelines. As a consequence, a Cochrane review came to the conclusion that because of the controversial findings in mainly retrospective studies, no formal recommendation could be given.[100] Detailed data on the frequency of early or late seizures caused by CSDH are not available to date. However, posttraumatic or postoperative epilepsy is thought to have a low incidence in patients with CSDH.[134] In a retrospective analysis of their own patient data and data obtained from a literature survey, Rubin and Rappaport found a 5.6% incidence of preoperative seizures versus 3% in the literature and a 4.3% incidence of postoperative seizures versus 1.8% in the literature.[101] This is in accordance with a generally low standardized incidence ratio of between 1.5 and 2.8 for epilepsy in patients with mild head injury.[135] From a pathophysiologic point of view, epileptic foci develop mainly from cortical injuries.[136] Subdural hematoma in the chronic state, however, is an exclusively extracerebral lesion in the majority of cases. Pathoanatomically, a fibrous visceral membrane separates potentially epileptogenic blood degradation products within the hematoma from the cerebral cortex.[101] Presumably, a higher risk for seizures might exist in cases in which the inner membrane was opened during surgery. Other risk factors are alcohol abuse and age older than 65 years.[101,135]

Patient posture in the early days after surgery was also thought to influence the rate of recurrence. In the first prospective study no difference was found with regard to recurrence and outcome.[137] A recent randomized controlled trial, however, found an increased incidence of CSDH recurrence when patients did not maintain a flat position in the first 3 days after surgery. The number of adverse events caused by the flat position was equal in both groups. No effect on final outcome was demonstrated.[138]

Postoperative reexpansion of the brain was found early on to be a factor associated with recurrence and hence considered to influence outcome. Generous hydration of patients with intravenous fluids postoperatively was thought to increase the brain's volume and decrease the risk for recurrence. However, attention

FIGURE 38-6 A, T2-weighted axial magnetic resonance image of a left-sided chronic subdural hematoma. There is only limited compression of the left ventricle despite considerable thickness of the hematoma. The hematoma appears hyperintense but has signal inhomogeneity, which might indicate different stages of blood degradation. The subarachnoidal space is still present. A small contralateral hematoma is also demonstrated. **B,** T1-weighted coronal magnetic resonance image of the same patient. The hematoma appears homogeneously hyperintense.

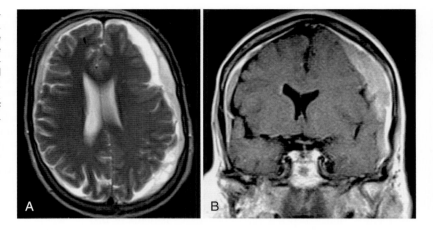

must be paid to elderly patients because postoperative hyperemia in areas of cortex that were covered by hematoma was demonstrated in up to 41% of patients older than 75 years after rapid decompression of CSDH.[139] Hyperemia might be one reason for postoperative subcortical hemorrhage[140-145] or postoperative hyperperfusion syndrome in agitated or delirious patients.[126]

Surgical Treatment

Surgical treatment of CSDH in symptomatic patients is still the "gold standard" of therapy because it allows immediate decompression of the space-occupying lesion and significantly improves outcome.[106] However, a standardized approach to the treatment of CSDH does not exist,[5] in part because of the fact that until recently, the advances in determining the pathophysiology of CSDH discussed earlier were of little practical relevance for treatment.

CSDH is still one of the most frequent problems encountered in neurosurgery. The progress in its surgical treatment is not comparable, however, to the sophisticated development of treatment concepts and surgical techniques in other subspecialities of neurosurgery, such as functional, spinal, or vascular neurosurgery. Unfortunately, even in light of the relatively frequent occurrence of unilateral and bilateral CSDH, there has been no definitive study or studies to define the best primary treatment. The number of randomized controlled trials on topics concerning CSDH has increased since the beginning of the 21th century, but there is still a surprisingly low level of scientific evidence for the different surgical approaches used for the treatment of CSDH.[5] All these studies report successful resolution of hematomas, albeit in a varying number of cases, and there are two possible explanations. First, resolution of hematomas occurs independently of the treatment chosen. Second, CSDH is not a uniform entity, and different manifestations of the disease might demand different approaches. If the latter is true, it offers the possibility of tailoring treatment to an individual patient. One challenge, therefore, is to characterize individual cases according to relevant parameters.

Parameters identified thus far aim at predicting risk for recurrence and complications. Both risks were appreciated by the appearance of CSDH on cross-sectional images. However, to date, the specificity of parameters is not high enough to allow more precise prediction of outcome or to tailor treatment on the basis of these parameters. Furthermore, to the best of our knowledge, no study has compared different approaches for different appearances of CSDH on cross-sectional imaging. Moreover, the very definition of recurrence may vary substantially from site to site. For example, Torihashi and colleagues defined a recurrent

CSDH as one in which the increased hematoma volume resulted in a neurological deficit.[146] Many neurosurgeons would intervene earlier for recurrence, before the development of a neurological deficit, if the patient suffered severe and progressive headache, which correlates with reaccumulation of fluid and a mass effect in the subdural space. Finally, the issue of recurrence cannot be considered in an isolated fashion. One must also consider the complication rate and morbidity associated with the various treatments, and given the lack of large controlled studies, this is quite difficult. We have therefore tried to treat the problem according to the principles of evidence-based medicine while always keeping in mind that such medicine is not "cookbook medicine"[147] and what appears to be the best treatment for a patient population is not necessarily the best option for an individual patient.

A systematic review of 48 publications from the MEDLINE database and from reference lists was conducted. The articles were written in English or German. Pediatric series and series with more than 10% of patients lost to follow-up were not included. The articles were classified as providing class I, class II, or class III evidence according to the criteria of the American Academy of Neurology.[148] The various surgical treatment options are summarized in Table 38-5 and range from single-needle trephination without intraoperative irrigation or postoperative drainage to large craniotomies with marsupialization of the membranes.[55,58-61,105,148-187] No study met the criteria for class I evidence, and six studies provided class II evidence. For analysis and comparison of results, the following uniform criteria were defined: morbidity—any complication during or after surgery other than recurrence; mortality—any death reported between surgery and discharge from the hospital; recurrence—clinical or radiologic deterioration requiring further surgery; and cure—complete patient autonomy after surgery (grade 0 or 1 in the classification of Markwalder and associates[116] or Bender and Christoff[103] and grade 5 in the Glasgow Outcome Scale).[188] Morbidity and mortality can be considered as a measure of the safety of a procedure, whereas the cure rate reflects the efficiency of a particular surgical method.

As with other analyses on topics such as unruptured aneurysms[189] or Parkinson's disease,[148] there are several methodologic problems inherent in such types of systematic review. Publication bias is related to the arbitrary selection of language and by primarily selecting manuscripts from a database such as MEDLINE, which yields papers that are more likely to report on positive results. Furthermore, the lack of any studies providing class I evidence and the paucity of studies providing class II evidence preclude the application of statistical procedures for meta-analysis. In the following section we briefly summarize the results

TABLE 38-5 Overview of Contemporary Neurosurgical Treatment Options for Chronic Subdural Hematoma in the Elderly

			NO. OF STUDIES (REFERENCES)
Craniotomy	Irrigation	Drainage	6 (55, 58, 61, 149-151)
Craniotomy	No irrigation	No drainage	4 (149, 152-154)
Bur hole	No irrigation	No drainage	2 (149, 155)
Bur hole	Irrigation	No drainage	7 (109, 153, 156-160)
Bur hole	No irrigation	Drainage	4 (149, 154, 161, 162)
Bur hole	Irrigation	Drainage	28 (55, 58, 59, 61, 105, 109, 116, 150, 151, 162-180)
Bur hole, drainage, continuous inflow and outflow irrigation			2 (58, 172)
Twist drill	No irrigation	No drainage	2 (60, 181)
Twist drill	No irrigation	Drainage	4 (174, 182-184)
Bur hole and CO_2			1 (185)
Twist drill and O_2			1 (186)
Endoscopy			1 (187)
Subdural-peritoneal shunt			1 (152)

of our analysis and provide "the best available external clinical evidence from systematic research."[147]

Surgical Approach

The principal techniques used for the treatment of CSDH at present are TDC (up to a diameter of 5 mm),[60,174,181-184,186] BHC or enlarged BHC (between 5 and 30 mm in diameter),* and craniotomy (larger than 30 mm in diameter).[55,58,61,147,150-154] The term *craniostomy* is an artificial descriptive term that was established in the past. It underlines the miniaturization of the surgical approach. Additional measures such as intraoperative irrigation and postoperative drainage increase the number of neurosurgical treatment options. During the search for reduction of recurrence rates it was also suggested that the hematoma cavity be filled with 100% oxygen[186] or carbon dioxide.[185] In single studies, subdural-peritoneal shunting was used.[152] Recurrent hematomas were successfully treated via BHC under endoscopic guidance.[187] The variety of strategies reflects the dilemma of the search for the optimal procedure (see Table 38-5).

No significant difference in mortality rates was found with the three principal techniques (Fig. 38-7). Craniotomy was burdened with the highest morbidity rate (12.3%), but it is conceivable that selection bias may have resulted in a somewhat distorted picture of the morbidity of craniotomy inasmuch as series involving primary craniotomy in general included patients who were presumed to be at higher risk for recurrence or who had less satisfactory performance preoperatively.[150-153]

The three principal techniques also do not differ significantly in cure rates. BHC and craniotomy are the most efficacious techniques and provide the lowest recurrence rates. Thus, it can be concluded that BHC shares the advantages of TDC, a high cure rate and safety, and the advantage of primary craniotomy, high efficiency. These results were supported by a recently published series that directly compared BHC and TDC in 62 patients. The authors demonstrated the superiority of BHC in terms of postoperative computed tomographic findings and the number of recurrences (7% versus 64%).[190] TDC and BHC can be performed under local anesthesia, but a cooperative patient is mandatory. Implementation of rigid fixation of the head during

craniotomy for recurrent CSDH strongly favors performing the operation under general anesthesia. The number of bur holes needed to drain CSDH successfully is still a matter of debate. Although many CSDHs appear to be loculated on CT, it was demonstrated with fiberoptic endoscopy that communication exists in the majority of cases.[187,191] A recent publication based on retrospective data, however, found a negative correlation between the number of bur holes and the rate of recurrence.[192]

Irrigation

The purpose of irrigation is to remove the hematoma completely or at least dilute its contents. Only a few articles allowed comparison of the results of patients treated with irrigation or without irrigation. Irrigation in conjunction with bur-hole techniques did not demonstrate a significant reduction in the recurrence rate.[162,169,177] In TDC, however, irrigation resulted in a significant decrease in recurrences.[181] Although often stated, the rate of infection was not increased with the use of irrigation.[5]

Two papers reported on the use of continuous inflow and outflow irrigation after surgical decompression of CSDH. Both described fewer recurrences with postoperative irrigation; however, a significant difference was seen in one publication only because of the small number of recurrences in the other paper.[58,172]

Drainage

The most convincing data on the treatment of CSDH refer to the use of a drain after BHC. Four of six studies with class II evidence were concerned with the question of whether drainage systems should be used; they highlighted different aspects of drainage systems. The use of a drain after BHC significantly reduced the number of recurrences.[178] One series reported faster recovery in patients treated with a closed system drainage, but ultimate outcome per se was not affected.[158] A frontal position of the drain was correlated with a reduced rate of recurrence.[171] Postoperative drainage volume less than 200 mL was associated with a higher recurrence rate, thus supporting the concept of a beneficial effect of total or subtotal evacuation of the hematoma.[168] One recently published paper on a consecutive series of 500 patients with subacute subdural hematoma or CSDH confirmed that recurrences were avoided when drains were used.[193]

*See references 55, 58, 59, 61, 105, 109, 149-151, 153-174, 176-180, 185.

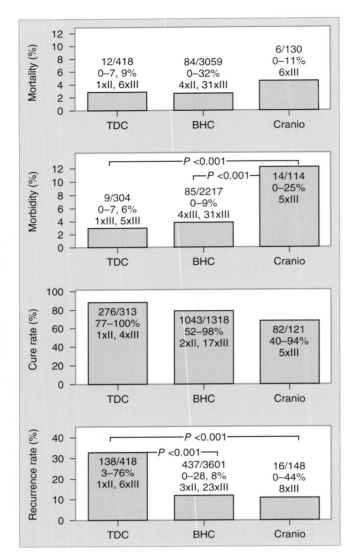

FIGURE 38-7 Comparison of the three principal surgical techniques for the treatment of CSDH. Mortality, morbidity, cure rate, and recurrence rate are compared for twist drill craniostomy (TDC), bur-hole craniostomy (BHC), and craniotomy (Cranio). The columns show the relative percentage of summarized data of corresponding treatment groups from different publications. The legends in the columns show absolute numbers, the range of relative values, and the number of studies that provided statistical data with their classes of evidence. *(Adapted from Weigel R, Schmiedek P, Krauss JK. Outcome of contemporary surgery for chronic subdural haematoma: evidence based review. J Neurol Neurosurg Psychiatry. 2003;74:937.)*

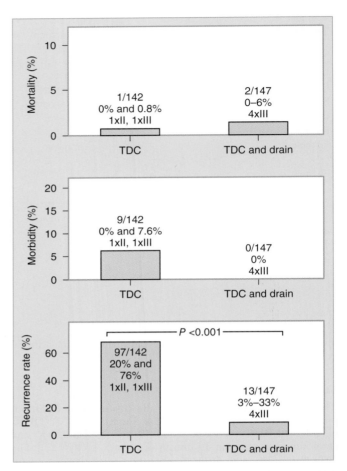

FIGURE 38-8 Effect of drainage in twist drill craniostomy (TDC). The figure compares mortality, morbidity, and the recurrence rate for simple TDC and TDC with drainage. The columns show the relative percentage of summarized data of corresponding treatment groups from different publications. The absolute numbers are shown in the legend within the columns. In addition, the range of relative values and the number of studies that provided statistical data are listed with their classes of evidence. *(Adapted from Weigel R, Schmiedek P, Krauss JK. Outcome of contemporary surgery for chronic subdural haematoma: evidence based review. J Neurol Neurosurg Psychiatry. 2003;74:937.)*

successful in 106 of 151 recurrences (70%). In 35 patients, a bur-hole procedure was chosen for reoperation (23%), and in 10 patients (7%) a craniotomy was the most useful procedure. For BHC, data on recurrences from 20 publications were available.* A total of 190 of 229 patients (83%) were successfully treated by the same procedure as previously, and 32 patients (14%) underwent craniotomy. Three patients died (1.3%). It seems that BHC is more effective than TDC in treating recurrent hematoma. Craniotomy is considered the treatment of last choice. Occasionally, interventional techniques were used in which the blood supply of the outer membrane was reduced by embolization of the middle meningeal artery.[83]

Pragmatic Recommendations for Surgery

In our personal experience with more than 500 treated cases of CSDH (JKK; RW), one bur hole most frequently sufficed to treat CSDH in the majority of cases (see Fig. 38-5A to D). An alterna-

With TDC the situation is less clear. Because we found no data on direct comparison of TDC alone and TDC with drainage, we pooled the available data from six publications.[60,174,182-184,194] There was a significant reduction in recurrences with closed system drainage (Fig. 38-8).

Treatment of Recurrences

A major concern is determining the best possible treatment of recurrence and how one can reduce the risk for recurrence, perhaps by altering the primary treatment used. Detailed information on recurrence after TDC was available from seven publications.[60,174,182-184,186,194] Repeating TDC once or twice was

---

*See references 59, 61, 116, 150, 153, 156, 158, 160, 163, 164, 166, 167, 172, 174, 175, 178-180, 187, 195.

tive is to place two bur holes just a few centimeters apart. We use a ventricular catheter to irrigate the cavity with warm saline in all directions until clear fluid exits. Several strategies can be used to minimize the amount of intracranial air after surgery. Some recommend that the patient's head be fixed so that the bur hole is located at the highest point and that the cavity be filled with saline before closing the wound. Others work with a drain located frontally and another located occipitally. The cavity is filled through the occipital drain after closing the wound tightly until no more air leaves the cavity through the frontal drain. After this maneuver the occipital drain can be removed, and the frontal drain is left in place for at least 3 days. While removing the drain, special care must be taken to avoid entrance of air into the cavity. In bilateral hematomas, it might be useful to connect both drains to only one reservoir to avoid a major pressure gradient between both sides, which can lead to a devastating midline shift. Continuous large drainage volumes do not argue against removing a drain. Theoretical considerations show that 7% of hematoma fluid is renewed every day[196] from an average volume of 90 mL.[110] Drainage volumes of greater than 50 mL/day are seen frequently, which argues for tearing of the inner membrane to allow CSF to escape via the drain.

Residual fluid within the subdural space on early postoperative CT is common and disappears on follow-up examinations in the majority of patients. In cases in which the hematoma increases and causes neurological deterioration or persistent or progressive headache, repeated treatment is recommended. Comparison of the architecture of the hematoma on follow-up CT with the preoperative appearance helps in deciding whether a second bur hole is useful. Reaccumulation of hematoma is commonly seen after TDC and seems to be the price for miniaturization of surgery. For practical purposes, a hierarchical treatment algorithm is suggested in which recurrence after TDC is decompressed via one or two bur holes. Recurrence after single–bur-hole surgery might require a second bur hole. Multiple recurrences are treated by craniotomy with careful and meticulous membrane stripping. Shunting of re-recurrent hematoma might be an alternative treatment option.

FUTURE PERSPECTIVES

It remains to be seen whether angiogenic activity inside the hematoma cavity and its surrounding tissue is just an epiphenomenon or is relevant to hematoma enlargement. If so, the armamentarium for treatment could be enhanced by the use of antiangiogenic therapy. Nevertheless, surgery will always be the first-line treatment option in cases in which immediate decompression is mandatory. Therefore, it might be useful to define parameters that allow the extent of surgery to be tailored to the individual patient.

In view of the surgical preferences of individual surgeons, the likelihood that a multicenter randomized trial will be successfully carried out seems low. Consequently, it is likely that we will continue to rely on either meta-analysis or retrospective single-center studies.

SUGGESTED READINGS

Bender MB, Christoff N. Nonsurgical treatment of subdural hematomas. *Arch Neurol.* 1974;31:73.

Benzel EC, Bridges RM Jr, Hadden TA, et al. The single burr hole technique for the evacuation of non-acute subdural hematomas. *J Trauma.* 1994;36:190.

Chen JC, Levy ML. Causes, epidemiology, and risk factors of chronic subdural hematoma. *Neurosurg Clin N Am.* 2000;11:399.

Friede RL, Schachenmayr W. The origin of subdural neomembranes II. Fine structure of neomembranes. *Am J Pathol.* 1978;92:69.

Glover D, Labadie EL. Physiopathogenesis of subdural hematomas. Part 2: Inhibition of growth of experimental hematomas with dexamethasone. *J Neurosurg.* 1976;45:393.

Hamilton MG, Frizzell JB, Tranmer BI. Chronic subdural hematoma: the role for craniotomy reevaluated. *Neurosurgery.* 1993;33:67.

Heckmann JG, Ganslandt O. Images in clinical medicine. The Mount Fuji sign. *N Engl J Med.* 2004;350:1881.

Hohenstein A, Erber R, Schilling L, et al. Increased mRNA expression of VEGF within the hematoma and imbalance of angiopoietin-1 and -2 mRNA within the neomembranes of chronic subdural hematoma. *J Neurotrauma.* 2005;22:518.

Hosoda K, Tamaki N, Masumura M, et al. Magnetic resonance images of chronic subdural hematomas. *J Neurosurg.* 1987;67:677.

Ito H, Yamamoto S, Saito K, et al. Quantitative estimation of hemorrhage in chronic subdural hematoma using the ^{51}Cr erythrocyte labeling method. *J Neurosurg.* 1987;66:862.

Lee KS, Bae WK, Doh JW, et al. Origin of chronic subdural haematoma and relation to traumatic subdural lesions. *Brain Inj.* 1998;12:901.

Loew F, Kivelitz R. Chronic subdural hematomas. In: Vinken PJ, Bruyn GW, eds. *Handbook of Clinical Neurology.* vol 24, part 2. Amsterdam: North Holland Publishing Company; 1976:297.

Markwalder TM. Chronic subdural hematomas: a review. *J Neurosurg.* 1981;54:637.

Nakaguchi H, Tanishima T, Yoshimasu N. Factors in the natural history of chronic subdural hematomas that influence their postoperative recurrence. *J Neurosurg.* 2001;95:256.

Rubin G, Rappaport ZH. Epilepsy in chronic subdural haematoma. *Acta Neurochir (Wien).* 1993;123:39.

Sambasivan M. An overview of chronic subdural hematoma: experience with 2300 cases. *Surg Neurol.* 1997;47:418.

Stroobandt G, Fransen P, Thauvoy C, et al. Pathogenetic factors in chronic subdural haematoma and causes of recurrence after drainage. *Acta Neurochir (Wien).* 1995;137:6.

Tabaddor K, Shulmon K. Definitive treatment of chronic subdural hematoma by twist-drill craniostomy and closed-system drainage. *J Neurosurg.* 1977;46:220.

Tokmak M, Iplikcioglu AC, Bek S, et al. The role of exudation in chronic subdural hematomas. *J Neurosurg.* 2007;107:290.

Virchow R. Das Hämatom der Dura mater. *Verh Phys Med Ges Würzburg.* 1857;7:134.

Wakai S, Hashimoto K, Watanabe N, et al. Efficacy of closed-system drainage in treating chronic subdural hematoma: a prospective comparative study. *Neurosurgery.* 1990;26:771.

Weigel R, Hohenstein A, Schlickum L, et al. Angiotensin converting enzyme inhibition for arterial hypertension reduces the risk of recurrence in patients with chronic subdural hematoma probably by an angiogenic mechanism. *Neurosurgery* 2007;61:788.

Weigel R, Schmiedek P, Krauss JK. Outcome of contemporary surgery for chronic subdural haematoma: evidence based review. *J Neurol Neurosurg Psychiatry.* 2003;74:937.

Full references can be found on Expert Consult @ www.expertconsult.com

PART 4

Infection

CHAPTER 39

Basic Science of Central Nervous System Infections

Jeffrey M. Tessier ■ W. Michael Scheld

The central nervous system (CNS) is protected from infections by a wide variety of pathogens by virtue of the blood-brain barrier (BBB), humoral immune factors, and resident and circulating immune cells. *Neurotropic* pathogens possess specific features that allow them to overcome these protective mechanisms, invade the CNS, and cause disease (e.g., *Streptococcus pneumoniae*). *Opportunistic* pathogens are organisms that are normally unable to invade the CNS independently but may cause an infection when the protective mechanisms are impaired (e.g., *Staphylococcus epidermidis*). Infections of the CNS by these broad categories of pathogens are not mutually exclusive, but a discussion based on these categories illustrates the important features of host-pathogen interactions relevant to CNS infections.

ROUTES OF CENTRAL NERVOUS SYSTEM INFECTION, OR "IT'S NOT WHO YOU KNOW, IT'S HOW YOU GET THERE"

A basic tenet of infectious disease pathogenesis is coined "the route of infection," which is a major determinant in the development of all infections, including those of the CNS. The principle is simple: the host has a finite number of entry points for pathogenic organisms, some naturally present and some introduced iatrogenically. Those naturally present are predominantly mucosal surfaces such as the nasopharynx, respiratory tree, and gastrointestinal tract, but also included is the cutaneous barrier; entry through this structure is usually via minor damage to the watertight epidermis. Iatrogenic routes are more relevant to the neurosurgeon for obvious reasons. These routes include perioperative breeches in structural barriers protecting the CNS (scalp, cranium, meninges), implantation of foreign bodies (e.g., cerebrospinal fluid [CSF] shunts, dural implants, electrodes, spinal hardware), and breeches in mucosal defenses (e.g., intubation, intravenous or intra-arterial catheterization, urinary catheterization, stress ulceration in the gastrointestinal tract). Alterations involving mucosal barriers are a common route for pathogens to enter the CNS and cause infection. Pathogens using mucosal routes gain *indirect* entry into the CNS by hematogenous spread or *direct* entry via contiguous anatomic structures such as the cranial nerves, penetrating veins, or sinus structures. Generally, direct routes into the CNS bypass the BBB, thus circumventing a major defense against infection in the CNS, whereas indirect routes (e.g., hematogenous spread) involve pathogens that must find pathways through or around the BBB to gain entry into the CNS.

ROLE OF THE BLOOD-BRAIN BARRIER IN CENTRAL NERVOUS SYSTEM INFECTIONS

The BBB is generally composed of the blood-parenchyma barrier and the blood-CSF (or blood-ependymal) barrier, both referred to here collectively as the BBB. The structural and functional properties of the BBB are addressed in more detail elsewhere in this textbook, but several salient features pertaining to infection and the BBB are highlighted here.

The BBB is composed of a specialized layer of microvascular endothelial cells, pericytes, and astrocyte foot processes (or ependymal cells in the case of the blood-ependymal barrier). Brain microvascular endothelial cells (BMECs) form monolayers with high transendothelial electrical resistance and highly selective macromolecular permeability, properties largely attributable to two features: (1) the formation of highly organized intercellular tight junctions and (2) a low rate of transcytosis relative to other endothelial subtypes.[1] These features restrict the movement of pathogens from the intravascular space across the BBB into the brain parenchyma or CSF. However, many pathogens have developed strategies to cross the BBB despite these elaborate defenses. Three major pathways are used by pathogens to gain entry to the CNS across the BBB: (1) transcellular passage (e.g., *Escherichia coli*, group B streptococci [GBS]), (2) paracellular passage (e.g., protozoa), and (3) carriage within a transmigrating leukocyte, known as the "Trojan horse" mechanism (e.g., *Listeria monocytogenes*, *Streptococcus suis*, *Mycobacterium tuberculosis*, human immunodeficiency virus [HIV]). Most of these pathways across the BBB are poorly characterized for the vast majority of pathogens associated with CNS infection. Among the best characterized CNS-invasive pathogens with respect to passage across the BBB is *E. coli*. The following section discusses mechanisms involved in *E. coli* traversal of the BBB to highlight the complex interactions occurring between host and pathogen during the early stages of CNS infection. Additionally, established features of GBS passage across the BBB are highlighted to broaden the scope of mechanisms reviewed here.

Escherichia coli at the Blood-Brain Barrier Interface

E. coli is a gram-negative bacterium implicated in the majority of cases of neonatal meningitis. In vitro studies of infection of human brain microvascular endothelial cells (HBMECs) by *E. coli*

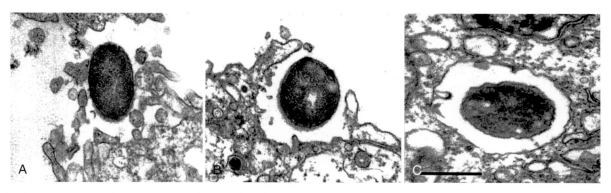

FIGURE 39-1 Transmission electron micrographs of *Escherichia coli* K1 strain RS 218 undergoing attachment (**A**) and internalization (**B** and **C**) into human brain microvascular endothelial cells. Scale bar, 1 μm. *(From Kim KS. Microbial translocation of the blood-brain barrier. Int J Parasitol. 2006;36:610.)*

K1, an encapsulated strain responsible for most cases of neonatal meningitis, have shown that *E. coli* K1 interacts with these cells in a unique manner involving both host- and pathogen-specific structures and signaling pathways. These interactions lead to alterations in the host actin cytoskeleton, membrane protrusion and ruffling around bacteria, and endocytosis of bacteria into membrane-bound vacuoles, where bacterial determinants act to prevent lysosome fusion and influence intracellular vacuole trafficking to achieve transcytotic passage.[2] Several bacterial determinants have been identified as part of the initial binding and invasion of HBMECs, including type 1 fimbriae, outer membrane protein A (OmpA), Ibe proteins, and cytotoxic necrotizing factor-1 (CNF-1).[2] Type 1 fimbriae are adhesins that bind to α-D-mannosides on the surface of host cells, thereby allowing binding and interaction of the bacterium with the host cell. Type 1 fimbriae have been shown to play an important role in the binding of *E. coli* K1 to HBMECs; deletion of *fimH*, the gene for the major adhesin protein of type 1 fimbriae, significantly decreases binding of *E. coli* K1 to HBMECs, a finding that is reversed by genetic complementation of *fimH* in deletion mutants.[3] OmpA also facilitates binding of *E. coli* K1 to HBMECs via interaction with surface glycoproteins containing *N*-acetyl-glucosamine residues.[4] In vivo studies using an experimental neonatal rat model of meningitis have shown that deletion mutants of *ompA* are impaired in their ability to enter the CNS in comparison to the parent K1 strain, and *N*-acetylglucosamine oligosaccharides are able to block penetration of the CNS by wild-type *E. coli* K1 in the same animal model.[5]

Once binding has occurred, the process of cellular invasion must take place for *E. coli* K1 to ultimately infect the CNS. Invasion of HBMECs is dependent on the host actin cytoskeleton; *E. coli* K1 invasion can be completely inhibited in vitro by using inhibitors of the actin cytoskeleton such as cytochalasin D.[6] Entry of *E. coli* K1 into membrane-bound vacuoles in HBMECs involves the formation of membrane projections, described as zipper-like structures, and subsequent membrane ruffling before internalization (Fig. 39-1).[7] These events are related to several important signal transduction pathways in the host cell known to be involved in the regulation of endocytosis, cell membrane interactions, and the actin cytoskeleton. In particular, *E. coli* K1 leads to activation of focal adhesion kinase (FAK) and phosphorylation of paxillin, a cytoskeletal protein that interacts with and regulates the actin cytoskeleton.[8] The exact mechanisms underlying FAK activation by *E. coli* K1 are unknown but appear to play a role in HBMEC invasion because overexpression of a dominant-negative form of FAK significantly inhibits HBMEC invasion by *E. coli* K1.[8]

Another important signal pathway involved in *E. coli* K1 invasion of HBMECs is the family of phosphatidylinositol-3′-kinases (PI3Ks), which lie downstream of FAK activation. Pharmacologic inhibition of PI3Ks with LY-294002 significantly limits HBMEC invasion by *E. coli* K1.[9] Akt/protein kinase B, a downstream effector of PI3K, is increased during *E. coli* K1 invasion of HBMECs.[9] These observations indicate a role for the PI3K/Akt pathway in *E. coli* invasion of HBMECs, although the exact roles that these kinases play in the process have yet to be described.

Rho family guanosine triphosphatases (GTPases) have been shown to regulate a diverse array of processes that affect the actin cytoskeleton, cell motility, and cell-cell/cell-matrix interactions.[10] *E. coli* strains associated with urinary tract infections and meningitis have been shown to produce CNF-1, an AB-type toxin with deaminase activity that targets this family of GTPases.[11] CNF-1 activates Rho GTPases and increases the in vitro uptake of bacteria by nonprofessional phagocytes such as epithelial and endothelial cells.[11] Deletion of the *cnf1* gene from *E. coli* K1 significantly decreases the invasion of HBMECs, and this deletion is associated with decreased activation of RhoA and Cdc42, GTPases that are activated during *E. coli* K1 invasion of these cells.[11]

Once *E. coli* K1 bacteria have been internalized in membrane-bound vacuoles within HBMECs, these organisms must survive the internal hostile milieu and avoid destruction in the lysosome to gain entry into the CNS. The K1 capsule appears to play a very important role in preventing the normal maturation of endosomes and fusion of vacuoles with the lysosome. K1 isogenic deletion mutants (K1⁻) have been shown to traffic through the endosomal system and colocalize with cathepsin D, thus confirming fusion of the lysosome with the vacuoles containing these bacteria.[12] The exact mechanisms underlying the K1 capsular effect on endosomal trafficking have yet to be elucidated, however.

In summary, a neuroinvasive strain of *E. coli* uses specific tools to gain entry into the CNS by binding/uptake into HBMECs and subsequent diversion of the normal protective trafficking of endosomal compartments to the lysosome (Fig. 39-2). These events allow *E. coli* K1 strains to cross the highly selective BBB and cause meningitis. The next section reviews the most recent information pertaining to crossing the BBB by GBS, gram-positive bacteria that remain a prominent cause of sepsis and meningitis in neonates and infants.

Group B Streptococci: If You Can't Beat Them, Join Them

GBS (i.e., *Streptococcus agalactiae*) are highly effective at colonizing the human female genitourinary tract and are responsible for significant morbidity and mortality in neonates and infants, predominantly in the form of pneumonia, sepsis, and meningitis.

FIGURE 39-2 Summary diagram of *Escherichia coli* K1 binding and invasion of the blood-brain barrier. CNF-1, cytotoxic necrotizing factor-1; FAK, focal adhesion kinase; GTPase, guanosine triphosphatase; OmpA, outer membrane protein A; PI3K, phosphatidylinositol-3′-kinase.

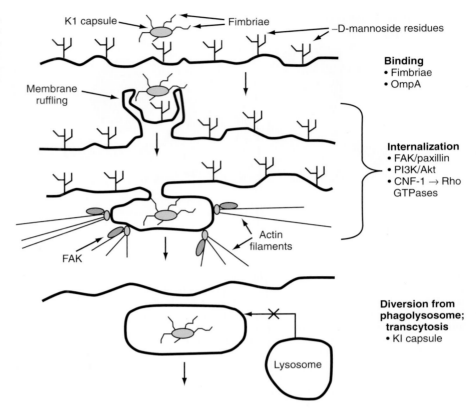

GBS use both similar and different strategies to gain entry into the CNS when compared with *E. coli* K1; these strategies are discussed here to highlight the diversity of virulence factors and pathogenic mechanisms used by neuroinvasive pathogens.

Like *E. coli* K1 strains, GBS express a polysaccharide capsule that serves many functions in the process of host invasion, including protection from opsonization, complement-mediated lysis, antibody-mediated clearance, and phagocytosis.[13] Nine distinct GBS capsular serotypes have been identified, with serotype III strains dominating the clinical isolates associated with meningitis.[13] Virulent strains of GBS have terminal sialic acid residues coating the surface of the polysaccharide capsule; GBS strains lacking these residues are less virulent than isogenic counterparts carrying these sialic acid groups.[14] Many host glycoproteins have the same terminal sialic acid residues ($\alpha 2 \rightarrow \alpha 3$ *N*-acetylneuraminic acid), so the presence of these residues on the GBS capsule may provide the bacterium with some protection from immune surveillance via molecular mimicry.[13] These residues also inhibit activation of the alternative complement pathway, thus preventing opsonophagocytosis of GBS.[13]

Like *E. coli* K1, GBS must bind to the luminal surface of BMECs to initiate invasion of the CNS. Importantly, GBS are able to bind to several components of the extracellular matrix, including fibrinogen, laminin, and immobilized but insoluble fibronectin. ScpB, a C5 peptidase anchored in the GBS membrane, has been identified as a selective fibronectin-binding protein that differentially associates with bound fibronectin.[13] FbsA is a surface-anchored protein that binds fibrinogen, and the gene *fbsA* is regulated by RogB, a transcriptional regulator that positively regulates several genes involved in binding to the extracellular matrix.[13]

Recently, GBS pili have been shown to play a role in GBS interactions with HBMECs, and targeted deletion of the gene for the pilus accessory surface protein PilA significantly reduces the ability of GBS to adhere to HBMECs, whereas deletion of *pilB*, the gene encoding the major pilus structural protein, does not affect adherence but significantly reduces HBMEC invasion by GBS.[15]

The dissociation of adherence and invasion observed with the pili mutants just described supports the hypothesis that these events, adherence and invasion, are mediated by distinct virulence factors expressed by GBS. Other invasion mediators that have been identified for GBS and HBMECs include a gene involved in modification of lipoteichoic acid (LTA), expression of a β-hemolysin/cytolysin, and factors that alter host cell signaling pathways. LTA is a major structural component of the surface of gram-positive bacteria and may mediate amphiphilic interactions with host cell membrane phospholipids. Allelic exchange of a glycosyltransferase homologue in GBS, *iagA*, reduces LTA anchoring in the GBS cell wall and significantly reduces HBMEC invasion in vitro and the development of meningitis in a murine in vivo model.[16] β-Hemolysin/cytolysin is a pore-forming exotoxin expressed by GBS that is known to promote GBS invasion of HBMECs at sublytic concentrations and cause HBMEC cytolysis at higher concentrations.[17] β-Hemolysin/cytolysin also induces HBMEC synthesis of interleukin-8 (IL-8), an extremely potent neutrophil chemoattractant, and promotes neutrophil transmigration across HBMEC monolayers.[17] Mice hematogenously infected with a GBS mutant lacking this exotoxin had lower brain bacterial counts and lower mortality than did mice infected with the parent wild-type strain expressing this toxin.[17]

As with *E. coli* K1, GBS have been shown to modulate a number of host signaling pathways to facilitate passage across the BBB. In fact, the FAK/paxillin/PI3K pathway is a common target involved in both *E. coli* K1 and GBS invasion of HBMECs. Inhibition of FAK signaling via a dominant-negative form of FAK and pharmacologic inhibition of PI3K with LY-294002 both significantly inhibit GBS invasion of HBMECs.[18] Another shared pathway involved in *E. coli* K1 and GBS invasion of HBMECs involves RhoA GTPase; RhoA levels are increased during GBS invasion of HBMECs, as are levels of Rac1.[19] Inhibition of RhoA and Rac1 with a geranylgeranyl transferase I inhibitor, GGTI-288, and expression of dominant-negative forms of these GTPases both result in significantly reduced HBMEC invasion by GBS.[19]

In summary, GBS take advantage of cloaking, molecular mimicry, exotoxin synthesis, and usurpation of host signaling pathways to bypass the BBB and cause meningitis. The common theme of modulating FAK and Rho GTPase signaling pathways during HBMEC invasion by *E. coli* K1 or GBS may provide future therapeutic targets for the prevention or treatment of CNS infections caused by these pathogens.

INNATE IMMUNITY IN THE CENTRAL NERVOUS SYSTEM

Once pathogens have entered the CNS, either by gaining entry across the BBB or by direct routes that bypass the BBB, they encounter cellular and humoral elements of the innate immune system present within the CNS. The next section addresses the interactions of pathogens with this "inner defense." Despite the common perception of the CNS as an immunologically inert compartment, an array of resident cells, including microglia, astrocytes, perivascular macrophages, and meningeal macrophages, participate in initiating a rapid, but relatively nonspecific response to invading pathogens. In addition to providing an initial defense, these cells actively recruit immune effectors from outside the CNS and provide a bridge to the development of a more specific adaptive immune response within the CNS. It is the evolution of this immune response in the CNS that largely dictates the ultimate clinical outcome of a patient with a CNS infection.

Microglia: Ramón y Cajal's "Third Element"

Santiago Ramón y Cajal (1852-1934) divided the histology of the brain into "elements," including neurons (*first element*), astrocytes (*second element*), and a third category of non-neuronal, nonastrocytic cells that he termed the *third element*. This third element contained cells later identified as oligodendrocytes, as well as a group of small, highly branched cells that were morphologically distinct from other cells in the CNS. These cells were eventually termed *microglia* by Pio del Rio Hortega (1882-1945), who went on to further characterize these cells as a distinct entity in the brain parenchyma.[20] Like monocytes and macrophages, these cells are derived from the bone marrow and share many features of monocytes/macrophages with respect to immune modulation.[20]

Microglia can exist in several different states, as defined by surface markers, morphology, migration status, and function. Resting microglia are small cells with few surface markers and prominent thin branches that are constantly reorganizing and sampling the microenvironment of the brain parenchyma.[21] A large number of stimuli activate resting microglia, with the nature of the stimulus influencing the structural and functional changes that occur during activation. Cellular debris from CNS damage, particularly free adenosine triphosphate, activates microglia and induces a morphologic change from a small, ramified cell to an ameboid cell capable of phagocytosing such debris in a manner similar to macrophages.[21] Microglia, like macrophages, express a large number of receptors associated with various mediators of the inflammatory response to tissue damage, pathogens, and immune stimuli. A major family of receptors expressed by microglia includes pathogen-associated molecular pattern (PAMP) receptors known as the Toll-like receptors (TLRs). Eleven TLRs (TLR1 to TLR11) have been identified to date in humans. Microglia express TLR1 to TLR9, which allows them

to detect and respond to a huge array of PAMPs; LTA (TLR2), double-stranded RNA (TLR3), lipopolysaccharide (LPS; TLR4), flagellin (TLR5), single-stranded RNA (TLR7), and unmethylated CpG DNA (TLR9) are examples.[22] Engagement of these receptors by cognate ligands triggers signal transduction of multiple intracellular pathways responsible for the inflammatory response. LPS-induced activation of TLR4 has been well characterized in microglia and leads to activation of nuclear factor κB (NF-κB), cytokine production (interferon-β [IFN-β]), tumor necrosis factor-α (TNF-α)], signal transducer and activator of transcription-1α (STAT-1α), production of reactive oxygen species (ROS), and production of nitric oxide (•NO, or NO).[23] Flagellin-mediated activation of TLR5 on microglia has been shown to upregulate expression of TLRs 1, 2, 4, and 5, as well as IL-6.[24] TLR3 activation in microglia has been demonstrated in response to HIV, and TLR9 activation in microglia leads to the production of multiple cytokines and chemokines (TNF-α, IL-1β, IL-6, IL-12, macrophage inflammatory protein-1α [MIP-1α], MIP-1β).[25,26]

Activation of microglia by invading pathogens has many consequences, some beneficial to the host and some detrimental. Microglia, like other members of the monocyte lineage, are capable of NO synthesis and a respiratory burst, processes directed at producing oxidative damage to the offending pathogen. Microglia produce NO via inducible nitric oxide synthase (iNOS, NOS-2), which leads to the formation of peroxynitrite (ONOO$^-$), a highly toxic product capable of damaging both host and pathogen.[27]

Microglia also possess the metabolic machinery (reduced nicotinamide adenine dinucleotide phosphate oxidase) necessary for the generation of superoxide anion (•O$_2^-$), an extremely reactive oxygen species that can damage nucleic acids, lipids, and proteins.[28] Pathogens expressing superoxide dismutase are able to neutralize this effective defense. Microglia also function as phagocytes in the CNS under both physiologic and pathophysiologic conditions. Microglia are the major scavengers of cell debris in the CNS and interact, in part, with apoptotic bodies expressing externalized phosphatidylserine.[29] The orphan receptor TREM-2 (triggering receptor expressed on myeloid cells-2) is important in transforming microglia into phagocytes, and activation of TREM-2 enhances phagocytosis while suppressing the production of proinflammatory cytokines, events that may be important for prevention of the autoimmune responses to the autoantigens present in apoptotic bodies.[30]

Microglia also regulate the response of other CNS cells to injury or infection and recruit cells from outside the CNS via the production of a wide variety of cytokines, chemokines, and lipid mediators. Table 39-1 lists some of the cytokines and chemokines known to be generated by microglia in response to a number of activating stimuli.[31] Microglia also produce factors that support glial and neuronal cells in their microenvironment, including nerve growth factor, NT-3, brain-derived neurotropic factor, glial-derived neurotropic factor, and basic fibroblast growth factor.[31] Many potent lipid mediators are synthesized by microglia, including prostaglandins (D$_2$, E$_2$, F$_{2\alpha}$, thromboxane B$_2$), leukotriene B$_4$, and platelet-activating factor.[32,33] Several of these lipid mediators serve an autocrine role; the EP2 receptor on microglia participates in the activation of microglia, and antagonism of this receptor may have a neuroprotective effect by preventing excessive microglial neurotoxicity.[34] The critical role of microglia in orchestrating the innate immune response has been established, and experimental evidence for this role is expanding rapidly; an extensive review of this evidence can be found elsewhere.[31,35,36]

In addition to initiating the innate immune response to a variety of pathogens in the CNS, microglia also function as antigen-presenting cells and are able to prime CD4$^+$ T cells to initiate the adaptive immune response. Various TLR ligands (LPS,

TABLE 39-1 Cytokines and Chemokines Produced by Microglial Cells

CYTOKINES	CHEMOKINES (CHEMOATTRACTANT CYTOKINES)
IL-1α/IL-1β	CXCL1 (growth-regulated oncogene-α)
IL-1 receptor antagonist	CXCL2/3 (MIP-2)
IL-3	CXCL8 (IL-8)
IL-4	CXCL10 (IP-10)
IL-6	CCL2 (MCP-1)
IL-10	CCL3 (MIP-1α)
IL-12	CCL4 (MIP-1β)
IL-13	CCL5 (RANTES)
IL-15	CCL22 (macrophage-derived chemokine)
IL-18	
TNF-α	
TGF-β	
M-CSF	

IL, interleukin; IP-10, interferon-γ–inducible protein-10; MCP-1, monocyte chemoattractant protein-1; M-CSF, macrophage colony-stimulating factor; MIP-1α, macrophage inflammatory protein-1α; RANTES, regulated on activation, normal T cell expressed and secreted; TGF-β, transforming growth factor-β; TNF-α, tumor necrosis factor-α.
Data from Hanisch UK. Microglia as a source and target of cytokines. *Glia.* 2002;40:140-155.

peptidoglycan, polyinosinic-polycytidylic acid [poly-I:C], CpG DNA) and infection with Theiler's murine encephalomyelitis virus result in increased expression of major histocompatibility class II complexes and costimulatory molecules on microglia, events that favor efficient antigen presentation and development of an adaptive immune response.[26] Cytomegalovirus (CMV), a gamma herpes virus capable of invading the human CNS, elicits CXCL10 (IFN-γ–inducible protein-10 [IP-10]) production from primary microglia but not from astrocytes (see later).[37] CXCL10 is an important chemokine involved in IFN-γ–induced T-cell recruitment, a process critical for control of CMV infection.[37] Remarkably, astrocytes infected with CMV produce the viral homologue of IL-10, UL111a, which suppresses the production of CXCL10 from activated microglia.[37] Thus, CMV is able to suppress T-cell recruitment in the CNS by subverting the production of an important antiviral chemokine by microglia.

Microglia, as potent regulators of the proinflammatory response to CNS injury and infection, are also able to downregulate these proinflammatory responses. Microglia express anti-inflammatory cytokines (IL-4, IL-10, IL-13, transforming growth factor-β [TGF-β]) and actively phagocytose apoptotic T cells after stimulation by IFN-β and IFN-γ.[31,38,39] Production of IL-4 and IL-13 ultimately triggers microglial apoptosis via autocrine receptor engagement, thereby providing a means of balancing inflammation in response to a specific CNS insult.[40]

Microglia are clearly multifunctional cells that serve as central regulators of the innate and adaptive immune response in the CNS. However, these cells do not act in a vacuum and interact with both immune and nonimmune cells to coordinate the events surrounding CNS injury or invasion. One important cell type included in this response is the astrocyte. The next section briefly addresses the importance of astrocytes in the CNS during various stages of infection.

Astrocytes: Stellar Actors in Central Nervous System Immunopathogenesis

Astrocytes are resident glial cells derived from neuroectoderm and are often thought of as "nurse" cells for neurons in the brain parenchyma. These cells compose a large portion of the brain parenchyma and can be identified by their star-shaped morphology and expression of glial fibrillary acidic protein (GFAP). In addition to maintaining the BBB, astrocytes also participate in the immunologic processes that are associated with CNS injury and infection. The overt histologic response of astrocytes to CNS damage is termed *reactive astrogliosis* and is manifested as an increase in the amount of GFAP expressed by resident astrocytes at the site of insult. However, these observations are a small reflection of the complex responses of astrocytes to CNS injury or infection.

Like microglia, astrocytes express several TLRs, but to a more limited degree, which allows them to participate in the initial innate immune response to CNS invasion. The close proximity of astrocyte foot processes to BBB tight junctions and the huge surface area presented by the brain endothelium also highly favor early interaction between astrocytes and invading pathogens. TLRs expressed by astrocytes include 1, 3, 4, 5, and 9, with little or no TLRs 2, 6, 7, 8, or 10.[22,41] Among the expressed TLRs, TLR3 levels are the most prominent by quantitative real-time polymerase chain reaction (PCR).[41] TLR3 ligation in astrocytes (by poly-I:C) triggers the production and release of IFN-β, CXCL10, and IL-6, as well as an increase in the expression of TLRs 1 to 5 and 9 mRNA by quantitative real-time PCR.[41] Astrocytes are the main source of IL-6 production in the CNS; IL-6 is a multifunctional cytokine with diverse biologic activities, including neurotropism, protection of neurons from glutamate toxicity and ischemic injury, astrocyte proliferation, inflammation, and modulation of Fas/FasL expression in astrocytes.[42] This latter effect on Fas/FasL expression may affect the general immunologic state of the CNS in that astrocytes normally express both elements of the Fas apoptosis apparatus yet do not succumb to this autocrine signaling.[43] The lack of astrocyte apoptosis despite Fas/FasL expression has been attributed to low-level expression of procaspase-8, whereas FasL expression by astrocytes is thought to provide a molecular barrier to circulating lymphocytes entering the CNS, cells that are highly sensitive to Fas/FasL-induced apoptosis.[44,45]

In addition to the production of important immunologically active cytokines and chemokines, astrocytes also respond to chemokines through expression of chemokine receptors. Multiple chemokine receptors have been identified in astrocytes, and ligation of these receptors has many downstream effects on astrocyte function, including regulation of chemokine production and receptor expression (Table 39-2).[46] Of note, astrocytes express CXCR4, the receptor for stromal cell–derived factor-1α (SDF-1α), a chemokine with autocrine activity leading to influx of Ca^{2+} and chemostasis of astrocytes. Both CCR5 and CXCR4 serve as CD4-associated coreceptors for HIV. Although astrocytes lack CD4 receptors, CXCR4 binds to the gp120 glycoprotein of HIV, an event that leads to activation of the mitogen-activated protein kinases (MAPKs) extracellular signal–regulated kinase-1 (ERK-1) and ERK-2.[46] HIV also infects astrocytes via a CD4-independent mechanism, which results in a restricted (i.e., nonlytic, nonproductive) infection with incorporation of the HIV provirion into genomic DNA. Nonetheless, this restrictive infection alters astrocyte functions: increased expression of immunomodulatory molecules such as monocyte chemotactic protein-1 (MCP-1), complement factor 3 (C3), and iNOS and decreased glutamate uptake (see later).[47] The decreased glutamate uptake and increased iNOS expression by HIV-infected astrocytes probably contribute to the neurotoxicity observed with HIV infection of the CNS.

TABLE 39-2 Select Astrocyte Chemokine Receptors and Ligands and Astrocyte Responses to Receptor Activation

CHEMOKINE RECEPTOR	LIGAND	ASTROCYTE RESPONSE
CCR1	CCL3	Chemotaxis, chemokine synthesis
	CCL4	Ca^{2+} mobilization, chemokine synthesis, chemostasis
CCR2	CCL2	Chemotaxis
	CCL11	Inhibition of forskolin-induced cAMP production, chemotaxis
CCR3	CCL3	Chemotaxis, chemokine synthesis
CCR5	CCL5	Ca^{2+} mobilization
CXCR2	CXCL2/3	Chemokine synthesis
	CXCL8	Complement protein 3 synthesis
CXCR4	CXCL12	Ca^{2+} mobilization, inhibition of forskolin-induced cAMP production, phosphorylation of ERK-1/2

cAMP, cyclic adenosine monophosphate; ERK, extracellular signal–regulated kinase.
Data from Dorf ME, Berman MA, Tanabe S, et al. Astrocytes express functional chemokine receptors. *J Neuroimmunol.* 2000;111:109-121.

One of the major functions of astrocytes is uptake of glutamate at synaptic junctions in the CNS. Glutamate is an excitatory neurotransmitter that is highly neurotoxic, mainly via two mechanisms: (1) hyperactivation of neurons and (2) inhibition of cysteine uptake leading to oxidative damage to neurons through glutathione depletion. Astrocytes "soak up" glutamate in the CNS via excitatory amino acid transporters and rapidly convert glutamate to nontoxic glutamine by expression of the enzyme glutamine synthase.[48] This glutamine is then exported from astrocytes, taken back into neurons, and converted back to glutamate via a mitochondrial-based glutaminase for use as a neurotransmitter.[48] Pathogen-associated factors or inflammatory mediators released in the CNS during infection, or both, can alter the ability of astrocytes to control the CNS glutamate concentration and result in glutamate-induced neurotoxicity as a by-product of infection. For example, HIV gp120 has been shown to reduce astrocyte expression of glutamine synthase, and patients with HIV-associated dementia have higher brain glutamate levels than do nonaffected controls.[49,50] Glucocorticoid-induced expression of glutamine synthase is inhibited by IL-1β and TNF-α.[51]

Astrocytes also contribute to the balance of CNS protection/destruction during infection by secretion of matrix metalloproteinases (MMPs). MMPs are a family of proteases produced in a wide range of tissues, including the CNS, and are discussed in the next section, with particular attention on their roles in bacterial meningitis.

Matrix Metalloproteinases, "You Can't Have Your Cake and Eat It Too!"

MMPs are a subgroup of the metzincin family of proteases that share a common Zn^{2+} binding site in their catalytic domain (...HExxHxxGxxH..., where x is any amino acid) and an associated methionine within a β turn, biochemical elements important

for proteolytic activity.[52] There are 24 members of the MMP group in mammals, and they can be further subdivided according to their domain structure (additional details can be found in the review by Yong[52]). Most MMPs are secreted from cells, although some may be associated with cell surface molecules such as integrins (e.g., pro-MMP-2) or the hyaluronan receptor (active MMP-9) or are linked to the cell membrane via a glycophosphatidylinositol link.[52] MMPs degrade a wide variety of substrates, including extracellular matrix components, receptors, growth factors, and adhesion molecules.[52] As a consequence, MMPs must be tightly regulated to prevent extensive tissue destruction or unintended biologic sequelae. The first level of control involves the transcriptional regulation of MMP genes based on specific activation signals. MMPs may also undergo posttranslational modification and are highly compartmentalized within cells, thereby allowing further intracellular control of MMP activity.[52] The second level of MMP regulation is based on secretion of these enzymes as zymogens, or proenzymes, which require additional cleavage to become active proteases. Finally, specific inhibitors, known as tissue inhibitors of metalloproteinases (TIMP-1 to TIMP-4), are expressed in tissues to counteract MMPs.[52]

MMPs have been implicated as playing a role, either beneficial or detrimental, in many different diseases affecting the CNS, including infections, ischemic or traumatic injury, and autoimmune disorders.[52] The cellular sources of these MMPs vary depending on the specific pathologic condition but generally include cellular elements of the CNS (microglia, astrocytes, neurons), endothelial cells, and infiltrating leukocytes, especially neutrophils and macrophages.[52] Neutrophils, in particular, represent an important early source of MMP-9 because these cells are among the "first responders" of the innate immune response to injury or infection and contain preformed stores of this MMP.[52] In general, MMPs can have complex effects on the inflammatory state of the CNS. The BBB is rich in potential substrates for MMPs, including type IV collagen, fibronectin, and laminin; MMP degradation of the BBB may favor transmigration of leukocytes, as well as the movement of macromolecules and water, thus contributing to brain edema. Injection of heat-killed *Neisseria meningitidis* results in BBB disruption and increased intracranial pressure (ICP), phenomena that are inhibited by the administration of batimastat, an MMP inhibitor.[53] MMPs also modify or degrade cytokines and chemokines relevant to this inflammatory state. For example, MMP-9 cleaves six amino acids from the N-terminal of IL-8 to produce a truncated form of IL-8 that is more potent with respect to neutrophil chemoattraction.[54] In contrast, MMPs degrade IL-1β, thus demonstrating anti-inflammatory activity.[55]

CNS infections in which MMPs have specifically been shown to play a role include pneumococcal, gram-negative bacterial, and tuberculous meningitis, as well as viral infections such as HIV, human T-cell lymphotropic virus type I, and mumps and parasitic infections such as cerebral malaria and *Angiostrongylus*-associated meningoencephalitis.[56-61] We focus here on the MMPs and pneumococcal meningitis as an example of the complex roles played by MMPs in CNS infection.

Streptococcus pneumoniae is a gram-positive bacterium responsible for a number of infections in humans, including pneumonia, otitis media, sinusitis, sepsis, and meningitis. A rabbit model of experimental pneumococcal meningitis demonstrated a positive correlation between MMP-9 levels and CSF leukocyte counts and total protein levels.[62] MMP-9 activity, as measured by gelatin zymography, localized predominantly to the intrathecal compartment and not to brain parenchyma, thus supporting the conclusion that the increase in MMP-9 activity during meningitis is derived from infiltrating leukocytes.[62] MMP-9 may become activated during pneumococcal infection by ROS, as shown by the inhibition of MMP-9 activity in but not release from rat brain slices or neutrophils exposed to heat-inactivated pneumococci in the presence of ROS inhibitors.[63] Pneumococci can directly activate MMP-9 via production of ZmpC, a pneumococcal zinc metalloproteinase.[64] Interestingly, MMP-9 knockout mice (MMP-9[-/-]) do not develop different CNS pathology than wild-type controls when *S. pneumoniae* is injected directly into the brain parenchyma, but these mice are less able to clear systemic bacteremia, which suggests that MMP-9 expression may play a more important role in clearing systemic pneumococcal infection.[65] Infant rat pups with experimental pneumococcal meningitis demonstrated a peak in brain parenchymal MMP-2 and MMP-9 levels 20 hours after infection and a peak in TIMP-1 levels 24 hours after infection.[66] The MMP-9/TIMP-1 ratio was significantly elevated during the first 20 hours of infection, thus supporting an imbalance in proteinase and inhibitor levels.[66] The elevation in MMP-9 was associated with proteolysis of collagen type IV in the meninges, perivascular spaces, and brain parenchyma, and parenchymal gelatinolytic activity correlated well with the degree of cortical damage.[66] In a rat model of pneumococcal meningitis, brain levels of MMP-9 increased in infected rats treated with ceftriaxone but not in saline-injected rats, whereas treatment with ceftriaxone plus dexamethasone reduced MMP-9 levels in comparison to untreated controls or animals treated with just ceftriaxone.[67] Glucocorticoids are known to inhibit MMP expression, and these findings are consistent with a potential protective effect of dexamethasone during pneumococcal meningitis. Tetracyclines inhibit the proteolytic activity of many MMPs, as well as the activity of TNF-α–converting enzyme (TACE), another proteolytic enzyme implicated in propagating CNS damage during meningitis.[68] Infant rats with pneumococcal meningitis that were treated with ceftriaxone plus doxycycline had lower mortality, less cortical damage, and less BBB disruption than did rats treated with ceftriaxone alone.[68] Both groups had sterile CSF by 40 hours after infection, with no differences in the time-kill curves between these groups during this time frame, thus suggesting that the effect of doxycycline was not due to enhanced bacterial clearance from CSF.[68] These animal models provide evidence that MMPs, particularly MMP-9, play a pathophysiologic role in bacterial meningitis and that targeting MMPs with inhibitors may reduce mortality and cortical damage without significantly altering sterilization of the CNS.

Data regarding MMPs in human disease also exist and are consistent with the observations described in animal models. In 27 children with bacterial meningitis, 91% and 97% had elevated CSF levels of MMP-8 and MMP-9, respectively, when compared with uninfected control children.[69] The majority of these children were infected with *Haemophilus influenzae* (*n* = 14) or *N. meningitidis* (*n* = 11), with only 2 infected with *S. pneumoniae.* However, elevated MMP-9 levels in CSF were associated (*P* < .05) with an increased risk for neurologic sequelae, including hearing loss and postinfection seizures.[69] In 19 adults with bacterial meningitis (*n* = 7 with *S. pneumoniae*), all had elevated MMP-9 activity, as measured by gelatin zymography, in comparison to uninfected controls or patients with Guillain-Barré syndrome.[53] Patients with bacterial meningitis also demonstrated increases in CSF TIMP-1 levels, and the MMP-9/TIMP-1 ratio was significantly elevated when compared with noninfected controls.[53] MMP-9 levels in the infected patients correlated with CSF protein concentrations but not CSF leukocyte counts, whereas TIMP-1 levels correlated with CSF leukocyte counts but not protein levels.[53] An investigation of 111 paired CSF and serum samples from patients with a range of neurological disorders, including both aseptic and bacterial meningitis, found that a CSF leukocyte count greater than 5/μL correlated well with elevated CSF MMP-9 activity by zymography (Spearman *r* = .755, *P* < .0001).[70] A more recent study examined the correlation between serum MMP-2 levels and the α₂-macroglobulin (α2M) index as a marker of increased BBB permeability in patients with infectious meningitis. The α2M index was defined as the ratio of α2M (CSF/serum) to albumin (CSF/serum). This study found that serum MMP-2 levels, as measured with an enzyme immunoassay, correlated well (*r* = .64, *P* < .0001) with the α2M index and were higher in patients with bacterial meningitis than in those with viral or fungal meningitis.[70]

In summary, MMPs contribute to the pathogenesis of bacterial meningitis by degrading components of the BBB, a process that favors the formation of brain edema and propagation of the inflammatory response via leukocyte transmigration across the impaired BBB. MMPs also have more complex actions on other components of the immune response to infection, including modulation of cytokines and chemokines involved in balancing a successful immune response to infection in the CNS. These proteinases are potential targets for therapeutic interventions aimed at minimizing the collateral damage that occurs during the immunologic assault on CNS pathogens. A major component of this collateral damage involves brain edema, the development of ischemia, and neurotoxicity from elements of the immune response and from the invading pathogens themselves. The next section addresses mechanisms in the development of brain edema, increased ICP, and neurotoxicity during CNS infections.

BRAIN EDEMA AND NEUROTOXICITY: CONSEQUENCES OF CENTRAL NERVOUS SYSTEM INFECTION

The severity of a CNS infection is dependent on many factors: the pathogenicity of the invading organism (i.e., the propensity of a pathogen to damage the host), the susceptibility of the host, the host immune response, and the timing and effectiveness of external interventions (e.g., antimicrobial agents, glucocorticoids, surgical therapies). Common mechanisms of injury to the CNS as a result of infection include brain edema and neurotoxicity. Brain edema can lead to increased ICP, decreased cerebral blood flow, ischemia, and herniation (Fig. 39-3). Specific infections can lead to increased ICP or herniation, or both, through a mass effect independent of the presence of brain edema, such as brain abscess or subdural empyema, or through effects on CSF drainage, such as cryptococcal or tuberculous meningitis. Neurotoxicity includes direct cytotoxic insults to neurons from pathogen-derived factors (e.g., pneumolysin from *S. pneumoniae*) or direct infection of neurons, as well as indirect cytotoxicity via immune system activation or altered neurophysiology (e.g., glutamate excitotoxicity). Earlier chapters discuss brain edema and the physiology of ICP in depth; this section addresses these issues as they relate to CNS infections.

Brain Edema and Central Nervous System Infections

Many factors contribute to the development of brain edema during the course of CNS infection, but most share a common final target, the BBB. The major cellular element of the BBB is the brain microvascular endothelium, a monolayer of overlapping endothelial cells connected by organized tight and adherens junctions and exhibiting little transcytosis, unlike the capillary endothelium in other tissues. BMECs behave much more like epithelial layers with respect to low paracellular permeability to macromolecules and cells, a feature that helps protect the brain parenchyma from unregulated fluid shifts based solely on Starling's forces, such as oncotic or hydrostatic pressure. Alterations in BBB permeability occur during CNS infection when pathogen- or host-derived factors influence the complex machinery responsible for maintaining low BBB permeability. During infection of the CNS by viruses, bacteria, fungi, or parasites, the innate and adaptive immune responses induce influx of leukocytes into the CNS, a

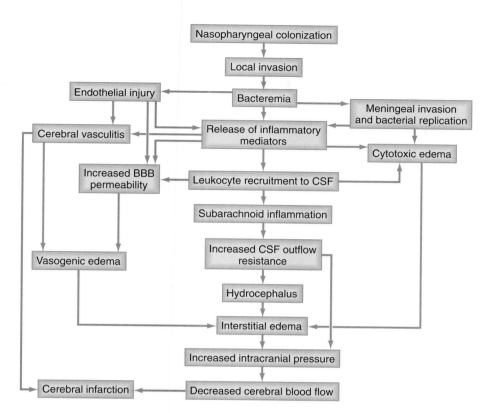

FIGURE 39-3 Schematic diagram of the pathogenesis of bacterial meningitis. BBB, blood-brain barrier; CSF, cerebrospinal fluid. *(Adapted from Tunkel AR, Scheld WM. Pathogenesis and pathophysiology of bacterial meningitis. Clin Microbiol Rev. 1993;6:119.)*

process associated with increased BBB permeability. This increase in BBB permeability is the sum of many individual, complex and interacting processes that involve leukocytic infiltration of the CNS, but changes in BBB permeability are not always dependent on leukocytes. Myriad proinflammatory and anti-inflammatory mediators are associated with this leukocyte infiltration and change in BBB permeability. Figure 39-3 provides a schematic view of the complex processes involved in the initiation and propagation of brain edema and neurotoxicity during bacterial meningitis; this scheme can also be applied to infection caused by nonbacterial meningitis. Some examples of specific pathogens and the mechanisms underlying alteration of the BBB during infection with these pathogens are discussed in the following sections.

Viruses Invading the Central Nervous System

A well-recognized feature of HIV-associated dementia is chronic breakdown of the BBB, a phenomenon attributed to immune dysregulation in the CNS via chronic activation of microglia, infiltration of the CNS by activated peripheral macrophages, and viral components such as gp120 and Tat.[71] Both these proteins downregulate components of tight junctions, the major barrier to the paracellular pathway between BMECs.[72,73] Tat possesses a cellular attachment domain that contains many positive charges, a feature that allows Tat to bind and cross cellular membranes. Exposure of BMECs to Tat leads to a number of important changes in BMEC physiology, including increased oxidative stress, expression of the early adhesion molecule E-selectin, and upregulation of inflammatory cytokines such as IL-6.[74] Tat also decreases claudin-1 and claudin-5 localization to tight junctions; claudin-5, in particular, is an important component of tight junctions, and loss of this protein increases paracellular permeability across tight junctions significantly.[73] The HIV envelope protein gp120 has been shown to decrease the expression of tight junc-

tion proteins.[72] A recent study has demonstrated gp120-induced, proteasome-mediated degradation of zona occludens-1 (ZO-1) and ZO-2, important components of tight junctions in BMECs, but not degradation of other structural tight junction components such as occludin or claudin-1.[75] This process is inhibited by lactacystin, a proteasome inhibitor, and enhanced by downregulation of the scaffold protein 14-3-3τ.[75] Thus, HIV invasion of the CNS results in increased BBB permeability via several mechanisms, a process that allows continued viral invasion and progression of CNS disease.

West Nile virus (WNV), a single-stranded RNA flavivirus, causes severe, even fatal encephalitis in susceptible hosts. The mechanism by which WNV crosses the BBB is not fully elucidated, but inflammation appears to play a critical role. TLR3-deficient mice infected with WNV are significantly more resistant to WNV-related mortality (40% survival rate versus 0%) and demonstrate little or no infection of the CNS despite an increased viral load in the periphery.[76] TLR3 recognizes double-stranded RNA and initiates an inflammatory response to cognate ligands. The lack of CNS involvement in WNV-infected, TLR3-deficient mice supports a role for TLR3-mediated inflammation in breakdown of the BBB and entry of WNV into the CNS. A recent study demonstrated that interference with the proinflammatory actions of macrophage migration inhibitory factor (MIF) in WNV-infected mice by antibodies, small molecule inhibitors, or MIF gene deletion results in a significant reduction in viral neuroinvasion, CNS leukocyte infiltration, and BBB breakdown.[77] These data indicate that the innate immune response to WNV infection causes increased BBB permeability and facilitates entry of WNV into the CNS.

Herpes simplex virus (HSV) is the most common cause of sporadic viral meningoencephalitis in the United States. Brain edema is a common feature of this viral CNS infection, but the mechanisms underlying the edema are unclear. A recent study examined changes in aquaporin (AQP) expression in the brains of mice with experimental HSV encephalitis.[78] AQPs are a family of protein water channels that are critical for water homeostasis in most organ systems, including the CNS. The predominant AQPs expressed in the CNS include AQP-1, which plays a role in CSF formation, and AQP-4, which is expressed heavily in astrocytes, especially at the BBB.[79] AQP-4–deficient mice demonstrate less severe cerebral edema in models of bacterial meningitis, thus suggesting that AQP-4 is involved in the modulation of brain edema during CNS infection (see later).[80] In mice with experimental HSV encephalitis, AQP-4 mRNA is significantly downregulated in the acute phase of disease (day 7 after inoculation), whereas AQP-1 and AQP-4 mRNA are both upregulated 6 months after inoculation.[78] The initial downregulation of AQP-4 may be a protective response to prevent excessive brain edema, and therapies directed at AQP-4 regulation may prove beneficial in a wide variety of CNS infections associated with brain edema.

Bacterial Infections of the Central Nervous System

Increased permeability of the BBB most often occurs after bacteria have crossed this barrier and are already present in the CNS. Accordingly, a reduction in the BBB is not a prerequisite for initiation of a CNS infection but is a common consequence of infection and probably facilitates further invasion of the CNS by the offending organism. Bacterial products and the immunologic responses to bacteria both contribute to an increase in BBB permeability. Perhaps equally as important as the increased permeability of the BBB is the decreased clearance of CSF that occurs during meningitis. Scheld and colleagues monitored cerebrospinal hydrodynamics in rabbits during experimental meningitis by using a pressure device in direct continuity with the supracortical subarachnoid space.[81] Rabbits were infected with either S. pneumoniae or E. coli (K1) to produce experimental meningitis, and a subgroup of animals were treated with penicillin G or methylprednisolone to assess the impact of antimicrobial or steroid therapy on CSF hydrodynamics. CSF outflow resistance increased 26-fold, from a baseline of 0.26 ± 0.04 mm Hg/µL per minute to 6.77 ± 3.52 mm Hg/µL per minute, during experimental meningitis and remained elevated up to 15 days later despite penicillin treatment. Administration of methylprednisolone early during pneumococcal meningitis reduced CSF outflow resistance 11.5-fold to 0.59 mm Hg/µL per minute. These observations highlight the extremely impaired drainage of CSF during bacterial meningitis, a process that itself promotes brain edema.

LPS, a common structural element of gram-negative bacterial outer membranes, is recognized by TLR4 on innate immune cells, such as microglia in the CNS, and triggers a proinflammatory response. TLR4 knockout mice demonstrate impaired leukocyte recruitment to the CNS after intracerebral LPS injection.[23] Intracisternal injection of LPS from H. influenzae type b (Hib) into rats produces increased BBB permeability, as measured by the accumulation of radiolabeled albumin in CSF, in a dose-dependent fashion (2 to 20 ng), although at higher doses (500 to 1000 ng) there is attenuation of the inflammatory response.[82] The LPS-induced increase in BBB permeability does not occur in leukopenic rats, thus supporting the hypothesis that leukocytes are responsible for LPS-induced alterations in BBB permeability.[82] However, an in vitro model of the rat BBB in which isolated primary rat cerebral microvascular endothelial monolayers were used demonstrated an increase in radiolabeled albumin flux across monolayers exposed to Hib LPS.[83] The absence of leukocytes in this in vitro model indicates that LPS may increase BBB permeability independent of leukocytes through a direct effect on endothelial cells. Murine brain endothelial monolayers exposed to LPS secrete IL-1α, IL-6, IL-10, granulocyte-macrophage colony-stimulating factor, and TNF-α.[84] These cytokines are released in a polarized fashion that favors secretion on the luminal side of the endothelial monolayer, and IL-6 production is further enhanced when the monolayer is exposed to LPS from the abluminal surface (akin to parenchymal exposure).[84] LPS also triggers the expression of E-selectin and P-selectin on BMECs, as well as vascular cell adhesion molecule-1 (VCAM-1) and intercellular adhesion molecule (ICAM).[85] The selectins are critical to the initiation of leukocyte margination and rolling, which allows these cells to slow down and interact with adhesion molecules that facilitate leukocyte transmigration across the BBB, such as VCAM-1, ICAM, and integrins. When rats are injected intracisternally with encapsulated or unencapsulated isogenic strains of Hib, an increase in BBB permeability is noted in both groups, but differences are noted in clearance of Hib from CSF.[86] Rats injected with unencapsulated bacteria are able to clear these bacteria from CSF more rapidly than are animals injected with encapsulated bacteria, a finding anticipated because of the known antiphagocytic properties of the capsule. Interestingly, when encapsulated or unencapsulated Hib is injected into leukopenic rats, an increase in BBB permeability is still observed despite reduced CSF pleocytosis in comparison to normal rats, and the degree of BBB permeability correlates with the CSF bacterial load, not the degree of CSF pleocytosis.[86] These data suggest that leukocytes are not an absolute requirement for the increase in BBB permeability noted during Hib meningitis; additional host or bacterial factors are involved in reducing the barrier function of the BBB during Hib meningitis. Consistent with this hypothesis is the finding that Hib peptidoglycan (PGN) also induces meningeal inflammation and an increase in BBB permeability when injected intracisternally into rats, probably via TLR2 signaling and the associated inflammatory response.[87]

N. meningitidis is a gram-negative coccus responsible for epidemic outbreaks of bacterial meningitis, most commonly among human populations in developed countries sharing close living conditions, such as college students and military recruits. A murine brain endothelial cell line (MB114En) exposed to meningococcal whole cell lysates rapidly produces a large amount of NO via expression of iNOS (or NOS-2), a series of events that actually results in the death of endothelial cells and is prevented by an inhibitor of NOS-2 (L-NNA) or an inhibitor of poly(ADP-ribose) polymerase (3-aminobenzamide).[88] This process is mediated by TLR2 and TLR4 and activation of the MAPK p38/NF-κB pathway.[89]

Although these studies have identified elements of gram-negative bacteria as modulators of BBB permeability, alterations in BBB permeability have also been shown with components of gram-positive bacteria. An in vitro model of the BBB was developed by using bovine BMECs cocultured with rat primary glial cells and subsequently exposed to the gram-positive cell wall components LTA and muramyl dipeptide (MDP, a subunit of PGN).[90] Exposure of glial cells to purified LTA (10 µg/mL) from Staphylococcus aureus or S. pneumoniae led to an increase in barrier permeability to fluorescein isothiocyanate (FITC)-inulin after 72 hours as opposed to complete loss of the BBB after 24 hours of exposure to LPS (10 µg/mL).[90] The increase in BBB permeability noted with LTA was augmented by the addition of MDP to LTA.[90] The changes in BBB permeability associated with glial activation by LTA with or without MDP were associated with glial production of TNF-α, IL-1β, and NO. In this model, an increase in BBB permeability to FITC-albumin and a decrease in transendothelial electrical resistance could be produced by exposure of endothelial monolayers to TNF-α or IL-1β and blocked by the addition of antibodies against TNF-α and IL-1β to LTA-activated glial cells. Addition of an iNOS inhibitor to activated glial cells also partly reversed the reduction in transendothelial electrical resistance associated with LTA.[90] These data indicate that glial cells contribute significantly to the increase in BBB permeability associated with LTA by the production of proinflammatory cytokines and NO.

The role of NO in BBB permeability has been examined further in vivo in a rat model of Hib meningitis. The CSF nitrite level, an indirect measure of NO production, increases significantly during the course of experimental Hib meningitis from basal levels to peak levels over the first 18 hours after intracisternal inoculation with live bacteria, but with no significant change in serum nitrite levels.[91] The CSF nitrite level correlates well with increased BBB permeability, as measured by accumulation of radiolabeled albumin in the CSF from serum ($r = .84$, $P = .018$), and administration of a systemic NOS inhibitor, N-nitro-L-arginine methyl ester, reduces CSF nitrite levels and the degree of CSF pleocytosis associated with intracisternal Hib lipooligosaccharide.[91]

NO can also interact with other mediators to produce alterations in BBB permeability. Intrathecal administration of LPS to induce experimental meningitis in rats leads to a rapid increase in NO and prostaglandin E_2 (PGE_2) levels in the CSF that peaks about 6 to 8 hours after LPS administration.[92] These increases in NO and PGE_2 were temporally associated with an increase in BBB permeability, as measured by ^{14}C-sucrose accumulation in brain parenchyma, thus supporting a role for these mediators in altering the BBB during meningitis.[92]

NO, in addition to myriad physiologic functions, can also react chemically with the ROS species $\bullet O_2^-$ (superoxide) to form peroxynitrite ($\bullet NO + \bullet O_2^- \rightarrow OONO^-$), an extremely reactive oxidant capable of damaging a wide variety of biomolecules. Peroxynitrite produces an increase in BBB permeability in response to experimental rodent viral CNS infections (Borna disease virus, rabies virus) via a TNF-α–independent mechanism, thus providing an additional mechanism for NO synthesis to modulate the BBB and immune response in the CNS.[93,94]

Alterations in BBB permeability as measured by leakage of macromolecules into the CSF during in vivo experimental meningitis correspond to morphologic changes in the cellular elements of the BBB. Experimental infection of rats with the encapsulated bacteria commonly responsible for human meningitis, S. pneumoniae, E. coli, or Hib, induces early changes in brain microvascular endothelium as examined by transmission electron microscopy.[95] An early (4 hours after infection) and sustained increase in pinocytotic vesicles (10 and 18 hours after infection) was noted with all these bacterial species (Fig. 39-4A).[95] The duration of infection is also associated with an increased observation of separation of intercellular junctions between BMECs (Fig. 39-4B).[95]

Functional changes in BBB permeability have micromolecular (changes in junctional protein levels, activation states, altered intracellular signaling pathways, and so on) and macromolecular (toxic injury to endothelial cells, endothelial apoptosis, altered endothelial migration, and so on) mechanisms that can and have been studied extensively. For example, an in vitro model of the human BBB using HBMECs examined changes in intercellular junctional regulation after exposure to E. coli K1.[96] HBMEC monolayers exposed to E. coli K1 exhibit decreased transendothelial electrical resistance before traversal of these bacteria across the monolayer, but only when these bacteria are expressing OmpA. OmpA interacts with a 95-kD endothelial glycoprotein expressed only in brain microvascular endothelium and induces actin cytoskeletal rearrangements before bacterial internalization, a process dependent on protein kinase C-α (PKC-α).[96] Activated PKC-α phosphorylates a specific protein at the adherens junction, vascular endothelial cadherin, which leads to dissociation of β-catenin from the adherens junction, decreased adherens junction intercellular adhesion, and increased paracellular permeability at the BBB.[96] This entire process of PKC-α activation, β-catenin dissociation, and increased BBB permeability can be prevented by antibodies directed against E. coli K1 OmpA or its glycoprotein receptor.[96]

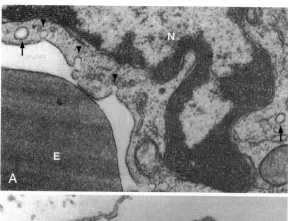

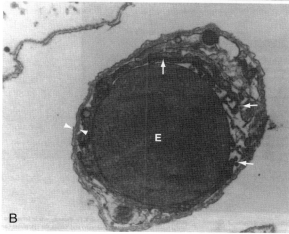

FIGURE 39-4 Transmission electron micrographs of rat cerebral capillary endothelium during bacterial meningitis. **A,** *Arrowheads* highlight pinocytotic vesicles forming at the luminal membrane, whereas *arrows* demonstrate fully formed vesicles in the cytoplasm 18 hours after intracisternal inoculation of *Escherichia coli* K1. E, intraluminal erythrocyte; N, endothelial nucleus. Magnification ×60,000. **B,** The *side arrows* highlight the wide separation between two cerebral capillary endothelial cells that share an intact intercellular junction elsewhere (*top arrow*) 18 hours after intracisternal inoculation with *Haemophilus influenzae. Arrowheads* demonstrate an intact basement membrane. E, intraluminal erythrocyte. Magnification ×15,000. *(From Quagliarello VJ, Long WJ, Scheld WM. Morphologic alterations of the blood-brain barrier with experimental meningitis in the rat. J Clin Invest. 1986;77:1087-1088.)*

In addition to functional changes in brain endothelium, bacteria often produce toxins capable of directly damaging endothelial cells and thereby destroying the BBB via cellular loss. S. pneumoniae, the most common bacterial cause of meningitis, produces a pore-forming toxin called pneumolysin. Pneumolysin is a member of the family of cholesterol-dependent cytolysins (CDCs), a group of gram-positive bacterial toxins that share a carboxy-terminal undecapeptide sequence that binds to cholesterol in the membranes of eukaryotic cells and leads to oligomerization and pore formation.[97] The CDC family includes proteins produced by many gram-positive human pathogens; some examples are streptolysin O (*Streptococcus pyogenes*), perfringolysin O (*Clostridium perfringens*), listeriolysin O (*L. monocytogenes*), and anthrolysin O (*Bacillus anthracis*). Pneumolysin lacks an amino-terminal signal sequence, which suggests that it is not secreted from pneumococci and requires autolysis for release.[98,99] Pneumolysin is highly cytotoxic to HBMECs, and pneumococci unable to produce pneumolysin do not alter the permeability of HBMEC monolayers in vitro.[100] Pneumolysin also plays a major role in neuronal damage during pneumococcal meningitis, as discussed in more detail later with respect to neurotoxicity.

Hemolytic-uremic syndrome, the leading cause of acute renal failure in children, is highly associated with infection by Shiga toxin (Stx1 or Stx2)-producing *E. coli* strains, and severe manifestations of this disease are complicated by CNS malfunction.[101] Stx1 and Stx2 are AB-type protein toxins composed of five B subunits and one A subunit.[102] The B subunits are responsible for binding to a cell surface glycolipid, globotriaosylceramide (Gb3), which results in endocytosis of Stx1/2 and retrograde transport of toxin to the cytosol of eukaryotic cells expressing Gb3.[102] Once in the cytosol, Stx1/2 inactivates ribosomes by removal of the adenine at position 4342 of the 28S RNA of the 60S ribosomal subunit, a reaction that inactivates protein synthesis.[102] Stx1 induces apoptosis of HBMECs, especially in the presence of TNF-α, and Stx2 induces apoptosis in HBMECs via upregulation of C/EBP homologue protein/growth arrest (CHOP) and caspase-3 activation.[103,104]

Neurotoxicity

In addition to alterations in BBB permeability, inflammation, brain edema, and increased ICP, CNS infections are associated with damage to or death of neurons, a process termed *neurotoxicity*. Neurotoxicity can result from direct infection of neurons, from collateral damage secondary to the immune response, or from pathogen-derived factors that damage neurons during the infection. Two particular pathogens that have been extensively studied with regard to neurotoxicity are HIV and *S. pneumoniae*, and they will be used as examples to highlight the mechanisms underlying infection-associated neurotoxicity.

Human Immunodeficiency Virus–Associated Neurotoxicity

Many investigations into the neurotoxic effects of HIV infection have been performed since the clinical recognition that patients with HIV/acquired immunodeficiency syndrome manifest a range of neurological maladies from mild cognitive impairment to full-blown dementia. Early investigations focused on target cells in the CNS, given the hypothesis that HIV was able to infect neurons directly. This hypothesis has been demonstrated in multiple studies to be incorrect; HIV does not infect human neurons directly, but invasion of the CNS clearly occurs, and this anatomic site can serve as a sequestration site for HIV latency.[105] Our understanding of how HIV damages CNS neurons is currently incomplete, but many aspects have been elucidated and reveal a complex interplay among the virus, the immune response, and resident glial cells such as astrocytes and microglia. Once HIV has invaded the CNS, an event that occurs very early after primary infection of the host, infected monocytes, macrophages, microglia, and lymphocytes provide sources of lytic viral reproduction, accompanied by nonproductive infection of astrocytes. Several protein components of the HIV virion have been shown to influence neuronal survival, including Vpr, gp120, and Tat. HIV-1 Vpr, a viral regulatory protein, has been shown to form ion channels in the membranes of rat hippocampal neurons and induces caspase-8 activation with subsequent apoptosis of both undifferentiated and fully differentiated NT2 cells, a neuron-like cell line.[106,107] Gp120, the HIV envelope glycoprotein, also induces apoptosis in NT2 cells and has been shown to significantly increase the production of ROS from glial cells in vitro by release of IL-1β, thereby leading to ROS-induced neurotoxicity.[107,108] Tat, a regulatory protein that *trans*-activates genes located in the HIV long terminal repeats, is secreted from HIV-infected cells and taken up by a wide variety of cell types, including astrocytes and neurons.[109] Exposure of neurons in vitro to Tat

results in neuronal apoptosis via TNF-α and activation of a non–*N*-methyl-D-aspartate (NMDA) receptor.[110] The direct neurotoxicity of Tat localizes to the carboxy-terminal portion of this protein, and a deletion mutant Tat protein lacking amino acids 31 to 61 (Tat$_{\Delta31-61}$) does not induce neurotoxicity in cultured human fetal neurons.[111] Although Tat$_{\Delta31-61}$ does not produce direct neurotoxicity in vitro, this deletion mutant is still capable of generating indirect neurotoxicity via TNF-α production from macrophages, thus indicating that Tat neurotoxicity occurs by direct and indirect mechanisms.[111] In contrast, both TNF-α and IL-1β upregulate expression of proteinase-activated receptor-2 (PAR-2) on neurons, and enhanced expression and activation of PAR-2 prevent the neurotoxicity associated with Tat.[112] PAR-2 is a member of the family of PARs, or G protein–coupled receptors that require proteolytic cleavage to remove biochemical constraints on a contiguous receptor ligand and allow activation of PAR.[113] In addition to activation by trypsin or mast cell tryptase, PAR-2 may also be activated by peptide sequences that mimic the intrinsic receptor ligand. Consistent with the protective role of activated PAR-2 on Tat-induced neurotoxicity, implantation of a PAR-2 peptide agonist in the mouse striatum prevented Tat-associated neurotoxicity in vivo.[112]

HIV also produces neuronal death via astrocytes and macrophages. Tat expression by astrocytes in vitro results in increased GFAP expression, a marker of astrocyte activation, and impairs glutamate uptake by astrocytes.[114] The culture supernates from Tat-expressing astrocytes cause neuronal death.[114] Additionally, HIV infection of human monocyte–derived macrophages increases macrophage glutamate synthesis via mitochondrial glutaminase, an enzyme present in macrophages that converts glutamine to glutamate.[115] HIV-infected macrophage media induces neuronal apoptosis via glutamate-induced neurotoxicity, a process that is significantly inhibited when macrophages are treated with a mitochondrial glutaminase inhibitor.[115]

In summary, HIV induces neurotoxicity by several mechanisms despite the absence of direct neuronal infection. These mechanisms are potentially cumulative, given their parallel nature, and probably explain the wide spectrum of clinical neurological disturbances observed in patients with HIV infection.

Neurotoxicity and Bacterial Meningitis

Despite advances in antimicrobial therapy for bacterial meningitis, neurological damage with resultant disabilities is a common outcome of bacterial meningitis, particularly when the causative organism is *S. pneumoniae*.[116] The mechanisms underlying the neurotoxicity associated with bacterial meningitis can be shared by a group of invading pathogens or may be unique to a specific pathogen. Some examples of broad neurotoxic mechanisms are discussed, followed by some examples of pathogen-specific mechanisms.

Unmethylated CpG motifs in DNA released from pathogens can activate microglial TLR9 and thereby lead to the production of NO and the synthesis and release of TNF-α.[117] Both NO and TNF-α are cytotoxic to neurons, and blockade of these mediators ameliorates the neurotoxicity associated with microglial activation via TLR9 ligation. Thus, this component of the innate immune response can result in neurotoxicity as a result of a wide array of invading pathogens whose DNA becomes available for TLR9 ligation. Similarly, components of the cell wall and outer membrane of bacteria are capable of eliciting an intense inflammatory response bearing all the hallmarks of the meningitis produced by the whole bacteria themselves. LTA activates both microglia and astrocytes via TLR2 ligation. In microglia, TLR2 activation by LTA results in the production and release of proinflammatory cytokines such as TNF-α, IL-6, and IL-1β, as well as upregulation of iNOS and increased production of NO.[118,119] Coculture of neurons with glial cells (astrocytes or microglia) exposed to LTA leads to neuron apoptosis, and this outcome is dependent on the presence of glial cells. Furthermore, inhibition of NO or superoxide synthesis or scavenging of peroxynitrite all prevented, partially or completely, the induction of neuron apoptosis after glial LTA exposure.[119] Nitrosative and oxidative damage to neurons secondary to activation of the innate immune effector cells in the CNS is a common mechanism involved in the neurotoxicity and neurodegeneration associated with CNS infections. In an infant rat model of GBS meningitis, treatment of the rats with a radical scavenger, α-phenyl-*tert*-butyl nitrone, at the onset of GBS infection abolished pathologic evidence of reactive oxygen intermediates, improved cerebral cortical blood flow, and prevented neuronal injury in both the cortex and dentate gyrus of the hippocampus.[120] Although microglia and infiltrating phagocytic cells (neutrophils, macrophages) develop an oxidative burst on activation, thus providing a host-derived source for the generation of reactive oxygen intermediates, bacteria also contribute to this pool of intermediates via production of hydrogen peroxide (H_2O_2). The pneumococcus produces H_2O_2 as a virulence factor, and H_2O_2 induces apoptosis in neurons by mediating the release of apoptosis-inducing factor (AIF) from the damaged mitochondria.[121] AIF is a flavoprotein with nicotinamide adenine dinucleotide oxidase activity, and its release from mitochondria and translocation to the nucleus result in chromatin condensation and DNA fragmentation in a caspase-independent manner.[122] AIF also plays a major role in the mechanism of pneumolysin-induced neuronal death and is discussed further later.

We have already mentioned the role of glutamate excitotoxicity in the context of HIV neurodegeneration, and glutamate is also involved in the neurotoxicity induced by bacterial meningitis. A common finding of pneumococcal meningitis in animal models is the loss of neurons in the dentate gyrus of the hippocampus, predominantly via apoptosis.[120] To investigate the contribution of glutamate to neuron apoptosis in the dentate gyrus, Tumani and associates examined glutamine synthetase activity in the brains of rabbits with pneumococcal meningitis.[123] Significant increases in glutamine synthetase protein concentration and enzyme activity were found in the frontal cortex of infected rabbits when compared with uninfected controls, but no changes in this protein concentration or enzyme activity were noted in the dentate gyri of infected animals. Intravenous administration of a glutamine synthetase inhibitor (L-methionine sulfoximine) to infected rabbits undergoing treatment with ceftriaxone significantly increased the density of apoptotic neurons in the dentate gyri of these animals when compared with rabbits receiving ceftriaxone alone.[123] These findings support an association between glutamate metabolism and apoptosis of neurons in the dentate gyrus during pneumococcal meningitis. Kynurenic acid, a by-product of L-tryptophan metabolism and an antagonist of excitatory neurotransmitters, inhibits necrosis and apoptosis of neurons in the cortex and hippocampus of rats with experimental GBS meningitis.[124] In contrast to these data, blockade of the NMDA receptor subunit NR2B, the subunit most highly expressed in the developing hippocampus, with a selective and potent antagonist (RO 25-6981) in infant rats with pneumococcal meningitis did not alter hippocampal neuron apoptosis, although this intervention did significantly reduce the frequency of seizures.[125]

Pneumolysin, a CDC released from *S. pneumoniae* after cell lysis, provides an excellent example of a pathogen-specific factor involved in neurotoxicity. Live pneumococci induce neuronal death, a process associated with influx of Ca^{2+} into neurons, mitochondrial damage, and translocation of mitochondrial AIF to the cell nucleus.[121] As mentioned previously, pneumococcal production of H_2O_2 accounts for some of these observations, but pneumococci lacking the ability to produce H_2O_2 are still able to kill primary neurons, whereas pneumococci lacking both H_2O_2

production and pneumolysin do not significantly affect neuronal survival.[121] Pneumolysin colocalizes with apoptotic neurons in the dentate gyrus of rats with pneumococcal meningitis, and pneumolysin is sufficient to induce neuronal death in vitro.[121] Pneumolysin has now been shown to act as a mitochondrial toxin that causes alterations in mitochondrial membrane potential and the release of AIF, thereby leading to neuronal death in a caspase-independent manner.[126] Pneumococci deficient in pneumolysin (Δply) or autolysin (LytA⁻), the protein effector of pneumococcal autolysis, demonstrate significantly reduced virulence in a rat model of experimental meningitis.[99] The contribution of autolysis to the pathogenesis of pneumococcal meningitis is relevant in the context of antibiotic-induced lysis of pneumococci in the CSF during meningitis. Grandgirard and coworkers examined differences in the inflammation associated with experimental pneumococcal meningitis treated with a lytic bactericidal antibiotic, ceftriaxone, and a nonlytic bactericidal antibiotic, daptomycin.[127] Inflammation was quantified in this study by measuring MMP-9 and TNF-α concentrations in CSF, as well as by examining cortical damage and assessing CSF bacterial counts. Infected rabbits treated with daptomycin demonstrated significantly reduced MMP-9 concentrations in comparison to those treated with ceftriaxone, as well as reduced cortical damage. These observations support the concept that release of bacterial products, through either autolysis or antibiotic lysis, contributes directly to the inflammatory damage associated with bacterial meningitis.

Many related and overlapping mechanisms come into play in ultimately producing the pathology observed in bacterial meningitis and other CNS infections. In addition to the neurotoxic effects described earlier, CNS infections can destroy or disturb CNS tissues and functions via digestion and mass effect on brain or spinal cord tissues. The next section addresses important basic science issues related to CNS infection more familiar to a neurosurgical audience, brain abscesses.

Brain Abscess—Pus in the Parenchyma

Brain abscesses are space-occupying purulent infections within the substance of the brain. The cause of brain abscess is most often related to infection outside the CNS and can be subdivided according to the following associations: (1) related to infection of the paranasal sinuses or otologic structures, (2) related to odontogenic infection, (3) related to thoracopulmonary infections (e.g., lung abscess, empyema), (4) hematogenous spread from other sites (e.g., endocarditis), (5) direct inoculation (e.g., trauma, neurosurgical procedures), and (6) cryptogenic (≈20%). The microbiology of brain abscess is predictably related to the primary source of the abscess; Table 39-3 lists microbes associated with specific primary sources. There is a predominance of streptococcal species and anaerobes associated with primary sources in the sinuses, mouth, and lung, whereas staphylococci and Enterobacteriaceae are commonly found in brain abscesses associated with direct inoculation from trauma or neurosurgical procedures.

The time course of brain abscess development in humans has been characterized by computed tomography and in animal models via necropsy and histology. Brain abscess begins as an early cerebritis (days 1 to 3), with edema formation, tissue necrosis, and neutrophil infiltration. This early phase is followed by an intermediate to late cerebritis with infiltration of macrophages and lymphocytes, and this process culminates in the formation of a capsule infiltrated with plasma cells and myofibroblasts.[128,129] Encapsulation allows isolation of the infection and is thought to be responsible for the lack of significant clinical symptoms in patients with chronic brain abscess.

Experimental study of the pathogenesis of brain abscess was significantly advanced with the development of a rat model of brain abscess.[130] Early studies involved stereotactic injection of a

TABLE 39-3 Specific Pathogens Associated with Anatomic Sources for Brain Abscesses

PREDISPOSING CONDITION	COMMON PATHOGENS
Otitis media or mastoiditis	Streptococci, *Bacteroides* spp., *Prevotella* spp., Enterobacteriaceae
Sinusitis	Streptococci, *Haemophilus* spp., Enterobacteriaceae, *Bacteroides* spp., *Staphylococcus aureus*
Dental infection	*Fusobacterium* spp., *Prevotella* spp., *Bacteroides* spp. streptococci
Direct inoculation (trauma, surgery)	*Staphylococcus* spp., Enterobacteriaceae, streptococci, *Clostridium* spp.
Lung infections (abscess, empyema), bronchiectasis	*Actinomyces* spp., streptococci, *Fusobacterium* spp., *Bacteroides* spp., *Prevotella* spp., *Nocardia* spp.
Endocarditis	*Staphylococcus aureus*, streptococci
Congenital heart disease	Streptococci, *Haemophilus* spp.
Unknown	Streptococci, *Staphylococcus* spp., *Haemophilus* spp., fastidious anaerobes

Adapted from Tunkel AR. Brain abscess. In: Mandell GL, Bennet JE, Dolin R, eds. *Principles and Practice of Infectious Diseases*, 6th ed. Philadelphia: Elsevier; 2005:1150-1163.

TABLE 39-4 Relative Potency of Different Bacteria Producing Experimental Brain Abscesses after Intraparenchymal Injection

BACTERIUM	ID_{50} (LOG_{10} COLONY-FORMING UNITS/mL) (95% CONFIDENCE INTERVAL)
Escherichia coli (K1 antigen positive)	2.44 (1.03-2.77)
E. coli (K1 negative)	3.64 (3.32-4.01)
Pseudomonas aeruginosa	4.92 (4.63-5.35)
Staphylococcus aureus	5.15 (4.45-5.67)
Streptococcus pyogenes	5.88 (2.34-6.68)
Candida albicans	6.24 (4.58-6.48)
Bacteroides fragilis	7.66 (7.31-8.95)

Data from Costello GT, Heppe R, Winn HR, et al. Susceptibility of brain to aerobic, anaerobic, and fungal organisms. *Infect Immun.* 1983;41:535-539.

mixture of bacteria, including aerobes and anaerobes, to simulate the known microbiology of brain abscesses in humans.[130-132] An important study by Costello and associates demonstrated that injecting microaerophilic or obligate anaerobic bacteria alone did not produce brain abscess, whereas the injection of facultative anaerobic organisms such as *E. coli*, *S. aureus*, or *Streptococcus pyogenes* produced abscesses, albeit with differences in potency (Table 39-4).[132] The *E. coli* strains in this study were more virulent with respect to abscess formation than were the gram-positive organisms tested, and the K1-encapsulated strain was more virulent than the nonencapsulated *E. coli* strain. These important experiments demonstrate that microaerophilic and obligate anaerobes are probably not involved in the initiation of brain abscess despite the common isolation of these organisms from abscesses derived from different primary processes. The authors point out that this experimental model may not adequately reflect the initiation of brain abscesses in humans inasmuch as many of them are associated with mixed facultative aerobe/obligate anaerobe infections of the paranasal sinuses or dental structures, thereby leading to chronic exposure of the brain to mixed bacteria. Mixed facultative aerobe/obligate anaerobe infections are known to be synergistic in establishing infections at other sites in the body, and the clinical picture in human brain abscess probably reflects this synergistic advantage in establishing a brain abscess in normal human brain tissue.

Before development of the rat brain abscess model, rhesus macaques (*Macaca mulatta*) were used to investigate the development and characteristics of brain abscesses in primates.[131] *S. epidermidis* was injected either intracerebrally (*n* = five macaques) or intra-arterially via the carotid artery (on silicone cylinders, *n* = eight macaques); brain abscesses developed in five of five macaques injected intracerebrally as opposed to six of eight macaques injected with contaminated cylinders intra-arterially. Interestingly, abscesses in the animals injected intracerebrally developed thick capsules with an exuberant inflammatory response, beneficial prognostic features, whereas abscesses caused by "septic emboli" developed thin capsules, features historically associated with poorer clinical outcomes. Figure 39-5 displays the coronal sections of abscesses from intracerebral injection and septic embolization.[131] Only recently have experiments begun to address the immunopathogenesis of brain abscesses, although in rodent models such as mice or rats as opposed to primates.

Kielian and Hickey published the first study that examined the host cytokine response to rat brain abscesses induced by direct inoculation of *S. aureus*.[133] Using RNase protection assays and reverse transcriptase PCR, they found early induction of mRNA for IL-1α, IL-1β, IL-6, and TNF-α. Within 24 hours of *S. aureus* injection there was an increase in mRNA for KC, the murine homologue of IL-8, as well as increases in MCP-1 and MIP-1α. The increase in KC correlated histopathologically with the appearance of neutrophils at the injection site, and the increases in MCP-1 and MIP-1α heralded the influx of macrophages and lymphocytes. Additionally, the authors noted an increase in the expression of ICAM-1 and platelet endothelial adhesion molecule in microvessels at 24 and 48 hours after injection. These cytokine/chemokine/adhesion molecule changes agree well with the progression of brain abscess from an early, neutrophil-predominant cerebritis to an organizing lesion infiltrated with macrophages and lymphocytes.

The importance of chemokines and neutrophils in the early inflammatory response to brain abscess was highlighted in a study using an *S. aureus* mouse brain abscess model.[134] Depletion of neutrophils from mice before the implantation of *S. aureus*–laden beads in the cerebral cortex led to higher bacterial counts and more severe abscesses than seen in control infected mice, thus supporting a role for neutrophils in the rapid containment of bacteria in brain parenchyma. Several chemokines were upregulated within 6 hours of *S. aureus* injection, including CCL1 to CCL4, CXCL1, and CXCL2; CXC1 and CXC2 are major neutrophil chemoattractants and share a common receptor, CXCR2. When CXCR2 knockout mice were injected with *S. aureus*–laden beads, the animals demonstrated poor neutrophil extravasation at the site of abscess formation, as well as an increased bacterial burden in these abscesses. As in the rat brain abscess model, IL-1 and TNF-α have been shown to play an important "containment" role in regulating the inflammatory response to *S. aureus*

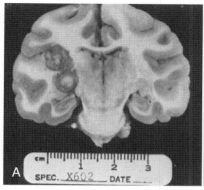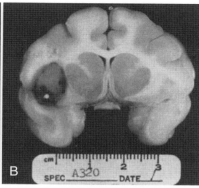

FIGURE 39-5 Coronal brain sections from rhesus macaques with experimental brain abscesses. **A,** Abscesses from intracerebral injection of *Staphylococcus epidermidis*. Note the thick abscess walls and associated shift of the midline structures away from the abscesses. **B,** Abscess from septic embolization of *S. epidermidis*–coated silicone cylinders. Note the thin abscess wall with cavitation of infarcted tissue and the lack of a midline shift. *(From Wood JH, Lightfoote WE, Ommaya AK. Cerebral abscesses produced by bacterial implantation and septic embolisation in primates. J Neurol Neurosurg Psychiatry. 1979;42:65.)*

in the murine brain abscess model.[135,136] TNF-α knockout mice injected intracerebrally with *S. aureus* have a higher mortality rate (54% versus 0%), higher bacterial loads, and higher inflammatory infiltrates, as well as delayed bacterial clearance rates, when compared with infected isogenic control mice.[136]

The expression of proinflammatory cytokines and chemokines is commonly triggered by engagement of TLRs, and this has been demonstrated in the murine brain abscess model. TLR2 and TLR4 are both important for the innate immune response to *S. aureus* brain abscess, as shown by the significantly delayed clearance of bacteria and increased mortality in TLR2 or TLR4 knockout mice injected intracerebrally with this bacterium.[137] Interestingly, the TLR2 and TLR4 receptors share a common intracellular adaptor molecule, MyD88, and MyD88 knockout mice are also subject to more severe brain abscesses, with significantly increased tissue necrosis, than infected isogenic control mice are.[138] However, unlike TLR2 or TLR4 knockout mice, MyD88 knockout mice do not have significantly increased bacterial loads, thus suggesting that MyD88 plays an important role in the containment of brain abscesses but not in clearance of bacteria from the initial cerebritis.

In addition to recruitment and activation of immune cells from outside the CNS, injection of *S. aureus* into cerebral cortex leads to the activation of astrocytes and microglial cells.[130,133,139] The involvement of astrocytes in the pathogenesis of brain abscess is highlighted by the observation that mice lacking GFAP, an intermediary filament upregulated in activated astrocytes, demonstrate poor containment of primary *S. aureus* cerebritis and exhibit severe inflammation, increased bacterial loads, ventriculitis, vasculitis, and contralateral cerebral leukocyte infiltration.[140] A major downregulator of microglia and astrocyte activation is the peroxisome proliferator–activated receptor-γ (PPAR-γ), and agonists of this nuclear regulator may modulate the inflammatory evolution of *S. aureus* brain abscesses in the murine model.[141] In vitro studies of PPAR-γ agonists (15-deoxy-Δ[12,14]-prostaglandin J₂, ciglitazone) on primary microglia or astrocytes do indeed demonstrate downregulation of proinflammatory cytokines, chemokines, and membrane inflammatory markers in these CNS cell types, although these effects in astrocytes were independent of PPAR-γ.[142,143] Administration of ciglitazone to mice 3 days after injection of *S. aureus* intracerebrally was associated with reduced bacterial loads secondary to enhanced microglial phagocytosis; reduced expression of TNF-α, IL-1β, CXCL2, CCL3, and iNOS; and enhanced abscess encapsulation.[143] These remarkable effects support the concept that effective control of brain abscesses requires a balance between proinflammatory and anti-inflammatory processes; factors favoring inflammation lead to excessive tissue damage, whereas impairment of specific inflammatory processes (e.g., CXCR2 knockout) leads to uncontrolled infection.

More evidence to support this "balance" hypothesis comes from observations on the effects of minocycline on experimental murine brain abscess. Minocycline has been shown to exert a number of neuroprotective effects, including modulation of microglial activation, inhibition of CNS cell apoptosis, and inhibition of proinflammatory signal transduction cascades.[144] Kielian and colleagues injected mice intracerebrally with a minocycline-resistant strain of *S. aureus* to induce brain abscess and then administered minocycline to these mice at various time points.[145] Minocycline administration, even as long as 3 days after injection, was associated with a reduction in brain abscess size, reduced mortality in the first 24 hours, transient reductions in IL-1β and CCL2 expression, and reduced astrocyte and microglial activation. Thus, the clinical effects of drugs such as ciglitazone and minocycline on human brain abscesses deserve further investigation as adjuncts to surgical and chemotherapeutic interventions.

Cerebrospinal Fluid Shunt Infections—The Role of Biofilms

We finish this chapter with a discussion of a sticky problem for neurosurgeons, bacterial biofilms. As biotechnology progresses, more and more patients will have the privilege of experiencing "bionic" medicine in the form of implanted prosthetic devices. We will use CSF shunt devices as an example of a neurosurgical prosthetic device that can become infected, a complication that offers many diverse challenges for the neurosurgeon and patient alike.

CSF shunts come in many different varieties, each specifically designed to specialize in specific methods to drain excess CSF from the CNS. Despite their variety, CSF shunts become contaminated with bacteria through a limited number of mechanisms:

1. Perioperative contamination—either at the time of primary implantation or via manipulation at later times
2. Wound dehiscence over the shunt—with direct contamination at the erosion site and along the shunt tract
3. Hematogenous seeding—most clearly with intravascular devices, but it can occur with nonvascular devices
4. Distal port contamination—especially with ureteral drainage devices, but also with intraperitoneal and externalized devices

Regardless of the mechanism of contamination, a common process that prevents subsequent sterilization of the shunt and often prompts removal of the device is the formation of bacterial biofilm. Biofilm formation occurs with both infection and colonization of prosthetic medical devices, and many features of bacterial communities living in biofilm present major challenges for device sterilization: (1) most bacteria in biofilms are in a

FIGURE 39-6 A and **B,** *Staphylococcus epidermidis* biofilm formation on a catheter surface. Note the deposition of extracellular matrix, manifested as a complex web of material around and between microcolonies. Magnification ×3600 (**A**); ×18,000 (**B**). *(From Yassien M, Khardori N. Interaction between biofilms formed by* Staphylococcus epidermidis *and quinolones.* Diagn Microbiol Infect Dis. *2001;40:79-89.)*

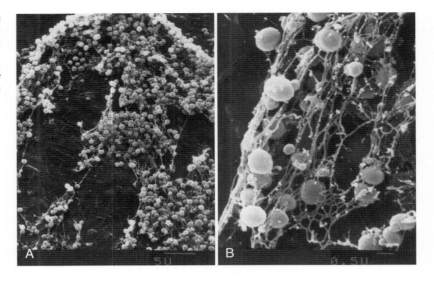

stationary phase of growth, thus making them less susceptible to antibiotics whose mechanism depends on active division; (2) biofilms are much less permeable to most antibiotics than the surrounding milieu; and (3) prosthetic devices lack a vascular supply, thus impairing delivery of immune effectors and antibiotics to the site of colonization.

Coagulase-negative staphylococci (CoNS) are common pathogens involved in the colonization and infection of CSF shunt devices, and these bacteria are notorious for their ability to form biofilm on prosthetic devices (Fig. 39-6). Several factors probably play a role in the initial adherence of CoNS to CSF shunt devices, including the surface materials of the shunt that interact with host tissues or fluids and bacterial virulence factors such as adhesins. Soon after placement, bioprosthetic materials are coated with host proteins, and these proteins may serve as receptors for adhesion molecules expressed by bacteria. These adhesion molecules are collectively known as "microbial surface components recognizing adhesive matrix molecules," or MSCRAMMs.[146] CoNS and *S. aureus* appear to adhere more readily to bioprosthetic material than do *S. pneumoniae* and *E. coli*, and the staphylococci adhere better to Teflon than to silicone.[147] Live bacteria may not be necessary to initiate bacterial adherence to CSF shunt material; "dead" biofilm on sterile, unused silicone CSF shunt devices has been shown to facilitate the adherence of bacteria, with subsequent new biofilm formation.[148] Once adherence has occurred, CoNS initiate the process of biofilm formation almost immediately. Biofilms are complex surface structures consisting of sessile bacteria embedded in an extracellular matrix that is permeated by water channels.[149] Regulation of the transition state between planktonic (free-living) bacteria and sessile bacteria in biofilms is very often dependent on a phenomenon known as quorum sensing. Quorum sensing itself is a complex set of processes that allow bacteria in a community to regulate the gene expression and phenotypes of other bacteria in the same community. Biofilm formation by *S. epidermidis* is a process associated with phase variation and regulation of a DNA sequence known as the intercellular adhesion (*ica*) gene cluster.[146] The *ica* gene cluster is organized as a four-gene operon (*icaADBC*) and encodes for the machinery necessary to synthesize a polysaccharide intercellular adhesin (PIA) that forms the extracellular matrix of *S. epidermidis* biofilms. PIA is composed of polymeric *N*-acetylglucosamine and accounts for the bulk of the extracellular matrix in CoNS biofilms.[146] The *icaADBC* operon is under the transcriptional control of several systems in staphylococci,

including repressors such as IcaR, TcaR, and the LuxS system, a quorum-sensing apparatus active in CoNS. Additionally, σ^B, a global stress regulator, acts as a positive regulator of biofilm formation in *S. epidermidis*, but not in *S. aureus*.[146] More recent studies have also identified PIA-independent mechanisms of biofilm formation in staphylococci; an excellent and extensive review of staphylococcal biofilm regulation can be found in the review by O'Gara.[146] Future advances in bioprosthetic device design, such as adhesion-resistant materials, antibiotic-impregnated devices, and devices designed to interfere with quorum sensing or transcriptional regulation of biofilm formation, may significantly reduce the infection rates associated with implanted bioprosthetic devices. Additionally, new chemotherapeutic interventions are needed; examples include bactericidal antimicrobials that penetrate biofilm and have a high threshold for the development of resistance, compounds that interfere with quorum sensing or transcriptional regulation of biofilm formation, or with both, and compounds that regulate phase variation among bacteria and drive sessile, biofilmed bacteria into the more susceptible planktonic form.

SUGGESTED READINGS

Albrecht J, Sonnewald U, Waagepetersen HS, et al. Glutamine in the central nervous system: function and dysfunction. *Front Biosci.* 2007;12:332-343.

Aravalli RN, Peterson PK, Lokensgard JR. Toll-like receptors in defense and damage of the central nervous system. *J Neuroimmune Pharmacol.* 2007;2:297-312.

Britt RH, Enzmann DR, Yeager AS. Neuropathological and computerized tomographic findings in experimental brain abscess. *J Neurosurg.* 1981;55:590-603.

Costello GT, Heppe R, Winn HR, et al. Susceptibility of brain to aerobic, anaerobic, and fungal organisms. *Infect Immun.* 1983;41:535-539.

Dorf ME, Berman MA, Tanabe S, et al. Astrocytes express functional chemokine receptors. *J Neuroimmunol.* 2000;111:109-121.

Fux CA, Quigley M, Worel AM, et al. Biofilm-related infections of cerebrospinal fluid shunts. *Clin Microbiol Infect.* 2006;12:331-337.

Hanisch UK. Microglia as a source and target of cytokines. *Glia.* 2002;40: 140-155.

Jack CS, Arbour N, Manusow J, et al. TLR signaling tailors innate immune responses in human microglia and astrocytes. *J Immunol.* 2005;175:4320-4330.

Kielian T, Hickey WF. Proinflammatory cytokine, chemokine, and cellular adhesion molecule expression during the acute phase of experimental brain abscess development. *Am J Pathol.* 2000;157:647-658.

Kim KS. Microbial translocation of the blood-brain barrier. *Int J Parasitol.* 2006;36:607-614.

Krantic S, Mechawar N, Reix S, et al. Apoptosis-inducing factor: a matter of neuron life and death. *Prog Neurobiol.* 2007;81:179-196.

Lehmann GL, Gradilone SA, Marinelli RA. Aquaporin water channels in central nervous system. *Curr Neurovasc Res.* 2004;1:293-303.

Meli DN, Christen S, Leib SL, et al. Current concepts in the pathogenesis of meningitis caused by *Streptococcus pneumoniae*. *Curr Opin Infect Dis*. 2002;15:253-257.

O'Gara JP. ica and beyond: biofilm mechanisms and regulation in *Staphylococcus epidermidis* and *Staphylococcus aureus*. *FEMS Microbiol Lett*. 2007;270:179-188.

Rock RB, Peterson PK. Microglia as a pharmacological target in infectious and inflammatory diseases of the brain. *J Neuroimmune Pharmacol*. 2006;1: 117-126.

Rosado CJ, Kondos S, Bull TE, et al. The MACPF/CDC family of pore-forming toxins. *Cell Microbiol*. 2008;10:1765-1774.

Rubin LL, Staddon JM. The cell biology of the blood-brain barrier. *Annu Rev Neurosci*. 1999;22:11-28.

Tunkel AR, Scheld WM. Pathogenesis and pathophysiology of bacterial meningitis. *Clin Microbiol Rev*. 1993;6:118-136.

Wood JH, Lightfoote WE, Ommaya AK. Cerebral abscesses produced by bacterial implantation and septic embolisation in primates. *J Neurol Neurosurg Psychiatry*. 1979;42:63-69.

Yong VW. Metalloproteinases: mediators of pathology and regeneration in the CNS. *Nat Rev Neurosci*. 2005;6:931-944.

Full references can be found on Expert Consult @ www.expertconsult.com

CHAPTER 40

Postoperative Infections of the Head and Brain

Christopher J. Farrell ■ Mary L. Pisculli ■ Frederick G. Barker II

Before Lister's 1867 introduction of surgical antisepsis, nearly 80% of operations were followed by infections at the surgical site and almost half of the patients died after operation.[1] Despite considerable advances in our understanding of the pathogenesis of surgical infection, the introduction of rigorous aseptic practices within the operating room, and the use of prophylactic antibiotics for clean operations, infection after neurosurgical intervention remains an all too frequent occurrence. Although mortality rates have decreased markedly, postcraniotomy infections commonly require prolonged antibiotic treatment and additional surgical interventions for successful eradication and frequently result in significant morbidity, prolonged hospitalization, and increased health care expenses. The economic burden of postoperative infections is significant: the estimated average cost of a surgical site infection (SSI) attributable to methicillin-resistant *Staphylococcus aureus* (MRSA) is almost $100,000,[2] and the overall cost of SSIs is believed to account for up to $10 billion annually in health care expenditures.[3]

The diagnosis of infection after craniotomy is often challenging. Many of the typical correlates of infection are nonspecific in the postoperative setting, and recognition of infection may frequently be delayed. An accurate understanding of the clinical, laboratory, and radiographic manifestations of postcraniotomy infection is critical to enable timely medical and surgical intervention and to limit the neurological sequelae of infection. This chapter examines these manifestations and discusses the tenets of effective therapy. The epidemiology of postcraniotomy infections is also discussed, along with a review of the factors conferring an increased risk for infection and the strategies that have proved to decrease the incidence of postoperative infection. Infections related to cerebrospinal fluid (CSF) shunting procedures are not included in this chapter.

EPIDEMIOLOGY AND ETIOLOGY

Postoperative infections are typically categorized according to anatomic site. The Centers for Disease Control and Prevention (CDC) defines superficial incisional infections as those limited to the skin and subcutaneous tissue, whereas deep incisional infections may involve the subgaleal space and bone flap. Deep organ space infections include subdural empyema, brain abscess, and meningitis/ventriculitis. According to data from the CDC's National Nosocomial Infection Surveillance (NNIS) program, superficial infections are responsible for 60% of SSIs after craniotomy. Meningitis is the most common deep organ space infection and represents 22% of postcraniotomy infections, whereas other intracranial infections, including subdural empyema and brain abscess, account for 14% of infections.[4] Estimating the infection rate after craniotomy from the neurosurgical literature is difficult because of differences in definitions and methodology. Several large prospective studies have reported infection rates ranging from 1% to 8%.[4-10] McClelland and Hall reviewed the postoperative courses of 1587 patients who underwent elective cranial operations over a 15-year period performed by a single

surgeon and found an impressively low rate (0.8%) of postoperative infection.[7]

In accord with other studies,[11,12] McClelland and Hall identified *S. aureus* as the causative agent for approximately half of the infections that develop after craniotomy.[7] Data from the NNIS also demonstrated *S. aureus* to be the most common pathogen after craniotomy, followed by coagulase-negative staphylococci. Other bacteria frequently causing postcraniotomy infection included enterococci, *Streptococcus* spp., *Pseudomonas aeruginosa*, *Acinetobacter* spp., *Citrobacter* spp., *Enterobacter* spp., *Klebsiella pneumoniae*, *Escherichia coli*, miscellaneous other gram-negative bacilli, and yeast; each of these organisms accounted for less than 10% of episodes.[13,14] Although direct spread from contiguous areas of infection is common, the causative agents tend to vary depending on the site of infection. Yang and colleagues retrospectively identified 31 patients with brain abscesses after neurosurgical procedures and found gram-negative bacilli and polymicrobial infections to be the most frequent pathogens isolated.[15] Gram-negative bacilli are also the most common cause of postoperative meningitis and account for 29% to 38% of nosocomial episodes.[16,17] Isolation of *Propionibacterium acnes*, an anaerobic gram-positive bacillus, from neurosurgical specimens has been dismissed as a contaminant because it is commensal scalp flora. However, the role of *P. acnes* as a causative agent of postcraniotomy infections is increasingly being recognized. Earlier reports probably underestimated its pathologic role because of its often indolent clinical manifestation, as well as difficulties associated with microbiologic isolation of the organism, specifically the need for anaerobic culture held for 10 days.[18]

RISK FACTORS FOR INFECTION AND PREVENTIVE STRATEGIES

Multiple factors combine to affect the risk for development of an SSI after craniotomy. Although it is unlikely that all postoperative infections can be completely prevented, many of the factors influencing the development of infection may be modifiable, including those attributable to the patient and those related to the surgical intervention itself. The majority of postsurgical infections are due to contamination of the wound with bacteria from the patient's skin. Although the magnitude of contamination and the virulence of the contaminating organism certainly contribute to the rate of infection, all surgical wounds become inoculated with bacteria to some extent at the time of surgery, but in only a small percentage of patients does this contamination lead to clinical infection.[19] Host defense mechanisms represent the primary barrier to establishment of infection, and these defenses may be impaired in patients undergoing craniotomy. Low levels of antibody and complement contribute to make the brain less efficient than other organs of the body at eradicating infection, and many of the underlying pathologies leading to neurosurgical intervention may significantly impair immune function. For example, patients with malignant gliomas express a variety of immune defects, including increased secretion of immunosuppressive cytokines and an increased fraction of regulatory T cells.[20] Additionally, many of the adjunctive therapies used for treating brain tumors, such as corticosteroids, chemotherapy, and radiation, may result in immune compromise. Other frequent indications for craniotomy, such as trauma, have also been shown to be profoundly immunosuppressive.[21] General surgical and infection control studies have identified other host factors that influence the risk for SSI, including advanced age, obesity, hypoalbuminemia, diabetes mellitus, and poor functional status.[3,22-25] Gianotti and associates demonstrated the importance of nutritional status in oncologic surgery by showing that malnourished patients had improved resistance to infection after as little as 5 days of enteral nutrition.[26] The increased rate of SSIs associated with these factors has been attributed to nonspecific deficits in host defense. Even though earlier reports suggested an increased rate of postoperative infection after general surgical procedures in patients infected with human immunodeficiency virus (HIV),[27,28] several more recent retrospective studies performed since the advent of highly active antiretroviral therapy (HAART) have failed to demonstrate an association between SSI rates and HIV infection.[29-31] Although the influence of these intrinsic factors on the rate of SSI after neurosurgical intervention has not been established in prospective studies, optimization of immune function through minimization of corticosteroid use, adequate nutritional support, and optimized perioperative glucose control may all be potentially helpful in the prevention of postcraniotomy infections.

Several factors specific to craniotomy have been identified as increasing the risk for postoperative infection. In a prospective multicenter trial, Korinek identified postoperative CSF leakage and early subsequent reoperation as independent risk factors for SSI, thus suggesting that careful attention to closure techniques and meticulous hemostasis may potentially result in lower rates of postoperative infection.[5] Several other studies confirmed CSF leakage as a major risk factor for infection.[8,32-35] Additionally, Korinek identified four independent predictors of postoperative infection after craniotomy: surgery lasting longer than 4 hours, emergency surgery, clean-contaminated and contaminated surgery, and neurosurgical intervention in the preceding month.[5] Valentini and coworkers also observed an increased relative risk of 24.3 for postoperative infection in elective clean craniotomies lasting longer than 3 hours.[36] The association between longer duration of surgery and infection has not been defined precisely, but plausible explanations include greater complexity of the surgery and prolonged exposure of the wound to bacterial contamination.[37]

A variety of other risk factors associated with infection after craniotomy have been less reliably demonstrated, including placement of drains or intracranial pressure monitors, poor neurological status, paranasal sinus entry, diabetes mellitus, and foreign body implantation (other than shunts).[5,8,38] Synthetic dural substitutes are foreign bodies and might represent a potential risk factor for infection in comparison to autologous graft materials such as pericranium, temporalis fascia, or fascia lata. Actual evidence demonstrating increased rates of infection with their use, however, is limited. Malliti and coauthors reported a nonsignificantly increased incidence of deep wound infections after craniotomy with the use of a nonresorbable polyester urethane synthetic dural graft (Neuro-Patch, B. Braun, Boulogne, France).[39] Postoperative CSF leaks were also significantly more frequent when using the synthetic dural substitute, thus limiting the ability of this study to determine whether use of the Neuro-Patch independently increased the risk for infection. The presence of nonresorbable dural substitutes may also impair the potential for an infected wound to be successfully treated because these grafts may become chronically colonized and could require removal to eradicate the infection.[40] A variety of nonautologous, resorbable collagen dural substitutes are currently available, and

their relationship to surgical infection has not been well explored. McCall and coworkers reported the uncomplicated use of several of these materials in a small number of patients in the setting of contaminated wounds, a finding suggesting that they may not impede clearance of infection.[40] The use of Gliadel wafers (MGI Pharma, Inc., Bloomington, MN), which contain 1,3-bis-(2-chloroethyl)-1-nitrosurea, for the treatment of malignant gliomas has also been associated with an increased incidence of postoperative infection. McGovern and coauthors reported a 29% rate of infection in cases associated with insertion of Gliadel wafers between 1996 and 1999.[41] Subsequent reports with larger patient populations, however, have not revealed statistically significant differences in the rate of infection with Gliadel use.[41,42]

Multiple prospective randomized clinical studies and a meta-analysis have validated the effectiveness of preoperative antibiotics in reducing the incidence of SSIs after craniotomy.[11,33,34,43,44] Hugh Cairns described the first trial of a modern prophylactic antibiotic in neurosurgery in 1947 when he reported sprinkling a "light frosting" of penicillin powder directly onto the brain in 670 patients and thought that the results were superior to those of historical controls.[45,46] In 1979, Malis demonstrated the ability of a prophylactic antibiotic regimen (vancomycin and an aminoglycoside) to reduce the incidence of SSI after craniotomy.[47] Since these initial reports, a variety of antibiotic regimens have been used for effective surgical prophylaxis, and the choice of agent should be guided by individual institutional data on frequently recovered pathogens and their resistance profiles. In general, the antibiotic chosen for prophylaxis should be safe, provide an appropriate narrow spectrum of coverage against relevant bacteria, and be administered for a defined, brief course. The Surgical Infection Prevention (SIP) project has recommended three performance measures for monitoring appropriate antimicrobial prophylaxis use: selection of an appropriate antibiotic, administration within 1 hour before incision (2 hours is allowed for the administration of vancomycin and fluoroquinolones), and discontinuation of the antibiotic within 24 hours after surgery is completed.[48] Antibiotics with short half-lives such as cefazolin should be readministered every 3 to 4 hours during surgery to ensure adequate drug levels throughout the operation, including the time of wound closure.[49] Prolonged use of antibiotics beyond 24 hours postoperatively has not shown a greater benefit, may increase the risk for other nosocomial infections, and might encourage the emergence of multidrug-resistant pathogens.[50,51] Despite wide acceptance of these basic measures, compliance with them continues to remain poor in the United States.[52] Prophylactic antibiotics for craniotomy are covered in more detail elsewhere in this book.

Additional perioperative factors that may potentially reduce the risk for postoperative infection include maintenance of normothermia and supplemental oxygenation. Several prospective randomized trials evaluating active warming of patients during colorectal surgery to maintain normothermia have shown decreased rates of infectious complications; the proposed mechanism of action is support of adequate blood flow and tissue oxygenation at the surgical site.[53-55] Supplemental administration of oxygen may also assist in preventing infection by increasing tissue oxygen levels and facilitating oxidative killing of bacteria by neutrophils. Belda and colleagues conducted a prospective trial to evaluate the postoperative infection rate in patients randomized to receive either 30% oxygen or 80% oxygen during elective colorectal surgery.[56] The group receiving 80% oxygen had a 54% reduction in wound infections. Studies evaluating the role of supplemental oxygen or temperature control for neurosurgical interventions have yet to be performed.

Other perioperative risk reduction considerations include surgical site preparation and environmental control within the operating room. Although no evidence has been found that preoperative hair removal reduces the incidence of postoperative infection, any hair removal that is performed should be done as close to the time of surgery as possible and clippers used rather than a razor to minimize the number of bacteria that colonize the inevitable small cuts and abrasions that develop from shaving.[57-60] Several antiseptic skin preparations have been used (chlorhexidine, iodophor compounds, alcohol), but no agent has been shown to be more effective than another.[61] To provide effective antisepsis, these agents must remain on the skin until they dry naturally, with avoidance of any pooling. Theoretically, adhesive barrier drapes with antiseptic embedded within the adhesive may prevent regrowth of bacteria at the surgical site throughout the operative procedure; however, their ability to reduce the incidence of SSI has not been proved.[62] Similarly, preoperative bathing or showering with an antiseptic skin product has no evidence in support of it.[63] The operating room environment represents another important consideration in the reduction of SSIs. The number of health care workers within the operating room and traffic throughout the procedure should be kept to a minimum because bacterial shedding increases with activity and can potentially result in increased airborne contamination.[58] Ensuring adequate ventilation minimizes the particulates and bacteria in the perioperative environment, and the use of high-efficiency particulate air (HEPA) filters has been shown to reduce the rate of SSI development after orthopedic implant surgery.[52]

PRINCIPLES OF TREATMENT

Immune defenses within the brain are rarely adequate to control infection once it has been established. Postoperative infections tend to be particularly difficult to resolve because of the complex anatomic changes resulting from craniotomy and the frequent involvement of virulent organisms. Early and decisive intervention is critical to limit morbidity, and the keystone of successful treatment is effective source control (i.e., drainage of abscesses and infected fluid collections and débridement of necrotic tissue).[64] Once source control has been achieved, initiation of appropriate antibiotic therapy is necessary to eliminate any residual local infection.

The ability of antimicrobials to treat postcraniotomy infections successfully is a function of multiple factors. Selection of an antibiotic regimen should be based on the capacity of the antibiotic to penetrate the infected tissue effectively and to exhibit activity against the suspected pathogen. Bactericidal rather than bacteriostatic agents are generally preferred because of the inefficient opsonization and phagocytic capabilities within the brain.[65] Maximal bactericidal activity is achieved only when the peak antibiotic concentration at the site of infection exceeds the minimal inhibitory concentration of the causative organism by at least 5- to 10-fold.[66,67] Most antibiotic agents enter the CNS predominantly by passive diffusion down a concentration gradient, with physical barriers such as the blood-brain and blood-CSF barriers functioning as the primary determinants of drug distribution. Inflammation at the site of infection may facilitate entry of drugs across these barriers and into the brain, but not all postoperative infections are accompanied by marked inflammation, and concomitant treatment with corticosteroids may further impair drug entry.[68] Other inherent physiochemical properties of the antimicrobial agent may affect its penetration into the CNS, including molecular weight, lipophilicity, protein binding, and ionization state. Optimal antibiotic administration and dosing rely on an understanding of the pharmacodynamic properties of the agent and the susceptibility profile of the microorganism. In the absence of data from prospective randomized clinical trials evaluating the success rates of specific antibacterial agents, recommendations for the treatment of postcraniotomy infections are based largely on the results of previous experience, along with consideration of the complex physiologic, bacteriologic, and pharmacologic factors involved.

Empirical treatment of postoperative infections should include broad coverage for the full spectrum of potential pathogens, including resistant gram-positive organisms (e.g., MRSA) and gram-negative bacilli (e.g., *Pseudomonas* and *Acinetobacter* spp.). Failure to include an antibacterial agent with activity against the responsible bacterium may result in severe neurological sequelae or death.[65] Suitable empirical regimens for postcraniotomy infections typically include a combination of vancomycin and a second drug such as a third- or fourth-generation cephalosporin having antipseudomonal activity (e.g., ceftazidime, cefepime) or a carbapenem (e.g., meropenem). Antibiotic selection can be tailored once speciation and susceptibility testing from a microbiologic specimen are available.

Vancomycin has weaker activity against staphylococcal infections relative to β-lactams[69] and decreased penetration into the CNS because of its large molecular weight (1449 daltons).[65] Even in the presence of significant inflammation, concentrations of vancomycin may be critically low at the site of infection,[70] and substitution of a β-lactamase–resistant penicillin (e.g., nafcillin, oxacillin) for vancomycin is appropriate, except in the setting of resistance or hypersensitivity. First-generation cephalosporins (e.g., cefazolin) have relatively poor CNS penetration and are not recommended for the treatment of deep wound infections.

Third-generation cephalosporins (specifically cefotaxime, ceftriaxone, and ceftazidime) are often used for the treatment of CNS and postcraniotomy infections because of their low toxicity, good CNS penetration, and excellent in vitro activity against many of the responsible bacterial pathogens. Administration of these agents in high doses achieves therapeutic concentrations within brain abscess cavities.[71,72] Carbapenems such as imipenem (with cilastatin) and meropenem also cover a broad antimicrobial spectrum and have been used successfully for the treatment of bacterial brain abscesses.[73-75] These agents, principally imipenem-cilastatin, are associated with an increased seizure risk, and their use in patients with postcraniotomy infections should be considered primarily for resistant pathogens. From a pharmacokinetic viewpoint, fluoroquinolones (levofloxacin, ciprofloxacin, moxifloxacin) are attractive agents for the treatment of CNS infection because of their lipophilicity and low molecular mass. The usefulness of these agents, however, is limited by a high rate of bacterial resistance, increased seizure potential (albeit modest), and a relative paucity of data regarding their clinical effectiveness for postoperative CNS infections.[76]

Newer agents that may prove useful for the treatment of resistant staphylococcal infections include linezolid and daptomycin. Linezolid has bacteriostatic activity against both MRSA and vancomycin-resistant enterococci and bactericidal activity against most streptococci. Linezolid may be administered intravenously or orally and has excellent bioavailability. Experience with this agent for the treatment of postcraniotomy infections is limited, and potential side effects include reversible myelosuppression and irreversible peripheral neuropathy.[69] Daptomycin is a novel cyclic lipopeptide antibiotic that shows better in vitro microbicidal activity against MRSA than either vancomycin or linezolid and has been used primarily for the treatment of skin and soft tissue infections. Animal models of meningitis suggest that it may be an effective therapeutic agent in a setting of meningeal inflammation[77-79]; human studies to date are lacking.

Rifampin is a broad-spectrum antimicrobial that may have a role in the adjunctive treatment of infections associated with foreign body implantation or bone flap osteomyelitis. These types of infections are notoriously difficult to eradicate because of their resistance to host defense mechanisms and poor penetration of antimicrobials. Most foreign body infections are caused by staphylococci growing in biofilms consisting of bacteria clustered together in an extracellular matrix attached to the foreign body.[80] Depletion of metabolic substances within the biofilm causes the microbes to enter a slowly growing (sessile) state, which renders them up to 1000 times more resistant to most antimicrobial agents than their free-living (planktonic) counterparts.[69,81-84] Rifampin is one of just a few agents that can effectively penetrate biofilms and kill organisms in the sessile phase of growth. Because of the rapid emergence of resistance, rifampin must always be used in combination with a second active agent. In vitro data, experimental animal models, and several randomized clinical trials suggest that dual therapy that includes rifampin may be better than monotherapy for orthopedic hardware–related staphylococcal infections in terms of bone sterilization and cure rates.[69,85,86] This experience makes adjunctive therapy with rifampin an attractive consideration for difficult postcraniotomy staphylococcal infections associated with retained hardware or osteitis. Caution must be used with rifampin therapy because of its very large number of drug interactions. Through cytochrome P-450 enzyme induction, rifampin increases the metabolism of many substrates, including antiseizure drugs, anticoagulants, and immunosuppressive and chemotherapeutic agents.[87]

Aminoglycosides have excellent activity against aerobic gram-negative bacilli, including *P. aeruginosa*, as well as synergistic activity with β-lactams against aerobic gram-positive cocci. Systemic use of aminoglycosides is limited by their toxicity profile and a narrow therapeutic window. Penetration into CSF and across the blood-brain barrier is poor.[88] Polymyxins (e.g., colistin) also have activity against a broad array of gram-negative bacilli but fell out of favor because of nephrotoxicity.[89] As a result of the retained activity of polymyxins against multidrug-resistant gram-negative bacilli, including *P. aeruginosa* and *Acinetobacter baumannii*, this class again plays a role in difficult to treat infections. Similar to the aminoglycosides, the distribution of systemically administered polymyxins to CSF is poor. Intraventricular antibiotic administration bypasses the blood-brain barrier, can achieve much higher CSF concentrations than with systemic administration, and has been used successfully in multiple case reports.[90-92] Intraventricular antibiotic dosing has been associated with neurotoxicity, however, in experimental animal models and a small number of case reports.[93,94] Currently, there are no well-established data to support adjunctive intraventricular administration when a systemically delivered antimicrobial can achieve adequate microbicidal concentrations in CSF.

SUPERFICIAL INFECTIONS AND BONE FLAP OSTEOMYELITIS

Clinical Manifestations

Superficial infections after craniotomy comprise a collection of anatomically distinct infections that may extend from the skin to the epidural space. The potential for these infections to extend through the dura mandates that they be effectively treated and the response to therapy closely monitored to ensure resolution of infection. Bone flap osteomyelitis is typically included in this category, and the development of infection within the devascularized bone flap presents increased challenges for treatment.

Superficial infections are the most frequent infectious complication after craniotomy. Although every surgical patient is at risk for postoperative infection, a variety of factors may contribute to create an environment that is suboptimal for wound healing and more favorable for infection, including repeat operative intervention, poor tissue quality, impaired vascular supply, radiation injury, nutritional deficiencies, and the presence of foreign bodies. The role of foreign material in facilitating infection was first reported by Elek and Conen, who demonstrated a 10,000-fold increased risk for skin abscesses in the presence of suture material.[95,96] Continuous activation of granulocytes by foreign bodies may lead to local impairment of phagocytic ability, thereby reducing the amount of bacterial contamination needed to establish infection.[18,66]

Superficial infections are typically manifested as local erythema, swelling, and tenderness at the craniotomy site or as wound breakdown and suppurative drainage. With progressive infection, systemic signs such as malaise, fever, or chills may develop. The presence of neurological symptoms such as meningismus, altered mental status, or new focal deficits strongly suggests the coexistence of deep wound infection. The most common pathogenic agents of superficial wound infections are gram-positive cocci, including *S. aureus*, coagulase-negative staphylococci, and *P. acnes*.[35,53,58,97] Infection of the bone flap most often results from either direct bacterial inoculation at the time of surgery or extension of infection from the adjacent subgaleal or epidural compartments.

Diagnostic Imaging and Laboratory Data

The presence of superficial wound infection is often clinically apparent; however, imaging studies can frequently assist in defining the anatomic extent of infection (especially extension through the dura), as well as possible precipitating factors, such as entry into the mastoid air cells or paranasal sinuses during craniotomy. Computed tomography (CT) or magnetic resonance imaging (MRI) may reveal fluid collections in the subgaleal or epidural spaces that require surgical evacuation or extension of infection beyond the dura and into the subdural space or brain parenchyma. Imaging studies may also show evidence of bone flap destruction suggestive of osteomyelitis. Unfortunately, diffusion-weighted imaging, which is very sensitive to spontaneous intracerebral abscesses, is frequently unreliable in diagnosing the presence of superficial infection after craniotomy.[98]

Measurement of the erythrocyte sedimentation rate (ESR) or C-reactive protein (CRP) level may provide some assistance in detecting infection and monitoring the response to therapy. These acute-phase reactants are normally elevated after craniotomy and return toward baseline levels by the fifth postoperative day.[99] Although these markers are highly nonspecific, prolonged elevation or a secondary increase in their levels may indicate the development of bone flap infection. Failure of the ESR or CRP level to decline after institution of therapy may signify persistent infection and the need for prolonged antibiotic therapy or further diagnostic imaging to detect recurrence.

Treatment

Treatment of superficial wound infections depends on the extent of infection. Superficial cellulitis, a spreading infection of subcutaneous tissue without deeper infection of the subgaleal space or bone flap, is generally treated with oral or intravenous antibiotic therapy. Oral agents typically used to treat gram-positive bacteria include first-generation cephalosporins (e.g., cefazolin) or β-lactamase–resistant penicillins (e.g., dicloxacillin). In patients with rapidly spreading infection, prominent systemic symptoms, or significant comorbidity, initial antibiotic administration should be by the intravenous route until the symptoms improve and fever abates.[100]

Devitalization and devascularization of the bone flap at the time of craniotomy present a unique challenge in the treatment of infection because of impaired delivery of host defense mechanisms and antibacterial agents. Treatment options include antibiotic therapy alone, débridement with replacement of the bone flap, or surgical débridement with removal of the bone flap. Prolonged antibiotic therapy may control the clinical manifestations of infection but rarely leads to complete eradication, with frequent recrudescence after discontinuation of the antibio. Removal of the infected bone flap followed by delayed cranioplasty allows the best chance of clearing the initial infection; however, this treatment approach entails multiple surgical interventions and at least temporary cosmetic deformity while predisposing to the possibility of subsequent brain injury with a long-term risk for cranioplasty infection.[13,101-103] Several small case series have reported clinical resolution of infection with preservation of the bone flap. Bruce and Bruce reported salvage of the bone flap in 11 of 13 patients simply by mechanical débridement of the bone flap to remove any necrotic or purulent debris and soaking the bone in antibiotic-containing solution and povidine.[104] Closed suction antibiotic solution irrigation systems have also been used to treat bone flap osteomyelitis with varying degrees of success.[102,105] In selecting a therapeutic approach for each patient, the risks associated with salvaging the bone flap must be weighed against the hazards of the infection itself.

Hyperbaric oxygen (HBO) therapy is sometimes used to treat complicated superficial infections, including those involving the bone flap. HBO therapy increases oxygen tension in infected tissues, thereby improving oxidative killing of aerobic bacteria by phagocytic cells and providing a direct bactericidal effect on anaerobic organisms such as *P. acnes*. Larsson and associates used HBO to treat postcraniotomy infections successfully without removing the bone flap in 15 of 19 patients and in 3 of 6 patients with acrylic cranioplasties.[106] HBO therapy may also prove useful in the treatment of poorly healing, secondarily infected wounds such as those frequently associated with radiation injury.[107] Irradiation may impair wound healing by multiple mechanisms, including microvascular injury and ischemic damage, fibroblast dysfunction, and alterations in the synthesis of growth factors.[108] In addition to helping clear the infection, HBO therapy may also promote neoangiogenesis and reverse the vascular compromise present at the wound.[6,109] Limitations of HBO therapy include the cost of treatment and the need for multiple sessions. The possibility of increased tumor growth with the use of HBO in patients with malignancy has been raised as a potential concern, although clinical and experimental evidence of a tumor stimulatory effect is lacking.[110-114] The use of local rotational or pedicled flaps or vascularized myocutaneous free flaps represents another potential treatment option for chronic postoperative infections that cannot be eradicated with conventional surgical débridement and bone flap removal.[115]

SUBDURAL EMPYEMA

Clinical Manifestations

Although spontaneously occurring subdural empyemas are typically accompanied by fever and headache, followed by the rapid development of focal neurological deficits, altered mental status, and seizures, this fulminant manifestation is rarely seen in patients in whom subdural empyema develops after craniotomy.[97,116] Hlavin and associates reviewed their experience in 27 patients with postoperative subdural and epidural empyemas and found that only a third were febrile and 85% were without headache.[16] The most common findings were evidence of superficial wound infection and the presence of diffuse encephalopathy. In almost half of the patients, the subdural empyema occurred more than 1 month after the craniotomy. Seizures were present in 25% of patients with postoperative subdural empyema.

Diagnostic Imaging and Laboratory Data

Sterile extra-axial fluid collections are commonly noted on postoperative imaging studies, and differentiation from infected purulent fluids (empyema) may be difficult in the absence of overt clinical signs. In subdural empyema, non–contrast-enhanced CT typically demonstrates a crescent-shaped fluid collection that is slightly more dense than CSF and located beneath the craniotomy flap or adjacent to the falx. Increased signal intensity is usually seen on T1-weighted and fluid-attenuated inversion recovery (FLAIR) MRI sequences because of the increased protein concentration of an empyema relative to CSF. Peripheral enhancement of the fluid collection is common (Fig. 40-1). Unfortunately, these imaging characteristics are nonspecific and may also be seen with postoperative hematomas or sterile effusions. The presence of restricted diffusion on MRI may be helpful, although the absence of restricted diffusion does not exclude the presence of infection; 29% of confirmed postoperative subdural infections did not demonstrate diffusion abnormalities in one study.[98] Progressive enlargement of the fluid collection or unexplained edema in adjacent cerebral cortex may be helpful in identifying the existence of infection.

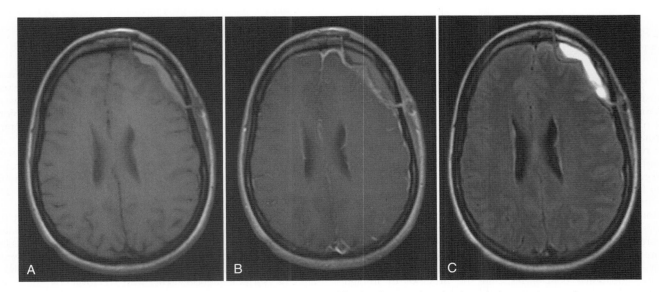

FIGURE 40-1 A, T1-weighted axial MRI reveals a hyperintense subdural fluid collection that developed after craniotomy for aneurysm repair. The fluid collection enhances peripherally with gadolinium (**B**) and exhibits increased signal intensity on fluid-attenuated inversion recovery (FLAIR) sequences (**C**) relative to CSF because of increased protein content. A craniotomy was performed to drain the collection, and frank purulence was encountered in the subdural space.

Laboratory data findings in patients with subdural empyema are typically nonspecific. Hlavin and colleagues found an elevated white blood cell count in 63% of their patients with postoperative infections, whereas ESR values were often within the normal range.[16] CSF findings may be normal or show evidence of a parameningeal reaction but rarely yield definitive evidence of infection. Additionally, lumbar puncture is frequently contraindicated in the setting of subdural empyema because of the possibility of cerebral herniation. In one study of 280 patients with spontaneous subdural empyemas who underwent lumbar puncture, 33 were thought to have experienced neurological deterioration as a direct result of the procedure.[117]

Treatment

Although postoperative subdural empyemas tend to have a more insidious course than spontaneous infections, early diagnosis and aggressive treatment are necessary to prevent spread of infection intraparenchymally and to avoid complications such as thrombophlebitis and venous infarction. Surgical drainage is usually necessary because antimicrobial agents do not reliably sterilize the empyema.[116] The goals of surgery are to evacuate the purulent collection completely and achieve adequate decompression of the brain when significant edema is associated with the infection. Although the optimal surgical approach (craniotomy versus burhole drainage) is debated, craniotomy is generally advocated because it ensures maximal drainage of the collection and allows inspection of adjacent anatomic areas and removal of the bone flap if necessary.

Empirical antibiotic therapy should be started as soon as material for culture has been obtained or earlier if surgical intervention must be delayed. The antibiotics chosen should be active against both skin flora and gram-negative bacilli because the latter have been shown to account for about half of subdural empyemas after craniotomy.[16] Vancomycin plus a third-generation cephalosporin with good activity against *Pseudomonas*, such as ceftazidime, is a frequently used empirical regimen, with adjustment according to individual institutional profiles of resistance. The duration of antibiotic therapy is typically 4 to 6 weeks. The role of imaging, especially diffusion imaging, in the evaluation of response to therapy or duration of therapy has been only minimally explored.[118,119]

BRAIN ABSCESS

Clinical Manifestations

Localized intraparenchymal abscesses may develop after craniotomy as a result of direct bacterial seeding or by extension of more superficial infection through an incompetent dura. Although the development of a brain abscess after craniotomy is rare, it is likely that common postoperative sequelae, such as small fluid collections or compromised areas of contused or ischemic brain, serve as a nidus for abscess formation. Once infection has been established, abscess development begins as a localized area of cerebritis characterized by perivascular inflammation and edema formation. It then progresses to a discrete focus of necrotic, purulent material surrounded by a well-vascularized capsule composed of fibroblasts and reactive collagen.[120]

Clinically, the classic triad of headache, fever, and focal neurological deficit is rarely present, and the signs and symptoms of postoperative abscess are frequently nonspecific. Fever is present in only about half of affected patients, and its absence should not be used to exclude the diagnosis.[15,72,121-123] Symptoms are often related to the presence of an expanding, irritative mass lesion and include altered level of consciousness, nausea, vomiting, and seizures. In a series of 31 patients with nosocomial brain abscess after neurosurgical intervention, Yang and coauthors reported that 17 had a disturbance in consciousness.[15] The prognosis is much poorer in patients with significant alterations in mental status or rapid progression of symptoms, and a high degree of suspicion is necessary to recognize the existence of infection as early as possible.[72,124] Seizures develop in about 20% of patients with spontaneous brain abscess and appear to occur at a similar rate with postoperative abscesses.[15,122,125]

Abrupt worsening of preexisting headache accompanied by new onset of meningismus may indicate rupture of a brain abscess into the cerebral ventricle, a condition associated with a high mortality rate that may require more aggressive medical and surgical intervention. Intraventricular rupture of a brain abscess (IVROBA) may also be manifested clinically by sudden neurological deterioration with obtundation or coma (Fig. 40-2). The pathophysiology of this decline is probably multifactorial, including both the development of severe widespread meningoencephalitis and alterations in CSF flow causing an increase in intracranial pressure. Zeidman and colleagues, in an extensive review of the literature from 1950 to 1993, identified 129 reported cases of IVROBA with a combined mortality rate of 85%.[126] Furthermore, although the overall mortality for brain abscesses decreased significantly over successive decades, the mortality rate for IVROBA remained consistent throughout this period. Lee and coauthors reported the most recent data on IVROBA outcome in a series of 62 patients treated between 1986 and 2005.[127] Their mortality rate was 27%; however, the overall rate of poor neurological outcome, including severe disability, persistent vegetative state, or death, was nearly 50%. Clinical and radiographic prediction of patients at increased risk for intraventricular rupture should prompt more urgent surgical intervention and decrease the incidence of IVROBA and its sequelae. Neither the specific infecting organism nor abscess size is associated with risk for rupture, although multiloculated abscesses have been correlated with increased risk.[127] Not surprisingly, decreased distance from the abscess capsule to the ventricular wall has also been demonstrated to correlate with the rate of intraventricular rupture.[127,128] These data correspond to findings in pathologic studies revealing that abscess capsule formation tends to be more complete on the cortical side of a brain abscess than on the ventricular side, which probably contributes to the increased rate of intraventricular rupture with deep-seated abscesses.[129] The presence of localized ventricular enhancement on CT has also been shown to herald impending intraventricular rupture and clinical deterioration.[130] Once IVROBA has occurred, radiographic imaging often reveals diffuse ependymal and meningeal enhancement and the presence of debris within the ventricles (see Fig. 40-2). Hydrocephalus accompanies IVROBA in about 50% of cases, and septation of the ventricles may occur as a delayed complication of intraventricular rupture.[127,131] Takeshita and colleagues found that all 20 of their patients with IVROBA reported prodromal symptoms of severe headache and meningeal irritation before the onset of their rapid clinical decline.[130] Decreased morbidity seems to be associated with IVROBA in patients taking antibiotics or with sterile abscesses at the time of rupture, thus suggesting that antimicrobial therapy should be instituted rapidly in patients exhibiting prodromal symptoms or with abscesses adjacent to the ventricular system.[128,130]

Diagnostic Imaging and Laboratory Data

Because of the often nonspecific clinical symptoms associated with brain abscess and the frequent absence of fever, neuroimaging typically plays a dominant role in the diagnosis of postoperative intraparenchymal infection. Imaging studies can also help define the anatomic extent of infection to guide surgical intervention and assist in evaluating the response to therapy. The radiographic features of brain abscess depend on its stage of progression.

FIGURE 40-2 Purulent drainage developed after craniotomy for a left frontal cavernous malformation. T1-weighted axial MRI with gadolinium (**A**) demonstrated enhancement within the extra-axial space and the resection cavity. A craniotomy with drainage of purulent material from the epidural and subdural compartments was performed, and treatment with intravenous antibiotics was started. Five days later, severe headache and worsened mental status developed. MRI (**B**) showed rupture of the intraparenchymal abscess into the adjacent lateral ventricle.

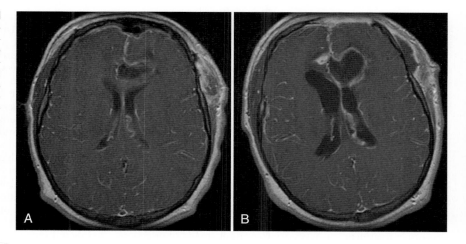

During the cerebritis stage, CT reveals a poorly defined area of low attenuation with a mass effect and significant edema. As a capsule begins to form around the infection, peripheral enhancement increases and the center of the lesion becomes progressively hypodense. Cerebritis typically appears on MRI as an area of high T2-weighted signal with patchy enhancement.[132] Subsequent capsule development is characterized on T1-weighted images as a ring of gadolinium enhancement surrounding a necrotic cavity of low signal intensity (Fig. 40-3). Concurrent treatment with corticosteroids, radiation therapy, and chemotherapy may alter the radiographic progression of abscess development.[133] Corticosteroids have been shown to reduce the thickness of the abscess capsule and the extent of contrast enhancement on both CT and MRI.[76] Additionally, the presence of peripheral enhancement

FIGURE 40-3 One month after resection of a right frontal glioma, this patient exhibited confusion and lethargy. T1-weighted axial MRI before (**A**) and after (**B**) gadolinium administration demonstrated enhancement of the resection cavity and surrounding meninges, and the FLAIR sequence (**C**) showed significant surrounding edema. Abnormal restricted diffusion (**D**) suggested infection. Craniotomy confirmed the presence of purulent material in the subdural and intraparenchymal locations.

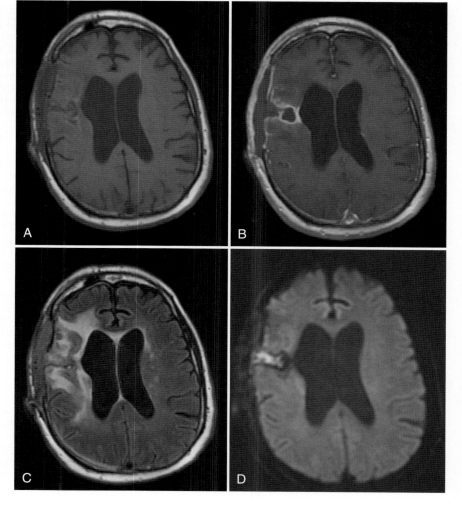

around a resection cavity is often nonspecific in the postcraniotomy setting and may reflect residual or recurrent tumor, treatment effect, infarction, or resolving hematoma. Diffusion-weighted MRI has demonstrated a high degree of specificity and sensitivity in differentiating spontaneous abscess from other ring-enhancing lesions, and its application to the diagnosis of postoperative brain abscess may prove useful. In a retrospective analysis we reviewed the diffusion-weighted findings in 50 patients with microbiologically confirmed postoperative infections and found evidence of abnormally restricted diffusion in all patients with intraparenchymal infection; much higher false-negative rates on diffusion-weighted imaging were found with more superficial infections such as epidural or subgaleal abscesses.[98] Importantly, the presence of restricted diffusion is not specific for infection, and correlation with apparent diffusion coefficient and T2-weighted MRI sequences or CT is necessary to evaluate for blood products that may cause a "T2 shine-through effect" in which the infection appears bright on diffusion-weighted images. The role of other advanced MRI sequences potentially useful for the diagnosis of infection, such as spectroscopy or perfusion imaging, has largely been unexplored in the postoperative setting.[134]

Similar to the nonspecific clinical and radiographic manifestations of postcraniotomy brain abscess, there are no laboratory findings that definitively establish the diagnosis. Peripheral leukocytosis is frequently absent, and although the ESR and CRP level are usually elevated, normal values may occur in patients with proven infection.[135,136] Blood cultures seldom yield a causative organism but should be performed to assess for a possible hematogenous source of infection. CSF analysis is rarely helpful and typically reveals only a nonspecific elevation in protein level and cell count, and lumbar puncture is frequently contraindicated because of increased intracranial pressure and risk for cerebral herniation.[123]

Treatment

The approach to treatment of postoperative brain abscesses is similar to that for spontaneous abscesses, although the increased frequency of multiantibiotic-resistant bacterial pathogens and the extension of infection into adjacent anatomic compartments in the postoperative setting may complicate treatment. The general goals of treatment are to relieve the mass effect, improve clinical symptoms, and fully resolve the infection. In most cases, a combination of surgical drainage and a prolonged course of intravenous antibiotics is required. Surgical options include open operative drainage or excision of the lesion and stereotactic aspiration. Both options have been used successfully in the treatment of postcraniotomy abscess, although stereotactic aspiration of brain abscesses is associated with a higher incidence of recurrence and the need for repeat surgical intervention.[109,137] Additionally, postcraniotomy abscesses are often multiloculated, which predicts a higher chance of recurrence after initial drainage.[138] Open surgical excision also allows débridement of any associated parameningeal infection and removal of necrotic debris or foreign bodies.

Once specimens have been obtained for culture, empirical antibiotic therapy should be started based on Gram stain results and institutional data regarding the probable causative agents and their antibiotic resistance patterns. Typically, vancomycin and a third- or fourth-generation cephalosporin with antipseudomonal activity (e.g., ceftazidime, cefepime) are appropriate initial choices, although studies comparing the relative efficacy of various treatment regimens have not been performed. Metronidazole may be added to the empirical regimen for coverage of anaerobic organisms if an otic, paranasal sinus, or mastoid source of infection is suspected based on the surgical intervention performed. In critically ill patients in whom urgent surgical drainage is not possible, initiation of broad-spectrum antibiotic therapy

before culture results are available may be necessary. Mampalam and coworkers reported, however, that 30% of patients who received antibiotics preoperatively had sterile cultures, thus potentially resulting in inappropriate medical treatment or the need for prolonged therapy with multiple antibiotics.[139]

High-dose intravenous antibiotics have conventionally been administered for 6 to 8 weeks in patients with brain abscesses. Frequently, this is followed by a course of oral antibiotic therapy if a suitable agent is available, although the efficacy and necessity of this approach have not been established.[72] Shorter course therapies have also been reported to be effective,[137,140] and length of treatment should be guided by the virulence of the causative organism, clinical therapeutic response, and serial neuroimaging findings. Progressive enlargement of the abscess or failure of the abscess to become smaller despite treatment of a susceptible organism with an appropriate antibiotic should prompt repeat surgical drainage and microbiologic reassessment. Several reports have also advocated placement of drains into the abscess for postsurgical drainage and intracavitary administration of antibiotics for difficult to treat infections[72,141,142]; however, this form of therapy should be used with caution given the minimal evidence in support of its efficacy and the potential for neurotoxicity, including seizures.[13] Brain abscesses associated with intraventricular rupture may also require more aggressive treatment to reduce morbidity and mortality. Intraventricular administration of antibiotics may be considered for the treatment of bacterial agents that are susceptible only to antibacterials with poor blood-CSF penetration. Multiple reports have demonstrated increased CSF antibiotic concentrations, successful clearance of ventricular infection, and minimal toxicity after intraventricular administration of antibiotics, most commonly vancomycin, aminoglycosides, and colistin.[90,143-147]

Adjunctive corticosteroid treatment may be indicated in patients with significant cerebral edema related to cerebral infections with signs of impending herniation. Additionally, given the high incidence of seizures associated with brain abscess, administration of seizure prophylaxis should be considered until the infection has resolved.

BACTERIAL MENINGITIS

Clinical Manifestations

Bacterial meningitis is relatively uncommon after neurosurgical procedures and complicates less than 1% of craniotomies.[7,12] Although the clinical course of nosocomial meningitis tends to be less fulminant than that of community-acquired meningitis, rapid diagnosis and implementation of antimicrobial therapy are critical because the mortality rate may exceed 20% if treatment is delayed.[68,148] The typical symptoms of meningitis tend to be present in patients with postoperative bacterial meningitis, including fever, headache, and neck stiffness; however, these symptoms may also occur in patients without infection after craniotomy, especially of the posterior fossa.

Complicating the diagnosis of postoperative meningitis is the clinically similar condition of a sterile postoperative meningitis presumed to be due to chemical irritation, as first described by Cushing and Bailey in 1928.[149] Subsequent authors have shown that aseptic (chemical) meningitis is responsible for 60% to 75% of all cases of postoperative clinical meningitis and that it occurs most frequently in children and after posterior fossa surgery.[148,150] Despite its frequent occurrence, the etiology of aseptic meningitis remains incompletely understood, but it is presumed to be caused by irritation from blood breakdown products or from factors released by surgical materials such as dural substitutes. Diagnosis of aseptic meningitis requires negative CSF Gram staining and cultures, and the patient must recover fully without the administration of antibiotics. Corticosteroids typically provide symptomatic relief in patients with aseptic chemical meningitis.

Diagnostic Imaging and Laboratory Data

Unfortunately, differentiation between chemical and bacterial meningitis is frequently problematic, and no single clinical sign or diagnostic test distinguishes between the two entities with certainty. Neuroimaging studies rarely assist in the diagnosis of postoperative meningitis because the characteristic imaging sign of meningeal enhancement can also be seen in up to 80% of postcraniotomy patients who do not have infections.[151] CT or MRI may, however, reveal secondary complications of meningitis, including hydrocephalus, parameningeal abscess, or ischemia/infarction related to vasculitis and thrombosis of superficial vessels.

CSF culture data remain the "gold standard" for diagnosis of postoperative bacterial meningitis, although the definition of nosocomial meningitis used by the U.S. Centers for Disease Control and Prevention does allow the diagnosis of meningitis to be made without and Prevention positive CSF cultures under certain circumstances only if a physician institutes "appropriate antimicrobial therapy."[152] CSF Gram staining is highly insensitive for infection. Several studies have shown that Gram staining is positive in only 25% to 50% of cases of culture-confirmed bacterial meningitis.[17,153] CSF hypoglycorrhachia and pleocytosis with neutrophilic predominance are common findings in both aseptic and bacterial meningitis, although one study found that CSF white blood cell counts greater than 7500 cells/μL and glucose concentrations lower than 10 mg/dL were not present in any patient with aseptic meningitis.[153] Unfortunately, laboratory findings within this range were not very common in patients who did have confirmed bacterial infections.

A variety of alternative diagnostic tests have been investigated to better distinguish between these two entities, with several retrospective studies identifying CSF lactate concentrations greater than 4 mmol/L and IL-1β levels greater than 90 ng/L predicting the presence of bacterial meningitis with good sensitivity and specificity in postsurgical patients.[154,155] Elevated CSF lactate probably results from a combination of bacterial production, anaerobic glycolysis, and metabolism by CSF leukocytes,[156] whereas IL-1β is a key inflammatory mediator in the response to meningeal infection.[157] Although data regarding the clinical utility of these newer assays are promising, until they have been well validated in prospective studies, the recommendation remains that all patients with clinical and laboratory features consistent with postoperative meningitis receive empirical antibiotic treatment until CSF culture results are confirmed to be sterile.[13,158]

Treatment

The choice of empirical coverage depends on local bacterial infection and resistance patterns; however, typically the combination of vancomycin and a third-generation cephalosporin with antipseudomonal activity (e.g., ceftazidime) is appropriate. If the patient is not deteriorating clinically, CSF culture results remain sterile, and the treating clinician believes the original clinical syndrome to have been consistent with aseptic chemical meningitis, antibiotics may be discontinued after several days, provided that antibiotic therapy had not been started before CSF was obtained for culture. Using this algorithm, Zarrouck and colleagues demonstrated that the duration of antibiotic treatment of aseptic meningitis could be decreased from a mean of 11 days to 3.5 days, with no cases of diagnosed aseptic meningitis later proving to be misdiagnosed bacterial meningitis.[148] However, the possibility of misdiagnosis suggests that the patient should be kept under close clinical observation for a time after treatment with antibiotics is stopped.

Once the infecting pathogen has been isolated and its susceptibility profile determined, antibiotic therapy can be modified for optimal treatment. The duration of treatment may depend on the offending organism and its antibiotic susceptibility pattern, as well as other complicating factors such as the presence of parameningeal foci or the patient's underlying immune status. Clinicians may wish to add corticosteroids to the regimen, given the evidence that they are beneficial in many cases of sporadic bacterial meningitis; however, no trials have evaluated their use for postoperative bacterial meningitis specifically. Failure to improve after the institution of appropriate antibiotic therapy for a susceptible organism should prompt further CSF evaluation and measurement of CSF antibiotic concentrations.

CONCLUSION

The development of infection after craniotomy is a relatively rare occurrence, and prospective, randomized data evaluating the relative efficacy of various medical and surgical interventions are limited. Because the management of postcraniotomy infections continues to become increasingly complex with the emergence of highly resistant bacteria and implantation of foreign devices, close cooperation among neurosurgeons, infectious disease specialists, and hospital infection control services is critical in achieving the best possible outcomes and reducing neurological morbidity.

SUGGESTED READINGS

Alexander JW. The contributions of infection control to a century of surgical progress. *Ann Surg.* 1985;201:423.

Barker FG 2nd. Efficacy of prophylactic antibiotics for craniotomy: a meta-analysis. *Neurosurgery.* 1994;35:484.

Bruce JN, Bruce SS. Preservation of bone flaps in patients with postcraniotomy infections. *J Neurosurg.* 2003;98:1203.

Darouiche RO. Treatment of infections associated with surgical implants. *N Engl J Med.* 2004;350:1422.

Durand ML, Calderwood SB, Weber DJ, et al. Acute bacterial meningitis in adults. A review of 493 episodes. *N Engl J Med.* 1993;328:21.

Farrell CJ, Hoh BL, Pisculli ML, et al. Limitations of diffusion-weighted imaging in the diagnosis of postoperative infections. *Neurosurgery.* 2008;62:577.

Forgacs P, Geyer CA, Freidberg SR. Characterization of chemical meningitis after neurological surgery. *Clin Infect Dis.* 2001;32:179.

Hlavin ML, Kaminski HJ, Fensternaker RA, et al. Intracranial suppuration: a modern decade of postoperative subdural empyema and epidural abscess. *Neurosurgery.* 1994;34:974.

Korinek AM. Risk factors for neurosurgical site infections after craniotomy: a prospective multicenter study of 2944 patients. The French Study Group of Neurosurgical Infections, the SEHP, and the C-CLIN Paris-Nord. Service Epidemiologie Hygiene et Prevention. *Neurosurgery.* 1997;41:1073.

Korinek AM, Golmard JL, Elcheick A, et al. Risk factors for neurosurgical site infections after craniotomy: a critical reappraisal of antibiotic prophylaxis on 4,578 patients. *Br J Neurosurg.* 2005;19:155.

Kurz A, Sessler DI, Lenhardt R. Perioperative normothermia to reduce the incidence of surgical-wound infection and shorten hospitalization. Study of Wound Infection and Temperature Group. *N Engl J Med.* 1996;334:1209.

Larsson A, Engstrom M, Uusijarvi J, et al. Hyperbaric oxygen treatment of postoperative neurosurgical infections. *Neurosurgery.* 2002;50:287.

Lee TH, Chang WN, Su TM, et al. Clinical features and predictive factors of intraventricular rupture in patients who have bacterial brain abscesses. *J Neurol Neurosurg Psychiatry.* 2007;78:303.

Lutsar I, Friedland IR. Pharmacokinetics and pharmacodynamics of cephalosporins in cerebrospinal fluid. *Clin Pharmacokinet.* 2000;39:335.

Malis LI. Prevention of neurosurgical infection by intraoperative antibiotics. *Neurosurgery.* 1979;5:339.

Mangram AJ, Horan TC, Pearson ML, et al. Guideline for prevention of surgical site infection, 1999. Hospital Infection Control Practices Advisory Committee. *Infect Control Hosp Epidemiol.* 1999;20:250.

Mathisen GE, Johnson JP. Brain abscess. *Clin Infect Dis.* 1997;25:763.

McClelland S 3rd, Hall WA. Postoperative central nervous system infection: incidence and associated factors in 2111 neurosurgical procedures. *Clin Infect Dis.* 2007;45:55.

Nau R, Sorgel F, Prange HW. Pharmacokinetic optimisation of the treatment of bacterial central nervous system infections. *Clin Pharmacokinet.* 1998;35:223.

Seydoux C, Francioli P. Bacterial brain abscesses: factors influencing mortality and sequelae. *Clin Infect Dis.* 1992;15:394.

Takeshita M, Kagawa M, Izawa M, et al. Current treatment strategies and factors influencing outcome in patients with bacterial brain abscess. *Acta Neurochir (Wien).* 1998;140:1263.

Tanner J, Woodings D, Moncaster K. Preoperative hair removal to reduce surgical site infection. *Cochrane Database Syst Rev.* 2006;3:CD004122.

Zarrouk V, Vassor I, Bert F, et al. Evaluation of the management of postoperative aseptic meningitis. *Clin Infect Dis.* 2007;44:1555.

Zeidman SM, Geisler FH, Olivi A. Intraventricular rupture of a purulent brain abscess: case report. *Neurosurgery.* 1995;36:189.

Full references can be found on Expert Consult @ www.expertconsult.com

CHAPTER 41

Postoperative Infections of the Spine

Michael A. Finn ■ Meic H. Schmidt

Postoperative infections in patients undergoing spine surgery are unfortunate complications that significantly contribute to patient morbidity. Although infection in the general spine surgery population is relatively infrequent, with rates between 1% and 5.4% usually being reported,[1-7] specific subpopulations, such as trauma or cancer patients, may have much higher infection rates.[4,8-10] The cost of treating postoperative infections was estimated at $100,000 per patient in 1996 in the United States,[11] but it is difficult to estimate the physical and social impact on the patient, who may be subjected to repeat washout and revision procedures and prolonged courses of intravenous antibiotic treatment. Modern surgical techniques, antisepsis, and antibiotic prophylaxis have made significant inroads into the problem of postoperative infection, but surgeons must be continually vigilant for this complication. Familiarity with current state-of-the art diagnostic tests, imaging evaluation, and treatment methods is essential.

INCIDENCE

Infections of the spinal column have been reported to occur both spontaneously and iatrogenically after surgical or other invasive intervention (e.g., after diskography, lumbar puncture). This chapter focuses on spinal infections resulting from open surgery. This group of infections represents a subgroup of all spinal infections, and it may be further divided into several smaller subgroups. The risks, symptoms, and treatment of spinal infection may be stratified according to whether the surgery involved the use of instrumentation and what approach was used.

Noninstrumented Spinal Procedures

Noninstrumented spinal procedures include anterior and posterior decompressive surgeries and are usually confined to short stretches of the spinal column, most often with only a single level treated. Although noninstrumented procedures may include fusions, most fusion procedures are now supplemented with instrumentation.

Lumbar diskectomy is one of the most common spinal procedures and is associated with highly successful clinical outcomes.[12] Fortunately, these procedures have an extremely low rate of infection, with most large series reporting an incidence of 1% or less.[13,14] Newer series of endoscopic minimally invasive diskectomy have achieved even lower rates of infection,[15,16] with one study reporting no infections in the treatment of 262 patients.[16] Infections after lumbar disk surgery can be manifested as superficial wound infections or as diskitis, with increasing back pain 2 weeks to several months postoperatively in conjunction with fever and laboratory and radiographic abnormalities.

Patients undergoing laminectomy without fusion may also enjoy a low incidence of infection, although slightly higher than that for patients undergoing diskectomy alone. Infection rates of approximately 2% are commonly reported in the literature for this procedure.[17] Laminoplasty techniques have been associated with a higher rate of infection and are probably more appropriately considered instrumented procedures because most involve the placement of some type of implant.[18]

Noninstrumented posterior spinal fusion is associated with a higher rate of infection than is simple laminectomy or lumbar diskectomy,[4,19] a factor attributable to longer operating times, more blood loss, greater soft tissue destruction, and placement of devascularized allograft.

Although most noninstrumented spinal surgeries involve a posterior approach, anterior cervical diskectomy and fusion procedures can be and often are performed without instrumentation, especially when only a single level is treated. Infection rates for the anterior cervical approach, however, are extremely low with and without the use of instrumentation,[20] thus making it difficult to discern any real difference between these two groups.

Finally, relatively limited interventional procedures such as chemonucleolysis and diskography are associated with an infection rate of up to 4% in the absence of preoperative antibiotics. Fortunately, this incidence can be dramatically decreased with the use of prophylactic antibiotics.[21-24]

Instrumented Spinal Procedures

The use of instrumentation in posterior spinal procedures increases the incidence of postoperative infection to approximately 3% to 7% in most series.[2,25-28] Spinal instrumentation increases the risk for infection by acting as a *locus minoris resistentiae* for organisms rather than as a source of inoculation.[29] In fact, one study demonstrated that 11 of 21 patients undergoing hardware removal for noninfectious reasons had positive bacterial growth on cultures.[30] Although most infections occur in the immediate postoperative period, there are multiple reports of delayed infections occurring years after surgery.[31-34] It is thus likely that colonization of implants is commonplace and that clinical infection occurs either when bacteria are sufficiently pathogenic or when host factors predispose to infection.

The type of instrumentation may affect the probability of clinical infection. Older steel implants tend to be uniquely implicated in the development of late spinal infections.[34] Corrosion and fretting at cross-connector sites have been associated with foreign body reactions and the development of a local environment favorable for the growth of endogenous or low-virulence bacteria.[32,34-36] This has not been reported with newer titanium implants, which are resistant to corrosion and thought to be relatively bacteria resistant.

Anterior instrumented spine surgeries are associated with extremely low rates of infection; when infections do occur, they tend to be superficial.[20,37-39] The low incidence of infections with the anterior approach is probably attributable to the use of avascular planes in dissections and minimization of soft tissue trauma and necrosis. Although the anterior approach itself is associated with a low risk for infection, the highest rates of infection are encountered with combined anterior and posterior approaches to the spine,[40] a finding probably attributable to the greater length and complexity of these cases.

An emerging category of spine surgery is minimally invasive surgery. The goal of minimally invasive spine surgery is to minimize soft tissue trauma and blood loss and thereby hasten patient recovery and decrease the risk for infection. Although several authors have realized good results with minimally invasive techniques,[41,42] most series are small and no reduction in wound infection rates has been conclusively demonstrated.[43] Further experience with these techniques will clarify the exact extent of the reduced infection risk with these methods.

Finally, the implantation of intrathecal drug delivery systems and spinal cord stimulators is associated with an approximately 5% risk for infection.[44,45] Infection with these devices occurs in the pump or stimulator pocket in most cases, although infection of the intraspinal component can lead to meningitis or epidural abscess.[44-46] These infections tend to occur early, usually within the first 2 postoperative months.

INFECTION RISK FACTORS

Although the type of surgery plays a large role in determining a patient's risk for infection, numerous patient-, surgery-, and disease-specific factors have been elucidated (Table 41-1).

Patient Factors

Important among patient factors are medical comorbid conditions, including increasing age, obesity, diabetes, poor nutritional status, and alcohol and tobacco use.[6,40,47-50] Other factors associated with an increased risk for postoperative infection include steroid use, rheumatoid disease, and an immunocompromised state.[40,51,52]

Obesity is a frequent comorbidity in the spine surgery population. Several studies have demonstrated an increased risk for infections in obese patients undergoing spine surgery.[40,49,51,53,54] Obese patients are subject to longer operative times; greater amounts of retraction, which, in turn, causes increased soft tissue necrosis; greater amounts of poorly vascularized fatty tissue with decreased oxygen tension; decreased immune defense in adipose tissue; and poor tissue concentrations of prophylactic antibiotics.[29,55-57] Finally, obesity predisposes the patient to diabetes.

Malnutrition is a well-known factor that predisposes patients to infection. It has been demonstrated to impair immune response and wound healing. Klein and coauthors reported that 25% of patients undergoing elective lumbar surgery had positive indices of malnutrition and that 11 of 13 infections occurred in these patients.[47] Other authors have also reported a high rate of infection in malnourished patients undergoing spine surgery,[58] as well as the development of malnutrition in some spine surgery patients during their hospital stay, a particular concern for those undergoing staged procedures.[59] Commonly used indices of malnutrition are serum albumin level and the total lymphocyte count, with values of less than 3.5 mg/dL and 1500/mL, respectively, being considered abnormal.[60] Other indices, including skinfold thickness, transferrin levels, arm muscle circumference, and weight-height ratio, can also be used to assess nutritional status.[61] Malnutrition may be associated with malignancy and trauma, two conditions known to be related to high rates of infection.

Diabetes impairs wound healing and predisposes to wound infection in spine and other surgeries.[6,40,62-64] Postoperative wound infections have been reported to occur in up to 24% of diabetic patients undergoing spine surgery.[40,63] Proposed mechanisms by which diabetes contributes to infection risk include increased glucose concentrations in wound fluids, the presence of dysfunctional polymorphonuclear neutrophils and macrophages, impaired lymphocyte chemotaxis, and delayed wound re-epithelialization.[65-68] Impaired glucose tolerance without overt diabetes has additionally been correlated with this complication in the spine.[6,51] Although studies of deep sternal surgical site infection in cardiothoracic procedures have demonstrated an ability to reduce this risk with strict perioperative glucose control, such a study in the spine is lacking.[69,70]

Tobacco use has been demonstrated to be a risk factor for wound infection in several studies.[71-73] Hypothesized mechanisms include deprivation of oxygen to tissues and impaired wound healing and neutrophil defense.[74-76]

Surgical Factors

Several surgical variables other than those discussed earlier have been identified that may predispose patients to infection. Many of these variables appear to correlate with the magnitude of the surgery itself. It is therefore not surprising that the number of levels treated, length of the surgery, procedural complexity, and amount of blood loss have all been associated with an elevated risk for infection.[2,25,49,62,77,78] Operative times longer than 5 hours have been associated with an increased rate of infection, as has blood loss of 1000 mL.[62,77]

The use of a cell saver system has been inconsistently correlated with infection risk. Although blood that has been processed by the cell saver system has been shown to be contaminated in 37% of various surgical procedures, no contamination was found in neurosurgical procedures.[79] Additionally, even though use of the cell saver system was correlated with infection in series of spinal patients,[31] no increased risk has been noted in other specialties.[80] The use of blood transfusion, however, has been correlated with infection in numerous studies, and this risk may be independent of the amount of blood loss.[31,80,81]

Other surgical risk factors include revision surgery, the use of allograft material, and surgery extending to the sacral region, the latter of which may be attributable to urine and fecal contamination.[25,82,83] Finally, the presence of two or more resident surgeons being involved in the procedure has been correlated with increased infectious risk in one study.[51] Although not completely explored, this variable may be a reflection of the length and complexity of the procedure rather than a truly independent risk factor.

TABLE 41-1 Risk Factors for Infection

TYPE OF FACTOR	CONDITION	INCREASED RISK
Patient specific	Age	>20 years
	Diabetes mellitus	Glucose intolerance
	Malnutrition	Albumin <3.5 mg/dL
		Total lymphocyte count <1500/mL
	Obesity	
	Alcoholism	
	Tobacco use	
	Urinary/fecal incontinence	
Disease specific	Immunocompromised state	Steroid use
		Rheumatoid disease
	Malignancy	
	Trauma	Spinal cord injury
Surgery specific	Posterior approaches	Staged anterior-posterior procedures
	Length of surgery	>5 hr
	Number of levels	
	Estimated blood loss	>1 L
		Blood transfusion
	Postoperative stay in an intensive care unit	
	Preoperative hospital stay	

Disease-Specific Factors

Infection risk has repeatedly been demonstrated as significantly altered by the disease state of the patient. The presence of malignancy appears to be associated with the highest incidence of infection, reported to be higher than 20% in some series.[4,8] This rate has been reported to be even higher in patients undergoing radiation therapy in conjunction with open surgery.[84-87] The high rate of postoperative infection in this population is probably multifactorial, however, with poor nutritional status, the long and complex surgical procedures necessary for spine reconstruction, and use of adjunctive therapies such as corticosteroids all contributing to the dramatically elevated risk for infection.

Traumatic spinal injury is also associated with a significantly higher risk for infection, especially in the presence of a complete neurological injury.[9,10] Again, the elevated risk in this group may be multifactorial, with prolonged stay in the intensive care unit, urinary or fecal incontinence, and large procedures all playing a role.[6]

Prolonged presurgical hospitalization and postoperative stay in the intensive care unit are also risk factors for wound infection. Blam and associates reported that patients staying in the intensive care unit for more than 1 day had a 6- to 13-fold greater risk for postoperative infection than did patients who did not stay in the intensive care unit.[9] Wimmer and coworkers showed that extensive presurgical hospital stay was significantly associated with infection.[62]

CLINICAL FINDINGS

The signs and symptoms of spinal infection depend on whether the infection is superficial or deep. Superficial infections occur above the lumbodorsal fascia in the dermis and subcutaneous tissue and are usually manifested in the immediate postoperative period as erythema, purulent drainage, and local tenderness. Patients may have low-grade fever, and laboratory evaluation may reveal elevated erythrocyte sedimentation rate (ESR), elevated C-reactive protein (CRP) level, and leukocytosis. The presence of these indices is variable, however. For example, Levi and coauthors reported an average temperature of 37.5° C and a white blood cell (WBC) count of 10.2×10^6 cells/mL in 17 patients with postoperative infections.[2] If the wound is open or purulence is expressible, Gram stain and cultures are often useful in revealing the pathogen and targeting treatment (Fig. 41-1).

Deep infections have a much more variable manifestation. They may develop in the immediate postoperative period, with some authors reporting most occurring 2 to 3 weeks postoperatively, or in a significantly delayed fashion several months to several years after surgery.[32,34] Patients with an acute manifestation are often symptomatic with significant pain, fever, anorexia, and night sweats. The wound overlying a deep infection can appear completely normal or, if the infection tracks superficially, can be purulent. Patients with a delayed manifestation often have increasing back pain, wound drainage, and erythema but may lack fever altogether.[34,88]

Spinal epidural abscess is a rare complication of spine surgery that may occur in an acute or delayed fashion and cause increased back pain, fever, and neurological deficit.[89,90] Patients with spinal epidural abscess may have a rapid neurological decline, and the presence of any neurological deficit should raise concern for this process.[91]

EVALUATION

Both laboratory evaluation and imaging are important in the assessment of postoperative spine infections. Laboratory evaluation should include a WBC count, ESR, CRP levels, and cultures and Gram staining if there is purulent drainage or an open wound. The WBC evaluation may be and often is normal, especially in patients with a delayed manifestation, but it can be useful if elevated.[88,92] The ESR is reliably elevated in the setting of infection, but a high ESR can be difficult to interpret in the immediate postoperative period. ESR values normally rise to a maximal value of 102 mm/hr after spine fusion surgery and 75 mm/hr after disk surgery on postoperative day 4 before declining to normal levels 2 to 4 weeks postoperatively.[92] Patients with infection have persistently elevated ESRs, usually more than 2 SD greater than the mean.[92] Infections with low-grade pathogens such as *Propionibacter* may, however, be associated with low or normal ESR values.[93] Obtaining serial ESRs can additionally be useful in tracking the response to treatment of infection. CRP values may be of added benefit in the diagnosis of infection, as well as in monitoring treatment response. A normal elevation of CRP is also seen in the immediate postoperative period; however, this elevation is more rapid and returns to baseline more quickly than does the rise in ESR, although complete normalization may take up to 2 weeks (Fig. 41-2).[94,95]

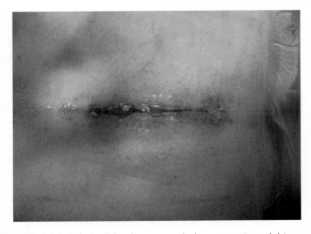

FIGURE 41-1 Infected lumbar wound demonstrating dehiscence, surrounding erythema, and purulence.

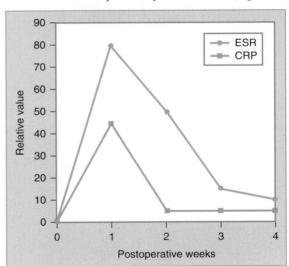

FIGURE 41-2 Graph showing normal postoperative spikes in the erythrocyte sedimentation rate (ESR) and C-reactive protein (CRP). Note that the decline in ESR is variable, with normalization taking between 2 and 4 weeks.

Additionally, CRP values are elevated more frequently than ESRs in the setting of infection with low-grade pathogens.[93]

Accurate diagnosis of bacterial pathogens is critical in the treatment of postoperative infections. Antibiotic therapy should be withheld until after specimens are taken for Gram staining and culture. These specimens are easily obtained from draining or open wounds, but care should be taken to prepare the skin carefully before specimen collection to prevent being misled by normal skin flora. If débridement is planned, specimens should be taken from both superficial and deep parts of the wound. Blood cultures can aid in the diagnosis of a pathogen when obtaining a direct specimen is difficult. Alternatively, computed tomography (CT)-guided or open biopsy of infected tissue may be helpful, with a diagnosis being obtained more than 50% of the time.[96-98]

Imaging Diagnosis

Use of appropriate imaging modalities may aid in the diagnosis of infection, as well as in assessing the adequacy of spinal instrumentation and fusion, which may be compromised with infection. Imaging during the immediate postoperative period may be difficult to interpret, however, because normal postoperative inflammatory changes mimic those found in infection. Imaging in this setting thus acts as an aid to diagnosis and can be valuable when considered in the context of clinical examination and laboratory findings.

Plain Radiographs and Computed Tomography

Plain radiographs are useful in the assessment of spine alignment, local soft tissue reaction to infection, and bony response to infection but have limited utility in the immediate postoperative period. Early bony changes in response to infection are manifested approximately 2 to 3 weeks postoperatively by evidence of disk space narrowing, bony destruction, and blurring of end plates. These findings may be followed by vertebral body collapse or sclerosis of end plates and bony ankylosis in the more chronic setting (Fig. 41-3).[99] Increased swelling noted in soft tissues, especially in the retropharyngeal space after anterior spine surgery, may indicate the presence of an abscess. Finally, plain radiographs are useful for evaluation of the integrity of spine hardware, with lucency around screws being associated with loosening and failure.

CT imaging reveals a sequence of bony changes similar to that seen in radiographs but provides improved anatomic detail and can better detect paraspinal masses and epidural collections.[99] When performed with contrast enhancement, CT can accurately delineate the presence of an abscess and provide a useful aid in surgical planning or can be used to guide percutaneous biopsy of infected bone or soft tissues.[100] CT myelography may be useful in aiding the diagnosis of epidural or subdural empyema when magnetic resonance imaging (MRI) is unavailable or contraindicated.[101]

Nuclear Imaging

Technetium 99m–labeled methylene diphosphonate bone scans can be used to help diagnose and localize an infection, but this technique suffers from limited sensitivity and specificity given that other conditions, such as trauma, tumor, or vascular insult, may have increased uptake and that uptake may be negative in photopenic areas where there is decreased blood flow or bone tissue.[99,102] A three-phase bone scan may increase the sensitivity and specificity of this test.[103] An indium 111– or technetium 99m–labeled leukocyte scan may help in diagnosing infection in settings where other factors, such as fracture, may cause false-positive results on bone scanning.[103,104]

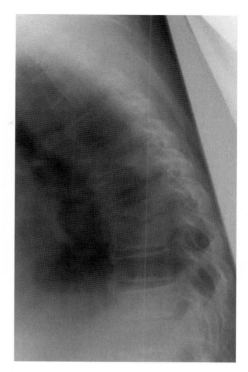

FIGURE 41-3 Lateral radiograph of a patient with chronic thoracic diskitis. Note the end-plate sclerosis, vertebral body collapse, and focal kyphosis.

Recent experience with ^{18}F-fluorodeoxyglucose positron emission tomography (PET) shows some promise, with the major caveat being the inability to differentiate tumor from infection.[105,106] PET may be particularly useful in the postoperative setting, however, where a negative PET scan can rule out infection.[107]

Magnetic Resonance Imaging

MRI is the imaging modality of choice when evaluating spine infections and enjoys a sensitivity and specificity of approximately 95% in the diagnosis of various spine infections, including osteomyelitis.[108-110] Early MRI findings in the setting of infection include bone marrow edema signal manifested as hypointensity on T1-weighted sequences and hyperintensity on T2/STIR (short tau inversion recovery) signals.[110,111] Although these findings are somewhat nonspecific, the observation of end-plate erosion with loss of the low signal intensity line, disk space narrowing, and disk space hyperintensity on T2-weighted sequences dramatically increases the sensitivity for infections.[112] Loss of the normal low-intensity disk space cleft on T2-weighted sequences is another clue to the presence of infection.[99] The addition of contrast enhancement is useful in confirming the presence of infection, delineating the extent of infection, and differentiating infection from solid granulation tissue, with the latter most often having a homogeneous pattern of enhancement (Fig. 41-4).[111-114] Finally, MRI is also useful in detecting the presence of soft tissue masses associated with infection, such as paraspinal or epidural abscesses. Identification of such an associated mass increases the likelihood of infection being present to 98%.[112]

Some of these MRI findings, including vertebral body edema signal and contrast enhancement, may be present in the postoperative setting in the absence of infection.[115,116] The presence of an adjacent soft tissue mass in this setting, however, strongly

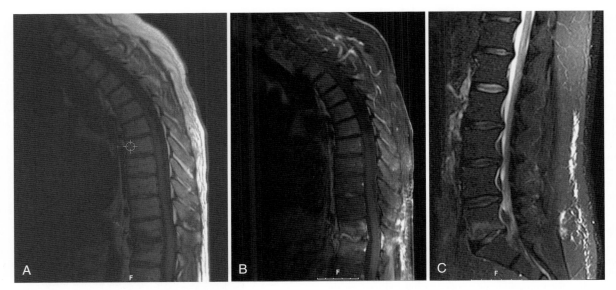

FIGURE 41-4 Sagittal T1-weighted non–contrast-enhanced (**A**) and contrast-enhanced (**B**) magnetic resonance images of thoracic diskitis. Note the hypointense signal intensity in the vertebral bodies and avid enhancement with the administration of contrast. **C,** Sagittal T2-weighted magnetic resonance image in a patient with postoperative L5-S1 diskitis. Note the hyperintense signal in adjacent end plates.

supports the diagnosis of infection. Moreover, absence of the MRI findings just listed strongly correlates with the absence of infection.[116]

BACTERIOLOGY

Skin flora are the most common causative organisms in postoperative spine infection, with staphylococcal species, particularly *Staphylococcus aureus*, being the most frequently detected.[2,27,52,117] Methicillin-resistant *S. aureus* (MRSA), gram-negative organisms, and mixed flora are detected in sufficient frequency, however, to recommend withholding antibiotics until adequate culture specimens have been obtained and then providing treatment with broad-spectrum antibiotics until the culture results are available. Delayed infections are most frequently caused by bacteria of low virulence, with *Propionibacterium* and *Staphylococcus epidermidis* being common offenders.[34,93,118] Isolation of *Propionibacterium* in culture specimens can take up to a week, and recent reports indicate that this bacterium might play a role in acute infections as well.[93]

TREATMENT

Treatment of postoperative spinal infections is not standardized, and there is much debate in the literature concerning infection management, much of which is centered on the need to remove instrumentation and on the use of newer treatment modalities, such as vacuum-assisted closure (VAC), continuous irrigation systems, and implanted antibiotic beads. Despite these ongoing discussions, it is clear that optimal outcome requires prompt diagnosis and aggressive treatment.

Nonoperative Treatment

Many superficial wound infections can be treated without surgical intervention. In the absence of wound breakdown, purulent drainage, or fluctuance, empirical antibiotic treatment aimed at skin flora may be adequate. Careful follow-up should be undertaken, however, to ensure that symptoms resolve with treatment.

Postoperative diskitis can most often be treated nonoperatively. The diagnosis of infecting pathogens should be made by blood cultures, which are positive in just more than half of patients,[119] or by tissue biopsy before the institution of antibiotic therapy. Broad-spectrum antibiotics should be used until culture results are available to guide targeted antibiotic therapy. If culture results do not indicate the causative organism, broad-spectrum antibiotics with good staphylococcal coverage should be used.[120] Although evidence-based recommendations for the duration of antibiotic therapy are lacking, a course of 6 weeks of intravenous antibiotics followed by 6 weeks of oral therapy is commonly used, along with an orthotic brace for comfort. Medical treatment is usually successful, although surgical treatment is indicated in patients with a poor clinical response to medical treatment, continued back pain, or instability. The surgical goal in such instances should be thorough débridement of infected tissue, including infected bone, and stabilization with bone graft and titanium instrumentation. Thoracic diskitis or osteomyelitis requiring débridement often requires an anterior approach, which may be difficult in patients with significant medical comorbid conditions. Thoracoscopic approaches are now used more often in this regard and have been reported to be effective in treating thoracic infections with acceptable morbidity.[121,122]

Surgical Débridement

Wounds that have broken down, have purulent drainage, or are fluctuant or otherwise concerning for deep extension usually require operative exploration with the goals of (1) diagnosis of the infective agent, (2) débridement of nonviable tissue, and (3) assurance of stabilization. Preoperative antibiotics are withheld until adequate culture specimens have been obtained and the entire length of the wound is opened. Preoperative imaging is helpful in determining the extent of débridement, with evidence of deep infection mandating opening of the lumbodorsal fascia. Although some authors recommend opening the fascia in all cases,[29] we believe that it can be left closed when it is intact and only superficial infection and wound breakdown are likely based on preoperative imaging and intraoperative findings. Alternatively, it has been suggested that the subfascial compartment be aspirated with a needle and an intraoperative Gram stain obtained, with the results guiding the need to open this layer.[25,78] If the lumbodorsal fascia is opened, it should be done only after thorough débridement and irrigation of the superficial compartment. Specimens for culture from the deep compartment should be taken and labeled separately.

Aggressive débridement should be undertaken in each open compartment. Loose bone fragments, Gelfoam or fibrin sealant remnants, and necrotic muscle and fat should be removed meticulously. All areas involved in the operation should be inspected. If the disk space was instrumented, it should be viewed, samples harvested for culture, and débridement performed. At the conclusion of débridement, healthy soft tissue as evidenced by adequate vasculature and perfusion should be exposed.

The issue of instrumentation removal has been a significant controversy in the setting of infection, with some authors recommending removal in all or most cases[1,33,34,93,117,118,123] and others reporting successful treatment with the instrumentation maintained.[27,28,78,124-127] Some authors even purport that the added stability endowed by maintenance of instrumentation may help clear the infection.[127] Recurrent infections with retention of hardware are often reported in the setting of delayed infections in the treatment of scoliosis in which old steel constructs that may predispose the patient to continued infection were used. Newer titanium implants are not associated with this problem and have been used with success in stabilizing the infected spine.[126,128] Furthermore, removal of the hardware in an unstable spine is not a viable option, and we therefore recommend maintenance of the hardware in all cases in which spine stability or fusion maturation are in question.

On completion of débridement, the integrity of the fusion construct should be confirmed by visual inspection and manual manipulation. If the instrumentation is found to be loose, it must be removed and alternative means of fixation used. In the case of pedicle screw fixation, a larger diameter screw can be used in a rescue fashion. Structural allograft used in the initial construct may also be left in place, but loose chips of bone should be removed.[126,129] If the infection has occurred in a delayed fashion and the fusion is solid, however, the surgeon can consider removing the instrumentation.[7] Careful follow-up should ensue in these cases because loss of correction has been observed with removal of instrumentation despite solid bony fusion.[34,118,123,130] It should also be noted that the presence of infection is associated with an increased rate of pseudarthrosis, and this complication, despite not strictly being correlated with a negative clinical outcome, should be watched for in follow-up examinations.[78,131]

Before closure, the wound should be thoroughly irrigated. We often use a low-pressure pulsatile irrigator with copious amounts (9 L) of antibiotic solution.[132,133] Primary wound closure should be attained if possible. Although some authors recommend closing wounds in a delayed fashion or allowing healing to occur by secondary intention,[125,134,135] this may mandate a return trip to the operating room and exposes the wound to a risk for secondary infection.[28] The wound should be closed in layers around a drain to eliminate dead space. Some authors have additionally proposed the performance of a routine review procedure 2 to 3 days postoperatively.[29] We have found this practice to be unnecessary in most patients and use clinical examination and laboratory findings to guide this decision.

Treatment of Intrathecal Pump and Spinal Cord Stimulator Infection

Treatment of intrathecal pump and spinal cord stimulator infections typically involves removal of the hardware and initial treatment with broad-spectrum antibiotics, with gradual narrowing of antibiotic coverage once culture results have been obtained.[44]

Removal of intrathecal drug delivery devices is, however, associated with a risk for drug withdrawal symptoms,[44] and this has prompted the generation of several reports on the nonoperative treatment of such infections, even in the setting of meningitis.[45,136-138] Although novel techniques such as injection and infusion of antibiotics into the drug delivery system are appealing in this setting, the efficacy of such measures has not been firmly established, and further experience is needed before routine nonsurgical treatment of neuroprosthetic devices can be recommended.

Adjuvant Surgical Techniques

Vacuum-Assisted Closure

Although there have been numerous reports of the efficacy of VAC in the general, orthopedic, and plastic surgery literature,[139-141] the application of VAC in the closure of spinal wounds has only recently been reported. VAC is a technique in which negative pressure is applied to the wound, which aids in closure via mechanisms of edema removal, improvement of blood flow, stimulation of angiogenesis, stimulation of granulation tissue development, and reduced bacterial load.[142-145] The VAC device is composed of a polyurethane sponge, a plastic sealant drape, and a negative-pressure suction device. The sponge should be placed within the confines of the wound bed, with care taken to ensure that it contacts all areas of the wound, thereby leaving no dead space, while at the same time avoiding skin contact. The sealant should cover an adequate amount of the surrounding area to prevent suction leak, and the device is then activated with approximately 125 mm Hg of suction. VAC dressings are then replaced every 2 to 4 days, as needed, by a skilled nurse or in the operating room. When the infection has been eradicated and the wound edges appear healthy, the patient can be returned to the operating room for delayed primary wound closure.

Although a randomized controlled trial has yet to prove the efficacy of this technique in spine surgery, potential advantages include more rapid resolution of infection, fewer trips to the operating room for wound washout, negation of the need for frequent dressing changes in open wounds, and decreased likelihood of reliance on closure by secondary intention.[146] Potential complications include significant blood loss, hypoalbuminemia, toxic shock syndrome, and retained sponges.[147]

Irrigation-Suction Technique

Application of an irrigation-suction apparatus has also been reported sporadically in the literature.[2,148] This technique involves closure of the wound over irrigation catheters and drains placed separately in both the deep and superficial compartments of the wound. An antibiotic solution, chosen according to Gram stain and culture results, is irrigated through the wound at a rate of up to 50 mL/hr, and the suction catheter is attached to a medium-pressure Hemovac. The drains are left in place for 5 to 7 days, at which point the irrigation drains are removed, with removal of the Hemovac a day later.

Although no randomized controlled trial has proved the efficacy of this technique, it is appealing in that it provides continuous antibiotic irrigation of the wound bed and does not necessitate leaving the wound open or require numerous return trips to the operating room.

Other Techniques

Other surgical adjuncts for the treatment of infection are the use of antibiotic beads and muscle flaps. The use of antibiotic beads placed in the surgical bed has been reported in the treatment of spinal infections with promising results.[78] High local concentrations of antibiotic are provided with this technique, which has also been shown to be effective in the treatment of open and contaminated fractures.[149,150]

In severe cases of wound breakdown, muscle flaps may be necessary to cover the wound and aid in wound healing by reducing dead space and enhancing antibiotic and oxygen delivery. Potential donor sites for spinal coverage include the latissimus, trapezius, gluteus, and paraspinal muscles. The assistance of a plastic surgeon is usually required for such reconstructions.[151-153]

ANTIBIOTIC THERAPY

Treatment with broad-spectrum antibiotics should be started after adequate specimens for culture have been obtained. Antibiotic choice should be appropriate to cover skin pathogens and take into account local resistance patterns. A Gram stain can guide initial therapy, but broad coverage should be used until final culture results are obtained. Once cultures are finalized, the choice of antibiotic is tailored to treat the specific organism or organisms. There are currently no standardized length-of-treatment recommendations for postoperative spine infections, but most authors recommend 4 to 6 weeks of intravenous antibiotic therapy, variably followed by a course of oral antibiotic therapy. An infectious disease specialist should be enlisted to guide appropriate therapy. Response to treatment is monitored by clinical examination, with increasing back pain and persistent fever being indicative of possible failure, and by laboratory evaluation. ESR, CRP, and WBC values are checked weekly and should trend to normal with effective therapy. Serial imaging is used in cases of suspected instability or neural compression, but caution should be exercised when evaluating infectious response to antibiotics because imaging findings lag behind treatment response by several months.

PREVENTION

The most effective way of dealing with postoperative infections is prevention. A comprehensive preoperative, intraoperative, and postoperative approach to prevention must be undertaken to minimize the risk of this devastating and costly complication.

Preoperative optimization of controllable risk can aid in the reduction of infection, especially in elective cases. Preoperative smoking cessation has been linked to a decreased risk for surgical complications, although the length of cessation needed to have an effect is not clear.[154] Because nutritional status is a major risk factor for the development of infection, consideration should be given to assessing indices of this variable preoperatively.[47,48] Easy tests include serum albumin or the total lymphocyte count. Abnormal values may prompt a delay in elective surgery, whereas deficiencies are corrected with the aid of a nutritionist or internist.[155-161] The presence of concomitant infections should be identified and treatment undertaken before surgery if possible. The presence of a common urinary tract or pulmonary infection may increase the risk for operative wound infection, especially in the setting of instrumentation.

The issue of hair shaving in skin preparation has received much attention in the cranial literature, and one recent randomized trial in the spine literature showed a significantly increased risk for infection in patients shaved preoperatively.[162] Potential mechanisms by which skin shaving may increase infection risk include the loss of protective skin flora and the creation of microabrasions that facilitate bacterial colonization.[162,163] If the presence of hair will interfere with the surgical approach, it should be removed with clippers and not a razor to reduce microtrauma to the skin.

The use of prophylactic antibiotic medications in spine surgery has been considered a standard of care since the mid-1970s when Horwitz and Curtin reported a significant decrease in postoperative infection with the use of prophylactic antibiotics.[19] Six subsequent randomized studies have examined the efficacy of antibiotics in preventing infection. Although none of them found a significant benefit alone, all have trended toward reduced infection with prophylaxis,[164-169] and when collective data were pooled in a meta-analysis, a significant overall reduction in infection rate from 5.9% to 2.2% was obtained.[170] Prophylactic antibiotics should cover skin flora and take into account local resistance patterns, as well as the history of patient reactions to antibiotics. Some authors additionally recommend screening even low-risk patients for MRSA preoperatively.[171] First-generation cephalosporins, such as cefazolin, are typically used prophylactically because they are effective against gram-positive skin flora and more frequent gram-negative offenders such as *Escherichia coli*. The use of second- and third-generation cephalosporins should be reserved for the treatment of infection rather than prophylaxis.[172] Patients who are MRSA positive or allergic to cephalosporins should be given a glycopeptide, such as vancomycin, and gentamicin. Antibiotics should be administered approximately 30 minutes to 1 hour before skin incision to ensure that adequate blood levels are achieved at skin incision and readministered at half the dose every 4 hours or with every 1500 mL of blood loss during surgery if cephalosporins are used or every 8 hours if a glycopeptide and gentamicin are given.[51,173-175] Doses should take into account patient body habitus, with those weighing more than 80 kg, for example, receiving 2 g cefazolin preoperatively.[51,173]

Patients undergoing procedures involving the disk space, such as diskography or diskectomy, should also receive antibiotic prophylaxis, although the optimal choice of drug is unclear. Several animal and human studies indicate that β-lactam antibiotics and cephalosporins have poor penetration into the disk and nucleus, but clindamycin, aminoglycosides, and glycopeptides have been shown to have good penetration.[24,155-161] Additionally, good results have been reported in retrospective studies in which antibiotics have been instilled directly into the disk space at the time of the procedure, either mixed with contrast material for diskography or delivered with a sponge at diskectomy.[21,176] Although randomized trials have not been conducted to validate the efficacy of either method of prophylaxis, careful thought should be given to each method by the treating physician.

Several intraoperative measures may play a role in reducing infectious risk. Maintenance of strict aseptic technique is critical, involves participation of the entire operating room staff, and requires minimization of operating room traffic. Periodic release of tissue retractors may reduce ischemic damage to the paraspinal musculature.[177,178] This may, in turn, reduce tissue necrosis, which may contribute to wound-healing issues and infection. Double gloving is highly recommended in spine procedures, especially those requiring instrumentation. Yinusa and colleagues recorded glove puncture in 63.6% of spine operations, the highest for any subspecialty of orthopedic surgery.[179] Glove puncture rates for the inner glove in those who double-gloved was significantly less than the rates for single gloves.

Intraoperative irrigation of the wound has frequently been cited as a prophylactic measure. The use of bacitracin irrigation has been shown to offer benefit over saline irrigation in a contaminated canine osseous tissue model.[180] Antibiotic irrigation has demonstrated promising results in general and orthopedic surgical procedures and is used widely.[181-184] The most robust evidence to date is that of Chang and associates,[185] who performed a prospective randomized trial using dilute (0.35%) povidone-iodine (Betadine) solution to irrigate tissues before bone grafting. They reported a reduction in the rate of infection from 3.4% with saline irrigation to 0% with Betadine irrigation without any adverse effects. Although this trial has not been replicated, use of Betadine irrigation is simple, and the results of this trial are strong enough to recommend routine use in posterior spinal cases. Care should be taken, however, to irrigate the spinal wound before decortication because bacitracin and Betadine have been noted to have a cytotoxic effect on osteoblasts at higher concentrations.[186]

Several postoperative measures have been proposed for decreasing the risk for infection, although none have proved their efficacy in randomized controlled trials. Use of a drain is controversial, with the authors of some studies reporting a decrease in infection, others reporting an increased incidence of infection, and still others reporting no change.[31,187] If a drain is used, prophylactic antibiotic use for the duration of drainage has not been shown to be beneficial.[171] Other postoperative measures that may reduce the risk for infection are the application of a sterile dressing, strict glucose control,[6,51,69] and aggressive maintenance of nutritional status.[8,47]

The use of postoperative antibiotics is also controversial. A recent retrospective study reported no difference in infection rates when postoperative antibiotics were continued for just the day of surgery versus continuation for 5 to 7 days. Infections occurring in the setting of prolonged administration were, however, more likely to involve resistant organisms.[172]

SUGGESTED READINGS

Chang FY, Chang MC, Wang ST, et al. Can povidone-iodine solution be used safely in a spinal surgery? *Eur Spine J*. 2006;15:1005.
Fraser RD, Osti OL, Vernon-Roberts B. Iatrogenic discitis: the role of intravenous antibiotics in prevention and treatment. An experimental study. *Spine*. 1989;14:1025.
James SL, Davies AM. Imaging of infectious spinal disorders in children and adults. *Eur J Radiol*. 2006;58:27.
Klein JD, Hey LA, Yu CS, et al. Perioperative nutrition and postoperative complications in patients undergoing spinal surgery. *Spine*. 1996;21:2676.
Lee MC, Wang MY, Fessler RG, et al. Instrumentation in patients with spinal infection. *Neurosurg Focus*. 2004;17(6):E7.
Levi AD, Dickman CA, Sonntag VK. Management of postoperative infections after spinal instrumentation. *J Neurosurg*. 1997;86:975.
Mangram A, Horan T, Pearson M, et al. Guideline for prevention of surgical site infection, 1999. Center for Disease Control and Prevention (CDC) Hospital Infection Control Practices Advisory Committee. *Am J Infect Control*. 1999;27:96.
Mehbod AA, Ogilvie JW, Pinto MR, et al. Postoperative deep wound infections in adults after spinal fusion: management with vacuum-assisted wound closure. *J Spinal Disord Tech*. 2005;18:14.
Olsen MA, Mayfield J, Lauryssen C, et al. Risk factors for surgical site infection in spinal surgery. *J Neurosurg*. 2003;98:149.
Olsen MA, Nepple JJ, Riew KD, et al. Risk factors for surgical site infection following orthopaedic spinal operations. *J Bone Joint Surg Am*. 2008;90:62.
Rubinstein E, Findler G, Amit P, et al. Perioperative prophylactic cephazolin in spinal surgery: a double-blind placebo-controlled trial. *J Bone Joint Surg Br*. 1994;76:99.
Weinstein MA, McCabe JP, Cammisa FP Jr. Postoperative spinal wound infection: a review of 2,391 consecutive index procedures. *J Spinal Disord*. 2000;13:422.
Wimmer C, Gluch H. Management of postoperative wound infection in posterior spinal fusion with instrumentation. *J Spinal Disord*. 1996;9:505.
Wimmer C, Gluch H, Franzreb M, et al. Predisposing factors for infection in spine surgery: a survey of 850 spinal procedures. *J Spinal Disord*. 1998;11:124.

Full references can be found on Expert Consult @ www.expertconsult.com

CHAPTER 42

The Use and Misuse of Antibiotics in Neurosurgery

Koijan Kainth ■ Matthew A. Hunt ■ Stephen J. Haines

THE IMPORTANCE OF ANTIBIOTICS IN NEUROSURGERY

Few neurosurgeons would be willing to practice modern neurosurgery without the ready availability of antibiotics. They have made it possible to treat infections of the brain, meninges, and surgical site effectively and to salvage excellent results from what would otherwise be devastating complications of neurosurgical operations. Although some still argue based on the extraordinary results of Harvey Cushing, who reported one infection in 149 patients (0.7%), that careful technique overcomes almost all sources of infection, a very special understanding of the available evidence is required to deliberately omit perioperative antibiotic prophylaxis in modern neurosurgical practice.[1] Antibiotics are an integral part of the daily life of the neurosurgeon.

Antibiotics, like all other neurosurgical interventions, however, carry with them cost and risk. A superficial understanding of their use and the evidence underlying their applications can lead to excessive use, ineffective use, and other forms of misuse that should be avoided if excellence in practice is to be achieved. In this chapter we review appropriate use and discuss common misuses of antibiotics in neurosurgical practice.

RISKS ASSOCIATED WITH ANTIBIOTIC ADMINISTRATION

Antibiotic therapy in neurosurgical patients is implemented in various situations, including prophylaxis for procedures, empirical treatment of a presumed infection, or treatment of a specific infection. Administration of antibiotics is not without consequence, however. Adverse drug reactions that may result include central nervous system (CNS) toxicities, systemic toxicities, allergic reactions, side effects, and drug-drug interactions. Moreover, there is the potential for antibiotic resistance with careless administration. The emergence of antibiotic resistance is a growing and potentially catastrophic problem that should not be taken lightly. Drug toxicity is a consequence of either excessive dosing or impaired drug metabolism, the latter possibly being due to hepatic or renal insufficiency. An allergic drug reaction is a hypersensitivity reaction to a medication that may be immunologically mediated and can result in urticaria, bronchospasm, anaphylactic shock, or angioedema. Side effects are other adverse drug reactions that are neither due to drug toxicity or to a hypersensitivity reaction. In this section, commonly used antibiotics in neurosurgery are addressed, along with their local toxicity, systemic toxicity, side effects, drug-drug interactions, and potential for resistance. Hypersensitivity reactions are discussed briefly and only in regard to specific antibiotics. Table 42-1 summarizes the most important neurotoxicities encountered with current antibiotic use. Table 42-2 summarizes selected drug interactions of importance to the neurosurgical patient.

Sulfonamides

Sulfonamide neurotoxicity can occur in the premature and newborn period because sulfonamides have the potential to displace bilirubin from albumin, with the resultant free bilirubin being deposited in the basal ganglia and subthalamic nuclei and resulting in kernicterus.[2] Moreover, there are reports in the literature of other CNS toxicities, including ataxia, depression, and psychosis with associated visual and auditory hallucinations.[3,4]

Quinolones

The incidence of neurotoxicity from quinolones ranges from 1% to 2%, and symptoms may include headache, dizziness, and insomnia.[5-8] Additionally, instances of delirium, acute psychosis, and seizures have been reported.[5,6,9] Moreover, there have been reports of the development of demyelinating polyneuropathy,[10] exacerbation of myasthenia gravis,[11-15] and peripheral sensory disturbances[16] with fluoroquinolone use. Signs of pseudotumor cerebri may develop in infants and young children with high doses of nalidixic acid, the first quinolone to be introduced.[17] These CNS effects should generally resolve with the discontinuation of therapy.

Penicillins

Neurotoxicity after parenteral administration of penicillin G is most likely to occur in patients with renal insufficiency, intracranial lesions, or alteration of the blood-brain barrier (BBB).[18] This toxicity can occur when the concentration of penicillin G in cerebrospinal fluid (CSF) exceeds 10 µg/mL and may be manifested as lethargy, confusion, twitching, multifocal myoclonus, or seizures.[18] Arachnoiditis and encephalopathy may follow the intrathecal injection of penicillin G, and therefore intraventricular and intrathecal administration should be avoided.[18] The development of symptoms that may resemble panic attacks or acute psychosis with seizures or hallucinations is known as Hoigne's syndrome and can follow the intravascular injection of penicillin.[19,20] Furthermore, ampicillin may exacerbate weakness in patients with myasthenia gravis.[21]

Cephalosporins

Many cephalosporins have been associated with neurotoxicity, and ceftazidime, in particular, has been reported to cause hallucinations,[22] confusion, encephalopathy,[23] and status epilepticus.[22,24] There have also been published reports of cephalosporin-associated recurrent aseptic meningitis.[25]

A hypersensitivity reaction is the most common side effect of cephalosporin administration and may be manifested as anaphylaxis, bronchospasm, urticaria, fever, or maculopapular rash.

Carbapenems

The most common adverse events encountered with carbapenem administration are nausea and vomiting.[26] Other frequent adverse

TABLE 42-1 Antibiotic Neurotoxicity

ANTIBIOTIC	SEIZURE	CNS	PNS	OTHER
Sulfonamides		Kernicterus in infants		Psychiatric syndromes*
Quinolones	X	Headache	Polyneuropathy	Psychiatric syndromes
		Dizziness	Exacerbation of myasthenia gravis	Pseudotumor
		Insomnia		
Penicillins	X	Encephalopathy	Exacerbation of myasthenia gravis (ampicillin)	Psychiatric syndromes
				Arachnoiditis (intrathecal)
Cephalosporins	X	Encephalopathy		Psychiatric syndromes
Carbapenems	X			
Polymyxins	X (intrathecal)	Encephalopathy	Neuromuscular blockade	
Vancomycin		Ototoxicity		
		Vestibular toxicity		
Tetracyclines		Vestibular toxicity	Neuromuscular blockade	Pseudotumor cerebri
			Exacerbation of myasthenia gravis	
Macrolides		Ototoxicity	Exacerbation of myasthenia gravis	Psychiatric syndromes
Linezolid			Peripheral and optic neuropathy	
Rifampin		Headache, confusion, ataxia	Numbness, weakness	

*Psychiatric syndromes include depression, hallucinations, anxiety attacks, psychosis, and other symptoms.
CNS, central nervous system; PNS, peripheral nervous system.

events include diarrhea, rash, fever, and laboratory abnormalities, such as elevated liver enzyme levels, eosinophilia, thrombocytopenia, and increased prothrombin time.[26] Patients at risk for seizures are those with preexisting renal insufficiency or an intracranial mass lesion who are given high doses of imipenem.[27] Furthermore, there are reports that concomitant administration of imipenem with theophylline, quinolones, metronidazole, ganciclovir, or cyclosporine may reduce the seizure threshold.[28-30] In contrast to imipenem, meropenem is less likely to induce seizures.[31-34]

Aminoglycosides

The most important and serious side effects of aminoglycosides are nephrotoxicity and ototoxicity. The other dose-related adverse effect of clinical importance is neuromuscular blockade, which occurs rarely and is usually related to an underlying condition.[35] The first signs of ototoxicity may be seen histologically, with the outer hair cells of the cochlea affected first, followed by the inner hair cells.[36] Damage to the hair cells results in high-frequency hearing loss, followed by progressive loss of hearing at lower frequencies.[35] After degeneration of the hair cells, there can also be damage to nerve fibers.[37] The first clinical symptom of cochlear damage is often high-pitched and continuous tinnitus.[38] In regard to the vestibular apparatus, hair cell damage occurs along with deterioration of the otoconial membrane and otolith structures.[39,40] Clinical signs and symptoms of vestibular damage include disequilibrium, ataxia, transient positional vertigo, and oscillopsia.[35,38] In rare instances, aminoglycosides have the potential to cause neuromuscular blockade and paralysis.[35] Patients with preexisting myasthenia gravis are at a higher risk for the development of neuromuscular blockade.[41] Risk factors for ototoxicity include renal insufficiency, preexisting impaired hearing, old age, sepsis, dehydration, fever, previous aminoglycoside exposure, and concomitant use of vancomycin, cisplatin, or carboplatin.[35] Anosmia after aminoglycoside therapy has also been described in the literature, with the sense of smell returning after time.[42,43] Intrathecal or intraventricular administration is used rarely because it may cause local inflammation and can result in aseptic meningitis.[44]

TABLE 42-2 Selected Drug Interactions

ANTIBIOTIC	WARFARIN	ANTICONVULSANTS	OTHER
Quinolones	Potentiate		Potentiate theophylline and caffeine
Carbapenems			Potentiate theophylline, quinolone, metronidazole, ganciclovir, or cyclosporine seizure threshold reduction
Chloramphenicol	Potentiates	Prolongs half-life of phenytoin, phenobarbital	Prolongs half-life of cyclosporine
Macrolides (erythromycin)	Potentiate	Prolong half-life of carbamazepine	Prolong half-life of theophylline, alfentanil, triazolam, midazolam, digoxin
Rifampin	Antagonizes		Speeds catabolism of oral contraceptives, cyclosporine, itraconazole, digoxin, verapamil, nifedipine, simvastatin, midazolam, and human immunodeficiency virus–related protease inhibitors

Polymyxins

The major adverse drug effects of polymyxins are nephrotoxicity, neurotoxicity, and neuromuscular blockade. Renal insufficiency and giddiness may result when polymyxins are used parenterally, and pain, numbness, paresthesias, confusion, coma, and convulsions may result when they are used intrathecally.[45-47]

Neurotoxicity from parenteral polymyxin B and colistin is seen most frequently in patients with compromised renal function, with an overall incidence of approximately 7.3%.[48] With increasing doses of polymyxin, patients may experience circumoral paresthesias, convulsions, apnea, distal paresthesias, ptosis, diplopia, dysphagia, dysphonia, areflexia, ataxia, and dizziness.[49-51] Intrathecal dosages greater than 50,000 U/day have been reported to cause chemical meningitis.[18,52]

Vancomycin

Neurotoxicity with the administration of vancomycin can include both vestibular damage and cochlear damage, which can result in tinnitus and sensory hearing loss.[53,54] Tinnitus may be an early symptom and can indicate the development of deafness.[55] Ototoxicity in the early stages, characterized by tinnitus and dizziness, appears to be reversible.[56] However, by the time that the patient experiences a noticeable hearing deficit, the toxicity is often irreversible.[57] The mechanism by which vancomycin causes ototoxicity is thought to be direct damage to the auditory nerve, which leads to irreversible loss of the sensory hairs in the cochlea that initially affects high-frequency sensory hearing.[57] Subsequently, lower frequencies are affected, and eventually, total hearing loss may result.[58]

Tetracyclines

Neurotoxicity is a well-recognized side effect of tetracycline therapy, and there are several reports in the literature documenting increased intracranial pressure with medium- to long-term use.[59-62] In infants, a bulging fontanelle may be apparent but resolves on discontinuation of the therapy.[63] Vestibular symptoms are also reported with tetracycline administration and may include dizziness and ataxia.[64-66] Additionally, tetracyclines are thought to block the neuromuscular junction by both prejunctional and postjunctional effects that depress the sensitivity of muscle to acetylcholine.[3,67] This neuromuscular blockade has been reported to exacerbate myasthenia gravis.[18]

Chloramphenicol

Neurotoxic effects of chloramphenicol administration are rare. Optic neuropathy and peripheral neuropathy have been cited in the literature in children with cystic fibrosis.[68-71] Symptoms of visual toxicity may include blurred vision followed by loss of visual acuity and impaired red-green color discrimination, whereas peripheral nerve toxicities result in burning, tingling, or numbness of extremities.[3] The aforementioned symptoms generally resolve after discontinuation of the therapy.[3] Additionally, there have been reports of chloramphenicol-induced encephalopathy that can progress to delirium.[72]

The most feared toxicities of chloramphenicol administration include bone marrow suppression, aplastic anemia, and gray baby syndrome.[73]

Macrolides

Neurotoxicity is mostly associated with erythromycin and may result in neuropsychiatric symptoms or ototoxicity.[74] The neuropsychiatric symptoms that have been reported in the literature include confusion, hysteria, anxiety, and nightmares, all of which disappeared after therapy was terminated.[75,76] The ototoxicity that is induced by erythromycin is a result of high doses, or it can occur in patients with preexisting hepatic or renal insufficiency.[74,77] In contrast to aminoglycosides, the hearing loss with macrolides is reversible with cessation of the drug.[78] There are also reports cited in the literature of the potential for erythromycin to exacerbate weakness in patients with myasthenia gravis.[79,80]

Linezolid

Neurotoxicity can result in peripheral neuropathy with prolonged use of linezolid.[81-83] Most cases of peripheral neuropathy have occurred when linezolid is used beyond the maximal recommended duration of therapy of 28 days.[83] Additionally, there have been several reports documenting linezolid-associated optic neuropathy.[84-86]

Rifampin

The neurotoxic effects of rifampin may include ataxia, confusion, dizziness, numbness, muscular weakness, inability to concentrate, and headache.[18,87]

The adverse reactions most commonly reported include rash, fever, headache, general malaise, gastrointestinal symptoms, nausea, and vomiting.[88,89]

GENERAL PRINCIPLES OF ANTIBIOTIC USE

Neurosurgeons are involved in the treatment of infections not only of the CNS itself but also of the surrounding tissues. These areas encompass multiple diverse compartments, including the cranial soft tissues, skull, paranasal sinuses, paraspinal soft tissues, and the spine itself, including bones, soft tissues, and intervertebral disks, as well as the tissues and body cavities used for the insertion of prostheses such as shunt hardware, electrodes, batteries, and pumps. Fortunately, many of the infections that neurosurgeons must deal with are extradural. This fact simplifies treatment in that delivery of antibiotics does not depend on the physiology of the brain barriers: the BBB and the blood-CSF barrier (BCSFB). The BBB and BCSFB provide protection to the CNS from substances circulating through the blood and help facilitate transfer of important nutrients to the CNS. However, these brain barriers present an obstacle to the entry of antibiotics and require special consideration when contemplating how to treat an infection inside these barriers. Treating infections such as meningitis or brain abscesses requires that adequate amounts of antibiotic cross the BBB and BCSFB into the CSF or the extracellular space of the CNS.

The Blood-Brain and Blood–Cerebrospinal Fluid Barriers

The BBB is formed by endothelial cells of the cerebral vasculature, supported by astroglia and pericytes, with tight junctions between the endothelial cells and minimal fenestrations or bulk transport across the cells. For the BCSFB, this barrier is located at the epithelial layer of the choroid plexus, not at the endothelium, but is similar in character, with tight junctions between the epithelial cells. For both barriers, active influx and efflux transporters located on the endothelial/epithelial cell surface may drastically alter the distribution of an antibiotic into the desired compartment.[90,91] Many factors can contribute to the permeability of any substance across the BBB:

- Molecular weight
- Lipophilicity (i.e., octanol/water partition coefficient)
- Ionization

- Presence of transport mechanisms (influx or efflux)
- Plasma protein binding
- Inflammation
- pH
- Metabolism at the barrier

Each of these factors affects a substance's ability to cross the brain barriers and reach its intended site of action. Increasing molecular weight, ionization, plasma protein binding, and metabolism at the barrier and the presence of efflux transporters decrease the permeability of substances across the brain barriers.[91,92] Increased lipophilicity, influx transporters, and inflammation can increase the permeability of the barriers to antibiotics.[93] The inflammation associated with infections may decrease over the course of and in response to treatment. Antibiotics may cross into the CSF or brain parenchyma more readily at the initiation of treatment, but as the inflammatory response to the infection abates, either from the antibiotic treatment or from the administration of other medications such as dexamethasone, the ability of an antibiotic to cross the brain barriers diminishes.[94,95] However, this effect may not alter outcome.[96-100]

The overall goal of antibiotic treatment is to deliver an adequate concentration of the drug to the proper compartment. Antibiotics that are bactericidal are generally preferred for the treatment of CNS infections as well because of the low concentration of immunologic proteins such as complement and immunoglobulins and the relatively low numbers of phagocytic cells, although this contention may be changing.[101-103] This goal may be accomplished in several ways. First, the dose of the drug may be increased. This method is helpful for drugs with low systemic toxicity and relatively low permeability across the brain barriers, such as β-lactam antibiotics. Second, the choice of antibiotic may be changed to a drug that has greater penetration into the CNS, such as chloramphenicol or quinolones. Third, antibiotics may be delivered directly across the brain barriers (usually by indwelling ventricular or lumbar catheters). This method is especially helpful when using antibiotics that have higher systemic toxicity and poor permeability across the brain barriers, which may limit the systemic dose that can be administered; such drugs include vancomycin and aminoglycosides. For example, administration of chloramphenicol via an intraventricular route does not provide the same advantage that intraventricular administration of vancomycin does because chloramphenicol's penetration of the brain barriers already exceeds that needed to provide a therapeutic concentration. In addition, bypassing the brain barriers does not provide a significant advantage because chloramphenicol also needs to be hydrolyzed to be effective, which is usually done in the liver. Although hydrolysis has been shown to occur in the CSF, intraventricular administration is probably not necessary.[104] Alternatively, using higher doses of β-lactam antibiotics to reach bactericidal concentrations is easily accomplished and generally associated with minimal systemic toxicity. Intraventricular administration of β-lactams is probably more toxic than systemic administration, although whether the source of the toxicity is the antibiotic or the underlying infection is not clear.[104]

Pharmacokinetics of Antibiotic Delivery

To achieve effective antibiotic dosing, the pharmacokinetics of antibiotic administration must be understood. For infections occurring outside the barriers of the CNS, the principles of systemically administering antibiotics are less complicated. Peak concentrations depend on bioavailability, the amount delivered, the volume of distribution, and elimination via metabolism and excretion.[103] However, the pharmacokinetics of antibiotic administration to the CNS depends on both systemic pharmacokinetics and the behavior of the antibiotic in its access to and elimination from the CNS. The sum of these factors can be ascertained by experimentally determining the proportion of antibiotic that reaches the CNS. Most data relating to antibiotic pharmacokinetics in the CNS come from studies on CSF and meningitis. Much less data exist on these parameters for the brain parenchyma itself.[105,106]

In determining this proportion, careful interpretation of experimental data is required. Many studies looking at the proportion of antibiotic reaching the CNS use simple plasma-CSF ratios at a single time point. These ratios can vary widely during a dosing cycle and can be quite misleading.[106,107] The most useful data are derived from using plasma-CSF AUC (*AUC* is the area under the drug concentration–versus–time curve) ratios in intermittent dosing or steady-state concentrations during continuous infusion. For β-lactam antibiotics, the AUC ratio generally ranges from 0.01 to 0.1. Less hydrophilic antibiotics, such as rifampicin, trimethoprim-sulfamethoxazole, and the fluoroquinolones, have ratios that range from 0.1 to 0.9. Vancomycin and the aminoglycosides also exhibit low penetration into CSF, with ratios of less than 0.1.[106,108] However, data suggest that these ratios may be different in the treatment of infections of the brain parenchyma (i.e., brain abscess). One study showed equivalent levels of antibiotic in abscess fluid and plasma 6 hours after administration; however, these are also point ratios, not AUC ratios.[109] Whether the antibiotics are as effective in abscess fluid is a separate consideration. Concentrations of antibiotics throughout the CSF are not constant. Ventricular CSF will have a lower concentration of protein and antibiotic than will lumbar CSF because the CSF produced in the ventricles has not yet mixed with exuded extracellular fluid from the brain parenchyma. Therefore, CSF concentrations of antibiotics rely on the permeability of both the BBB and the BCSFB. Penetration of antibiotics through the blood-lesion barrier (specifically, the blood-abscess barrier) will vary with the stage of formation of the abscess, the relative vascularity of the lesion, and even the cause of the lesion. However, it is impossible to differentiate the individual contributions of the blood-lesion barrier and the surrounding BBB to antibiotic concentrations by measuring antibiotic levels within abscesses.[105,109-111]

The half-life of the antibiotic in CSF is also an important consideration. Most antibiotics are not metabolized in CSF. Elimination is achieved either by diffusion back through the BBB and BCSFB or from turnover of the CSF. Generally, the CSF half-life of antibiotics is significantly longer than the plasma half-life. The CSF half-life of antibiotics may also be increased in CNS infections because of decreased turnover of CSF. Conversely, in patients with CSF shunts or external CSF drains, the CSF half-life may be quite variable because the circulation of CSF is altered by the presence of the shunt or drain.[112,113]

Central Nervous System Toxicity of Antibiotic Therapy

Antibiotics may be toxic to the CNS when administered systemically, as discussed earlier, or when administered directly into the CNS via an intrathecal route or by means of antibiotic irrigation.

Intrathecal antibiotics may also have significant neurological toxicities, although the most commonly used intrathecal antibiotics, vancomycin and gentamicin, appear to have relatively low toxicity when administered intrathecally. Additionally, discerning these effects may be difficult in patients with a coexisting serious CNS infection. Intraventricular vancomycin appears to be relatively free of toxicity, even at high CSF levels.[114] Intraventricular gentamicin may lead to CNS toxicity and cause ototoxicity or epilepsy; however, these effects are not clearly related to CSF levels of gentamicin.[115,116] Other antibiotics less commonly used intraventricularly, such as the β-lactam antibiotics, may cause similar effects, especially seizures, as when they are administered systemically.[117,118]

ANTIBIOTIC PROPHYLAXIS

Systemic Antibiotic Prophylaxis

Antibiotic prophylaxis should be considered in terms of the inherent risk for infection associated with the procedure being contemplated. The standard approach to estimating risk for infection at the surgical site is the classification endorsed by the Centers for Disease Control and Prevention (Table 42-3).[119]

Expected infection rates range from less than 1% in clean wounds with antibiotic prophylaxis to 6% to 10% in dirty wounds, even with antibiotic treatment.[120]

Clean wounds in neurosurgery are generally subdivided into those with and without implantation of a substantial foreign body. The prototypical neurosurgical foreign body is the shunt. Clean shunt implantations with antibiotic prophylaxis have approximately an 8% to 10% infection rate, a rate much higher than that for non–foreign body operations.[121]

The use of antibiotics in contaminated and dirty wounds is considered therapeutic, not prophylactic. A full therapeutic course is recommended. Limiting antibiotics to perioperative use in these wound categories would be considered misuse.

Clean Neurosurgical Procedures

The value of systemic antibiotic prophylaxis in clean neurosurgical operations is supported by level I evidence from multiple randomized clinical trials and high-quality meta-analysis.[122] The same is true of systemic antibiotic prophylaxis for shunt operations.[123,124] Additional meta-analyses have supported its value in preventing meningitis after craniotomy[125] and in spine neurosurgery.[126]

The value of systemic antibiotic prophylaxis in clean-contaminated operations has not been adequately studied to allow a confident conclusion to be reached. The current accepted practice in transnasal surgery varies from limited perioperative use[127] to use as though the procedure were contaminated (i.e., therapeutic doses for a therapeutic duration).[128]

It is not feasible to study the differential effectiveness of different antibiotics. If one antibiotic reduces the expected infection rate to 1% and another is twice as good (infection rate of 0.5%), a study consisting of more than 5000 patients would be required to have a reasonable chance (power of 0.8) of finding that result to be statistically significant ($P \leq .05$). Although the duration of prophylactic antibiotic administration in neurosurgery has not

been specifically studied in a randomized trial, the general principles of systemic prophylactic antibiotic administration are well established in many disciplines[119]:

- Use an antibiotic directed at the most common organisms implicated in postoperative infections for the specific operation in the institution in which the operation takes place.
- Administer the antibiotic intravenously and time it so that a bactericidal level is obtained at the time of incision.
- Repeat the antibiotic dose at intervals so that bactericidal serum levels are maintained during the operation.
- Do not continue the antibiotic more than a few hours after the end of the operation.
- Vancomycin should be avoided unless no other antibiotic meets the aforementioned criteria.[129]

The value of systemic antibiotic prophylaxis in reducing the rate of infection after neurosurgical operations is well established with evidence of the highest quality. Failure to use antibiotics in this way requires justification with evidence of similar quality.

External Ventricular Drains

There is insufficient evidence to support a firm conclusion about the value of systemic antibiotic prophylaxis in reducing infections associated with external ventricular drains.[130] One underpowered trial compared systemic antibiotic prophylaxis with placebo for ventriculostomy and found no difference in the infection rate.[131] A single trial compared short-term and long-term antibiotic administration and suggested that long-term use reduced infection rates but selected for resistant organisms.[132] The infection rates in this study were high (extracranial infection rates of 40% with short-term use and 20% with long-term use). This is an area in which further study could be useful.

Cerebrospinal Fluid Fistula

A recent Cochrane Systematic Review examined the value of systemic antibiotic prophylaxis in preventing meningitis in patients with basilar skull fracture and confirmed the long-held view that the practice is ineffective.[133]

Topical Antibiotic Prophylaxis

The topical use of antibiotics during neurosurgical procedures to prevent postoperative infection has a long history but has not been studied with sufficient rigor to produce a definitive conclusion about its effectiveness. Two reviews have been published.[134,135]

TABLE 42-3 Classification of Surgical Site infection

WOUND CLASS	DESCRIPTION	EXAMPLES
Clean	Uninflamed, uncontaminated, no trauma or infection, primarily closed with no break in sterile technique	Craniotomy for tumor Microlumbar diskectomy
Clean-contaminated	Entry into the alimentary, respiratory, or genitourinary tract under controlled circumstances; no contamination; minor break in sterile technique	Transnasal hypophysectomy
Contaminated	Nonpurulent inflammation, recent trauma, gastrointestinal tract contamination, major break in sterile technique	Depressed skull fracture with overlying laceration Dropped bone flap
Dirty	Purulent inflammation, perforated viscus, fecal contamination, trauma with devitalized tissue, foreign bodies or other gross contamination	Open depressed skull fracture with in-driven foreign bodies Epidural abscess Brain abscess

When antibiotics first became available, they were sprinkled into the wound in powdered form. Pennybacker and coauthors reported a reduction in infection rates to modern levels (0.9%),[136] but a large review of practice at Massachusetts General Hospital did not confirm this benefit.[137] A report by Malis in 1979, however, renewed enthusiasm for the practice (now with antibiotic solutions rather than powder).[138] Subsequent case series have supported the concept, although a randomized comparison of systemic plus topical antibiotic prophylaxis against systemic antibiotics alone has not been done.[135,139,140]

The principles of topical antibiotic prophylaxis are similar to those for systemic antibiotic prophylaxis:

- Bactericidal concentrations of antibiotic in solution should be used.
- The antibiotic should be active against the most likely infecting organisms in the institution in which it is used.
- Vancomycin should be avoided unless no other active antibiotic is available.
- Toxicity should be minimized.

The issue of toxicity requires special consideration for topical administration. The tendency of penicillin to produce seizures when applied to the cerebral cortex is well known, therefore topical penicillins should be avoided.[141] Limited study of the effect of topical application on the cerebral cortex suggests that bacitracin and metronidazole have the lowest likelihood of producing epileptiform activity.[142] pH is likely to be an important parameter, and topical solutions applied directly to the nervous system should be adjusted to physiologic pH when possible.

Cerebrospinal Fluid Shunts

Topical antibiotic prophylaxis is commonly used during CSF shunt procedures in two ways: wound irrigation plus filling the shunt with antibiotic solution and the use of antibiotic-impregnated shunt catheters. The topical use of solutions has the same quality of evidence as it does for other neurosurgical procedures (see earlier). A recent Cochrane Systematic Review of the prevention of CSF shunt infection examined the evidence regarding antibiotic-impregnated shunt catheters and concluded that the evidence did support their effectiveness in reducing shunt infection rates.[123]

ANTIBIOTIC TREATMENT

This section details the treatment of common neurosurgical infections. A review of the literature reveals that there is a lack of properly designed randomized controlled studies evaluating the different treatment regimens. Therefore, the majority of the evidence regarding the effectiveness of the different antibiotic therapies is classified as only level III evidence. The recommendations come from the experiences of individuals and groups who have found success in the way that they manage a certain infection.

Soft Tissue Infections

Initial treatment in most cases should be directed against staphylococci and streptococci. Oral antibiotic therapy with a semisynthetic penicillin, a first-generation cephalosporin, clindamycin, or erythromycin should be considered.[143] If methicillin-resistant *Staphylococcus aureus* is suspected, vancomycin should be used until cultures prove otherwise. The duration of antimicrobial therapy is dictated by how the infection responds but should typically continue for 7 to 10 days.

Necrotizing Soft Tissue Infections

Because of the polymicrobial nature of necrotizing soft tissue infections, empirical treatment with broad-spectrum antibiotics is often initiated. A number of different regimens may be used to achieve broad-spectrum coverage, the most common of which include the following[144]:

1. Penicillin or ampicillin plus anaerobic coverage (clindamycin or metronidazole)
2. Vancomycin plus anaerobic and gram-negative coverage (an aminoglycoside, aztreonam, or third-generation cephalosporin)
3. Ampicillin/sulbactam with additional gram-negative coverage
4. Imipenem with additional coverage

The most common antibiotic prescribing error is inadequate coverage of *Enterococcus*, which optimally requires ampicillin or vancomycin plus an aminoglycoside.[144]

Meningitis

Antibiotic therapy for neurosurgical patients with postoperative bacterial meningitis is initially empirical. Practice guidelines for the initial empirical antimicrobial treatment of bacterial meningitis have been published by the Infectious Disease Society of America along with recommended dosages (Table 42-4). First-line empirical therapy includes a third-generation cephalosporin such as cefotaxime or ceftriaxone and vancomycin.[145] In suspected cases of *Pseudomonas aeruginosa*, ceftazidime should be used. Unfortunately, there have been reports of the emergence of resistant gram-negative bacilli (i.e., resistant *Enterobacter*[146-149] and *Acinetobacter*[150-152] species) with plasmid-encoded or inducible chromosomal β-lactamases that hydrolyze extended-spectrum cephalosporins.[153] In these cases, amikacin can be added, although this does not always prevent the development of resistance, as Chow and associates reported in their study.[154] Therefore, for β-lactamase–producing Enterobacteriaceae or *Acinetobacter* species, an extended-spectrum carbapenem such as meropenem may be used because these organisms tend to be resistant to multiple antibiotics. Moreover, Parodi and coauthors reported good clinical and microbiologic responses with carbapenems for *Enterobacter* meningitis.[155] Judicious use of this antibiotic needs to be ensured because carbapenem-resistant *Enterobacter* strains have been reported.[156] For resistant *Acinetobacter* meningitis, Nguyen and colleagues demonstrated that intravenous imipenem and amikacin with or without intrathecal amikacin could be used successfully with the caveat that all patients have their ventriculostomy catheters removed as part of the treatment.[151] Although their study consisted of a small number of cases, Rodriguez Guardado and coworkers demonstrated that intravenous and intrathecal colistin is an option and is as safe and effective as carbapenems for the treatment of nosocomial meningitis caused by *Acinetobacter*.[157] Furthermore, a review by Falagas and associates documented that therapy with intraventricular and intrathecal polymyxins alone or in combination with systemic antimicrobial agents is effective against gram-negative meningitis.[52]

As mentioned previously, gram-negative bacilli have the potential to become resistant to β-lactam antibiotics, therefore CSF needs to be sampled at regular intervals to ensure that it is being sterilized. When the response to systemic antibiotic treatment is poor during the treatment of gram-negative meningitis, the use of intraventricular antibiotics in combination with intravenous antibiotics should be considered early. The most commonly used intraventricular agents include gentamicin, amikacin, and polymyxin E (colistin) (Table 42-5).[104,153]

TABLE 42-4 Recommendations for Empirical Antimicrobial Therapy for Purulent Meningitis Based on Patient Age and Specific Predisposing Condition (A-III)

PREDISPOSING FACTOR	COMMON BACTERIAL PATHOGENS	ANTIMICROBIAL THERAPY
Age		
<1 mo	*Streptococcus agalactiae, Escherichia coli, Listeria monocytogenes, Klebsiella* species	Ampicillin plus cefotaxime or ampicillin plus an aminoglycoside
1-23 mo	*Streptococcus pneumoniae, Neisseria meningitidis, S. agalactiae, Haemophilus influenzae, E. coli*	Vancomycin plus a third-generation cephalosporin*†
2-50 yr	*N. meningitidis, S. pneumoniae*	Vancomycin plus a third-generation cephalosporin*†
>50 yr	*S. pneumoniae, N. meningitidis, L. monocytogenes,* aerobic gram-negative bacilli	Vancomycin plus ampicillin and a third-generation cephalosporin*†
Head trauma		
Basilar skull fracture	*S. pneumoniae, H. influenzae,* group A β-hemolytic streptococci	Vancomycin plus a third-generation cephalosporin*
Penetrating trauma	*Staphylococcus aureus,* coagulase-negative staphylococci (especially *Staphylococcus epidermidis*), aerobic gram-negative bacilli (including *Pseudomonas aeruginosa*)	Vancomycin plus cefepime, vancomycin plus ceftazidime, or vancomycin plus meropenem
Neurosurgery	Aerobic gram-negative bacilli (including *P. aeruginosa*), *S. aureus,* coagulase-negative staphylococci (especially *S. epidermidis*)	Vancomycin plus cefepime, vancomycin plus ceftazidime, or vancomycin plus meropenem
Cerebrospinal fluid shunt	Coagulase-negative staphylococci (especially *S. epidermidis*), *S. aureus,* aerobic gram-negative bacilli (including *P. aeruginosa*), *Propionibacterium acnes*	Vancomycin plus cefepime,‡ vancomycin plus ceftazidime,‡ or vancomycin plus meropenem‡

*Ceftriaxone or cefotaxime.
†Some experts would add rifampin if dexamethasone is also given.
‡In infants and children, vancomycin alone is reasonable unless Gram stains reveal the presence of gram-negative bacilli.
Adapted from Tunkel AR, Hartman BJ, Kaplan SL, et al. Practice guidelines for the management of bacterial meningitis. *Clin Infect Dis.* 2004;39:1267.

TABLE 42-5 Recommended Dosages of Antimicrobial Agents Administered by the Intraventricular Route (A-III)

ANTIMICROBIAL AGENT	DAILY INTRAVENTRICULAR DOSE (mg)
Vancomycin	5-20*
Gentamicin	1-8†
Tobramycin	5-20
Amikacin	5-50‡
Polymyxin B	5§
Colistin	10
Quinupristin/dalfopristin	2-5
Teicoplanin	5-40¶

NOTE: There are no specific data that define the exact dose of an antimicrobial agent that should be administered by the intraventricular route. Virtually all intrathecal use of antibiotics is considered "off label."
*Most studies have used a 10- or 20-mg dose.
†The usual daily dose is 1 to 2 mg for infants and children and 4 to 8 mg for adults.
‡The usual daily intraventricular dose is 30 mg.
§The dosage in children is 2 mg daily.
¶Dosage of 5 to 10 mg every 48 to 72 hours.
Adapted from Tunkel AR, Hartman BJ, Kaplan SL, et al. Practice guidelines for the management of bacterial meningitis. *Clin Infect Dis.* 2004;39:1267.

As results from cultures are confirmed for susceptibility, the antibiotic treatment should be adjusted accordingly. Practice guidelines for pathogen-specific antimicrobial treatment of bacterial meningitis have been published by the Infectious Disease Society of America along with recommended dosages (Tables 42-6 and 42-7). The length of treatment when treating gram-negative bacilli is most often 2 weeks after culture results have been negative.[158,159] Other authors have recommended a treatment duration between 2 and 4 weeks.[153,160,161] When treating *S. aureus*, 2 weeks of treatment is reasonable. However, the duration of therapy should always be individualized based on the patient's clinical response to treatment.

Empyema

Antibiotic treatment is initially broad spectrum and is directed against streptococci, staphylococci, and anaerobes. Empirical therapy includes a third-generation cephalosporin, vancomycin, or penicillin and metronidazole, with the latter providing anaerobic coverage. The suggested duration of treatment includes 2 weeks of intravenous therapy with an additional 6 weeks of oral therapy.[162,163] Nathoo and colleagues use a regimen consisting of a penicillin, chloramphenicol, and metronidazole administered intravenously for 2 weeks followed by a 4-week oral course.[164] The antibiotic regimen will require appropriate modification to either narrow or broaden the coverage based on bacterial culture and susceptibility results.

TABLE 42-6 Recommendations for Specific Antimicrobial Therapy for Bacterial Meningitis Based on Isolated Pathogen and Susceptibility Testing

MICROORGANISM, SUSCEPTIBILITY	STANDARD THERAPY	ALTERNATIVE THERAPIES
Streptococcus pneumoniae		
Penicillin MIC		
<0.1 µg/mL	Penicillin G or ampicillin	Third-generation cephalosporin,* chloramphenicol
0.1-1.0 µg/mL[†]	Third-generation cephalosporin*	Cefepime (B-II), meropenem (B-II)
≥2.0 µg/mL	Vancomycin plus a third-generation cephalosporin*[‡]	Fluoroquinolone[§] (B-II)
Cefotaxime or ceftriaxone MIC ≥1.0 µg/mL	Vancomycin plus a third-generation cephalosporin*[‡]	Fluoroquinolone[§] (B-II)
Neisseria meningitidis		
Penicillin MIC		
<0.1 µg/mL	Penicillin G or ampicillin	Third-generation cephalosporin,* chloramphenicol
0.1-1.0 µg/mL	Third-generation cephalosporin*	Chloramphenicol, fluoroquinolone, meropenem
Listeria monocytogenes	Ampicillin or penicillin G[‖]	Trimethoprim-sulfamethoxazole, meropenem (B-III)
Streptococcus agalactiae	Ampicillin or penicillin G[‖]	Third-generation cephalosporin* (B-III)
Escherichia coli and other Enterobacteriaceae[¶]	Third-generation cephalosporin (A-II)	Aztreonam, fluoroquinolone, meropenem, trimethoprim-sulfamethoxazole, ampicillin
Pseudomonas aeruginosa[¶]	Cefepime[‖] or ceftazidime[‖] (A-II)	Aztreonam,[‖] ciprofloxacin,[‖] meropenem[‖]
Haemophilus influenzae		
β-Lactamase negative	Ampicillin	Third-generation cephalosporin,* cefepime, chloramphenicol, fluoroquinolone
β-Lactamase positive	Third-generation cephalosporin (A-I)	Cefepime (A-I), chloramphenicol, fluoroquinolone
Staphylococcus aureus		
Methicillin susceptible	Nafcillin or oxacillin	Vancomycin, meropenem (B-III)
Methicillin resistant	Vancomycin**	Trimethoprim-sulfamethoxazole, linezolid (B-III)
Staphylococcus epidermidis	Vancomycin**	Linezolid (B-III)
Enterococcus species		
Ampicillin susceptible	Ampicillin plus gentamicin	—
Ampicillin resistant	Vancomycin plus gentamicin	—
Ampicillin and vancomycin resistant	Linezolid (B-III)	—

NOTE: All recommendations are A-III unless otherwise indicated.
*Ceftriaxone or cefotaxime.
[†]Ceftriaxone/cefotaxime-susceptible isolates.
[‡]Consider addition of rifampin if the MIC of ceftriaxone is greater than 2 µg/mL.
[§]Gatifloxacin or moxifloxacin.
[‖]Addition of an aminoglycoside should be considered.
[¶]Choice of a specific antimicrobial agent must be guided by in vitro susceptibility test results.
**Consider addition of rifampin.
MIC, minimal inhibitory concentration.
Adapted from Tunkel AR, Hartman BJ, Kaplan SL, et al. Practice guidelines for the management of bacterial meningitis. *Clin Infect Dis.* 2004;39:1267.

Brain Abscess

Initial coverage should begin with vancomycin, a third-generation cephalosporin, and metronidazole for anaerobic coverage.[165] As cultures and sensitivities are reported, the antibiotic regimen should be tailored accordingly. *Proteus, Escherichia coli,* and *Serratia* species, which are common causes of cerebral abscesses in neonates, should be covered with a combination of cefotaxime and gentamicin or amikacin. If the infection is refractory to the aforementioned management, craniotomy with eradication of the primary foci should be undertaken.

The duration of therapy is still a point of debate. In most cases, parenteral treatment for 6 to 8 weeks is recommended.[166,167] Some authors advocate an additional course of oral antibiotics for 2 to 3 months to eliminate any residual foci.[167]

Ventriculitis

The initial antibiotic regimen should include broad-spectrum coverage for possible resistant gram-positive and gram-negative organisms. Appropriate antibiotic therapy may include vancomycin plus a cephalosporin with antipseudomonal coverage such as cefepime or ceftazidime. Alternatively, vancomycin can be combined with meropenem to achieve similar coverage. Intraventricular vancomycin has also been reported to be successful in the treatment of ventriculitis caused by *Staphylococcus* and *Enterococcus* species.[168,169]

Intravenous polymyxin E (colistin) may be an option for gram-negative organisms, such as *Acinetobacter* and *Pseudomonas,* that are resistant to first-line antibacterial treatments.[170] There have also been case reports documenting the success of intrathecal colistin in the treatment of resistant *Acinetobacter* ventriculitis.[171-173]

TABLE 42-7 Recommended Dosages of Antimicrobial Therapy in Patients with Bacterial Meningitis (A-III)

ANTIMICROBIAL AGENT	TOTAL DAILY DOSE (DOSING INTERVAL IN HOURS)			
	Neonates 0-7 Days of Age*	Neonates 8-28 Days of Age*	Infants and Children	Adults
Amikacin[†]	15-20 mg/kg (12)	30 mg/kg (8)	20-30 mg/kg (8)	15 mg/kg (8)
Ampicillin	150 mg/kg (8)	200 mg/kg (6-8)	300 mg/kg (6)	12 g (4)
Aztreonam	—	—	—	6-8 g (6-8)
Cefepime	—	—	150 mg/kg (8)	6 g (8)
Cefotaxime	100-150 mg/kg (8-12)	150-200 mg/kg (6-8)	225-300 mg/kg (6-8)	8-12 g (4-6)
Ceftazidime	100-150 mg/kg (8-12)	150 mg/kg (8)	150 mg/kg (8)	6 g (8)
Ceftriaxone	—	—	80-100 mg/kg (12-24)	4 g (12-24)
Chloramphenicol	25 mg/kg (24)	50 mg/kg (12-24)	75-100 mg/kg (6)	4-6 g (6)[‡]
Ciprofloxacin	—	—	—	800-1200 mg (8-12)
Gatifloxacin	—	—	—	400 mg (24)[§]
Gentamicin[†]	5 mg/kg (12)	7.5 mg/kg (8)	7.5 mg/kg (8)	5 mg/kg (8)
Meropenem	—	—	120 mg/kg (8)	6 g (8)
Moxifloxacin	—	—	—	400 mg (24)[§]
Nafcillin	75 mg/kg (8-12)	100-150 mg/kg (6-8)	200 mg/kg (6)	9-12 g (4)
Oxacillin	75 mg/kg (8-12)	150-200 mg/kg (6-8)	200 mg/kg (6)	9-12 g (4)
Penicillin G	0.15 mU/kg (8-12)	0.2 mU/kg (6-8)	0.3 mU/kg (4-6)	24 mU (4)
Rifampin	—	10-20 mg/kg (12)	10-20 mg/kg (12-24)[‖]	600 mg (24)
Tobramycin[†]	5 mg/kg (12)	7.5 mg/kg (8)	7.5 mg/kg (8)	5 mg/kg (8)
TMP-SMZ[¶]	—	—	10-20 mg/kg (6-12)	10-20 mg/kg (6-12)
Vancomycin**	20-30 mg/kg (8-12)	30-45 mg/kg (6-8)	60 mg/kg (6)	30-45 mg/kg (8-12)

*Smaller doses and longer intervals of administration may be advisable for very low-birth-weight neonates (<2000 g).
[†]Need to monitor peak and trough serum concentrations.
[‡]Higher dose recommended for patients with pneumococcal meningitis.
[§]No data on optimal dosage needed in patients with bacterial meningitis.
[‖]Maximum daily dose of 600 mg.
[¶]Dosage based on trimethoprim component.
**Maintain serum trough concentrations of 15 to 20 μg/mL.
TMP-SMZ, trimethoprim-sulfamethoxazole.
Adapted from Tunkel AR, Hartman BJ, Kaplan SL, et al. Practice guidelines for the management of bacterial meningitis. *Clin Infect Dis.* 2004;39:1267.

Shunt Infections

Initial antibiotic selection should be broad spectrum and include coverage for methicillin-resistant *S. aureus* and *Staphylococcus epidermidis*, along with coverage for resistant gram-negative organisms such as *Pseudomonas* species, which have a propensity to adhere to foreign material.[174] Recommended empirical antibiotic therapy should consist of vancomycin to cover gram-positive organisms along with a cephalosporin that has antipseudomonal activity, such as cefepime or ceftazidime.[175-177] Rifampin can also be added for gram-positive shunt infections that fail to clear with vancomycin monotherapy.[174] Intrathecal administration of vancomycin or aminoglycosides may need to be initiated for shunt infections that are difficult to eradicate and fail to clear with systemic therapy.[174] For the treatment of *Propionibacterium acnes*, small studies have documented success with intravenous penicillin combined with shunt externalization and replacement.[178]

An alternative treatment of gram-positive shunt infections is intravenous linezolid, which has been demonstrated to be successful in case reports.[179,180] Linezolid possesses many attractive features that may increase its use, such as excellent CSF penetration and broad-spectrum activity. Additionally, Cruciani and coworkers demonstrated that intraventricular administration of teicoplanin was effective in seven patients with staphylococcal neurosurgical shunt infections.[181]

The introduction of antibiotic-impregnated shunt catheters may prove beneficial. A randomized controlled study performed by Eymann and associates demonstrated that antibiotic-impreg-

nated shunt catheters reduce the infection rate significantly in both pediatric and adult populations.[182]

Infection with Spinal Instrumentation

Empirical antibiotic therapy should be directed against staphylococcal species along with gram-negative organisms. Initial treatment with vancomycin and a third-generation cephalosporin until culture and susceptibility results return is appropriate. In most cases, removal of hardware is not necessary and can potentially have devastating complications because of spine instability and lack of bony fusion. Retrospective reviews of clinical practice have suggested that titanium instrumentation does not interfere with the treatment of spinal infection to the extent that stainless steel or other foreign bodies do.[183] Therefore, instrumentation should be left in place.[184]

The duration of antibiotic therapy for postoperative infection after spinal instrumentation is still debated. Lonstein proposes intravenous antibiotics for 10 to 14 days followed by oral antibiotics for 3 to 6 months.[185] Perry and coauthors recommend antibiotic treatment until the fever and leukocytosis resolve or for a minimum of 10 days.[186]

Vertebral Osteomyelitis

Specific antibiotic treatment should be based on culture and susceptibility results. For methicillin-resistant S. *aureus*, combination therapy with rifampin and intravenous vancomycin is the preferred regimen,[187,188] whereas linezolid can serve as an alternative. Previous studies have recommended that antibiotics be administered for a minimum of 6 to 8 weeks.[189-191] Gasbarrini and colleagues recommend that a minimum of 6 weeks of intravenous antibiotics be administered followed by 6 weeks of oral antibiotics.[192] For tuberculous vertebral osteomyelitis, the current standard of practice is to initiate isoniazid and rifampin for a 6- to 9-month period.[193] Nussbaum and coworkers have recommended that the course of treatment be at least 12 months in duration and consist of at least two antituberculous drugs.[194]

Osteomyelitis of the Skull

Initial antibiotic therapy should be directed against staphylococci with vancomycin plus a third-generation cephalosporin to cover gram-negative bacilli. If there is concern about anaerobes, metronidazole should be initiated. Once culture and susceptibility results return, the antibiotic therapy can be modified. Intravenous antibiotic treatment should be continued for at least 4 weeks and possibly followed by an additional oral course of antibiotics.[195]

Diskitis

For antibiotic treatment of diskitis, Cushing recommends empirical treatment directed against methicillin-resistant *S. aureus* for 5 to 7 days, followed by oral therapy for 1 to 2 weeks.[196] An appropriate empirical regimen may include a combination of vancomycin and a third-generation cephalosporin. Jansen and associates recommend intravenous antibiotics for 4 to 6 weeks followed by oral antibiotics until the symptoms resolve.[197]

CONCLUSION

Antibiotics are essential to modern neurosurgical practice. Like all drugs, they have important risks and their misuse can lead to serious problems for individual patients. Irresponsible use by the profession can even lead to public health concerns. Judicious use and adherence to the basic principles of appropriate use optimize their value in the treatment of neurosurgical patients. Basic principles include the following:

1. Antibiotics should be used only for the prevention or treatment of susceptible infections.
2. The choice of antibiotic should be guided by the most likely infecting organisms and directed by culture results whenever possible.
3. Antibiotics should be used for their shortest effective duration.
4. The risks associated with antibiotic administration must be considered every time that they are used.
5. The dose and frequency of administration should be guided by principles of pharmacokinetics and, in serious infections, by measured antibiotic levels.

Failure to follow established basic principles can lead to antibiotic misuse ranging from embarrassing (using an antibiotic in a way that it cannot work) to harmful (superinfection with an organism resistant to all known drugs). The following is a list of a few such misuses of antibiotics in neurosurgery.

Intraventricular administration of chloramphenicol
- It penetrates the BBB very well.
- It requires hydrolysis in the liver to be active.

Routine use of vancomycin for prophylaxis
- Most infections are not caused by methicillin-resistant *S. aureus*.

- Vancomycin penetration into the CSF is variable and frequently poor in the absence of inflammation.
- Indiscriminant prophylactic use contributes to the emergence of vancomycin resistance, which threatens to become a major public health problem because alternative antibiotics for vancomycin-resistant organisms are not widely available.

Assuming that good CSF penetration in the presence of meningeal inflammation is equivalent to good penetration of the CNS in the absence of inflammation

It can't hurt
- See the list of toxicities and interactions.

More is better
- Excessive use leads to selecting resistant organisms, which makes treatment more difficult.
- Superinfections hurt patients (e.g., *Clostridium difficile*).

Adherence to basic principles and appropriate consultation with specialists in infectious disease can optimize the use of antibiotics in neurosurgical practice.

SUGGESTED READINGS

Barker FG. Efficacy of prophylactic antibiotics against meningitis after craniotomy: a meta-analysis. *Neurosurgery.* 2007;60:887.

Barker FG. Efficacy of prophylactic antibiotic therapy in spinal surgery: a meta-analysis. *Neurosurgery.* 2002;51:391.

Barker FG. Efficacy of prophylactic antibiotics for craniotomy: a meta-analysis. *Neurosurgery.* 1994;35:484.

Chow KM, Hui AC, Szeto CC. Neurotoxicity induced by beta-lactam antibiotics: from bench to bedside. *Eur J Clin Microbiol Infect Dis.* 2005;24:649.

Eymann R, Chehab S, Strowitzki M, et al. Clinical and economic consequences of antibiotic-impregnated cerebrospinal fluid shunt catheters. *J Neurosurg Pediatr.* 2008;1:444.

Falagas ME, Bliziotis IA, Tam VH. Intraventricular or intrathecal use of polymyxins in patients with gram-negative meningitis: a systematic review of the available evidence. *Int J Antimicrob Agents.* 2007;29:9.

Haines SJ, Walters BC. Antibiotic prophylaxis for cerebrospinal fluid shunts: a metaanalysis. *Neurosurgery.* 1994;34:87.

Kearney BP, Aweeka FT. The penetration of anti-infectives into the central nervous system. *Neurol Clin.* 1999;17:883.

Lee MC, Wang MY, Fessler RG, et al. Instrumentation in patients with spinal infection. *Neurosurg Focus.* 2004;17:E7(6).

Mangram AJ, Horan TC, Pearson ML, et al. Guideline for Prevention of Surgical Site Infection, 1999. Centers for Disease Control and Prevention (CDC) Hospital Infection Control Practices Advisory Committee. *Am J Infect Control.* 1999;27:97.

Nagarajan L, Lam GC. Tetracycline-induced benign intracranial hypertension. *J Paediatr Child Health.* 2000;36:82.

Nau R, Prange HW, Muth P, et al. Passage of cefotaxime and ceftriaxone into cerebrospinal fluid of patients with uninflamed meninges. *Antimicrob Agents Chemother.* 1993;37:1518.

Nau R, Sorgel F, Prange HW. Pharmacokinetic optimisation of the treatment of bacterial central nervous system infections. *Clin Pharmacokinet.* 1998;35:223.

Neuwelt EA. Mechanisms of disease: the blood-brain barrier. *Neurosurgery.* 2004;54:131.

Ratilal B, Costa J, Sampaio C. Antibiotic prophylaxis for surgical introduction of intracranial ventricular shunts: a systematic review. *J Neurosurg Pediatr.* 2008;1:48.

Ratilal B, Costa J, Sampaio C. Antibiotic prophylaxis for preventing meningitis in patients with basilar skull fractures. *Cochrane Database Syst Rev.* 2006;1:CD004884.

Snavely SR, Hodges GR. The neurotoxicity of antibacterial agents. *Ann Intern Med.* 1984;101:92.

Thomas RJ. Neurotoxicity of antibacterial therapy. *South Med J.* 1994;87:869.

Wagner C, Sauermann R, Joukhadar C. Principles of antibiotic penetration into abscess fluid. *Pharmacology.* 2006;78:1.

Wen DY, Bottini AG, Hall WA, et al. Infections in neurologic surgery. The intraventricular use of antibiotics. *Neurosurg Clin N Am.* 1992;3:343.

Full references can be found on Expert Consult @ www.expertconsult.com

CHAPTER 43

Brain Abscess

Allan R. Tunkel ■ W. Michael Scheld

Brain abscess is defined as a focal intracranial infection that is initiated as an area of cerebritis and evolves into a collection of pus surrounded by a vascularized capsule.[1] Given their location, the approach to brain abscesses often presents diagnostic and therapeutic challenges. The following sections review the epidemiology, pathogenesis, etiology, and diagnostic and management approach for this devastating infection.

EPIDEMIOLOGY

Incidence and Risk Factors

Before the advent of infection with human immunodeficiency virus (HIV), brain abscess was not common, with an incidence of 0.3 to 1.3 cases per 100,000 persons per year in the United States.[2] This translates to approximately 1500 to 2500 cases per year in the United States, with a higher incidence in developing countries.[3] There is a male preponderance of 2:1 to 3:1, and the median age at infection is between 30 and 40 years.[2,4] Differences in age are based on the primary site of infection—when the abscess is from an otitic focus, patients are generally younger than 20 years or older than 40 years, and when secondary to a focus in the paranasal sinuses, most patients are between 30 and 40 years of age. About 25% of brain abscess cases occur in children, mostly secondary to an otitic focus or in those with congenital heart disease; in one review from the University of Virginia Children's Hospital from 2000 to 2007, an average of only 1.5 children per year were admitted to the inpatient pediatric service with a primary diagnosis of brain abscess.[5] Brain abscess may occur after cranial operations. It was reported in only 0.2% of 1587 operations in one study[6] and in 10 of 16,540 cranial surgeries performed by 25 neurosurgeons in another review[7]; although rare, a small percentage of patients will require a repeat operation to treat the infection. In more recent series, brain abscess is more commonly reported in patients who are immunocompromised,[2,3] including those infected with HIV, receiving chemotherapy for cancer, receiving immunosuppressive therapy after organ transplantation, or after prolonged use of corticosteroids.

Pathogenesis

Organisms can reach the central nervous system (CNS) by spread from a contiguous source of infection (25% to 50% of cases), hematogenous dissemination (20% to 35% of cases), or trauma[1-5,8-16]; brain abscess is cryptogenic in about 10% to 35% of patients.[2,17] Sources from a contiguous focus of infection include infections in the middle ear, mastoid cells, or paranasal sinuses. Brain abscess that results from otitis media usually localizes to the temporal lobe or cerebellum; in one review, 54% were in the temporal lobe, 44% in the cerebellum, and 2% in both locations.[18] Recent series, however, have demonstrated that cases of brain abscess secondary to otitis media have been decreasing, although intracranial complications may be increased in patients in whom appropriate treatment of otitis media is neglected. In

patients with brain abscess secondary to paranasal sinusitis, the frontal lobe is the predominant site. When the abscess is a complication of sphenoid sinusitis, the temporal lobe or sella turcica is usually involved. Dental infections, particularly of the molar teeth, can lead to brain abscess, often in the frontal lobe, but temporal lobe extension has been reported.[19,20]

Hematogenous dissemination to the brain generally leads to multiple, multiloculated abscesses, which are associated with higher mortality than abscesses that result from contiguous foci of infection.[2-4] The most common sources in adults are chronic pyogenic lung diseases (especially lung abscess), bronchiectasis, empyema, and cystic fibrosis. Other distant sources of infection include wound and skin infections, osteomyelitis, pelvic infections, and intra-abdominal infections; they can also occur after esophageal dilation or sclerosing therapy for esophageal varices.[21-23] Cyanotic congenital heart disease (especially in patients with tetralogy of Fallot and transposition of the great vessels) is another predisposing factor that accounts for 5% to 15% of brain abscess cases. Even higher percentages are reported in pediatric series,[24,25] although advances in cardiovascular surgery have led to a decrease in patients with cyanotic congenital heart disease as a predisposing factor.[3] Brain abscess occurs in less than 5% of patients with infective endocarditis despite the presence of continuous bacteremia.[26-28] There is also a significant likelihood of brain abscess in patients with hereditary hemorrhagic telangiectasia, which is almost always observed in those with coexisting pulmonary arteriovenous malformations, perhaps by allowing septic emboli to cross the pulmonary circulation without capillary filtration[29-32]; the risk ranges from 5% to 9% and is 1000 times greater than in the general population.

Trauma can lead to brain abscess formation as a result of an open cranial fracture with dural breach or foreign body injury or as a sequela of neurosurgery.[33] The incidence of traumatic brain abscess in the civilian population ranges from 2.5% to 10.9%, and reports have included brain abscess secondary to compound depressed skull fractures, dog bites, rooster pecking, tongue piercing, and injuries from lawn darts and pencil tips.[34-36] Nosocomial brain abscess has been seen after halo pin insertion,[37] after electrode insertion to localize seizure foci,[38] and in malignant glioma patients treated by placement of Gliadel wafers in the tumor bed to release carmustine.[39] In military populations, the incidence of brain abscess after head trauma ranges from 3% to 17%, and they usually occur secondary to retained bone fragments or contamination of initially uninfected missile sites with bacteria from skin, clothes, or the environment.[40] However, the importance of retained bone fragments in the pathogenesis of infection has been questioned. In a study from Croatia of 160 war missile penetrating craniocerebral injuries in which 21 skull base injuries were treated surgically,[41] only the accessible retained bone or metallic fragments were removed; the retained foreign bodies did not seem to increase the infection rate except in patients who suffered an in-driven cluster of bone fragments or leakage of cerebrospinal fluid. These findings were confirmed in another retrospective study from Croatia in which 88 patients with brain missile wounds had only accessible bone or metallic fragments removed during intracranial débridement[42]; there were 9 cases of brain abscess and the presence of retained fragments was not responsible for an increased rate of infection. Similar results were found in another study of 43 patients who survived low-velocity missile injuries to the brain during military conflicts and had retained fragments; suppurative sequelae were seen in 6 patients and only 2 progressed to brain abscess.[43]

ETIOLOGY

Numerous infectious agents have been reported to cause brain abscess. The probable infecting pathogen depends on the pathogenesis of the infection (see earlier) and the presence of various predisposing conditions (Table 43-1). This chapter focuses on important bacterial and fungal causes of brain abscess. Protozoal and helminthic causes (e.g., *Trypanosoma cruzi*, *Taenia solium*, *Entamoeba histolytica*, *Schistosoma* spp., *Microsporidia* spp., and *Paragonimus* spp.) are discussed in other chapters of this book. The most important protozoal cause of brain infection is *Toxoplasma gondii*, which is seen primarily in patients infected with HIV; this organism and the approach to CNS mass lesions in patients infected with HIV are also discussed in other chapters of this book.

Bacteria

The most common bacterial causes of brain abscess are streptococci (aerobic, anaerobic, and microaerophilic), which are isolated in up to 70% of cases.[2,10,44] They include organisms in the *Streptococcus anginosus* (*milleri*) group, which normally reside in the oral cavity, appendix, and female genital tract. *Staphylococcus aureus* is isolated in 10% to 20% of cases, most commonly after cranial trauma or infective endocarditis.[2] Enteric gram-negative bacilli (e.g., *Proteus* spp., *Escherichia coli*, *Klebsiella* spp., *Pseudomonas aeruginosa*, and *Enterobacter* spp.) are isolated in 23% to 33% of patients; predisposing factors include otitis media, bacteremia, neurosurgical procedures, and the immunocompromised state.[2,45,46] Anaerobes (especially *Bacteroides* and *Prevotella* spp.) have more often been isolated after proper culture techniques and are found in 20% to 40% of patients, frequently in mixed culture.[2,47,48] Multiple organisms are cultured in 14% to 28% of those with positive culture results.[2,9-12] The incidence of negative cultures has ranged from 0% to 43%[2,3,9-13,15,18,47,49]; previous use of antimicrobial therapy may account for these negative culture results.

Other species are less commonly isolated in patients with bacterial brain abscess but should be considered in those with certain underlying conditions. For example, brain abscess caused by *Listeria monocytogenes* is uncommon (<1% of cases) but accounts for about 10% of cases of CNS listeriosis[50,51]; *Listeria* should be considered in patients who are immunocompromised (e.g., leukemia, lymphoma, HIV infection, and conditions requiring corticosteroids or other agents that cause immunosuppression). *Salmonella* species may cause brain abscess in patients who are bacteremic or in the presence of some compromise of the reticuloendothelial system.[52] Brain abscess caused by *Nocardia* species may occur as part of a disseminated infection in patients with cutaneous or pulmonary disease; most have defects in cell-mediated immunity such as corticosteroid therapy, organ transplantation, HIV infection, or neoplasia.[53,54] Rare cases of *Nocardia* brain abscess have also been seen in pregnant women. Other bacteria that cause brain abscess include *Streptococcus pneumoniae*, *Haemophilus influenzae*, *Burkholderia pseudomallei*, and *Actinomyces* species.[2,16,55,56] When meningitis is caused by certain facultative gram-negative organisms (e.g., *Citrobacter diversus*), concomitant brain abscess is observed in more than 75% of cases.[1,57,58] *Mycobacterium tuberculosis* and nontuberculous mycobacteria have increasingly been observed to cause brain abscess,[1,2,59] with most cases reported in patients with HIV infection[60,61]; when the caseous core of a CNS tuberculoma liquefies, a tubercular abscess will result.[62]

Fungi

In recent years, the incidence of fungal brain abscess has been rising as a result of the increased use of corticosteroid therapy, broad-spectrum antimicrobial therapy, and immunosuppressive agents.[63-66] *Candida* species have been the most prevalent fungi but are often not discovered until autopsy; these fungi cause microabscesses, macroabscesses, noncaseating granulomas, and diffuse glial nodules. Risk factors for candidal brain abscess include the use of broad-spectrum antimicrobial agents, corticosteroids, and hyperalimentation; premature birth; malignancy; neutropenia; chronic granulomatous disease; diabetes mellitus; thermal injury; and the presence of a central venous catheter.

CNS aspergillosis is reported in 10% to 20% of patients with invasive disease.[63,65,67,68] The lungs are the usual primary site of infection, with dissemination to the CNS occurring by direct extension from an area that is anatomically adjacent to the brain.

TABLE 43-1 Predisposing Conditions and Probable Etiologic Agents in Brain Abscess

PREDISPOSING CONDITION	POSSIBLE MICROBIAL CAUSES
Otitis media or mastoiditis	Streptococci (aerobic or anaerobic), *Bacteroides* spp., *Prevotella* spp., Enterobacteriaceae
Sinusitis (frontoethmoidal or sphenoidal)	Streptococci, *Bacteroides* spp., Enterobacteriaceae, *Haemophilus* spp., *Staphylococcus aureus*
Dental infection	Mixed *Fusobacterium*, *Prevotella*, *Actinomyces*, and *Bacteroides* spp.; streptococci
Penetrating trauma or secondary to neurosurgical procedure	*Staphylococcus aureus*, Enterobacteriaceae, *Clostridium* spp.
Lung abscess, empyema, or bronchiectasis	*Fusobacterium*, *Actinomyces*, *Bacteroides*, and *Prevotella* spp.; streptococci; *Nocardia* spp.
Bacterial endocarditis	*Staphylococcus aureus*, streptococci
Congenital heart disease	Streptococci, *Haemophilus* spp.
Immunocompromised state	
Neutropenia	Aerobic gram-negative bacilli, *Aspergillus* spp., Mucorales, *Candida* spp., *Scedosporium* spp.
Transplantation	Enterobacteriaceae, *Listeria monocytogenes*, *Nocardia* spp., *Aspergillus* spp., *Candida* spp., Mucorales, *Scedosporium* spp., *Toxoplasma gondii*
HIV infection	*Listeria monocytogenes*, *Nocardia* spp., *Mycobacterium* spp., *Cryptococcus neoformans*, *Toxoplasma gondii*

The most important underlying immune defect in patients with invasive aspergillosis is neutropenia (i.e., in those who have an underlying malignancy), but it may also be seen in patients with hepatic disease, diabetes mellitus, chronic granulomatous disease, Cushing's syndrome, HIV infection, injection drug use, organ transplantation, and bone marrow transplantation, as well as after craniotomy and in patients receiving chronic corticosteroid therapy.

CNS infections caused by the Mucorales group are among the most fulminant infections known. Diabetes mellitus, usually associated with acidosis, is the most common predisposing condition (≈70% of cases), but disease may also be seen in patients with acidemia from profound systemic illness (e.g., sepsis, severe dehydration, severe diarrhea, chronic kidney disease), hematologic neoplasms, renal transplantation, injection drug use, and use of deferoxamine.[65,69] CNS disease results from direct extension from the rhinocerebral form, after open head trauma, or after hematogenous dissemination. Bilateral involvement of the basal ganglia has been reported in injection drug users. *Rhizopus arrhizus* is the most common isolate.[70]

Scedosporium species may cause CNS disease in immunocompetent and immunocompromised hosts.[65,71-75] These organisms may enter the CNS by direct trauma, hematogenous dissemination, or direct extension from infected sinuses. An association between near-drowning and subsequent CNS infection has been reported because these organisms are present in contaminated water and manure.

Many other fungal species have been reported to cause brain abscess, including *Cryptococcus neoformans*, the endemic mycoses (*Coccidioides* spp., *Histoplasma* spp., and *Blastomyces dermatitidis*), and many of the dematiaceous fungi. It is beyond the scope of this chapter to review all fungal causes of brain abscess, and more detail can be found from other sources.[65]

EXPERIMENTAL MODELS OF INFECTION

Numerous animal models have been developed to study the pathogenesis and pathophysiology of brain abscess.[76] Some large-animal models were created by direct implantation of bacteria into the brain; however, these models were limited by lack of reproducibility, they required multiple steps and an agar vehicle to initiate infection, and they were quite expensive. Another method used embolization of contaminated pliable cylinders implanted into the carotid artery but required concomitant cerebral injury for abscess formation, and the accompanying brain infarction caused a high mortality rate even in uninfected control animals.

A better animal model involved the use of mice or rats and consisted of a simple, one-step, easily reproducible procedure for consistent production of brain abscess. Infection was produced by the injection of 1 μL of saline containing a fixed inoculum of bacteria through a bur hole and into the frontal lobe of the brain.[77,78] With this model, brain abscess was achieved in a one-step process at a specific site with the injection of bacteria alone, the inoculum could be regulated in terms of both volume and number of organisms, the number of injected bacteria and the number of bacteria that remain viable in the tissue could be quantified at a later time, and there was precise control of the injection site, thereby reducing tissue trauma with minimal (or no) infection in the subarachnoid space. This model also simulated human infection in that the abscess was produced in the white matter at the white and gray matter junction and migrated toward the ventricle, a shift in intracranial contents occurred, and there was minimal histologic evidence of meningitis; the abscess capsule was asymmetric by being more complete on the cortical than on the ventricular side, perhaps because the increased vascularity of normal cortical gray matter allowed greater fibroblast proliferation and collagen helix formation. In addition, develop-

ment of the abscess paralleled clinical disease with the initial development of cerebritis and massive white matter edema followed by encapsulation.

In another animal model, brain abscess was produced in a rat by direct intracerebral injection of agarose beads laden with *S. aureus*.[79] This method was also easy, reproducible, effective, and associated with a low mortality rate, and the histologic features of these experimental abscesses were similar to those observed in other animal models and in humans. These models have been useful in delineating the early events in brain abscess formation with respect to bacterial virulence factors and the host defense mechanisms involved in brain abscess formation; these concepts are reviewed in greater detail subsequently.

Initiation of Infection

The brain appears to be significantly more sensitive to infection than many other tissues. In a rat model of experimental brain abscess, injection of 10^4 colony-forming units (CFUs) of *S. aureus* or 10^6 CFUs of *E. coli* failed to cause infection in the skin, but abscess formation in brain tissue was induced by a level as low as 10^2 CFUs of either organism.[80] The brain may also be more susceptible to infection by different organisms; in the experimental rat model, strains of *E. coli* were more virulent (i.e., led to abscess formation at lower inocula) than *P. aeruginosa*, *S. aureus*, or *Streptococcus pyogenes*.[81] In addition, *E. coli* strains possessing the K1 antigen were more infective than strains without this antigen, thus indicating that certain encapsulated strains may be more virulent in brain abscess formation. Furthermore, inoculation of *Bacteroides fragilis* or streptococci such as *S. intermedius* failed to lead to abscess formation in rats even though these organisms account for a high percentage of isolates from brain abscesses in humans; this may be explained by the fact that brain abscess is often the result of a contiguous focus of infection and the synergistic infectivity of mixed populations of anaerobes plus a facultative organism may be necessary to establish infection.[82,83] In an experimental dog model of brain abscess formation, inoculation of *B. fragilis* with *Staphylococcus epidermidis* in mixed culture caused a virulent reaction,[84] although each organism was not tested separately. The role of other bacterial virulence factors in the pathogenesis of brain abscess formation has not been elucidated. However, the role of virulence factor production in the development of brain abscess was demonstrated by the inability of heat-inactivated *S. aureus* to induce proinflammatory cytokine or chemokine expression in an experimental mouse model; alpha toxin was identified as a key virulence factor for survival of *S. aureus* in the brain and subsequent development of brain abscess.[85]

Brain abscess may also develop in patients with bacterial meningitis, a rare complication except in human neonates with meningitis caused by *C. diversus*.[45,46] Pathologically, there is cerebral necrosis and liquefaction, along with vasculitis of small vessels and hemorrhagic necrosis of adjacent tissue with a propensity for contiguous inflammation in the cerebral white matter, which may reflect the effects of endotoxin in the small penetrating vessels in this area; the typical abscess with capsule formation was not present. The pathogenesis was investigated in an infant rat model in which infection was initiated with the production of a high-grade bacteremia, infiltration of the leptomeninges, and subsequent development of ventriculitis.[86] Brain abscesses were found exclusively in the periventricular white matter, apparently from disruption of the ventricular ependymal lining with direct extension of the infection into the parenchyma. The virulence factors responsible for the propensity of this organism to cause brain abscess are undefined, although a minor 32-kD outer membrane determinant may be a marker for strains that are more likely to produce ventriculitis and brain abscess[87]; strains that lacked the 32-kD outer membrane protein caused more bacteremia, meningitis, and death.

Stages of Infection

The temporal course and pathologic consequences of brain abscess were examined in a canine model of infection after inoculation of α-hemolytic streptococci. Four stages of infection were identified (Table 43-2): early cerebritis, late cerebritis, early capsule formation, and late capsule formation.[88] These stages are somewhat arbitrary but are useful in the classification and comparison of virulence between different organisms in the production of brain abscess. Similar neuropathologic findings were described in an experimental model of anaerobic brain abscess,[84] but capsule formation could not be divided into early and late stages because of delayed encapsulation. *S. aureus* was found to be more virulent than α-hemolytic streptococci, with a greater amount of necrosis and total area of involvement and a longer course of progression to resolution, time to reach a stable size, and time to contain the necrotic region within a collagenous capsule.[89] Inflammation with histologic evidence of extension of inflammation, necrosis, and edema beyond the capsule was also observed, similar to findings after inoculation with *B. fragilis*. In all these studies, capsule formation was less prominent on the ventricular than on the cortical surface,[84,88,89] perhaps because differences in vascularity between the cortical gray and white matter allow greater fibroblast proliferation, which probably explains the tendency for brain abscesses to rupture into the ventricular system rather than into the subarachnoid space. In contrast, the histopathologic sequence of brain abscess formation was examined in an experimental rat model after inoculation of *E. coli*[90]; the histopathologic findings supported an alternative hypothesis that brain abscesses tend to rupture intraventricularly because the infectious process is directed along the major white matter tracts (areas of lower tissue resistance) rather than as a result of asymmetric collagen deposition. However, the question of rupture of brain abscess requires further study.

The histopathologic findings in brain abscesses after direct implantation differ from those produced by intracarotid embolization because metastatic abscesses induced only transient midline displacements, inflammatory cell infiltration was reduced, and collagen formation was retarded around proliferating capsular vessels; this may have patient care implications because a lower degree of encapsulation contributes to mortality.

Host Defense Mechanisms

In the experimental models just described, bacteria were inoculated directly into the brain, thus bypassing the brain's normal host defense mechanisms. Although the brain is generally protected from infection by an intact blood-brain barrier, once infection is established, immune defenses are usually inadequate to control the infection. Local opsonization in the brain is deficient, which allows encapsulated bacteria such as *B. fragilis* and *E. coli* to escape efficient phagocytosis; phagocytosis of *Bacteroides* species also requires heat-labile serum factors such as complement and lysozyme, and these factors are probably absent in the CNS.[91,92] The outer membrane components of *Bacteroides* species may also be important in the inhibition of neutrophil chemotaxis, thereby reducing the host response to brain abscess caused by this organism.[93]

As shown in Table 43-2, the border around the initial area of inoculation is composed of acute inflammatory cells during the early cerebritis stage, accompanied by the rapid development of a perivascular infiltrate consisting of neutrophils, plasma cells, and mononuclear cells.[84,88,89] In an experimental rat model of brain abscess formation, production of the proinflammatory cytokines interleukin-1α (IL-1α), IL-1β, IL-6, and tumor necrosis factor-α (TNF-α) occurred as early as 1 to 6 hours after exposure to *S. aureus*.[94] This was followed by enhanced concentration of the CXC chemokine KC, which correlates with the appearance of neutrophils in the abscess. The importance of neutrophils in the initial containment of *S. aureus* in the brain was established by the fact that mice transiently depleted of neutrophils, before the implantation of bacteria-laden beads, had higher CNS bacterial burdens than did control animals.[95] Both macrophage inflammatory protein-2 (MIP-2) and KC/CXCL1, two neutrophil-attracting CXC chemokines, were significantly elevated in the brain after *S. aureus* exposure, thus indicating the importance of the CXCR2 ligands MIP-2 and KC, as well as neutrophils, in the acute host response. The continued release of proinflammatory

TABLE 43-2 Histopathologic Findings in the Stages of Brain Abscess Formation

	EARLY CEREBRITIS (DAYS 1-3)	LATE CEREBRITIS (DAYS 4-9)	EARLY CAPSULE FORMATION (DAYS 10-13)	LATE CAPSULE FORMATION (DAY 14 AND LATER)
Necrotic center	Acute inflammatory cells; bacteria present on Gram stain	Enlarging necrotic center reaching maximal size	Decrease in necrotic center	Further decrease in necrotic center
Inflammatory border	Acute inflammatory cells	Inflammatory cells, macrophages, and fibroblasts	Increased numbers of fibroblasts and macrophages	Further increase in number of fibroblasts
Cerebritis and neovascularity	Rapid perivascular infiltration of neutrophils, plasma cells, and mononuclear cells	Maximal extent of cerebritis; rapid increase in new vessel formation	Maximal degree of neovascularity	Cerebritis restricted to outside of collagen capsule; reduced neovascularity
Collagenous capsule	Reticulin formation begins by day 3	Appearance of fibroblasts with rapid formation of reticulin	Evolution of mature collagen	Capsule completed by end of second week
Reactive gliosis and cerebral edema	Marked cerebral edema	Prominent cerebral edema; appearance of reactive astrocytes	Regression of cerebral edema; increase in reactive astrocytes	Regression of cerebral edema; marked gliosis outside capsule by third week

Data from Tunkel AR, Scheld WM. Pathogenesis and pathophysiology of bacterial infections. In: Scheld WM, Whitley RJ, Durack, DT, eds. *Infections of the Central Nervous System*, 2nd ed. Philadelphia: Lippincott-Raven; 1997;297-312; and Britt RH, Enzmann DR, Yeager AS. Neuropathological and computerized tomographic findings in experimental brain abscess. *J Neurosurg.* 1981;55:590-603.

mediators by activated glia and infiltrating peripheral immune cells may potentiate the subsequent recruitment and retention of newly recruited inflammatory cells and glia,[96] thereby perpetuating the antibacterial inflammatory response. Recent studies support this persistent immune activation associated with experimental brain abscess in which increased concentrations of IL-1α, TNF-α, and MIP-2 were detected between 14 and 21 days after *S. aureus* exposure,[97] thus suggesting that intervention with antiinflammatory compounds, subsequent to bacterial neutralization, might minimize damage to the surrounding brain parenchyma. Although Toll-like receptor 2 (TLR2) has an important role in mediating *S. aureus*–induced activation, additional receptors are also involved in glial responses to *S. aureus*. With progression to the late cerebritis stage, the acute inflammatory cells become mixed with macrophages and fibroblasts, and reticulin formation surrounds the necrotic center. As the capsule begins to form, increased numbers of fibroblasts and macrophages infiltrate the periphery, and mature collagen is deposited to form a capsule. The necrotic center then continues to decrease in size while marked gliosis develops outside the capsule.

Despite the presence of virulence factors of the organism that resist host defense mechanisms, the host inflammatory response is important in containment of the abscess, as has been examined with the use of immunosuppressed animals. Initial studies in a dog model of experimental brain abscess with *S. aureus* or *Proteus mirabilis* demonstrated that the administration of dexamethasone slowed, but did not fully impair, capsule formation.[98] In contrast, there was no evidence of capsule formation when dexamethasone was given at the same time as inoculation of either *S. pyogenes* or *S. aureus* in another study.[99] In an experimental rat model of *E. coli* brain abscess,[90] dexamethasone administration led to a reduction in macrophage and glial responses, collagen deposition, and host survival, with demonstration of an increased number of viable bacteria in the brain abscess. Coadministration of dexamethasone also impaired the lymphocytic and fibroblastic response in a rat model of experimental *S. aureus* brain abscess,[100] although it did not entirely halt the encapsulation or reduce the associated cerebral edema.

Another study in dogs, who were immunosuppressed with azathioprine and prednisone 7 days before the intracerebral inoculation of α-hemolytic streptococci, demonstrated that the immunosuppressed animals manifested a decreased inflammatory response that was characterized by a reduction in neutrophils and macrophages in the lesion, a decrease and delay in collagen deposition, and persistence of viable organisms into the late capsule stage.[101] Reduction of neutrophils, plasma cells, lymphocytes, and

macrophages in the areas surrounding the necrotic center of the abscess was observed, and cerebritis was also decreased outside the developing capsule. However, gliosis was markedly increased in the area surrounding the collagenous capsule in these immunosuppressed dogs. Although the decreased inflammatory response and edema initially resulted in less mass effect, the eventual size and area of the abscess may have become larger as a result of the diminished host response.

CLINICAL FINDINGS

The clinical manifestations of brain abscess may run the gamut from indolent to fulminant; most are related to the size and location of the space-occupying lesion within the brain and the virulence of the infecting organism.[1-3,8-17] Common symptoms and signs are presented in Table 43-3. Headache is generally observed in 70% to 75% of patients; sudden worsening of the headache, accompanied by new onset of meningismus, may signify rupture of the abscess into the ventricular space.[102,103] In one study of 33 consecutive patients with intraventricular rupture of brain abscess, severe headaches and signs of meningeal irritation were prominent findings before rupture, followed by rapid clinical deterioration within 10 days.[104] Intraventricular rupture appears to be more likely if the abscess is deep-seated, multiloculated, and in close proximity to the ventricular wall[102]; a 1-mm reduction of the distance between the ventricle and the abscess increased the rupture rate by 10%. The classic triad of fever, headache, and focal neurological deficits is seen in less than 50% of patients with brain abscess. The specific neurological findings of brain abscess are also defined by location within the CNS (Table 43-4).[1-3,9-16,105,106]

TABLE 43-3 Initial Symptoms and Signs in Patients with Brain Abscess

SYMPTOM OR SIGN	FREQUENCY RANGE (%)
Headache	49-97
Fever	32-79
Focal neurological deficits*	23-66
Altered mental status	28-91
Seizures	13-35
Nausea and vomiting	27-85
Nuchal rigidity	5-41
Papilledema	9-51

*The specific deficit depends on the central nervous system location of the abscess (see Table 43-4).
Data from references 1, 2, 8, 9-17, 102.

TABLE 43-4 Possible Initial Findings in Patients with Brain Abscess Based on Intracranial Location

INTRACRANIAL LOCATION	FINDING
Parietal lobe	Headache
	Visual field deficits (ranging from inferior quadrantanopia to homonymous hemianopia)
	Endocrine disturbances
Frontal lobe	Headache
	Drowsiness
	Inattention
	Personality change
	Mental status deterioration
	Hemiparesis
	Motor speech disorder
Temporal lobe	Ipsilateral headache
	Aphasia or dysphasia (if in the dominant hemisphere)
	Visual field deficit (ranging from upper quadrant homonymous quadrantanopia to complete homonymous hemianopia)
Cerebellum	Headache
	Nystagmus
	Ataxia
	Vomiting
	Dysmetria
	Meningismus
	Papilledema
Brainstem	Cranial nerve involvement
	Deficits of ascending and descending pathways

In immunocompromised patients, the clinical findings may be masked by the diminished inflammatory response.

The clinical manifestations of brain abscess may also be defined by the infecting pathogen. For example, patients with nocardial brain abscess may have concomitant pulmonary, skin, or muscle lesions[53,54,107]; however, the CNS findings are more often nonspecific and associated with fever, headache, and focal neurological deficits defined by location. Patients with *Aspergillus* brain abscess commonly manifest signs of a stroke syndrome as a result of ischemia or intracerebral hemorrhage, or both, that is referable to the involved areas of the brain.[65,67,68] Patients who are severely immunocompromised usually have nonspecific findings shortly before death, whereas those who are less immunocompromised are more likely to have headache and focal neurological deficits, but evidence of aspergillosis in other organ systems is usually apparent.

Patients with rhinocerebral mucormycosis initially have symptoms referable to the eyes or sinuses and complaints of headache, facial pain, diplopia, lacrimation, and nasal stuffiness or epistaxis.[65,69] With continued infection and spread to contiguous structures, necrotic lesions appear in the turbinates, nose, paranasal skin, or hard palate; chemosis, proptosis, and external ophthalmoplegia may also occur. Cranial nerve involvement is common, and blindness may occur as a result of invasion of the cavernous sinus, ophthalmic artery, and orbit. Because the organism has a proclivity for blood vessel invasion, thrombosis is a striking feature of the disease. Far advanced disease is suggested by focal deficits such as hemiparesis, seizures, or monocular blindness. In patients with the nonrhinocereb form, fever, headache, and focal neurological deficits are present in more than half the patients. In one review of 22 cases, half the patients were injection drug users and the basal ganglia was the most commonly involved site.[70]

Scedosporium apiospermum brain abscess tends to occur in immunocompromised patients or in individuals 15 to 30 days after an episode of near-drowning.[72,73] The location tends to be in the cerebrum, cerebellum, or brainstem. Clinical findings include seizures, altered consciousness, headache, meningeal irritation, focal neurological deficits, abnormal behavior, and aphasia.

DIAGNOSIS

Magnetic resonance imaging (MRI) is the diagnostic neuroimaging procedure of choice in patients with brain abscess; it is more sensitive than computed tomography (CT) and offers significant advantages in the early detection of cerebritis, more conspicuous spread of inflammation into the ventricles and subarachnoid space, and earlier detection of satellite lesions (Figs. 43-1 and 43-2).[17,108] On T1-weighted images, the abscess capsule often appears as a discrete rim that is isointense to mildly hyperintense; administration of gadolinium-diethylenetriaminepentaacetic acid helps clearly differentiate the central abscess, surrounding enhancing rim, and cerebral edema. On T2-weighted images, the zone of edema that surrounds the abscess demonstrates marked high signal intensity in which the capsule now appears as an ill-defined hypointense rim at the margin of the abscess. On diffusion-weighted images, restricted diffusion (bright signal) may be seen and may distinguish abscesses from necrotic neoplasms.[3] Proton MR spectroscopy is another diagnostic modality that may assist in differentiating between malignant tumors and cerebral abscesses; when combined with diffusion-weighted imaging, MR spectroscopy can significantly increase the diagnostic accuracy of conventional MRI.[109] In patients who cannot undergo MRI, CT with and without intravenous contrast enhancement is recommended; there is characteristically a hypodense center with peripheral uniform ring enhancement after the intravenous injection of contrast material.[110-112] Other findings include nodular areas and regions of low attenuation without enhancement, the

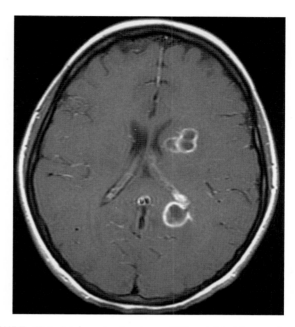

FIGURE 43-1 Axial contrast-enhanced T1-weighted image demonstrating two rim-enhancing masses of the left periventricular white matter that represent abscesses. The intraventricular enhancement is suggestive of ventriculitis. *(Courtesy of Stanley Lu, MD, Monmouth Medical Center, Long Branch, NJ.)*

latter finding seen in the early cerebritis stage before abscess formation. In later stages, contrast material no longer differentiates the lucent center, and the CT appearance is similar to that of the early cerebritis stage.

Neuroimaging may be quite sensitive in defining the findings in patients with fungal brain abscess.[65] In patients with CNS aspergillosis, there may be the finding of a cerebral infarct, which typically develops into either single or multiple abscesses; in immunocompromised patients, there may be little or no contrast enhancement on MRI.[68] Characteristic changes may be seen on MRI in patients with rhinocerebral mucormycosis, including sinus opacification, erosion of bone, and obliteration of deep fascial planes; cavernous sinus thrombosis may also be apparent. The lack of contrast enhancement in patients with mucormycosis is a poor prognostic sign because it indicates failure of host defense mechanisms to control the offending agent.

A major advance is the ability to perform stereotactic MRI- or CT-guided aspiration to facilitate microbiologic diagnosis.[3] Current techniques afford the surgeon rapid, accurate, and safe access to virtually any intracranial point, including those in deep critical areas of the CNS (i.e., the brainstem, cerebellum, and diencephalic structures adjacent to the ventricles). At the time of aspiration, specimens should be sent for Gram stain, routine aerobic and anaerobic culture, modified acid-fast smears, acid-fast smears and culture, and fungal smears and culture. In patients with histopathologic and Gram stain findings suggestive of a bacterial brain abscess but in whom cultures are negative, 16S ribosomal RNA gene sequencing and amplification may be an important adjunct,[113] although more data are needed. In patients with *Aspergillus* brain abscess, appropriate stains may reveal the presence of septate hyphae with acute-angle, dichotomous branching, whereas in patients with mucormycosis, tissue specimens may reveal irregular hyphae with right-angle branching. Histologic preparations of brain abscess specimens caused by *Scedosporium* species are indistinguishable from those caused by *Aspergillus* species. The hyphae of dematiaceous fungi may be brownish on hematoxylin-eosin staining but are not distinguishable from those of other molds.

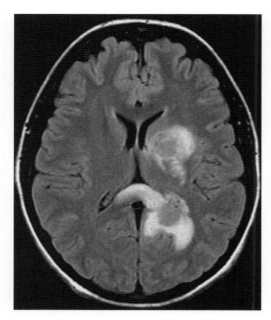

FIGURE 43-2 Axial fluid-attenuated inversion recovery (FLAIR) image in the same patient in Figure 43-1 demonstrating vasogenic edema surrounding each lesion. *(Courtesy of Stanley Lu, MD, Monmouth Medical Center, Long Branch, NJ.)*

TABLE 43-5 Predisposing Conditions and Empirical Antimicrobial Therapy in Patients with Presumed Bacterial Brain Abscess

PREDISPOSING CONDITION	ANTIMICROBIAL THERAPY
Otitis media or mastoiditis	Metronidazole + a third-generation cephalosporin*
Sinusitis (frontoethmoidal or sphenoidal)	Metronidazole + a third-generation cephalosporin* + vancomycin[†]
Dental infection	Penicillin + metronidazole
Penetrating trauma or secondary to a neurosurgical procedure	Vancomycin + a third- or fourth-generation cephalosporin[‡]
Lung abscess, empyema, or bronchiectasis	Penicillin + metronidazole + a sulfonamide[§]
Bacterial endocarditis	Vancomycin + gentamicin
Congenital heart disease	Third-generation cephalosporin*
Unknown	Vancomycin + metronidazole + a third- or fourth-generation cephalosporin[‡]

*Cefotaxime or ceftriaxone; may also use the fourth-generation cephalosporin cefepime.
[†]Add if infection caused by methicillin-resistant *Staphylococcus aureus* is suspected, pending results of in vitro susceptibility testing.
[‡]Use ceftazidime or cefepime if infection with *Pseudomonas aeruginosa* is suspected.
[§]Trimethoprim-sulfamethoxazole; include if infection caused by *Nocardia* species is suspected.

MANAGEMENT

The initial approach to management of a patient with a suspected brain abscess is a multidisciplinary one that involves a neuroradiologist, neurosurgeon, and infectious disease specialist.[114] After neuroimaging, if single or multiple ring-enhancing lesions are found, the patient should be taken to surgery and all lesions larger than 2.5 cm excised or aspirated under stereotactic guidance; for abscesses in the early cerebritis stage or if all lesions are 2.5 cm or smaller in diameter, the largest lesion should be aspirated for definitive diagnosis and identification of the organism.[115] After aspiration of abscess material and submission of specimens for special stains, histopathologic examination, and culture, empirical antimicrobial therapy should be initiated. The empirical approach to antimicrobial therapy in patients with bacterial brain abscess is based on stains of the aspirated specimen and the probable pathogenesis of infection (Table 43-5).[2] The combination of metronidazole plus a third-generation cephalosporin is commonly used[14,115,116]; in patients in whom *S. aureus* is also considered a probable pathogen, vancomycin is added pending identification of the organism and in vitro susceptibility testing.[117] In patients in whom gram-negative bacilli such as *P. aeruginosa* is likely, either ceftazidime, cefepime, or meropenem can be used. In patients with no clear predisposing factors, a reasonable regimen to administer is the combination of vancomycin, metronidazole, and a third- or fourth-generation cephalosporin. Once the infecting pathogen is isolated, antimicrobial therapy can be modified for optimal treatment (Table 43-6); recommended dosages of agents in patients with normal renal and hepatic function are shown in Table 43-7.

Bacterial Brain Abscess

The principles of antimicrobial therapy for bacterial brain abscess are to use agents that are able to penetrate the abscess cavity and have in vitro activity against the isolated pathogen.[1,2,4,8,47,118-120] Few studies have examined the penetration of specific antimicrobial agents into brain abscess pus, and some antimicrobial agents that penetrate may be inactivated in a purulent environment. It is also important to note that depending on the pathogenesis, a mixed infection may be present even though only one organism was isolated, thus necessitating the use of more than one antimicrobial agent for therapy. An important agent in the treatment of brain abscess is metronidazole, which has excellent in vitro activity against strict anaerobes, an excellent pharmacokinetic profile, and good oral absorption and penetration into brain abscess cavities[116]; metronidazole, however, must always be used in combination with an agent effective against streptococci because polymicrobial infections are common in patients with bacterial brain abscess. Vancomycin has also achieved excellent penetration into brain abscess fluid after prolonged therapy, with concentrations that are 90% of those in serum.[117] The third-generation cephalosporins are another class of antimicrobial agents that are useful, given their excellent in vitro activity against many etiologic agents that cause brain abscess and their demonstrated success in small clinical studies[121,122]; when combined with metronidazole and used with surgical therapy (see later) in one study, high doses of cefotaxime were used effectively in the treatment of bacterial brain abscess.[123] Imipenem has been used successfully for the treatment of pyogenic and nocardial brain abscess,[124,125] although it has been associated with an increased risk for seizures, thus limiting the utility of imipenem in patients with brain abscesses. Meropenem has been efficacious in isolated cases of brain abscess, including one patient with a brain abscess caused by *Enterobacter cloacae*,[126] so this agent may be especially valuable in patients with infections caused by resistant pathogens. The fluoroquinolones have also been used in isolated brain abscess cases given their good CNS penetration[127]; further studies are needed to demonstrate their efficacy, however.

TABLE 43-6 Antimicrobial Therapy for Brain Abscess Based on Isolated Pathogen

ORGANISM	STANDARD THERAPY	ALTERNATIVE THERAPIES
BACTERIA*		
Actinomyces spp.	Penicillin	Clindamycin
Bacteroides fragilis	Metronidazole	Clindamycin
Enterobacteriaceae[†]	Third- or fourth-generation cephalosporin	Aztreonam, meropenem, fluoroquinolone, trimethoprim-sulfamethoxazole
Fusobacterium spp.	Penicillin G	Metronidazole
Haemophilus spp.	Third-generation cephalosporin[‡]	Aztreonam, fluoroquinolone, trimethoprim-sulfamethoxazole
Listeria monocytogenes	Ampicillin[§] or penicillin G[§]	Trimethoprim-sulfamethoxazole
Mycobacterium tuberculosis	Isoniazid + rifampin + pyrazinamide + ethambutol	
Nocardia spp.[∥]	Trimethoprim-sulfamethoxazole	Minocycline, imipenem, meropenem, a third-generation cephalosporin, amikacin
Prevotella spp.	Metronidazole	Clindamycin, cefotaxime
Pseudomonas aeruginosa	Ceftazidime,[§] cefepime,[§] or meropenem[§]	Aztreonam,[§] fluoroquinolone[§]
Staphylococcus aureus (methicillin sensitive)	Nafcillin or oxacillin	Vancomycin
Staphylococcus aureus (methicillin resistant)	Vancomycin	Trimethoprim-sulfamethoxazole,[†¶] daptomycin[¶]
Streptococcus anginosus (*milleri*) group, other streptococci	Penicillin G	Third-generation cephalosporin,[‡] vancomycin
FUNGI		
Aspergillus spp.	Voriconazole	Amphotericin B deoxycholate, liposomal amphotericin B, amphotericin B lipid complex, itraconazole,** posaconazole**
Candida spp.	Amphotericin B deoxycholate,[††] liposomal amphotericin B,[††] amphotericin B lipid complex[††]	Fluconazole
Cryptococcus neoformans	Amphotericin B deoxycholate,[††] liposomal amphotericin B,[††] amphotericin B lipid complex[††]	Fluconazole
Mucorales	Amphotericin B deoxycholate, liposomal amphotericin B, amphotericin B lipid complex	Posaconazole**
Scedosporium spp.	Voriconazole	Itraconazole,** posaconazole**

*Depending on the pathogenesis of brain abscess formation (see Table 43-1), combination therapy should be continued for the possibility of a mixed aerobic/anaerobic infection.
[†]Use of a specific agent depends on in vitro susceptibility testing of the isolated organism.
[‡]Cefotaxime or ceftriaxone.
[§]Addition of an aminoglycoside should be considered.
[∥]Combination therapy may be required in immunocompromised patients or in those failing standard therapy (see text).
[¶]No data on the efficacy of these agents in patients with methicillin-resistant *S. aureus* brain abscess.
**Consider for use as salvage therapy in nonresponding patients or those intolerant of amphotericin B–based therapies.
[††]Addition of flucytosine should be considered.

Surgical therapy is often required for the optimal approach to patients with bacterial brain abscess.[5,16,17,49,115,128] Procedures include aspiration after bur-hole placement or complete excision after craniotomy, although no prospective trial comparing these two procedures has ever been performed. Aspiration may be performed under stereotactic neuroimaging guidance, which affords the neurosurgeon rapid, accurate, and safe access to virtually any intracranial point.[122,129-132] Stereotactic aspiration is a useful approach for abscesses located in eloquent or inaccessible regions[133]; repeat aspiration should be considered if the initial aspiration proves ineffective or partially effective. Intraoperative ultrasound guidance is also helpful for the aspiration of small abscesses and can delineate abscess pockets,[134] although endoscopic aspiration is said to be more effective. In one series of 142 patients with brain abscess,[13] there were no significant differences in outcome in those who were treated by excision, craniotomy with drainage, or stereotactic drainage, thus indicating that therapy must be individualized for each patient. Recurrence rates after stereotactic aspiration range from 0% to 24%. Complete excision by craniotomy is now infrequently performed because of the success of aspiration and closed drainage techniques, although it may be required for patients with multiloculated abscesses in whom aspiration techniques have failed, for abscesses containing gas, or for abscesses that fail to resolve. Excision is usually required for posttraumatic abscesses that contain foreign bodies or retained bone fragments to prevent recurrence, for abscesses that result from fistulous communications (e.g., secondary to trauma or congenital dermal sinuses), and for those localized to one lobe of the brain and contiguous with a primary focus.[17] It has also been suggested that excision is

TABLE 43-7 Recommended Dosages of Antimicrobial Agents in Adults with Brain Abscess and Normal Renal and Hepatic Function*

ANTIMICROBIAL AGENT	TOTAL DAILY DOSAGE (DOSING INTERVAL IN HOURS)
Amikacin[†]	15 mg/kg (8)
Amphotericin B deoxycholate[‡]	0.6-1 mg/kg (24)
Amphotericin B lipid complex	5 mg/kg (24)
Ampicillin	12 g (4)
Aztreonam	6-8 g (6-8)
Cefepime	6 g (8)
Cefotaxime	8-12 g (4-6)
Ceftazidime	6 g (8)
Ceftriaxone	4 g (12-24)
Ciprofloxacin	800-1200 mg (8-12)
Fluconazole	400-800 mg (24)
Flucytosine[§]	100 mg/kg (6)
Gentamicin[†]	5 mg/kg (8)
Isoniazid[§]	300 mg (24)
Itraconazole	400 mg (12)
Liposomal amphotericin B	5 mg/kg (24)
Meropenem	6 g (8)
Nafcillin	9-12 g (4)
Oxacillin	9-12 g (4)
Penicillin	24 million units (4)
Posaconazole[§]	800 mg (6-12)
Pyrazinamide[§]	15-30 mg/kg (24)
Rifampin[§]	600 (24)
Tobramycin[†]	5 mg/kg (8)
Trimethoprim-sulfamethoxazole[‖]	10-20 mg/kg (6-12)
Vancomycin[¶]	30-45 mg/kg (8-12)
Voriconazole[**]	8 mg/kg (12)

*Unless indicated, therapy is administered intravenously.
[†]Need to monitor peak and trough serum concentrations.
[‡]Doses up to 1.5 mg/kg per day may be required in patients with aspergillosis or mucormycosis.
[§]Oral administration.
[‖]Dosage based on trimethoprim component.
[¶]Need to monitor trough serum concentrations (maintain at 15 to 20 µg/mL).
[**]Load with 6 mg/kg every 12 hr for two doses.

the preferred method of surgical treatment of cerebellar abscesses in children,[135,136] given that worse outcomes have been seen in those treated only by aspiration. In patients with intraventricular rupture of a purulent brain abscess who have dilated ventricles and ventriculitis,[102,104] rapid evacuation and débridement of the abscess cavity via urgent craniotomy and ventricular drainage should be undertaken, along with intravenous or intrathecal administration of appropriate antimicrobial agents.

Although the optimal approach to brain abscess most often requires a combined medical and surgical approach, certain groups of patients may be treated with medical therapy alone.[106,137-139] Such groups include those with medical conditions that increase the risk associated with surgery, multiple abscesses, abscesses in a deep or dominant location, the presence of coexisting meningitis or ependymitis, early reduction of the abscess with clinical improvement after antimicrobial therapy, and abscess size

less than 3 cm. However, in one series, no abscess larger than 2.5 cm resolved without surgical therapy.[137]

The optimal duration of medical treatment of bacterial brain abscess is unclear but has traditionally been 6 to 8 weeks of high-dose intravenous antimicrobial therapy,[1,2,17,138] which is often followed by oral antimicrobial therapy for 2 to 3 months if appropriate agents are available; however, the efficacy and necessity for additional oral antimicrobial therapy have not been established. In one study, the authors thought that a combination of surgical aspiration or removal of all abscesses larger than 2.5 cm in diameter, 6 weeks or more of antimicrobial therapy, and weekly neuroimaging to document abscess resolution should lead to cure rates of greater than 90%.[140] Courses of 3 to 4 weeks of antimicrobial therapy may be adequate for patients who have undergone surgical excision of the brain abscess, whereas longer courses (up to 12 weeks with parenteral agents) may be required in patients treated with antimicrobial therapy alone. The Infection in Neurosurgery Working Party of the British Society for Antimicrobial Therapy recommends that intravenous therapy be used for 1 to 2 weeks for bacterial brain abscess[141]; depending on the clinical response, change to an oral regimen can be considered. Although this approach has been used in several series,[14,142,143] it cannot be considered standard therapy in most patients with bacterial brain abscess. Repeat neuroimaging studies performed biweekly for up to 3 months after completion of therapy has been suggested to monitor for reexpansion of the abscess or failure of resolution.[17,114]

Nocardial Brain Abscess

In patients with *Nocardia* brain abscess, a sulfonamide, with or without trimethoprim, is recommended.[54,144-146] Alternative agents with in vitro activity against *Nocardia* include minocycline, imipenem, amikacin, third-generation cephalosporins, and linezolid,[147-150] although in vitro activity may not always correlate with clinical efficacy. In immunocompromised patients or those in whom therapy fails, combination treatment with regimens containing a third-generation cephalosporin or imipenem, along with a sulfonamide or amikacin, should be considered.[1,151-155] In patients with brain abscess caused by *Nocardia farcinica*, a species that may be highly resistant to various antimicrobial agents, successful treatment has included moxifloxacin alone or combined with another agent.[156-158]

Craniotomy with total excision is difficult in patients with *Nocardia* brain abscess because these abscesses are often multiloculated.[107] In one review of 11 patients with nocardial brain abscess, aspiration alone was effective in 9 patients.[159] In contrast, in another series of 3 patients, cure was achieved only after neurosurgical enucleation,[160] thus suggesting that an aggressive surgical approach should be used. The duration of therapy in patients with nocardial brain abscess is usually 3 to 12 months,[54,161] but it should probably be continued up to 1 year in those who are immunocompromised. Careful follow-up is necessary to monitor for relapse.

Fungal Brain Abscess

Patients with fungal brain abscess, especially those who are immunocompromised, have a high mortality rate despite combined medical and surgical therapy. In patients with candidal brain abscess, recommended therapy is an amphotericin B preparation plus 5-flucytosine[65]; the efficacy of fluconazole has not been evaluated, but this agent has been used successfully in combination therapy in isolated case reports.[162]

The therapy of choice for *Aspergillus* brain abscess is voriconazole.[163] In one review that included 19 patients with aspergillosis and cerebral disease, 3 had a partial response to treatment.[164] In more recent series, however, the response rate was approximately

35%.[68,163] Alternative agents include an amphotericin B preparation, posaconazole, and itraconazole.[165-167] Although itraconazole has in vitro activity against *Aspergillus* species and high-dose therapy has resulted in success in some patients, its unreliable absorption and the modest reported experience in treatment of patients with *Aspergillus* brain abscess make use of itraconazole more promising as an extension of successful treatment rather than as primary therapy. One patient with an *Aspergillus* brain abscess was successfully treated with amphotericin B, itraconazole, and interferon gamma, with amphotericin B discontinued after the first 3 weeks of therapy.[167] Combination therapies that have shown efficacy are voriconazole in conjunction with either caspofungin or amphotericin B.[168-170] Excisional surgery or drainage is a key factor in the successful management of CNS aspergillosis.[68,163,171]

Patients with CNS mucormycosis should be treated with amphotericin B deoxycholate or a lipid formulation of amphotericin B[65,172,173]; correction of the underlying metabolic derangements and aggressive surgical débridement are also critical to successful therapy. Because the etiologic agents of mucormycosis invade blood vessels, tissue infarction occurs and impairs the delivery of antifungal agents to the site of infection; this often leaves surgery as the only modality that may effectively eliminate the infecting microorganism. In patients not responding to or intolerant of an amphotericin B formulation, posaconazole can be used as salvage therapy.[174] In addition to surgery, hyperbaric oxygen therapy has been reported to be a useful adjunct,[175,176] although no randomized, prospective studies have been performed to assess its efficacy.

Surgery is the cornerstone of therapy for brain abscesses caused by *Scedosporium* species.[72] Given the inherent resistance of this organism to amphotericin B, voriconazole is the agent of choice.[177] In one review that included 21 patients with CNS disease caused by *Scedosporium*, 43% had a therapeutic response.[178] Combination therapy with voriconazole and terbinafine was also successful in 1 patient with chronic granulomatous disease and a brain abscess caused by *Scedosporium prolificans*.[179] One patient with acute lymphoblastic lymphoma and multiple *S. apiospermum* brain abscesses who did not respond to itraconazole, amphotericin B, and ketoconazole combined with neurosurgical drainage was successfully treated with posaconazole.[180]

Adjunctive Therapy

Therapy with corticosteroids should be initiated in brain abscess patients who have associated edema and mass effect, progressive neurological deterioration, or impending cerebral herniation.[2,3,17,115] Although use of corticosteroids has not been studied in well-controlled randomized trials and they may lead to a reduction in host defense mechanisms and decrease penetration of some antimicrobial agents into the brain abscess cavity, they may result in improvement of neurological symptoms and signs. High-dose corticosteroid therapy (e.g., dexamethasone, 10 mg every 6 hours) is generally administered initially and then tapered once the patient has stabilized. The use of prolonged courses of corticosteroids is discouraged. These agents may also decrease contrast enhancement of the abscess capsule in the early stages of infection, thereby being a false indicator of radiologic improvement.[3]

OUTCOME

Mortality rates in patients with brain abscess in the pre-antibiotic era and into the 1970s were unacceptably high and ranged from 30% to 80%.[2,4,8] Since the 1970s, case fatality rates have ranged from 0% to 24%, results attributable to the availability of more effective antimicrobial therapy and the availability of neuroimaging (i.e., CT and MRI), which allows early diagnosis and monitoring of response to therapy.[181] In recent series, mortality rates have ranged from 8% to 25%.[9-14,115] Factors associated with a poor prognosis include a low Glasgow Coma Scale score and the presence of certain underlying diseases and other comorbid conditions. A more favorable outcome was noted in one study of 142 patients when the Glasgow Coma Scale score was higher than 12 and the patients had no evidence of sepsis.[12] One important complication that has been associated with poor outcome is intraventricular rupture of the abscess, for which mortality rates have ranged from 27% to 85%.[102] In patients who survive the episode of brain abscess, the incidence of neurological sequelae has ranged from 20% to 70%; the prognosis is determined by the rapidity of progression and the patient's mental status on initial evaluation.[182] Long-term sequelae include hemiparesis, persistent visual field defects, cognitive dysfunction, learning disorders, hydrocephalus, and seizures[2,3,5]; the latter is a long-term risk in approximately 30% to 50% of patients with brain abscesses.

CRANIAL SUBDURAL EMPYEMA AND EPIDURAL ABSCESS

Epidemiology and Etiology

Cranial subdural empyema refers to a collection of pus between the space of the dura and arachnoid, and it accounts for 15% to 20% of all intracranial infections. The most common predisposing conditions are otorhinologic infections, especially of the paranasal sinuses, which are affected in 40% to 80% of patients.[183-189] The mastoid and middle ear are affected in 10% to 20% of patients, who are usually living in geographic locales where patients with otitis media are not properly treated. Other predisposing conditions are skull trauma, neurosurgical procedures, and infection of a preexisting subdural hematoma.[190] In one 20-year review of cases of subdural empyema in children,[191] it developed in approximately 20% after head trauma or neurosurgery. The infection is metastatic in 5% of cases, usually from a pulmonary source. Meningitis is an important predisposing condition in infants with cranial subdural empyema, which occurs in 2% to 10% of those with bacterial meningitis.[187]

The etiologic agents in patients with cranial subdural empyema are usually microbial flora from those with chronic sinusitis, and such agents include aerobic streptococci (25% to 45%), staphylococci (10% to 15%), aerobic gram-negative bacilli (3% to 10%), and anaerobic streptococci and other anaerobes (33% to 100% in some series in which careful culturing for anaerobes was performed).[185-188,192,193] If the predisposing condition is postoperative or posttraumatic, the usual pathogens are staphylococci and aerobic gram-negative bacilli. *Propionibacterium acnes* may be isolated from patients after trauma, neurosurgical procedures, or dural allografts.[194-196] Operative cultures are reported to be negative in 7% to 53% of patients.[189]

Cranial epidural abscess refers to a localized collection of pus between the dura mater and overlying skull; because the abscess can cross the cranial dura along emissary veins, an accompanying subdural empyema may also be present.[183,197] Therefore, the pathogenesis and bacterial etiology are usually identical to that described in patients with cranial subdural empyema (see earlier).

Clinical Findings

The clinical manifestation of patients with cranial subdural empyema may be rapidly progressive, with symptoms and signs related to increased intracranial pressure, meningeal irritation, or focal cortical inflammation.[183-187,189,198] Most patients have fever and headache; vomiting is common as intracranial pressure increases. Altered mental status can occur and progress rapidly to obtundation and coma if the infection is not treated. Focal neurological signs (e.g., hemiparesis and hemiplegia, ocular palsies, dysphasia, homonymous hemianopia, dilated pupils, and cerebellar signs) appear in 24 to 48 hours and progress rapidly, with eventual involvement of the entire cerebral hemispheres, although in one series no focal signs were observed in 41% of 699 patients.[187] Seizures occur in 25% to 80% of patients.[189] Signs of meningeal irritation are seen in about 80% of patients. In untreated patients, there is rapid neurological deterioration with signs of increased intracranial pressure and cerebral herniation. However, these clinical findings may not be seen in patients in whom subdural empyema develops after cranial surgery or trauma, in those who have previously received antimicrobial therapy, in patients with infected subdural hematomas, or in those with metastatic infection to the subdural space.

The clinical manifestation of cranial epidural abscess may be insidious and is usually overshadowed by the primary focus of infection (whether sinusitis or otitis media).[183,197] The findings are generally insidious because the dura is closely opposed to the inner surface of the cranium such that the abscess usually enlarges too slowly to produce a sudden onset of major neurological deficits, as is seen in patients with cranial subdural empyema (see earlier), unless there is deeper intracranial extension. The usual complaints are fever and headache, but the patient may not appear acutely ill, thereby leading to a delay in diagnosis. Eventually, however, focal neurological signs and seizures may develop, and as the abscess enlarges, papilledema and signs of increased intracranial pressure may develop in untreated patients. If the location of the epidural abscess is near the petrous bone, Gradenigo's syndrome may develop, a condition characterized by the involvement of cranial nerves V and VI and manifested clinically as unilateral facial pain and weakness of the lateral rectus muscle.

Diagnosis

The diagnosis of cranial subdural empyema should be suspected in any patient with meningeal signs and a focal neurological deficit.[183-187] MRI is the diagnostic imaging procedure of choice and usually demonstrates a crescentic or elliptical area of hypointensity (on T1 images) below the cranial vault or adjacent to the falx cerebri.[189,198,199] Depending on the extent of disease, there may also be an associated mass effect with displacement of midline structures. MRI is superior to CT because it provides better clarity of morphologic detail and may detect the presence of a subdural empyema that is not seen on CT; it is particularly helpful in detecting a subdural empyema at the base of the brain, along the falx cerebri, or in the posterior fossa.

MRI is also the diagnostic imaging procedure of choice in patients with cranial epidural abscess; it usually demonstrates a superficial, circumscribed area of diminished intensity with pachymeningeal enhancement.[197] CT is used for imaging bone or if MRI is not available, although MRI is superior in identification and delineation of the collection and is able to differentiate epidural abscesses from sterile effusions or hematomas that may be present in patients who have undergone cranial surgery or suffered head trauma.

Management

Cranial subdural empyema is a surgical emergency because antimicrobial therapy alone does not reliably sterilize the empyema. The goals of surgical therapy are to achieve adequate decompression of the brain and to evacuate the empyema completely.[183,198,200,201] The optimal surgical approach is controversial. When comparing craniotomy drainage with drainage after placement of bur holes, some studies have demonstrated a lower mortality rate in patients who have undergone craniotomy, although it may be that the patients who underwent drainage via bur-hole

placement were more ill and had a greater surgical risk. If bur-hole drainage is performed, multiple bur holes may be required to allow extensive irrigation. For patients undergoing craniotomy, wide exposure is needed to permit surgical exploration of all areas where empyema is suspected. In a large series of 699 patients in which the efficacy of drainage after CT-guided bur holes was compared with craniectomy or craniotomy drainage,[202] mortality rates were higher in patients treated by only drainage via bur holes (23.3%) than in those who underwent craniectomy (11.5%) or craniotomy (8.4%). Patients who underwent drainage via bur holes or craniectomy required more frequent operations to drain recurrent or remaining pus and exhibited higher mortality rates and worse outcomes. Drainage via bur holes or craniectomy is therefore recommended only for patients in septic shock, those with localized parafalcine collections, and children with subdural empyema secondary to meningitis because there is usually no brain swelling and the pus is thin. Despite the surgical approach, however, repeat surgery was required in half the patients treated by bur-hole drainage and a fifth of those initially treated by craniotomy.[203]

Regardless of the method of drainage, once purulent material is aspirated, initial antimicrobial therapy should be based on the results of Gram staining and the pathogenesis of the infection.[189,198] If *S. aureus* is suspected, vancomycin should be initiated but changed to nafcillin if the organism is found to be susceptible to methicillin. For suspected anaerobes, metronidazole is recommended. If aerobic gram-negative bacilli are suspected, empirical therapy with either ceftazidime, cefepime, or meropenem can be used. Cultures (both aerobic and anaerobic) are needed to guide the use of specific antimicrobial therapy. Depending on the clinical response, antimicrobial therapy should be continued for 3 to 4 weeks after drainage; longer periods of therapy (intravenous or oral) may be needed if the patient has accompanying osteomyelitis. Antimicrobial therapy alone can be considered for patients with cranial subdural empyema who have minimal or no impairment of consciousness, no major neurological deficit, limited extension of the empyema with no midline shift, and early improvement with antimicrobial therapy,[186,200] although these patients need careful clinical and neuroimaging monitoring and may require longer courses of antimicrobial therapy.

Management of cranial epidural abscess also requires a combined medical and surgical approach.[183,197,200,204] Empirical antimicrobial therapy is similar to that for cranial subdural empyema. For surgical drainage, craniotomy or craniectomy is generally preferred over bur-hole placement or aspiration of purulent material through the scalp. Antimicrobial therapy is usually continued for 3 to 6 weeks or longer (i.e., 6 to 8 weeks) after drainage if the patient also has underlying osteomyelitis.

SUGGESTED READINGS

Cavusoglu H, Kaya RA, Turkmenoglu ON, et al. Brain abscess: analysis of results in a series of 51 patients with a combined surgical and medical approach during an 11-year period. *Neurosurg Focus.* 2008;24(6):E9.

Dupuis-Girod S, Giraud S, Decullier E, et al. Hemorrhagic hereditary telangiectasia (Rendu-Osler disease) and infectious diseases: an underestimated association. *Clin Infect Dis.* 2007;44:841-845.

Eckburg PB, Montoya JG, Vosti KL. Brain abscess due to *Listeria monocytogenes*: five cases and a review of the literature. *Medicine (Baltimore).* 2001;80:223-235.

Erdogan E, Cansever T. Pyogenic brain abscess. *Neurosurg Focus.* 2008;24(6):E2.

Hagensee ME, Bauwens JE, Kjos B, et al. Brain abscess following marrow transplantation: experience at the Fred Hutchinson Cancer Center, 1984-1992. *Clin Infect Dis.* 1994;19:402-408.

Hakan T. Management of bacterial brain abscesses. *Neurosurg Focus.* 2008;24(6):E4.

Infection in Neurosurgery Working Party of the British Society for Antimicrobial Chemotherapy. The rational use of antibiotics in the treatment of brain abscess. *Br J Neurosurg.* 2000;14:525-530.

Jansson AK, Enbland P, Sjolin J. Efficacy and safety of cefotaxime in combination with metronidazole for empirical treatment of brain abscess in clinical practice: a retrospective study of 66 consecutive cases. *Eur J Clin Microbiol Infect Dis.* 2004;23:7-14.

Kocherry XG, Hegde T, Sastry KVR, et al. Efficacy of stereotactic aspiration in deep-seated and eloquent-region intracranial pyogenic abscesses. *Neurosurg Focus.* 2008;24(6):E13.

Lee GYF, Daniel RT, Brophy BP, et al. Surgical treatment of nocardial brain abscesses. *Neurosurgery.* 2002;51:668-672.

Lee TH, Chang WN, Thung-Ming S, et al. Clinical features and predictive factors of intraventricular rupture in patients who have bacterial brain abscess. *J Neurol Neurosurg Psychiatry.* 2007;78:303-309.

Lu CH, Chang WN, Lin YC, et al. Bacterial brain abscess: microbiological features, epidemiological trends and therapeutic outcomes. *Q J Med.* 2002;95:501-509.

Mamelak AN, Mampalam TJ, Obana WG, et al. Improved management of multiple brain abscesses: a combined surgical and medical approach. *Neurosurgery.* 1995;36:76-86.

Mampalam TJ, Rosenblum ML. Trends in the management of bacterial brain abscesses: a review of 102 cases over 17 years. *Neurosurgery.* 1988;23:451-458.

Mathisen GE, Johnson JP. Brain abscess. *Clin Infect Dis.* 1997;25:763-781.

McClelland S III, Hall WA. Postoperative central nervous system infection: incidence and associated factors in 2111 neurosurgical procedures. *Clin Infect Dis.* 2007;45:55-59.

Nathoo N, Nadvi SS, Gouws E, et al. Craniotomy improves outcomes for cranial subdural empyemas: computed tomography–era experience with 699 patients. *Neurosurgery.* 2001;49:872-878.

Nathoo N, Nadvi SS, van Dellen JR, et al. Intracranial subdural empyemas in the era of computed tomography: a review of 699 cases. *Neurosurgery.* 1999;44:529-535.

Osborn MK, Steinberg JP. Subdural empyema and other suppurative complications of paranasal sinusitis. *Lancet Infect Dis.* 2007;7:62-67.

Pandey P, Umesh S, Bhat D, et al. Cerebellar abscesses in children: excision or aspiration? *J Neurosurg Pediatr.* 2008;1:31-34.

Peleg AY, Husain S, Qureshi ZA. Risk factors, clinical characteristics, and outcome of *Nocardia* infection in organ transplant recipients: a matched case-control study. *Clin Infect Dis.* 2007;44:1307-1314.

Seydoux C, Francioli P. Bacterial brain abscess: factors influencing mortality and sequelae. *Clin Infect Dis.* 1992;15:394-401.

Stephanov S. Surgical treatment of brain abscess. *Neurosurgery.* 1988;22:724-730.

Tseng JH, Steng MY. Brain abscess in 142 patients: factors influencing outcome and mortality. *Surg Neurol.* 2006;65:557-562.

Walsh TJ, Anaissie EJ, Denning DW, et al. Treatment of aspergillosis: clinical practice guidelines of the Infectious Diseases Society of America. *Clin Infect Dis.* 2008;46:327-360.

Full references can be found on Expert Consult @ www.expertconsult.com

CHAPTER 44

Meningitis and Encephalitis

Ian E. McCutcheon

Meningitis, defined as inflammation of the leptomeninges, can be caused by almost any microbial pathogen that afflicts humans. However, some pathogens are much more frequently seen than others. The typical symptoms of headache and fever are each shared by a host of other diseases, and thus detecting meningitis requires both a degree of clinical wisdom and a willingness to perform the ultimate diagnostic test—lumbar puncture—when appropriate. Even in the era of advanced antibiotics, meningitis remains a serious disease that continues to impose both morbidity and mortality on neurosurgical patients. Because operations on the central nervous system (CNS) afford the opportunity for bacterial ingress whenever the cerebrospinal fluid (CSF) spaces are breached, meningitis is a potential complication with many neurosurgical procedures. It may also accompany disease processes that prompt neurosurgical consideration before the performance of any surgery. In addition, noninfectious forms of meningitis can produce clinical syndromes that overlap those of infectious meningitis and will be considered in this chapter, as will encephalitis, which represents inflammation of the brain and whose pathogens are quite different from those usually seen in meningitis. Overlap between the two (called *meningoencephalitis*) is also possible and will be addressed as well.

Ventriculitis is focal or diffuse inflammation of the ependymal lining of the cerebral ventricular system. It has no specific clinical syndrome to distinguish it from meningitis, and a diffuse encephalitis usually reaches the ependyma. Infection within the subarachnoid space can find its way to the ventricles, but this requires retrograde movement of bacteria against CSF flow. Thus, the best place to sample CSF for maximal diagnostic yield is the lumbar subarachnoid space. The only circumstance in which ventriculitis can be considered in isolation is a "chemical ventriculitis" caused by inflammation induced by blood released during or after a neurosurgical operation that breaches the ventricular wall.

BACTERIAL MENINGITIS

Pathophysiology

Pyogenic infections of the meninges originate either by hematogenous spread of bacteria or infected thrombi or by direct extension from bacterially colonized cranial structures adjacent to the meninges. Typical sources of direct extension include surgical or traumatic breaches of the paranasal sinuses or mastoid air cells, osteomyelitic foci within the skull, or congenital sinus tracts.[1] Iatrogenic infection via an infected shunt, intraoperative contamination, or even a lumbar puncture needle is also possible. In animal models of bacteremia, placement of a needle into the subarachnoid space causes clustering of bacteria at the site of injury. It is tempting to extend this by analogy to humans, although there is no proof that this occurs in systemic human bacterial infection.

Cerebral tissue itself is relatively resistant to infection, and direct injection of virulent bacteria into the brains of animals seldom yields abscess formation. Some coincident infarction of brain tissue either by venous or arterial occlusion or by direct injury is the usual (and possibly requisite) antecedent event. Bacteria in the CSF, however, attract a robust inflammatory response and require no such additional injury. Parameningeal foci of infection, whether lodged in meningeal or superficial cerebral vessels or in adjacent sinus cavities or bone, simply require a physical breach in the arachnoid membrane to initiate bacterial colonization of CSF and result in frank meningitis. When septic material embolizes from an infected lung or congenital heart lesion or when it extends directly from the ears or sinuses, more than one type of bacterium can be found in the CSF. By contrast, hematogenous infections usually permit only one bacterial type to gain entry into the subarachnoid space. Bacterial pathogens differ by age of the patient (Table 44-1), and therapy initiated before identification of the pathogen is generally chosen to cover the typical pathogens found within the age group of the patient. Once bacteria enter the CSF space, they initiate a cascade of events within that space that extends throughout its reach. Thus, meningitis starting in the spine can easily cause cranial nerve dysfunction, and the converse is equally true. CSF within the ventricles is not spared because bacteria may enter it (and cause ventriculitis) either directly from infective emboli to the choroid plexus or by reflux of bacteria through the foramina of Magendie and Luschka.

The first effect of bacteria within the CSF is hyperemia of the meningeal vessels, followed rapidly by migration of neutrophils into the subarachnoid space. The exudates increase quickly and extend to the sheaths of cranial and spinal nerves and into the perivascular spaces of the cortex. At first, neutrophils predominate, but over the next few days lymphocytes and histiocytes show a gradual increase. Exudation of fibrinogen and other proteins from blood continues while the meningitis is active and leads to the typical increase in CSF protein seen in spinal taps performed during the acute phase of bacterial meningitis. Toward the end of the second week plasma cells appear, and thereafter they increase as well. On a microscopic level, the exudate disperses into two layers, with the outer one immediately beneath the arachnoid consisting of neutrophils and fibrin and the inner one adjacent to the pia consisting of lymphocytes, macrophages, and plasma cells. Eventually, the exudate organizes and arachnoid fibrosis ensues with loculation of small pockets of cellular exudate that may allow recrudescence of the meningitis if antibiotic treatment is not prolonged.

During resolution of meningitis, the inflammatory cells disappear in the same order in which they came. The last to go are lymphocytes, macrophages, and plasma cells, which disappear more slowly than neutrophils and may remain for several months in decreasing numbers. Infections controlled early may leave no trace on arachnoid structure, whereas those treated after the infection has become solidly established may leave behind a thickened, cloudy, and adherent arachnoid membrane. The presence of this cellular immune reaction within the CSF also leads to changes in the small blood vessels on the cortical surface. Within 2 to 3 days of the onset of infection, endothelial swelling

TABLE 44-1 Bacterial Pathogens Causing Meningitis

AGE	TYPICAL PATHOGENS
Neonates (0 to 4 wk)	*Escherichia coli*
	Listeria monocytogenes
	Streptococcus (group B)
Infants (4-12 wk)	*Escherichia coli*
	Haemophilus influenzae
	Listeria monocytogenes
	Streptococcus (group B)
	Streptococcus pneumoniae
Children (3 mo to 18 yr)	*Haemophilus influenzae*
	Neisseria meningitidis
	Streptococcus pneumoniae
Adults (18-60 yr)	*Neisseria meningitidis*
	Streptococcus pneumoniae
Elderly adults (>60 yr)	Gram-negative bacilli
	Haemophilus influenzae
	Listeria monocytogenes
	Streptococcus pneumoniae

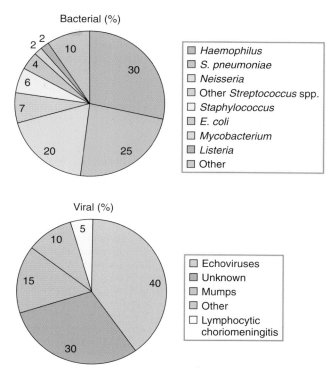

CAUSES OF ACUTE MENINGITIS
(WORLDWIDE, ALL AGES)

Bacterial (%)

- Haemophilus
- S. pneumoniae
- Neisseria
- Other Streptococcus spp.
- Staphylococcus
- E. coli
- Mycobacterium
- Listeria
- Other

Viral (%)

- Echoviruses
- Unknown
- Mumps
- Other
- Lymphocytic choriomeningitis

FIGURE 44-1 Causes of acute meningitis worldwide and for all ages combined.

occurs and compromises the diameter of the vascular lumen, and the adventitia is infiltrated by neutrophils. Occasionally, necrosis of the arterial wall develops and may result in subarachnoid bleeding. The vessels ultimately demonstrate subintimal fibrosis, which is seen with any long-standing infection of the meninges but most typically with tuberculous meningitis. A similar process occurs in the veins, although the subintimal cellular infiltration is not seen; rather, the immune cells tend to infiltrate the entire wall diffusely. This can lead to necrosis of the wall, mural thrombus formation, and infectious thrombophlebitis by the end of the second week of infection. Ultimately, such vascular changes can culminate in ischemia and stroke.

Dysfunction of cranial and spinal nerves occurs as the purulent exudate surrounds the nerves and then, over a period of several days, infiltrates the perineurial sheaths. The endoneurium is typically not infiltrated, and the nerve fibers themselves are not usually damaged. Disruption of nerve function is also promoted by the vascular changes alluded to earlier should they affect the vasa nervorum and cause ischemia within the nerves.

Infection does not generally spread outward from the subarachnoid space to the subdural space. Occasionally, however, a subdural effusion is produced, more often in infants than in adults. Because they tend to resolve spontaneously as the infection fades with medical therapy, these effusions are tapped only if they produce a significant mass effect on adjacent brain tissue.[2]

In the spine, fibrinopurulent exudate can accumulate around the spinal cord and roots of the cauda equina in sufficient quantity to block the spinal subarachnoid space (and cause chronic root pain). Blockage of the foramina of Magendie and Luschka or the basal cisterns can lead to hydrocephalus through interference with the normal circulatory pattern of CSF. Here, too, treatment of the hydrocephalus is generally deferred unless it is significant enough to produce symptomatic intracranial hypertension and endanger neurological function; it is usually mild in degree and will settle as the infection and inflammation subside and CSF flow is reestablished.

The effects of meningitis on the brain itself are minimal in the early stages, but an increase in cortical microglia and astrocyte numbers occurs after several days because of either diffusion of bacterial toxins from the meninges or disturbances in blood flow (but not the presence of bacteria within the brain parenchyma). The encephalopathy that ensues, as well as any associ-

ated seizures, should be considered indirect effects of the infection and probably associated with cerebral edema or changes in local vascular permeability and flow. In like fashion, bacteria within the ventricles initially show little effect on the ependyma and subependymal zone, but analogous changes are seen at later stages. The concomitant hydrocephalus, with resulting disruption of ependymal integrity, probably promotes subependymal proliferation of microglia and astrocytes.

Types of Bacterial Meningitis

The three most common bacteria causing meningitis are *Haemophilus influenzae*, *Neisseria meningitidis*, and *Streptococcus pneumoniae*, which together account for 75% of cases (Fig. 44-1). Less frequently seen are *Staphylococcus aureus*, *Staphylococcus epidermidis*, and *Streptococcus* group A, which usually occur after head trauma or neurosurgical procedures or with a brain or epidural abscess; *Streptococcus* group B, which is seen in newborns; and the Enterobacteriaceae (*Klebsiella*, *Proteus*, and *Pseudomonas* spp.), which occur after lumbar puncture or shunt placement.

Pneumococcal, *Haemophilus*, and meningococcal meningitides have a seasonal pattern, with the majority of cases occurring in fall, winter, and spring and with a male preponderance. Because of the overuse of antibiotics prevalent in medicine today, drug-resistant strains occur increasingly, and it is important to know the patterns of drug resistance in general and the resistance of the bacterium in question in particular to form an effective therapeutic plan. Meningococcal meningitis occurs most often in children and adolescents but can be seen in adulthood until the age of 50, after which it sharply declines in incidence.[3,4] Pneumococcal meningitis and *Haemophilus* meningitis both predominate in the very young and in elderly adults.

These three most common meningeal pathogens colonize the nasopharynx in a significant percentage of the general population and need not be eradicated if found on routine nasal culture. Antecedent viral infection of the upper respiratory tract may predispose the patient to hematogenous spread to the meninges, but this is by no means certain. Certainly, these three microorganisms have a tropism for the meninges not shared by other bacteria.

Clinical Features

Adults and Older Children

Early manifestations of bacterial meningitis include fever, headache (typically severe), generalized seizures, and impaired sensorium. Neck stiffness on flexion is common but may be abrogated in a patient already taking steroids. The older Kernig sign (inability to extend the legs completely) and Brudzinski sign (hip and knee flexion in response to neck flexion) are sometimes seen but are less reliable. Some patients even have abdominal pain because of initial onset of infection in the spine with effect on the thoracolumbar spinal roots. These symptoms are seen in any type of bacterial meningitis, but certain features suggest one or another type.[5] During epidemics of meningitis, meningococcus should be suspected if evolution is rapid, if a petechial rash or ecchymosis accompanies the onset of symptoms, or when circulatory collapse occurs. The rash in particular should drive immediate therapy for *N. meningitidis* because in such cases time is critical and death can ensue within 2 days. In patients with preexisting infection of the lungs, sinuses, or ears or in those who have disorders of the heart valves, pneumococcus should be suspected. It is also more common in alcoholics and in patients who have dermal sinus tracts, sickle cell anemia, basal skull fracture, or previous splenectomy. The most common scenario for *Haemophilus* meningitis is after an upper respiratory or ear infection in a child.

In a young patient or in a comatose adult, signs of meningeal irritation may be absent. The use of steroids may also lessen the intensity of such stiffness and provide symptomatic relief to patients.

Infants

Infants have a greater incidence of meningitis than adults do because of their less developed immune system. The signs are nonspecific and shared by many illnesses and include fever, irritability, drowsiness, vomiting, seizures, and a bulging fontanelle. Neck stiffness can occur but usually develops late in the course of the illness. The key to successful treatment is early diagnosis, and a key to early diagnosis is maintenance of a high index of suspicion and a low threshold for lumbar puncture. Neonatal meningitis is more common in males than females by a 3 : 1 ratio. Infants in whom meningitis develops early are more likely to have

been born prematurely or after prolonged labor. One significant factor promoting neonatal meningitis is infection of the mother, often a urinary tract infection sharing the same bacterium as the meningitis.

Clinical Testing

Lumbar puncture is the key test in diagnosing meningitis.[6] This test should be done *before* instituting antibiotic therapy, and a positive diagnostic yield is increased by multiple taps. Those with bleeding disorders should, if possible, have hematologic correction of their coagulopathy before lumbar puncture. Those with increased intracranial pressure should undergo computed tomography (CT) or magnetic resonance imaging (MRI) of the head before lumbar puncture. Some will have hydrocephalus sufficient to require a ventriculostomy, and CSF can be acquired by that route rather than by a redundant lumbar puncture. In general, the fear of herniation when a spinal tap is performed in the presence of an intracranial mass lesion is much overstated. It is actually very unusual for transtonsillar herniation to occur when small amounts of CSF are withdrawn from the lumbar cistern. However, it is wise to use a small (25-gauge) needle in preference to a large-bore needle when intracranial pressure is elevated because this will permit more gradual removal of CSF and may further lessen the chance of such herniation.

The CSF findings in the various types of meningitis are shown in Table 44-2. Spinal fluid pressure is typically elevated, and a normal pressure in a patient strongly suggests that meningitis is not present. Pleocytosis is the most diagnostic finding, with the typical white blood cell count in CSF ranging from 1000 to 10,000 cells/mm³. A very high count (>50,000) should raise the possibility of a bacterial abscess that has ruptured into the ventricles. Such patients will be very ill and may require intraventricular as well as intravenous antibiotics. In bacterial (as opposed to viral or fungal) meningitis, a neutrophilic predominance is seen (85% to 95% of the total cell population), but later in the course of the illness the percentage of mononuclear cells rises.

Protein levels are high in 90% of patients, in the range of 100 to 500 mg/dL. Glucose levels fall to a level of less than 40 mg/dL. In hyperglycemic patients, the diagnostic finding is a drop in glucose to less than 40% of the blood glucose level measured simultaneously. Gram stain of spinal fluid sediment may show the bacterium in patients who have not previously been treated with antibiotics. It is invariably negative in those who have been so treated. CSF samples for culture are always best obtained before treatment because they too will be affected by the presence of previously administered circulating antibiotic. In untreated cases, cultures should be expected to be positive in 20% to 90% of patients. In culture-negative patients, counterimmunoelectrophoresis may help detect bacterial antigens that linger after the bacteria themselves have disappeared. Other adjunctive methods include radioimmunoassay and enzyme-linked immunosorbent assay (ELISA), also done to detect bacterial antigens,

TABLE 44-2 Cerebrospinal Fluid Findings in the Various Types of Meningitis

	CSF PRESSURE	WBC COUNT (cells/mm³)	DIRECTION OF DIFFERENTIAL SHIFT	PROTEIN (mg/dL)	GLUCOSE (mg/dL)
Normal (no meningitis)	Normal	0-5	Mononuclear cells	15-45	45-80
Bacterial meningitis	Elevated	500-100,000	Neutrophils	Elevated	Low
Viral meningitis	Elevated	5-500	Mononuclear cells	15-100	Normal
Tuberculous meningitis	Normal to elevated	50-500	Mononuclear cells	Elevated	Low
Fungal meningitis	Elevated	25-500	Lymphocytes	Elevated	Low

CSF, cerebrospinal fluid; WBC, white blood cell.

and polymerase chain reaction (PCR) amplification of nucleic acid sequences specific for bacterial species.[7]

Additional measurements may include lactate dehydrogenase (LDH) in CSF, which consistently rises in patients with bacterial meningitis. LDH isozymes 4 and 5 contribute the most to this rise. In patients who sustain brain injury from meningitis, LDH isozymes 1 and 2 rise sharply; they are only slightly elevated in those without such injury and thus can be used to predict neurological outcome. Lactic acid may also be measured because it is consistently elevated in meningitis caused by bacteria or fungi but remains normal in viral meningitis. Levels of lactic acid in CSF higher than 35 mg/dL are considered elevated.

Blood cultures should always be done because they are positive in 40% to 70% of patients with *Haemophilus*, meningococcal, and pneumococcal meningitis. If CSF cultures are negative, blood cultures may provide the only clue to the bacterial etiology. Cultures of the nasopharynx are occasionally helpful in that the absence of *Haemophilus* or meningococcus in a patient's nose makes it unlikely that the meningitis is caused by either of these bacteria.

Radiologic Studies

Radiographs of chest, skull, and sinuses are useful in any patient suspected of having bacterial meningitis without a known source. CT of the skull base may also be useful in showing sinus infection or mastoiditis. Both CT and MRI will allow the diagnosis of hydrocephalus, infarction, brain abscess, or subdural empyema (or effusion), and such a scan should be performed at some point during the hospital stay of any patient being treated for bacterial meningitis.

Postcraniotomy Meningitis

The risk of CSF contamination leading to meningitis begins during surgery, but seeding of bacteria can occur after surgery in patients with either controlled CSF drainage or uncontrolled CSF leakage. The most common organisms cultured in patients after craniotomy have been *S. aureus* and *S. epidermidis*, with gram-negative organisms also being common.[8,9] Patients have fever, neck stiffness, and altered levels of consciousness, as do those with standard meningitis. However, those in whom meningitis develops after surgery have an increased risk for stroke secondary to venous infarction, an event precipitated by septic thrombophlebitis and encouraged by the dehydration that is often present. A lumbar puncture can be done safely in most postoperative patients, particularly those from whom a mass lesion has been resected and in whom the brain has been decompressed. CSF should be evaluated in the usual fashion for cell count, protein, and glucose. One study of meningitis in the postoperative period defined it (somewhat arbitrarily) as 100 white cells/mm³ with a minimum of 50% polymorphonuclear cells or 400 white cells/mm³ regardless of the polymorphonuclear percentage.[10] However, normal lumbar puncture parameters have never been defined for specific times after craniotomy and would additionally depend on the nature of the disease for which the craniotomy was performed. It is likely that the measurements are changed by the operation itself, by anesthesia, by the use of steroids, and by the disruption of cerebral tissue that occurs. In the absence of precise information for each type of craniotomy, interpretation of the CSF results should not rely on borderline values or on one parameter alone but must be a synthesis of all relevant measurements. Gram stain of CSF can help guide selection of antibiotics because culture may take 2 or more days to yield bacterial identity and sensitivity to treatment. In patients in whom the clinical symptoms and signs point to meningitis, treatment is instituted after a spinal tap is performed. If subsequent cultures show the meningitis to be aseptic, antibiotic administra-

tion may be stopped. However, it is common to continue them because perioperative administration of antibiotics may interfere with CSF cultures done in the first few days after craniotomy.

The role of prophylactic antibiotics in preventing meningitis after craniotomy remains controversial. A study by Barker, a meta-analysis of six trials involving 1729 patients, showed that meningitis accounted for 32% of the 102 infections reported after craniotomy.[11] The incidence of meningitis in antibiotic-treated patients was 1.1% versus 2.7% in untreated controls. Because statistical analysis suggested no heterogeneity among the different trials, the author concluded that antibiotics conferred significant benefit in preventing meningitis after surgery. A second study by Korinek and associates drew a different conclusion.[12] In a series of 6243 consecutive craniotomies they showed an overall 1.5% incidence of meningitis and identified the presence of CSF leakage, concomitant infection of the surgical incision, and surgical duration to be independent risk factors. Antibiotic prophylaxis reduced incisional infection by half but did not change the incidence of meningitis. Such conflicting results leave the question of prophylaxis for meningitis unsettled, but it is widely accepted that prophylaxis should be used to prevent postcraniotomy infection in a more general sense. The main issue would seem to be the choice of antibiotics to allow suppression of the broadest possible range of types of postoperative infection.

Recurrent Meningitis

Meningitis will recur if the source of the bacteria remains active after treatment and suppression of the meningitis itself. Such recidivism should raise suspicion of an ongoing CSF leak through a previous basilar skull fracture or surgical procedure affecting the frontal, sphenoid, or ethmoid sinuses or the cribriform plate (Fig. 44-2). In the absence of previous trauma, a congenital fistula between the nasal sinuses and subarachnoid space may be suspected. In either case, CT with thin cuts through the skull base on bone windows is very helpful. Difficult cases are those in which the CSF leak is intermittent or very slow. We have found the best method of detecting small leaks to be injection of radioactive tracer (typically ^{99}Tc or ^{111}In) into the lumbar subarachnoid space with placement of nasal pledgets.[13] The patient is then imaged over the next 24 to 48 hours to observe gradual movement of the tracer to the head (and if leak is present, into the nose and stomach). The pledgets are removed after the first day and also scanned; if a very slow leak is present, they may be the only source of positive detection. Finally, the kinetics of disappearance in CSF have been determined in normal patients, and an overly quick decay of tracer activity beyond the normal range suggests that a leak is present even if anatomic localization is lacking.[14] Ultimately, if a fistula is found that is causing repeated bouts of meningitis, it should be closed surgically.[15]

Treatment

Treatment of specific pathogens is presented in Table 44-3. The antibiotics suggested are only starting points because ongoing evolution of bacterial resistance to antibiotics has changed the patterns of antibiotic use significantly over the past 20 years.[16] In all cases the best antibiotics are those with good penetration into CSF, a penetration that in some instances is enhanced by the presence of meningeal irritation. Selection of an antibacterial agent should take into consideration the need for bactericidal activity and for adequate penetration into CSF. The antibacterial concentration should be at least 10 to 20 times the minimal bactericidal concentration of the agent in question. Penetration of CSF by antibiotics is enhanced by a low molecular weight and simple chemical structure of the drug, low degree of ionization at physiologic pH, high lipid solubility, and low degree of protein binding. Initial therapy is empirical according to the most likely

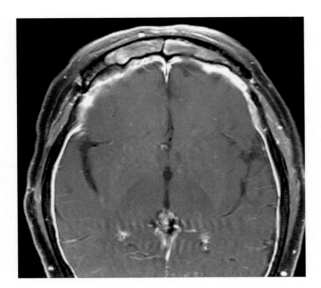

FIGURE 44-2 Recurrent meningitis caused by persistent leakage of cerebrospinal fluid (CSF) through the skull base. This 53-year-old woman with Cushing's disease underwent subtotal resection through a transbasal approach for tumor resection, and then a CSF leak developed 1 month later. This leak persisted over the next 9 months, during which time she suffered three separate bouts of meningitis, the first of which was culture positive for *Streptococcus intermedius*. This magnetic resonance image (axial T1 weighted, contrast enhanced) was obtained during the third episode. It shows diffuse enhancement over the brain convexities and falx cerebri, a classic finding with active bacterial meningitis. The expanded extracerebral space is consistent with ongoing intracranial hypotension from the loss of CSF. Of note, the frontal sinus shows mucosal thickening and enhancement consistent with paranasal sinusitis. However, there is no breach in the posterior wall allowing direct contact between the sinus cavity and intracranial compartment, and the meningitis must be ascribed to the ongoing CSF leak.

TABLE 44-3 Treatment of Specific Pathogens Causing Meningitis

ORGANISM	DRUG OR DRUGS COMMONLY USED
STANDARD BACTERIAL SPECIES	
Streptococcus pneumoniae	
MIC < 0.06 µg/mL	Penicillin G or ampicillin
MIC 0.1 to 1.0 µg/mL	Third-generation cephalosporin
MIC ≥ 2 µg/mL	Vancomycin
Neisseria meningitidis	Penicillin G or ampicillin
Haemophilus influenzae	
β-Lactamase negative	Ampicillin with chloramphenicol
β-Lactamase positive	Ceftriaxone or cefotaxime
Listeria monocytogenes	Penicillin G or ampicillin
Streptococcus group B	Penicillin G or ampicillin
Pseudomonas aeruginosa	Ceftazidime (if sensitive), consider adding an aminoglycoside
Enterobacteriaceae	Third-generation cephalosporin
Staphylococcus	
Methicillin sensitive	Nafcillin or oxacillin
Methicillin resistant	Vancomycin
OTHER MICROBIAL SPECIES	
Mycobacterium tuberculosis	3-4 antituberculosis drugs (isoniazid, rifampin, ethambutol, pyrazinamide)
Fungi	Amphotericin B or voriconazole
Naegleria fowleri	Amphotericin B plus rifampin
Spirochete	
Borrelia burgdorferi	Ceftriaxone or penicillin G
Treponema pallidum	Penicillin G

MIC, minimal inhibitory concentration.

organism suspected for the age of the patient.[17] The duration of therapy should be 10 to 14 days for those with bacterial meningitis in general and 21 days for patients with gram-negative bacteria and *Listeria*. If a shunt is present, it will typically require externalization or removal, or both, with reinsertion done only when the meningitis has been completely treated. Thus, prolonged ventriculostomy drainage will be needed in patients in whom meningitis develops but who are heavily shunt dependent. The ventricular drains should be changed at least weekly because their rate of infection (thereby perpetuating the meningitis) goes up after that time point.[18] When a persistent parameningeal focus of infection is present, this too must be cleared (medically or surgically) before the patient's meningitis can be declared cured. Treatment is invariably by intravenous administration, and in refractory cases or in those with profound ventriculitis, intraventricular therapy may additionally be needed.[19] It is not necessary to repeat lumbar puncture at intervals during therapy as long as progressive clinical improvement suggests that the disease is clearing. CSF glucose in particular remains low after other signs of infection have disappeared and must be interpreted in the context of the patient's clinical status.

The use of dexamethasone for meningitis has been controversial, with most data acquired from children.[20] It diminishes the inflammatory response in the subarachnoid space and decreases the production of tumor necrosis factor and interleukin-1. It also reduces cerebral edema and production of CSF without attenuating bacterial killing. In adults, studies have shown a decreased incidence of sensorineural hearing loss and a decrease in mortality.[21] We recommend using dexamethasone in patients of any age

at a dose of 0.15 mg/kg every 6 hours during the first 4 days of antibiotic therapy. Anticonvulsants should be given when seizures are present but need not be given prophylactically. Serum sodium levels should be checked frequently because they may fall and require the institution of fluid restriction. Ventricular enlargement seen on scans may indicate postmeningitic hydrocephalus but need not be treated unless the ventriculomegaly worsens. Clearly, if a shunt is needed because of the presence of transependymal fluid flow or symptoms of increased intracranial pressure in a patient with active meningitis, a ventriculostomy drain is used rather than an indwelling shunt.

Prevention

Strategies for prevention include active immunization, passive immunization with immunoglobulins, and chemoprophylaxis. The most effective vaccine is that against *Haemophilus*, which decreases *Haemophilus* meningitis in children and is commonly given to them; consequently, many cases now occur in unvaccinated adults. The *Haemophilus* vaccine is recommended for high-risk individuals with complement deficiency, which predisposes them to such meningitis. Vaccines for meningococcus have also been developed and are being used with increasing frequency.[22] Meningococcal meningitis is associated with a high risk of secondary infection in household members, who have 500 times the risk for infection that the general population does. Thus, rifampin (10 to 20 mg/kg per day orally for 4 days to a maximal dose of

600 mg daily) should be given to those who have had close contact with the patient in the 2 weeks before the diagnosis of meningitis. Ciprofloxacin has been shown to be effective in eradicating the meningococcal carrier state in adults, but chemoprophylaxis for other types of meningitis is not recommended. The exception is patients with posttraumatic CSF fistulas. Although a number of studies individually have not shown a significant difference in the incidence of meningitis with antibiotic prophylaxis in such patients, a meta-analysis that grouped six studies for analysis did show a 2.5% incidence of meningitis in those who received antibiotics versus 10% in those who did not, a difference that supports antibiotic use in that group.[23]

Prognosis

Bacterial meningitis is commonly fatal when untreated. Currently, the mortality rate for treated *Haemophilus* and meningococcal meningitis is 5% to 15% and has remained so for many years. Pneumococcal meningitis has a somewhat higher mortality rate of 15% to 30%. Fulminant meningococcemia is possible with or without meningitis and has a very high mortality rate from vasomotor collapse associated with adrenocortical hemorrhage (Waterhouse-Friderichsen syndrome).[24] In neonates the mortality rate from this phenomenon is 40% to 75%, and at least half who recover have serious neurological injury. The prognosis for bacterial meningitis is worse in those who have proven bacteremia, coma, seizures, and such concomitant disease as alcoholism and diabetes mellitus. Death occurs for a variety of reasons, including vascular collapse from septic shock, cerebral edema leading to transtonsillar herniation, respiratory failure secondary to aspiration pneumonia in an obtunded patient, and uncontrolled seizures. Those who recover from meningococcal meningitis usually show no residual deficits, but neurological injury occurs in 25% or more of children with *Haemophilus* meningitis and up to 30% of those with pneumococcal meningitis. In one study that monitored children after meningitis, 31% of those with pneumococcal meningitis had persistent sensorineural hearing loss, whereas the figures for meningococcal and *Haemophilus* meningitis were 10% and 6%, respectively.[25,26] *Haemophilus* meningitis in infants leaves only 50% entirely normal, with the remainder having either behavioral problems or significant ongoing neurological deficits.

TUBERCULOUS MENINGITIS

The incidence of tuberculous meningitis is very low because only 1% of patients with tuberculosis contract this extrapulmonary form of the disease.[27] It accounts for about 2500 cases per year in the United States. However, in developing countries, tuberculosis remains a very significant medical problem, and the lowering of barriers to immigration together with the increasing incidence of multidrug-resistant mycobacterial strains suggests that the case numbers are likely to rise in North America.

Pathogenesis

Tuberculous meningitis is caused by *Mycobacterium tuberculosis* in most patients and very occasionally by *Mycobacterium bovis*. Typically, it begins with bacterial seeding of the brain with the formation of tubercles that subsequently rupture and seed mycobacteria into the adjacent subarachnoid space. Such meningitis can be the terminal event in patients with miliary tuberculosis or occur less dangerously in the context of generalized tuberculosis with a single area of brain involvement.[28]

The usual location for tuberculous meningitis is the basal meninges, with little involvement of the cerebral convexities. The accompanying exudate obliterates the basal cisterns and forms small white tubercles scattered throughout this area. The ependyma and choroid plexus within the ventricles may also be studded with minute tubercles, and the exudate extends to the CSF space around the spinal cord. This inflammatory exudate is not confined to the subarachnoid space, as is the case with bacterial meningitis, but spreads along pial vessels to invade adjacent brain tissue. Thus, the disease is more of a meningoencephalitis than a true meningitis.

Clinical Features

Tuberculous meningitis occurs at any age and is currently more frequent in adults than children in the United States. Headache afflicts more than half the patients, a stiff neck is found in 75%, and lethargy, confusion, and fever are typical. The symptoms evolve more slowly in tuberculosis than in bacterial meningitis, usually over a period of 1 to 2 weeks, but sometimes longer. This chronicity leads to frequent cranial nerve involvement, present in 20% of patients at the time of admission to the hospital. Spinal symptoms are uncommon, and both infarction and increased intracranial pressure are seen occasionally.

Most patients with tuberculous meningitis have active tuberculosis elsewhere, although in some only inactive pulmonary lesions are found. Alcoholism is a common companion of this disease. In patients who die, the outcome is fatal within 1 to 2 months of onset.

Lumbar puncture is the paramount test for making the diagnosis. The main distinction lies in the glucose level, which is reduced but not usually to the very low levels seen with bacterial meningitis. Indeed, CSF glucose falls slowly in tuberculous meningitis and may be detected as low only several days after admission. Mycobacteria can be stained by the Ziehl-Neelsen method in the CSF sediment and can be cultured, but cultures take longer than 1 month to show positive results; greater amounts of CSF will enhance the chance of recovering the organism. Currently, the diagnostic examination of choice is demonstration of mycobacterial gene sequences by PCR technology, which provides much quicker demonstration of the microbe. MRI is typically performed and will often show hydrocephalus, as well as enhancement within the basal cisterns, subpial cortex, and subependymal areas. Occasionally, a frank tuberculoma can be seen.

A more self-limited meningitis known as "serous meningitis" will develop in a few patients with a cerebral tuberculoma. In such patients, CSF shows a modest pleocytosis, normal or elevated protein levels, and normal glucose levels. The meningeal signs are mild and the symptoms tend to clear over a period of several weeks. However, it is possible for serous meningitis to progress to a more generalized (and fatal) tuberculous meningitis.

Treatment of tuberculous meningitis always requires a combination of drugs, three at a minimum, with capacity to penetrate the CNS.[29] Administration is prolonged and continues for 18 to 24 months. The single most effective drug is isoniazid, but it has side effects (neuropathy and hepatitis) that can be disabling in alcoholics who may have these conditions from the outset. Neuropathy can be prevented by giving pyridoxine concomitantly, but hepatitis is not treatable except by discontinuing use of the drug. In patients taking ethambutol, optic neuropathy occasionally develops, so those receiving long-term ethambutol treatment should be screened at intervals for visual acuity and color discrimination. Corticosteroids are not generally used. At times, an intracerebral tuberculoma requires resection if there is a mass effect or if it fails to shrink with drug therapy. Mortality is lower when treatment is started early, but it reaches 50% in patients in whom the condition is diagnosed while in coma. Neurological impairment is found in 20% to 30% of survivors.

Despite the basal cistern loss caused by tuberculous meningitis, the associated hydrocephalus can be treated successfully in 70% of cases by endoscopic third ventriculostomy.[30]

TREPONEMAL (SYPHILITIC) MENINGITIS

The incidence of neurosyphilis has decreased dramatically over the past 50 years, but cases still linger within the general population and are seen from time to time, particularly in those immunocompromised by human immunodeficiency virus (HIV) or other causes. Meningitis develops in about 25% of patients with syphilis, but it is generally asymptomatic and discoverable only by lumbar puncture. Rarely, it is manifested symptomatically as cranial nerve palsies, seizures, and increased intracranial pressure. Invasion of the CNS takes place 3 to 18 months after the initial infection. If the CNS shows no involvement 2 years after inoculation, as proved by a negative spinal tap, neurosyphilis will subsequently develop in just 5% of patients and in only 1% after 5 years has elapsed. Such meningitis may persist in the asymptomatic state or may subside spontaneously. If it persists, it may cause parenchymal damage even after years have elapsed. Neurosyphilis always begins as a meningitis, but not all such meningitis progresses to vascular syphilis and the classic late phases of general paresis and tabes dorsalis. Syphilis is the most chronic form of meningitis affecting humans, and many of its associated pathologic changes may simply reflect the chronicity of the meningeal reaction. Factors leading to a transition from asymptomatic syphilitic meningitis to more symptomatic parenchymal neurosyphilitic forms are not known. However, treatment of asymptomatic syphilis is generally successful and will prevent such transformation. Thus, detection of the CSF changes in an asymptomatic patient is quite important, and any patient known to have syphilis should have a CSF examination soon after diagnosis. The course of the disease is quite variable from person to person, and presumably undefined immunologic factors temper the course of the disease.

The abnormalities of spinal fluid seen in syphilitic meningitis include a pleocytosis of 200 to 300 cells/mm^3, mainly lymphocytes and other mononuclear cells; elevation of total protein to 40 to 200 mg/dL; normal glucose content; and positive serologic tests. Serology includes use of the older Venereal Disease Research Laboratory (VDRL) flocculation technique, which if positive is diagnostic for syphilis. Seronegativity is common, however, and in patients clinically suspected of having syphilis with negative VDRL findings, a more specific test is available, the fluorescent treponemal antibody absorption (FTA-ABS) test. The pleocytosis and elevated protein may become apparent before serology becomes positive, and positive serology is the last component of the CSF testing to normalize when the disease goes into remission. Indeed, CSF serology may remain positive in the face of therapy and subsidence of disease activity.

When they occur, symptoms are similar to those of other meningitides, and hydrocephalus may occur. However, unlike other forms of meningitis, patients with syphilitic meningitis are afebrile. Meningovascular syphilis is a more advanced form of the disease that usually occurs 6 to 8 years after the original infection. It should be considered when a relatively young person has one or more cerebral infarcts. CSF will show positive serology and pleocytosis, and the disorder includes not only meningeal but also arterial inflammation with fibrosis leading to arterial occlusion and thus ischemia.

Treatment still involves administration of penicillin as the drug of choice for all varieties of neurosyphilis, regardless of whether symptoms are present.[31] Ideally, crystalline penicillin G is given at high doses intravenously for 2 weeks. If at 6 months the patient is symptom free and the CSF abnormalities have normalized, no further treatment is necessary, but a second lumbar puncture at 1 year is advisable. If, however, at 6 months pleocytosis or elevated protein is still present in CSF, another course of penicillin should be given.

MENINGITIS FROM LYME DISEASE

Lyme disease, named after the town in Connecticut where it was first recognized, is a tick-borne multisystem disease associated with relapsing fever and caused by spirochetes of the genus *Borrelia*. As in syphilis, the *Borrelia* spirochete invades the CNS early and causes asymptomatic meningitis, with later manifestation of more profound neurological abnormality in a smaller proportion of patients.[32] Also as in syphilis, the neurological complications mainly derive from the effects of chronic meningitis, but in Lyme disease a peripheral neuropathy may likewise produce neurological symptoms and make explication of the symptoms more complex. The disease starts as a tick bite with associated rash. Weeks to months later, neurological symptoms appear in 15% of patients. The neurological involvement takes the form of a fluctuating meningoencephalitis or peripheral neuritis, or both. The meningitis is manifested as headache, stiff neck, nausea and vomiting, malaise, and chronic fatigue and fluctuates over a period of weeks to months. In CSF a lymphocytosis is seen with counts of up to 3000 cells/mL and protein levels of up to 300 mg/dL. The glucose level is usually normal. Cognitive and behavioral changes sometimes occur, as do seizures, ataxia, and choreiform movements, and cranial neuropathy is seen in half of patients, most frequently a facial palsy. CSF testing with ELISA is positive in 50% of those in the early stage and 100% of those in the later stage. Recommended treatment is high-dose penicillin (20 million units intravenously daily for 10 days) or ceftriaxone.

FUNGAL MENINGITIS

Meningitis of fungal origin is far less common than bacterial meningitis, but it causes similar pathophysiologic and clinical effects. Although many fungi can involve the nervous system, only a few do so with regularity and are listed in this section. They enter the CNS either by a hematogenous route or through infected paranasal sinuses.[33] Although fungal meningitis may have no apparent predisposing cause, it usually occurs in the context of immunosuppression from another disease, such as diabetes mellitus, hematopoietic malignancy, prolonged immunosuppression in transplant patients, or chronic steroid therapy (Fig. 44-3). Patients with leukopenia are particularly susceptible. The course of onset and the symptom profile of fungal meningitis are much like that of tuberculous meningitis, and the onset is insidious. As in other chronic meningitides, these patients are often afebrile and may have cranial nerve involvement, arteritis with thrombosis and infarction, and hydrocephalus. The spinal fluid alterations also mirror those of tuberculous meningitis. CSF pressure is elevated with a moderate pleocytosis of lymphocytic predominance. CSF protein is elevated and glucose is low. The diagnosis is made from KOH preparation of CSF smears, from culture of CSF, and by antigen recognition tests or PCR amplification. Specific subtypes are summarized in the following text.

Cryptococcosis is one of the more frequent fungal infections. *Cryptococcus* is a fungus of the soil commonly carried by birds and transmitted to humans through the lungs or skin. The meningitis is granulomatous in nature, with granulomas containing fibroblasts, giant cells, areas of necrosis, and the organisms themselves. Its evolution is subacute, much like that of tuberculosis, but it may be fatal within a few weeks if left untreated.[34] Headache, fever, and a stiff neck are usually but not always seen, and patients often have symptoms of gradually increasing intracranial pressure, ataxia, or a confusional state. Because this is not a basal meningitis, cranial nerve palsies are infrequent. Meningovascular involvement may lead to stroke. In some patients the course may be chronic, with the disease persisting for years in a waxing and waning course. To diagnose cryptococcal meningitis, the organism must be found in CSF, large volumes of which are needed to find it. The classic test is the India ink preparation, which is

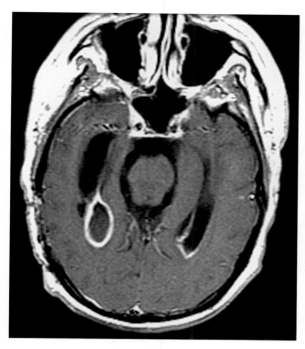

FIGURE 44-3 Bacterial meningitis followed by fungal ventriculitis with ventricular loculation. Immunocompromised patients can contract central nervous system infection by multiple microbial forms. This 34-year-old man with multiple previous resections for anaplastic astrocytoma also underwent radiotherapy, cytotoxic chemotherapy, and prolonged steroid use. Three months before this magnetic resonance image (MRI, axial T1 weighted, contrast enhanced), he underwent placement of an Ommaya reservoir for management of a tumor-associated cyst. The reservoir became infected with *Enterobacter aerogenes*, meningitis and ventriculitis developed, and the reservoir was removed. After a prolonged course of intravenous antibiotics, he improved clinically and then relapsed with further fever and obtundation. This MRI shows linear enhancement along the posterior wall of the left lateral ventricle and a loculated cyst filling the trigone of the right lateral ventricle and trapping the anterior portion of that ventricle, which is disproportionately enlarged. This was aspirated stereotactically and proved to contain *Cryptococcus neoformans*. Treatment with amphotericin B resulted in clinical stabilization, but he remained neurologically devastated and required long-term institutional care.

positive in only 60% of proven cases. Fungal cultures will often yield the organism, but in some the only evidence of infection is *Cryptococcus* serology by a latex agglutination test. Treatment of this and indeed most fungal meningitides is amphotericin B given intravenously. Nephrotoxicity is the main side effect of therapy, but even with treatment the mortality is 40%. In some cases, voriconazole has also proved effective.[35]

Candidiasis is the most frequent opportunistic fungal infection, but it causes meningitis only rarely. When candidiasis involves the CNS, it generally takes the form of parenchymal abscesses and noncaseating granulomas, with meningitis being less frequent. The diagnosis is often made post mortem. The mortality rate, with or without treatment, is very high, but occasional successes do occur.[36]

Coccidioidomycosis progresses from the typical influenza-like illness with pulmonary infiltration to the disseminated form of the disease in very few individuals. Meningitis is sometimes part of that dissemination (Fig. 44-4). The organism is difficult to recover from CSF and is more easily cultured from lymph nodes or skin lesions. The meningitis is again clinically much like that associated with tuberculous meningitis.[37]

Other chronic meningitides occasionally complicate histoplasmosis, blastomycosis, and actinomycosis. No specific clinical features distinguish these forms from cryptococcal meningitis. Treatment is amphotericin B for all except actinomycosis, which fortunately remains sensitive to penicillin.

UNCOMMON MENINGITIDES RARELY ENCOUNTERED

Amebas of the genus *Naegleria*, typically found in the southeastern states, cause a meningoencephalitis that patients acquire by swimming in ponds colonized by the organism. After a rapid onset characterized by severe headache, fever, nausea and vomiting, and a stiff neck, the disease progresses quickly to coma with a fatal outcome in most patients. CSF shows findings similar to those of acute bacterial meningitis, but it may also yield viable trophozoites in a wet preparation of unspun fluid. Culture is unhelpful. Treatment with antiprotozoal agents does not work, but with amphotericin B instituted quickly a few patients will recover.[38]

Trypanosomiasis, a common disease in the equatorial regions of Africa and South America, can cause a diffuse meningoencephalitis much slower in onset than the amebic form. The African variety, caused by *Trypanosoma brucei* and transmitted by the tsetse fly, begins with a chancre at the site of entry on the skin and regional lymphadenopathy. Subsequent dissemination of the parasite, typically in the second year of the infection, causes meningoencephalitis manifested as progressive cranial neuropathies, seizures, apathy, and ultimately coma. In South America the parasite is *Trypanosoma cruzi*, transmitted by reduviid bugs. The clinical picture is the same, and treatment for both is with pentavalent arsenical agents.

Toxoplasmosis, caused by the obligate intracellular parasite *Toxoplasma gondii*, typically affects the CNS in immunosuppressed patients. The most common scenario occurs in patients with HIV infection. The neurological manifestations of toxoplasmosis may be attributed to the background disease causing the immunosuppression, with the diagnosis being delayed and having a negative impact on outcome. The overall clinical picture includes rash, myocarditis, and polymyositis, with neurological symptoms being quite variable.[39] Most often a meningoencephalitis occurs with seizures, confusion, coma, and in the CSF, increased protein and lymphocytic pleocytosis.[40] Lesions are scattered throughout the brain, and presumably those adjacent to the subarachnoid space cause the meningitis component of the meningoencephalitis. The diagnosis can be made by finding organisms in CSF or in stereotactic biopsy specimens of brain lesions.[41] However, treatment with sulfadiazine and pyrimethamine (with leucovorin given as well to abrogate the antifolate effect of the latter drug) is now given to any immunocompromised patient with brain lesions consistent with *Toxoplasma*. A positive response to medical treatment is considered diagnostic. When the immune system compromise is expected to persist, long-term treatment is advisable.

VIRAL MENINGITIS AND ENCEPHALITIS

Viral infections of the CNS are invariably complications of more generalized viral infections, with invasion of the nervous system being a relatively infrequent occurrence. The systemic illnesses may themselves be relatively insignificant, but when the CNS is breached, destructive sequelae may follow. The route of entry of viruses is either through the respiratory passages (mumps, measles, varicella), through the gastrointestinal system (polioviruses and other enteroviruses), through the oral or genital mucosa (herpes simplex), or by inoculation through the skin (arboviruses). Once in the body, the virus multiplies, creates a viremia,

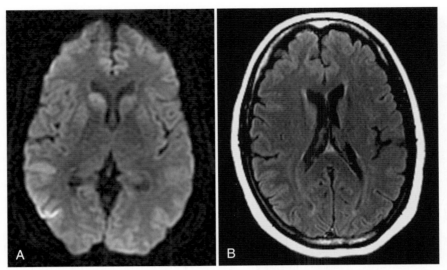

FIGURE 44-4 Fungal meningoencephalitis. The devastation of meningoencephalitis is exemplified in this 58-year-old woman with previous invasive ductal carcinoma of the breast. She underwent mastectomy uneventfully and then 6 weeks later began to have blurring of vision and imbalance of gait. Serial examination showed rapid loss of visual acuity and the onset of left homonymous hemianopia. Initial magnetic resonance imaging was negative, and electroencephalography (EEG) showed focal dysfunction in the right temporal region (polymorphic nonrhythmic delta activity). Performed 1 week after the first scan, these images include diffusion-weighted (**A**) and fluid-attenuated inversion recovery (**B**) sequences. In **A**, cortical hyperintensity from restricted diffusion is seen over the posterior right temporal convexity. In **B**, very subtle cortical hyperintensity is seen in the same area and extends to the frontal convexity as well. Initial diagnostic considerations included vasculitis and Creutzfeldt-Jakob disease given the findings on EEG and the patient's employment in a blood bank. Open biopsy of the right temporal cortex and white matter revealed branching hyphae, and cerebrospinal fluid serology was positive for *Coccidioides immitis*. She was treated with amphotericin B, voriconazole, and caspofungin without improvement and at discharge to long-term care was mute, agitated, and blind.

and may then (or may not) go on to invade the CNS through capillaries in the brain and choroid plexus. Neurotropic infection is also thought possible through retrograde movement of virus up the axons of cranial or peripheral nerves; the classic neurotropic virus is rabies, but herpes simplex may also follow this route. The diversity of viral effects on the CNS stems from the variety of cell populations that it contains with differential susceptibility to infection by different viruses. Viral infection of a cell requires the presence on the cell membrane of a specific receptor protein to which the virus attaches before entering the cell. When the virus attacks the cells of the leptomeninges, a benign ("aseptic") meningitis results. When the cells of the brain are targeted, the more serious disorder of encephalitis ensues. Once inside the cell, the virus commandeers its genetic apparatus to transcribe and translate viral proteins and replicate viral DNA, thereby allowing assembly and release of new viral particles.

The effects of viruses on infected cells vary. Acute encephalitis shows neuronal invasion by virus, with subsequent neuronophagia and lysis of cells leading to an inflammatory reaction and gliosis. In herpes zoster and some cases of herpes simplex, the virus stays latent within neurons for prolonged periods until the immune defenses falter as a result of either age or more active instances of immunosuppression. The basic clinical syndromes relevant here are (1) aseptic meningitis and (2) acute encephalitis or meningoencephalitis.

ASEPTIC MENINGITIS

The clinical syndrome of aseptic meningitis includes fever, headache, and mild neck stiffness. The most frequent symptom is headache; a variable degree of lethargy or irritability may occur, but confusion and coma are not generally seen. Photophobia is common but the neck stiffness is slight. Additionally, sore throat or rashes occur as more general manifestations of the causative virus.

CSF findings include a mononuclear pleocytosis and a slight rise in CSF protein. Cultures are negative, hence the term *aseptic* meningitis. CSF glucose is normal, which rules out other more serious meningitides linked with lymphocytic pleocytosis (e.g., tuberculous meningitis). However, a slight depression of CSF glucose may occur in meningitis caused by mumps, varicella-zoster, lymphocytic choriomeningitis, or herpes simplex type 2.

Aseptic meningitis is fairly common, with the majority of cases being due to viral infection, most commonly from the enterovirus family (Fig. 44-5; also see Fig. 44-1). Such organisms include

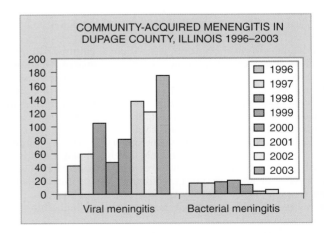

FIGURE 44-5 Incidence of community-acquired acute meningitis in DuPage County, Illinois, 1996 to 2003. Viral (aseptic) meningitis is much more common than the bacterial form, but the latter occurs more within a hospital setting as a complication of ongoing disease and may be underreported. Year-to-year variation is significant for the viral etiology, but less so for the bacterial, in this relatively wealthy suburban area near Chicago.

echovirus, coxsackievirus, and nonparalytic poliovirus, which together cover 80% of cases in which a specific virus is identified. The next most common cause is mumps virus, followed by herpes simplex type 2, lymphocytic choriomeningitis virus, and adenovirus.[42] These viruses, together with leptospirosis, cause 95% of cases of aseptic meningitis. Very occasional cases are caused by Epstein-Barr virus or sometimes occur in conjunction with *Mycoplasma pneumoniae*. Patients with HIV infection can also have acute, self-limited aseptic meningitis.

The enteroviruses are by far the most common cause of viral meningitis.[43] They occur most often in children, and outbreaks in families are typical because of spread by the fecal-oral route. The peak incidence is in the months of August and September. Meningitis from mumps can occur at any time during the year, but most often in the late winter and spring. Males are afflicted 3 times more often than females, and other manifestations of mumps infection are not always present. Because a previous attack of mumps confers lifelong immunity, a past history of the disease excludes this cause. Lymphocytic choriomeningitis virus infection occurs through contact with infected hamsters or food contaminated by mouse feces. Respiratory symptoms precede the onset of meningitis, and the infection is most common in late fall and winter when mice tend to congregate indoors. A previous sore throat with generalized lymphadenopathy and a transient rash may suggest infectious mononucleosis caused by Epstein-Barr virus, which occasionally causes aseptic meningitis.

Leptospira is actually a spirochete rather than a virus, but the clinical syndrome of leptospirosis is indistinguishable from that of viral meningitis. The infectious agent is transmitted through human contact with soil or water contaminated with the urine of rats, which act as the reservoir of the disease. The disease occurs in any season but peaks in August and may be accompanied by conjunctivitis and pulmonary infiltrates.

Few laboratory tests are helpful other than CSF analysis. Although the advent of PCR technology has increased detection of viruses such as enterovirus, cytomegalovirus, and herpesvirus in CSF, many still escape detection. The diagnosis of aseptic meningitis remains a diagnosis of exclusion, and CSF cultures should always be done to confirm that bacterial meningitis is not present in mild form. Most cases of viral meningitis are not treated with antiviral drugs but resolve on their own; symptom management is the main form of therapy. However, if herpesvirus or varicella-zoster is suspected, treatment with acyclovir is commonly recommended.

The nonviral forms of aseptic meningitis fall into four categories that cause a lymphocytic or mononuclear reaction in the leptomeninges with negative CSF cultures:

1. Bacterial infection adjacent to the meninges, commonly referred to as a parameningeal focus of infection, is the first group, a classic example of which is mastoiditis or sinusitis.
2. Specific meningeal infections in which the organism is difficult to isolate form the second group, important members of which include syphilis, cryptococcosis, and tuberculosis, as described earlier in this chapter. Brucellosis is another uncommon disease that is sometimes manifested as acute meningitis or meningoencephalitis with the CSF findings of culture-negative acute meningitis. The organism can rarely be cultured, and detection depends on antibody titers in serum and CSF ELISA.
3. The third group includes leptomeningeal carcinomatosis, formerly termed *carcinomatous meningitis*, a term now discarded because of its infectious implication. Such cases are generally identifiable by cytologic analysis of CSF to identify the presence of malignant cells. The most common cancers causing leptomeningeal involvement are leukemias and lymphomas, which may be accompanied by a pleocytosis of lymphocytic nature and thereby cause diagnostic confusion.

4. The final category is associated with autoimmune diseases, among which Behçet's disease is the one most commonly accompanied by aseptic meningitis. The classic triad in this disease includes relapsing iritis, ulcers of mouth and genitalia, and meningitis, but other symptoms, including ulcerative colitis and polyarthritis, also form part of its spectrum. Neurological manifestations occur in 30% of patients and include recurrent meningoencephalitis, as well as recurring episodes of dysfunction of the brainstem and diencephalon mimicking vascular insufficiency. A brisk pleocytosis is found in the CSF when neurological symptoms are active, along with elevated protein and normal glucose.

ACUTE ENCEPHALITIS/MENINGOENCEPHALITIS

The distinction between encephalitis and meningoencephalitis is too fine to make effectively, and indeed there is sometimes overlap with aseptic meningitis. The encephalitic syndrome consists of an acute febrile illness with meningeal involvement and some combination of confusion, delirium, seizures, dysphasia, hemiparesis, involuntary movements, cranial nerve palsies, and coma. Between 5% and 15% of patients with acute viral encephalitis will die, and lasting neurological impairment is seen in an additional 20% to 35%. Mortality is, however, worse in some subtypes, 40% with herpes simplex encephalitis, and half the survivors of that disease have ongoing neurological dysfunction.

Encephalitis may be caused by virus, but also by a postinfection allergic reaction and in a few cases by bacteria. Most cases of viral encephalitis are caused by a small group of viruses with geographic and seasonal associations. Eastern equine encephalitis typically occurs in New England in early autumn, western equine encephalitis occurs west of the Mississippi, and St. Louis (contrary to its name) encephalitis occurs nationwide but centers on the Mississippi River and usually comes in late summer. Venezuelan equine encephalitis occurs in South and Central America and thus in the United States in the southwestern region and in Florida. California virus encephalitis occurs in the northern Midwest and northeastern states. Such regional variation means that national statistics may not apply to a given locality. Other causative viruses include West Nile virus, Epstein-Barr virus, and herpes simplex, all three of which carry no special geographic distribution.

All the viruses just named are arboviruses with the exception of herpes simplex and Epstein-Barr. Arboviruses are "arthropod borne," a mode of transmission (in most cases by mosquitoes) from which their name derives. Thus, most have a seasonal incidence that peaks in summer and early fall, when mosquitoes are most active. The clinical manifestations of the various arboviruses are fairly uniform and have been detailed earlier. CSF findings are similar to those of aseptic meningitis, and the fever and neurological signs subside in 1 to 2 weeks in patients who survive. However, brain involvement is sometimes severe and destructive, particularly with eastern equine encephalitis. The usual pathologic changes in patients with arboviral encephalitides include degenerative changes in nerve cells with scattered foci of inflammation and necrosis through both gray and white matter. Other hallmarks of viral encephalitis are perivascular cuffing by lymphocytes, monocytes, and plasma cells and a patchy infiltration of the meninges by a similar cell population. The worst of the arboviral encephalitides is eastern equine encephalitis, from which two thirds of those afflicted die or remain severely disabled. Luckily, it is the least frequent of the arboviral infections, and mortality with the other types varies from 2% to 10%, with a similar incidence of residual neurological dysfunction.

Herpes simplex encephalitis is the most common form of acute encephalitis and the most likely to come to neurosurgical attention when brain biopsy is requested. Between 30% and 60% of cases are fatal, and the majority of patients who survive retain significant brain impairment. It is the only common encephalitis that lacks seasonal variation, and it occurs throughout the world in patients of all ages. Type 1 virus (the causative agent of the well-known herpetic lesions of the oral mucosa) is almost always the viral form provoking encephalitis. Type 2 virus causes acute encephalitis only in neonates in conjunction with transmission from a genital herpetic infection in the mother, yet exceptions to this dichotomy occasionally surface. When type 2 virus causes meningitis in adults, it is aseptic and of mild severity and short duration.

Symptoms of herpes simplex encephalitis evolve over a period of several days and resemble those of the other acute encephalitides. Occasional premonitory symptoms, including temporal lobe seizures, personality changes, anosmia, or olfactory or gustatory hallucinations, match the tendency of this disease to involve the inferomedial portions of the frontal and temporal lobes (Fig. 44-6). Changes in memory are usually identified only during the convalescent phase. In severe cases, temporal lobe edema and status epilepticus can cause uncal herniation and subsequent coma and death.[44]

Lumbar puncture shows increased CSF pressure with pleocytosis in the range of 10 to 500 cells/mm³. The cells are largely lymphocytes, but neutrophils may be seen as well. Because the lesions are often hemorrhagic, CSF can be xanthochromic and include many red cells. Protein content is increased, and CSF glucose is either normal or slightly reduced. Occasionally, the virus can be isolated from CSF, but PCR technology is the preferred method today for demonstrating viral DNA. Pathologically, there is an intense hemorrhagic necrosis in the fronto-orbital area of the brain and in the inferomedial temporal lobes unilaterally or bilaterally.

Making the diagnosis can be difficult even with CSF analysis and characteristic MRI findings showing an appropriate geographic location of the hemorrhagic lesions. Electroencephalographic findings suggest the disease but are not specific for it and include periodic high-voltage sharp waves in the temporal area.

As the disease progresses, a rising antibody titer can be demonstrated, but this does not generally become apparent early enough to affect therapy. The most certain way of diagnosing herpes simplex encephalitis is by viral culture of brain tissue obtained by brain biopsy or by immunohistochemical staining for viral antigens on such tissue. PCR analysis can also be performed, particularly if the specimen is obtained stereotactically and thus is small in volume. Biopsy can be performed either by stereotactic methods or, to increase diagnostic yield, by a small open craniotomy in which the cortical surface is exposed and a volume of tissue measuring 1 cm³ is removed from the inferior temporal region.[45] Because the temporal lobe may be particularly hemorrhagic, meticulous hemostasis is required with such biopsies, and care should be taken to maintain the integrity of the specimen during its removal to avoid a crush artifact, which hinders histologic analysis.

The treatment of choice is acyclovir, which in the body is converted to acyclovir triphosphate, a potent inhibitor of the herpes simplex DNA polymerase needed for viral replication.[46] The drug is given intravenously and has relatively few serious side effects, but its dose should be decreased in patients with renal dysfunction. It can cause phlebitis and gastrointestinal disturbance and is considered safe for use during pregnancy. Because most relapses occur within 3 months of completing the initial course of intravenous acyclovir, prolonged therapy with an oral antiviral agent (such as valacyclovir) has been suggested. The role of steroids in treating this disease remains unclear. Although steroids help limit the cerebral edema associated with the infectious process, they may also suppress the immune responses necessary to inhibit viral replication. Animal studies have suggested benefit without evidence of increased viral dissemination,[47] and a nonrandomized retrospective study in humans has shown an improved outcome at 3 months in the steroid-treated group.[48] Treatment should be given for 2 weeks to minimize relapse. Outcomes are better in patients younger than 30 years, in whom a mortality of 25% is noted, and only 10% of survivors escape neurological damage if treatment begins after the onset of coma.

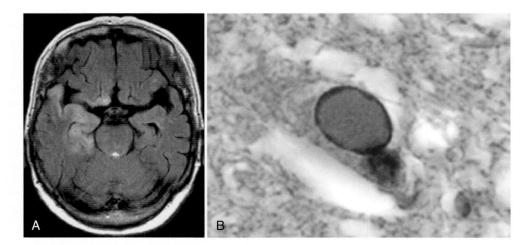

FIGURE 44-6 Herpes simplex encephalitis. This 71-year-old woman had an onset of olfactory hallucinations and confusion over a 1-week period. She was febrile, lethargic, and confused on examination but showed no focal deficits. Cerebrospinal fluid analysis revealed the following: protein, 64 mg/dL; glucose, 67 mg/dL; and white blood cell count, 175 cells/mm³. Electroencephalography showed paroxysmal lateralized epileptiform discharges, a classic finding in this condition. **A,** Magnetic resonance imaging (axial, fluid-attenuated inversion recovery sequence) is the most sensitive for showing areas of cerebral involvement and the resulting inflammatory changes. Here, hyperintensity is seen in the right temporal lobe and is affecting the uncus and insular cortex, as well as the subfrontal cortex. Although not present in this patient, foci of hemorrhage are frequent, and uncal herniation and neurological decline from a mass effect are the result if the disease expands in this location. This patient underwent open biopsy of the temporal cortex and white matter within the area of scan abnormality, which revealed the typical findings of microglial nodules and cytoplasmic and intranuclear inclusion bodies (**B**). After treatment with acyclovir, this patient recovered to a normal state.

In some patients with meningoencephalitis and severe cerebral edema, decompressive craniectomy can yield good results. In one report of three patients so treated by either bifrontal craniectomy or hemicraniectomy, two survived without residual focal deficit, and others have reported similar success with this procedure.[49,50] In addition, temporal lobectomy has been reported with good outcome in a child with refractory brain edema from herpes encephalitis.[51]

BACTERIAL ENCEPHALITIS

Three systemic bacterial infections are commonly complicated by encephalitis or meningoencephalitis. The first is legionnaires' disease caused by the gram-negative bacillus *Legionella pneumophila*. This disease shows a variety of neurological abnormalities, yet CSF is entirely normal, as are scans of the brain. Serum antibodies for the bacillus peak at 7 to 10 days after the onset of disease in most patients with neurological involvement, and generally the CNS disorder resolves rapidly and completely. This disease is usually treated with erythromycin. *M. pneumoniae* also provokes a variety of neurological syndromes, among which are aseptic meningitis, acute disseminated (postinfectious) encephalomyelitis, and acute hemorrhagic leukoencephalitis. Antibody titers can be determined in CSF, which usually contains increased protein and a mild pleocytosis of lymphocytes and other mononuclear cells. At the time of onset of CNS involvement there may be no sign of pneumonia. Finally, *Listeria monocytogenes* meningoencephalitis occurs in immunosuppressed or elderly patients and is also a well-known cause of neonatal meningitis. Although meningitis is the typical neurological manifestation, encephalitis is not uncommon. Cultures of blood and CSF will disclose the organism, and treatment consists of ampicillin with an aminoglycoside. Recovery is more likely in the absence of serious intercurrent medical disease, but in immunocompromised patients an attack is often fatal.

SPECIAL CIRCUMSTANCES

Acquired Immunodeficiency Syndrome

HIV infection has a number of neurological consequences. Its specific link to meningitis and encephalitis comes through opportunistic infection by such entities as cerebral toxoplasmosis, which does not infect immunocompetent individuals. Primary CNS lymphoma develops in about 5% of patients infected with HIV and can be difficult to distinguish from toxoplasmosis clinically or radiologically. In such cases of diagnostic confusion, when CSF cytology is negative, a brain biopsy (typically done stereotactically) may be needed. Because the response to radiotherapy and corticosteroids is short-lived, the prognosis of such patients is poor. In HIV-positive patients, varicella-zoster infection is generally more severe. In addition, mycobacterial infection is more frequent in patients with HIV than in the unaffected population.[52] Such infection can be caused by either *M. tuberculosis* or *Mycobacterium avium-intracellulare*. Here too the response to treatment is less than ideal, and grossly destructive cerebral lesions are more likely to be present. Both syphilitic meningitis and meningovascular syphilis have an increased incidence in patients with acquired immunodeficiency syndrome (AIDS), as do opportunistic infections caused by cytomegalovirus and *Cryptococcus*.[53] At autopsy a third of patients with AIDS are found to be infected with cytomegalovirus, but the clinical relevance of this finding is uncertain. Cryptococcal infections may take the form of meningitis or a solitary cryptococcoma and are the most frequent fungal agents complicating HIV disease. Clear symptoms of meningitis or encephalitis may be absent, however, with little CSF abnormality. With the current widespread use of retroviral therapy and multidrug cocktails providing much better long-term suppression of HIV, such secondary afflictions are somewhat less common but remain part of the overall burden of a patient infected with HIV.[54]

Chemical Meningitis

Chemical meningitis refers to meningeal inflammation caused by a noninfectious agent. This typically takes the form of release of blood or cyst contents into CSF from a lesion adjacent to the subarachnoid space. Such lesions include craniopharyngiomas, Rathke's cleft cysts, epidermoid and dermoid cysts, and cholesteatomas.[55] Release of the irritative element often occurs repeatedly, and the result is a chronic headache syndrome relieved by resection of the offending lesion. This is a form of aseptic meningitis, although one without a viral etiology. In Mollaret's meningitis, a syndrome consisting of recurrent bouts of fever and the signs and symptoms of aseptic meningitis, recovery is rapid and spontaneous. Although no cause has been definitively identified, it has been ascribed to an occult reservoir of herpes simplex virus type 1, but this association is not conclusive.

SUGGESTED READINGS

Brouwer MC, Tunkel AR, van de Beek D. Epidemiology, diagnosis, and antimicrobial treatment of acute bacterial meningitis. *Clin Microbiol Rev*. 2010;23:467-492.

Davis LE, Beckham JD, Tyler KL. North American encephalitic arboviruses. *Neurol Clin*. 2008;26:272-757.

DeGaudio M, Chiappini E, Galli L, et al. Therapeutic management of bacterial meningitis in children: a systematic review and comparison of published guidelines from a European perspective. *J Chemother*. 2010;22:226-237.

Hall WA, McCutcheon IE, eds. *Infections in Neurosurgery*. Park Ridge, Illinois: American Association of Neurological Surgeons; 1999.

Kastrup O, Wanke I, Maschke M. Neuroimaging of infections of the central nervous system. *Semin Neurol*. 2008;28:511-522.

Logan SA, MacMahon E. Viral meningitis. *BMJ*. 2008;336:36-40.

Full references can be found on Expert Consult @ www.expertconsult.com

CHAPTER 45

Acquired Immune Deficiency Syndrome

M. Kelly Nicholas ■ Rimas V. Lukas ■ Koen van Besien

Acquired immunodeficiency syndrome (AIDS) is caused by infection with human immunodeficiency virus (HIV) and is defined by the Centers for Disease Control and Prevention as occurring in any HIV-infected individual with a helper T-cell (CD4+) count less than 200/μL blood.[1] Before adoption of this definition, HIV-positive individuals with either opportunistic infections or rare malignancies associated with immunocompromise were said to have developed an AIDS-defining illness. This terminology persists, and AIDS-defining illnesses are often found coincident with CD4+ T-cell counts that meet the criteria for the definition of AIDS.

HIV is a retrovirus that infects cells by docking and binding at two essential sites on a target cell: the CD4 receptor and one of two chemokine receptors (CCRs), CCR5 or CXCR4.[2] Although the primary cell of focus in HIV infection is the T lymphocyte, it is important to know that other cell types, including resident cells of the brain, are also susceptible. Once an individual is infected, CD4+ T lymphocytes are gradually depleted until cell-mediated immunity finally deteriorates and AIDS develops. The latency between HIV infection and the development of AIDS may be many years. The symptoms and signs of HIV infection are protean and may go unrecognized as being related to HIV. This, along with the stigma associated with HIV infection, leads to frequent delays in diagnosis and treatment, thereby further spreading the virus and compromising the health of infected individuals.[3]

Effective HIV treatment, in the form of highly active antiretroviral therapy (HAART), now exists, and as a result in some communities AIDS has become a chronic illness.[4,5] Accordingly, AIDS patients may require neurosurgical intervention for any number of conditions affecting the population at large. The risk of exposure to HIV by surgeons and allied health care workers during diagnostic procedures is real but small.[6] In the early days of the AIDS epidemic, when the mechanisms of disease transmission were unknown, many justified reluctance to perform invasive procedures because of this risk. The poor prognosis associated with the condition was used to bolster this claim. Today, decisions regarding the need for and timing of neurosurgical procedures are dictated by an understanding of AIDS itself. Biopsy or resection of intracranial lesions that might be performed in otherwise healthy individuals is often delayed in an AIDS patient pending response to trials of medical therapy for conditions commonly encountered. However, cases must be approached individually and be based on an understanding of risk-benefit ratios in this population.

In this chapter we focus on the neurological manifestations of HIV/AIDS and the role of the neurosurgeon in their diagnosis and management. Because the neurosurgeon may often be called on to consult on HIV/AIDS patients, an understanding of HIV infection and its consequences on the nervous system will help guide practice.

The neurological complications of HIV/AIDS can be divided into four areas: (1) consequences of HIV infection itself, (2) opportunistic (and other) infections, (3) AIDS-related malignancies (primary and metastatic), and (4) complications of HIV treatment. These categories often coexist in a given patient and complicate diagnosis and treatment. Some HIV-associated neurological complications are associated with more than one of these categories. For example, peripheral neuropathy may be caused by the virus itself, by opportunistic infections, or by antiretroviral therapies. In these cases, the reader may be referred to different sections, as appropriate. We consider each in turn in the following sections.

HUMAN IMMUNODEFICIENCY VIRUS INFECTION OF THE NERVOUS SYSTEM

Both the central nervous system (CNS) and the peripheral nervous system can be directly affected by HIV. Although controversy still exists regarding the extent to which CNS cells (excluding microglia) can harbor HIV, immunologic responses to HIV-infected cells in the CNS probably account for many of the neurological complications associated with HIV/AIDS. These complications include many of the more elusive disorders causing difficulties in diagnosis and treatment, as outlined in Table 45-1.

Acute Retroviral Syndrome

Acute HIV infection results in an acute retroviral syndrome in the majority of those exposed.[7] Although these symptoms are often systemic in nature, aseptic meningitis occurs in almost 25% of infected individuals.[8] Other neurological manifestations of acute HIV infection include facial nerve palsies, radiculopathy, and acute demyelinating polyneuropathy.[9] These symptoms are usually manifested within 2 to 6 weeks of infection and may be the primary reason that an infected individual seeks medical attention after HIV infection.

The neurological signs and symptoms of acute retroviral syndrome are probably distinct from the infection of CNS tissue itself. Nevertheless, HIV infection of the CNS is an early event that is thought to occur through trafficking of infected monocytes/macrophages and CD4+ T lymphocytes into the brain. Microglia, or resident CNS macrophages, are early reservoirs of HIV infection. Furthermore, astrocytes can also be infected by HIV.[10] Astrocyte infection is CD4+ lymphocyte independent and results in nonproductive virus. However, the presence of HIV within them may account for many of the chronic effects of CNS infection by HIV, especially in the pediatric population.[11]

Human Immunodeficiency Virus–Associated Encephalopathy

HIV infection of the brain is associated with a spectrum of clinical findings often referred to as either HIV-associated encephalopathy (HAE) or HIV-associated dementia.[12] The disorder is manifested differently in children and adults.[13] HAE in adult patients is characterized by a gradual decline in cognitive

TABLE 45-1 Common Neurological Conditions Associated with HIV Infection (Independent of Subsequent Opportunistic Infection, AIDS-Associated Malignancies, and Treatment-Related Toxicities)*

NEUROLOGICAL CONSEQUENCES OF PRIMARY HIV INFECTION	CLINICAL MANIFESTATIONS	IMAGING	CSF FINDINGS	ANCILLARY TESTS	TREATMENT
Acute retroviral syndrome	Aseptic meningitis, cranial neuropathy, polyradiculopathy, AIDP	Usually normal; meningeal enhancement may occur	Lymphocytic pleocytosis (aseptic meningitis), cytoalbumic dissociation in AIDP	Electrical studies consistent with neuropathic process	Symptomatic medications for neuropathy, immune modulation for AIDP
HIV-associated encephalopathy	Gradual decline in cognition (adults); developmental delay, often progressive (children)	Progressive atrophy with periventricular white matter changes	Mild elevation of proteins, lymphocytic pleocytosis	Diffuse slowing on EEG	HAART (but CNS resistance occurs)
Myelopathy	Spasticity, weakness, sensory ataxia, incontinence	Cord atrophy, high signal intensity lesions on T2-weighted images	Often normal, elevated protein, pleocytosis (rare)	Abnormal SSEPs	HAART (CNS resistance occurs)
Stroke	Acute neurological change consistent with stroke	Findings consistent with stroke (no distinguishing features)	Normal	None	Risk reduction, rehabilitation
Neuropathy	Distal, symmetrical, sensory > motor, often painful	None	Normal	Reduced nerve conduction velocity and amplitude	Symptomatic (WHO analgesic ladder); correct nutritional deficiencies
Myopathy	Proximal > distal weakness	None	Normal	Elevated serum creatine kinase, myopathic changes on EMG	Immune modulation, discontinuation of offending medications, steroids

*See text for details.

AIDP, acute inflammatory polyradiculopathy; CNS, central nervous system; EEG, electroencephalogram; EMG, electromyogram; HAART, highly active antiretroviral therapy; SSEP, somatosensory evoked potentials; WHO, World Health Organization.

functioning, often occurring long after the initial infection. Motor slowing is usually evident, sometimes coincident with but often after the onset of cognitive decline. Both are progressive, and behavioral changes may also become apparent. Neuroimaging reveals diffuse atrophy. Nonenhancing periventricular white matter changes may also be seen, and the electroencephalogram usually shows diffuse slowing. Cerebrospinal fluid (CSF) evaluation often reveals a mild lymphocytic pleocytosis and protein elevation. Focal lesions on imaging or more extreme findings on CSF evaluation should prompt evaluation for other or coexisting illnesses.

HAE in children is similar to that in adults in many ways, but because the infection occurs during brain development, some differences may be seen. Specifically, evidence for more widespread infection of astrocytes and even neurons may be found.[14,15] Developmental delay may be the first sign of HIV infection and can be manifested as either motor or language delay. Behavioral consequences may also be seen. Frequently, these manifestations exist together. Again, comorbid conditions associated with AIDS may be present and should be ruled out before a diagnosis of HAE is made.

Myelopathy

The spinal cord is commonly involved in HIV infection. The characteristic lesion in adults consists of vacuolar changes, predominantly in the lateral and posterior columns of the thoracic cord, although any level may be affected.[16] Even though present in up to 50% of autopsy cases, clinical manifestations of myelopathy are much less frequently described, either because they are less pronounced than other neurological symptoms (i.e., those of dementia and neuropathy) or because they are attributed to some other cause.[17] Common symptoms include spasticity, weakness, sensory ataxia, urinary incontinence, and erectile dysfunction. The disorder is usually a late manifestation of AIDS. Although also common in children, the nature of the myelopathic changes differs from that commonly seen in adults.[18]

The cause of vacuolar myelopathy remains poorly understood, but HIV-infected macrophages are often seen. There is no compelling evidence for overt HIV infection of spinal cord tissue itself. Two hypotheses, not mutually exclusive, that might explain the pathologic features include (1) toxicity associated with proinflammatory cytokine production by infected macrophages and

(2) impaired intraspinal methylation essential for myelination and neurotransmitter metabolism.[19] Pathologic examination reveals a symmetrical axon-sparing process initially, which in advanced cases may disrupt axons and appear more symmetrical.

The diagnosis is usually clinical, but findings on magnetic resonance imaging (MRI) include atrophic changes of the thoracic cord with occasional increased signal on T2-weighted and fluid-attenuated inversion recovery (FLAIR) sequences.[20] CSF is often normal. Occasionally, a mild lymphocytic pleocytosis and protein elevation are observed.[17] Somatosensory evoked potentials are frequently abnormal even before clinical symptoms develop.[20]

HIV-associated vacuolar myelopathy tends to be insidious in onset. There is no effective treatment. Therefore, in any patient with a rapidly progressive myelopathic disorder, especially one associated with focal back pain or marked CSF abnormalities, alternative diagnoses should be sought because treatments may be available.[17] Other possibilities include disorders caused by other retroviruses (human T-cell lymphotropic virus types I and II), cytomegalovirus (CMV), herpes simplex virus type 2, and herpes zoster. Less common causes include those associated with malignancies, especially lymphoma and myeloma. Ischemic myelopathies are rarely reported.

Human Immunodeficiency Virus–Associated Stroke

HIV infection is associated with an increased risk for stroke.[21] However, attribution of HIV itself as being causative of stroke is problematic. HIV infection has been associated with the presence of both antiphospholipid antibodies and protein S deficiency in HIV-positive stroke patients.[22,23] HIV has also been associated with vasculitis.[24] Although rare in children, stroke should be considered in those with HIV and an acute onset of neurological symptoms because cerebrovascular disease is well documented.[25] In addition, dyslipidemia, a common side effect of HAART therapy, carries an increased risk for stroke. To date, however, no compelling evidence for a strong association between HAART and an increased incidence of stroke has been documented.[21] In conclusion, stroke must be considered in the differential diagnosis of any HIV-positive individual with an abrupt onset of neurological symptoms.

Human Immunodeficiency Virus–Associated Neuropathy

Peripheral neuropathy is often encountered in HIV/AIDS patients and is considered the most common neurological manifestation of the disease.[26] Acute HIV infection may result in acute inflammatory polyradiculopathy either in isolation or as part of the acute retroviral syndrome described earlier.[9] A painful distal symmetrical polyneuropathy is present in many AIDS patients at diagnosis. It is thought to be due to the direct effects of HIV on peripheral nerves or the neurotoxic effects of proinflammatory cytokines that result from viral infection.[27] Related metabolic and nutritional deficiencies may also contribute to distal symmetrical polyneuropathy. Patients complain of numbness and burning of the feet, which are exquisitely sensitive to touch. The hands may be involved as well, but this is usually a late complication. Weakness is rare. Distal reflexes are diminished relative to proximal reflexes in a symmetrical fashion. Electrical studies demonstrate reduced nerve conduction velocities or amplitudes, or both, along with evidence of denervation and reinnervation distally.[28] Rarely is evaluation of the CSF or nerve/muscle biopsies indicated. Later in the course of the disease, opportunistic infections may cause radiculopathies and mononeuritis multiplex. Finally, many

of the agents included in HAART are known neurotoxins (see later).

Acute inflammatory polyradiculopathy is treated by immunomodulation, most often either plasmapheresis or intravenous immune globulin. Treatment of distal symmetrical polyneuropathy includes identifying and correcting any comorbid nutritional or infectious factors as well as the use of many medications, including analgesics of all classes, anticonvulsants, anesthetic agents, and select antidepressants. An "analgesic ladder" has been constructed by the World Health Organization to aid in the treatment of symptoms from distal symmetrical polyneuropathy, but many reports suggest that pain is inadequately treated in these patients.[29]

Human Immunodeficiency Virus–Associated Myopathy

Symmetrical and proximal myopathy is a common finding in those with HIV/AIDS.[30] Its etiology is unknown but it is found in those without underlying explanations, such as opportunistic infection or myopathy-causing therapies, including HAART. Presumed causes include HIV itself, as well as associated inflammatory cytokines. The process affects the hip flexors and neck muscles disproportionately. Serum creatine kinase is frequently elevated, and electrical studies show classic myopathic changes.[31] Muscle biopsies are characterized by degeneration of myofibers. Inflammation may or may not be present. Management includes identifying and treating any underlying causes (including HAART) and administration of steroidal and nonsteroidal antiinflammatory agents and intravenous immune globulin.

INFECTION

Infections of many kinds are common in those with HIV/AIDS, and the nervous system is frequently involved. Impaired cell-mediated immunity predisposes HIV-infected individuals to opportunistic infections rarely encountered in the population at large. Opportunistic infections encountered in the CNS of persons with HIV/AIDS are outlined in Table 45-2 and are the focus of this section. As noted earlier, the clinical manifestations and radiographic features of various opportunistic infections can be quite similar, and they can also mimic other AIDS-associated conditions (i.e., malignancies and nonopportunistic infections such as *Treponema pallidum* or *Bartonella*, which are common in patients with HIV/AIDS). Furthermore, several processes may coexist and thus complicate diagnosis and treatment. As a result, histologic confirmation of a suspected infectious process may be warranted. Serologic studies, cell culture, and molecular techniques such as polymerase chain reaction (PCR) are also commonly used.

Toxoplasmosis

The parasite *Toxoplasma gondii* and the fungus *Cryptococcus neoformans* are the most common causes of opportunistic brain infections in HIV/AIDS patients. They cause a constellation of neurological symptoms and findings that can be very difficult to differentiate from each other, from lymphoma, and from tuberculosis.

T. gondii, a ubiquitous parasite, is the most common. Human exposure occurs through contact with oocytes shed by its definitive host, the cat, and the risk for AIDS-related CNS toxoplasmosis is related to the prevalence of *Toxoplasma* exposure in a particular population or area.[31] After infection, persistent and asymptomatic cysts form in both the brain and muscle. Reactivation occurs as a consequence of impaired cellular immunity and often causes an encephalitis without significant meningeal

TABLE 45-2 Diagnostic Findings in HIV-Associated Central Nervous System Opportunistic Infections

OPPORTUNISTIC INFECTION	CD4+ COUNT	MRI	ENHANCEMENT	CSF	SERUM	RESPONSE TO EMPIRICAL THERAPY
PARASITIC						
Toxoplasmosis	<100/µL	Parenchymal Multiple With or without bleeding Decreased T2 signal, but surrounding edema with increased T2 signal Variable DWI	Ring enhancement Decreases with lower CD4+ count	PCR Tachyzoites on cytology	Increased IgG but may be negative PCR	Often significant radiographic response
FUNGAL						
Cryptococcus	<200/µL	Cryptococcoma Meningitis Encephalitis Dilated perivascular spaces	Meningeal enhancement With or without ring enhancement Decreases with lower CD4+ count	Cell count normal India ink Cryptococcal Ag Culture	Culture Cryptococcal Ag	May respond
Aspergillus	<50/µL	Vasculitis, CVA with ICH Cerebritis Abscess Meningitis	With or without ring enhancement Dural enhancement	Fungal culture Low sensitivity	Fungal culture Low sensitivity Galactomannan assay	Not typically
BACTERIAL						
Mycobacterium tuberculosis	250-400/µL	Tuberculoma multiple or single with no mass effect T2 isointense with occasionally increased T2 center Abscess usually single with mass effect/edema May be multiloculated	Ring enhancement of both tuberculoma and abscess Meningeal enhancement	Culture AFB stain AFB PCR Increased WBC count, protein Decreased glucose Increased viscosity	Culture	Not typically
Mycobacterium avium complex	<50/µL	Tuberculoma multiple or single, no mass effect T2 isointense with occasionally increased T2 center Abscess usually single with a mass effect/edema May be multiloculated	Ring enhancement of both tuberculoma and abscess Meningeal enhancement	Culture AFB stain AFB PCR Increased WBC count protein Decreased glucose Increased viscosity	Culture	Not typically
Treponema pallidum		CVAs Gummas Increased T2, decreased T1 signal	Meningeal enhancement Gummas enhance	Increased protein, WBC count CSF VDRL FTA-ABS MHA-TP PCR	RPR/VDRL FTA-ABS MHA-TP	
Bartonella	<100/µL	May be normal	Variable	Antibodies positive in a third Culture PCR	Culture	

Continued

TABLE 45-2 Diagnostic Findings in HIV-Associated Central Nervous System Opportunistic Infections—cont'd

OPPORTUNISTIC INFECTION	CD4+ COUNT	MRI	ENHANCEMENT	CSF	SERUM	RESPONSE TO EMPIRICAL THERAPY
VIRAL						
JC virus	50-100/μL	Multiple, asymmetric, subcortical No mass effect Increased T2 signal	Nonenhancing	Rare increased WBC count Increased protein Normal glucose JC virus PCR	Low CD4+ count High viral load	HAART may result in IRIS
Cytomegalovirus	<50-200/μL	Diffuse white matter hypodensity Ependymal enhancement No periventricular calcifications	Meningeal/nerve root enhancement, cord enhancement Rarely ring enhancing	CMV PCR or antigen Increased WBC count Protein, glucose normal	CMV PCR or CMV Ag CMV antibodies are not specific	

AFB, acid-fast bacilli; Ag, antigen; CD4, typical CD4 count below which infection is common; CMV, cytomegalovirus; CSF, cerebrospinal fluid; CVA, cerebrovascular accident; DWI, diffusion-weighted images; FTA-ABS, fluorescent treponemal antibody, absorbed; HAART, highly active antiretroviral therapy; ICH, intracranial hemorrhage; IRIS, immune reconstitution inflammatory syndrome; MHA-TP, microhemagglutination—*Treponema pallidum*; MRI, magnetic resonance imaging; PCR, polymerase chain reaction; RPR, rapid plasmin reagin; VDRL, Venereal Disease Research Laboratory; WBC, white blood cell.

involvement. Multiple lesions can develop subacutely in the brain and cause location-dependent symptoms.

In typical cases of toxoplasmosis, both computed tomography (CT) and MRI reveal varying numbers of nodular or ring-enhancing lesions with surrounding edema (Fig. 45-1). The degree of enhancement varies and may be less pronounced in those with advanced AIDS and weaker immune responses.[32] The lesions are most common at the gray-white interface and in the basal ganglia and thalamus.[33] Although signal characteristics vary, the lesions are often hyperintense on T2-weighted sequences. The center of the lesion may be hypointense on diffusion-weighted imaging, with the surrounding edema being hyperintense.[34]

The differential diagnosis of ring-enhancing lesions includes lymphoma and other infections, especially tuberculosis and cryptococcosis. Although the lesions in lymphoma can be nodular and ring enhancing, a homogeneous pattern of enhancement is more common. Small parenchymal hemorrhages are common in toxoplasmosis and infrequent in lymphoma.[35] Diffusion-weighted imaging may also help differentiate between toxoplasmosis and lymphoma in that the latter is often characterized by a uniformly restricted pattern.[36] Periventricular and callosal involvement is more common in lymphoma as well.

Serum and CSF studies may help in determining the etiology of CNS lesions, but many caveats exist. Antibody titers for *Toxoplasma* are not very helpful in immunocompromised individuals.[37-39] Serum or CSF PCR, in contrast, is associated with good specificity and reasonable sensitivity.[40] CSF cytology can occasionally demonstrate the *Toxoplasma* organisms.[41]

Because of the high incidence of toxoplasmic encephalitis in HIV-infected patients and the difficulty in establishing a diagnosis by noninvasive means, empirical treatment is often initiated in patients with characteristic enhancing mass lesions. Toxoplasmosis often responds rapidly to therapy with pyrimethamine and sulfadiazine. Radiologic improvement is usually apparent within 2 to 4 weeks, but in rare cases, it may take up to 6 months to see a response.[42]

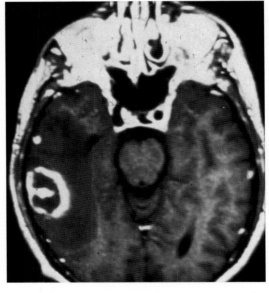

FIGURE 45-1 T1-weighted gadolinium-enhanced image demonstrating a ring-enhancing lesion with surrounding edema, typical of toxoplasmosis.

In cases of failed diagnosis or failed response to empirical treatment of presumed toxoplasmosis, the neurosurgeon may be called to perform a biopsy. Biopsy specimens of toxoplasmotic tissue are often necrotic, and when histopathologic evaluation fails to reveal organisms, other means of establishing the diagnosis are necessary,[42,43] including isolation of active *T. gondii* from cultured biopsy specimens. *Toxoplasma* infection can also be established by identification of *Toxoplasma*-specific DNA by PCR performed on either fresh or formalin-fixed, paraffin-embedded tissue.[42,44]

Toxoplasmosis is usually responsive to treatment.[45] Unfortunately, treatment does not affect the dormant bradyzoite form of the infection, and there is a high potential for reactivation. In the event of suspected recurrence or progression because of drug resistance, repeat biopsy may be warranted.

Fungal Infections

C. neoformans infection, like toxoplasmosis, is endemic. The organism is found in bird excrement and infects humans via inhalation, although overt pulmonary infection and pneumonia are rare.[46,47] In the setting of HIV infection, both meningoencephalitis and isolated encephalitis may occur, usually in those with CD4+ T-cell counts less than 200 cells/μL. The clinical manifestations probably represent reactivation of latent infection.[47] The symptoms and signs of cryptococcal meningitis develop over a period of weeks to months. Because of an impaired immune response to infection, the findings may be more subtle and insidious in onset in HIV-infected patients. Cranial neuropathies are common because of the predilection for meningeal involvement at the base of the brain. Hydrocephalus is also common, and strokes sometimes occur. Direct involvement of the brain parenchyma, when present, may be either focal or diffuse, and symptoms and signs vary according to the area or areas affected.[48]

Radiologic findings in cryptococcosis are relatively nonspecific. Occasionally, ring-enhancing lesions occur and can be difficult to differentiate from toxoplasmosis. Less commonly, cryptococcosis causes pseudocysts in the CSF spaces, which are seen as dilated perivascular spaces.[42] Sputum culture is unreliable because of fungi colonizing the upper respiratory tract. Blood cultures are often positive for cryptococcosis in HIV-positive patients with CNS involvement.[49] Positive serum cryptococcal antigen by latex agglutination may also help support the diagnosis.[47,50] CSF cell counts are frequently unremarkable in HIV/AIDS patients infected with *Cryptococcus*.[51,52] Therefore, India ink stains, cryptococcal antigen assay, and fungal culture are useful in making the diagnosis. These studies have high specificity, but their sensitivity is variable. CSF culture is positive in 56% to 99% of all patients with cryptococcal meningitis, India ink staining in 75% to 98%, and latex agglutination in 80% to 98%.[53,54]

On histopathologic review, cryptococcomas reveal chronic granulomatous changes with only a few organisms. Occasionally, these lesions are surrounded by more profound inflammation. In cryptococcosis, thickening and opacification of the meninges is commonly seen. India ink and mucicarmine stains of the meninges may reveal budding yeast. If biopsy is performed on the brain parenchyma, pseudocysts may be found. These gelatinous dilations of the perivascular spaces are described as "soap bubbles." They are most common in the basal ganglia but can be found elsewhere in the parenchyma as well.[42]

HIV-associated CNS cryptococcal infection, if untreated, is fatal. Treatment often consists of fluconazole or amphotericin B (or one of its lipid derivatives). The majority of patients respond to treatment, but as with toxoplasmosis, the relapse rate is high.[51,54-56] The mortality associated with cryptococcal meningoencephalitis remains 10% to 30%.[57,58] Because hydrocephalus is a common problem, the neurosurgeon may often be consulted to place a ventricular shunt.

Aspergillus is another fungal infection commonly encountered in HIV/AIDS patients. It is a septate hyaline mold found in plants and soil that causes severe sinopulmonary infections in immunocompromised hosts. From there it can spread either hematogenously or by direct invasion from the sinuses to the CNS.[59] Most patients with CNS aspergillosis will also have evidence of ongoing or previous sinopulmonary infection. *Aspergillus* can cause diffuse cerebritis, focal abscesses, or meningitis. It can also cause a vascular invasion and result in stroke.[60] Biopsy may be required to establish a definitive diagnosis in these severely immunocompromised patients.

Mycobacterial Infections

The prevalence of *Mycobacterium tuberculosis* is high in the developing world and increasing in the United States and other developed nations. HIV/AIDS patients are particularly prone to reactivation of tuberculosis and to extrapulmonary infection.[61] In cases of CNS involvement, patients often have a history of pulmonary tuberculosis.[62] The atypical mycobacteria *M. avium* and *M. intracellulare* are endemic in the environment, found in water, soil, and animal hosts. In profoundly immunocompromised AIDS patients (CD4+ T-cell counts <50 cells/μL), they cause a systemic syndrome classified as *Mycobacterium avium* complex (MAC). CNS involvement, when present, mimics tuberculosis and is difficult to distinguish from it.[63]

Meningitis is the most common manifestation of tubercular infection of the CNS in both immunocompetent and immunocompromised individuals. In immunocompromised patients, typical meningeal signs can be absent.[64,65] Tubercular meningitis, like fungal meningitis, may be associated with stroke.[66] Parenchymal brain lesions are less common, but two types are seen: fibrotic tuberculomas and tubercular abscesses containing actively dividing mycobacteria.[62]

The radiologic features of tubercular meningitis are indistinguishable from those associated with fungal infections. Leptomeningeal thickening may be noted, particularly in the area at the base of the skull. MRI may be helpful in distinguishing tuberculomas from tubercular abscesses. Tuberculomas may be single or multiple. Like abscesses, they more commonly appear in the supratentorial space and can often be found at the gray-white interface. On T2-weighted MRI sequences they are isointense, frequently with a low-signal center.[42] On contrast-enhanced studies they are at times described as "target lesions." There may be ring enhancement with a small area of enhancement or calcification in the center of the lesion.[33] A mass effect is not usually present.[66] Although tubercular abscesses are also most commonly found in the supratentorial space, they have a number of unique imaging characteristics. These abscesses are often solitary. They are generally larger and can appear multiloculated on imaging studies.[33] They usually enhance, cause a mass effect, and are surrounded by significant edema. Magnetic resonance spectroscopy (MRS) can be used to help differentiate these lesions from neoplasms. Tubercular abscesses will have elevated lipid and lactate peaks without a significant increase in cell membrane markers such as choline.[67]

Purified protein derivative skin tests for *M. tuberculosis* are unreliable in patients with HIV. CSF cultures are positive in approximately a third to two thirds of patients with tubercular meningitis, and it may be weeks before they turn positive.[64,68] Acid-fast bacillus staining is often negative. Acid-fast bacillus PCR has higher sensitivity, but a negative PCR result does not rule out *M. tuberculosis* in the CNS. CSF typically demonstrates an elevated white blood cell count with a lymphocytic predominance. This is less pronounced in the setting of HIV.[69] CSF protein and CSF viscosity are also elevated. CSF glucose is typically decreased.

Tubercular meningitis only rarely requires a biopsy for diagnosis, but it may cause obstructive hydrocephalus requiring placement of an extraventricular drain or shunt by the neurosurgeon. *M. tuberculosis* brain abscesses, however, frequently require surgical drainage. These multiloculated lesions typically have pus with abundant acid-fast bacilli that can be easily cultured. Vascular granulation tissue may be present at the periphery of the lesions. Histologic evaluation of parenchymal lesions in patients with MAC demonstrates poorly formed granulomas with the greatest concentration of organisms located perivascularly. Necrosis and parenchymal infarctions can also be found.[70,71]

CNS tuberculosis in the setting of HIV is treated with multidrug regimens. Treatment duration varies but can extend to a year or more. The role of steroids in treating tubercular meningitis in the setting of HIV/AIDS is unknown.[72] The standard of care for the parenchymal tubercular CNS lesions in AIDS patients is even less firmly defined. Steroids may be added to the treatment regimen to decrease inflammation and the mass effect. In addition to establishing a diagnosis, surgical decompression for a significant mass effect or increase in intracranial pressure may be necessary.[73] Treatment of CNS MAC in HIV patients involves HAART in addition to a multidrug regimen that includes ethambutol and macrolide antibiotics. Mortality, however, is higher, with a large proportion of patients dying of this disease.[74,75]

Viral Infections

Progressive Multifocal Leukoencephalopathy

JC virus is a ubiquitous DNA polyomavirus that infects most individuals before adulthood. It remains latent in B lymphocytes, monocytes-macrophages, hematopoietic stem cells (CD34+), and renal epithelial cells. Reactivated in the setting of immune suppression, progressive multifocal leukoencephalopathy (PML) is usually diagnosed in HIV-positive patients when CD4+ T-cell counts fall to less than 100 cells/µL. Once reactivated, JC virus can spread via B lymphocytes to the CNS, where it replicates in oligodendrocytes and leads to their death. Demyelination follows. Subacute neurological decline with focal symptoms develops, depending on the location of the lesions. Seizures may occur. The disease progresses and is often fatal. In the pre-HAART era, evidence of PML was found in up to 5% of HIV-positive patients at autopsy,[76] but the incidence has decreased significantly during the HAART era.[77] MRI reveals areas of increased signal in the white matter on T2/FLAIR sequences, with corresponding decreased signal intensity on T1-weighted images (Fig. 45-2) This is most pronounced posteriorly but can be found anywhere in the brain, including the posterior fossa. The lesions are often multifocal and have an asymmetric distribution. Because of the blunted immune response, enhancement, edema, and a mass effect are frequently absent. Enhancement after contrast administration, although rare, is associated with improved survival.[78] There is less atrophy than is typically associated with HAE.[42] Unlike some opportunistic infections, which may improve radiographically with treatment, PML rarely does. Correlative imaging studies such as MRS are seldom helpful.

Anti–JC virus antibodies are present in up to 75% of healthy adults in developed countries.[79] JC virus is detected in serum by PCR in 2% to 3% of the population, and its detection is not pathognomonic for JC disease.[80] PML is often associated with a decreased CD4+ T-cell count and elevated viral load.[77] CSF rarely demonstrates pleocytosis. Protein is elevated in approximately half of the patients, but there is usually no decrease in glucose.[77] The lack of inflammatory findings in the CSF correlates with the lack of meningeal signs in the patient. CSF PCR for JC virus is highly specific, but the sensitivities reported have been quite variable (57% to 90%).[81,82] For unclear reasons, the sensitivity of CSF JC virus PCR appears to be decreasing during the HAART era.[83]

With the low sensitivity of CSF studies and the lack of radiographic response to empirical therapy, brain biopsy plays an important role in this setting. Approximately half of the patients who undergo biopsy because of negative CSF PCR have a diagnosis of PML on biopsy. Histologic examination reveals demyelination accompanied by "bizarre"-looking astrocytes with pleomorphic nuclei, as well as enlarged oligodendrocyte nuclei containing virions on electron microscopy. The spherical and filamentous virion particles are sometimes described as "spaghetti and meatballs." There is only scant evidence of perivascular inflammation.[42] Immunohistochemistry can be performed to evaluate for the presence of the JC virus capsid protein VP-1 in oligodendrocyte nuclei. JC virus PCR can also be performed on the biopsy tissue.

No specific treatment of PML is available. There have been some reports of the viral DNA inhibitor cidofovir being used.[84,85] The mainstay of treatment has been immune reconstitution via HAART. In the HAART era, survival has increased to a median of greater than 1 year. This is particularly likely if the CD4+ count is greater than 50 at the time of initial PML diagnosis.[77] One of the potential side effects of treatment with HAART is an exacerbated immune response in the CNS. This immune reconstitution syndrome is discussed in greater depth later in this chapter.

Cytomegalovirus

The majority of adults in the United States are infected with CMV, a herpesvirus. Its prevalence is even greater in the developing world. CMV remains latent and asymptomatic in immunocompetent individuals but can reactivate when immunity wanes, as in HIV patients with CD4+ T-cell counts lower than 50 cells/µL.

CMV can cause myriad neurological syndromes, including encephalitis, myelitis, polyradiculopathy, and polyneuropathy. Encephalitis often involves the periventricular tissue and the brainstem, tends to occur concomitantly with meningitis, and

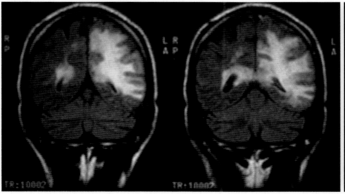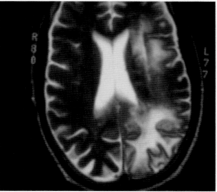

FIGURE 45-2 MRI features of progressive multifocal leukoencephalopathy. Large multifocal areas of high signal intensity are seen on FLAIR sequences (*left*) and T2-weighted image (*right*).

may be associated with stroke. The myelitis is subacute in onset and can resemble similar syndromes found in patients with autoimmune disorders or other infectious conditions. It has been hypothesized that both direct viral infection of the spinal cord and a misdirected immune attack play roles in the development of this syndrome.[86] The polyradiculopathy associated with CMV most commonly affects the lumbar spinal nerve roots. Patients have bilateral lower extremity weakness and bowel and bladder symptoms. Sensory symptoms include numbness and paresthesias. Neurological examination reveals a decrease in reflexes consistent with a lower motor neuron syndrome.[87] Finally, patients may also have a subacute syndrome of sensory and lower motor symptoms secondary to a multifocal polyneuropathy.

MRI in patients with encephalitis may demonstrate focal findings, particularly increased signal on T2/FLAIR images, with rare enhancement in the ependymal region, the periventricular white matter, and elsewhere in the brain or brainstem. The periventricular calcifications of congenital CMV infection are not seen in HIV.[33] If there is a meningeal component, leptomeningeal enhancement may be noted. Myelopathy exhibits similar findings in the spinal cord. Patients with radiculopathy may demonstrate enhancement of the nerve roots. A high percentage of the population has previously been exposed to CMV and is seropositive, so antibody titers are not helpful. CSF may reveal increased protein and glucose levels, as well as white blood cells. CMV grows very slowly in culture, which has largely been superseded by CMV antigenemia and PCR-based assays. Both have high sensitivity and specificity in HIV-positive individuals with encephalitis.[88] However, CMV PCR positivity is not sufficient by itself for diagnosis because CSF CMV PCR may also be positive in individuals with systemic CMV infection in the absence of neurological syndrome.[89] Histologic evaluation, when performed, reveals eosinophilic intranuclear inclusions with surrounding halos. Specific treatment of CMV consists of ganciclovir or foscarnet, or both. HAART may also help reconstitute the immune system. Unfortunately, the mortality rate is high, with death often occurring within weeks.

Treponema pallidum and Bartonella

Infection by the bacterium *T. pallidum*, the cause of syphilis, is common in HIV/AIDS patients and should be considered in the differential diagnosis of those with neurological symptoms. The manifestations of the disease differ in HIV-infected individuals as a consequence of their immunocompromised condition. The tertiary stage of syphilis is associated with diffuse systemic involvement, including the CNS. Syphilitic meningitis[90] or meningovasculitis,[33] the symptoms of which resemble many of the other opportunistic infections of the CNS discussed earlier, commonly develop in patients with HIV. A third CNS syphilitic syndrome that appears more frequently in HIV-infected patients is subacute polyradiculopathy.[91] The classic manifestations of tertiary syphilis, such as general paresis of the insane, tabes dorsalis, and cerebral gummas, are less common in the HIV/AIDS setting.[92]

The gram-negative bacteria *Bartonella henselae* and *Bartonella quintana* are the causative agents of cat-scratch disease and bacillary angiomatosis, respectively. Usually self-limited in immunocompetent individuals, systemic disease with florid meningoencephalitis is much more common in AIDS patients. The diagnosis should be suspected in those with typical skin lesion or lymphadenopathy.[93-95]

ACQUIRED IMMUNE DEFICIENCY SYNDROME–RELATED MALIGNANCIES

Malignancies associated with HIV/AIDS include Kaposi's sarcoma, Hodgkin's lymphoma, non-Hodgkin's lymphoma (NHL), squamous cell carcinoma, plasmacytoma, and leiomyosarcoma.[96,97] When encountered in the AIDS population, these tumors are frequently associated with viral infections, which are presumed to play a role in their pathogenesis. Direct involvement of the CNS by these tumors is rare, with one exception: primary central nervous system lymphoma (PCNSL). It should be remembered that other primary and metastatic CNS tumors also occur at high frequency in HIV-positive patients, especially with the advent of HAART and the prolongation of life associated with its use.[98] In the following section we review AIDS-related PCNSL, followed by a discussion of other AIDS-related malignancies.

Primary Central Nervous System Lymphoma

PCNSL is a rare NHL that accounts for less than 5% of primary CNS tumors.[99] Before the emergence of HIV/AIDS, PCNSL was most often seen either in the setting of known immunocompromised status or with advanced age. The emergence of the AIDS epidemic was mirrored by a rise in the incidence of PCNSL, and it soon became an AIDS-defining illness. Unlike PCNSL in the population at large, the AIDS-associated variant is relatively resistant to treatment and usually follows an aggressive course. Fortunately, with the advent of HAART, it has become less common and may be more amenable to treatment. In approximately 2% of HIV-infected individuals in the developed world, PCNSL will be diagnosed in their lifetime, but autopsy series suggest that the incidence may be as high as 10%.[100]

The clinical manifestations of PCNSL are highly variable and depend on the CNS site or sites involved. The tumor is often but not always multifocal and occupies white matter spaces preferentially. Symptoms range from nonspecific (i.e., nonlocalizing headache, mild encephalopathy, delirium) to those associated with discrete lesions in so-called eloquent areas of the brain. PCNSL is second only to cerebral toxoplasmosis as a cause of space-occupying CNS disease in the developed world and needs to be considered in any HIV-infected patient with either a single or multiple contrast-enhancing lesions.

PCNSL usually demonstrates homogeneous contrast-enhanced lesions with either a hypodense appearance (on CT) or low signal intensity (on T1-weighted MRI) (Fig. 45-3). The lesion or lesions are frequently concentrated in the periventricular regions. The use of metabolic imaging, especially single-photon emission spectroscopy after thallium administration, may show avid uptake of the radiotracer in areas of contrast enhancement.[101] Other metabolic imaging techniques, including positron emission tomography and MRS, have been less widely used, and their sensitivity and specificity remain unclear.

The entire neuraxis (eyes, brain, spinal cord, and CSF spaces) must be evaluated for the presence of PCNSL if suspected. With the exception of the eyes, all these spaces are commonly affected in AIDS-related PCNSL. Because ophthalmologic involvement requires special treatment considerations, a careful slit-lamp evaluation to rule out vitreal tumor should be performed despite its infrequency. CSF should be examined (when safe to obtain) and a large volume sent for cytopathologic evaluation in addition to routine tests. It is possible to make the diagnosis with CSF alone in some cases, thus avoiding the need for brain biopsy. We suggest review of the Wright stain used for routine cell count by hematopathologists, as well as review of the Papanicolaou stain by cytopathologists. Flow cytometry on a CSF sample containing a predominant lymphocyte population may be useful to confirm clonality.

A strong association exists between AIDS-associated PCNSL and infection with Epstein-Barr virus (EBV).[101] The potential mechanisms responsible for EBV transformation of lymphoid cells in this setting include coinfection with both EBV genotypes, the presence of particular deletions in EBV-associated membrane

FIGURE 45-3 T1-weighted contrast-enhanced (*left*) and T2-weighted (*right*) coronal images of a patient with primary central nervous system lymphoma affecting the corpus callosum and right cerebellar hemisphere (*arrows*).

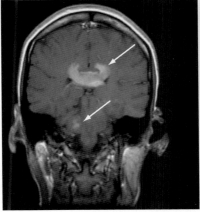
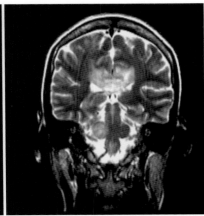

proteins, and aberrant regulation of EBV-associated gene promoters and enhancers.[102,103] For this reason, attempts to diagnose suspected PCNSL from CSF by PCR, even in the absence of suspicious cells, are ongoing.[104,105] Because EBV infection is common, the presence of EBV-specific DNA in CSF alone should not be considered diagnostic of PCNSL.

The neurosurgeon will often be called on to biopsy suspected PCNSL because the course of the disease is aggressive and treatment delays can result in significant morbidity. The diagnosis itself (usually by stereotactic biopsy) has high specificity in most cases.[106,107] Exceptions occur, especially when patients have received corticosteroids before biopsy because these drugs are acutely lympholytic and may transiently obscure the diagnosis. As with all PCNSL, there is no role for surgical intervention beyond diagnostic biopsy in AIDS patients.

Although PCNSL is fairly common, similar lesions caused by infectious agents in individuals with HIV/AIDS are more common. Worldwide, toxoplasmosis accounts for the majority of these lesions (see earlier). In some regions of the developing world, cerebral tuberculosis is also commonly encountered. Positive CSF cultures and stains for either of these conditions do not exclude the coexistence of PCNSL. Nevertheless, empirical treatment of these conditions often precedes attempts at biopsy in many cases. Despite its high specificity, biopsy in HIV/AIDS patients carries an increased risk for morbidity and mortality over that in the general population.[108] Risks for infection, bleeding, and death are increased. Thus, many advocate the use of empirical antimicrobial treatment for a defined period in conjunction with close clinical observation for signs of either improvement or deterioration. The majority of patients with cerebral toxoplasmosis show signs of clinical improvement within 3 days of treatment, and improvement on neuroimaging follows within 7 to 10 days. In the case of suspected tuberculosis, improvement occurs less rapidly. Therefore, if this approach is adopted, careful clinical assessment must be maintained, and biopsy should be performed in any person with early deterioration after the initiation of empirical treatment of presumed infectious disease.

Treatment of AIDS-related PCNSL is difficult because immune suppression plays a central role. In the pre-HAART era, survival after diagnosis rarely exceeded 3 months, even with treatment, although palliation of symptoms was often achieved.[109] Whole-brain radiotherapy (WBRT) has played an important role in the treatment of AIDS-related PCNSL. Before the use of HAART, chemotherapy—a mainstay of treatment in immunocompetent patients—was associated with high morbidity and mortality. Survival after WBRT alone in PCNSL patients is approximately 15 months[110,111] and decreases to 2 to 5 months in AIDS patients.[112] The addition of HAART to this regimen results in improved survival over the use of WBRT alone.[113] Protease inhibitors, an important component of HAART, may enhance the effects of radiation.[114,115]

Methotrexate-based chemotherapy regimens, the standard of care in immunocompetent patients, are being used with greater frequency in those with AIDS-related PCNSL. HAART has rendered more AIDS patients suitable for chemotherapy and has led to cautious optimism in improving survival.[115] Furthermore, treatment strategies that also target EBV are under way and may improve survival.[116] Despite these advances, AIDS-related PCNSL remains difficult to treat, and improved survival outcomes remain an elusive goal for many.

Other Acquired Immune Deficiency Syndrome–Related Malignancies

Both Kaposi's sarcoma[117] and leiomyosarcoma[118-120] are known to develop in the brains of HIV-infected individuals, but they are rare. Systemic NHL can involve the leptomeninges and, in some series, has been observed in the majority of cases.[120,121] The use of HAART has dramatically decreased the incidence of meningeal involvement from systemic NHL.[121] As shown in Figure 45-4, meningeal involvement can be extensive and cause significant neurological morbidity. Finally, lung cancer is also increased in patients with HIV and is a frequent cause of NS metastasis.[98]

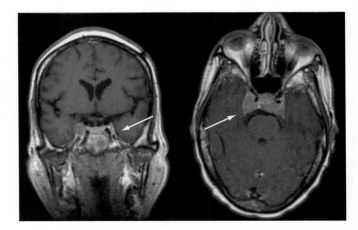

FIGURE 45-4 T1-weighted contrast-enhanced coronal (*left*) and axial (*right*) magnetic resonance images showing an enhancing mass (non-Hodgkin's lymphoma) involving the parasellar region with involvement of the clivus and cavernous sinus (*arrows*). The patient had ophthalmoplegia characterized by bilateral lateral rectus paresis and right ptosis. Cerebrospinal fluid cytology was positive.

HUMAN IMMUNODEFICIENCY VIRUS TREATMENT–RELATED NEUROTOXICITIES

The value of HAART in the treatment of HIV/AIDS is unquestionable. As with all therapies, however, side effects can be dose limiting. The predominant neurological consequence of HAART therapy is peripheral neuropathy. The nucleoside analogues, a critical component of HAART therapy, are associated with a dose-dependent distal sensory polyneuropathy.[122,123] More recently, protease inhibitors have also been implicated.[124] The incidence of distal sensory polyneuropathy has decreased as awareness of this effect has led to lower doses in contemporary HAART regimens. As noted earlier, the causes of peripheral neuropathy in HIV-positive persons may be multifactorial and include HIV infection itself, opportunistic infection, and nutritional deficiencies.

Restoration of immune competence as a result of HAART can paradoxically cause clinical deterioration because of innocent bystander–like effects. Immune responses directed against infectious agents may also damage the tissues involved. This syndrome is known by a number of names, including immune reconstitution inflammatory syndrome (IRIS), immune reconstitution syndrome, and immune restoration disease. Our discussion here is limited to its role in the CNS.

IRIS has been described in the CNS in the setting of many opportunistic infections, including PML, CMV, *M. tuberculosis*, MAC, and *Cryptococcus*.[125-127] The risk for development of this syndrome appears to be higher when initiating HAART. It also appears more likely when multiple infections are present.[125,128,129]

The neurological symptoms of IRIS, like those of the opportunistic infections and HIV-associated malignancies, are protean and largely dependent on location. Generalized symptoms can occur (e.g., impaired concentration and somnolence) and might also be the result of proinflammatory cytokines and other irritants on nervous system tissue. The onset of symptoms typically occurs within 2 months of initiating HAART.[125]

Imaging studies often reveal contrast enhancement. When opportunistic infection does not cause significant enhancement, such as in PML, imaging can be of significant value in differentiating infection from IRIS.[130] Unfortunately, many opportunistic infections are also associated with radiographic enhancement, sometimes obscuring the difference between treatment effect and progressive disease. The neurosurgeon may be called on to perform a biopsy to help determine the cause of the clinical deterioration. Histologic evaluation in patients with IRIS generally reveals diffuse cytotoxic T-cell infiltrates.[130] Residual histologic characteristics of the opportunistic infection might also be present.

Management of IRIS is problematic. The overarching goal of HAART—control and prevention of AIDS-associated illnesses—must be balanced against the short- and long-term consequences of bystander immune effects. Seldom should HAART be discontinued in the setting of IRIS. Some authors have suggested using steroids to dampen the immune response, particularly if significant cerebral edema or a mass effect is present.[130]

CONCLUSION

The neurological manifestations of HIV/AIDS and its treatment are many. The clinician must consider the possibility of multifactorial causes, many with similar clinical and radiographic features. Proper management of AIDS patients requires a team approach, ideally with an AIDS-experienced physician at the helm. The role of the neurosurgeon in treating those with HIV/AIDS varies tremendously with individual circumstances and may range from routine neurosurgical procedures in the chronically infected to emergency diagnostic procedures in the acutely ill. In this chapter we have attempted to provide a framework for understanding the ways in which the nervous system can be affected by HIV/AIDS, with a goal of aiding the neurosurgeon in decision making when consulted on these challenging cases. We have attempted to avoid dogmatic paradigms and schemata in addressing patient management because practice patterns are evolving and vary significantly between the developed and developing world. It is our goal to provide the reader with a comprehensive knowledge-based approach to HIV/AIDS patients applicable across a variety of practice settings.

SUGGESTED READINGS

Black KE, Baden LR. Fungal infections of the CNS: treatment strategies for the immunocompromised patient. *CNS Drugs.* 2007;21:293.

Cherry CL, McArthur JC, Hoy JF, et al. Nucleoside analogues and neuropathy in the era of HAART. *J Clin Virol.* 2003;26:195.

Collazos J. Opportunistic infections of the CNS in patients with AIDS: diagnosis and management. *CNS Drugs.* 2003;17:869.

Cornblath DR, Hoke A. Recent advances in HIV neuropathy. *Curr Opin Neurol.* 2006;19:446.

Di Rocco A. Diseases of the spinal cord in human immunodeficiency virus infection. *Semin Neurol.* 1999;19:151.

Dorsey SG, Morton PG. HIV peripheral neuropathy: pathophysiology and clinical implications. *AACN Clin Issues.* 2006;17:30.

Engsig FN, Hansen AB, Omland LH, et al. Incidence, clinical presentation, and outcome of progressive multifocal leukoencephalopathy in HIV-infected patients during the highly active antiretroviral therapy era: a nationwide cohort study. *J Infect Dis.* 2009;199:77.

Hamlyn E, Easterbrook P. Occupational exposure to HIV and the use of post-exposure prophylaxis. *Occup Med (Lond).* 2007;57:329.

Kastrup O, Wanke I, Maschke M. Neuroimaging of infections of the central nervous system. *Semin Neurol.* 2008;28:511.

Marra CM. Bacterial and fungal brain infections in AIDS. *Semin Neurol.* 1999;19:177.

Mitsuyasu RT. Non–AIDS-defining malignancies in HIV. *Top HIV Med.* 2008;16:117.

Offiah CE, Turnbull IW. The imaging appearances of intracranial CNS infections in adult HIV and AIDS patients. *Clin Radiol.* 2006;61:393.

Ortiz G, Koch S, Romano JG, et al. Mechanisms of ischemic stroke in HIV-infected patients. *Neurol.* 2007;68:1257.

Shelburne SA III, Hamill RJ. The immune reconstitution inflammatory syndrome. *AIDS Rev.* 2003;5:67.

Skiest DJ, Crosby C. Survival is prolonged by highly active antiretroviral therapy in AIDS patients with primary central nervous system lymphoma. *AIDS.* 2003;17:1787.

Smith AB, Smirniotopoulos JG, Rushing EJ. From the archives of the AFIP: central nervous system infections associated with human immunodeficiency virus infection: radiologic-pathologic correlation. *Radiographics.* 2008;28:2033.

Travis J, Varma A, duPlessis D, et al. Immune reconstitution associated with progressive multifocal leukoencephalopathy in human immunodeficiency virus: a case discussion and review of the literature. *Neurologist.* 2008;14:321.

Van Rie A, Harrington PR, Dow A, et al. Neurologic and neurodevelopmental manifestations of pediatric HIV/AIDS: a global perspective. *Eur J Paediatr Neurol.* 2007;11:1.

Wadhwa A, Kaur R, Bhalla P. Profile of central nervous system disease in HIV/AIDS patients with special reference to cryptococcal infections. *Neurologist.* 2008;14:247.

Whiteman M, Espinoza L, Post MJ, et al. Central nervous system tuberculosis in HIV-infected patients: clinical and radiographic findings. *AJNR Am J Neuroradiol.* 1995;16:1319.

Full references can be found on Expert Consult @ www.expertconsult.com

CHAPTER 46

Parasitic Infections

Oscar H. Del Brutto ■ Juan J. Figueroa ■ Hector H. Garcia

Parasitic diseases of the central nervous system (CNS) affect millions of people in the developing world, where most infections are linked to poverty and related conditions. In addition, increased tourism and immigration have turned some formerly geographically restricted parasitic infections into widespread conditions.[1] Parasites are divided primarily into protozoa and helminths. Protozoa are simpler unicellular microorganisms, whereas helminths are multicellular organisms with functional structures and complex life cycles that usually involve two or more hosts. Helminth parasites include nematodes (roundworms), trematodes (flukes), and cestodes (tapeworms). Infection of the CNS by parasites causes pleomorphic and nonspecific clinical syndromes, including seizure disorders, subacute or chronic meningitis, acute or subacute encephalitis, space-occupying brain lesions, stroke, and myelopathy.[2] In this chapter we review the most common parasitic infections of the CNS.

PROTOZOAL INFECTIONS

Malaria

Plasmodium infections have a complex biologic cycle. Humans are infected when the sporozoite forms of the parasite are inoculated through the skin during a blood meal by a female *Anopheles* mosquito. Sporozoites are carried to the liver of the host, where they hide and mature into tissue schizonts that liberate many merozoites, or products of asexual division. Merozoites enter the bloodstream, parasitize red blood cells, mature into trophozoites, and again divide to produce schizonts, which will rupture and simultaneously release many merozoites into the circulation. These merozoites invade a new group of red cells and the cycle continues. A proportion of trophozoites transform into male or female gametocytes. The life cycle is completed when the mosquito ingests gametocytes in infected human red blood cells and they reproduce sexually in the mosquito to form sporozoites.[3] Of the four species of malaria parasites that can infect humans, only *Plasmodium falciparum* causes cerebral malaria.

Clinical Manifestations

Cerebral malaria is a major cause of mortality in the world, mostly in Africa. The current definition of cerebral malaria requires all of the following: (1) unarousable coma, (2) evidence of acute infection with *P. falciparum*, and (3) no other identifiable cause of coma.[3] Fever is the initial complaint. This is followed by progressive somnolence associated with seizures, extensor posturing, and disconjugate gaze. Retinal hemorrhages suggest a poor prognosis. Some patients, particularly children, have focal signs related to cerebral infarcts or hemorrhage. Hypoglycemia, pulmonary edema, renal failure, bleeding diathesis, and hepatic dysfunction may complicate the course of the disease.[4] Up to 25% of patients die despite medical care. Permanent sequelae, more common in children, include mental retardation, epilepsy, blindness, and motor deficits.[5]

Diagnosis

P. falciparum may be seen by examining thin and thick blood smears with Giemsa stain; repeated examinations may be needed because the parasitemia is cyclic. Although cerebrospinal fluid (CSF) is usually normal, routine CSF examination is mandatory to exclude other causes of encephalopathy. Neuroimaging studies may show brain swelling or small hemorrhages in severe cases.[6]

Pathology

Brain edema and small ring hemorrhages in the subcortical white matter are found in almost 80% of fatal cases. The hemorrhaging is caused by extravasation of erythrocytes as a result of endothelial damage. The erythrocytes that form the ring hemorrhages are not parasitized, thus suggesting that the damage to blood vessels is related to the liberation of cytokines and vasoactive substances (humoral hypothesis). Capillaries and venules are plugged by clumped, parasitized erythrocytes, which causes brain damage because of obstruction of the cerebral microvasculature, reduced cerebral blood flow, increased concentrations of lactic acid, and ischemic hypoxia (mechanical hypothesis).[7] The brains of patients who survive the acute phase of the disease have granulomatous lesions (Dürck's nodules) at the site of the ring hemorrhages.

Treatment

Because of chloroquine-resistant strains of *P. falciparum*, quinine is the drug of choice for cerebral malaria. After an initial loading dose (20 mg/kg), the maintenance dose of quinine should be adjusted according to plasma concentrations to prevent accumulation. Quinidine may be used when quinine is not available. More recent clinical trials have shown that artemether, an artemisinin derivative, is equally as effective as but less toxic than quinine for the treatment of cerebral malaria.[8] Artesunate, another artemisinin derivative, can reduce mortality by more than a third in comparison to quinine.[9] Systemic complications must be recognized and treated. Symptomatic measures include anticonvulsants, sedatives, and osmotic diuretics. Corticosteroids are harmful to comatose patients with cerebral malaria.[10]

Toxoplasmosis

After the acquired immunodeficiency syndrome (AIDS) epidemic, toxoplasmosis has become a highly common parasitic disease of the CNS.[11] *Toxoplasma gondii* is a protozoan acquired by the ingestion of contaminated cat feces or by eating undercooked meat. In AIDS patients, CNS toxoplasmosis most often results from reactivation of a dormant infection with *T. gondii*. CNS toxoplasmosis may also develop in immunocompetent hosts during acute infections, and fetuses may be involved as a result of placental transmission of tachyzoites from women who acquire the disease during pregnancy.

Clinical Manifestations

Neurological symptoms rarely develop in immunocompetent hosts, although an acute encephalitis with fever, irritability, seizures, and drowsiness progressing to coma occurs in some cases. Immunocompromised hosts are also susceptible to an acute encephalitic syndrome or, more frequently, a subacute disease characterized by focal signs associated with seizures and signs of intracranial hypertension.[12,13] Apparently, this focal form predominates in AIDS patients who contracted latent infection before the depletion of CD4+ cells, whereas the diffuse encephalitic form, in which multiple parasite-containing microglial nodules are disseminated through the brain, is more common in those who became infected after they were immunosuppressed.[14] Meningeal signs rarely occur in patients with cerebral toxoplasmosis because the pathologic lesions are usually confined to the brain parenchyma and do not disseminate through the subarachnoid space.[14] In AIDS patients, the clinical picture is usually complicated because of concurrent infections.

Diagnosis

In normal hosts, a fourfold rise in serum antibody titer is a sensitive indicator of acute infection. The sustained persistence of specific IgM antibodies and high IgG titers in a significant proportion of individuals in the general population complicates the serologic interpretation for discrimination between latent infection and active infection, regardless of their human immunodeficiency virus serologic status.[15-17] There is controversy regarding the positive predictive value of high IgG titers for presumed CNS toxoplasmosis in AIDS patients.[18,19] The role of serology in AIDS patients is to establish at-risk status for active disease. Absence of antibodies in AIDS patients with CNS toxoplasmosis is rarely seen and should raise the possibility of an alternative diagnosis.[15,20] Neuroimaging studies show ring-enhancing lesions surrounded by edema; the lesions are usually multiple and may be located in the subcortical white matter, the basal ganglia, or the brainstem.[21] However, ring-enhancing lesions are not pathognomonic for cerebral toxoplasmosis because they may be observed in other diseases affecting AIDS patients, so definitive diagnosis requires histologic demonstration of the parasite. Empirical therapy followed by repeated neuroimaging studies at 3 weeks has been proposed as an alternative to biopsy in AIDS patients. Polymerase chain reaction (PCR) techniques have been introduced with promising results for the detection of T. gondii DNA from the CSF of patients with cerebral toxoplasmosis.[22]

Pathology

T. gondii may produce a focal or diffuse necrotizing encephalitis associated with perivascular inflammation. Cerebral abscesses may also occur and are most often located at the corticosubcortical junction, basal ganglia, and upper brainstem.[23] They consist of a necrotic center and a periphery in which multiple tachyzoites and cysts are seen together with patchy areas of necrosis and perivascular cuffing of lymphocytes. Glial nodules composed of astrocytes and microglial cells are common in the surrounding brain tissue.

Treatment

The combination of pyrimethamine (100 to 200 mg the first day, followed by 50 to 75 mg/day for 6 weeks) and sulfadiazine (4 to 6 g/day for 6 weeks) is the therapy of choice for CNS toxoplasmosis.[24] Clindamycin, clarithromycin, trimetrexate, piritrexim, and atovaquone are alternative drugs in patients in whom skin reactions to sulfadiazine develop.[25] In AIDS patients, permanent maintenance therapy with pyrimethamine and sulfadiazine is usually advised to decrease the risk for relapse.

African Trypanosomiasis

There are two different Trypanosoma diseases in humans, sleeping sickness or African trypanosomiasis, caused by Trypanosoma brucei, and Chagas' disease or American trypanosomiasis, caused by Trypanosoma cruzi. T. brucei enters the human body by direct inoculation through a bite of its vector, the tsetse fly.

Clinical Manifestations

T. brucei invades the CNS very shortly after inoculation and remains latent for a long time.[26,27] Thereafter, the disease enters into a stage in which the symptoms—fever, hepatosplenomegaly, and cervical lymphadenopathy (Winterbottom's sign)—suggest activation of the reticuloendothelial system. Somnolence, apathy, involuntary movements, and rigidity then appear. The neurological manifestations progress to dementia, stupor, coma, and death.

Diagnosis

T. brucei may be isolated from blood smears and from CSF, lymph node, and bone marrow aspirates. Repeated examinations and concentration techniques may be necessary. CSF examination may reveal lymphocytic pleocytosis, increased protein, and the typical Mott cells (plasma cells filled with eosinophilic inclusions of IgM). Demonstration of motile trypanosomes in CSF confirms CNS involvement. Chronic disease may be diagnosed by immune tests performed with serum or CSF. Neuroimaging findings are nonspecific and include diffuse changes in white matter, hyperintensity in the basal ganglia, and ventricular enlargement.[28,29]

Pathology

Autopsy studies have shown diffuse meningoencephalitis with infiltrates of macrophages, hypertrophied lymphocytes, and plasma cells (Mott cells) involving the meninges, perivascular spaces, and brain parenchyma. Perivascular demyelination of subcortical white matter and brain edema are seen is most cases. Hemorrhagic leukoencephalopathy may also occur.

Treatment

When CNS symptoms and signs of CSF inflammation have appeared, therapy requires the use of melarsoprol. This arsenic drug produces a severe reactive encephalopathy in about 10% of patients, half of whom die of it. The role of pretreatment with corticosteroids to prevent this reaction is unclear.[30]

American Trypanosomiasis

Triatomine bugs ("kissing bugs"), found mostly in the genus Triatoma, are the vector for T. cruzi. These insects infect humans by biting them to feed on their blood and defecating in the area. T. cruzi parasites in the insect's feces are then exposed to the bite wound or facial mucosae (eyes, mouth), usually by the bitten person when scratching. More rarely, infection can be acquired through uncooked food contaminated with infected bug feces, from blood/organ donation, or congenitally from an infected mother. An estimated 10 to 12 million people are currently infected with T. cruzi in Latin America, approximately 30% of whom, or 3 to 4 million, have or will eventually have consequent life-threatening cardiac or gastrointestinal disease, or both.[31-33] CNS disease is rare and occurs mostly in immunocompromised individuals.

Clinical Manifestations

Unilateral orbital edema (Romaña's sign) is considered the typical sign of acute Chagas' disease and reflects the site of a bite. The edema is associated with mild constitutional symptoms, although early invasion of the CNS by trypanosomes may cause a diffuse encephalopathy, particularly in infants and patients with AIDS.[34] Chronic disease is not usually associated with primary neurological complications; however, cardioembolic brain infarcts develop in some patients as a result of chagasic dilated cardiomyopathy. In addition, immunocompromised patients can experience reactivation of chronic infections, which results in a rapidly fatal meningoencephalitic syndrome similar to that observed in acute infections.[35]

Diagnosis

During the acute phase, diagnosis is possible by demonstration of *T. cruzi* in blood smears or CSF samples or by xenodiagnosis. Chronic disease is confirmed by serologic testing. PCR may also be used to support the diagnosis.

Pathology

The brains of patients with Chagas' disease involving the brain show multiple areas of hemorrhagic necrosis, glial proliferation, and perivascular infiltrates of inflammatory cells.[36]

Treatment

Antitrypanosomal drug therapy with either nifurtimox or benznidazole can cure most, if not all, congenitally infected infants when treated early in life, as well as 60% or more of infected children. The earlier the treatment in the course of infection, the higher the probability of cure. Chronic Chagas' disease has no specific treatment. Nevertheless, recent studies suggest that adults with clinical signs of early chronic Chagas' disease may also benefit from specific drug therapy.[37] However, antitrypanosomal drug therapy requires prolonged administration of one of the only two available drugs, both with significant side effects and elevated cost.

Free-Living Amebae

Free-living amebae of the genera *Acanthamoeba*, *Balamuthia*, and *Naegleria* may invade the CNS.[38] *Acanthamoeba* spp. and *Balamuthia mandrillaris* are opportunistic pathogens that affect mainly immunocompromised patients, and they invade the CNS by the hematogenous route from a primary infection of the skin or the respiratory tract. In contrast, *Naegleria fowleri* infection occurs in normal hosts and is acquired during swimming in warm fresh water; the parasites enter through the nasal cavity and migrate through olfactory nerves to the CNS.

Clinical Manifestations

Acanthamoeba spp. and *B. mandrillaris* produce a subacute disease called *granulomatous amebic encephalitis* characterized by low-grade fever, focal signs, seizures, intracranial hypertension, and behavioral changes; the disease runs a progressive course over a 2- to 8-week period.[38-40] *Balamuthia* infection is usually manifested initially by a centrofacial skin lesion, which allows the diagnosis. *N. fowleri* causes primary amebic meningoencephalitis, a fulminant disease carrying a grim prognosis that resembles acute bacterial meningitis.[38,41]

Diagnosis

Neuroimaging studies usually show multiple ring-enhancing lesions in patients infected with *Acanthamoeba* spp. and *B. mandrillaris* and diffuse edema in those infected with *N. fowleri*.[42] Examination of fresh CSF may reveal mobile trophozoites in patients with *N. fowleri* encephalitis. In contrast, the diagnosis of infection with *Acanthamoeba* spp. and *B. mandrillaris* usually rests on the demonstration of parasites in biopsy specimens.

Pathology

CNS infection by *Acanthamoeba* spp. and *B. mandrillaris* results in the formation of hemorrhagic brain abscesses surrounded by a granulomatous inflammatory infiltrate. Invasion of arterial walls by trophozoites causes a necrotizing angiitis that may lead to cerebral infarcts.[39,40] *N. fowleri* induces purulent meningitis associated with diffuse hemorrhagic necrosis of the brain parenchyma; involvement is more prominent in the frontal lobes and the olfactory bulbs, around the portal of entry of the microorganisms.[41]

Treatment

Amebic infections of the brain are highly fatal diseases with mortality exceeding 90%. Amphotericin B and rifampin may be used for *N. fowleri* infections, whereas surgery and metronidazole are advised for *Acanthamoeba* and *B. mandrillaris* brain abscesses.[43]

Amebiasis by *Entamoeba histolytica*

The intestinal parasite *E. histolytica* normally causes dysenteric diarrhea or liver abscesses. It may invade the CNS from the colon or liver in patients with severe infections (usually in the setting of advanced systemic amebiasis) and produce a multifocal encephalopathy.[43] Neuroimaging studies generally show multiple ring-enhancing lesions. The diagnosis of *E. histolytica* amebiasis is made by demonstration of parasites in biopsy specimens. Pathologic examination of tissue infected with *E. histolytica* shows multiple ill-defined brain abscesses formed by a central hemorrhagic area and a rim of necrotic tissue.[43] Surgery and metronidazole are advised for *E. histolytica* brain abscesses.[43]

HELMINTHIC INFECTIONS

Cysticercosis

Cysticercosis occurs when humans become intermediate hosts of *Taenia solium* by ingesting its eggs from contaminated food or through contact with the feces of *T. solium* carriers. After ingestion, the eggs mature into oncospheres, which are then carried into the tissues of the host, where cysticerci develop. Invasion of the parasites into the CNS causes neurocysticercosis (NCC).[44]

Clinical Manifestations

Epilepsy is the most common manifestation of NCC,[45] but a variety of focal neurological signs have also been described in patients with NCC. These manifestations usually follow a subacute course, thus making it difficult to differentiate NCC from neoplasia or other infections of the CNS. Hydrocephalus, mass effect, and cysticercotic encephalitis are the most common causes of intracranial hypertension in patients with NCC.[46,47] As a result of intense inflammation around cysticerci and diffuse cerebral edema, cysticercotic encephalitis is a particularly severe form of NCC characterized by headache, vomiting, generalized seizures, decreased visual acuity, and clouding of consciousness.[47] Manifestations of spinal cysticercosis include motor and sensory deficits, which vary according to the level of the lesion.[48]

Diagnosis

Accurate diagnosis of NCC is possible with proper interpretation of clinical data together with neuroimaging findings and results of immunologic tests.[49] Neuroimaging studies provide objective evidence about the location of lesions and the degree of the host inflammatory response against the parasites. The most typical findings are cystic lesions showing the scolex and parenchymal brain calcifications.[50] Other neuroimaging findings in NCC, such as ring-enhancing lesions, abnormal enhancement of the leptomeninges, hydrocephalus, and cerebral infarctions, are nonspecific because many other conditions cause similar changes on neuroimaging studies.[51] CSF may be normal in patients with parenchymal NCC. In the subarachnoid and ventricular forms of the disease, CSF analysis demonstrates a lymphocytic pleocytosis, an increased protein concentration, and a normal glucose concentration. The most accurate serologic test is immunoblotting.[52] However, false-positive results occur in patients who have cysticerci outside the CNS or antibodies arising from exposure only, and false-negative results are common in patients with a single cyst.[53]

Pathology

Within the CNS, cysticerci may be located in the brain parenchyma, subarachnoid space, ventricular system, or spinal cord. Parenchymal brain cysts usually lodge in the cerebral cortex or the basal ganglia. Subarachnoid cysts are most commonly located in the sylvian fissure or in the cisterns at the base of the brain. Ventricular cysticerci may be attached to the choroid plexus or may be floating free in the ventricular cavities. Spinal cysticerci may be found in both the cord parenchyma and the subarachnoid space.[54] Cysticerci may remain viable within the CNS for years and elicit few inflammatory changes in the surrounding tissue. In other cases, cysticerci enter the CNS and prompt a complex immune attack from the host that results in a process of degeneration ending with death of the parasite. The inflammation around cysticerci induces changes in cerebral tissues, including edema, gliosis, thickening of the leptomeninges, entrapment of the cranial nerves, angiitis, hydrocephalus, and ependymitis. Calcified cysticerci have been seen as inert lesions that do not cause further neuropathologic changes in the CNS. However, there is growing evidence that periodic remodeling of calcifications may be associated with the release of cysticercal antigens into the brain, which in turn may induce recurrent inflammatory reactions and relapsing symptoms.[55]

Treatment

Therapeutic approaches to patients with NCC include the use of cysticidal agents, as well as anticonvulsants and other symptom-relieving drugs. Surgical procedures are needed in some cases.[56] Praziquantel and albendazole have been used with success to treat NCC; these drugs destroy 60% to 80% of parenchymal brain cysticerci after a course of therapy. The most accepted regimens of cysticidal drugs are albendazole, 15 mg/kg per day for 1 week, and praziquantel, 50 mg/kg per day for 2 weeks.[57,58] It seems that patients with giant subarachnoid cysts require higher doses of albendazole or longer courses of therapy.[59] Although cysticidal drugs have changed the prognosis of most patients with NCC, the anecdotal nature of the first studies on these drugs generated criticism about their usefulness. Some authors claimed that cysticidal drugs do not modify the natural course of the disease. In a recent double-blind, placebo-controlled trial, albendazole was found to be safe and effective for the treatment of viable parenchymal brain cysticerci.[60] In this study, treated patients had better seizure control than the placebo group did, as reflected by a 67% reduction in the number of seizures. In addition, the number of cystic lesions that resolved was significantly higher in patients receiving albendazole. A recent meta-analysis of randomized trials of cysticidal drug therapy evaluated the effect of cysticidal drugs on neuroimaging and clinical outcomes of NCC.[61] According to this meta-analysis, cysticidal drug therapy results in better resolution of both colloidal and vesicular cysticerci, a lower risk for recurrence of seizures in patients with colloidal cysticerci, and a reduction in the rate of generalized seizures in patients with vesicular cysticerci.

Patients with cysticercotic encephalitis should not receive cysticidal drugs because they may exacerbate symptoms in this form of the disease. These patients must be managed with high doses of corticosteroids and osmotic diuretics.[47] Cysticidal drugs must be used with caution in patients with giant subarachnoid cysticerci because the host inflammatory response to destruction of the parasites may occlude small leptomeningeal vessels surrounding the cyst. In such cases, concomitant corticosteroid therapy is mandatory.[62] Patients with calcifications alone should not receive cysticidal drugs because these lesions represent dead parasites.

Hydrocephalus secondary to cysticercotic arachnoiditis requires placement of a ventricular shunt. The main complication of a ventricular shunt is the high incidence of shunt dysfunction. The high mortality rate (up to 50%) associated with the development of hydrocephalus from NCC is related to the number of surgical interventions for revision of the shunt.[63] A shunt that functions at a constant flow rate and does not allow spinal CSF to enter the ventricular system has been developed to treat these patients.[64] Inversion of CSF transit is the most important cause of shunt dysfunction because it allows parasitic debris to enter the ventricular system. The efficacy of this new shunt was compared with that of a conventional Pudenz-type shunt. After 1 year of follow-up, withdrawal of the shunt was necessary in 45% of patients with the Pudenz-type shunt but in only 30% of those with the new shunt.[65]

Although albendazole destroys many ventricular cysts, the inflammatory reaction may cause acute hydrocephalus if the cysts are located within the fourth ventricle or near the interventricular foramina of Monro. Ventricular cysts can be removed more safely by surgical excision or endoscopic aspiration.[66] The surgeon must consider the possibility of cyst migration between the time of diagnosis and the surgical procedure, and such migration must be ruled out with a neuroimaging study before surgery to avoid unnecessary craniotomies.[67] Shunt placement should follow or even precede the excision of ventricular cysts associated with ependymitis.

Echinococcosis (Hydatid Disease)

There are two main forms of echinococcosis: cystic hydatid disease (caused by *Echinococcus granulosus*) and alveolar hydatid disease (caused by *Echinococcus multilocularis*). In the cycle of hydatid disease, a herbivore usually harbors the larvae, mostly in the viscera, and a carnivore becomes infected with the adult tapeworm by eating raw viscera. In turn, the herbivore intermediate host acquires a larval infection by ingesting tapeworm eggs in pasture. Humans acquire the infection when they become intermediate hosts of these tapeworms by accidental ingestion of the eggs of *Echinococcus* spp.[68] After entering the body, the eggs transform into cysts that grow in the liver, lungs, heart, and CNS. In the latter, cysts may also result from metastatic dissemination of a visceral cyst.

Cystic Hydatid Disease (Echinococcus granulosus)

Clinical Manifestations

Cystic hydatid disease results in seizures or increased intracranial pressure of subacute onset and has a progressive course, often in

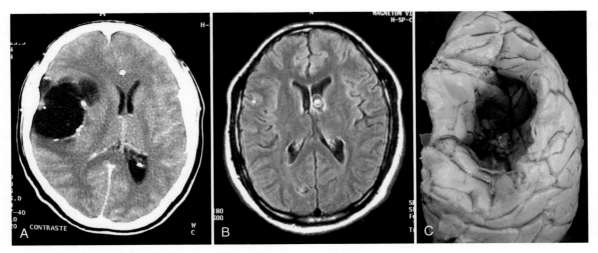

FIGURE 46-1 A, "Giant" cysticercal cyst in the right sylvian fissure. **B,** Intraventricular cysticercus. **C,** Brain impression after surgical excision of a hydatid cyst. *(Courtesy of the Neuropathology Museum, Instituto de Ciencias Neurologicas, Lima, Peru.)*

association with focal neurological deficits.[69] Orbital involvement in patients with cystic hydatid disease is manifested as proptosis and ophthalmoplegia.[70]

Diagnosis

On neuroimaging studies, cystic hydatid disease is characterized by a large nonenhancing vesicle that is well demarcated from the surrounding brain parenchyma (Fig. 46-1). Some lesions may be calcified.[71] Cystic lesions located in the subarachnoid space may be multiple and confluent. Intracranial or spinal epidural cysts have a biconvex shape or a multilocular appearance and may be associated with bone erosion. Immunologic diagnosis of cystic hydatid disease by enzyme-linked immunosorbent assay (ELISA) or enzyme-linked immunoelectrotransfer blot (EITB) is not accurate because of cross-reactions with other parasitic diseases. Moreover, these tests yield false-negative results in up to 50% of patients with intact brain cystic hydatid lesions.

Pathology

E. granulosus cysts are large, spherical, and well demarcated from surrounding tissue.[72] Within the CNS, these cysts may be located in the brain parenchyma, ventricular system, subarachnoid space, epidural space, orbits, and both the epidural and subarachnoid spaces in the spinal canal; epidural cysts tend to be associated with vertebral bone erosion.[73] Primary hydatid disease of the heart may be the source of an embolic cerebral infarction, usually in the territory of the middle cerebral artery.

Treatment

Current therapy for hydatid disease of the CNS is largely empirical, and experience is limited to anecdotal cases and uncontrolled studies. Surgical resection has been the classic approach to most hydatid cysts of the CNS.[74] Antiparasitic drugs are usually given before surgical resection in the case of intraoperative rupture of cysts or postoperatively to treat recurrent hydatid disease.[75] Therapy for hydatid disease of the CNS is differentiated into three categories: cystic hydatid disease of the brain, cystic hydatid disease of the spine, and alveolar hydatid disease.

CYSTIC HYDATID DISEASE OF THE BRAIN

Most hydatid cysts are removed with Dowling's technique, which consists of hydrostatic expulsion of the entire cyst by irrigation of saline solution between the lesion and the surrounding nervous tissue.[76] The aim of this technique is to remove the cyst without damaging its walls; however, accidental intraoperative rupture of the cyst occurs in 25% of cases.[74] Such rupture is associated with spillage of the cyst's contents (including the protoscolices), which may in turn cause an allergic reaction or recurrent hydatid disease.[76] Other complications associated with the Dowling technique include subdural effusions and intracranial hemorrhages. To avoid these complications, some surgeons puncture the cyst, aspirate its contents, irrigate the cyst with a hypertonic saline solution, and then remove the shrunken cyst. This is a modification of the percutaneous aspiration, injection, and reaspiration (PAIR) technique that is the currently accepted approach for removal of most hydatid cysts of the liver. Albendazole at doses ranging from 10 to 15 mg/kg per day, given for several 1-month cycles with therapy-free intervals of 14 days between cycles, cured 28% of patients and improved the condition of 51% of the 72% of remaining patients. Albendazole may be used in patients who are not candidates for surgical resection of lesions, as prophylactic therapy for those at risk for accidental rupture of the cysts perioperatively, or to treat recurrent cystic hydatid disease after surgery.

Praziquantel is not effective against hydatid cysts; however, the drug has protoscolicidal activity at doses of 40 mg/kg once per week and may have a role in the prevention of secondary reactions related to accidental spillage of protoscolices during surgery. Two trials suggested that combined albendazole and praziquantel therapy may be more effective than albendazole alone for preoperative prophylactic treatment of hydatid cysts.[77,78]

CYSTIC HYDATID DISEASE OF THE SPINE

The surgical approach to patients with spinal hydatid disease usually includes a combination of decompressive laminectomy, removal of cysts, excision of involved bone, and stabilization of the spine.[79] Almost 50% of these lesions may rupture during surgery because of the narrow space in which the surgeon has to work. Moreover, involvement of adjacent bone and multiplicity of lesions make complete removal of spinal cysts difficult. Hydatid disease recurs after surgery in up to 40% of patients, and this complication is associated with neurological deterioration. The use of albendazole, in a regimen similar to that recommended for patients with intracranial cystic hydatid disease, is advised to reduce such complications.[80]

Alveolar Hydatid Disease (Echinococcus multilocularis)

Clinical Manifestations

The neurological manifestations progress more rapidly and are more severe with alveolar hydatid disease than with cystic hydatid disease. Alveolar hydatid disease is characterized by focal neurological deficits, seizures, and intracranial hypertension.[81] Spinal cord involvement, associated with root pain and motor or sensory deficits below the level of the lesion, is more common in cystic hydatid disease than in alveolar hydatid disease, but it may be observed in both.

Diagnosis

On neuroimaging studies, alveolar hydatid disease is characterized by multiple lesions surrounded by edema, with ring-like enhancement mimicking other infectious or neoplastic diseases of the CNS.[82] Alveolar hydatidosis of the spinal canal may be visualized by magnetic resonance imaging (MRI), although the findings are nonspecific; computed tomography (CT) is better than MRI for demonstrating lytic lesions in vertebral bodies. Immunologic diagnosis is better with alveolar echinococcosis than with cystic hydatid disease. ELISA using purified and recombinant antigens (Em2 and II/3-10 ELISA) is the test of choice.[83]

Pathology

E. multilocularis cysts are small, group in clusters, elicit a severe inflammatory reaction from the host, and tend to metastasize both locally and distantly. They are usually located within the brain parenchyma.[81] Primary hydatid disease of the heart may be the source of an embolic cerebral infarction that is generally located in the territory of the middle cerebral artery.

Treatment

Alveolar hydatid disease is invasive, and total surgical removal usually requires resection of adjacent tissue. This approach may cause neurological deficits from cysts located in eloquent cerebral areas. Administration of albendazole should follow or even precede the surgical procedure, or it may be used as primary therapy in patients with inoperable alveolar hydatid disease.[84] The drug is given in regimens similar to those described for cystic hydatid disease. With a combination of surgery and cysticidal therapy, 50% of lesions regress, 40% remain static, and 10% continue to grow.[85]

Paragonimiasis

Paragonimiasis is caused by flukes of the genus *Paragonimus*. Humans acquire the infection by ingesting metacercariae in undercooked crustaceans. Metacercariae liberate larvae, which cross the intestinal wall and migrate to the lungs, where they mature into adult worms. Erratic migration of worms along the jugular veins and carotid arteries or hematogenous dissemination of larvae results in CNS involvement.[86]

Clinical Manifestations

Most patients have acute meningitis associated or not with focal neurological signs as a result of cerebral infarction secondary to arteritis.[86] Other patients with parenchymal brain granulomas have seizures, focal neurological deficits, and intracranial hypertension. Cerebral hemorrhages may occur along tracks of larval migration or as a result of the necrotizing vasculitis that occurs during granuloma formation.[87] Spinal paragonimiasis is associated with radicular pain, weakness, and sensory disturbances.[88]

Diagnosis

In patients with meningitis, analysis of CSF reveals a mild eosinophilic pleocytosis with increased protein concentration and normal glucose levels. Neuroimaging abnormalities include cystic or ring-enhancing parenchymal lesions, hemorrhages, or multiple calcifications that are typically located in the occipital and temporal lobes, are closely related to each other, and have the appearance of "soap bubbles."[89,90] The diagnosis rests on the demonstration of specific antibodies in blood and CSF or by finding *Paragonimus* eggs in sputum or adult worms in tissue samples.[86]

Pathology

The CNS lesions associated with paragonimiasis include necrotic tracks in the brain parenchyma, cystic lesions, granulomatous reactions, diffuse arachnoiditis, and obstructive hydrocephalus.[86] Parenchymal brain lesions predominate in the occipital and temporal lobes. Spinal lesions may be located in both the subdural and epidural spaces.[91]

Treatment

There is scant experience with the use of antiparasitic drugs in patients with cerebral paragonimiasis. Bithionol (40 mg/kg every other day for 1 month) improved the neurological status of 9 of 24 patients with different forms of cerebral involvement.[92] This study was performed before the availability of CT, and the results are difficult to interpret. Praziquantel (75 mg/kg per day for 2 days) has also been used with success in a few patients.[86] Corticosteroids are the primary form of therapy for patients with arachnoiditis to prevent further cranial nerve and blood vessel damage. Corticosteroids also reduce the edema surrounding active lesions and ameliorate the adverse effects related to destruction of parasites by praziquantel or bithionol. Antiepileptic drugs must be used in patients with cystic lesions and parenchymal brain calcifications who have seizures.

Surgical resection of intracranial lesions has a limited role in management of this disease.[91] The large size and multiplicity of lesions make radical resection difficult without damaging the surrounding brain parenchyma. Patients with calcified "soap bubble" lesions should not undergo surgery because resection of these lesions is rarely associated with clinical improvement.[93] Surgery is useful to remove cystic lesions located in the spinal subdural and epidural spaces and to decompress the spinal cord.[91] A ventricular shunt for relief of hydrocephalus may be necessary in patients with arachnoiditis.

Schistosomiasis (Schistosoma mansoni, haematobium, and japonicum)

Schistosomiasis, or infection with the flukes *S. mansoni*, *S. haematobium*, or *S. japonicum*, affects approximately 200 million individuals, mostly in sub-Saharan Africa; 10% have severe liver or urinary disease and 100,000 die per year. Schistosomiasis is endemic in most of sub-Saharan Africa, Asia, and Latin America. Other less frequent species include *Schistosoma mekongi* and *Schistosoma intercalatum*.[94]

CNS infection, a rare complication of schistosomiasis, is caused by aberrant location of eggs transported by the circulatory system. Among the different species. *S. japonicum* is associated more often with this rare complication (2% to 5% of cases), which contributes to seizures and epilepsy. CNS symptoms include seizures, focal neurological deficits, mass effect, or diffuse encephalitis. Nodular, ring-enhancing intraparenchymal lesions are seen on CT or MRI. Occasionally, eggs in the medulla may cause transverse myelitis as a result of granulomatous lesions (*S. mansoni*). Treatment involves the administration of praziquantel or oxamniquine. Surgery may be required for refractory epilepsy.[94,95]

Toxocariasis (*Toxocara canis* and *cati*)

Toxocariasis is a cosmopolitan nematode infection caused by *T. canis* or *T cati*. Most infected humans are asymptomatic, as shown by multiple seroepidemiologic studies demonstrating antibody prevalence ranging from 20% to 55%.[96] Human disease is mostly related to allergic, lung, or liver complications of larval migration. Larvae (measuring less than 0.5 mm) originate from the intestine and migrate through the circulatory system to the liver, lungs, and other locations (visceral larva migrans) or the eye (ocular larva migrans). Apparently, symptomatic CNS invasion is infrequent. It has, however, been associated with seizures, motor and sensory problems, meningitis, encephalitis, and other neurological syndromes.[96-98] Treatment with anti-inflammatory or anthelmintic drugs may be considered for severe complications of the brain. Given the scarce number of proven cases, there are no controlled trials to define therapy. Benzimidazoles and diethylcarbamazine seem to be the more useful regimens. As with other brain parasites (e.g., cysticercosis), in the initial days of treatment an intense inflammatory response may occur along with a subsequent increase in symptoms after liberation of antigen from the injured larvae. There are also some reports of successful management with corticosteroids, with or without specific anti-larval therapy. Surgery is rarely if ever required.

SUGGESTED READINGS

Carod-Artal FJ. Neurological complications of *Schistosoma* infection. *Trans R Soc Trop Med Hyg*. 2008;102:107-116.

Cobo F, Yarnoz C, Sesma B, et al. Albendazole plus praziquantel versus albendazole alone as a pre-operative treatment in intra-abdominal hydatidosis caused by *Echinococcus granulosus*. *Trop Med Int Health*. 1998;3:462-466.

Del Brutto OH, Roos KL, Coffey CS, et al. Meta-analysis: cysticidal drugs for neurocysticercosis: albendazole and praziquantel. *Ann Intern Med*. 2006;4:43-51.

Del Brutto OH, Santibañez R, Noboa CA, et al. Epilepsy due to neurocysticercosis: analysis of 203 patients. *Neurology*. 1992;42:389-392.

Derouin F, Leport C, Pueyo S, et al. Predictive value of *Toxoplasma gondii* antibody titres on the occurrence of toxoplasmic encephalitis in HIV infected patients. *AIDS*. 1996;10:1521-1527.

Dondorp A, Nosten F, Stepniewska K, et al. Artesunate versus quinine for treatment of severe falciparum malaria: a randomized trial. *Lancet*. 2005;366:717-725.

Duma RJ, Ferrell HW, Nelson EC, et al. Primary amebic meningoencephalitis. *N Engl J Med*. 1969;281:1315-1323.

Finsterer J, Auer H. Neurotoxocarosis. *Rev Inst Med Trop Sao Paulo*. 2007;49:279-287.

Garcia HH, Pretell EJ, Gilman RH, et al. A trial of antiparasitic treatment to reduce the rate of seizures due to cerebral cysticercosis. *N Engl J Med*. 2004;15:249-258.

Gottstein B, Jacquier P, Bresson-Hadni S, et al. Improved primary immunodiagnosis of alveolar echinococcosis in humans by an enzyme-linked immunosorbent assay using the Em2plus antigen. *J Clin Microbiol*. 1993;31:373-376.

Kennedy PG. Human African trypanosomiasis of the CNS: current issues and challenges. *J Clin Invest*. 2004;113:496-504.

Kirchhoff LV. Changing epidemiology and approaches to therapy for Chagas disease. *Curr Infect Dis Rep*. 2003;5:59-65.

Kusner DJ, King CH. Cerebral paragonimiasis. *Semin Neurol*. 1993;13:201-208.

Mohamed AE, Yasawy MI, Al Karawi MA. Combined albendazole and praziquantel versus albendazole alone in the treatment of hydatid disease. *Hepatogastroenterology*. 1998;45:1690-1694.

Phillips RE, Warrell DA. The pathophysiology of severe falciparum malaria. *Parasitol Today*. 1986;2:271-282.

Porter SB, Sande MA. Toxoplasmosis of the central nervous system in the acquired immunodeficiency syndrome. *N Engl J Med*. 1992;327:1643-1648.

Proaño JV, Madrazo I, Avelar F, et al. Medical treatment for neurocysticercosis characterized by giant subarachnoid cysts. *N Engl J Med*. 2001;345:879-885.

Raffi F, Aboulker J, Michelet C, et al. A prospective study of criteria for the diagnosis of toxoplasmic encephalitis in 186 AIDS patients. *AIDS*. 1997;11:177-184.

Viotti R, Vigliano C, Lococo B, et al. A. Long-term cardiac outcomes of treating chronic Chagas disease with benznidazole versus no treatment: a nonrandomized trial. *Ann Intern Med*. 2006;144:724-734.

Warrell DA, Looareesuwan S, Warrell MJ, et al. Dexamethasone proves deleterious in cerebral malaria. A double-blind trial in 100 comatose patients. *N Engl J Med*. 1982;306:313-319.

Full references can be found on Expert Consult @ www.expertconsult.com

CHAPTER 47

Surgical Risk of Transmittable Diseases

Donald E. Fry

The first reports of transmission of blood-borne pathogens from patients to surgeons occurred more than 50 years ago.[1,2] These early reports of "serum hepatitis" were generally viewed with a detached attitude by surgeons as something that occasionally happened, and these events did not arouse concern about occupational risks. With the recognition of hepatitis A virus (HAV) and hepatitis B virus (HBV) as distinct viral pathogens and the development of specific antibody detection methods, the scope of HBV infection in patients and surgeons was appreciated. Surgeons had a disproportionately higher prevalence of HBV positivity than did the population in general, and it was rapidly appreciated that transmission of the infection from patients to surgeons (and other health care workers [HCWs]) was a far more common event than had been appreciated. Moreover, a nonserotyped hepatitis was identified, and this indicated that yet another form of transmissible hepatitis existed after blood transfusion and other forms of percutaneous blood exposure.[3] This nonserotyped hepatitis was labeled non-A, non-B hepatitis (NANBH).[4] During the 1970s, evidence was mounting that surgeons and other HCWs worked in an environment with multiple potential hepatitis viruses, but an attitude of indifference persisted with respect to these risks.

In 1981, acquired immunodeficiency syndrome (AIDS) was first identified,[5] and subsequent investigations then characterized human immunodeficiency virus (HIV) as the putative agent. HIV infection was associated with blood transfusion and other mechanisms of percutaneous exposure to contaminated blood. During the 1980s, it became apparent that nearly 1 million individuals in the United States had HIV infection and that clinical AIDS was a uniformly fatal disease.[6] Furthermore, it became apparent that HIV infection was a latent disease that otherwise healthy-appearing individuals carried for a number of years before AIDS was evident clinically.[7] Events surrounding the recognition of AIDS led to great concern and anxiety in the surgical profession about the occupational risks for both AIDS and hepatitis infection.

More than 25 years has passed since the first AIDS cases were reported, and many events have temporized the great fears that surfaced about the occupational risks of this infection in the 1990s. The risk of occupational transmission has been proved to be very uncommon. The development of highly active antiretroviral therapy (HAART) has not eradicated HIV infection but has provided long-term quality life for many of these patients,[8] and by virtue of reduced circulating viral loads in these patients receiving treatment, HAART has further reduced the risks of transmission. On the hepatitis front, a highly effective HBV vaccine has been developed from recombinant technology that has dramatically reduced the risk of occupational HBV infection for surgeons. Unfortunately, these developments have created an environment of lassitude and indifference once again about occupational infection in the operating room.

HEPATITIS

The past 20 years have yielded a dramatic expansion in our understanding of the world of hepatitis infection. Currently, six distinct hepatitis viruses have been identified (Table 47-1). There

remains a probability that at least one additional virus remains to be characterized. At present, only HBV and hepatitis C virus (HCV) appear to be of great occupational concern to surgeons. The majority of the following discussion is limited to HBV and HCV infection.

HAV is transmitted by the fecal-oral route and is usually acquired after the ingestion of contaminated water or food products.[9] It is an RNA virus that causes an acute and frequently severe hepatitis syndrome. Infected individuals with the hepatitis syndrome (jaundice, malaise, and so on) are acutely ill, but seldom is the outcome of the infection lethal. Importantly, once HAV clinical infection has resolved, there is no state of chronic infection in the aftermath of the acute infection. The absence of a chronic state of infection and the infrequently identified transmission of HAV from blood or blood products do not make this a virus of occupational concern in health care.

Hepatitis E virus is identified primarily in Southeast Asia and is infrequently seen in the United States.[10] It too is transmitted by the fecal-oral route, and like HAV, there is no chronic infection after resolution of the acute infection. It is mentioned only for completeness.

Hepatitis D virus, also known as the delta agent, is an incomplete RNA virus that cannot cause infection or replicate without the coexistence of concurrent acute or chronic HBV infection.[11] It is seen principally in the intravenous drug abuse population. Infection with hepatitis D virus amplifies the severity of the underlying HBV infection. It is a blood-borne pathogen and theoretically could be an occupational infection for HCWs if preexistent HBV infection were present. Effective vaccination against HBV infection eliminates this risk.

Hepatitis G virus is the most recently identified agent (hepatitis F was putatively identified but has not been validated).[12] It is considered the same as the GB virus, where the "GB" initials came from the index infected surgeon who was the source of the virus used in early studies. It is blood borne and found commonly with HBV and HCV infection, and it has genetic homology to HCV. Hepatitis G virus is infrequently found as the sole agent in clinical hepatitis. It is present in as many as 1.4% of blood donors and persists in a chronic state for many years.[13] The full scope of its clinical relevance and its risk for occupational transmission continue to be debated.

Hepatitis B

HBV infection is the most thoroughly studied of the blood-borne hepatitis events in humans. HBV is a DNA virus that is very efficiently transmitted by exposure to blood or blood products. Before the era of effective vaccination, HBV infection was the most common and most serious of occupational infections for surgeons. A single hollow-needle percutaneous injury is associated with a 25% to 30% risk of transmission to a naïve host.[14] In society, intravenous drug abuse with shared needles has been a major source of transmission of the infection. The virus is a sexually transmitted disease, which has led to a national initiative to vaccinate the pediatric and adolescent populations against HBV.[15] Effective screening of the blood supply has virtually eliminated

TABLE 47-1 Specific Features of the Known Hepatitis Viruses That Have Currently Been Identified*

TYPE OF HEPATITIS	GENOME	VIRAL FAMILY	ROUTE OF TRANSMISSION	OCCUPATIONAL RISK
A	RNA	Picornaviridae	Fecal-oral	No chronic infection; no risk for occupational infection
B	DNA	Hepadnaviridae	Blood borne	More than 1 million chronically infected patients in the United States; documented vaccination eliminates the risk for new infection
C	RNA	Flaviviridae	Blood borne	About 3 million chronically infected patients in the United States; no vaccination; avoiding exposure is the only preventive strategy
D	RNA	Viroid	Blood borne	Not identified as an occupational risk; requires coexistent HBV infection; no risk with HBV vaccination
E	RNA	Caliciviridae	Fecal-oral	No chronic disease; not common in the United States; no occupational risk
G	RNA	Flaviviridae	Blood borne	Commonly called GBV-C; not associated with infection; not considered an occupational risk

*Only hepatitis B and hepatitis C are considered occupational pathogens.

contaminated units of transfused blood as a source of new cases of HBV infection.

Access of the HBV virus to the host results in binding and internalization of the virus within hepatocytes. Viral replication occurs at varying rates after infection. In only about 25% of acute infections is there a clinically discernible hepatitis syndrome.[16] The majority of cases either are characterized by a mild malaise without jaundice or have a completely indolent character. Among all acute infections, about 5% of cases result in chronic sustained infection that persists indefinitely.[17] The incidence of chronic infection is not related to whether acute infection was identified, which means that many individuals with chronic disease are unaware of the disease. This chronic state of infection is associated with sustained damage to the liver, although selected cases may have a persistent viremia without evidence of continued liver damage. Hepatocellular carcinoma, portal hypertension, and end-stage liver disease from hepatic cirrhosis are the consequences of the chronic disease for many patients.[18] An individual with chronic HBV infection is a reservoir of virus for the infection of others. It is currently estimated that more than 1 million individuals in the United States have chronic HBV infection,[19] and the numbers in the international community are many millions more.

HBV infection in surgeons in the era before the availability of a vaccine was quite common. In a 1996 study, about a third of surgeons in practice for more than 10 years had serologic evidence of previous HBV infection.[20] About a third had been vaccinated, but a third were serologically devoid of antibody and remained vulnerable to acute infection. It was estimated in the late 1980s by the Centers for Disease Control and Prevention (CDC) that 250 HCWs die annually from the consequences of occupationally acquired chronic HBV infection that had obviously been contracted many years previously.[21] A more recent analysis has attributed 75 to 250 deaths to occupationally acquired HBV infection for the year 2002.[22]

In the 1980s, a highly effective HBV vaccine was developed by using attenuated virus from infected patients.[23] Recombinant technology rapidly emerged and resulted in the development of an equally effective vaccine that was not derived from other persons. The vaccine is administered in three doses, with the second and third doses being given 1 and 6 months after the initial administration. About 95% of individuals will have an appropriate antibody response to the surface antigen of HBV. Documentation of antibody response is essential, with revaccination being necessary for those who do not seroconvert from the initial immunization effort. Revaccination after a failed initial attempt has a 30% to 50% probability of being successful.[24] Vaccination of all surgeons and HCWs is necessary, and not being vaccinated is unacceptable.

Hepatitis C

HCV was identified in 1989 and has for the most part been the virus responsible for NANBH.[25] HCV is an RNA virus with multiple different serotypes. It is a source of occupational infection for surgeons and HCWs, but it is less efficiently transmitted than HBV. A percutaneous needlestick from a hollow needle has about a 2% risk of transmission of the infection.[26] HCV shares many of the same epidemiologic characteristics of HBV with respect to high-risk populations of patients and means of infection within society.[27] Screening of the blood supply for antibody to the virus has dramatically reduced the risk for transfusion-associated infection.

The clinical sequelae after infection of the hepatocyte follow patterns similar to those of HBV. Like HBV, the majority of acute infections are clinically indolent and not associated with a clinical picture of hepatitis.[28] However, unlike HBV infection, rates of chronic infection are 60% to 80%.[29] The natural history of chronic disease is highly variable, with some patients progressing to end-stage liver disease or hepatocellular carcinoma and others having chronic antigenemia but not an evolving pattern of liver damage.[30] Still others may have spontaneous resolution of the infection at a later time. It has an unpredictable time course. Individuals who are antigen positive are infectious to others. There are 3 to 4 million persons in the United States who have chronic HCV infection,[31] and HCV has become the primary cause of disease leading to hepatic transplantation.[32]

There is no vaccine for HCV, although progress has been made with antiviral treatment of this infection.[33] HCV infection results in a circulating antibody that is believed to ineffectively neutralize the virus. There are multiple different serotypes of the virus, and reinfection can occur with the same viral type in patients who actually cleared the initial infection. The prospects for a vaccine are challenging when even acute infection does not confer protective immunity for the host against future infection. The antibody response may be delayed for up to 6 months after acute infection, which makes HCV detection in the blood supply more difficult in donors with recent acute infection.

HUMAN IMMUNODEFICIENCY VIRUS

HIV is a retrovirus. It is an RNA virus, and as a consequence of the enzyme reverse transcriptase, a complementary DNA (cDNA) is produced from the RNA template after the virus invades the target cell. Incorporation of viral cDNA into the host cell genome becomes the basis for the synthesis of viral proteins and replication of new viral units. The CD4+ lymphocyte becomes the major target of the virus, with lysis and loss of these cells being a fundamental issue in the immunodeficiency state that evolves, with subsequent clinical AIDS. Acute infection may be characterized by a modest and nonspecific viral syndrome or by no discernible symptoms at all. Without treatment, HIV infection progresses for 10 years or longer before AIDS emerges.

HIV infection is transmitted by sexual contact and by intravenous drug abuse. Vertical transmission from infected mothers to newborns has been dramatically reduced in frequency in the United States by the use of antepartum antiretroviral therapy.[34] Transmission secondary to blood transfusion has essentially been eliminated with effective screening procedures in the United States and western Europe. HIV infection remains an international pandemic, especially in the African continent, where preventive strategies have been ineffective and treatment of established infection has been unavailable. At present, about 750,000 people are living with HIV infection in the United States, and nearly 600,000 have died since recognition of the disease.[35]

Considerable effort has been extended in the evaluation and prevention of occupational HIV infection in HCWs. A serologic survey of more than 3000 orthopedic surgeons at a national meeting identified only 2 cases of HIV infection, both of which occurred in individuals with nonoccupational risks for infection.[36] Prospective evaluation of mucous membrane and percutaneous exposure events in HCWs has documented 57 cases of occupational infection (Table 47-2).[37] The rate of transmission to HCWs from percutaneous exposure is thought to be 0.3%.[38] Epidemiologic evaluation of HCWs in whom HIV infection has developed but who do not have nonoccupational risk factors for the disease has resulted in the identification of 139 cases of probable occupational transmission (Table 47-3).

At this time, no documented infections have been transmitted from patient to surgeon in the United States from percutaneous exposure events in the operating room. Epidemiologic evaluation has identified six probable infections in surgeons. When compared with HBV and HCV, the efficiency of transmission in the health care setting is much less with HIV. Long-term survivors with successful treatment of HIV infection are being seen with greater frequency, although concern has been expressed about the emergence of resistant strains as a result of long-term antiretroviral treatment. Much work has been, and is currently being, undertaken in an effort to prevent HIV infection with a vaccine. The changing antigenic manifestation of the virus from the constant mutation process has made stable antigen targets for vaccine development quite elusive.

PREVENTION OF OCCUPATIONAL INFECTION

Occupational infection with one of the viruses discussed previously has been the result of percutaneous or mucous membrane exposure to contaminated blood. Transmission events have generally occurred in the setting of exposure to blood when the infectious status of the patient was unknown. Because patients themselves may not be aware of their own infectious status and social risk factors for infection are not commonly discovered during the preoperative evaluation of a surgical patient, it is generally recommended that standard preventive measures be used in the care of all patients. Application of enhanced or relaxed preventive measures based on the surgeon's presumption of patient risk is not dependable and is discouraged. Preventive strategies are grouped into (1) personal protective barriers, (2) technical considerations, and (3) prompt response to exposure events. Of greatest importance is vigilance and constant

TABLE 47-2 Number of Patients with Documented Seroconversion to HIV after a Specific Exposure Incident*

OCCUPATION	NO. DOCUMENTED OCCUPATIONAL HIV INFECTIONS
Nurses	24
Clinical laboratory workers	16
Physicians, nonsurgical	6
Nonclinical laboratory workers	3
Housekeeping/maintenance workers	2
Surgical technician	2
Embalmer/morgue technician	1
Health aide/attendant	1
Respiratory therapist	1
Dialysis technician	1
Total	**57**

*All patients had negative serology at the time of the exposure event and then seroconverted to a positive HIV status after the event.

TABLE 47-3 Number of Health Care Personnel Who Are Thought to Represent Possible Seroconversions for Occupational HIV Infection*

OCCUPATION	NO. POSSIBLE OCCUPATIONAL HIV INFECTIONS
Nurses	35
Clinical laboratory workers	17
Health aide/attendants	15
Housekeeping/maintenance workers	13
Nonsurgical physicians	12
Emergency medical technicians	12
Other technicians/therapists	9
Surgical physicians	6
Dental workers/dentists	6
Dialysis technicians	3
Surgical technicians	2
Embalmers/morgue technicians	2
Respiratory therapists	2
Others	5
Total	**139**

*These cases were identified from the epidemiologic evaluation of health care workers reported to the Centers for Disease Control and Prevention with HIV infection but who were determined after case evaluation not to have nonoccupational risk factors for the infection.

awareness when using sharp instruments in the operating room. Many injuries are due to carelessness and could have been prevented by the surgeon having a keen appreciation of the dangers of avoidable behavior that leads to a percutaneous injury to self or a colleague.

Personal Protective Barriers

Much has been made of the value of using eye shields and double gloving to prevent contact of blood with the skin or mucous membranes of the surgeon. Every surgeon has had the experience of an arterial or irrigation spray in the face during an operation. Protective eyewear and face shields are available in every operating room and are mandated by the Occupational and Safety Health Administration (OSHA).[39] Observations in many operating rooms today will give testimony to the lassitude about occupational infection when one sees inadequate or no eye protection during operations where eye exposure is a real risk.

Double gloving has been shown in many studies to prevent blood contact by the hands of surgeons.[40-42] If surgeons wash their hands with isopropyl alcohol after a lengthy craniotomy or a major spine procedure, all of the stinging about the cuticles and elsewhere will be validation that nonintact skin is present. Sustained blood contact by hands with nonintact skin means that occupational infection is a potential risk. Double gloving will prevent blood contact, and the use of indicator systems permits prompt recognition when the glove barrier has been breeched.[43]

In a previous study, 90% of blood contact with the skin of the operating room team occurred on the hands and forearms (Table 47-4).[44] Reinforcement of the forearms with sleeve covers combined with double gloving extending above the level of the seam of the glove cuff of the surgical gown provides a double layer of protection to the area of the body most vulnerable to blood contact during operations. Use of these sleeves is most appropriate for operations involving the chest or abdomen, but they are certainly worth considering during craniotomy for trauma and major spine procedures, where significant blood loss can be anticipated. Wearing a plastic apron underneath the surgical gown and trauma boots that cover the feet up to the level of the knee are also options when intracranial hematomas are being managed surgically.

Technical Considerations

Safe surgery means a zero tolerance for avoidable behavior that leads to percutaneous injury. Sharp instruments must be handled with respect. Blunt-needle technology has been shown to reduce injuries[45] and has been endorsed by the American College of Surgeons (ACS)[46] and by the National Institute for Occupational Safety and Health (NIOSH).[47] Use of the surgical "way" station (e.g., Mayo stand) for the passage of loaded needle holders will prevent injury to the surgeon and scrub personnel from direct hand-to-hand exchanges.[48] Use of an electrocautery instead of a scalpel may reduce risks from knife injury. Some have advocated that selected common procedures be done without sharp instruments of any kind in the surgical field.[49] Towel barriers to cover bony edges of the cranial vault or spicules of bone in spine procedures can minimize inadvertent abrasions, glove tears, and punctures from these structures. Drills, saws, and rongeurs are all part of selected procedures and require attention to avoid injury. Avoidance of injury in the operating room is more attitude than technique.

Response to Exposure

Exposure events will occur. They should be recognized promptly and managed at an opportune moment. Blood contamination of the hand or forearm should ideally be managed by a surgical scrub of the site, but events at the time of the exposure commonly make this practice impractical. Glove violations or needle punctures require, at a minimum, removal of the glove, irrigation of the site with povidone-iodine or isopropyl alcohol, and then regloving. Exposed eyes should be rinsed promptly with sterile saline solution. Blood break-through of the surgical gown should result in removal of the gown, irrigation of the exposed skin, and regowning.

When exposure from a patient with known or suspected infection has occurred, a specific course of action is necessary. Current serologic testing for the index viruses must be performed for the exposed surgeon to document that preexistent disease is not present.[50] For HBV exposure, the current antibody status of the surgeon is important. Previous vaccination with a positive antibody response for the HBV surface antigen means that nothing

TABLE 47-4 Frequency of Blood Contact with the Skin of Personnel in the Operating Room or Blood Exposure from either a Percutaneous or Mucous Membrane Event in a 4-Week Prospective Study of Surgical Care at the University of New Mexico Hospital

TYPE OF OPERATION	TOTAL CASES STUDIED	NO. BLOOD CONTACT CASES	TOTAL PERSONNEL WITH BLOOD CONTACT	NO. PERSONNEL WITH BLOOD EXPOSURE
Orthopedic	201	56 (28%)	71	19
Gynecologic	81	24 (30%)	32	8
General surgery	75	19 (25%)	25	7
Otolaryngology	58	10 (17%)	13	1
Pediatric surgery	50	11 (22%)	22	3
Trauma/burn	45	21 (47%)*	37	7
Neurosurgery	43	11 (26%)	16	6
Cardiothoracic	26	15 (58%)†	36	6
Cesarean section	25	12 (48%)*	25	5
Others	80	11 (14%)	16	1
Total	**684**	**190 (28%)**	**293**	**63**

*$P < .05$.
†$P < .025$.
From Popejoy SL, Fry DE. Blood contact and exposure in the operating room. *Surg Gynecol Obstet.* 1991;172:480.

further needs to be done. If the serology indicates a weak reaction or no antibody response, a dose of HBV immune globulin and a dose of HBV vaccine should be given. If the exposed individual has not had a previous course of full vaccination, a dose of HBV immune globulin and HBV vaccine should be administered. The exposed surgeon should complete the full 6-month course of vaccination. If a surgeon is positive for the *core antibody* of HBV, that surgeon has previously had HBV infection. If this is a new finding for the surgeon, the presence of the core antigen for HBV needs to be evaluated because the surgeon may be one with unrecognized chronic infection. With the increased emphasis on HBV vaccination, it is hoped that there will be very few chronic HBV infections discovered after an exposure event in the operating room.

Because there is no vaccine for HCV, the exposed individual should have convalescent sera drawn to document whether seroconversion has occurred. Repeat serologic testing may be done 3 to 6 months after exposure. No prophylactic HCV antiviral treatment is recommended until evidence of active infection is documented. Exposure to patients with known HCV infection creates considerable anxiety, and early serologic testing at 10 to 12 weeks is commonly done. A test for HCV RNA may also be performed at the earlier time frame if potentially earlier diagnosis is desired. Because HCV seroconversion may occur later, a 6-month serologic evaluation for HCV infection is recommended.

There is no vaccine for HIV, but some epidemiologic evidence suggests that prophylactic antiretroviral therapy should be administered for known or suspected exposure.[51] The treatment should be continued for a full course with three drugs and serologic evaluation for seroconversion then completed.[52]

What should be the response to a severe exposure event when preexistent infection is not suspected? A safe course of action is to request serologic testing of the index patient. Most patients will give permission, especially if they know that the surgeon is also being tested. When serologic information about the index patient is not available for whatever reason, the surgeon may be advised to have appropriate serologic follow-up. Relative to HIV infection, the surgeon will have to make the decision for antiretroviral therapy. Indeed, surgeons engaged in invasive procedures with significant rates of exposure to patient blood (e.g., intracranial trauma, spine surgery) or those treating populations with high prevalence rates of infection (e.g., trauma patients) need to know their serologic status for all viral pathogens of concern and have it repeated on an annual basis.

THE INFECTED SURGEON

A great source of debate during the 1990s was whether surgeons who had contracted one of the blood-borne viral infections, by whatever means, should continue to engage in invasive procedures. Some have argued for routine testing of physicians and surgeons and recommend suspension of privileges for those who are positive. Others have pointed to an absence of evidence demonstrating that infected surgeons are a risk to their patients. The identification of a Florida dentist who apparently transmitted HIV infection to several of his patients, presumably by intention, really ignited the controversy.[53,54] Many states passed laws requiring various levels of action if physicians were known to harbor HBV or HIV infection. Although the intensity of the debate has receded, many punitive laws about infected surgeons remain.

There have been many clusters of HBV infection that have been transmitted from infected surgeons and dentists to patients.[55-57] The common feature for transmission is that the surgeon has had a high concentration of viral units per milliliter of blood. The "e" antigen of HBV has been a marker to identify such surgeons. The e antigen of HBV is a degradation product of the viral nucleocapsid and is seen in patients with active viral replication in the liver.[58] Because an epitope of the HBV virus has been identified that is not associated with the e antigen,[59]

actual viral counts in blood are considered a better predictor of the risk for transmission to patients. A nonsurgical group has recommended that surgeons who are e antigen positive should not continue in the surgical care of patients.[60] An e antigen–positive surgeon known to have chronic HBV infection should adhere to the recommendations of the ACS and have an expert local panel convened to make recommendations about future surgical practice (Table 47-5).[61]

Although many cases of HBV transmission to patients from infected surgeons have been identified, only four surgeons have been associated with transmission of HCV infection to patients. The most notable case was from Spain.[62] A cardiac surgeon with high viral blood counts (10^7 viruses/mL) was identified as transmitting infection to at least five patients. Single surgeon-to-patient transmissions of HCV infection have been reported from

TABLE 47-5 Key Points for Emphasis from the Statement on the Surgeon and Hepatitis by the American College of Surgeons*

POINT OF EMPHASIS ON HEPATITIS INFECTION	COMMENT
Surgeons have an ethical obligation to care for patients with HBV or HCV infection.	Hepatitis infection is not covered by the Americans with Disabilities Act. The moral imperative remains while exercising appropriate standards of infection control in the health care setting.
Surgeons should know their HBV and HCV infection status.	Significantly improved antiviral chemotherapy for these infections is currently available. Future additional therapies are being pursued.
HBV "e" antigen–positive surgeons are at potential risk for transmission to their patients.	These surgeons should be evaluated by an expert panel to make recommendations about the prevention of infection in patients.
All surgeons should know their antibody status for HBV infection and should be immunized against HBV infection.	Surgeons must all be vaccinated against HBV infection. Documentation of an antibody response to vaccination is important.
HCV-infected surgeons can safely continue to practice surgery.	A surgeon with HCV infection should adhere to all standards of infection control in the care of patients. It is advisable to seek expert advise about currently available treatment of the infection.
Surgeons should seek expert consultation when documented or suspected exposure to a chronic HBV- or HCV-infected patient has occurred.	The surgeon should confer with local experts.†

*http://www.facs.org/fellows_info/statements/st-22.html.
†National Clinicians' Postexposure Prophylaxis Hotline at 1-888-448-4911 or visit the website at http://www.nccc.ucsf.edu/Hotlines/PEPline.

TABLE 47-6 Key Points for Emphasis in the Statement on the Surgeon and HIV Infection from the American College of Surgeons*

POINT OF EMPHASIS ON HIV INFECTION	COMMENT
Surgeons have an ethical obligation to give care to HIV patients.	It is the law that a health care provider must provide care for HIV-infected patients based on the Americans with Disabilities Act.
Contemporary standards of infection control practice should be used in all venues of patient care.	In the era of other nosocomial pathogens that can be transmitted in the course of patient care, infection control practice is a must in all patient contacts.
HIV-infected surgeons may continue to practice with invasive procedures under the provision that standards of infection control are used and the surgeon is physically fit to practice.	HIV-infected surgeons, especially when given highly effective antiretroviral chemotherapy, should have privileges to practice in the same context as those with diabetes or hypertension. Functional considerations of health should dictate. When there are questions, the surgeon's personal physician or a locally convened group of experts in HIV should provide recommendations about the continuation of surgical practice.
Postexposure prophylaxis with antiretroviral chemotherapy is recommended.	Although the data are not completely convincing, exposure to an HIV-infected patient or an unusually severe event involving exposure to a patient of unknown serology should initiate the triple-drug prophylaxis regimen.
All surgeons should know their HIV status.	Because effective treatment is available, surgeons should be tested. The attitude of the early 1990s, when treatment was less effective and restrictions of practice loomed in the background, has passed.
All surgeons and the leadership in U.S. surgery must remain sensitive to the issues of patient safety and workplace risks for HIV infection.	Individual surgeons and the national organizations that represent them should maintain an interest in all developments surrounding HIV, its treatment, and transmission. All should maintain interest for patient safety.

*http://www.facs.org/fellows_info/statements/st-13.html.

a cardiac surgeon from the United Kingdom,[63] and single transmissions involving a gynecologist[64] and an orthopedic surgeon have been reported from Germany.[65] No occupational infection has been identified at this time from a neurosurgeon to a patient.

Surgeons and other physicians have been vectors in the transmission of infection even though they may not be infected with HCV themselves. Several clusters of nosocomial HCV infection in patients have resulted from contaminated multidose vials,[66,67] contaminated radiopharmaceuticals,[68] unsafe injection practices,[69] reused needles and syringes,[70] and poor hand hygiene.[71]

To date, no occupational transmission of HIV infection has occurred in the United States except for the dental cases noted earlier. A single case report from France identified a potential transmission from an HIV-infected orthopedic surgeon.[72] Studies of patients from the practices of surgeons with HIV infection have not identified evidence of transmission.[73] The position of the ACS with respect to HIV-infected surgeons continues to be a valid one (Table 47-6).[74] It is important for HIV-positive surgeons to know that they are infected so that effective treatment can be given.

LEGAL ISSUES

It is understandable that issues of transmissible infection passing from surgeons or other HCWs to patients would generate some legal issues. The legal and political issues were triggered by recommendations from the CDC for the prevention of HIV and HBV infection during "exposure-prone invasive procedures."[75] Among these recommendations, it was advised that "exposure-prone procedures should be identified by medical/surgical/dental organizations and institutions at which the procedures are performed." Moreover, "HCWs who are infected with HIV or HBV (and are e-antigen positive) should not perform exposure-prone

procedures unless they have sought counsel from an expert review panel and been advised under what circumstances, if any, they may continue to perform these procedures. Such circumstances would include notifying prospective patients of the HCWs' seropositivity before they undergo exposure-prone invasive procedures." This led to passage of Public Law 102-141 by Congress in October 1991, which required states to implement the CDC's recommendations, or their equivalent, as a condition for the receipt of Public Health Service funds. All states complied, although laws were very different from state to state. Although the furor and passion about this subject have waned, fines and imprisonment remain in the law of many states for surgeons who do not follow the requirements established by the CDC in 1991.

A more serious issue for neurosurgeons and for surgeons in general is the Americans with Disabilities Act (ADA).[76] The ADA was passed in 1990 and prohibits discrimination on the basis of a person's disability, which specifically includes HIV/AIDS patients. It explicitly prohibits private providers of public accommodations (dental/medical services) from discrimination based on the defined disability. The Supreme Court of the United States ruled in favor of a lawsuit filed by an HIV-positive patient in 1998 in *Bragdon v Abbott*.[77] In this case a dentist refused to fill a cavity for this patient in his office, but rather chose to do it in the hospital because of concerns of safety from HIV infection. The Supreme Court ruled that the patient posed no direct threat to the dentist and that damages were incurred in the discriminatory expense of having the dental work performed at a hospital.

In yet another case, a private neurosurgery group was required to pay $40,000 in monetary compensation and a $10,000 civil penalty to the United States.[78] A neurosurgeon in the group allegedly refused to provide care for a patient with a back condition who was HIV positive. An Assistant Attorney General stated,

Basic Science of Epilepsy

Epilepsy Surgery Overview

Guy M. McKhann II ▪ Matthew A. Howard III

Neurological surgery has played an important role in the management of patients with epilepsy throughout the history of our specialty.[1] The types of operative procedures performed and the indications for surgical intervention have evolved and changed in parallel with technical and scientific advances in multiple related disciplines. The chapters in this section are organized to provide a comprehensive review of these topics and are authored by leading investigators and neurosurgeons in their respective fields. In this introduction to the section on epilepsy surgery we provide a brief overview of the topics that will be covered and the rationale for their inclusion.

The history of epilepsy surgery has been strongly influenced by the dynamic balance between the perceived values of surgical procedures and medical treatments. The risk-benefit calculation for epilepsy surgery is affected by multiple factors, many of which are difficult to rigorously quantify and extrapolate across large patient populations and may not be directly related to the surgical treatment itself. The probability of a seizure-free outcome after surgery, for example, is dependent on the ability to accurately characterize a patient's seizure disorder.[2-6] Thus, technologic advances in nonsurgical disciplines that have an impact on the presurgical evaluation process (e.g., magnetoencephalography [MEG]) have the potential to indirectly alter the surgical risk-benefit assessment. On the medical management side, enormous resources have been committed over a period of many decades to research and develop new antiepileptic drugs (AEDs). In the past, the actual effectiveness of AEDs or the anticipated usefulness of new AEDs in the development pipeline provided a rationale for treating physicians to not explore surgical treatment options.

In the modern era, the epilepsy surgical decision-making calculus has changed significantly. Contemporary clinical reports, including a landmark prospective study of epilepsy surgery versus best medical management for intractable temporal lobe seizures, provide incontrovertible evidence of the safety and efficacy of epilepsy surgery.[7-11] It is also now widely accepted that neuronal cell loss occurs with persistent seizures and that uncontrolled epilepsy can be associated with progressive, irreversible loss of brain functions.[7,8,12] Hopes that new AEDs would prove to be markedly more effective than older generation drugs have largely been unrealized to date.[13,14] The side effects of newer AEDs are better tolerated by some patients, but the complex underlying pathophysiology of refractory seizure disorders continues to resist a medical "magic bullet." For these and other reasons, it is now widely accepted that patients with intractable seizures should

be evaluated for possible epilepsy surgery after a circumscribed period of expert medical management. Persistent seizures should not be tolerated if a viable surgical option exists. The probability of a new drug succeeding in eliminating a patient's seizure disorder when other drugs have failed is exceedingly low.[7,14]

Contemporary reviews of bench epilepsy research and experimental animal models are included in this section because of their direct relevance to epilepsy surgery. Much of this research is designed to gain new insights into the neurophysiologic and molecular mechanisms of epilepsy that can be used to develop more effective AEDs. However, information gained from this research also guides the design and implementation of new, nonablative functional neurosurgical applications. As an example, drugs that are demonstrated to disrupt pathologic epileptic circuitry in animal models but have unacceptable side effects when given systemically to humans at the desired concentration could be delivered in a brain site–specific manner by using stereotactically implanted catheters and drug pumps.[15,16] Knowledge of the fine details of abnormal epileptic discharges and the effects of precisely timed electrical stimulation of the abnormal medial temporal lobe circuitry set the stage for ongoing clinical trials of patterned electrical stimulation through implanted electrodes as a new neurosurgical treatment.[17-19] In these and other examples, the concept of bench-to-bedside translational research has had a direct impact on the treatment of epilepsy patients.

The vast majority of epilepsy surgery procedures are performed at major centers that have the resources to support a comprehensive multidisciplinary program.[20] One of the main tasks of this group is to correctly identify patients who will probably benefit from epilepsy surgery. In most instances, neurologists, neuropsychologists, and neuroradiologists gather and perform the primary analysis of the data that are used to make this determination. The epilepsy surgeon, however, must have a thorough understanding of the strengths and limitations of these preoperative examinations. Preoperative evaluation topics are addressed in sections throughout many of the chapters in this section. Technical advances in areas such as functional brain imaging have had an impact on the preoperative evaluation process, with some caveats. One of the most difficult diagnostic challenges is to identify brain activation patterns that typify a patient's seizure-onset patterns. This necessitates measuring brain activity during a seizure, and in most instances, because of technical constraints, it is not feasible to obtain functional magnetic resonance imaging (fMRI), MEG, or positron emission tomography (PET) data during these ictal events. Functional brain imaging data provide valuable information that influences clinical decision making; however, well-established electroencephalography (EEG)-based diagnostic methods that can be used in both the interictal and ictal states continue to play a preeminent role in the preoperative evaluation process.[2,5,21,22]

A wide range of surgical strategies are used for the treatment of medically refractory epilepsy. The indications, techniques, risks, and results of these procedures are included in this section. Although the specific techniques used vary somewhat across centers, all contemporary epilepsy procedures can be grouped into clearly identifiable categories. The most commonly performed resective procedure is temporal lobectomy. A variety of methods are used to plan the extent of resection, and different technical approaches can be used to access the mesial portions of the temporal lobe. Irrespective of the approach used, seizure control outcomes are excellent in properly selected patients with temporal lobe epilepsy.[7,9,11] Approximately 60% to 80% of patients are seizure free on long-term follow-up, as opposed to less than 10% of refractory patients who continue to be managed with medical treatment alone.

Seizure disorders localized to brain regions outside the temporal lobe represent a more difficult surgical challenge. This heterogeneous group of disorders typically requires a more extensive presurgical evaluation than needed for temporal lobe cases. Even when seizure onsets appear to be accurately localized to noneloquent brain regions, extratemporal lobe resections are associated with only approximately 50% to 60% seizure-free outcome rates.[23] In cases in which the seizure focus localizes to eloquent brain regions, such as primary motor or sensory cortex or language critical sites, resective surgery often cannot be performed safely. In this setting, multiple subpial transection (MST) surgery is a treatment option.[24-26] As with extratemporal resective surgery, seizure-free outcome rates after MST are significantly lower than after temporal lobe procedures. The rationale for pursuing these treatment options, despite the high rate of persistent seizures after surgery, is that the alternative of continued medical management is associated with an even higher incidence of persistent seizures and progressive neurological decline.

As with all neurosurgical procedures, the potential benefits of surgery must be weighed against the potential risks. In the case of epilepsy surgery, the risk variable is particularly important and is specifically addressed in a chapter devoted to this topic. Most patients who undergo resective surgery have results on neurological examination that are grossly normal or are in a state of chronic compensation for a long-standing deficit. With the exception of SUDEP (sudden unexplained death in epilepsy), the condition being treated surgically is not usually life-threatening in the conventional sense. Although major neurological complications, such as stroke causing hemiplegia, are rare, when they do occur, the functional consequences for the patient can be devastating. In addition, because of the nature of the brain regions being removed and the preexisting chronic neurological injury caused by frequent seizures, some patients will experience significant procedure-related morbidity even when no complications occurred during surgery. Such morbidity includes loss of memory function and depression.[15,27-31] Epilepsy surgeons and their patients must thoroughly understand the avoidable and unavoidable risks before electing a surgical treatment option.

In many patients with refractory epilepsy, the results of the presurgical evaluation will reveal that they are poor candidates for resection surgery. A typical scenario in this setting is one in which the patient is found to have multiple seizure foci that localize to widely distributed brain regions. In the past, there was no viable surgical treatment option for these patients. Now, many of them can be helped by implantation of a vagal nerve stimulator.[32-34] This is a low-risk procedure that reduces the frequency of seizures in more than half of the patients implanted, but it rarely results in a seizure-free outcome. As described earlier, other nonablative surgical interventions are also under development, including chronic electrical brain stimulation and local drug infusion methods.

Another unique aspect of the subspecialty of epilepsy surgery is the opportunities that it affords to study normal human brain functions. Safe and effective epilepsy surgery is predicated on the ability of the surgical team to accurately localize seizure activity and map the normal functions of the human brain. For this reason, many epilepsy operations and all chronic extraoperative monitoring procedures are performed on awake subjects. This provides a unique opportunity not only to examine the pathophysiology of epilepsy but also to study normal human brain functions by using invasive research techniques that do not increase the risks associated with epilepsy surgery. The strategy of using epilepsy surgery patients to perform basic neuroscience research was pioneered by Wilder Penfield and colleagues at the Montreal Neurological Institute.[35-39] Even with the development of powerful noninvasive brain research methods such as fMRI, answers to certain important neuroscience questions can still be answered only with direct, invasive methods. For this reason, multidisciplinary basic research teams throughout the world have incorporated this investigative approach into their overall human brain research strategy.[40-43] The range of research activities being pursued, along with specific examples, are presented in the chapter devoted to this topic. Well-trained neurosurgeon-scientists are critical members of these teams, and future prospects for young neurosurgeons who wish to pursue this career path have never been brighter.

Full references can be found on Expert Consult @ www.expertconsult.com

CHAPTER 49

Electrophysiologic Properties
of the Mammalian Central Nervous System

Guy M. McKhann II ▪ Damir Janigro

The study of excitable cells is, for a number of reasons, a fascinating one. Interest in electrophysiology and neuronal function spans many medical specialties because these excitable cells are those by which we move, think, and perform complex yet automatic tasks such as cardiovascular regulation. It is for these reasons that electrophysiologic studies have attracted the foremost physiologists in this century. Despite these outstanding contributions, several fundamental issues in neuroscience remain unresolved. Traditionally, clinical electrophysiology has used a more holistic approach than nonclinical neurophysiology has. Clinical insight into brain function (or dysfunction) is commonly achieved today by increasingly sophisticated imaging techniques that allow real-time observations. The booming advancement in molecular biology, as well as its fundamental contribution to medicine in general and neuroscience in particular, has unveiled an incredible level of ordered complexity in neuronal function. Basic scientists are producing a large quantity of molecular data, spanning from investigation of the role of a single protein in the electrical behavior of neurons to genetic markers of neurological disease. Despite the immense popularity of these approaches, it is important to remember that the electrical properties of individual neurons and the neuronal environment are the final effectors of brain activity and that diseases of the brain derive from the cellular level. It is thus foreseeable that recording of electrophysiologic signals will continue to provide a reliable method for in-depth investigation of central nervous system (CNS) function.

CNS function is dependent on homeostatic mechanisms that precisely regulate the extracellular level or concentration of neurotransmitters, ions, pH, and other variables. The neuronal cell membrane is a complex biochemical entity that interfaces between the cell and its environment. Its functions include directional transport of specific substances and maintenance of chemical gradients, particularly electrochemical gradients, across the plasma membrane. These ion gradients can be of high specificity (e.g., sodium versus potassium ions) and of great functional significance (e.g., in the production of action potentials). In addition, CNS function is supported by numerous non-neuronal mechanisms responsible for the control of extracellular and intracellular homeostasis (glial cells, cerebral vasculature). It has become increasingly evident that pathophysiologic changes in ion channel function play a major role in the etiology of certain disorders of the nervous system.

The following brief introductory chapter on CNS electrophysiology does not attempt to explain in detail the complex biophysical properties underlying communication between individual neurons or transduction of environmental and sensory signals into electrical activity in specific regions of the brain or spinal cord. Several excellent textbooks deal with specific aspects of CNS function and electrophysiology, and recent publications have described in a concise yet comprehensive manner the complex properties of the ion currents responsible for neuronal excitation. This chapter provides the reader with succinct background information on the electrical properties of neurons and additionally focuses on other aspects of brain function relevant to modern understanding of the pathophysiologic changes occur-

ring in diseased brain. Such aspects include description of some of the mechanisms involved in brain homeostasis, the genesis of synchronous activity by electrotonic and ephaptic interactions, and the molecular changes in ion channels underlying neurological diseases. Because complete referencing of such a broad topic would entail a bibliography of thousands of references, relevant recent reviews, textbooks, and a nonexhaustive compilation of representative work are included.

ELECTRICAL PROPERTIES
OF MAMMALIAN CELLS

Matter is composed of atoms, which consist of positively charged nuclei and negatively charged electrons. Electrical phenomena occur whenever charges opposite in sign are separated or moved in a given direction; static electricity is the accumulation of electric charge. An electric current results when these charges flow across a permissive material, called a *conductor*. An *ion current* is a particular type of current carried by charges present on atoms or small molecules flowing in an aqueous solution. Separation of charges in an aqueous solution can be achieved by inserting an impermeable membrane in the solution itself. In mammalian cells, these membranes coincide with the plasma membrane, and its lipophilic composition ensures a remarkable level of electrical isolation for cells and tissues. Excitable as well as most nonexcitable cells are characterized by an asymmetric distribution of electric charges across the plasma membrane.

The biophysical bases for maintenance of this electric potential have been extensively investigated experimentally and modeled by mathematical simulations. Under normal resting conditions, mammalian cells allow transmembrane ion currents such that the internal portion of the cell is negatively charged; the presence of nonpermeant anions such as proteins also contributes to the maintenance of transmembrane potentials. This relatively stable state results in a net transmembrane potential of several millivolts and is commonly referred to as the resting membrane potential (RMP) (Fig. 49-1).

Most of what we know about the physiology of excitable cells was derived from electrical measurements (Fig. 49-2). Our knowledge of the complex properties of the CNS is based on the application to neuronal cells of simple physical rules governing the movement of charged particles. The physical principles of cell electrophysiology can be thus be compared with the biophysical rules governing flow of electric current through a so-called RC circuit (see Fig. 49-2), where electrons flow through a *resistive* component (in the case of living cells, represented by ion channels) set in parallel with a *capacitive* component (represented by the poorly conductive phospholipid bilayer). Ohm's law describes the relationship between current flow (I) and the resulting voltage drop (E) across a resistor when no capacitive component is present. This is, of course, an abstract situation, in particular when dealing with ion fluxes across biologic membranes, but it allows one to understand the basic principles governing flow of electric current.

The following relationship constitutes Ohm's law (or principle):

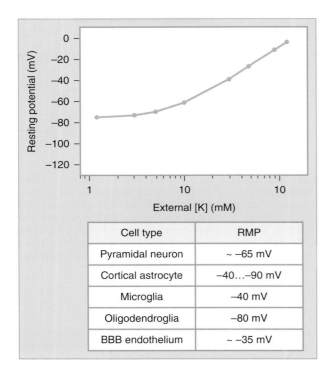

Cell type	RMP
Pyramidal neuron	~ −65 mV
Cortical astrocyte	−40...−90 mV
Microglia	−40 mV
Oligodendroglia	−80 mV
BBB endothelium	~ −35 mV

FIGURE 49-1 Relationship between resting potential and $[K^+]_{out}$. The *line* represents the "ideal" case predicted by the Nernst equation (see Equation 3). Experimental measurements show a significant departure from a linear dependency at physiologic $[K^+]_{out}$ values. Resting potential values for excitable and nonexcitable central nervous system cells are shown. BBB, blood-brain barrier; RMP, resting membrane potential.

$$E = IR \tag{1}$$

where I represents the current flowing through a resistance (R) when voltage is applied. In a hypothetical cell, this relationship can be written as follows:

$$E_m = I_m \times R_m \tag{2}$$

where E_m represents the difference in voltage (in millivolts) between the inside and the outside of the cell, I_m represents the *net* current flowing at that particular time across the cell membrane, and R_m is the total membrane resistance. An important consequence of this relationship is that small *changes* in current will significantly affect cell RMP only when R_m is large. This is particularly important for inhibitory synaptic currents; for instance, in the case of γ-aminobutyric acid receptor A (GABA$_A$) activation, inhibition is achieved not only by hyperpolarizing cell RMP further away from the firing threshold but also by greatly increasing postsynaptic conductance,* thus reducing the synaptic efficacy of concomitant excitatory signals.

A mathematical derivation of Ohm's law useful for studies of biologic membranes was first formulated by Nernst,[1] who described the relationship between intracellular and extracellular ion concentrations and changes in transmembrane potential attributable to permeation of an ion. In the case of potassium ions, the Nernst equation can be written as follows:

$$E_K = RT/ZF \ln[K^+]_{in}/[K^+]_{out} \tag{3a}$$

where R and F are constants, T is the temperature at which the observation is performed, and Z is the charge of the permeant ion. Note that if the charge (sign, or "Z" in Equation 3) of the permeant ion is changed (e.g., if we look at the Nernst equation for chloride), the direction of the gradient is changed as well. The logarithm of the ratio between intracellular and extracellular K^+ dominates the right side of the equation because RT/ZF is constant under most biologic conditions when temperature can be maintained within a few degrees. This equation predicts, as expected from Ohm's law, that net potassium flux will approach zero when intracellular and extracellular potassium levels are isosmolar, that is, when $E_K = 0$ mV. Under physiologic conditions ($[K^+]_{out} = 3.5$ mM; $[K^+]_{in} = 135$ mM), the transmembrane potential at which potassium flux will be nil is around −90 mV.* This value constitutes the *potassium equilibrium potential* at these concentrations. Note that small changes in the extracellular potassium concentration will cause relatively large changes in the fraction of total membrane currents attributable to potassium ions. Because permeability to potassium is essential for maintenance of RMP, a net increase in extracellular potassium will cause a significant departure from RMP (see Fig. 49-1).

In practical form, the Nernst equation for potassium can be rewritten by converting to $\log_{10}$ and calculating RT/ZF at 20°C. This rearrangement leads to

$$E_K = -58 \text{ mV} \ln[K^+]_{in}/[K^+]_{out} \tag{4}$$

It can be seen that a 10-fold change in the concentration gradient for potassium can produce a 58-mV change in membrane potential. Because under normal conditions there is an almost 40-fold outward gradient for potassium ions and a 12-fold inward gradient for sodium ions, the resulting equilibrium potentials are −92 mV and +65 mV, respectively. Since the membrane at rest is much more permeable to potassium than to sodium (see later), RMP is closer to E_K than to E_{Na}.

Two additional considerations can help us understand the genesis of cell RMP: (1) if the membrane is exclusively permeant to K^+ and no active, electrogenic transport of ions occurs, the cell potential will tend toward E_K and only small movements of K^+ will be sufficient to maintain RMP at −92 mV, and (2) if the membrane potential is clamped at E_K, net potassium flux will be zero (as predicted by the fact that E_K is the equilibrium potential for potassium). If the membrane potential is held positive with respect to E_K, outward potassium currents will develop; conversely, if RMP is held at potentials negative with respect to E_K, inward potassium fluxes will develop. Interestingly, the notion that cell RMP is controlled by potassium ions was first derived independently from direct observations: Julius Bernstein in 1902 correctly predicted that in most mammalian cells, potassium ions govern the transmembrane voltage difference.[2] Direct experimental evidence was achieved only half a century later when a microelectrode could be placed into cells to directly measure RMP and the effects of changing $[K^+]_{out}$. Bernstein also proposed that selective potassium permeability was lost during the process of excitation, during which numerous "pores" opened to allow entry of other small ions (Cl⁻ and Na⁺).[2] This theory explained several features of the regulation of RMP and generation of action potentials, including the depolarizing effects of $[K^+]_{out}$.

In fact, a prediction of the formalism just presented is that RMP changes linearly with $[K^+]_{out}$. As shown in Figure 49-1, experimental evidence contradicts this notion, at least in the case of mammalian neurons.[†] Most neurons depolarize significantly

---

*Because one is most commonly interested in *permeation* (or flux) of charges across the membrane rather than its nonconductive properties, the term *conductance* (G_m, which equals $1/R_m$) is used instead of R_m.

---

*The reader should bear in mind that ionic concentrations are not always constant. In reality, large changes occur during sustained neuronal activation or in pathologic states in which ion homeostasis is impaired (e.g., ischemia).
†A linear dependence of RMP on $[K^+]_{out}$ is found in other CNS cells, such as glia and brain microvascular endothelium.

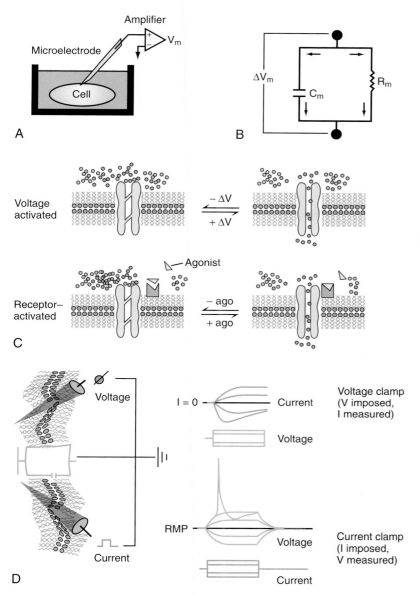

FIGURE 49-2 Methodologies commonly used for the investigation of mammalian central nervous system physiology. **A,** Neuronal and non-neuronal cells are investigated in vitro and in vivo by patch clamp recording. The electrophysiologic properties of the cell ("whole-cell configuration") and of individual membrane channels ("cell-attached configuration") can be investigated. **B,** The corresponding electric circuit for a cell is shown (see text). **C,** Voltage-activated channels are frequently studied by investigating the changes in channel and cellular properties that result from applied hyperpolarization and depolarization, whereas receptor-activated channels are usually studied by the application of appropriate receptor agonists and antagonists. **D,** The differences between voltage clamp and current clamp recordings are shown. Voltage clamp recordings allow the study of ion currents and their modulation by voltage, or transmitters/second messengers, whereas current clamp experimentation is commonly used to determine resting properties and the excitability of cells.

after large changes in extracellular potassium, whereas changes around physiologic potassium concentrations do not significantly affect neuronal RMP. This can only be due to concomitant participation of other conductances. Although the exact nature of the ionic conductances contributing to the regulation of neuronal RMP varies between different neurons, a generic set of equations predict how these "parallel" conductances may affect E_m. The most illustrious of these equations was provided by Goldman, who described the expected RMP in a cell endowed with more than one ion current mechanism as

$$E_m = (RT/ZF) \ln \frac{(g_K[K]_i + g_{Na}[Na]_i + g_{Cl}[Cl]_o)}{(g_K[K]_o + g_{Na}[Na]_o + g_{Cl}[Cl]_i)} \tag{5}$$

where G_K, G_{Na}, and G_{Cl} represent the conductances for potassium, sodium, and chloride.[5] Note that these conductance values are multiplied by the relative chemical concentration gradient for each ion, thus combining the "passive" electro-osmotic tendency for ion permeation with the average conductance of the membrane for a particular ion. Note also that if G_{Cl} and G_{Na} are close

to zero, the transmembrane potential is governed almost exclusively by potassium ions and their conductance. This condition is common at resting potential in most neurons and glial cells, where I_K (and to some extent I_{pump}) determines RMP (Fig. 49-3).

In 1949, Alan Hodgkin and Bernard Katz first applied the Goldman equation systematically to changes in membrane potentials evoked by altering external ion concentrations in the squid giant axon.[4] They measured changes in RMP induced by changes in $[K^+]_{out}$, $[Na^+]_{out}$, and $[Cl^-]_{out}$. They discovered that although changes in extracellular potassium dramatically changed RMP, comparable changes in $[Na^+]_{out}$ had little effect. Changing $[Cl^-]_{out}$ had an intermediate effect. The following permeability ratios were obtained at rest:

$$P_K/P_{Na}/P_{Cl} = 1.0{:}0.4{:}0.45 \tag{6a}$$

When the measurements were performed at the peak of the action potential, however, these values changed dramatically to yield

$$P_K/P_{Na}/P_{Cl} = 1.0{:}200{:}0.45 \tag{6b}$$

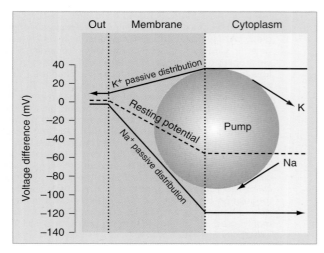

FIGURE 49-3 Maintenance of neuronal resting membrane potential. At rest, passive movement of potassium out of the cell is balanced by movement of sodium into the cell. The ion fluxes are the product of the electrochemical gradient and the membrane conductance for each ion. The high gradient but low conductance of sodium influx is balanced by the lower gradient (at resting membrane potential) but higher conductance of potassium efflux. To prevent the dissipation of ionic gradients over time, the electrogenic sodium-potassium adenosine triphosphate (Na^+,K^+-ATPase) pump extrudes three sodium ions in exchange for two potassium ions per molecule of adenosine triphosphate expended, thereby further hyperpolarizing the membrane.

Therefore, when the predominant membrane conductance is P_K, the Goldman equation can be reduced to the Nernst equation for potassium:

$$E_K = RT/ZF \log[K^+]_{in}/[K^+]_{out} = ca. -70 \text{ mV} \quad (3b)$$

whereas when P_{Na} predominates, the following applies:

$$E_K = RT/ZF \log[Na^+]_{in}/[Na^+]_{out} = +55 \text{ mV} \quad (3c)$$

which is approximately the peak value of action potential overshoot. Direct measurement of changes in the relative permeability for Na^+ and K^+ contradicted one of the hypotheses formulated by Bernstein, who incorrectly predicted that neuronal excitation was due to *loss* of potassium permeability rather than *activation* of an inward sodium current (Table 49-1). Had this hypothesis been correct, the maximum depolarizing value reached during the action potential would have been around 0 mV and not at +30 mV as experimentally determined by Hodgkin and Katz.

It has become apparent more recently that I_{Na} is not the only ionic current that can generate action potentials; calcium ions also play an important role in neuronal excitability. Similarly, I_K is not the exclusive component of the electrical regulation of cell resting properties inasmuch as several other conductances are involved in the control of neuronal resting potential.

ION CHANNELS IN NEURONS AND GLIA

Ion channels are protein channels in cell membranes that allow ions to pass from the extracellular solution to the intracellular solution and vice versa. Similarly, transporters are specialized enzymes that carry specific ions or molecules across otherwise impermeant membranes or against electro-osmotic gradients. Not surprisingly, from a purely thermodynamic (or energetic) point of view, ion channels are less "expensive" to operate, whereas pumps or exchangers require considerable consumption of energy. Most ion channels and pumps are selective in that they allow only certain ions to pass, and an individual cell has ion channels with various ion selectivity. In the context of studies of biologic cell membranes, the term *ion selectivity* refers to the ability of all cell membranes to distinguish between various ions such as Na^+, K^+, Ca^{2+}, and Cl^-. We will focus on Na^+, K^+, and Ca^{2+} channels. All of these voltage-gated channels are made up of one or more pore-forming α subunits and variable numbers of accessory subunits, denoted β, γ, and so on. The α subunits determine ion selectivity and mediate the voltage-sensing functions of the channel. This ion selectivity involves specific pores or channels in the cell membrane, with certain channels being specific for certain ions and the opening or closing (gating) of channels depending on conditions and various interactions with ligands binding to receptors. These receptors are in some cases part of the channel itself and in other cases neighboring entities that control channel dynamics. The selectivity of an ion channel can be "gated," with the channel effectively opened or closed, and ion channels are said to be voltage gated or ligand gated, depending on how the change in selectivity is provoked. A summary of the most studied CNS ion channels is presented in Table 49-2.

TABLE 49-1 Glossary of Commonly Used Electrophysiologic Terms

Inward current	Positive charges enter the cell (e.g., I_{Na} responsible for the action potential upstroke)
Outward current	Positive charges leave the cell (e.g., I_K during action potential repolarization)
Depolarization	Change in RMP to less negative values (e.g., EPSP)
Hyperpolarization	Change in RMP to more negative values (e.g., IPSP)
Inward-going rectification	Tendency of some ionic currents to allow passage of inward-flowing but not outward-flowing ions (inward rectifier potassium currents)
Outward-going rectification	Tendency of some currents to allow passage of outward-flowing but not inward-flowing ions (most other potassium currents activated by depolarization)
Voltage clamp	Electrophysiologic technique allowing the study of ion currents and their modulation by voltage, or transmitters/second messengers
Current clamp	Technique used during intracellular recordings to determine the resting properties and excitability of cells
Single-channel recording	Modern variation (patch clamp) that allows study of the electrophysiologic properties of a single ion channel/protein
Multi–single-unit recording	Extracellular recording from a neuron or a cluster of neighboring neurons

EPSP, excitatory postsynaptic potential; IPSP, inhibitory postsynaptic potential; RMP, resting membrane potential.

TABLE 49-2 Classification of the Most Studied Central Nervous System Ion Channels Based on the Nature of the Physiologically Permeant Ion

ION	ION CHANNEL	LOCALIZATION	PHYSIOLOGIC SIGNIFICANCE
Na$^+$	Fast Na current (I$_{Na}$)	All neurons	Generation of action potential
		Astrocytes*	
	Slow Na current	Pyramidal neurons	Depolarization of afterpotentials; firing rate
K$^+$	Delayed rectifier (I$_{DR}$)	All neurons	AP repolarization
			K$^+$ homeostasis (glia)
			GABA$_B$ inhibition (neurons)
	Inward rectifier (K$_{IR}$)	Most glial cells, some neurons	Presynaptic effects of adenosine
	I$_{HERG}$	Astrocytes	K$^+$ homeostasis
	M-channel (I$_M$)	Neurons	Firing threshold, RMP (modulated by ACh)
	K$_{ATP}$ channel	Neurons, glia, BBB	Couples intracellular metabolism to electrical activity
Cl$^-$	**I$_{GABA}$**	Neurons, glia	GABA$_B$ inhibition (neurons)
			Unknown in glia
Ca^{2+}	I$_{Ca}$ T-type	Neurons	Firing threshold
	I$_{Ca}$ L-type	Neurons	Neurotransmission
	I$_{Ca}$ N-type	Neurons	Synaptic release
		I$_{Ca}$ not found in glia, BBB endothelium	
Mixed (K$^+$, Na$^+$)	Anomalous rectifier (I$_h$)	Neurons, glia, BBB endothelium	Neuronal firing rate; firing threshold
			Homeostasis (?)
	I$_{AMPA}$	Most neurons, glia	Synaptic transmission
Mixed (K$^+$, Na$^+$, Ca^{2+})	**I$_{NMDA}$**	Most neurons	Synaptic transmission, LTP and LTD

Receptor-operated ion channels are indicated in bold.
*Only in diseased tissue.
ACh, acetylcholine; AP, action potential; AMPA, α-amino-3-hydroxy-5-methyl-4-isoxazolepropionate; ATP, adenosine triphosphate; BBB, blood-brain barrier; GABA, γ-aminobutyric acid; LTP, long-term potentiation; LTD, long-term depression; NMDA, N-methyl-D-aspartate; RMP, resting membrane potential.

Genesis of Fast Sodium Action Potentials and Properties of Sodium Channels

Neuronal cells use a single type of signaling based on all-or-nothing action potentials. Sodium action potentials such as those recorded in axons or cell bodies are relatively invariant in normal tissue, and thus the shape and duration of these electrical signals do not change significantly within neuronal subtypes in the nervous system. Calcium action potentials are similarly predictable, but the underlying ionic mechanism can be rather complex, depending on the cell type and its topographic location within the cell (see later). The terms *sodium action potential* and *calcium*

action potential refer to the initial (depolarizing) phase of these rapid changes in membrane polarity. Although genetic or molecular alteration of I$_{Na}$ and I$_{Ca}$ can significantly affect neuronal firing and, ultimately, central and peripheral nervous system neurophysiology, it must be remembered that gross changes in neuronal excitability may also result by altering the *repolarization* phase of individual action potentials.

Action potentials have a characteristic shape once a certain threshold is reached. In normal tissue, stereotyped electrical events follow the initial depolarization (Fig. 49-4). The sequence can be described as follows: (1) RMP moves from an initial negative value (−65 to −80 mV for most neurons) toward the so-called

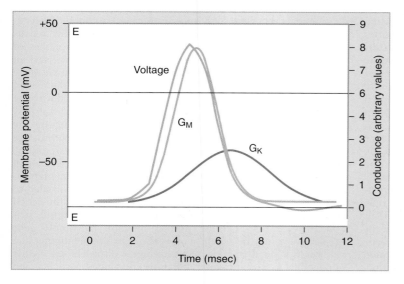

FIGURE 49-4 Changes in conductance during generation of an action potential.

threshold for activation of sodium channels (around −40 mV). This change can be slow and may occur spontaneously as a result of fluctuations in RMP; the threshold is reached rapidly when the initial depolarization is triggered by a synaptic potential (or a summation of synaptic potentials). (2) After reaching the threshold value, an extremely rapid (1 to 2 msec) depolarization occurs because of opening of sodium channels and massive influx of sodium ions into the cell. (3) Termination of the "upstroke" phase depends on a combination of factors: *voltage- and time-dependent inactivation* of I_{Na} and a concomitant decrease in the driving force for sodium occurring in parallel with *voltage-dependent activation* of I_K. (4) Further increases in the permeability to potassium ions restore the pre–action potential RMP values and force the membrane toward E_K. (5) Under most circumstances, an *undershoot* of cell resting voltage occurs (a few millivolts from RMP) as a result of residual activation of I_K and the contribution of the electrogenic sodium-potassium adenosine triphosphatase (Na^+,K^+-ATPase) extruding 3 Na^+ ions in exchange for 2 K^+. The return to pre–action potential voltage favors the so-called *removal of inactivation*, a necessary step that allows a subsequent cycle of depolarization-induced action potential firing. This stereotyped and relatively simple sequence of events is typically recorded in axons; other more complex interactions of various I_{Na} and I_K values may lead to slightly different voltage profiles.

From a functional standpoint, it is important to remember that the genesis of fast sodium action potentials is a hallmark of neuronal function, to the degree that during neurophysiologic recordings, the presence or absence of Na^+ spikes is frequently used to determine the neuronal or glial cell type. Recently, this notion has been challenged, and glial "action potentials" have been reported with increasing frequency. These responses, however, appear to usually be associated with pathologic conditions (brain tumors, epilepsy), and the old perception that neuronal cells are the exclusive tenants of sufficient I_{Na} density to promote active responses is still generally accepted. Within the same neuronal cell, Na^+ channels involved in the generation of action potentials can be located heterogeneously, and it is common for clusters of channels to be located at specific and crucial membrane segments. The most commonly encountered clustering of Na^+ channels occurs at the node of Ranvier of myelinated axons, but clustering also occurs at synaptic contacts, dendrites, and cell bodies, in proximity to the initial segment of axons.

Early pharmacologic studies attempting to elucidate the ionic correlates of the action potential greatly benefited from the availability of naturally occurring toxins that specifically and powerfully block I_{Na}. The magic bullet for sodium channels was tetrodotoxin (TTX),[5] a lethal poison produced by a selected species of puffer fish (*Fugu*). TTX is present in large quantities in the liver and female genital organs, but the real culinary treat is the testes of this hermaphroditic animal. Separation of the toxic portions is paramount to survival of the consumer. The sea anemone toxin (ATX) and α-scorpion toxin are also powerful blockers of I_{Na}. TTX and other natural toxins block the external portion of the ion channel. Interestingly, although most sodium channels are blocked by micromolar concentrations of TTX, genetic ablation of one amino acid (Tyr or Phe) in the sequence of the ion channel protein confers relative resistance to TTX because binding of the toxin is restricted to this region.[6] The amazing specificity of TTX binding suggested that normally occurring variation in the amino acid sequence of ion channels may prove to be an extremely important determinant of not only the pharmacologic properties of the channels but also their inactivation/activation/voltage dependency. In fact, although the poisonous actions of TTX are primarily due to direct blockade of Na^+ fluxes through the channel's pore, ATX and α-scorpion toxin bind to a portion responsible for channel inactivation.

Mutations in these regions cause faulty inactivation, a condition linked to neuropathogenesis.

The biophysical correlates of Na^+ channel function are well understood today. The general scheme of

$$Closed \rightarrow Open \rightarrow Inactivated \rightarrow Closed$$

explains the properties of whole-cell I_{Na} recorded from neurons. The voltage dependency of each process justifies the initial depolarization required to promote the opening of channels; the consequent depolarization induced by sodium current promotes further opening of channels, the process being terminated by time- and voltage-dependent closure of the channels. The passage from closed to open (and visa versa) is referred to as activation (deactivation), whereas the passage from open to inactivated is called inactivation. Removal of inactivation occurs when the channel returns to its closed state.

From a structural point of view, Na^+ channels are constituted by αβ1β2 heterotrimers, often with four repeated domains each with six-membrane–spanning subunits. The voltage sensor is located on the fourth transmembrane domain. Different subunits are represented differently in the central and peripheral nervous systems. According to the recent literature, the following tissue-specific localization and pharmacology can be derived: for α subunits, SCN1A is primarily expressed in brain tissue and is blocked by TTX and saxitoxin (SXT). The most abundant brain α subunit is encoded by SCN2A1; this subunit is also found in peripheral nerves, in the initial axonal segment, and in the nodes of Ranvier (TTX and SXT sensitive). SCN2A2 and SC2NA3 are predominantly expressed in the brain, whereas SCN4A encodes channels found in muscle. In addition to TTX, these channels are sensitive to ω-conotoxins (GIIIA, GIIIB, GIIIC). Mutations of these channels are responsible for hyperkalemic periodic paralysis, paramyotonia, and myotonia. The SCN5A subunit is expressed in the heart and in denervated skeletal muscle; in the heart, these channels are responsible for upstroke of the action potential. These subunits are resistant to blockade by TTX and SXT; mutations of these genes are involved in subtypes of long QT syndrome, a cardiac condition that is sometimes associated with epileptic seizures. SCN6A (uterus), SCN10A, SCN11A, and SCN9A (dorsal root ganglion) are all sensitive to TTX. The molecular nature of glial sodium channels and the contribution of a specific α subunit are not fully understood at present. β Subunits are bound covalently to α subunits and provide inactivation kinetics to Na^+ channels. Mutations of these SCN1B and SCN1A subunits have been linked to generalized epilepsy with febrile seizures (see Catterall and colleagues[7] and Gambardella and Marini[8] for review of voltage-gated ion channel–related hereditary diseases).

The fact that even slight mutations cause profound deficits in sodium channel function and that these mutations result in neurological diseases leads to the hypothesis that replacement of defective channels by *gene therapy* may repristinate the loss of function caused by the initial genetic deficit. If a single gene mutation is responsible (as in cystic fibrosis and in a number of neurological disorders) and if the tissue to be transfected with the repair mechanism is accessible (such as skeletal muscle), it is possible that viral delivery of genetic products may alleviate the consequences of faulty ion channels. A positive outcome with this approach is somehow dependent on the pathogenesis of the disease itself. If the observed deficit is the consequence solely of the inherited mutation, replacement by a normal genotype is likely to be successful. If, however, the initial deficit has led to extensive rearrangement of neuronal connections or if the deficit causes extensive neuronal cell death (such as in epilepsy), it is unclear whether restoring normal function by simple gene replacement may be beneficial. It is also worth remembering that although a small fraction of neurological disorders are clearly imputable to a single gene mutation affecting a particular ion

TABLE 49-3 Summary of Characteristics of Voltage-Gated Calcium Channels

	I_{Ca}— LOW VOLTAGE ACTIVATED		I_{Ca}—HIGH VOLTAGE ACTIVATED		
Additional names	T	N	L	P	R, Q
Threshold (mV)	−60	−40	−40		
Pharmacologic antagonists	Nickel Mibefradil Kurtoxin	ω-conotoxin MVIIC	Dihydropyridines (nimodipine) Phenylalkylamines (verapamil) Benzodiazepines (diltiazem)	ω-AGA$_{IVA}$ ω-Conotoxin GIVA	ω-Conotoxin MVIIC (Q) SNX-482
Second messengers			cAMP/PK-G$_s$		
Neurotransmitters			Somatostatin, ACh, ATP, ADO		
Cell type/subcellular localization	Neuronal and cardiac	Presynaptic	Skeletal muscle: α$_{1S}$ Brain (neuronal soma and proximal dendrites): α$_{1B}$ Cardiac muscle: α$_{1C}$ Neuroendocrine: α$_{1D}$ Retina: α$_{1F}$	High concentration of α subunit in cerebellum, Purkinje cells, neuromuscular junctions	Cerebellar granule cells; hippocampal pyramidal neurons (Q) Neuronal presynaptic
Function	"Pacemaker" potentials in cardiac muscle and neurons	Transmitter Release	Excitation-contraction coupling Dendritic action potentials	Transmitter release	

ACh, acetylcholine; ADO, adenosine; ATP, adenosine triphosphate; cAMP, cyclic adenosine monophosphate; PK, protein kinase.

channel, the most common forms of disease result from a complex interaction of initial genotypic changes followed by adaptive responses, including apoptosis or necrosis. Finally, given that mutations of crucial ionic mechanisms such as I_{Na} affect cardiac, neuronal, and muscular function, it is possible that a large number of mutations are nonvital and that the vital mutations are possible because of redundancy of gene expression or compensatory over-expression of similar ion channel proteins.

Phenotypic changes caused by relatively minor alterations in ion channel gating sometimes become clinically relevant when concomitant deficits not necessarily associated with action potentials are present. This is the case, for example, in mutations of the SCN4A subunit leading to hyperkalemic periodic paralysis. For the paralytic symptoms to occur, patients must concomitantly experience variations in plasma potassium (by either K^+ intake or exercise followed by rest). This leads to opening of Na^+ channels that switch to a non-inactivating mode, thereby leading to the development of a persistent inward Na^+ current. The ensuing depolarization of muscle membrane will further increase $[K^+]_{out}$ via loss through voltage-dependent K^+ channels and thus aggravate the initial trigger. Furthermore, the persistent depolarization causes inactivation of normal Na^+ channels, which leads to rapid loss of tissue excitability and paralysis. This example demonstrates the complex interactions between normal and abnormal ion channels expressed in a certain cell type, the importance of the extracellular milieu in biophysical signaling via ion channels, and the difficulties associated with the diagnosis of altered ion channel phenotypes.

Calcium Action Potentials and Calcium Channels

The mechanism of calcium action potentials is somewhat different, but it follows the general principles of threshold for activation and rapid gating mechanisms. As is the case with sodium channels, Ca^{2+} channels are distributed heterogeneously in the CNS, and even within the same cells different subspecies of Ca^{2+} channels may be found. This inhomogeneous expression is func-

tionally significant in that it allows Ca^{2+} influx to perform several different cellular tasks, including depolarization of dendrites and propagation of signals to the cell body, synaptic release of neurotransmitter, contraction, and second messenger function. As for sodium channels, membrane depolarization is the most common trigger for opening of channels; the kinetic properties of Ca^{2+} channels, however, are characterized by longer time constants. This kinetic behavior underlies the different durations of neuronal/axonal action potentials (I_{Na}, 1 to 3 msec) versus cardiac action potentials (several hundreds of milliseconds; large inward currents carried by I_{Ca}).* An additional difference between Na^+ and Ca^{2+} action potentials (or the underlying ion channel mechanisms) is the fact that the threshold for I_{Ca} activation varies greatly between different Ca^{2+} channel families. *Low-threshold* Ca^{2+} channels (or low voltage activated) are also characterized by relatively rapid opening and closing and are also referred to as "T-type" (transient) currents. *High-threshold* Ca^{2+} channels (or high voltage activated) can be further subdivided into neuronal (N), L, and P types. The pharmacologic properties of the calcium channel families are equally complex (Table 49-3).[9,10] Although sodium action potentials are typically triggered by depolarization *and* terminated by depolarization (inactivation of I_{Na} and voltage-dependent activation of I_K), an additional mechanism is involved in repolarization: activation by intracellular Ca^{2+} channels that act as powerful terminators of cell depolarization. Ca^{2+} channels are modulated by important intracellular signals such as cyclic adenosine monophosphate (cAMP; cAMP-dependent protein kinases) and G proteins. These modulatory signals arise from receptor stimulation, thus coupling the activity of postsynaptic (or presynaptic in the case of presynaptic receptors) Ca^{2+} channels to the activity of neighboring cells.

Ca^{2+} channels contain four or five distinct subunits: α subunits display different tissue and peptide specificity. They are constituted by transmembrane-spanning proteins and act in both voltage sensor and selectivity filter capacities. The

---

*The overall duration of action potentials is also determined by other factors, such as the duration of repolarizing potentials.

dihydropyridines verapamil and nifedipine bind to α_1 subunits. In Lambert-Eaton myasthenic syndrome, the autoimmune component of the disease is due to IgG binding to α_{1A} subunits. In the majority of cases, P/Q-type channels are involved; in a small percentage of cases, the α_{1B} subunit constituting N channels mediates the autoimmune response. Other subunits increase the amplitude of Ca^{2+} currents and bind the antiepileptic drug gabapentin ($\alpha_{2\delta}$). The β subunit is localized in the cytoplasm, associates with α subunits that are membrane bound, has regulatory functions, and mediates the effects of cAMP; phosphorylation of cAMP-dependent protein kinase modifies current, voltage dependence, and activation-inactivation. γ Subunits are exclusively localized within the membrane and lack a cytoplasmic component. Similar to subunits in other channels, γ subunits modulate channel voltage dependency.

Not all calcium channels are involved in transmembrane fluxes of calcium. Ca^{2+} release channels are located ubiquitously in intracellular organelles and regulate the cytoplasmic Ca^{2+} content of virtually every mammalian cell type. These channels belong to two separate families, those sensitive to the alkaloid ryanodine and those activated by inositol 1,4,5-triphosphate (IP_3). Ryanodine-sensitive Ca^{2+} release is triggered by the activity of dihydropyridine-sensitive Ca^{2+} channels and therefore acts as a signal amplifier. These channels are located mainly in skeletal and cardiac muscle. Disorders resulting from changes in these channels include malignant hyperthermia and central core disease. The IP_3 receptors are located primarily in glial and neuronal endoplasmic reticulum membranes. In response to stimulation of cell surface receptors, intracellularly generated IP_3 binds to these receptors and causes intracellular Ca^{2+} stores to be released. Thus, although IP_3 receptors link changes in intracellular calcium to chemical transmission and act as second messengers, the ryanodine-sensitive mechanism is optimized to link the electrical activity promoted by Ca^{2+} action potentials to calcium mobilization.

Given the large number of Ca^{2+} channel families and their widespread distribution in the nervous system, it is not surprising that numerous neurological disorders have been linked to mutation, autoimmune inactivation, or altered expression of I_{Ca}. Disorders affecting the presynaptic terminal of motor axons cause the aforementioned Lambert-Eaton myasthenic syndrome, and mutations of the α_{1A} subunit are responsible for a form of episodic ataxia type 2. Lambert-Eaton myasthenic syndrome is an autoimmune disorder associated with an immunologically abnormal response to neoplasms, whereas type 2 ataxia is caused by defective production of ion channels. Familial hemiplegic migraine is associated with missense mutations in transmembrane segments, and progressive ataxia is caused by either trinucleotide repeat expansion in an intracellular region near the C-terminal or by missense mutation.[11]

Repolarization of Action Potentials and Maintenance of Resting Membrane Potential: Potassium Channels

There are many subtypes and functions of potassium channels in the mammalian CNS, with whole textbooks devoted to them. Different families of K^+ channels are found in the mammalian CNS, including (1) Kv channels, which are activated by a change in transmembrane voltage, and (2) inward rectifier channels (K_{IR} channels), which have high conductance for K^+ ions moving into a hyperpolarized cell (in contrast to K^+ ions moving out of a depolarized cell) and are often regulated by intracellular messengers. Kv channels are typically closed at RMP and open rapidly after membrane depolarization. They are variably spliced tetramers composed of four homologous α subunits that each contains a voltage sensor and a sequence that provides cation

selectivity for potassium. Kv channels are variably composed of alternative RNA splicing and subunit duplication of gene products from four subfamilies, Kv1 to Kv4, which correspond to the murine *Shaker*, *Shab*, *Shaw*, and *Shal*. Rates of channel inactivation vary dramatically between the different subtypes.

Potassium channels are the major contributor to both neuronal and glial RMP. As described earlier, neuronal membranes are predominantly permeable to potassium at rest, which results in cell RMP being near the potassium reversal potential E_K. Even more so than neurons, the majority of glial resting channels are K^+ permeable, which results in a relatively hyperpolarized RMP. Because of their lack of electrical excitability, a hyperpolarized RMP was previously a defining criterion during physiologic recordings from glia in situ. However, it has been demonstrated over the past several years that glial cells can have a wide range of RMPs, depending on the glial cell subtype, ion channel endowment, location within the nervous system, and developmental stage.[12,13]

Hodgkin and Huxley initially characterized the important role of (what are now termed) delayed rectifier Kv potassium channels in action potential repolarization.[14] These channels, which are blocked by tetraethylammonium (TEA), are similar to sodium channels in that the probability of channel opening is increased by membrane depolarization, with increased opening in proportion to the amount of membrane depolarization. However, delayed rectifier potassium channels differ from sodium channels in that they open more slowly and do not inactivate in the presence of persistently maintained depolarization. As discussed earlier, it is this sodium channel inactivation together with persistent activation of outward potassium channels (and inward chloride channels that produce an outward current by allowing negatively charged chloride ions to enter the cell) that results in action potential repolarization. After repolarization of the action potential, there is a refractory period during which the threshold for initiation of another action potential is elevated. The absolute refractory period, during which an action potential cannot be generated, is followed by a relative refractory period, during which an increased stimulus is necessary to generate an action potential. The refractory period results from residual sodium channel inactivation and potassium channel activation; it limits the maximum firing frequency of different classes of neurons.

The M channel has distinctly different properties from the Kv potassium channels that are responsible for repolarization of the action potential. Although activated by membrane depolarizations, these channels are inhibited by muscarinic acetylcholine receptor binding, as well as by a variety of other neurotransmitters and neuroactive compounds. Rates of channel opening and closing are approximately 100 times slower than delayed rectifier channels. Based on these different characteristics, M channels are thought to have divergent functions in the CNS. On the one hand, by means of their slow kinetics, they prevent repetitive neuronal discharges and hyperexcitability, whereas on the other hand, their inhibition by modulatory neurotransmitters results in local increases in excitation. Inhibition of these channels is thus a double-edged sword that promotes local increases in excitation important to such processes as learning and memory while also potentially rendering areas of the brain proepileptic. The M channel KCNQ1 is mutated in a subtype of long QT syndrome, whereas KCNQ2 and KCNQ3 are mutated in two different forms of benign familial neonatal convulsions.[15]

Several other potassium currents present in CNS neurons are beyond the scope of this chapter.[16] These include (1) channels that are opened by intracellular calcium ($I_{K(Ca)}$) and function in action potential repolarization and determination of the interspike interval between action potentials; (2) slowly hyperpolarizing currents (I_{AHP}), blockade of which promotes neuronal excitation; (3) mixed cation currents (I_{ha}) that are permeant to K^+ and Na^+ and are involved in rhythmic burst firing (see the later section "Expression of Ion Currents in Different Neuronal Populations"); (4) the transiently inactivating current I_A, which lengthens the interspike interval between action potentials; and (5) K_{ATP} channels, an inwardly rectifying subtype that opens in response to lowered intracellular adenosine triphosphate (ATP) and has been implicated in protection from ischemia, insulin-mediated hypothalamic neuronal glucose homeostasis, and glial potassium homeostasis.

By considering the clinical manifestation of diseases caused by altered expression of I_{Na}, I_K, and I_{Ca}, it is surprising that permanent changes in the normal endowment of ion channels can cause episodic diseases. This is true for a variety of inheritable cardiac conditions (arrhythmias), as well as neurological disorders such as episodic ataxia and epilepsy. How it is possible that most of the time patients affected by these disorders lack symptoms and what precipitates the clinical manifestations largely remains unknown. The modern techniques used to map and pinpoint the molecular mechanisms of diseases have thus far failed to determine the cofactors that transform a small ion channel deficit into a full-blown neurological disease. Understanding these coexisting conditions will perhaps provide information sufficient to chart an effective therapy. Channelopathies are summarized in Table 49-4.[17]

Glial Ion Channels and Glutamate Release

Glial potassium channels are the most common electrophysiologic feature of both cultured and in situ astrocytes and can be categorized as follows: channels that allow inward but not outward current flow (*inward rectifiers*, K_{IR}), channels that allow outward but not inward current flow (*delayed rectifier*, I_{DR}; *transient outward current*, I_A), and channels that are opened by intracellular calcium ($I_{K(Ca)}$). Glial potassium channels differ in their sensitivity to blockers: inward rectifiers are blocked by submillimolar concentrations of external cesium and barium, and outward I_{DR} and I_A are both sensitive to TEA and 4-aminopyridine (4-AP), but I_A blockade by TEA requires high concentrations.[18] Recently, a mixed cation channel (I_{ha}) permeant to K^+ and Na^+ and ether-a-go-go currents (HERG 1)[19] have been described in both cultured and in situ astrocytes and may assist in potassium homeostasis in the CNS.

Voltage-dependent, TTX-sensitive and TTX-insensitive sodium channels are also expressed in both cultured and in situ glial cells.[20] Although astrocytes are incapable of producing action potential–like responses, possibly because of the relatively low Na^+ current densities in these cells, a role of Na^+ channels in extracellular buffering of potassium has been proposed.

TABLE 49-4 Overview of Ion Channel Disorders Relevant to Neurological Surgery

DISORDER	ION CHANNEL	MUTATION(S)
Generalized myotonia (Becker's)	CLCN1 (skeletal muscle chloride channel)	Point mutations—reduced Cl^- conductance; increased membrane resistance; less current required for action potential, slower repolarization; more sensitive to K^+ concentration
Myotonia congenita (Thomsen's)	CLCN1 (skeletal muscle chloride channel)	Missense mutations and deletions—reduced Cl^- conductance; increased membrane resistance; less current required for action potential, slower repolarization; more sensitive to K^+ concentration
Sodium channel myotonia Paramyotonia congenita Periodic paralysis, type II (hyperkalemic)	SCN4A (skeletal muscle sodium channel)	Point mutations in regions involved in channel inactivation—impaired inactivation resulting in slowed decay of transient sodium current

DISORDER	ION CHANNEL	MUTATION(S)
NEUROLOGICAL		
Familial hemiplegic migraine	CACNL1A (α_1 voltage-sensitive calcium channel subunit)	Assorted mutations (α_1 voltage-sensitive calcium channel subunit)
Episodic ataxia type 2	CACNL1A	Assorted mutations (α_{1A} calcium channel subunit)
Spinocerebellar ataxia	CACNL1A	Expansion of trinucleotide repeat
Episodic ataxia type 1/partial complex seizures	Kv1.1/KCNA1 (delayed rectifier K^+ channel)	Multiple missense and stop codon mutations; rare human, severe mouse seizures
Benign neonatal convulsions	KCNQ2 and KCNQ3 (M-type potassium channel)	Multiple mutations, altering regulation of rapid neuronal firing
Generalized epilepsy with febrile seizures	SCNA1 and SCNB1	Multiple mutations

DISORDER	ION CHANNEL	CAUSE
ACQUIRED CHANNELOPATHIES		
Long QT syndrome	HERG K^+ channel	Antiarrhythmic medications class IA or III
Neurological effects prevented by BBB		HERG channel blockade
Myasthenia gravis	AChR	Autoimmune
Acquired myotonia	Voltage-gated K^+ channel	Autoimmune
Eaton-Lambert syndrome	Voltage-gated Ca^{2+} channel	Autoimmune

AChR, acetylcholine receptor; BBB, blood-brain barrier.

According to this hypothesis, Na$^+$ influx sustains the Na$^+$,K$^+$-ATPase pump, which results in net uptake of K$^+$. Finally, calcium channels are represented sparingly in glial cells and require either neuronal or otherwise differentiating factors for expression; whether I$_{Ca}$ can be recorded from in situ hippocampal astrocytes is still unknown, but release of calcium from intracellular stores in response to neurotransmitters acting on astrocytes has clearly been demonstrated. Relevant to potassium homeostasis, micromolar [Ca^{+2}]$_{in}$ can cause opening of I$_{K(Ca)}$ and may thus participate in the generation of outward potassium fluxes.

Astrocytes can release the excitatory transmitter glutamate, which acts on at least three families of receptors.[21-25] Astrocytic release of glutamate can occur through several mechanisms, some of which are specific to glia (e.g., reversal of glutamate uptake) or occur via Ca^{2+}-dependent exocytosis, which shares similarities to neurotransmission. In addition to glutamate, astrocytes can release a variety of neurotransmitters such as taurine and adenosine. Unlike synaptic transmission, which is specific for a post-synaptic site, release of glutamate by a single astrocyte affects several adjacent neurons, thereby simultaneously controlling the excitability of several neighboring pyramidal cells. This may constitute one of the mechanisms of neuronal synchronization in epilepsy.

If astrocytes release glutamate and have neurotransmitter receptors, what differentiates neurons from glia? Are these phenomena operating in vivo, or are these findings limited to slice preparations? For example, glial cells display intrinsic activity in the absence of neuronal stimulation, but this finding was observed only in vitro. Astrocytes greatly outnumber neurons, and the ratio of astrocytes to neurons is larger in more evolved brain. There is no question about the importance of non-neuronal cells to CNS function and human disease; however, the laboratory findings need to be confirmed in preparations in which artifacts are controlled and known. An important physiologic aspect of the astrocyte in situ is its proximity to capillaries and the perivascular space of arterioles.[26] Astrocytes influence maintenance of the blood-brain barrier, which in turn regulates brain ion homeostasis.[27] Whether astrocytes also release significant levels of vasodilators or constrictors remains to be proved in vivo in preparations in which the surrounding tissue is intact. However, a clear effect of astrocytes on small-diameter, capillary-like structures has been demonstrated.[28] This effect may be important when capillary perfusion pressure is altered by brain edema or other disruptors of brain homeostasis.

Expression of Ion Currents in Different Neuronal Populations

Morphologically distinct neuronal populations in different areas of the CNS are endowed with distinct mixtures of ion channels, which results in widely differing electrophysiologic properties such as RMP, intrinsic ionic conductance, and rhythmicity. Several different patterns of neuronal activity can be classified. Brainstem and spinal cord motor neurons generate single spikes of action potentials that form trains of activity in direct correlation with the degree of depolarization. In contrast to this nearly linear firing pattern is that exhibited by many hippocampal and cortical pyramidal cells that display spike frequency adaptation, in which trains of action potentials decrease in frequency over time. Other neuronal populations, such as thalamic relay neurons, inferior olivary neurons, and some pyramidal cells, have intrinsic rhythmicity that allows the generation of bursts of activity without afferent stimulation. Other cells such as many GABAergic inhibitory interneurons are specialized to generate a high firing frequency (>300 Hz) of short-duration (<1 msec) action potentials. A final type of pattern is that exhibited by cholinergic, serotoninergic, noradrenergic, and histaminergic cells, which

innervate large areas of the brain. These discrete cell populations carry out their modulatory function by spontaneously generating low firing frequencies (1 to 10 Hz).

This electrophysiologic heterogeneity affects the function of particular cell populations in the brain. Individual cell types possess particular combinations of the previously described Na$^+$, K$^+$, and Ca^{2+} currents that merge to result in the patterns of neuronal activity that are found in different areas of the CNS. These patterns can be investigated by in vitro isolated brain slice recordings, as well as by computer modeling simulations, to dissect the individual channel components. For example, relay neurons in the lateral geniculate nucleus that project to the visual cortex are characterized by an RMP of −70 mV during sleep versus −55 mV during the awake state, thus decreasing the transmission of information to the visual cortex during sleep. This sleep-wake variability is modulated by the low-threshold calcium current I$_T$, which together with the hyperpolarization-activated mixed cationic current I$_{ha}$ generates rhythmic bursts of action potentials in thalamic relay neurons. During slow-wave sleep, thalamic relay neurons have a relatively hyperpolarized RMP that de-inactivates low-threshold calcium currents and thereby results in I$_T$-generated slow spikes of activity. Between these spikes, a slowly depolarizing potential is generated by activation of I$_{ha}$. Together, these two currents result in spontaneous synchronized bursts of low-frequency action potentials. In contrast, the transition from slow-wave sleep to either wakefulness or rapid eye movement sleep is characterized by relative depolarization of thalamic relay neurons. This depolarization inactivates I$_T$ and I$_{ha}$, which results in conversion to a tonic action potential mode in which single spikes are produced one at a time in response to stimulation.[16]

INTERCELLULAR COMMUNICATION: ELECTRICAL AND CHEMICAL SYNAPTIC TRANSMISSION

The nervous system has the unique ability to communicate both locally and over large distances by using a combination of action potential–driven axonal conduction and interneuronal synaptic transmission. Synaptic transmission occurs in two forms: (1) electrical transmission of ion currents via gap junction channel pores that communicate directly with adjoining cells and (2) chemical transmission mediated by neurotransmitters across the synaptic cleft.

The different endowment of ion channels predictably leads to a broad variety of firing patterns (Figs. 49-5 and 49-6). Most of the traditional studies focused on cortical, cerebellar, and hippocampal neurons because of technical reasons (more densely packed neurons are easier to find) and also the popularity of brain-slicing technologies.[29] More recently, with the advent of surgical procedures for deep brain stimulation, it became possible to record from other human brain regions, such as the thalamus and the subthalamic nuclei. The examples shown highlight the different firing properties derived from extracellular unit recordings. The essential feature of the action potential phenotype shown consists of frequency of discharge within a certain period. Two extremes are shown, one depicting high-frequency, non–time-dependent firing and the other showing time-dependent changes in frequency in thalamic neurons.

Analysis of the data provided by these deep brain recordings has also resulted in the quest for novel quantitative approaches to describe neuronal behavior. In other words, the comparably sparse firing of hippocampal and cortical neurons can easily be described by plotting the digitized versions of the recordings themselves. Thus, if the application of stimuli is superimposed, the reader may quickly and easily derive the effect of any given

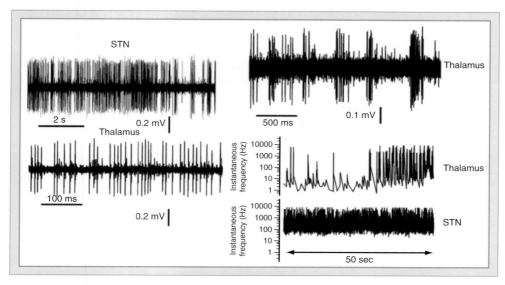

FIGURE 49-5 Firing properties of thalamic and subthalamic neurons. Note the distinct differences in firing properties, as also illustrated by the frequency plot. The ordinate axis (in hertz) depicts the instantaneous frequency, a variable that takes into account the "density" of events measured during a brief, millisecond-long interval. STN, subthalamic nucleus.

manipulation by limiting the presentation to the *time domain*. When dealing with recordings such as those in Figure 49-5, transformation of data in the *frequency domain* becomes necessary. This can be achieved with a variety of software of increasing complexity (and cost!). The results in Figure 49-6 show examples of this analysis. Data can be shown as either two- or three-dimensional plots. Fast Fourier transform (FFT) analysis reveals

time-dependent changes over a time interval, as well as the "FFT amplitude" of firings at a given range of frequency.

Electrical Synaptic Transmission

Because electrical synapses transmit current between cells directly coupled by gap junctions, there is minimal synaptic delay, and

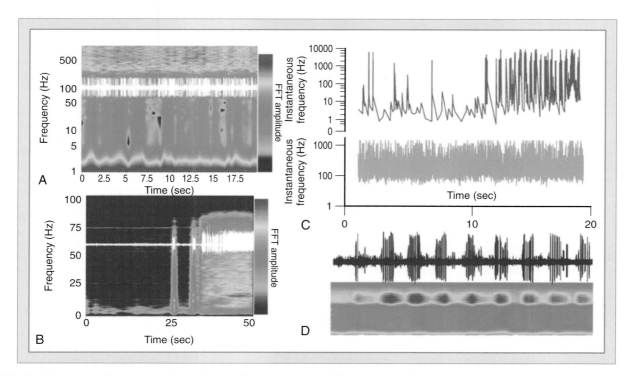

FIGURE 49-6 Examples of data analysis based on the *frequency* domain. The graph in **A** shows a trace of a unit recording (raw data, in *white*) superimposed on a frequency/amplitude plot. The colors depict the amplitude of the events occurring at a certain time and at a certain frequency. **B** shows the same protocol applied to an electroencephalographic signal recorded from a rat brain before and during a seizure. Again, the *white* trace refers to the raw data, whereas the color graph gives an overview of the frequency and intensity of spiking. The graph in **C** is the same as in Figure 49-5 but in color. **D** shows a ribbon trace (*bottom*) that has the same meaning and dimensions of the graph in **A.** The trace in *blue* is a recording from a bursting thalamic neuron. Data analysis was performed with DIADEM. FFT, fast Fourier transform.

intercellular transmission of current is nearly instantaneous. Gap junctions form a low-resistance pathway that allows electric current to flow from one cell to another, thereby resulting in depolarization of the postsynaptic cell. This depolarization can potentially trigger an action potential, thus linking electrical and chemical neurotransmission.

Intercellular electrical communication occurs through specialized channels called gap junctions. Each gap junction channel is made up of a pair of hemichannels contributed by the presynaptic and postsynaptic cell. The hemichannels together form an approximately 1.5-nm channel pore that directly communicates with the cytoplasm of the two cells and allows the passage of small molecules up to 1000 daltons, ions, and intercellular dyes to facilitate the study of gap junction function. Each hemichannel is composed of a connexon, which in turn consists of six identical connexin proteins. The cytoplasmic side of gap junction channels is sensitive to various modulators, including pH and intracellular calcium. Intracellular acidification and elevated intracellular calcium both result in closure of the gap junction channels by electrically uncoupling cells from one another. In contrast, alkalinization increases the degree of intercellular coupling. Electrical neurotransmission can be either bidirectional (nonrectifying) or directionally selective (rectifying), depending on whether the gap junction channels joining the two cells are voltage sensitive. The strength of electrotonic coupling between two cells can be changed by altering the shape or duration of the presynaptic impulse, the junctional conductance, or the conductance of nearby nonjunctional membrane.[30,31]

Electrical synaptic transmission is extremely rapid, which facilitates the synchronous firing of large groups of neurons. Although the degree of neuronal electrical synaptic activity is probably underappreciated at the present time, the functional importance of this form of intercellular communication is increasingly being recognized. For example, the normal development of neuronal columnar domains is dependent on gap junction–mediated intercellular signaling. Spontaneous excitation of one or a few trigger neurons subsequently activates other columnar cells via gap junctions. Gap junctions may also coordinate hippocampal CA1 oscillatory behavior. Parvalbumin-containing GABAergic interneurons in the rat hippocampal CA1 region, known to form a network by mutual axosomatic chemical synaptic contacts, also form another network connected by dendrodendritic gap junctions. Gap junctions linking this dendritic network may facilitate the synchronization of oscillatory activities generated in the interneuron network.[32,33]

Gap junction communication is found to a much larger degree between glial cells than between neurons in the adult mammalian brain. Glial cell gap junction signaling can be either homotypic (i.e., between two astrocytes) or heterotypic (between an astrocyte and an oligodendroglial cell). Astrocytes are extensively coupled by gap junctions, thus potentially forming a functional syncytium for the regulation of extracellular homeostasis of potassium ion concentration and pH. Neuronal stimulation causes an activity-dependent release of potassium, which results in a local increase in extracellular potassium ($[K^+]_{out}$). After a single action potential, $[K^+]_{out}$ increases by 0.01 to 0.02 mM. Despite the firing of large populations of neurons, $[K^+]_{out}$ is extremely tightly regulated and even during seizure activity in the hippocampus does not rise above a ceiling level of 12 mM. Additionally, $[K^+]_{out}$ returns to normal in a relatively short period. Experiments have suggested that glial uptake and distribution via gap junctions play a pivotal role in conditions in which there is massive $[K^+]_{out}$ accumulation, such as epilepsy. Gap junctional communication between glial cells also provides a pathway for long-range metabolite or second messenger signaling. In response to direct astrocytic or neuronal stimulation,

intercellular waves of Ca^{2+} can be generated in astrocytes. These waves spread from cell to cell by one of two mechanisms: either directly through gap junctions or via an extracellular route whereby ATP or glutamate released from astrocytes subsequently propagates via binding to P_2 purinergic or glutamatergic receptors.[30,31]

Chemical Synaptic Transmission

In contrast to the direct intercellular communication between cells coupled by electrical synapses, chemical synapses are anatomically separated by a 20- to 40-nm-wide synaptic cleft across which neurotransmitter travels from the presynaptic to the postsynaptic cell. The presynaptic cell contains a region of membrane specialized for neurotransmitter release at which synaptic vesicles are clustered, termed the *active zone*. When an action potential arrives at the presynaptic terminal, voltage-gated calcium channels open. The resultant rise in intracellular calcium results in fusion of the synaptic vesicles with the presynaptic membrane, and neurotransmitters are released into the synaptic cleft by exocytosis. The neurotransmitter molecules are then able to diffuse to receptors on the postsynaptic cell terminal, which results in ion channel opening and alterations in the membrane properties of the postsynaptic cell. The specific postsynaptic neurotransmitter receptors determine whether the result of neurotransmitter binding is excitation or inhibition of the postsynaptic cell. Neurotransmitter receptors can be either ionotropic receptors that directly gate ion channels or metabotropic receptors that indirectly gate ion channels through modulatory activity by second messenger cascades. The direct synaptic activity produced by ionotropic receptors lasts on the order of milliseconds, whereas metabotropic receptor–gated activity lasts seconds to minutes.

Perhaps the best studied example of ionotropic synaptic transmission is at the neuromuscular junction. In a specialized region of muscle membrane termed the *end plate*, the motor neuron axon innervates the muscle. The axon ends in varicosities termed *synaptic boutons*, each of which contains a specialized area of membrane termed the *active zone*. The active zone contains the synaptic vesicles filled with acetylcholine, as well as voltage-gated calcium channels. The synaptic boutons are each positioned over an area of postsynaptic muscle fiber containing a clustering of acetylcholine receptors termed the *junctional fold*. When the acetylcholine released by presynaptic cells binds to its receptors in the junctional zone, an end-plate potential is generated by flow of both sodium and potassium ions through the nicotinic acetylcholine receptor–gated ionotropic channel. The end-plate potential thus generated results in a depolarization that is large enough to activate voltage-gated sodium channels at the base of the junctional folds; the end-plate potential is then converted into an action potential that propagates along the muscle fiber. In contrast to the acetylcholine-gated channel, which is permeable to both sodium and potassium and blocked by α-bungarotoxin, the voltage-gated sodium channel is permeable only to sodium and is blocked by TTX.

Similar to the neuromuscular junction, most CNS neurons use ionotropic receptors for rapid intercellular signaling. However, in contrast to the monosynaptic excitatory input at the neuromuscular junction, CNS neurons are usually innervated by both excitatory and inhibitory input from multiple cells using both excitatory and inhibitory neurotransmitters. Input from a single excitatory neuron generates a depolarizing excitatory postsynaptic potential (EPSP), whereas inhibitory innervation generates a hyperpolarizing inhibitory postsynaptic potential (IPSP). Excitatory and inhibitory synapses are morphologically different, as summarized in Table 49-5.

TABLE 49-5 Morphologic Differences between Central Nervous System Synapses

GRAY TYPE I	GRAY TYPE II
Usually glutamatergic/excitatory	Usually GABAergic/inhibitory
Prominent round synaptic vesicles	Less prominent flattened synaptic vesicles
Larger synaptic cleft (30 nm) and active zone (1-2 μm)	Smaller synaptic cleft (20 nm) and active zone (<1 μm)

GABAergic, transmitting γ-aminobutyric acid.

MAINTENANCE OF EXTRACELLULAR HOMEOSTASIS

Contribution of Astrocytes to Regulation of Neuronal Excitability: Spatial Buffering

We will focus on CNS potassium homeostasis as an example of the importance of astrocyte function in the maintenance of extracellular homeostasis. The action potential generation of large-voltage signals is accompanied by an equally impressive accumulation/depletion of ions in the extracellular space (ECS) or in the cytosol. The region of accumulation is easily derived from the Nernst equation: depolarizing potentials generated by the influx of Na^+ or Ca^{2+} will cause an increase in $[Na]_{in}$ and $[Ca^{2+}]_{in}$, whereas repolarization mediated by K^+ movements will cause an extracellular increase in $[K^+]_{out}$. The concentration of potassium in the ECS (K_{ECS}) in the mammalian CNS increases measurably (from 3 to about 4 mM) during physiologic stimulation, to a larger extent (up to 12 mM) during seizures or direct, synchronous stimulation of afferent pathways, and to exceedingly high values (>30 mM) during anoxia or spreading depression. Despite these rapid and large changes in K_{ECS}, K^+ values return to normal levels in a relatively short period.

Neuronal excitability is regulated by a complex interaction of excitatory and inhibitory potentials. In pyramidal neurons, the depolarizing ion conductances involved in action potential generation are regulated primarily by the voltage-dependent activation/inactivation properties of Na^+ and Ca^{2+} channels; in addition, inward Na^+ and Ca^{2+} currents underlie the generation of EPSPs. Termination of these depolarizing potentials occurs through the voltage- and calcium-dependent activation of intrinsic potassium conductances and by activation of interneurons that release inhibitory neurotransmitters to produce IPSPs; the latter are mediated by postsynaptic activation of chloride and potassium currents. Although I_{Na}, I_{Ca}, and I_{EPSP} are, under physiologic conditions, relatively independent of modest changes in the driving force for the permeant ions (because E_{Na} and E_{Ca} are remote with respect to cell resting potential), both repolarizing potassium and IPSP conductances are critically affected by even modest changes in cell RMP, $[K^+]_{out}$, and $[Cl]_{in}/[Cl]_{out}$. Because neuronal RMP depends significantly, albeit not exclusively, on $[K^+]_{out}$, maintenance of homeostatic control of extracellular potassium plays a crucial role in the regulation of neuronal firing.

Several mechanisms have been suggested to explain the rapid clearance of K^+ from the ECS: passive diffusion through the ECS, active removal by blood flow, and neuronal reuptake. However, these mechanisms alone are not fast enough to account for the rapid removal of K^+ from the ECS seen under experimental conditions. Several lines of evidence suggest that brain glial cells support homeostatic regulation of the neuronal microenvironment. CNS astrocytes are strategically located in proximity to

excitable neurons and are sensitive to the changes in extracellular ion composition that follow neuronal activity.[34-39] Experiments have suggested that glial uptake plays a pivotal role in conditions in which there is massive K_{out} accumulation. In cortical regions, glial cells participate in genesis of the changes in extracellular field potential associated with neuronal depolarization and efflux of potassium in the ECS. The combination of potassium uptake into glial cells immediately followed by redistribution through electrotonically coupled glial gap junctions ("spatial buffering") provides a valid working hypothesis to explain some of the features of K^+ movement in the ECS (Fig. 49-7). Although a direct demonstration that K_{IR} or I_{ha} plays a role in CNS extracellular potassium homeostasis is still lacking, evidence from studies on cultured neocortical astroglia has demonstrated K^+-induced inward currents sensitive to K_{IR} blockers. In addition, recent work has demonstrated evidence of glial spatial buffering during slow sleep oscillations in spike wave seizures in rodents.[40]

It has long been known that in conditions involving high levels of neuronal activity (e.g., seizures), $[K]_{out}$ accumulation is accompanied by cell swelling. The swelling that accompanies epileptiform neuronal discharge is due to excessive activity of the ionic mechanisms normally involved in the control of ECS homeostasis. One of the several proposed mechanisms associated with cell swelling, the $Na^+/K^+/2Cl^-$ cotransporter, is also believed to participate in uptake of K^+ into glia. This transporter is blocked by the loop diuretic furosemide. Treatment of "epileptic" hippocampal slices (treated with bicuculline, 0 Ca^{2+}, or 4-AP) with furosemide has been shown to inhibit spontaneous burst discharge. It has been hypothesized that this mechanism is related to furosemide's blockade of the swelling induced by the large ionic (and water) shifts that accompany $Na^+/K^+/2Cl^-$ cotransporter activity.[41,42] More recent experimentation has suggested that furosemide-induced opening of glial inwardly rectifying potassium channels may contribute to the antiepileptic mechanism.[43]

Neuronal K^+ reuptake and part of the hyperpolarizing undershoot that follows the action potential are mediated in part by an energy-dependent process that requires Na^+,K^+-ATPase activity. Similarly, extracellular potassium accumulation in glia may depend on energy-dependent processes. Na^+,K^+-ATPase activity is regulated by both $[Na^+]_{in}$ and $[K]_{out}$. Thus, increases in extracellular potassium or influx of Na^+ will cause activation of this electrogenic uptake mechanism. As a result, glial cells will accumulate potassium and extrude Na^+, the net result being hyperpolarization. Whether Na^+,K^+-ATPase–dependent potassium uptake plays a significant role in K^+ buffering is still controversial, partially because of the fact that selective pharmacologic blockade of the glial pump has been difficult.

Loss of Brain Homeostasis and Resultant Effects

It has been recognized for many years that one of the most peculiar histologic features of the mammalian brain is the infinitesimal size of the ECS separating various parenchymal cells. Because permeation of ions across neuronal membranes results in depletion/accumulation of ions undergoing transmembrane movement, it is important to understand how the brain maintains a constant extracellular and intracellular milieu. The essential nature of the latter function becomes apparent if one considers the volumetric rigidity of the skeletal structure encompassing the brain and the limited amount of osmotic changes that such a structure can withstand. This, together with the lack of lymphatic drainage from the CNS, implies that even a small accumulation of ion and water in the CNS requires immediate and complete clearance by mechanisms other than circulation of lymph. For simplicity, the following discussion focuses on changes in extracellular potassium and on the control of potassium homeostasis;

FIGURE 49-7 Diagrammatic representation of the proposed "spatial buffering" mechanism underlying transcellular potassium movement across cortical astrocytes. Under resting conditions, both cells are bathed in similar $[K^+]_{out}$, and cell 1 is characterized by a resting potential close to E_K by virtue of its high potassium permeability. Cell 2 is similarly sensitive to changes in E_K but has a more depolarized resting membrane potential. Under these "resting" conditions, gap junctions are kept closed because of a relatively acidic pH_i (1). Increases in $[K^+]_{out}$ in proximity to cell 1 cause influx of potassium into cell 1; during this accumulation process, cell depolarization will occur as a result of the sudden shift in E_K (2). Escape of intracellular potassium in this cell cannot occur because of the exclusive presence of potassium currents characterized by inward-going rectification; furthermore, electrochemical communication with cell 2 is precluded by the low conductance of gap junctions. As a result, a net increase in intracellular potassium sufficient to depolarize the cell occurs (3). This results in depolarization-induced alkalization (DIA), subsequent opening of gap junctions, and transport of potassium to cell 2 (4). Finally, outflow of K^+ occurs from cell 2 (5). R_j represents the junctional resistance (100% at steady state, 50% decrease after DIA); R_e represents the resistance of the extracellular fluid. Only two cells of the syncytium are shown together with the equivalent electric circuit showing the resistive pathways involved in the transfer of extracellular potassium from the extracellular space close to cell 1 to cell 2; the final step implies restitution of potassium to the extracellular space, but other mechanisms, such as backward diffusion or passage across the blood-brain barrier (or both), may act in conjunction with spatial buffering.

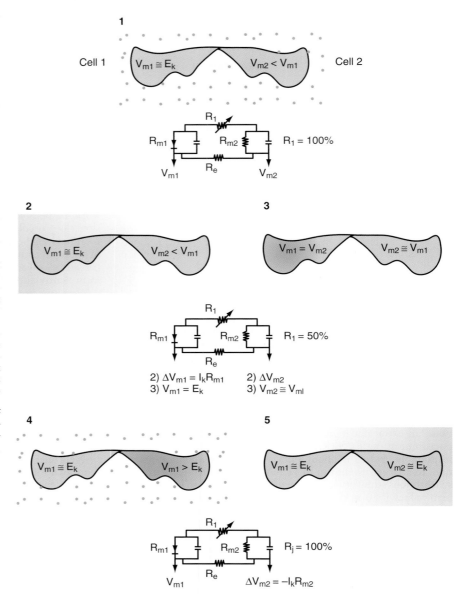

similar considerations, however, apply to other physiologically relevant ions (H^+, Ca^{2+}, Na^+, Cl^-).

Potassium ions play a fundamental role in the control of neuronal (and cardiac) excitability. Action potential repolarization is curtailed by increased $[K^+]_{out}$, and elevated potassium causes a dramatic decrease in some inhibitory potentials. The most direct effect of elevated extracellular potassium, however, consists of its direct depolarizing effects on neurons and neuronal terminals. Experimentally, the synaptic changes normally achieved by direct stimulation of presynaptic fibers (e.g., long-term potentiation) can be mimicked by small increases in potassium, whereas synchronous firing of thousands of cortical or hippocampal pyramidal cells is observed when $[K^+]_{out}$ is slightly elevated. The latter is commonly referred to as "potassium-induced epileptogenesis."

The delicate homeostatic electrophysiologic balance of the CNS is readily perturbed in association with or as a result of various pathologic conditions such as seizures, brain edema, and brain tumors. In various forms of epilepsy, alterations in neuronal and glial ion channel expression, ECS size, and intercellular astrocytic gap junction coupling may all contribute to the development or maintenance of seizure activity. In temporal lobe epilepsy, the most common surgically treated form of epilepsy, a number of pathologic features are characteristically found, including selective neuronal loss in the CA1, CA3, and hilar regions of the hippocampus, reactive gliosis in these same subfields, and sprouting of granule cell excitatory axon collaterals (mossy fibers). Epileptic granule cells are characterized by alterations in GABA receptors that increase their zinc sensitivity at a time when "mossy fiber sprouting" of zinc-positive granule cell axonal projections has occurred.[44,45] In addition, alterations in either glial or neuronal electrotonic gap junction coupling may promote seizure activity. Neuronal synchrony is enhanced in conditions of increased intercellular coupling, whereas uncoupling agents that block gap junctions may prevent neuronal synchronization.

Glial regulation of ECS size and $[K^+]_{out}$ may similarly contribute to epileptogenesis. Astrocytes from animal model or human limbic epilepsy are characterized by decreased expression of the inwardly rectifying potassium channel K_{IR}.[46] This channel alteration would be expected to result in raised $[K^+]_{out}$, as well as the need to use other glial mechanisms for potassium uptake such as the Na^+,K^+-ATPase pump and the $Na^+/K^+/2Cl^-$ cotransporter. Together, these changes would be expected to increase epileptogenicity both by increasing $[K^+]_{out}$ and by decreasing ECS size. These hypotheses have been confirmed in normal rodent tissue with pharmacologic blockade of the inwardly rectifying potassium channel K_{IR},[12] as well as in an animal model of traumatic brain injury.[47] Investigation is ongoing in human epileptic tissue.

Brain tumors are also associated with various electrophysiologic abnormalities. Gliomas are characterized both by selective expression of a chloride channel not expressed by normal astrocytes and by alterations in astrocytic mechanisms for the uptake of glutamate. The chloride currents expressed by glioma cells are volume activated and are proposed to contribute to the changes in cell shape and volume that are necessary for extracellular tumor cell migration.[48] Synaptically released glutamate and GABA are both removed from the ECS through the action of electrogenic Na^+-dependent transporters. In the case of glutamate, five transporter subtypes have been identified, including the astrocytic transporters GLAST and GLT-1, which are the most abundant glutamate transporters in brain. In glioma cells, there is very little expression of GLAST and mislocalization of GLT-1 to the nuclear rather than the cytoplasmic membrane. Rather than take scavenging neuronally released glutamate, glioma cells locally release internally generated glutamate, thereby resulting in increased neurotoxicity and invasiveness. Blockade of glioma glutamate release may hold promise as a novel therapy for malignant gliomas.[49]

ELECTROPHYSIOLOGIC TECHNIQUES IN NEUROSURGERY

Origin of Field Potentials in the Brain and Spinal Cord

Since the discovery of electroencephalographic (EEG) waves, the origin of extracellular field potentials underlying EEG activity has been studied intensively. There is general agreement that the generation, distribution, size, and polarity of extracellular recordings (or EEG recordings) are somehow related to the structural geometry of the CNS. Analogous to the heart and electrocardiogram, it has been assumed that extracellular potentials recorded with microelectrode techniques, scalp electrodes, or corticography are related to neuronal firing and that the polarity of the signals reflects both the distance from the generator cells and the "dipolar" nature of neuronal cells. At the present state of knowledge it is assumed that this explanation is valid only under particular circumstances. Two seemingly opposing points of view have been expressed to explain the origin of field potentials and their relationship to intracellularly recorded signals. For clarity, let us consider the characteristics and generators of each of the most commonly used extracellular recording techniques individually.

1. Single-unit recordings arise from firing of individual neurons. The contribution of other cell types (i.e., glia) is virtually nonexistent. The composition of the ECS where conduction of the signal occurs is also minimal because these signals are typically recorded only in close proximity (a few microns) to the cell.
2. Recordings of cortical field potentials are a common experimental paradigm, and both synaptically evoked and spontaneous signals can be detected. It has generally (and incorrectly) been assumed that both signals are a mirror reflection of changes in intracellular neuronal voltage. This assumption has been challenged experimentally, at least for recordings from the cerebral cortex. Although the rapid, transient changes recorded during synchronous *excitation* of presynaptic fibers

and postsynaptic neurons* are directly related to neuronal depolarization, the long-lasting changes that sometimes follow synchronous neuronal discharge appear to be due to a complex interplay of neuronal and glial cells; furthermore, these signals originate from depolarization of neurons secondary to opening of voltage-dependent Na^+ and Ca^{2+} channels *and* uptake of positively charged ions (mainly potassium) into the glial syncytium (see Fig. 49-7). It has been known for several years that the intracellular potentials recorded in glial cells run in parallel with changes in extracellular potential. Thus, although the *initiators* of slow changes in potential recorded extracellularly are neuronal elements, the polarity and amplitude of these changes are due to flow of current through the ECS and the glial cell syncytium.

Electrical EEG activity measured at the surface of the skull represents a summation of dendritic synaptic potentials in cortical neurons. The EEG rhythms seen are thus thought to represent waves of thalamocortical excitatory synaptic potentials. These field potential spikes of activity are the extracellular reflection of the synchronized activity of large numbers of neurons. Because of the scalp location of the EEG recording electrodes, the surface EEG recording predominantly reflects the activity of cortical neurons that are close to the electrodes rather than activity of deeper hippocampal, thalamic, or brainstem cells. The overall EEG signal is on the level of microvolts, as opposed to the millivolt recordings obtained from single neurons intracellularly, because of distortion and attenuation of the signal between the electrode and the underlying brain tissue. In addition, because the EEG recording is a summated signal from a large number of neurons, the individual contributions of the cells reflected at the surface electrode will depend on whether the contributing cells are more superficial or deeper in the cortex and whether they are receiving EPSPs or IPSPs.

Recording Methods in Neurosurgery

The different recording methods used in the neurosurgical treatment of epilepsy, movement disorders, and pain syndromes are summarized in Table 49-6. Although single-unit recordings carried out with microelectrodes are used for research purposes in epilepsy patients, the majority of epilepsy recordings are EEG recordings using scalp electrodes, subdural or epidural electrode arrays, or intracerebral targeted-depth electrodes. These techniques allow both the lateralization and localization that is required in medically refractory patients before focal cortical resection of their seizure focus. Intraoperative electrocorticography (ECoG) is often used in patients with lesional epilepsies, such as those caused by tumors, focal cortical dysplasia, or cavernous malformations with refractory seizures, to determine whether the epileptogenic zone extends beyond the borders of the pathologic lesion. The use of ECoG in mesial temporal lobe epilepsy to guide surgical resection is more controversial. Intraoperative hippocampal ECoG can potentially be used to determine how much hippocampus to remove to maximize seizure-free outcome. Neocortical ECoG has not been shown to be of clear benefit in the intraoperative management of mesial temporal lobe epilepsy.[50]

With the resurgence over the past several years of stereotactic surgery for the treatment of Parkinson's disease, essential tremor, dystonia, and other movement disorders, the use of intraoperative physiology has similarly increased. Intraoperative macrostimulation for deep brain mapping of the thalamus, as well as microelectrode recording of neuronal units in the thalamus, globus pallidus, and subthalamic nucleus, is commonly used to guide the placement of lesions or stimulating electrodes for the

---

*These potentials are commonly called field EPSP and population spike.

TABLE 49-6 Recording Methods in Neurophysiology

	TECHNIQUE	CELLULAR/PHYSIOLOGIC TARGET (SIGNAL SIZE)	RECORDING DEVICE
	Single-unit recording	Frequency of firing of individual neurons (<μV)	Metal/glass electrodes
	Corticography	Firing and spread of excitation along large segments of the cortex (several μV)	Multi-array electrodes
In vivo	Field potentials	Recordings of spontaneous or evoked discharges from discrete areas (μV to mV)	Microelectrode
	Electroencephalography	Similar to corticography, but with scalp electrodes (μV)	Multi-array electrodes
	Field potentials	Recordings of spontaneous or evoked discharges from discrete areas (usually mV)	Glass microelectrode
	Intracellular recording	Recordings from neurons or glia; voltage or current clamp (mV or nA)	Glass microelectrode
In vitro	Patch clamp (whole cell)	Similar to intracellular recording, but with large pipettes: allows access to cell cytoplasm (mV or nA)	Glass pipette
	Patch clamp (single channel)	Recordings from small membrane patches; allows measurement of currents through single channel proteins (pA)	Glass pipette

treatment of these movement disorders. For determining proper lesion or stimulator location in the thalamus of patients with essential tremor or tremor-predominant Parkinson's disease, thalamic "tremor" cells can be recorded in the ventrolateral motor thalamus. The firing pattern of these cells is synchronized with the tremor in the affected upper extremity, as recorded by electromyography. In addition, thalamic neurons with joint movement-activated (kinesthetic) receptive fields in the limb of interest are somatotopically organized in the target area. During the placement of lesions or stimulating electrodes in the globus pallidus interna or in the subthalamic nucleus in patients with Parkinson's disease, characteristic neuronal recordings are obtained with microelectrodes in conjunction with frame-based imaging to physiologically and anatomically identify the desired target. In addition, stimulation can be carried out through the microelectrode to confirm proper target location and to minimize potential side effects or complications. Further details of the specific neuronal patterns of recordings obtained and the anatomic pathways mapped during these movement disorder procedures are detailed in the section of this text on movement disorders.

ION CHANNELS IN NEUROLOGICAL DISORDERS

Excitotoxicity

Excitotoxicity refers to the ability of glutamate or other amino acid agonists at the glutamate receptors to mediate the death of central neurons. The most common excitotoxic mechanism consists of sustained exposure to large quantities of these agonists. Excitotoxic neuronal death is almost always a pathologic feature of CNS disorders and may contribute to the pathogenesis of human brain or spinal cord disease. Excitotoxicity has substantial cellular specificity and, in most cases, is mediated by glutamate receptors. N-Methyl-D-aspartate (NMDA) receptor activation is the most common signaling event that causes excitotoxicity, and NMDA triggers injury more rapidly than do α-amino-3-hydroxy-5-methyl-4-isoxazoleproprionate (AMPA) or kainate receptors

(Fig. 49-8). It is commonly accepted that this depends on NMDA's greater ability to induce calcium influx and subsequent cellular calcium overload. A good example of excitotoxicity is hippocampal sclerosis.[51,52] Hippocampal sclerosis is the most frequent pathologic finding in patients with temporal lobe epilepsy undergoing resective neurosurgery, and it is a common neuroimaging finding.[53]

Recent reports have overturned a series of dogmas that have been well entrenched in the neuroscience literature concerning NMDA-type glutamate receptors (NMDARs). The new data show that NMDARs exist on the myelin sheath formed by oligodendrocytes, that an uncompetitive NMDAR antagonist has successfully passed human clinical trials, and that NMDARs trigger multiple deleterious cascades to inflict cellular damage on both neurons and glia during cerebral ischemia (stroke). These recent findings bode well for clinical intervention with NMDAR antagonists in more neurological disorders than previously thought, including multiple sclerosis, cerebral palsy (periventricular leukomalacia), and spinal cord injury.

Epilepsy and Channelopathies

Epileptic seizures are electrical events that produce a complex behavioral response ranging from absence seizures to convulsions. Several investigators have studied the link between ion channels and seizure disorders. Animal data show that several features of epilepsy can be reproduced in rodents. Electrophysiologic recordings performed both in vivo and in vitro allowed the discovery of several important features that may contribute to the development of seizures. For example, the response to GABA and NMDA varies during development, and an attempt has been made to link abnormal GABA responses to infantile seizures.[54,55]

In addition to developmental changes, several insults that are cofactors in human epilepsy have been shown to cause similar effects in animal models. Virtually all animal models have shown either altered excitatory or altered inhibitory loops, but more recent research has revealed a significant role for non-neuronal cells. For example, a specific deficit in potassium channels involved in glial potassium buffering has been discovered in both

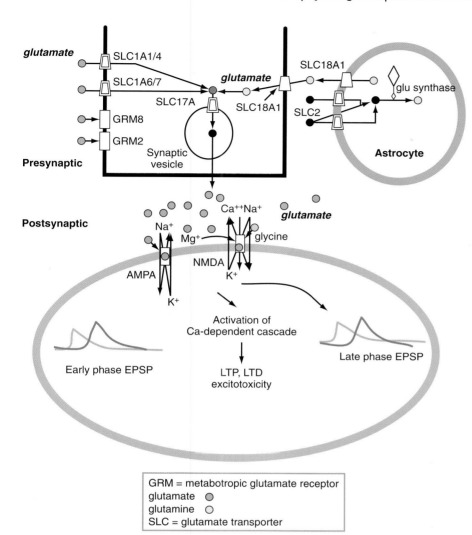

FIGURE 49-8 Complexity of synaptic transmission. Note the numerous sites that allow modulation of release, action, and metabolism of the excitatory mediator glutamate. AMPA, α-amino-3-hydroxy-5-methyl-4-isoxazolepropionate; EPSP, excitatory postsynaptic potential; LTD, long-term depression; LTP, long-term potentiation; NMDA, N-methyl-D-aspartate.

human tissue and animal model brain.[47,56,57] More recently, involvement of other members of the neurovascular unit has expanded the electrophysiologic mechanisms to other nonexcitable cells (e.g., blood-brain barrier endothelial cells).[58] Finally, it has to be emphasized that most of the work of the neurovascular unit consists of keeping the neuronal cells well nourished and living in a tightly controlled environment. As also mentioned in other sections of this chapter, altered potassium or calcium can have profound effects on neuronal firing.

A genetic contribution to the epilepsies has long been suspected, but progress in elucidating the specific genetic influences was relatively slow. A recent flurry of new experimental tools has allowed the discovery of several genetic features associated with epileptic disease. Among those that are most likely to influence neuronal discharges are "channelopathies," or conditions involving the altered electrical property of neuronal or glial cells. Thus far, almost all of the progress in discovering "epilepsy genes" has come from analysis of rare families with mendelian modes of inheritance, and all but two of these genes encode voltage-gated or ligand-gated ion channels. Among these are *KCNQ2* and *KCNQ3* for potassium channels; *SCN1A*, *SCN1B*, and *SCN2A* for sodium channels; and *GABRG2* for inhibitory chloride channels, among others. Genetic analysis of these genes is confounded by the numerous overlapping properties of ion channels. In other words, a specific mutation in a potassium channel may cause a variety of diseases in which seizures are not most prominent. On the other hand, it is possible that environmental or pharmacologic factors can mimic the genetic ablation of function even in the presence of a normal genotype. An example is the impotence drug Viagra (sildenafil), which acts on the KCNQ2 potassium channel. This compound acts as a specific phosphodiesterase type V inhibitor with a selective inhibitory effect on cyclic guanosine monophosphate (cGMP). Its enhancement of the release of nitric oxide (NO) leads to an increase in cGMP concentration, which is responsible for its main clinical effect, relaxation of smooth muscle in the corpus cavernosum. Sildenafil also affects KCNQ2 channels, which are regulated by cGMP/NO pathways. Not surprisingly, four instances of patients experiencing epileptic seizures during the clinical trials of sildenafil were reported, and anecdotal evidence supports the association between sildenafil and potassium channels expressed in the brain.[59]

SUGGESTED READINGS

Bordey A, Sontheimer H. Properties of human glial cells associated with epileptic seizure foci. *Epilepsy Res*. 1998;32:286-303.

Catterall WA, Dib-Hajj S, Meisler MH, et al. Inherited neuronal ion channelopathies: new windows on complex neurological diseases. *J Neurosci*. 2008;28:11768-11777.

Coulter DA. Epilepsy-associated plasticity in gamma-aminobutyric acid receptor expression, function, and inhibitory synaptic properties. *Int Rev Neurobiol*. 2001;45:237-252.

del Zoppo GJ. Virchow's triad: the vascular basis of cerebral injury. *Rev Neurol Dis.* 2008;5(suppl 1):S12-S21.

Goldman DE. Potential, impedance, and rectification in membranes. *J Gen Physiol.* 1943;27:37-60.

Hodgkin AL, Huxley AF. A quantitative description of membrane current and its application to conduction and excitation in nerve. *J Physiol (London).* 1952;117:500-544.

Hodgkin AL, Katz B. The effect of sodium ions on electrical activity of the giant axon of the squid. *J Physiol.* 1949;108:37-77.

Hugenaard J, McCormick DA. *Electrophysiology of the Neuron.* New York: Oxford University Press; 1994.

Oby E, Janigro D. The blood-brain barrier and epilepsy. *Epilepsia.* 2006;47:1761-1774.

Ransom BR, Sontheimer H. The neurophysiology of glial cells. *J Clin Neurophysiol.* 1992;9:224-251.

Rozental R, Giaume C, Spray DC. Gap junctions in the nervous system. *Brain Res Brain Res Rev.* 2000;32:11-15.

Full references can be found on Expert Consult @ www.expertconsult.com

CHAPTER 50

Animal Models of Epilepsy

Maria Elisa Calcagnotto ■ Scott C. Baraban

Epilepsy affects a sizable proportion of the population worldwide and is responsible for a heavy social and economic burden.[1] Given that epileptic disorders frequently result in uncontrolled and often medically intractable seizures, further experimental studies offer hope for a deeper understanding of the underlying pathophysiology and, ultimately, better treatments. To achieve these goals, human studies, albeit of great value, may not be sufficient because of both ethical and practical limitations.[2] Accordingly, it is not surprising that animal models were developed and have significantly contributed to the epilepsy research literature. A common concern with all animal models is how reliable they are in mimicking the human condition. Are the anatomic and electrophysiologic similarities with human epileptic disorders real or superficial? To what extent can findings in animal research be extended to humans? Furthermore and perhaps most important, what new insights can be gained from animal model studies that cannot be predicted from clinical studies? In the design and interpretation of animal models, it is important to remember that epilepsy is not a single disease, a syndrome, or a homogeneous entity. Although a common feature of epilepsy is the tendency to have spontaneous epileptic seizures,[3] the many ways in which seizures are generated (and manifested) are quite varied. Seizures can be motor, sensory, or autonomic and are caused by excessive and abnormal neuronal discharge. Causes of epilepsy range from genetic to acquired to "of unknown origin" (i.e., idiopathic).[4] Its symptoms are also many because they depend on the brain areas that are involved in a certain type of seizure and the stage of brain maturation. The type (or types) of seizures that one individual has and other symptoms that are also present can be used to define a specific *epileptic syndrome*. Because epilepsy involves many levels of structures and activity in the brain, be it from molecules to networks, with causes that range from genes to environmental insults, it is no surprise that many epilepsy models are needed.

A good model of epilepsy should reproduce as many salient aspects as possible for a specific type of human epilepsy.[5,6] Ideally, there should be evidence in a model for spontaneous behavioral seizures of the kind (e.g., partial, absence, tonic-clonic) that its human counterpart exhibits, as well as electroencephalographic (EEG; ictal and interictal discharges, focal or generalized) and structural (if any) abnormalities similar to the ones seen in the human epilepsy that it mirrors. The etiology (e.g., cortical malformation [CM], genetic predisposition, focal gliosis) should, if possible, be the same in the animal model as in the human condition. If the human epilepsy has a specific age at onset, the model should do the same. The animal model should have behavioral characteristics (such as memory deficits or developmental retardation) that parallel the human condition. Finally, the model in question should respond to antiepileptic drugs (AEDs) in a manner similar to the human condition after which it is modeled. Even though these goals are scientifically sound, few (if any) animal models actually fulfill all these criteria. Here we review animal models designed to mimic three broad classes of epileptic disorders: (1) temporal lobe epilepsy (TLE), (2) epilepsy associated with a brain malformation, and (3) other focal epilepsies.

TEMPORAL LOBE EPILEPSY

Seizures that arise from the temporal lobe are very common in humans and are often resistant to pharmacologic treatment. The most common type of TLE is that associated with hippocampal sclerosis.[7] Kindling, pilocarpine, and kainic acid (kainate) are the most common animal models of TLE.

Stimulus-Induced Model of Temporal Lobe Epilepsy

Kindling

Kindling has been used as a model of seizures and epilepsy for more than 3 decades. Initially, these animals were not used for epilepsy, but rather as a physiologic model of learning and memory.[8] This model is based on the kindling phenomenon, which involves the progressive development of EEG and behavioral seizures evoked by repeated electrical stimulation of certain brain structures. The first studies from the 1960s showed that repetitive electrical brain stimulation produces an increase in convulsive behavior and eventually generalized motor seizures.[8-10] The progression of motor seizures proceeds through several stages as defined by Racine for the amygdala kindling protocol.[11] With initial stimulation, there is an initial ictus with orofacial movements (stage 1) and head nodding (stage 2), which is associated with a focal EEG seizure. Further stimulation results in contralateral forelimb clonus (stage 3) and rearing (stage 4). Additional loss of balance, rearing, and falling (stage 5) are accompanied by tonic-clonic seizures involving all four limbs.[12] If the kindling stimulus continues to be applied to the focus after a stage 5 seizure is reached, the behavioral sequence evolves further to more severe seizures. Thus, the more advanced the animal in this process, the more intense the seizures and the more widespread and prolonged the electrical seizures or afterdischarges (i.e., the most sensitive parameter of focal seizure activity in kindled rats). Kindling occurs best in neuroplastic areas of the brain; the amygdala is the brain region most susceptible to kindling.[13]

Although other, but not all encephalic structures can be kindled, there are some differences between them regarding the speed of the kindling process and seizure manifestation.[14-16] Stimulation of the cerebellum and superior colliculus, for example, cannot start kindling. Kindling from the hippocampus produces seizures quite similar to but slower to develop than those induced by amygdala kindling. The profile of afterdischarges is different from amygdala kindling in that they recur daily during the kindling process until the seizures recruit other temporal areas.[14,17] One peculiar early behavioral response seen during hippocampal kindling in some rats is the so-called wet dog shakes, which start and progressively disappear during the kindling process before the expression of any Racine motor stages.

The neurological alterations associated with the types of kindling behavior seem to be permanent. Kindled animals that have not been stimulated for many months after stage 5 kindling often respond with full seizure behavior on repeat exposure to the original kindling stimulus.[8,18] Moreover, kindling of a second structure is usually achieved with fewer stimuli than needed for the primary kindled site.[8,19,20] This "transfer phenomenon" might be the physiologic basis for secondary epileptogenesis.[21-23] In contrast, if two different nonhomologous areas receive concurrent and alternate stimulation, only one of them undergoes a typical kindling progression, and seizure genesis in the other site is suppressed. This "kindling antagonism" may involve inhibitory mechanisms recruited by the seizure activity from the more dominant site[24,25] and could reflect the types of endogenous compensatory mechanisms that the brain has evolved to combat seizure activity.

When the amygdala or other brain areas such as the frontal and posterior cortex, entorhinal cortex, and perforant pathway are kindled, spontaneous seizures can develop in the animals after a period. However, just a few kindled animals reach this point.[26,27] Recent evidence from the laboratory of Dan McIntyre suggests that there may be a genetic explanation for this interesting observation. Over time, they isolated strains of "fast"- and "slow"-kindling rats, with the former being highly susceptible to kindling treatment and the latter more resistant.[28-30] These rats exhibit different seizure predispositions and behavior that might be attributed to differences in the expression of GABA$_A$ receptor subunits and in the kinetics of miniature inhibitory postsynaptic currents in different limbic structures.[28,31-33] Behaviorally, the fast-kindling rat strains are more prone than the slow-kindling strains to the development of seizures and appear much like humans with attention-deficit/hyperactivity disorder in that they show easy distraction, hyperactivity, and impulsivity.[32,34,35] Importantly, spontaneous seizures in kindled animals are not just a rat phenomenon inasmuch as epilepsy has developed in every animal tested thus far with this stimulation protocol: frogs, reptiles, mice, rats, rabbits, cats, dogs, rhesus monkeys, and baboons.[36-38] A persistent question with this model is whether a kindling-like phenomenon occurs in patients with epilepsy. This discussion was initiated by Gowers, who affirmed that "seizures do beget seizures." In other words, epilepsy could be a progressive condition wherein the chronic recurrence of seizures would increase the likelihood of new seizures, and they could come from new areas (e.g., homologous contralateral sites). There are some hints in epilepsy associated with brain tumors that secondary epileptogenesis does occur in humans.[23] Although deliberately causing kindling in humans would be ethically suspicious, to say the least, some reports of such do exist in the literature.[39]

As a model of epilepsy, the kindling model has been successfully used as a screening tool for AEDs. Lamotrigine, used as an AED in patients with partial and generalized seizures, has long-acting anticonvulsant effects on both amygdala- and hippocampal-kindled seizures in rats.[40] GABA uptake inhibitors, such as tiagabine, were also found to be highly effective in the kindling model,[41] consistent with the GABA receptor involvement described earlier. Another example is levetiracetam, a relatively new AED that is effective in the kindling, pilocarpine, and kainate models of TLE and in human TLE.[42-45] Interestingly, these three drugs are inactive against seizures induced by maximum electroshock (MES), a model of acute seizures in nonepileptic animals and additionally used to screen for potential AEDs.[41] More recently, amygdala kindling has also been proposed as an animal model for drug-resistant epilepsy.[46] Studies have shown that kindled seizures are less sensitive than primarily generalized seizures to anticonvulsant treatment, as demonstrated with the MES test.[41] The response to phenytoin, for example, differs in kindled rats (i.e., in some animals phenytoin has an anticonvulsant effect consistently and in others never).[47] Unfortunately, the preparation of kindled rats and drug testing in this model are both labor and time intensive, which limits its use in high-throughput drug discovery and development programs. Some less laborious models

are discussed in this respect, including corneal kindling, acute models of focal seizures (e.g., electrical induction of afterdischarges), and genetic models. However, when compared with conventional amygdala kindling, none of these models have been characterized sufficiently as yet to judge their usefulness for drug development.[48]

Finally, the kindling model offers some distinct advantages over systemically drug-induced models of TLE. With kindling, one knows precisely where the epileptogenesis begins (i.e., the site and intensity of the stimuli applied) and can track by numerous methods the progressive changes that occur during a very prolonged latent period, which ends with spontaneous seizures. Additionally, gross brain damage does not appear to be a prerequisite for the initial manifestation of spontaneous seizures.[26] After repeated secondary generalized seizures evoked by kindling, cumulative neuronal loss can be detected in the CA1 and CA3 subfields of the hippocampus and in the hilus of the dentate gyrus (DG), similar to classic human hippocampal sclerosis, which is associated with long-term seizure-induced memory dysfunction.[49-51] Although kindling does not result in a large loss of neurons, there is clear reorganization of the neuronal circuitry. This reorganization is based on synaptogenesis[52] or sprouting of mossy fibers (or both) in the inner molecular layer of the DG[53] and in the stratum oriens of the CA3 hippocampal area.[54] In addition, kindling-induced seizures result in changes in the morphology of astrocytes that (1) appear to be dependent on seizure intensity, (2) occur early in the kindling process, and (3) persist for weeks after the last seizure. An increase in astrocytic proliferation in the hippocampus, amygdala, and piriform cortex was also observed after kindling.[55] Some of these structural alterations induced by kindling are similar to those in the human epileptic temporal lobe, thus raising the possibility that mechanisms operative in kindling may play a role in the pathogenesis of human TLE associated with hippocampal sclerosis.[56] As one might expect, the seizure progression and structural changes are accompanied by progressive functional alterations in the kindled animal. These changes have been particularly well studied in the DG. When the first seizure is induced, there is an increase in excitability through N-methyl-D-aspartate (NMDA)-mediated synaptic transmission. Even though this increment is not permanent,[57] it appears to play an important long-term role by initiating structural and functional modifications that contribute to long-lasting seizure susceptibility in the hippocampal circuitry.[58] Neurochemical and neurophysiologic studies have indicated that the activity of the GABAergic projection from the striatum to the substantia nigra pars reticulata is reduced and the density of GABAergic striatal interneurons is increased in kindled rats.[59-62] In addition, GABAergic inhibition is altered in the piriform cortex of kindled rats.[63]

Chemical-Induced Models of Temporal Lobe Epilepsy

Pilocarpine and Kainate

Pilocarpine and kainate models replicate several phenomenologic features of human TLE, and both can be used as animal preparations to understand the basic mechanisms of epileptogenesis.[64-66] Pilocarpine is a cholinergic muscarinic agonist originally isolated from the leaflets of South American shrubs (*Pilocarpus jaborandi*). The first evidence that the brain damage produced by pilocarpine-induced status epilepticus (SE) could lead to spontaneous recurrent seizures (SRSs) in rats over a long-term period occurred in 1983.[67] Kainate is an excitatory amino acid extracted from seaweed (*Digenea simplex*) and has been used as a model of epilepsy since the late 1970s.[68,69] Local or systemic administration of either pilocarpine or kainate to rodents leads to a pattern of repetitive limbic seizures and SE that can last for several hours.[67,70,71] Systemic administration of a single dose of pilocarpine or repetitive low doses of kainate to rodents leads to a sequence of seizures that build progressively into a limbic SE lasting up to 24 hours (acute period). In these models, induction of SE is critical for the later development of SRSs. By managing the severity of SE one can decrease animal mortality without decreasing the development of recurrent epilepsy. For pilocarpine, this can be accomplished by using thionembutal or diazepam after the beginning of SE. Pretreatment with scopolamine also minimizes the peripheral cholinergic side effects of pilocarpine.[72,73] In some protocols, lithium is applied before pilocarpine to increase its effect and reduce mortality.[74] For kainate, a multiple low-dose protocol may decrease mortality and produce animals with robust SRSs.[75,76] SE induced by kainate can also be abolished by diazepam. However, some animals may die before the benzodiazepine injection, and this approach may lead to a lower percentage of animals in which robust and long-lasting convulsive SE and subsequent SRSs develop. Seizures during the acute period are similar with both drugs. After injection of pilocarpine, the animal begins with staring and facial automatisms, followed by motor limbic seizures with rearing, forelimb clonus, salivation, intense masticatory movements, and falls. This progression follows the Racine stages.[77] For kainate, the seizures are characterized by wet dog shakes, staring, searching, and gnawing, subsequently leading to forelimb clonus (stage 3 of Racine) and followed by Racine stages 4 and 5.[78] The electrographic pattern during the acute period is characterized by theta rhythm activity in the hippocampus and low-voltage fast activity in the cortex with progression to high-voltage fast activity with spikes in the hippocampus. Sequentially, spiking activity spreads to the cortex and evolves into electrographic recurrent seizures that build up to continuous epileptiform activity.[71,79] This acute period is followed by a "silent period" (seizure-free phase) with progressive normalization of EEG activity and behavior of variable extent that lasts from days to weeks. This sort of latent interval is believed to play an important role in "ripening of the focus," a process that renders the animal chronically epileptic.[80] After this latent period, animals begin to have frequent SRSs (chronic period).[67,70,73,81-83] The main features of the SRSs observed during the long-term period resemble those of human complex partial seizures.[66,67,79,84] SRSs are characterized by facial automatisms, head nodding, forelimb clonus, rearing, and falling and electrographically by paroxysmal hippocampal discharges that rapidly spread to cortical regions. The ensuing spontaneous seizures show gradual electrographic synchronization of cortical and hippocampal activities and a longer duration of ictal events. Forelimb clonus and rearing with falling (kindling stages 4 or 5) are the clinical hallmarks of this SRS phase.[71,79]

As models for temporolimbic epilepsy, the pilocarpine and kainate models are important instruments for screening new AEDs. Studies have shown that diazepam, phenobarbital, valproic acid, and trimethadione protect against acute pilocarpine-induced SE whereas phenytoin and carbamazepine are ineffective.[66] In contrast, during the chronic period, phenobarbital, carbamazepine, phenytoin, and valproic acid but not ethosuximide are able to control pilocarpine-induced SRSs. Valproic acid was likewise able to abolish SRSs in kainate-treated animals.[85] These AEDs can also control complex partial seizures in humans.[86] SRSs may thus be more reliable than acute seizure models for finding new AEDs with better efficacy against complex partial seizures. In the kainate model, a ketogenic diet also seems to be effective in reducing SRSs.[87]

In hippocampal tissue removed from patients with refractory TLE, neuronal loss is most prominent in the hippocampal formation, particularly in the DG and the CA1 and CA3 subfields.[88-90] Mossy fiber sprouting,[91,92] hippocampal gliosis,[88,89] cell dispersion

in the granular cell layer of the DG, and local ectopic areas[91] are additional neuropathologies. Although these morphologic changes are much more prominent in pilocarpine- and kainate-treated rats than in humans,[73] the structural changes in these models of epilepsy during the acute and chronic periods resemble the anatomic changes found in many patients with mesial TLE.[64,65,67,69,73,93-95] Morphologic analysis of the rodent brain during the acute period shows that both kainate- and pilocarpine-induced SE invariably leads to cellular loss and injury in the hippocampal subfields CA1 and CA3 and in the DG hilus. Cell loss is also often seen in the septum, olfactory tubercle, amygdala, piriform cortex, neocortex, thalamic nuclei, and substantia nigra.[67,96-98] In fact, the thalamus can exhibit severe atrophy in various nuclei.[99] Damage to subpopulations of GABAergic inhibitory neurons is also extensive throughout the hippocampus.[100] In the following months the cell damage tends to progressively involve other areas. In the chronic period, cell loss is often noted in the DG (mainly attributed to a decrement in GABAergic interneurons) and in the hippocampal subfields CA1 and CA3 (loss of pyramidal cells). The decreased subpopulation of interneurons in the DG is associated with a functional hyperexcitability.[65] In the kainate model, the CA3 area seems to be preferentially damaged in comparison to area CA1, which probably reflects the higher distribution of hippocampal kainate receptors in CA3. This differs from the typical hippocampal sclerosis in humans, in which CA1 is usually more damaged than CA3. As in humans, the DG and the CA2 area are relatively spared.[69,88,89,93] Cell dispersion is evident in the granule cell layer of the DG[101]; increased neurogenesis[102] and supragranular and intragranular mossy fiber sprouting[73,103,104] are also important features in these models during the period of SRSs. Interestingly, SRSs can occur in animals with complete absence of mossy fiber sprouting.[105,106] These morphologic changes seem more likely to represent a reactive response rather than a direct consequence of the initial insult. As observed in kainate-treated rats, axonal sprouting and synaptic reorganization take place not only in the DG but also in other hippocampal areas, such as CA1 and CA3.[107] These cellular and synaptic modifications are associated with neurochemical and cellular dysfunctions that lead to permanent hyperexcitability. For example, the decrease in GABAergic cells in the DG and entorhinal cortex in the pilocarpine model of epilepsy is associated with decreased inhibitory synaptic input to the granule cells and to the layer II stellate cells, respectively, with a consequent increase in network excitability. Reduced granule cell inhibition in the DG seems to precede the onset of SRSs by days to weeks.[108,109] Decreased expression of some postsynaptic GABA$_A$ receptor subunits,[110-116] loss of GABAergic interneurons in the entorhinal cortex, and changes in neuropeptide Y expression, including ectopic expression in the granule cells and mossy fibers, have also been observed in rats with pilocarpine-induced epilepsy.[117] Some of these changes precede the onset of SRSs by weeks and correlate with profound alterations in receptor function that contribute to the process of epileptogenesis. Increased glutamate release in the hippocampus was also observed during the acute period[118,119] and could further contribute to the epileptogenic process in this model. For example, constant activation of NMDA-type glutamate receptors, which leads to increased intracellular Ca^{2+} and consequent activation of lipases, proteases, and nucleases, can kill cells by necrosis, apoptosis, or both. Thus, activation of NMDA receptors plays an important role in SE and brain damage in these models.[120] The expression of proteins related to ionotropic NMDA and metabotropic glutamate receptors in the hippocampus is also modified in the pilocarpine model of epilepsy.[121,122]

As much as the pilocarpine and kainate effects in rats can resemble the human condition, species differences between rodents and primates are frequently used to explain existing discrepancies. To this end, developmental changes are often called on to explain features such as tectonic malformations[123] and DG cell dispersion[91] in humans even though these findings have been demonstrated to take place in adult epileptic rats.[101] As a means to more properly evaluate the extent to which rodent models mimic the human condition, pilocarpine has also been used in a nonhuman primate, the marmoset (*Callithrix jachus*).[124,125]

In seminal work by Luiz Mello and colleagues, administration of pilocarpine was used to induce SE in marmosets followed, after a silent period, by SRSs. It was observed from this model that prolonged SE is required to promote injury during the acute period and that the mortality rate is higher during SE in marmosets than in rats. That rodents seem to be more resistant to pilocarpine-induced SE (in wild types, 20% to 30% of animals will not reach full SE after drug administration) may be the reason that more damage is necessary for spontaneous seizures to develop. Different from the rodent pilocarpine and kainate models but similar to human TLE, brain damage is minimal during the chronic period in marmosets and generally limited to the limbic structures (mainly the hippocampus), and neurogenesis, exuberant in rodents,[102] is mild in this primate.[126] Cellular dispersion in the granular cell layer of the DG; neuronal loss in CA1, CA3, and the DG hilus; and supragranular mossy fiber sprouting were detected in marmosets with SRSs. Regarding morphology, one interesting observation in the marmoset pilocarpine model was the finding of tectonic malformations in the DG characterized by invaginations and lateral displacement of the granular cell layer, mainly in the posterior plates, similar to that described by Sloviter and coworkers in humans with TLE.[123] This new model of TLE in marmosets may have a greater resemblance to the alterations seen in human TLE and may provide a new tool to more properly evaluate the causes of and consequences associated with TLE.

CORTICAL MALFORMATIONS AND EPILEPSY

CMs are developmental neuronal disorders in humans characterized by (1) disorganization of cortical architecture or (2) the presence of abnormal, immature, and eventually nondifferentiated neurons (or both).[127-130] Genetic or environmental prenatal factors can lead to focal or diffuse CMs, or both, which are often associated with refractory epilepsy.[127-129] The anatomic features of CMs associated with epilepsy have been widely studied.[131-134] Although no single animal model can reproduce the precise anatomic disorganization and cell abnormalities observed in humans, these models have proved useful in studying the functional characteristics of dysplastic neuronal networks. Some CM models are based on induced injury in the immature brain (e.g., freeze, undercut, irradiation, teratogen exposure); others are based on spontaneous genetic mutations or on trangenesis that gives rise to abnormal cortical architecture. Here we review some of the injury-based and genetic models of CMs.

Injury-Based Models of Cortical Malformations

Brain malformation can be induced in animals by teratogenic compounds or by mechanical treatment. These models include prenatal exposure (embryonic days 14 to 16) to methylazoxymethanol acetate (MAM)[135] or to irradiation (γ- or x-rays)[136] and the neonatal application (postnatal days 0 to 2) of a freeze lesion in the cortical plate of rodents.[137,138] There are similarities in the embryonic development of the human and rat brain, and neurogenesis occurs in a relatively known spatiotemporal manner.[139] Deleterious agents applied at selected stages of development can reduce neuronal populations in the injured brain regions,[140] similar to those seen in some forms of CM in humans. This reduction and altered architecture subsequently lead to a focal or diffuse structural and functional impairment of the brain that contributes to epileptogenesis.

Methylazoxymethanol Acetate

MAM is an antimitotic methylating agent known since the 1960s to induce brain malformations[141-145] in rats when the exposure takes place at the beginning of the third week of intrauterine development. MAM has a short half-life and exerts an antiproliferative action on dividing, but not quiescent neuroepithelial cells via methylation of nucleic acids.[135,143] Prenatal injection of MAM into female rats at gestational day 15 selectively affects the proliferation of specific neuronal cell populations by disrupting the sequence of normal brain development. The offspring resulting from prenatal MAM exposure exhibit multifocal brain malformations, microcephaly,[141,146] loss of lamination, vascular abnormalities, and neuronal heterotopia in the hippocampal and periventricular locations.[147-153] The abnormal cell clusters (heterotopia) first appear postnatally in the hippocampus (postnatal days 1 to 2), and their appearance is preceded by a distinct sequence of perturbations in neocortical development.[154] These induced neuronal heterotopias possess many features of CMs associated with epilepsy in humans, such as focal cortical dysplasia, periventricular nodular heterotopia, and tectonic hippocampal malformations in patients with TLE.[123,148,155] In addition, heterotopic neurons have an abnormal synaptic network, with neurons communicating directly between the neocortex and hippocampus,[156] and they exhibit characteristics of neocortical cells. For example, molecular analysis has revealed that hippocampal heterotopic cells express mRNA markers normally found abundantly in layer II and III supragranular neocortical neurons and exhibit firing properties strikingly similar to those of supragranular cortical neurons.[157] MAM-treated rats have increased susceptibility to induced seizures in vivo,[158-160] and hyperexcitability in vitro is refractory to the commonly available AEDs.[161] This hyperexcitability can be attributed to a combination of different cellular mechanisms.[162,163] Functionally, heterotopic hippocampal cells (1) lack Kv4.2 A-type potassium channels,[162] which results in abnormal neuronal firing, and (2) exhibit changes in glutamate receptor function and expression.[164-166] The inhibitory synaptic system is also altered in hippocampal heterotopia, including changes in the inhibitory drive such as a prolonged duration of inhibitory synaptic events associated with a decrease in transporter-mediated GABA reuptake.[131] These alterations in GABAergic inhibition could represent some type of postnatal compensatory response to the intrinsic hyperexcitability of these animals because spontaneous electrographic seizures, although present, are rare in MAM-exposed rats.[165] Interestingly, some of these same deficits were found to occur in dysplastic tissue samples from patients with focal cortical dysplasia and epilepsy.[132]

Irradiation

Different radiation sources (x-rays, γ-rays) have been used to induce CMs in animal models, but the results have been similar in all cases. The histologic abnormalities in irradiated animals are attributed to the initial injury from irradiation associated with continued cortical development in an altered cellular environment. Immature, migrating neurons and radial glia are particularly sensitive to radiation.[136,167] Different CMs were produced in rats exposed to x-rays in utero (200 cGy)[168] and γ-irradiation (150 to 250 cGy). Pregnant rats exposed to external γ-irradiation on gestational day 16 to 17 produce offspring with various degrees of CMs and architectural abnormalities, depending on the dose of in utero radiation.[169] Timing of the exposure is also critical,[136] with exposure on gestational day 16 to 17 producing the most severe malformations. These abnormalities include microcephaly; diffuse CM with dyslamination and lack of columnar organization in multiple areas of the neocortex; subcortical, periventricular, and hippocampal neuronal heterotopias; and dysgenesis of the corpus callosum.[169-172] Not only do radiation-exposed rats exhibit epileptiform discharges, but spontaneous seizures also develop in vivo.[172-174] The epileptogenicity in vivo increased with mild to moderate radiation doses. However, high doses of in utero radiation leading to more severe pathologic changes in the neocortex and hippocampus are not associated with the occurrence of spontaneous seizures,[173,175,176] again suggesting potential compensatory mechanisms or widespread brain damage that could preclude the ability to generate network activity. Extracellular recordings from brain slices of in utero irradiated rats showed enhanced epileptiform activity in the dysplastic areas in vitro.[177] Anatomic reduction of GABAergic interneurons (parvalbumin- and calbindin-positive cells[178]) was associated with decreased inhibitory synaptic networks in the malformed cortical regions of irradiated animals[134]; reduced synaptic inhibition, measured in voltage-clamp experiments, was later confirmed in this model.

Freeze Lesion

Several studies reported on the development of focal cortical microgyria in the cortex of neonatal rats (up to 3 to 4 days postnatally) as a result of different types of injuries such as transcortical freeze lesions[137,138] and focal injection of ibotenate (glutamate agonist).[179] The induced microgyria in these models is characterized by four cortical layers instead of six, with an absence of layers V, VIa, and sometimes part or all of layer IV,[138,180-182] and it mimics all histologic aspects of human four-layered polymicrogyria.[183] One of the original models of focal CM is the neonatal freeze lesion model.[184] The polymicrogyria resulting from a lesion induced by the application of a deep-freeze probe to the skull of newborn rats is believed to be caused by cell death secondary to focal hypoxia rather than a migratory defect.[182,185] There is a correlation between the presence of layered polymicrogyria and hypoxic events occurring during the late stages of cortical migration.[183,186,187] Hyperexcitability in vitro has been recorded in the paramicrogyral zone[180,184,188-190] and is associated with an increase in NMDA-mediated excitation and a decrease in glutamatergic input onto inhibitory interneurons.[191] An anatomic substrate for this hyperexcitability could be the increased expression of NMDA receptors within the microgyrus and α-amino-3-hydroxy-5-methyl-4-isoxazoleproprionate (AMPA) receptors in both the microgyral and paramicrogyral zones.[192] An increase in excitatory glutamatergic projections from the thalamus has also been described in the area bordering the microgyrus.[192] This rearrangement of thalamic afferents is attributed to the absence of layer IV neurons (their normal target) in the microgyric area.[190,193] This excitatory input adjacent to the microgyrus may be increased as a result of abnormal circuitry in the paramicrogyral zone. In addition, variable decreases in inhibitory interneurons and GABA$_A$ binding[194] were observed within the microgyrus and in the paramicrogyral zone,[194,195] as well as widespread, regionally differential reduction of the GABA$_A$ receptor subunits α1, α2, α3, α5, and γ2,[196] thus suggesting a disturbance in excitation-inhibition balance. Although hyperexcitability was reported in the freeze lesion model, some studies failed to demonstrate epileptogenicity in vivo.[197] This illustrates one of the potential problems with a number of animal models of epileptic pathology: the dissociation between in vitro and in vivo epileptogenicity.

Genetic Models of Cortical Malformations

In recent years, a number of genes have been discovered that play critical roles in neurogenesis, neuronal migration, and differentiation. Not surprisingly, mutations in these genes provide insight into human CMs associated with epilepsy. Here we describe three animal models with gene mutations that affect normal brain development and seizure susceptibility.

Telencephalic Internal Structural Heterotopia (tish) Mutant Rat

The *tish* mutant rat is a genetic model with a CM similar to the subcortical band heterotopia seen in humans (double cortex syndrome).[198-200] These rats display a bilateral band of heterotopic neocortical neurons that extends dorsally from the frontal to the dorsoparietal neocortex.[199] The bilateral heterotopia is prominent below the frontal and parietal neocortices but is rarely observed in the temporal neocortex. Heterotopic cells exhibit neocortical-like morphology, have regional connectivity characteristic of the neocortex, and are composed of cells generated during the normal period of neocortical neurogenesis.[199] Double cortex syndrome in humans is linked to the X chromosome,[201,202] whereas the *tish* mutation is not. As in patients with subcortical band heterotopia, in which seizures arise from normotopic and heterotopic areas,[203] spontaneous seizures occur in most *tish* mutants and also appear to initiate simultaneously in normotopic and heterotopic neocortex.[204] However, normotopic neurons are more prone than heterotopic neurons to exhibit epileptiform activity in the *tish* cortex, and heterotopic neurons are recruited into spiking by activity initiated in normotopic neurons.[204] This distribution and initiation of epileptiform activity could be linked to the reported attenuation of GABAergic synaptic transmission in the *tish* cortex, mainly in normotopic cells, in association with a reduction in the presynaptic GABAergic terminals surrounding pyramidal cell somata in normotopic and heterotopic *tish* neocortex. This attenuation of inhibitory innervation was more prominent in normotopic neurons and was correlated with a reduction in a subset of GABAergic interneurons expressing parvalbumin.[205] From an anatomic point of view, embryos of *tish* mutant rats display a second ectopic proliferative zone external to the normal periventricular proliferative zone,[206] thus suggesting that band heterotopia could be a consequence of a neuronal migration disorder. Therefore, *tish* mutant rats seem to be a good model to study mechanisms involved in the formation of band heterotopia in humans.

The Reeler Mutant Mouse

During embryonic corticogenesis, Cajal-Retzius cells express reelin, an extracellular protein that regulates the radial migration of principal cortical neurons, in the marginal zone of the developing neocortex and hippocampus.[207-209] The *reeler* mutant mouse has an absence of reelin caused by an autosomal recessive mutation in the reelin locus (chromosome 5 in mice).[210,211] Consequently, homozygous mice exhibit severe layer disorganization in all cortical structures (e.g., neocortex, hippocampus, and cerebellum).[208,212-215] In the *reeler* cortex, principal neurons initiate their radial migration normally but fail to assemble into layers according to an inside-out mode of development. The neocortex of the adult *reeler* mutant is best described as "a reversed cortex," with the deeper layers assuming an external position.[210] In the cortex, neurons of all classes survive even though they may be in abnormal positions and some may be decreased in number.[216] In the hippocampus, the pyramidal cell layer is split (mainly CA1) and the DG is diffuse and disorganized. The cerebellum is hypoplastic in the *reeler* mouse.[217,218] It has also been shown that lack of reelin signaling results in abnormal positioning and altered morphology of forebrain interneurons.[219] Interestingly, a recent study demonstrated that homozygous *reeler* mice have enhanced seizure susceptibility that is, at least in part, intrinsic to the malformed neocortex and hippocampus.[220,221] In these studies, low thresholds and an increased incidence/severity of seizures induced by MES or isoflurane were detected in vivo; in vitro, prolonged periods of spontaneous epileptiform activity in the presence of bicuculline were recorded in neocortical and hippocampal slices.[221]

Similar, although milder, malformations reminiscent of *reeler* mutant mice have been also reported in the neocortex and hippocampus of mice with a hemizygous deletion of the *Lis1* gene[222,223] (see the next section) and in mice lacking *p35*, a neuronal-specific activator of cyclin-dependent kinase (Cdk5); such mice exhibit cortical lamination defects and seizures.[224,225] Mutation at the human gene encoding reelin has been identified in individuals with an autosomal recessive form of lissencephaly associated with cerebellar hypoplasia and epilepsy.[226]

Lis1

Classic or type I lissencephaly in humans is characterized by generalized agyria/pachygyria, four abnormal cortical layers, enlarged ventricles, generalized neuronal heterotopias, and corpus callosum defects.[227,228] The loss-of-function mutation in the microtubule-associated protein–encoding gene *PAFAH1B1* (encoding the Lis1 protein, or brain-specific noncatalytic subunit of platelet-activating factor acetylhydrolase 1b)[229,230] was identified from patient samples with informative deletions of 17p13.3.[231] Because Lis1 protein is important in the microtubule-based motor activity of cytoplasmic dynein,[228,231,232] which is vital for the proper migration of neuronal precursors,[233] an insufficient amount of Lis1 protein could cause migration problems with subsequent brain malformation.[234,235] Mutation of the human gene, which has its homologue *Lis1* in the mouse, is associated with embryonic lethality in homozygotes and disruption of neuronal migration across the cerebral parenchyma along with severe hippocampal dyslamination and hyperexcitability in heterozygotes.[222,223,236] A recent set of anatomic studies showed significant disruption of the supragranular zone of the DG in adult *Lis1*[+/−] mice and aberrant neurogenesis.[237] Although fiber termination patterns in the hippocampus are relatively normal, disorganization of hippocampal CA1-CA3 pyramidal cells and dispersion of granule cells are significant in the *Lis1*[+/−] mice.[238] In vitro extracellular recording of hippocampal slices from *Lis1*[+/−] mice showed a reduced threshold for potassium-induced epileptiform bursting and enhanced excitatory synaptic transmission in the *Lis1*[+/−] CA1 subfield,[222] which presumably contributes to the lowered threshold and intense epileptogenesis observed in the *Lis1*[+/−] mouse. Studies of embryonic slice cultures from *Lis1*[+/−] mice suggest that the nonradial migration of cortical and hippocampal interneurons is defectively slowed.[234] However, an increase in large-amplitude GABA-mediated synaptic events and enhanced glutamatergic excitation of hippocampal interneurons were noted in the dysplastic CA1 pyramidal cell region of these mice.[239] Further analysis of these anatomic and physiologic hippocampal defects may provide a better understanding of the neuronal basis for epileptogenesis associated with lissencephaly.

FOCAL EPILEPSIES

Aluminum Model

Focal epilepsies, or epilepsies whose seizures arise from a limited area within a hemisphere, are the most common form of epilepsy in humans. Since the 1940s, topical injection of alumina hydroxide onto the cortex of animals has been used as a model for partial seizures. Monkeys appear to be the best animal to use with this method, followed by dogs, cats, and guinea pigs. After cisternal or systemic injection of aluminum compounds, an encephalopathy with multifocal seizures can also be induced in rabbits, cats, and ferrets but not rats.[240]

After local alumina hydroxide application onto the cortex of the temporal lobe or rolandic area, focal SRSs develop in animals in 1 to 2 months and may persist for as long as several years. Sometimes SE can occur, especially when a large injection of alumina hydroxide is applied. This can probably be attributed to subpial spread of the drug. The symptomatology depends on the location of the injection. For example, after application to the sensorimotor cortex, seizures develop that are similar to simple partial seizures in humans, with rhythmic jerking of an extremity or the face contralateral to the inflicted lesion and occasional progression to generalization. In primates, seizure symptomatology is very similar to that in humans. Scalp EEG recordings from these animals show interictal and ictal spikes, and the seizures respond to AEDs such as phenobarbital and phenytoin.[241,242] The anatomic changes are characterized by cell loss, mainly GABAergic neurons (a potentially unifying theme in nearly all the animal models discussed here), and reactive gliosis at the site of injection.[243] The attractive aspect of this model is that it uses animals that are phylogenetically closer to humans and induces partial seizures similar to those in humans. The disadvantages of this model include a long and unpredictable latency period before clinical and electrographic onset of spontaneous seizures (4 to 8 weeks in cats; 6 to 12 weeks in rhesus monkeys), as well as heavy resource allocation, which limits the number of animals that can be studied in any given project.[5,244]

Ferrous Chloride Model

The focal application of ferrous chloride as a model of epilepsy arose from the observation that deposits of iron on brain tissue after head trauma or stroke can be a risk factor for the development of epilepsy.[245] In this model, ferrous chloride is injected into the cortex or amygdala of the rat. After 5 to 7 days, spontaneous seizures develop in more than 90% of the animals. Histologic analysis of the cortical lesions 6 weeks after the injection shows neuronal loss, activated astroglial cells, iron-positive macrophages, and fibroblasts surrounding the iron deposit. Some of the surviving layer V pyramidal neurons stain positive for iron, with loss of dendritic spines and decreased dendritic branching.[246] The latter anatomic findings have clear implications for synaptic excitability. Interestingly, most of the AEDs available are effective in controlling the SRSs induced by ferrous chloride.[247]

CONCLUSION

In this brief discussion of existing animal models of epilepsy, there is much that cannot be summarized. Space limitations preclude a more comprehensive analysis of animal models of febrile seizures; absence epilepsies; seizure syndromes associated with ion channel mutations; and emerging models in simple species such as *Drosophila*, *Caenorhabditis elegans*, and zebrafish. Indeed, there are several good textbooks devoted entirely to these topics, and they provide excellent reading for clinicians, clinician-scientists, or basic scientists interested in epilepsy research. The animal models of epilepsy described here highlight some of the fundamental insights that have emerged from this line of study, as well as specific alterations in excitatory or synaptic systems that may explain epileptogenesis. Further analysis of these models and the continued development of even better animal models are warranted and should continue to be a major thrust of the epilepsy research community.

SUGGESTED READINGS

Baraban SC, Wenzel HJ, Hochman DW, et al. Characterization of heterotopic cell clusters in the hippocampus of rats exposed to methylazoxymethanol in utero. *Epilepsy Res.* 2000;39:87-102.

Buckmaster PS, Dudek FE. Neuron loss, granule cell axon reorganization, and functional changes in the dentate gyrus of epileptic kainate-treated rats. *J Comp Neurol.* 1997;385:385-404.

Calcagnotto ME, Paredes MF, Baraban SC. Heterotopic neurons with altered inhibitory synaptic function in an animal model of malformation-associated epilepsy. *J Neurosci.* 2002;22:7596-7605.

Cavalheiro EA, Leite JP, Bortolotto ZA, et al. Long-term effects of pilocarpine in rats: structural damage of the brain triggers kindling and spontaneous recurrent seizures. *Epilepsia*. 1991;32:778-782.

Chevassus-au-Louis N, Baraban SC, Gaiarsa JL, et al. Cortical malformations and epilepsy: new insights from animal models. *Epilepsia*. 1999;40:811-821.

Dvorak K, Feit J, Jurankova Z. Experimentally induced focal microgyria and status verrucosus deformis in rats—pathogenesis and interrelation. Histological and autoradiographical study. *Acta Neuropathol*. 1978;44:121-129.

Fleck MW, Hirotsune S, Gambello MJ, et al. Hippocampal abnormalities and enhanced excitability in a murine model of human lissencephaly. *J Neurosci*. 2000;20:2439-2450.

Goddard GV. Development of epileptic seizures through brain stimulation at low intensity. *Nature*. 1967;214:1020-1021.

Houser CR. Granule cell dispersion in the dentate gyrus of humans with temporal lobe epilepsy. *Brain Res*. 1990;535:195-204.

Jacobs KM, Hwang BJ, Prince DA. Focal epileptogenesis in a rat model of polymicrogyria. *J Neurophysiol*. 1999;81:159-173.

Lee KS, Schottler F, Collins JL, et al. A genetic animal model of human neocortical heterotopia associated with seizures. *J Neurosci*. 1997;17:6236-6242.

Longo BM, Mello LE. Effect of long-term spontaneous recurrent seizures or reinduction of status epilepticus on the development of supragranular mossy fiber sprouting. *Epilepsy Res*. 1999;36:233-241.

Luhmann HJ, Karpuk N, Qu M, et al. Characterization of neuronal migration disorders in neocortical structures. II. Intracellular in vitro recordings. *J Neurophysiol*. 1998;80:92-102.

McIntyre DC, Kelly ME, Dufresne C. FAST and SLOW amygdala kindling rat strains: comparison of amygdala, hippocampal, piriform and perirhinal cortex kindling. *Epilepsy Res*. 1999;35:197-209.

Mello LE, Cavalheiro EA, Tan AM, et al. Circuit mechanisms of seizures in the pilocarpine model of chronic epilepsy: cell loss and mossy fiber sprouting. *Epilepsia*. 1993;34:985-995.

Nadler JV, Perry BW, Cotman CW. Intraventricular kainic acid preferentially destroys hippocampal pyramidal cells. *Nature*. 1978;271:676-677.

Parent JM, Yu TW, Leibowitz RT, et al. Dentate granule cell neurogenesis is increased by seizures and contributes to aberrant network reorganization in the adult rat hippocampus. *J Neurosci*. 1997;17:3727-3738.

Patrylo PR, Browning RA, Cranick S. Reeler homozygous mice exhibit enhanced susceptibility to epileptiform activity. *Epilepsia*. 2006;47:257-266.

Racine R, Rose PA, Burnham WM. Afterdischarge thresholds and kindling rates in dorsal and ventral hippocampus and dentate gyrus. *Can J Neurol Sci*. 1977;4:273-278.

Roper SN, Gilmore RL, Houser CR. Experimentally induced disorders of neuronal migration produce an increased propensity for electrographic seizures in rats. *Epilepsy Res*. 1995;21:205-219.

Sloviter RS, Kudrimoti HS, Laxer KD, et al. "Tectonic" hippocampal malformations in patients with temporal lobe epilepsy. *Epilepsy Res*. 2004;59:123-153.

Trotter SA, Kapur J, Anzivino MJ, et al. GABAergic synaptic inhibition is reduced before seizure onset in a genetic model of cortical malformation. *J Neurosci*. 2006;26:10756-10767.

Turski WA, Cavalheiro EA, Schwarz M, et al. Limbic seizures produced by pilocarpine in rats: behavioural, electroencephalographic and neuropathological study. *Behav Brain Res*. 1983;9:315-335.

Wang Y, Baraban SC. Granule cell dispersion and aberrant neurogenesis in the adult hippocampus of an LIS1 mutant mouse. *Dev Neurosci*. 2007;29:91-98.

Wenzel HJ, Robbins CA, Tsai LH, et al. Abnormal morphological and functional organization of the hippocampus in a p35 mutant model of cortical dysplasia associated with spontaneous seizures. *J Neurosci*. 2001;21:983-998.

Zhu WJ, Roper SN. Reduced inhibition in an animal model of cortical dysplasia. *J Neurosci*. 2000;20:8925-8931.

Full references can be found on Expert Consult @ www.expertconsult.com

CHAPTER 51

Malformations of Cortical Development

Gregory G. Heuer ■ Peter B. Crino

Malformations of cortical development (MCDs) are a heterogeneous group of disorders characterized by abnormal cerebral cortical cytoarchitecture. MCDs represent a spectrum of disorders from subtle microdysgenesis affecting a small area of the cortex to devastating lissencephaly in which the regional, gyral, and laminar patterning of the cortex is lost. A unifying feature of MCDs is their high association with intractable epilepsy and in many cases with cognitive disabilities, autism, or pervasive developmental disorders. With the routine use of magnetic resonance imaging (MRI), many subtle MCDs are being identified with greater frequency and with higher resolution,[1-7] although so-called minimal MCDs (mMCDs) often remain radiographically undetectable.

There is considerable variability in the molecular mechanisms and pathologic features of each MCD; those affecting broad areas of the cortex tend to have greater neurological manifestations, whereas more minor malformations are often associated with pharmacoresistant epilepsy. Infantile spasms can be associated with virtually any type of malformation. MCDs can occur as autosomal recessive, autosomal dominant, or X-linked disorders; however, many occur sporadically without a clear family pedigree or even as discordant findings in monozygotic twins. In contrast, some MCDs result from intrauterine toxins, such as exposure to cytomegalovirus, hypoxia-ischemia, or fetal alcohol exposure. Over the past 15 years rapid progress has been made in identifying single-gene defects associated with individual MCDs. The creation of animal models for some of these MCDs has generated significant insight into the molecular mechanisms of epilepsy and cognitive disabilities seen in patients.

CLASSIFICATION OF MALFORMATIONS OF CORTICAL DEVELOPMENT

The majority of patients with MCDs do not have a known specific genetic syndrome. Development of the normal six-layered human cortex results from a complex series of events, in large part controlled by known and as yet unknown genes.[8-11] Disruptions in these developmentally regulated genes can result in cortical malformations. A number of new genes have been discovered that cause certain forms of MCD (Table 51-1).[12-52] The specific malformation resulting from each mutation is related to the normal temporal and anatomic expression of the gene product that has been lost.

The dynamic process of cortical development can be disrupted at many time points by gene mutation or environmental events. Formation of the normal cerebral cortex extends from weeks 8 to 26 of human gestation and is orchestrated by a complex array of genes[5-11] that ultimately result in the correct cortical laminar organization. The cortex forms from neuroglial progenitor (stem) cells born in the ventricular and subventricular zones that undergo successive rounds of mitosis. Once exiting the cell cycle, neurons migrate via both radial and tangential pathways in response to various trophic and repulsive cues to form the cortical plate (the nascent cortex). Excitatory neurons follow a radial inside-out migratory gradient along radial glial cells from layer VI to layer II. Layer I is an early embryonic layer that predates the deeper layers. Inhibitory neurons are born in the ganglionic eminences and migrate by tangential pathways into the cortical plate. Cells arriving at their appropriate cortical laminar destination cease migration, begin to extend axons and dendrites, and form early functional synapses. Conceptually, normal corticogenesis can be broadly divided into three stages: proliferation, migration, and organization.

Based on the proposed steps for normal cortical development and the recent identification of single genes responsible for many MCDs, a classification scheme for abnormal cortical development (i.e., MCDs) was defined in 1996 and later modified in 2001 and 2004.[53-55] The MCD taxonomy is organized according to the putative cellular mechanisms that are disrupted in development. These groups include (1) disorders of cellular proliferation, (2) disorders of neuronal migration, (3) disorders of cortical organization, and (4) disorders with unknown mechanisms (Table 51-2). Functional in vitro studies have been used to mechanistically support parcellation of particular MCDs into each category.

Disorders of Cellular Proliferation

Malformations in this group include disorders that result in either increased or decreased growth or in increased or decreased apoptosis. These disorders are often manifested as abnormal brain size or localized areas of enlargement. Abnormalities in brain size can be manifested as microcephaly with a normal to thin cortex, microlissencephaly, microcephaly with polymicrogyria, or macrocephaly.[15,17,32,47]

Microcephaly is defined as a head circumference that is more than 2 SD smaller than normal.[56] Patients with this condition have a brain that may be up to 70% smaller than normal, but the brain has essentially normal cortical laminar architecture. In some cases of microcephaly, a simplified gyral folding pattern is observed on MRI. Because any process that interferes with brain growth can lead to reduced head/brain size, microcephaly is associated with a highly heterogeneous group of disorders. It can result from a number of prenatal insults, including hypoxia-ischemia and fetal alcohol exposure. Additionally, a number of genes (ASPM, MCPH1, CENPJ, and CDK5RAP2) have been shown to result in autosomal recessive forms of microcephaly.[15-17,32,57,58] Rare syndromic forms include Amish lethal microcephaly and Seckel's syndrome.[16,46] The ASPM (abnormal spindle-like microcephaly associated) gene is of particular interest because it is the single most common genetic mutation associated with microcephaly and has provided new insight into evolutionary mechanisms governing brain size across species. ASPM is an orthologue of a Drosophila gene that has been shown to be essential for normal mitotic spindle function in embryonic neuroblasts. When absent, neuroblasts are arrested in the cell cycle and fail to proliferate, which results in a reduction in the number of cells in the brain and consequently a smaller brain size. When the human ASPM gene sequence was compared with that of primates, there was a correlation between sequence

TABLE 51-1 Genetic Causes of Malformations of Cortical Development

SYNDROME	LOCUS	GENE	PROTEIN
Autosomal recessive periventricular heterotopia and microcephaly[1,17,32,47]	8p23	MCPH1	Microcephalin
	1q31	ASPM	Abnormal spindle-like microcephaly
	17q25.3	ARFGEF2	ARFGEF2
Autosomal recessive microcephaly[16]	9q32	CDK5RAP2	Cyclin-dependant kinase 5 regulatory-associated protein 2
	13q12.2	CENPJ	Centromere-associated protein J
Amish lethal microcephaly	17q25.3	SLC25A19	Nuclear mitochondrial deoxynucleotide carrier
Seckel's syndrome I[39]	3q22-q24	ATR	Ataxia-telangiectasia and Rad3-related protein
Isolated lissencephaly sequence[18,22,26,41-43,45]	Xq22.3-q23	DCX, XLIS	DCX, doublecortin
	17p13.3	LIS1	PAFAH1B1
Subcortical band heterotopia[27,28,38]	Xq22.3-q23	DCX, XLI	DCX, doublecortin
	17p13.3	LIS1	PAFAH1B1
Miller-Dieker syndrome[23,51]	17p13.3	Several genes	PAFAH1B1 and others
Lissencephaly with cerebellar hypoplasia[31]	7q22	RELN	Reelin
X-linked lissencephaly with abnormal genitalia[34,35]	Xp22.13	ARX	Aristaless-related homeobox protein
Fukuyama's congenital muscular dystrophy[36,48,49]	9q31	FCMD	FCMD, fukutin
Muscle-eye-brain disease[14,19,20]	1p33-34	POMGnT1	POMGnT1
	19q13.3	FKRP	Fukutin-related protein
Congenital muscular dystrophy[37,50]	19q13.3	FKRP	Fukutin-related protein
	22q12.3-q13.1	LARGE	
Walker-Warburg syndrome[13,14,21]	9q34.1	POMT1	O-Mannosyl-transferase 1
	19q13.3	FKRP	Fukutin-related protein
	9q31	FCMD	FCMD
Bilateral periventricular nodular heterotopia[25,47]	Xq28	FLNA	Filamin-A
	20q13.3	ARFGEF2	BIG2
	5p15	Unknown	Unknown
Tuberous sclerosis[24,29,30,33]	9q32	TSC1	Hamartin
	16p13.3	TSC2	Tuberin
Pretzel syndrome[44]	17q23.3	LYK5	Strad
Bilateral frontoparietal polymicrogyria[40]	16q13	GPR56	Unknown
Warburg's microsyndrome-1[12]	2q21.3	RAB3GAO	
Bilateral perisylvian polymicrogyria[52]	Xq28	Unknown	Unknown

Adapted from Barkovich AJ, Kuzniecky RI, Jackson GD, et al. A developmental and genetic classification for malformations of cortical development. *Neurology*. 2005;65:1873-1887; and Crino PB, Miyata H, Vinters HV. Neurodevelopmental disorders as a cause of seizures: neuropathologic, genetic, and mechanistic considerations. *Brain Pathol.* 2002;12:212-233.

and brain size.[59] Thus, *ASPM* appears to have played a central role in the genetic component of the evolutionary expansion in brain size from primates to *Homo sapiens*.

Macrocephaly, defined as measurable enlargement of the head (>2 SD), can occur in conjunction with a large number of syndromes and conditions that are not associated with MCDs, including hydrocephalus, autism, leukodystrophies, and organic acidurias.[60] Hemimegalencephaly (HME) is a malformation characterized by the abnormal enlargement of one entire hemisphere (Fig. 51-1); a variant of HME is lobar dysplasia, in which an entire brain lobe is enlarged. HME may be seen in isolation or in the setting of a known syndrome such as linear sebaceous nevus (of Jadassohn), hypomelanosis of Ito, tuberous sclerosis complex (TSC), or Proteus syndrome. HME is highly associated with intractable seizures and, frequently, infantile spasms. Pathologic analysis of HME brain demonstrates loss of cortical lamination, dysmorphic neurons, and cytomegalic cells similar to those seen in focal cortical dysplasia (FCD) and TSC (see later).[61-63] As yet, no specific gene has been associated with HME, although reports suggest an association with *PTEN* mutations in Proteus syndrome.[64-67]

In addition to changes across broad cortical areas, disorders of cellular proliferation can result in focal malformations or dysplasias. Such lesions include FCDs, in particular, cortical dysplasias containing balloon cells, tubers in TSC, and low-grade neoplastic lesions such as dysembryoplastic neuroepithelial tumor, ganglioglioma (Fig. 51-2), and gangliocytoma.[24,29,30,33,44,61-63,68] TSC results from mutations in *TSC1*, which encodes TSC1 or hamartin, or from mutations in *TSC2*, which encodes TSC2 or tuberin.[24,29,30,33] TSC1 and TSC2 are known modulators of the mammalian target of rapamycin (mTOR) pathway, which governs cell size and proliferation. Neurological manifestations of TSC include epilepsy, infantile spasms, cognitive disabilities, and autism.[69] Cortical tubers are focal areas of disorganized cortical lamination characterized by the presence of cytomegalic cells known as giant cells.[69,70] The number of tubers across patients is variable and does not seem to vary with mutation type, patient age, or necessarily, neurological phenotype.

FCD with balloon cells (so-called Palmini type 2B dysplasia; Fig. 51-3) is a sporadic condition for which no specific gene mutation has been found.[68,71] Like the tubers in TSC, FCD 2B consists of focal areas of cortical laminar disorganization

TABLE 51-2 Classification of Malformations of Cortical Development

GROUP	SUBGROUP	CONDITION
Disorders of cellular proliferation	Abnormal proliferation	Microcephaly
		Macrocephaly
		Cortical tubers (TSC)
		FCD with balloon cells
		Hemimegalencephaly
	Abnormal proliferation	Dysembryoplastic neuroepithelial tumor
	Neoplastic process	Ganglioglioma
		Gangliocytoma
Disorders of neuronal migration		Lissencephaly
		Heterotopia
	Muscular dystrophy	Congenital muscular dystrophy
		Muscle-eye-brain disease
		Walker-Warburg syndrome
Disorders of cortical organization		Polymicrogyria
		Schizencephaly

FCD, focal cortical dysplasia; TSC, tuberous sclerosis complex.
Adapted from Barkovich AJ, Kuzniecky RI, Jackson GD, et al. A developmental and genetic classification for malformations of cortical development. *Neurology.* 2005;65:1873-1887.

characterized histopathologically by neuronal dysmorphism and pathognomonic enlarged cells, known as balloon cells, that are similar to the giant cells found in TSC. In addition to appearance, balloon cells and giant cells share many immunohistochemical features.[62,70,72-74]

Disorders of Neuronal Migration

Disorders of migration are a heterogeneous set of syndromes characterized by altered gyral patterning and cortical laminar organization or the presence of ectopic neurons in the subcortical white matter or periventricular region. Such disorders include lissencephaly, subependymal/periventricular heterotopia, marginal glioneuronal heterotopia, subcortical band heterotopia, and

heterotopia syndromes.[75,76] Disorders of neuronal migration can exhibit various clinicopathologic phenotypes, depending on the timing and location of the migratory disruption.

Lissencephaly ("smooth brain") refers to a heterogeneous group of disorders characterized by loss of the normal gyral pattern and significant disorganization of cortical laminar cytoarchitecture (Fig. 51-4). Lissencephaly is separated into two

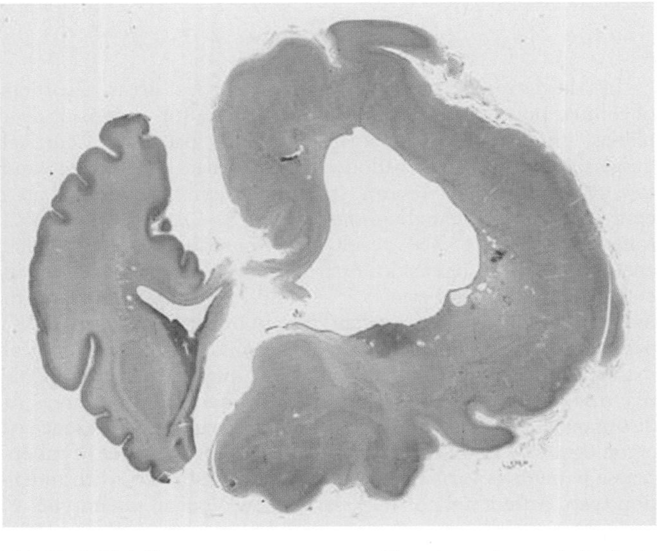

FIGURE 51-1 Postmortem specimen of hemimegalencephaly. Brain tissue stained with cresyl violet reveals massive enlargement of the left hemisphere.

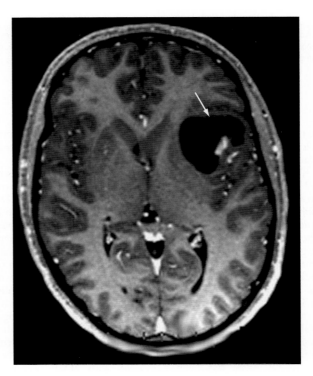

FIGURE 51-2 Magnetic resonance image depicting a left frontal ganglioglioma (*arrow,* T1-weighted image after intravenous gadolinium).

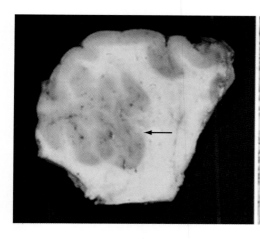 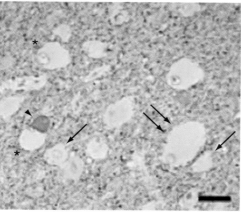

FIGURE **51-3** Histopathology of Palmini type II cortical dysplasia. **Left,** Fresh specimen demonstrating thickened cortex (*arrow*). **Right,** Balloon cells (*double arrows*), dysmorphic neurons (*single arrows* and *asterisk*), and glial cells (*arrowhead*) (labeled with glial fibrillary acidic protein).

pathologic subtypes: type 1 or classic and type II or cobblestone lissencephaly. In type I lissencephaly, the gyral patterning across the entire cortex is altered. Because of abnormal neuronal migration, neuronal progenitor cells fail to move to their correct laminar location and the normal six-layer cortex is reduced to a four-layered pattern.

Several autosomal recessive and X-linked forms of type I lissencephaly exist and result from mutations in the *LIS1, DCX, ARX,* or *RELN* genes.* These genes are believed to be involved in important cell processes, such as movement of the neuronal nucleus or dynamic changes in the neuronal cytoskeleton, that are required for neuronal progenitor cells to migrate properly from the ventricular zone into the cortical plate.[77-79] *LIS1* mutations are seen in isolated lissencephaly, as well as in association with Miller-Dieker lissencephaly syndrome.

Syndromic forms of type II or cobblestone lissencephaly are associated with rare congenital forms of muscular dystrophy, muscle-eye-brain disease, and Walker-Warburg syndrome.[12-14,19-21,36,37,48-50] In type II lissencephaly, the altered gyral patterning is more heterogeneously distributed across the cortical mantle. The combination of a muscular dystrophy and lissencephaly should prompt a search for one of these syndromes.

Subcortical band heterotopia (Fig. 51-5) and periventricular nodular heterotopia (Fig. 51-6) syndromes are X-linked disorders that are manifested as sexually dimorphic phenotypes. For

example, in females, mutations in the *DCX* (doublecortin) gene are associated with a type of subcortical band heterotopia in which a broad focal band of cortical neurons is trapped within the subcortical white matter bilaterally.[26,41,79,80] The band consists of neurons of both excitatory and inhibitory phenotypes and makes connections with the overlying cortices. In males, the *DCX* mutation is associated with lissencephaly. Periventricular nodular heterotopia is a disorder resulting from mutations in the filamin-1 (*FLN1*) gene in which focal nodules of cortical neurons are observed within the walls of the lateral ventricles. These collections are also composed of both excitatory and inhibitory neurons, and recent tensor tract imaging techniques have revealed that these cells make connections with the overlying cortex. *FLN1* mutations in males lead to embryonic lethality. It has been proposed that the differential mutational features in males and females reflect the effects of the mutation expressed on a single X chromosome in males versus the presence of both mutated and

*See references 18, 22, 23, 26, 31, 34, 35, 41-43, 45, 51.

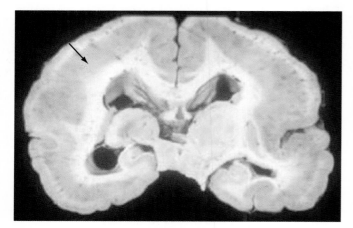

FIGURE 51-4 Unfixed specimen of lissencephaly. Note the thickened cortex (*arrow*) and absence of cortical gyri.

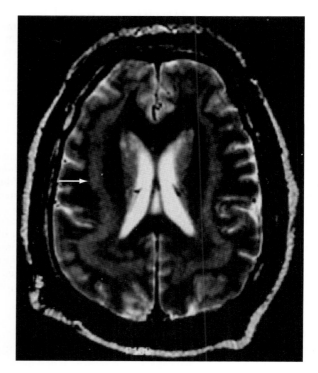

FIGURE 51-5 T2-weighted magnetic resonance image demonstrating subcortical band heterotopia (*arrow*). Note that the heterotopia extends within the white matter bilaterally.

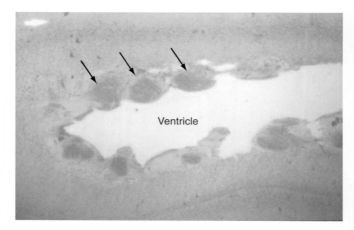

FIGURE 51-6 Periventricular nodular heterotopia. Note the small nodules (*arrows*) of hematoxylin-stained cells adjacent to the lateral ventricle (hematoxylin and eosin staining).

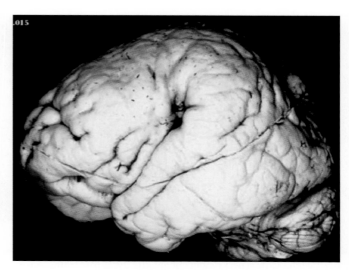

FIGURE 51-7 Whole-brain specimen depicting polymicrogyria. Note the many small and disorganized gyri across the surface of the hemisphere.

normal X chromosomes in females. The focal pathology in both disorders is hypothesized to be variable X chromosome inactivation in developing neural stem cells, which occurs in the affected female brain.[22,43]

Disorders of Cortical Organization

This group of disorders results from disruptions in late neuronal migration, neurite extension, synaptogenesis, and neuronal maturation. This group includes polymicrogyria, schizencephaly, FCD without balloon cells (Palmini type 1), and microdysgenesis.

Polymicrogyria is characterized by an excessive number of abnormally small gyri (Fig. 51-7). It can occur secondary to genetic mutations and has been hypothesized to result from prenatal infections or abnormal twinning.[40,52,81] There are rare case reports in which abnormal twin pregnancies resulted in cortical disruption and polymicrogyria.[82,83] Bilateral perisylvian polymicrogyria (BPP) is the most common type of polymicrogyria and is characterized clinicopathologically by bilateral polymicrogyria in the perisylvian region, pseudobulbar paresis, mental retardation, and epilepsy. BPP has been mapped to Xq27-28. Additionally, there are a number of congenital conditions in which polymicrogyria is part of the syndrome, including Joubert's, Delleman's, Adams-Oliver, and Galloway-Mowat syndromes.

Schizencephaly is characterized by a cerebral cleft that, unlike a porencephalic cyst, is lined by gray matter (Fig. 51-8).[84-88] The schizencephalic cleft extends from the surface of the cortex to the ventricle. The cleft can be filled with cerebrospinal fluid (the open-lipped form) or the two surfaces can be fused (the closed-lipped form). Schizencephaly is almost always associated with localized polymicrogyria around the cleft.

FCD without balloon cells (Palmini type 1 dysplasia) is a focal cortical malformation in which there is mild disorganization of cortical lamination and malpositioning of cortical neurons. Classic balloon cells are not observed. Type 1 cortical dysplasia is highly associated with focal intractable epilepsy. Microdysgenesis is a subtle malformation of the cerebral cortical architecture. Recent classifications have replaced this term with mMCD.

Disorders with Unknown Mechanisms

This group of MCDs includes disorders not associated with the other pathologic entities, such as sublobar dysplasias and malformations associated with inborn errors of metabolism. The genetic conditions include mitochondrial disorders, pyruvate metabolic disorders, and peroxisomal disorders.

SURGERY FOR MALFORMATIONS OF CORTICAL DEVELOPMENT

MCDs are the most common cause of intractable pediatric epilepsy.[89,90] For example, 70% to 90% of patients with TSC, HME, or lissencephaly suffer from seizures. In studies on epilepsy surgical samples, MCDs may be seen in 30% of cortical resections, and therefore these lesions and the conditions associated with

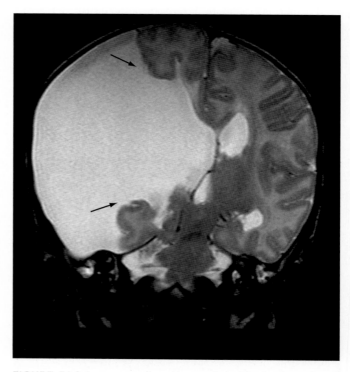

FIGURE 51-8 Large open-lip schizencephaly. The banks or lips of the schizencephaly (*arrows*) typically exhibit a malformed cortical cytoarchitecture.

them are particularly important for epilepsy surgeons. Untreated epilepsy in infants, such as infantile spasms, can result in profound developmental problems for the child.[91] Although surgery can be difficult in very young patients, surgical treatment of MCDs associated with intractable seizures can lead to cure and ameliorate some of the developmental problems.[92-97]

The surgical treatment of epilepsy associated with these lesions includes simple lesionectomy, lesionectomy and resection of the surrounding epileptic focus, resection of the lesion and the mesial temporal structures, and hemispherectomy. Each lesion and the treatment strategy are approached individually based on the extent of the malformation and the age of the patient. In addition, in the setting of long-standing seizures, the mesial temporal structures may be involved and must be resected along with the seizure focus.[98]

Patients undergo a phase I evaluation that includes an inter-ictal electroencephalogram (EEG), video-EEG, and MRI. In addition, patients can receive advanced imaging that may include functional MRI, magnetoencephalography, and interictal positron emission tomography. Patients often require phase II studies involving placement of strip, grid, or depth electrodes and neurobehavioral testing to define the location and laterality of higher order functions and regions of eloquent cortex. Moreover, invasive monitoring is often needed because patients may have multiple lesions, only some of which are causing seizures, and in many cases regions other than the obvious area containing the MCDs may be involved in the epileptogenic focus.

The outcome of surgical treatment of these disorders varies according to the condition. Even with significant advances in localization and surgical technique, surgical treatment of FCD results in cure in only 42% to 55% of patients, with around 70% having a good surgical outcome (Engel classes I and II).[99-101] Resection of glioneuronal tumors such as gangliogliomas results in freedom from seizures in 58% to 86% of patients.[102-106] Better surgical outcome was associated with a shorter duration of seizures, absence of generalized seizures, younger patient age, and total resection.[102]

Epilepsy surgery for TSC lesions results in freedom from seizures in 53% to 68% of patients and good seizure outcome in 64% to 92%.[107-109] Presurgical evaluation of patients with TSC is particularly important and is primarily directed at identifying the specific seizure-causing lesion. In the setting of a patient with multiple tubers, treatment may require invasive mapping to identify the seizure focus or may require multiple resections.[109,110] A worse outcome is associated with younger age at seizure onset, history of infantile spasms, and bilateral focal interictal discharges.[108]

HME is often treated by hemispherectomy, and both functional and anatomic methods have been described. HME may be associated with a worse outcome than other MCDs with regard to freedom from seizures or developmental outcome; however, the number of patients in most studies is small, and it is difficult to draw major conclusions from such studies.[111-114] In a study of 10 patients with HME, 60% were seizure free and 80% had a good outcome.[111] A study involving 9 infants with HME demonstrated freedom from seizures in 57% after hemispherectomy.[115] Anatomic resection may be preferable to disconnection procedures in the management of HME because disconnection procedures for this condition can be technically difficult with an increased risk for incomplete hemispheric disconnection.

In the limited number of series on schizencephalic lesions, surgery has been shown to be particularly effective, especially when the resection was tailored to the seizure focus and not just the schizencephalic region. However, studies on schizencephaly are limited to case reports and small case series, and it is difficult to draw major conclusions on outcomes after seizure surgery for this condition.[116-118]

In addition to surgical resection, other options for the treatment of epilepsy associated with MCDs include corpus callosotomy and vagal nerve stimulation. These options are used in patients in whom the seizure focus is in eloquent areas, is bilateral, or cannot be well defined or in patients who are poor surgical candidates for focal resection. Even though these treatments rarely result in cure, they can lead to a significant reduction in seizure frequency in patients with MCDs.[119-124]

CONCLUSION

MCDs are a diverse group of disorders that often result in profound neurological impairment. As is the case in other areas of neurosurgery, there have been significant advances in the molecular understanding of these conditions, both in their development and in their pathogenesis. There is great promise in developing new treatments of MCDs based on the genetics of these lesions.

SUGGESTED READINGS

Andermann F. Cortical dysplasias and epilepsy: a review of the architectonic, clinical, and seizure patterns. *Adv Neurol.* 2000;84:479-496.

Barkovich AJ, Kuzniecky RI, Jackson GD, et al. A developmental and genetic classification for malformations of cortical development. *Neurology.* 2005;65:1873-1887.

Bond J, Roberts E, Mochida GH, et al. *ASPM* is a major determinant of cerebral cortical size. *Nat Genet.* 2002;32:316-320.

Crino PB. Molecular pathogenesis of focal cortical dysplasia and hemimegalencephaly. *J Child Neurol.* 2005;20:330-336.

Cross JH. Functional neuroimaging of malformations of cortical development. *Epileptic Disord.* 2003;5(suppl 2):S73-S80.

Granata T, Freri E, Caccia C, et al. Schizencephaly: clinical spectrum, epilepsy, and pathogenesis. *J Child Neurol.* 2005;20:313-318.

Mathern GW, Andres M, Salamon N, et al. A hypothesis regarding the pathogenesis and epileptogenesis of pediatric cortical dysplasia and hemimegalencephaly based on MRI cerebral volumes and NeuN cortical cell densities. *Epilepsia.* 2007;48(suppl 5):74-78.

Olney AH. Macrocephaly syndromes. *Semin Pediatr Neurol.* 2007;14:128-135.

Palmini A, Najm I, Avanzini G, et al. Terminology and classification of the cortical dysplasias. *Neurology.* 2004;62:S2-S8.

Puffenberger EG, Strauss KA, Ramsey KE, et al. Polyhydramnios, megalencephaly and symptomatic epilepsy caused by a homozygous 7-kilobase deletion in *LYK5. Brain.* 2007;130:1929-1941.

Weiner HL, Carlson C, Ridgway EB, et al. Epilepsy surgery in young children with tuberous sclerosis: results of a novel approach. *Pediatrics.* 2006;117:1494-1502.

Zhang J. Evolution of the human *ASPM* gene, a major determinant of brain size. *Genetics.* 2003;165:2063-2070.

Full references can be found on Expert Consult @ www.expertconsult.com

Approach to the Patient

52

Diagnosis and Classification of Seizures and Epilepsy

Frank Gilliam

Epilepsy is perhaps the most complex neurological disorder from a clinical and pathophysiologic perspective. Many distinct molecular changes in neurons and glia can cause seizures,[1] and seizures occurring in specific neuronal networks manifest very different clinical symptoms and signs. In fact, there are many different epilepsy syndromes, each with multiple neurobiologic origins.[2] For example, juvenile myoclonic epilepsy is now understood to be associated with mutations on several different chromosomes.[3] Complex partial seizures of temporal lobe origin[4] may be caused by mesial temporal sclerosis,[5,6] developmental malformations,[7,8] brain injury, specific genetic mutations, or possibly a combination of these causes.[9] One of the major challenges of contemporary neuroscience is to better understand the ways in which the clinical manifestations of the epilepsies represent underlying structural, physiologic, and genetic alterations.

The epilepsies have importance for public health in that they are among the most common disabling neurological disorders occurring across the life span.[10-12] The prevalence of epilepsy is estimated to be about 1% of the U.S. population.[13] The World Health Organization reports that more than 100 million people are affected by epilepsy worldwide.[14] It is noteworthy that the Centers for Disease Control and Prevention emphasizes the lack of research on prevalence and incidence and recently stated that "epidemiological and surveillance data on epilepsy are limited" (www.cdc.gov/Epilepsy/).

Although earlier clinical studies suggested that more than 85% of patients with epilepsy have "adequate" seizure control with antiepileptic drugs,[15,16] more recent data indicate that in 35% to 40%, the available medications will not fully control the epilepsy.[13,17] In a Scottish study of more than 470 patients with recently diagnosed epilepsy, about 35% had a seizure during the most recent year of follow-up after a mean of 5 years of treatment. Furthermore, in only 11% was the epilepsy ever fully controlled with subsequent medications after the first antiepileptic drug failed.[17] A recent population-based study by the Centers for Disease Control and Prevention that included 120,000 people from 19 states found results that supported the Scottish data: 44% of patients with epilepsy who were currently taking medications had at least one seizure during the past 3 months.[13] Because the most important initial steps in effective treatment of epilepsy involve accurate diagnosis and subsequent selection of appropriate antiepileptic drugs based on seizure type, classification of the epilepsy based on precise history and supportive clinical testing is critical for optimal outcome.[18]

SEIZURE AND EPILEPSY CLASSIFICATION

The Commission on Classification and Terminology of the International League Against Epilepsy (ILAE) developed a widely used classification system based on review of videotaped seizures at commission workshops.[19] This classification system categorizes seizures in a format that facilitates diagnosis, treatment, and communication among medical professionals through standardized nomenclature.

Seizures are divided into two major categories—partial and generalized. Partial seizures are "those in which the first clinical and electrographic changes indicate initial activation of a system of neurons in one hemisphere and are subclassified based on the presence or absence of impairment of consciousness."[19] Simple partial seizures are associated with minimal change in awareness, as indicated clinically by the patient's complete recollection of the event. Complex partial seizures are characterized by alteration of awareness and amnesia for at least a portion of the seizure. Partial seizures may include signs or symptoms correlating with activation of any brain region—specifically, motor, autonomic, somatosensory, special sensory, or psychic, as elegantly demonstrated by Drs. Penfield and Jasper in their intraoperative stimulation studies of persons with epilepsy.[20] Both simple and complex partial seizures can propagate throughout the brain to become secondarily generalized seizures, typically with tonic or clonic motor features (or with both). Generalized seizures are "those in which the first clinical changes indicate initial involvement of both hemispheres."[19] The subclassification of generalized seizures includes absence, myoclonic, clonic, tonic, tonic-clonic, and atonic seizures. The generalized epilepsies, as opposed to generalized seizures, are often divided into primary (idiopathic) and secondary (symptomatic).[2] This distinction is useful because the seizures of primary generalized epilepsy are frequently genetic,[21,22] are usually limited to childhood or adolescence, and respond readily to certain anticonvulsant medications.[23]

Knowledge of the frequency of the common causes of epilepsy is necessary when assessing a patient with seizures. Cerebrovascular disease is the most frequently identified cause of epilepsy, followed by developmental disorders, head trauma, brain tumor, infection, and degenerative disorders.[24] The proportional incidence of the causes of seizures varies considerably with age, with cerebrovascular disease predominating in senior adults, head trauma and brain tumors more common in adolescents and adults, and developmental and infectious disorders proportionally most frequent in neonates and young children.[24]

Epilepsy syndromes are disorders associated with specific seizure types, clinical characteristics, and ages at onset. Similar to seizure classifications, the epilepsies are divided into two main categories: localization related and generalized. The ILAE classification system for epileptic syndromes is summarized in Table 52-1.[2]

DIAGNOSIS OF EPILEPSY

Epilepsy is often operationally defined as two unprovoked seizures occurring more than 24 hours apart. However, the ILAE recently proposed that "epilepsy is a disorder of the brain characterized by an enduring predisposition to generate epileptic seizures and by the neurobiologic, cognitive, psychological, and social consequences of this condition. The definition of epilepsy requires the occurrence of at least one epileptic seizure."[25] For the purposes of this chapter, we will consider epilepsy to be two unprovoked seizures or one unprovoked seizure with additional clinical evidence of increased risk for recurrent seizures. Hence, factors that influence the risk for seizure recurrence will be discussed as they relate to the diagnosis and especially to the decision for treatment to prevent subsequent seizures.

TABLE 52-1 International Classification of the Epilepsies and Epileptic Syndromes

1. Localization-related (focal, local, partial) epilepsies and syndromes
    1.1 Idiopathic with age-related onset. At present, two syndromes are established, but more may be identified in the future
        Benign childhood epilepsy with centrotemporal spikes (benign rolandic epilepsy)
        Childhood epilepsy with occipital paroxysms
    1.2 Symptomatic
        This category includes syndromes of great individual variability that will mainly be based on anatomic localization, clinical features, seizure types, and etiologic factors (if known)
2. Generalized epilepsies and syndromes
    2.1 Idiopathic, with age-related onset, listed in order of age
        Benign neonatal familial convulsions
        Benign neonatal convulsions
        Benign myoclonic epilepsy in infancy
        Childhood absence epilepsy (pyknolepsy)
        Juvenile absence epilepsy
        Juvenile myoclonic epilepsy (impulsive petit mal)
        Epilepsy with grand mal seizures on awakening
        Other generalized idiopathic epilepsies, if they do not belong to one of the above syndromes, can still be classified as generalized idiopathic epilepsies
    2.2 Idiopathic, symptomatic, or both, in order of age of appearance
        West's syndrome (infantile spasms, Blitz-Nick-Salaam-Krämpfe)
        Lennox-Gastaut syndrome
        Epilepsy with myoclonic-astatic seizures
        Epilepsy with myoclonic absences
    2.3 Symptomatic
        2.3.a Nonspecific etiology
            Early myoclonic encephalopathy
        2.3.b Specific syndromes
            Epileptic seizures may complicate many disease states
            Included under this heading are diseases in which seizures are an initial or predominant feature
3. Epilepsies and syndromes undetermined regarding whether they are focal or generalized
    3.1 With both generalized and focal seizures
        Neonatal seizures
        Severe myoclonic epilepsy in infancy
        Epilepsy with continuous spike waves during slow-wave sleep
        Acquired epileptic aphasia (Landau-Kleffner syndrome)
    3.2 Without unequivocal generalized or focal features
        This heading covers all cases in which clinical and electroencephalographic findings do not permit classification as clearly generalized or localization related, such as in many cases of sleep grand mal
4. Special syndromes
    4.1 Situation-related seizures
        Febrile convulsions
        Seizures related to other identifiable situations, such as stress, hormonal changes, drugs, alcohol, or sleep deprivation
    4.2 Isolated, apparently unprovoked epileptic events
    4.3 Epilepsies characterized by specific modes of seizure precipitation
    4.4 Chronic progressive epilepsia partialis continua of childhood

Adapted from Commission on the Classification and Terminology of the International League Against Epilepsy. A revised proposal for the classification of epilepsy and epileptic syndromes. *Epilepsia*. 1989;30:268-278.

The major factors to consider in confirming the diagnosis of epilepsy are the history of the experience of the seizure (especially the aura, or initial symptoms), description by a reliable witness, the physical examination, the electroencephalogram (EEG), and structural neuroimaging. Each of these factors will be discussed in the following sections.

Approach to the First Seizure

Acute Evaluation

A seizure after which mental status and the results of neurological examination quickly return to normal is not typically an emergency; this clinical situation is discussed in the next section. If mental status and the neurological examination have not normalized within minutes after the event appears to end, however, two questions must be answered as rapidly as possible. First, is there an underlying medical or neurological condition that requires immediate treatment? Second, has the seizure ended? These two questions must be addressed whether the patient is in an emergency room, intensive care unit, or ambulatory setting.

The urgent evaluation should include serum glucose, sodium, urea nitrogen, creatinine, and calcium and hepatic enzyme concentrations. Arterial blood pH, oxygen, and carbon dioxide are important to measure. A toxicology screen is necessary if no other cause is readily identified, especially for ethyl alcohol, cocaine, amphetamines, benzodiazepines, opioids, phencyclidine, tricyclic antidepressants, and antipsychotic drugs.[26] Hypothyroidism with myxedema coma has been associated with seizures in rare cases.[27]

Brain imaging, preferably computed tomography (CT) in view of its rapid availability at most centers, is necessary to exclude a structural cerebral abnormality such as hemorrhage, tumor, abscess, or contusion.[28] If significant temperature elevation, nuchal rigidity, leukocytosis, or other signs of possible central nervous system inflammation are present, a lumbar puncture is required to exclude infection or subarachnoid hemorrhage. If the patient has a possible history of seizures, anticonvulsant medications should be identified and serum concentrations determined.

Decreased responsiveness or unusual behavior may be the only indication of a persistent seizure.[29] An urgent EEG is therefore recommended for any patient whose mentation does not begin to normalize within minutes after a witnessed seizure. Furthermore, an EEG should be considered for any patient without a clearly defined cause of the altered mental status. If "subclinical" seizures are a possible cause of the confusion or abnormal behavior and the EEG is not diagnostic, intravenous injection of a short-acting benzodiazepine such as lorazepam may support the diagnosis if clinical improvement is observed soon after administration.[29] Change in the EEG pattern after injection does not confirm that a rhythmic or semirhythmic pattern was a seizure; in many cases, this can be determined only by correlative improvement in the mental status examination.[30]

Seizure Evaluation in the Ambulatory Setting

A patient being evaluated in an ambulatory setting with a history of a possible seizure is a common clinical situation. An acute evaluation such as that just described may have been performed in an emergency department before referral. If metabolic assessment was not performed previously, the serum studies described in the previous section should be considered. The subsequent evaluation aims at answering four questions: (1) Was the paroxysmal change in behavior or symptom a seizure? (2) What is the classification of the seizure? (3) Is there a cause that requires specific treatment? (4) What is the probability of another seizure?

A complete history of the event from both the patient and a witness is frequently the most helpful diagnostic tool.[31] An epi-gastric, olfactory, or experiential (psychic) aura suggests a partial seizure of temporal lobe onset,[32-35] for example, whereas generalized clonic activity immediately preceding the tonic-clonic phase may indicate a primary generalized epilepsy.[36] The clinical history may be ambiguous or suggest multiple possible diagnoses, however, including cardiac syncope, dysautonomia, conversion disorder, or panic attacks. In this situation, the physician must use diagnostic tests judiciously to make a definitive diagnosis and exclude progressive or potentially life-threatening disorders expeditiously. The two most helpful tests for achieving these goals in the ambulatory setting are the EEG and magnetic resonance imaging (MRI).[37] I recommend that an EEG be obtained for every patient in whom a seizure is a reasonable diagnosis. MRI is also recommended for these patients unless the clinical history, family history, and EEG strongly indicate a primary generalized epilepsy or a definite nontraumatic provocation such as transient hypoglycemia is known. If a cardiac cause is suspected, appropriate testing or referral should be requested.

The following sections focus on aspects of the seizure experience, seizure semiology or changes in behavior, and EEG and neuroimaging studies that facilitate the diagnosis, classification, and localization of epilepsy.

Components of the Seizure Experience

Before beginning the discussion of symptoms and changes in behavior (i.e., semiology) in patients with seizures arising from different regions of the brain, it is critically important to recognize that many patients are amnestic for at least a component of their seizures. Blum and colleagues initially reported that patients undergoing video-EEG monitoring were unable to state that they had experienced a seizure after 30% to 50% of partial seizures or generalized tonic-clonic seizures.[38] Although this is counterintuitive for many clinicians, the observation has now been replicated in subsequent studies.[39,40] These results indicate that self-reported seizure rates in the outpatient clinic can be as misleading as they are helpful in assessing the severity of the epilepsy or outcome after treatment. A thorough history of potential clues to seizure occurrences, supplemented by reports from family, friends, and coworkers, is required to optimize care.

Any paroxysmal symptom or change in behavior could represent a potential seizure. Another approach to defining the spectrum of the phenomenology of seizures is to emphasize that any experience that the brain can generate could be a component of a clinical seizure. The patient is often aware of the initial evolution of a seizure, which is commonly called an aura. Because an aura can define the early experience of a seizure, it may provide reliable clues to the region of onset within the brain.

Auras, or simple partial seizures, are often classified by the type of symptoms experienced during the ictal event. For example, the most common symptoms in patients with temporal lobe epilepsy are categorized as visceral/abdominal, psychic, autonomic, somatosensory, special sensory, and visual.[32-35,41] Specific examples are listed in Figure 52-1. The visceral symptoms may be an ascending sense of constriction or warmth in the abdominal region, which is sometimes described in the literature as an "epigastric rising sensation." This rising sensation may be difficult for some patients to describe, and the autonomic aspects of the feeling often lead to descriptions such as "I feel like I am dropping quickly in an elevator" or "it feels like the drop on a roller-coaster ride." The psychic symptoms are most often intense déjà vu, but patients may simply describe a sense that they know what is about to happen. Other psychic symptoms include a sense of dissociation from the environment, depersonalization, or a sense of never being in a familiar place (jamais vu). Common special sensory symptoms are olfactory or less frequently gustatory. Visual symptoms may be formed or unformed hallucinations or visual distortion such as change in size or apparent speed of

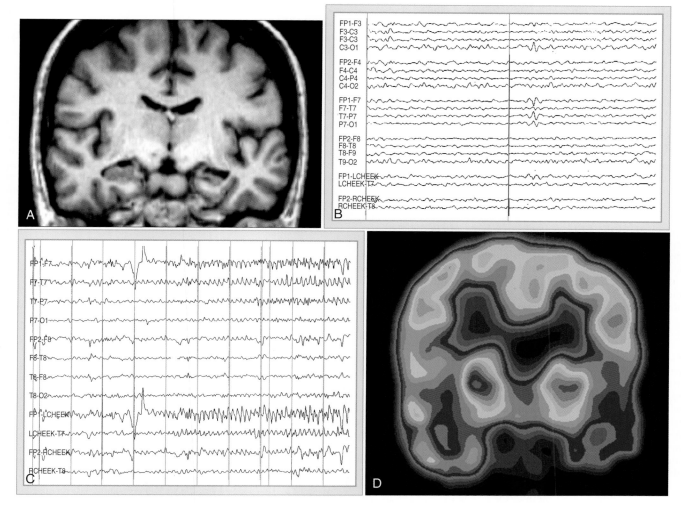

FIGURE 52-1 Results of T1-weighted magnetic resonance imaging (**A**), interictal electroencephalography (EEG) (**B**), ictal EEG (**C**), and fluoro-deoxyglucose positron emission tomography (**D**) in a 35-year-old man whose aura consisted of an epigastric rising sensation, déjà vu, and a sense of dissociation from the surrounding environment. Pathologic evaluation showed hippocampal sclerosis after selective left mesial temporal resection.

motion. It is important to understand that seizures arising from the region of the visual cortex my not have visual auras and that visual auras can occur with seizures beginning in areas other than the occipital lobe. An uncommon but well-described visual symptom is the sensation of watching a movie, which may localize to the mesial temporal region. Somatosensory auras are typically positive, such as a tingling or electrical sensation, and are contralateral to a parietal epileptogenic region; however, bilateral and ipsilateral somatosensory auras have been reported in patients with insular[42,43] and mesial frontal seizures.[44]

Clinical Semiology

Specific behavioral changes can be used to localize brain regions involved in a seizure.[45,46] For example, a common pattern of movements in a complex partial seizure of mesial temporal lobe origin is ipsilateral motor automatisms (e.g., tapping, patting, or rubbing movements) and contralateral dystonic flexor posturing of the wrist and hand.[47] Oral automatisms such as lip smacking, licking, or repetitive swallowing are also common in temporal lobe seizures. Complete behavior arrest is reportedly more frequently associated with temporal lobe than with frontal lobe seizures. Focal tonic or clonic motor seizures are typical of

lateral premotor seizures, and hypermotor/frenetic ("motor agitation") behavior is more common with orbitofrontal or frontopolar seizures.[45] Partial abduction of the arms with tonic stiffening is typical of supplementary sensorimotor area seizures, although fencer posturing has been considered a classic movement.[48]

Physical Examination

Although the findings on physical and neurological examination are frequently normal in persons with epilepsy, some neurological syndromes are often associated with seizures and specific physical abnormalities. For example, tuberous sclerosis complex has a prevalence of epilepsy of 78% and is characterized by facial angiofibromas, hypomelanotic macules, shagreen patches, ungual fibromas, and retinal hamartomas.[49,50] Patients with neurofibromatosis type 1 have an increased incidence of seizures (but lower than in patients with tuberous sclerosis) and clinical examination findings of café au lait spots, axillary freckling, cutaneous neurofibromas, and iris hamartomas (Lisch nodules).[49,50] A thorough cutaneous and retinal examination should therefore be performed at the initial evaluation of all persons with a history of a seizure or epilepsy.

An interesting, but frequently overlooked clinical finding in temporal lobe epilepsy is asymmetric facial movement with spontaneous smiling.[51,52] The asymmetry may not be present with volitional face movement and is accentuated with laughing. It is present on the side of the face contralateral to the epileptogenic region in more than 25% of persons with mesial temporal lobe epilepsy. The presumed mechanism of this finding is amygdala dysfunction resulting in an abnormal emotional motor response.[51]

Electroencephalography

EEG is an indispensable test to support the diagnosis of seizures, as well as accurately classify the epileptic syndrome. The typical EEG abnormalities seen in various seizure types are described in this section. The sensitivity of a single EEG recording for identifying specific epileptiform abnormalities is about 50%, but it increases to greater than 90% with the third recording.[53] The specificity of the EEG depends, to a large extent, on the interpreter; utmost care always should be taken to not misinterpret normal variants as epileptiform abnormalities.[54] A typical interictal sharp wave in localization-related epilepsy of mesial temporal origin is displayed in Figure 52-1. The reader is referred to more detailed review for additional information regarding EEG abnormalities in specific epilepsy syndromes.[55,56]

Neuroimaging

MRI has dramatically improved the imaging of normal and pathologic brain structures. Although CT remains a useful tool, especially in the acute setting or when imaging calcified structures, the limited resolution and bone artifact are problematic when assessing patients with focal seizures. The first goal of neuroimaging of patients with seizures is to exclude a progressive or dangerous lesion such as a tumor or vascular malformation. Several studies have shown MRI to be superior to CT in identifying small lesions[57-59]; MRI is therefore recommended, when available, for all patients with suspected partial seizures.

MRI is a dynamic, rapidly improving technology. The definition of the optimal MRI method for evaluation of patients with seizures is therefore changing continually. In general, T1-weighted scans with short repetition time/echo time (TR/TE) demonstrate anatomic relationships with superior resolution, whereas T2-weighted long TR/TE sequences are more sensitive for revealing focal pathology. New strategies such as "short flip angle" scans have been suggested to identify small calcifications or hemorrhages. Recent reviews are suggested for a more detailed discussion of MRI technology for imaging patients with epilepsy.[60-63]

Although broad anatomic coverage is necessary to maximize sensitivity in most MRI screening examinations, more detailed and specific imaging is useful in certain situations. Specifically, because the temporal lobe is the most frequent site of onset in the majority of patients with partial seizures, attention to the mesial temporal region is advantageous. Mesial temporal sclerosis (MTS) is the most common pathologic substrate found in patients with temporal lobe epilepsy. The amygdala appears to be variably involved.[64] When atrophy on T1-weighted images and increased signal intensity on T2-weighted images of the hippocampus are used to identify MTS, the sensitivity rages from 80% to 93%, with a specificity of between 86% and 93%.[57,65,66] Quantitative T2 relaxometry appears to be a useful technique as well.[67] Sensitivity and interobserver reliability are high when these criteria are determined by visual inspection, but quantitative volumetric analysis remains valuable for identifying bilateral MTS and for research studies.[68,69] High-resolution MRI may also demonstrate loss of definition of the internal architecture of the sclerotic hippocampus.[70] Figure 52-1 shows an example of T1-weighted and fluid-attenuated inversion recovery (FLAIR)

MRI of right hippocampal sclerosis. Imaging of neoplastic and vascular lesions is critically important for many persons with epilepsy, but specific aspects of these abnormalities are reviewed in other chapters.

CONCLUSION

Epilepsy is one of the most common neurological disorders, is often disabling, and is associated with increased mortality. Accurate diagnosis and treatment are therefore of the utmost importance at the initial evaluation. Classification of epilepsy syndromes is based on seizure type and supportive clinical information. The history of the event, especially when corroborated by a witness, is the most important aspect of the evaluation, but EEG is also essential. Serum studies, especially for glucose, sodium, calcium, and drugs, are required to exclude a metabolic or toxic provocation. MRI is necessary to exclude a lesion that may require urgent intervention, such as a vascular malformation or neoplasm, but it may not be required in certain idiopathic epilepsy syndromes such as childhood absence epilepsy.

SUGGESTED READINGS

Blum DE, Eskola J, Bortz JJ, et al. Patient awareness of seizures. *Neurology*. 1996;47:260-264.

Cascino GD, Jack CR Jr, Parisi JE, et al. Magnetic resonance imaging–based volume studies in temporal lobe epilepsy: pathological correlations. *Ann Neurol*. 1991;30:31-36.

Chang BS, Lowenstein DH. Epilepsy. *N Engl J Med*. 2003;349:1257-1266.

Commission on the Classification and Terminology of the International League Against Epilepsy. A revised proposal for the classification of epilepsy and epileptic syndromes. *Epilepsia*. 1989;30:268-278.

Commission on the Classification and Terminology of the International League Against Epilepsy. Proposal for revised clinical and electroencephalographic classification of epileptic seizures. *Epilepsia*. 1981;22:489-501.

Duncan JS. Imaging and epilepsy. *Brain*. 1997;120:339-377.

Gilliam F, Wyllie E. Diagnostic testing of seizure disorders. *Neurol Clin*. 1996;14:61-84.

Glauser TA, Sankar R. Core elements of epilepsy diagnosis and management: expert consensus from the Leadership in Epilepsy, Advocacy, and Development (LEAD) faculty. *Curr Med Res Opin*. 2008;24:3463-3477.

Harden CL, Huff JS, Schwartz TH, et al. Reassessment: neuroimaging in the emergency patient presenting with seizure (an evidence-based review): report of the Therapeutics and Technology Assessment Subcommittee of the American Academy of Neurology. *Neurology*. 2007;69:1772-1780.

Hoppe C, Poepel A, Elger CE. Epilepsy: accuracy of patient seizure counts. *Arch Neurol*. 2007;64:1595-1599.

Janati A, Nowack WJ, Dorsey S, et al. Correlative study of interictal electroencephalogram and aura in complex partial seizures. *Epilepsia*. 1990;31:41-46.

King MA, Newton MR, Jackson GD, et al. Epileptology of the first-seizure presentation: a clinical, electroencephalographic, and magnetic resonance imaging study of 300 consecutive patients. *Lancet*. 1998;352:1007-1011.

Kotagal P, Arunkumar G, Hammel J, et al. Complex partial seizures of frontal lobe onset statistical analysis of ictal semiology. *Seizure*. 2003;12:268-281.

Kotagal P, Lüders HO, Williams G, et al. Psychomotor seizures of temporal lobe onset: analysis of symptom clusters and sequences. *Epilepsy Res*. 1995;20:49-67.

Kuzniecky R, de la Sayette V, Ethier R, et al. Magnetic resonance imaging in temporal lobe epilepsy: pathological correlations. *Ann Neurol*. 1987;22:341-347.

Kwan P, Brodie MJ. Early identification of refractory epilepsy. *N Engl J Med*. 2000;342:314-319.

Manford M, Fish DR, Shorvon SD. An analysis of clinical seizure patterns and their localizing value in frontal and temporal lobe epilepsies. *Brain*. 1996;119:17-40.

Morris HH 3rd, Dinner DS, Lüders H, et al. Supplementary motor seizures: clinical and electroencephalographic findings. *Neurology*. 1988;38:1075-1082.

O'Brien TJ, Kilpatrick C, Murrie V, et al. Temporal lobe epilepsy caused by mesial temporal sclerosis and temporal neocortical lesions. A clinical and electroencephalographic study of 46 pathologically proven cases. *Brain*. 1996; 119:2133-2141.

O'Brien TJ, Mosewich RK, Britton JW, et al. History and seizure semiology in distinguishing frontal lobe seizures and temporal lobe seizures. *Epilepsy Res*. 2008;82:177-182.

Palmini A, Gloor P. The localizing value of auras in partial seizures: a prospective and retrospective study. *Neurology*. 1992;42:801-808.

Penfield W, Jasper H. *Epilepsy and the Functional Anatomy of the Human Brain*. Boston: Little, Brown; 1954.

Remillard GM, Andermann F, Rhi-Sausi A, et al. Facial asymmetry in patients with temporal lobe epilepsy. A clinical sign useful in the lateralization of temporal epileptogenic foci. *Neurology*. 1977;27:109-114.

Ryvlin P, Minotti L, Demarquay G, et al. Nocturnal hypermotor seizures, suggesting frontal lobe epilepsy, can originate in the insula. *Epilepsia*. 2006;47:755-765.

Salinsky M, Kanter R, Dasheiff RM. Effectiveness of multiple EEGs in supporting the diagnosis of epilepsy: an operational curve. *Epilepsia*. 1987;28:331-334.

Taylor DC, Lochery M. Temporal lobe epilepsy: origin and significance of simple and complex auras. *J Neurol Neurosurg Psychiatry*. 1987;50:673-681.

Tuxhorn IE. Somatosensory auras in focal epilepsy: a clinical, video EEG and MRI study. *Seizure*. 2005;14:262-268.

Van Paesschen W, King MD, Duncan JS, et al. The amygdala and temporal lobe simple partial seizures: a prospective and quantitative MRI study. *Epilepsia*. 2001;42:857-862.

Full references can be found on Expert Consult @ www.expertconsult.com

CHAPTER 53

Antiepileptic Medications: Principles of Clinical Use

Blaise F. D. Bourgeois

Several new antiepileptic drugs (AEDs) have been introduced since 1993, and there is now a relatively large number of drugs to choose from when treating a patient with newly diagnosed or uncontrolled seizures. Although the newer drugs have not solved the problem of intractable epilepsy, they offer a welcome addition to the therapeutic armamentarium of epilepsy. Several have advantages with regard to efficacy, safety, pharmacokinetics, or drug-drug interactions. The established, or older, drugs are no longer the drugs of first choice for the majority of seizure types because most physicians treating epilepsy are now more familiar with the newer drugs and have concerns about the short- and long-term adverse effects of the older drugs. Many newer AEDs offer the main advantages of relative safety, favorable pharmacokinetics and interaction profiles, or the absence of need for blood level or other routine laboratory monitoring.

This chapter presents a systematic review of the clinical pharmacology of each of the main established AEDs and the newer AEDs, including their pharmacokinetics, interactions, dosages, efficacy profile, and safety profile. The pharmacokinetic properties, as well as doses and therapeutic ranges of the AEDs to be discussed, are summarized in Table 53-1. The principles of drug treatment of epilepsy are discussed, such as the decision to initiate long-term prophylactic drug treatment, the sequence of drug choices for various seizure types or syndromes (Table 53-2), initiation and monitoring of antiepileptic therapy, and discontinuation of treatment.

CLINICAL PHARMACOLOGY OF ANTIEPILEPTIC DRUGS

Older Antiepileptic Drugs

Phenytoin

The use of phenytoin (PHT) has decreased, but it is still a widely used AED. In addition to its good efficacy against convulsive seizures and decades of experience with a good safety profile, PHT can be loaded rapidly without the need to titrate the dose slowly. This property is particularly valuable in neurosurgical practice. The volume of distribution of PHT is about 0.75 L/kg. A dose of 7.5 mg/kg given intravenously raises the level by 10 mg/L. Elimination of PHT is unique among AEDs because it is saturable at therapeutic concentrations[1] in all age groups.[2,3] This results in a nonlinear relationship between maintenance doses and steady-state concentrations. Especially in the upper therapeutic range, small increases in dosage can cause relatively large increases in levels. PHT does not have an elimination half-life because the time for the level to decrease by 50% becomes longer at higher levels. Steady-state levels are reached only after 2 to 3 weeks of a stable maintenance dose. To achieve average levels of about 15 mg/L, adult patients must usually take 5 to 6 mg/kg per day, which corresponds to 350 to 450 mg/day. The common dose of 300 mg/day often results in levels of 10 mg/L or less. PHT is a potent enzyme inducer and lowers the level of many other drugs. This affects other AEDs, such as carbamazepine, valproate, felbamate, lamotrigine, topiramate, zonisamide, and tiagabine, as well as many other drugs, including warfarin, oral contraceptives, and cyclosporine. PHT is highly protein bound and is displaced from serum proteins by valproate. Such displacement increases the free fraction of PHT and makes total serum levels unreliable.

The spectrum of activity of PHT includes partial seizures (simple or complex without or with secondary generalization), generalized convulsive seizures, status epilepticus,[4] and neonatal seizures.[5] Intravenous administration of PHT can cause bradyarrhythmia and hypotension, as well as skin necrosis.[6] This local irritation in particular can be avoided by using the prodrug phosphenytoin instead of PHT for intravenous administration. The rate of administration of phosphenytoin is up to 150 mg/min (or 3 mg/kg per minute) instead of 50 mg/min (or 1 mg/kg per minute) for PHT.

The dose-related central nervous system side effects of PHT are nystagmus, ataxia, and lethargy. PHT can cause various forms of hypersensitivity reactions,[7] as well as a hypersensitivity syndrome.[8] Chronic or delayed adverse effects include gingival hyperplasia, hirsutism, peripheral neuropathy, and bone demineralization secondary to reduced vitamin D levels.

Carbamazepine

Carbamazepine (CBZ) is gradually being displaced from its exclusive place as the drug of first choice for partial and secondarily generalized seizures. The elimination kinetics of CBZ is linear.[9] The characteristic feature of CBZ elimination is autoinduction of its metabolism,[10] which results in an increase in CBZ clearance during the first weeks of treatment unless the patient already is taking another enzyme-inducing drug, such as phenytoin, phenobarbital, or primidone. Accordingly, the elimination half-life of CBZ decreases from about 36 hours to 10 to 20 hours.[11] The practical consequence is that the dose of CBZ must be increased progressively during the first 3 to 4 weeks of treatment from 100 to 200 mg/day to 600 to 800 mg/day. Further increases in dosage may be needed and tolerated. Because of the relatively short half-life after induction, the regular CBZ preparations are best taken three times a day. Slow-release preparations are taken every 12 hours. CBZ is involved in many pharmacokinetic interactions. Similar to phenytoin, it is an enzyme inducer (see earlier). Other enzyme-inducing drugs, such as phenytoin, phenobarbital, and primidone, accelerate CBZ metabolism to a degree that exceeds CBZ autoinduction.

CBZ is effective against partial seizures without or with secondary generalization, as well as against generalized tonic-clonic seizures. Against partial and secondarily generalized seizures, phenytoin, CBZ, phenobarbital, and primidone are about equally effective in terms of seizure control.[12] There is no parenteral preparation for CBZ. Dose-related central nervous system toxicity is the most common side effect. This toxicity may subside with time, can be minimized by careful titration, and is closely related to CBZ serum levels.[13] Other side effects include neutropenia and

TABLE 53-1 Pharmacokinetic Parameters of Antiepileptic Drugs

	F (%)	T$_{max}$ (hr)	Vd (L/kg)	PROT. BIND. (%)	T$_{1/2}$ (hr)	T$_{ss}$ (days)	THER. RANGE (mg/L)	DOSE (mg/kg/day)
Carbamazepine	75-85	4-12	0.8-2	75	20-50* 5-20*	20-30*	3-12	10-30
Felbamate	>90	2-6	0.75	25	14-23	4	—	40-80
Gabapentin	30-60	2-3	0.85	0	5-9	2	—	30-40
Lamotrigine	>90	1-3	1.0	55	15-60	3-1	—	1-15
Levetiracetam	>95	1	0.5-0.7	0	6-8	2	—	30-60
Oxcarbazepine	>90	1-3	—	—	—	—	—	15-30
(10-OH-carbamazepine)		4-6	0.7-0.8	45	10-15	2	10-35	—
Phenobarbital	>90	0.54	0.55	45	65-110	15-20	10-30	2-5
Phenytoin	>90	2-12	0.75	90	10-60†	15-20	3-20	5-10
Primidone	>90	2-4	0.75	<10	8-15	—	—	10-20
Tiagabine	>90	1-2	1.4	96	2-9	1-2	—	0.1-1
Topiramate	>80	1-4	0.65	15	12-30	3-5	—	5-10
Valproate	>90	1-8‡	0.16	70-93†	5-15	2	50-100	15-30
Zonisamide	>90	2-5	1.5	40	50-70	10-15	15-40	4-12

*Steady-state values for half-life and serum levels are reached only after complete autoinduction.
†Concentration dependent.
‡Absorption of enteric-coated tablets is delayed.
F, bioavailability; Prot. Bind., protein binding, fracture bound to serum proteins; T$_{1/2}$, elimination half-time; Ther. Range, therapeutic range of serum concentration; T$_{max}$, time interval between ingestion and maximum serum concentration; T$_{ss}$, steady-state time; Vd, volume of distribution.

rare, severe blood dyscrasias,[14] hyponatremia, movement disorders, allergic rashes, and hypersensitivity syndrome.

Valproate

Valproate (VPA) is unique among the older AEDs because of its broad spectrum of activity against various seizure types. Absorption from enteric-coated VPA tablets can be delayed by several hours, but once it begins, it is rapid, as opposed to the slow release from extended-release tablets. Other oral preparations exhibit rapid and early absorption, except for enteric-coated sprinkles, which have an intermediate absorption pattern. VPA is highly bound to serum proteins and tends to displace other drugs, such as phenytoin. The elimination half-life of VPA varies as a function of comedication. In adults, the half-life is 13 to 16 hours in the absence of inducing drugs[15] and 9 hours in induced patients.[16] In addition to displacement from serum proteins, VPA is involved in two types of pharmacokinetic interactions: its metabolism is accelerated by inducing drugs such as phenytoin, carbamazepine, phenobarbital, and primidone, and VPA itself can prolong the elimination (and raise the levels) of other drugs, such as phenobarbital, ethosuximide, lamotrigine, and felbamate. The initial target dose of VPA is 15 mg/kg per day, which can be attained within a few days. Higher doses of 60 mg/kg per day or more may be necessary in certain patients, especially in children and those taking inducing drugs.

VPA has a broad spectrum of activity. In addition to being effective against partial seizures,[17] VPA is highly effective against absence seizures, generalized tonic-clonic seizures, and myoclonic seizures. It is a drug of first choice in patients with primary (idiopathic) generalized epilepsies. It can be helpful in the treatment of infantile spasms[18] and Lennox-Gastaut syndrome. VPA has several side effects that affect different systems and are of variable severity. Mild side effects include transient hair loss and dose-related tremor. VPA is not sedative, but drowsiness and lethargy may appear in some patients at levels around 100 mg/L, as well as idiosyncratic stuporous states at therapeutic levels.[19] Gastrointestinal upset is less common with enteric-coated tablets. Fatal hepatotoxicity[20] and pancreatitis[21] are the most serious complications of VPA treatment. Thrombocytopenia, in conjunction with other VPA-mediated disturbances of hemostasis, such as impaired platelet function, fibrinogen depletion, and coagulation factor deficiencies,[22] may cause excessive bleeding. The common practice of withdrawing VPA before elective surgery is recommended, although reports have found no objective evidence of excessive operative bleeding in neurosurgical patients maintained on VPA.[23,24] In women of childbearing age, concerns associated with VPA treatment include not only an increased risk for neural tube defects in the fetus but also an increased risk for polycystic ovaries and metabolic and endocrine disturbances.[25]

Phenobarbital and Primidone

The use of phenobarbital (PB) and primidone (PRM) for the treatment of seizures has declined steadily because of their central nervous system side effects. PB and PRM produce more sedative and behavioral side effects than most other AEDs do, but they have relatively little systemic toxicity. PB has excellent pharmacokinetic properties, can be administered intravenously and intramuscularly, is effective in patients with status epilepticus, and is inexpensive. The volume of distribution of PB is 0.55 L/kg, with an elimination half-life averaging 80 to 100 hours in adults and newborns and shorter in infants and children. Maintenance doses range from 2 to 5 mg/kg per day. Although treatment with PRM results in the accumulation of significant levels of PB, PRM has independent pharmacologic activity and probably is not just a prodrug. PRM itself has a much shorter half-life than PB. Daily dosage requirements of PRM are about five times higher than those of PB. As an enzyme inducer, PB causes pharmacokinetic interactions that are shared by other enzyme-inducing drugs and by PRM because of the derived PB. Other enzyme-inducing drugs, in particular phenytoin,[26] accelerate the conversion of PRM to PB, thereby increasing the PB-to-PRM serum level ratio.

PB and PRM are as effective against partial and secondarily generalized seizures as carbamazepine and phenytoin but were found to be associated with more treatment failures because of mostly early central nervous system side effects.[12] PB can be used

TABLE 53-2 Place of Newer Antiepileptic Drugs in the Treatment Sequence of Seizures and Epileptic Syndromes in Children

PARTIAL SEIZURES WITH OR WITHOUT SECONDARY GENERALIZATION

First choice	Oxcarbazepine, carbamazepine, levetiracetam
Second choice	Lamotrigine, valproate, gabapentin
Third choice	Topiramate, zonisamide, phenytoin, phenobarbital, primidone
Consider	Pregabalin, tiagabine, benzodiazepine, acetazolamide

GENERALIZED TONIC-CLONIC SEIZURES

First choice	Valproate, levetiracetam, lamotrigine
Second choice	(Ox)carbamazepine, topiramate, phenytoin
Third choice	Zonisamide, phenobarbital, primidone

ABSENCE SEIZURES

Before 10 years of age

First choice	Ethosuximide, valproate
Second choice	Lamotrigine
Consider	Methsuximide, benzodiazepine, levetiracetam, topiramate, zonisamide, acetazolamide

After 10 years of age

First choice	Valproate
Second choice	Lamotrigine
Third choice	Ethosuximide, methsuximide, levetiracetam, topiramate, zonisamide, benzodiazepine, acetazolamide

JUVENILE MYOCLONIC EPILEPSY

First choice	Valproate
Second choice	Levetiracetam, lamotrigine, topiramate, clonazepam
Third choice	Zonisamide, phenobarbital, primidone

LENNOX-GASTAUT AND RELATED SYNDROMES

First choice	Topiramate, lamotrigine
Second choice	Valproate
Third choice	Ketogenic diet, felbamate, zonisamide, rufinamide, benzodiazepine, phenobarbital
Consider	Ethosuximide, methsuximide, levetiracetam, steroids

Infantile Spasms

First choice	Adrenocorticotropic hormone, vigabatrin
Second choice	Valproate, topiramate, lamotrigine, zonisamide, benzodiazepine, ketogenic diet
Consider	Pyridoxine, levetiracetam, felbamate

BENIGN EPILEPSY WITH CENTROTEMPORAL SPIKES

First choice	Sulthiame, gabapentin
Second choice	Valproate, levetiracetam
Consider	Lamotrigine, topiramate, zonisamide, pregabalin

for the treatment of status epilepticus and neonatal seizures, as well as for the prophylaxis of febrile seizures. In addition to the well-known sedative and behavioral side effects, PB and PRM can cause allergic reactions. Use over many years may be associated with connective tissue disorders, such as Dupuytren's contracture and frozen shoulder.

Newer Antiepileptic Drugs

Felbamate

Because of potentially serious side effects, felbamate (FBM) is currently used only in special circumstances. FBM is involved in multiple pharmacokinetic interactions; its levels are decreased by enzyme-inducing drugs, and it raises levels of phenytoin and valproate. The recommended initial dose of FBM is 1200 mg/day (15 mg/kg per day) during the first week. This dose can be doubled at the beginning of the second week and tripled at the beginning of the third week. It is prudent to reduce the dose of

other AEDs by about a third when FBM is introduced. In double-blind studies, FBM was shown to be effective against partial onset seizures,[27,28] as well as in the treatment of Lennox-Gastaut syndrome.[29] Uncontrolled reports have suggested efficacy of FBM against absence seizures, juvenile myoclonic epilepsy, and infantile spasms.

The main common side effects of FBM have been nausea and vomiting, anorexia and weight loss, somnolence, and insomnia. Within 1 year after its marketing, it became evident that FBM was associated with a relatively high incidence of potentially fatal aplastic anemia[30] and hepatic necrosis.[31] Currently, the main indication for FBM is as a drug of third choice for the treatment of Lennox-Gastaut syndrome and focal onset seizures.

Gabapentin

Gabapentin (GBP) differs from previously used AEDs by the fact that it is eliminated entirely by the kidneys. As a consequence, it has no pharmacokinetic interactions. GBP absorption is saturable, and the daily dose should be divided into three or four fractions per day, especially with high doses.[32] Initial target doses of GBP are about 1800 mg/day (30 mg/kg per day). Doses higher than 3600 mg/day (60 to 100 mg/kg per day) are often well tolerated and may be necessary to achieve the maximum benefit.

GBP has been shown in double-blind trials to be effective against focal onset seizures.[33] It was found to be superior to placebo in a double-blind study in patients with benign epilepsy of childhood with centrotemporal spikes (rolandic epilepsy).[34] Serious side effects of GBP appear to be exceedingly rare.[35] However, excessive weight gain and behavioral problems in children are common.

Lamotrigine

Lamotrigine (LTG) has a relatively long half-life and can be administered two times a day. The pharmacokinetic interactions of LTG consist of a marked reduction of its levels by enzyme-inducing drugs and marked elevation of its levels by valproate.[36] As a consequence of these interactions, dosage requirements for LTG vary from patient to patient. Patients taking valproate should receive 25 mg/day or less (0.2 mg/kg per day) during the first 2 weeks of treatment. Patients taking enzyme-inducing drugs without valproate may start with higher doses. Slow titration with increases in dosage at 2-week intervals is important because it seems to reduce the risk for the potentially severe rash, or even Stevens-Johnson syndrome, associated with LTG.[37] Against focal onset seizures, LTG appears to be as effective as carbamazepine and phenytoin.[38,39] LTG has also been found to be effective in the treatment of Lennox-Gastaut syndrome,[40] absence seizures, generalized tonic-clonic seizures, and juvenile myoclonic epilepsy.

Topiramate

Topiramate (TPM) is also a broad-spectrum AED. It can be administered two times a day in most cases. The main pharmacokinetic interaction involving TPM consists of an approximately twofold increase in its clearance by enzyme-inducing AEDs.[41] TPM can reduce the efficacy of oral contraceptives. To reduce the incidence of early side effects, the dose of TPM needs to be titrated slowly. The initial dosage should be 25 to 50 mg/day (0.5 to 1.0 mg/kg per day) with weekly increases by the same amount to achieve an initial target dose of 200 to 400 mg/day (5 to 6 mg/kg per day). The efficacy of TPM was found to be relatively high against focal onset seizures in an analysis comparing trials of several newer AEDs.[42] TPM was also found to be effective in double-blind studies of patients with generalized tonic-clonic seizures[43] and in patients with Lennox-Gastaut syndrome.[44] The most common side effects of TPM include somnolence, impaired concentration, confusion, abnormal thinking, and impaired verbal memory. Other side effects include anorexia, weight loss, and nephrolithiasis, as well as metabolic acidosis and decreased sweating in children.

Tiagabine

Among the newer AEDs, tiagabine (TGB) has not found widespread use, mostly because of a narrow spectrum of activity and central nervous system side effects. TGB has a short half-life (see Table 53-1), which becomes shorter in the presence of enzyme-inducing drugs. There are no other pharmacokinetic interactions. When TGB is introduced, the dose should be titrated slowly with weekly increments.

Thus far, the known clinical efficacy of TGB is limited to partial onset seizures without or with secondary generalization.[45] TGB does not appear to have severe or potentially life-threatening side effects. The main side effects include dizziness, tremor, difficulty with concentration, nervousness, and emotional lability.[45]

Oxcarbazepine

Oxcarbazepine (OXC) is a derivative of carbamazepine and shares most of the clinical characteristics of carbamazepine. OXC is a prodrug and is rapidly metabolized to the active compound monohydroxycarbamazepine, which is measured in serum for therapeutic monitoring.[46,47] This metabolite has a half-life of 10 to 15 hours, and its level can be reduced by 30% to 40% in the presence of enzyme-inducing drugs such as phenytoin, carbamazepine, or phenobarbital. OXC is an enzyme inducer, but less so than phenytoin, phenobarbital, or carbamazepine. There is no parenteral preparation. The usual initial dose of OXC is 300 mg twice daily in adults and 5 to 10 mg/kg per day in children. The dose can be increased by that amount at weekly intervals to reach a target dose of 1200 to 1800 mg in adults and 20 to 30 mg/kg per day in children. A therapeutic range of 10 to 35 mg/L has been suggested.

OXC has the same narrow spectrum of efficacy as carbamazepine, with efficacy limited to partial onset and secondarily generalized seizures.[48] The side effects of OXC are similar to those of carbamazepine, although they may be somewhat milder. They consist mostly of somnolence, dizziness, ataxia, diplopia, and blurred vision. An allergic rash can occur, and cross-reactivity with carbamazepine is at least 25%. Hyponatremia is more common with OXC than with carbamazepine and is more frequent in adults, especially in the elderly, than in children.[49,50]

Levetiracetam

Despite its relatively short half-life of 6 to 8 hours, levetiracetam (LEV) is usually administered twice daily. The pharmacokinetics are linear, protein binding is low, and no pharmacokinetic interactions caused by or involving LEV have been identified.[51] The initial dose is 250 to 500 mg twice daily (500 to 1000 mg/day) in adults and 20 mg/kg per day in children. The maintenance dose is 1000 to 3000 mg/day in adults and 30 to 40 mg/kg per day in children. Higher doses may be needed and are tolerated. A therapeutic range of approximately 10 to 40 mg/L is probably appropriate in most patients, but levels of 40 to 80 mg/L may be beneficial and are well tolerated.

LEV has emerged as a broad-spectrum antiepileptic drug. It is approved for the treatment of partial and secondarily generalized seizures,[52] primarily generalized tonic-clonic seizures in idiopathic general epilepsies,[53] and myoclonic seizures in juvenile myoclonic epilepsy.[54] LEV has also been used for absence seizures, severe myoclonic epilepsy in infancy, progressive myoclonic epilepsy (Unverricht-Lundborg), rolandic epilepsy,[55] and posthypoxic and postencephalitic myoclonus. LEV has virtually no serious or life-threatening side effects. Its side effects may include somnolence, asthenia, dizziness, emotional lability, depression, and psychosis.[56] Behavioral problems are particularly common in children and include agitation, hostility, oppositional behavior, anxiety, and aggression. Allergic reactions, liver failure, and bone marrow suppression are exceedingly rare.

Zonisamide

Zonisamide (ZNS) has a long half-life, about 60 hours in adults, and can be administered once or twice daily.[57] Its pharmacokinetics is linear, and protein binding is 50% or less. Clearance of zonisamide is increased and levels of zonisamide are lowered by the addition of the following drugs (discontinuation of these drugs has an opposite effect): phenytoin, carbamazepine, phenobarbital, primidone, and valproic acid. ZNS has no known effect on the kinetics of other drugs. The initial dose is 100 mg/day in adults and 1.0 to 2.0 mg/kg per day in children. The initial target dose in adults is 100 to 600 mg/day (lower doses may be sufficient with monotherapy, and higher doses may be necessary with enzyme inducers). The initial target dose in children is 8 mg/kg per day with monotherapy and 12 mg/kg per day with enzyme inducers. Higher doses may be needed, particularly in infants and in patients comedicated with enzyme-inducing drugs.

ZNS is also a broad-spectrum drug.[58] It can be effective against partial and secondarily generalized seizures,[59] primarily generalized tonic-clonic seizures, Lennox-Gastaut syndrome, juvenile myoclonic epilepsy,[60] absence seizures, infantile spasms,[61] myoclonic astatic epilepsy (Doose's syndrome), and progressive myoclonic epilepsy. Side effects of ZNS include drowsiness, fatigue, ataxia, psychomotor slowing, behavioral or psychiatric side effects, anorexia and weight loss, and allergic rash. Other possible side effects are metabolic acidosis (lowered serum bicarbonate or CO_2, especially in children), hypohidrosis (decreased sweating, especially in children, may lead to hyperthermia),[62] nephrolithiasis (1% to 2%), and paresthesias.

Pregabalin

Pregabalin (PGB) is very similar to gabapentin in most aspects, except for the fact that PGB has better bioavailability than gabapentin does.[63] The elimination half-life of PGB is about 6 hours, which requires dosing twice or three times daily. PGB is not bound to serum proteins, is eliminated mostly unchanged in urine, and has no pharmacokinetic interactions. The usual dose in adults is 150 mg/day the first week, 300 mg/day the second week, 450 mg/day the third week, and 600 mg/day thereafter. A dosage schedule for children has not been established.

PGB, like gabapentin, has a narrow spectrum of activity that is limited to focal onset and secondarily generalized seizures.[64] Its most common side effects are dizziness, somnolence, dry mouth, peripheral edema, blurred vision, excessive weight gain,[65] and difficulty with concentration. PGB is a controlled substance because of a slight potential for recreational abuse and dependence.[66]

PRINCIPLES OF TREATMENT

Decision to Initiate Antiepileptic Drug Therapy

After a first seizure, the decision to treat or not to treat is based not only on the risk for seizure recurrence alone but also on the potential risks associated with seizure recurrence and those associated with chronic AED therapy. There is good overall agreement that routine treatment after a first unprovoked seizure is not indicated in all cases. The decision has to be individualized by taking into account all the available information on a given patient, as well as the patient's own preference. Certain factors have been associated with an increased risk for seizure recurrence, such as a remote symptomatic seizure, a focal onset seizure, a history of previous acute symptomatic seizures, epileptiform abnormalities on electroencephalography (EEG), a first seizure manifested as status epilepticus, and a first seizure followed by Todd's paralysis. Conversely, factors associated with a lower risk for seizure recurrence include an idiopathic generalized tonic-clonic seizure and the absence of epileptiform abnormalities on EEG. As a group, adults tend to have a higher risk for seizure recurrence after a first seizure and are more likely to be treated after a first seizure.

Antiepileptic Drug Selection by Seizure Type or Epilepsy Syndrome

When a decision to treat has been made, the first step is to determine the drug of first choice for the patient. The choice of an AED is based first on the seizure type or on the epileptic syndrome. Among the drugs available for a particular seizure type or syndrome, the choice is based mainly on the adverse effect profile while taking into consideration the patient's age and gender, as well preference. The place of any AED in the treatment sequence of epilepsy is not firmly established and not strictly scientifically determined because there have been no head-to-head comparisons of their efficacy against any given seizure type or epilepsy syndrome, especially for the newer drugs. With this concept in mind, Table 53-2 assigns places to AEDs in the treatment sequence of seizures. The listing of drugs as second and third choices applies only to patients whose seizures could not be controlled with a drug of first choice.

Basic Principles of Antiepileptic Drug Use

When the drug of first choice has been selected in an untreated patient, this drug almost always is used as monotherapy. An initial target dose is achieved, either rapidly or over the course of several weeks, depending on the drug. Further increases in dosage are dictated more by seizure control and side effects than by drug levels. The simple rule that the optimal drug dose is "as much as necessary, as little as possible" is too often disregarded. If the seizures do not come under control initially, the conclusion that the drug has failed should not be reached unless the maximal tolerated dose has been reached. The maximal tolerated dose, or subtoxic dose, is just below the dose at which dose-related side effects have appeared. Invariably, children, especially infants, have higher drug clearances and require significantly higher doses in milligrams per kilograms per day to achieve the same drug levels. In contrast, elderly patients often require lower doses, not only because they have lower clearances but also because they may be more sensitive to the side effects.

If the first drug fails to control the seizures at the maximal tolerated dose, a second drug is selected. When a therapeutic dose or level of the second drug has been reached, the first drug should be tapered. It is exceptional for a drug combination to provide better seizure control than adequate monotherapy with either one of the two drugs alone. If drug levels are available, they should be used judiciously, with the understanding that the therapeutic range provided by the laboratory is a rough guideline and should never replace clinical observation and judgment. While monitoring a patient being treated with an AED, it should be kept in mind that physicians invariably underestimate patients' lack of compliance with drug intake. Besides judiciously used drug levels, only a few AEDs require periodic monitoring of laboratory values: complete blood count with carbamazepine therapy and complete blood count and liver function tests with valproate and felbamate therapy. Discussing side effects of the medications and asking patients to report possible symptoms of adverse events are more important than laboratory monitoring.

Discontinuation of Antiepileptic Drug Therapy

Similar to the initiation of therapy, discontinuation is based on a risk-versus-benefit analysis. Factors shown to increase the risk for seizure recurrence after stopping AED therapy include a known remote cause, seizure onset after the age of 12 years, a family history of epilepsy in patients with idiopathic epilepsy, focal or generalized slowing on EEG before discontinuation, a history of atypical febrile seizures, and an IQ of less than 50. The 2-year risk for recurrence after drug discontinuation may vary from about 10% in patients with none of these risk factors to about 80% in patients with remote symptomatic seizures and three risk factors. Contrary to widespread belief, seizure control can almost always be reestablished with medication if seizures recur after discontinuation. In general, the decision to discontinue an AED is made after 2 years without seizures. Because there is usually no urgency, the drug dosage should be tapered slowly over a period of at least 3 months. In patients who have become free of seizures after epilepsy surgery, it is a common practice to reduce the number of AEDs after 1 year and to discontinue all drugs after 2 years.[67]

SUGGESTED READINGS

Andermann F, Bourgeois BF, Leppik IE, et al. Postoperative pharmacotherapy and discontinuation of antiepileptic drugs. In: Engel J, ed. *Surgical Treatment of the Epilepsies.* New York: Raven Press; 1993:679-684.

Anderson GD, Lin YX, Berge C, et al. Absence of bleeding complications in patients undergoing cortical surgery while receiving valproate treatment. *J Neurosurg.* 1997;87:252-256.

Asconapé JJ, Penry JK, Dreifuss FE, et al. Valproate-associated pancreatitis. *Epilepsia.* 1993;34:177-183.

Ben-Menachem E. Pregabalin pharmacology and its relevance to clinical practice. *Epilepsia.* 2004;45(Suppl 6):13-18.

Berkovic SF, Knowlton RC, Leroy RF, et al for the Levetiracetam N01057 Study Group. Placebo-controlled study of levetiracetam in idiopathic generalized epilepsy. *Neurology.* 2007;69:1751-1760.

Brodie M, Richens A, Yuen A. Double-blind comparison of lamotrigine and carbamazepine in newly diagnosed epilepsy. *Lancet.* 1995;345:476-479.

Brodie MJ, Duncan R, Vespignani H, et al. Dose-dependent safety and efficacy of zonisamide: a randomized, double-blind, placebo-controlled study in patients with refractory partial seizures. *Epilepsia.* 2005;46:31-41.

Brodie MJ, Perucca E, Ryvlin P, et al for the Levetiracetam Monotherapy Study Group. Comparison of levetiracetam and controlled-release carbamazepine in newly diagnosed epilepsy. *Neurology.* 2007;68:402-408.

Bryant A, Dreifuss FE. Valproic acid hepatic fatalities: III. U.S. experience since 1986. *Neurology.* 1996;46:465-469.

Dam M, Ekberg R, Lyning Y, et al. A double-blind study comparing oxcarbazepine and carbamazepine in patients with newly diagnosed, previously untreated epilepsy. *Epilepsy Res.* 1989;3:70-76.

Guberman A, Besag F, Brodie M, et al. Lamotrigine-associated rash: risk/benefit considerations in adults and children. *Epilepsia.* 1998;40:985-996.

Leiderman D. Gabapentin as add-on therapy for refractory partial epilepsy: results of five placebo-controlled trials. *Epilepsia.* 1994;35:S74-S76.

Leppik IE. Practical prescribing and long-term efficacy and safety of zonisamide. *Epilepsy Res.* 2006;68S:S17-S24.

Marescaux C, Warter JM, Micheletti G, et al. Stuporous episodes during treatment with sodium valproate: report of seven cases. *Epilepsia.* 1982;23:297-305.

Mattson RH, Cramer JA, Collins JF, for the Department of VA Epilepsy Cooperative Study No. 264 Group. A comparison of valproate with carbamazepine for the treatment of complex partial seizures and secondarily generalized tonic-clonic seizures in adults. *N Engl J Med.* 1992;327:765-771.

Mattson RH, Cramer JA, Collins JF, et al. Comparison of carbamazepine, phenobarbital, phenytoin and primidone in partial and secondarily generalized tonic-clonic seizures. *N Engl J Med.* 1985;313:145-151.

Nielsen OA, Johannessen AC, Bardrum B. Oxcarbazepine-induced hyponatremia, a cross-sectional study. *Epilepsy Res.* 1988;2:269-271.

O'Brien T, Cascino G, So E, et al. Incidence and clinical consequence of the purple glove syndrome in patients receiving intravenous phenytoin. *Neurology.* 1998;51:1034-1039.

Patsalos PN. Pharmacokinetic profile of levetiracetam: toward ideal characteristics. *Pharmacol Ther.* 2000;85:77-85.

Specchio LM, Gambardella A, Giallonardo AT, et al. Open label, long-term, pragmatic study on levetiracetam in the treatment of juvenile myoclonic epilepsy. *Epilepsy Res.* 2006;71:32-39.

Ward MM, Barbaro NM, Laxer KD, et al. Preoperative valproate administration does not increase blood loss during temporal lobectomy. *Epilepsia.* 1996;37:98-101.

Full references can be found on Expert Consult @ www.expertconsult.com

CHAPTER **54**

Continuous Electroencephalography in Neurological-Neurosurgical Intensive Care: Applications and Value

Hiba Arif ■ Jan Claassen ■ Lawrence J. Hirsch

Every year tens of thousands of patients are admitted to neurological-neurosurgical intensive care units (neuro-ICUs). Patients admitted to neuro-ICUs mainly consist of those with intracerebral hemorrhage (ICH), subarachnoid hemorrhage (SAH), traumatic brain injury (TBI), and ischemic stroke, as well as postsurgical patients, both neurosurgical and otherwise. The common reason for admission of a patient with any of these diagnoses to the neuro-ICU is for monitoring and for early detection and correction of potentially life-threatening changes in physiologic function. When a comatose, critically ill patient arrives in any ICU, the patient is connected to a pulse oximetry monitor, electrocardiographic monitor, respiratory monitor, blood pressure monitor, and possibly other devices for monitoring various cardiac and pulmonary indices—all in an attempt to provide physicians and nurses with real-time information about the patient's cardiopulmonary function. Similar monitoring for the brain, which is obviously dysfunctional in stuporous and comatose patients, has been unavailable to ICUs until recently. Typically, in most neuro-ICUs the patient may be serially examined every few hours for mental status, state of arousal, motor function, and the presence of brainstem reflexes, which provides only a snapshot of the patient's neurological status in time and assesses only a small subset of important brain functions. In comatose patients, examination findings are frequently limited to be sensitive enough for detection of worsening brain injury. Examination is often even more difficult in patients who are sedated, paralyzed, or both. Neuroimaging provides information primarily about structural brain injury, frequently after it is irreversible, and cannot reveal real-time changes in function, such as seizures and levels of sedation. In addition, neuroimaging often requires the transport of unstable patients. Multimodal monitoring such as microdialysis and brain tissue oxygenation are invasive and may limit other diagnostic options such as magnetic resonance imaging. As more interventions become available to prevent, treat, or reverse ongoing neurological injury, the need for real-time neurophysiologic monitoring for at-risk patients is increasing.

Electroencephalography (EEG) provides a noninvasive means of assessing brain function dynamically. Recent advances in computer technology, networking, and data storage have made continuous EEG (cEEG) monitoring at the bedside increasingly practical, and it is now a commonly used modality for diagnosing seizures and monitoring response to treatment in many neuro-

ICUs. Methods for analyzing and compressing the vast amounts of data generated by cEEG are now available and allow neurophysiologists to more efficiently review recordings from many patients monitored simultaneously and provide frequent, timely information for guiding treatment. In this chapter, we review current indications and potential uses for cEEG in the critically ill (summarized in Table 54-1) and identify future areas for research.

DETECTION OF NONCONVULSIVE SEIZURES AND STATUS EPILEPTICUS

Nonconvulsive seizures (NCSzs) are electrographic seizures with little or no overt clinical manifestations (Fig. 54-1). The EEG criteria for definite NCSzs are outlined in Table 54-2. They are an increasingly commonly recognized entity in neuro-ICUs, where 8% to 34% of comatose patients may have NCSzs, depending on the clinical setting.[1-11] Major studies investigating NCSzs in various patient populations are summarized in Table 54-3. Nonconvulsive status epilepticus (NCSE) occurs when NCSzs are prolonged; a commonly used definition is continuous or nearly continuous electrographic seizures of at least 30 minutes' duration.[12] Although some forms of NCSzs may occur in ambulatory patients (typically manifested as confusion and easily treated), our main focus in this chapter is on NCSzs in neuro-ICU patients, for whom the most common manifestation is a depressed level of consciousness.[12] Most patients with NCSzs have purely electrographic seizures,[8] but other subtle signs that have been associated with NCSzs include face and limb myoclonus, nystagmus, eye deviation, pupillary abnormalities (including hippus), and autonomic instability.[12-15] However, none of these clinical findings are highly specific for NCSzs, and cEEG is usually necessary to confirm or refute the diagnosis of NCSzs. A recent study showed that findings from cEEG monitoring in 287 patients led to a change in AED prescribing in 52% of all studies, with initiation of AED therapy in 14%, modification of AED therapy in 33%, and discontinuation of AED therapy in 5% of all studies. The detection of electrographic seizures led to a change in AED therapy in 28% of all studies.[15a]

The causes of NCSzs and NCSE in neuro-ICU patients may vary by age and patient group but in general are similar to the causes of convulsive seizures in these patients, including structural lesions, infections, metabolic derangements, toxins, drug

TABLE 54-1 Indications for Continuous Electroencephalographic Monitoring

1. Detection of nonconvulsive seizures and characterization of spells in patients with altered mental status and
   A history of epilepsy
   Fluctuating level of consciousness
   Acute brain injury, especially if supratentorial and either hemorrhagic or involving the cortex
   Recent convulsive seizure
   Stereotyped activity such as paroxysmal movements, twitching, jerking, or autonomic variability
   Abnormal eye movements, including eye deviation, nystagmus, and hippus
2. Monitoring of ongoing therapy
   Induced coma for elevated intracranial pressure or refractory status epilepticus
   Assessing the level of sedation
   Assessing cerebral perfusion/ischemia during induced hypertension, etc.
3. Detection of ischemia
   Vasospasm in patients with subarachnoid hemorrhage
   Cerebral ischemia in other patients at high risk for stroke
4. Prognosis
   After cardiac arrest
   After acute brain injury

Adapted with permission from Friedman D, Claassen J, Hirsch LJ. Continuous EEG monitoring in the intensive care unit. *Anesth Analg.* 2009;109:506.

withdrawal, and epilepsy, all of which are common diagnoses in critically ill patients.[16] However, nonconvulsive or subtle seizures are much more common than clinically overt seizures in critically ill patients (see Table 54-3). In this section we review the incidence of NCSzs/NCSE in neuro-ICU patients by diagnostic and demographic category.

Convulsive Status Epilepticus

In many patients with convulsive status epilepticus (SE), electrographic seizures can persist even when convulsive seizures have stopped.[17,18] In a prospective study, DeLorenzo and colleagues found that 48% of the patients monitored with cEEG for 24 hours after convulsive SE had stopped experienced NCSzs and 14% had NCSE.[19] In most of these patients, coma was the only clinical manifestation. Patients with NCSE after convulsive SE had a twofold greater mortality than did patients whose seizures ended when convulsive activity stopped in this study, as well as in the Veterans Affairs Cooperative Study.[18] Therefore, cEEG should be performed on any patient who does not quickly regain consciousness after a convulsive seizure to detect ongoing seizure activity. This includes patients who are sedated or paralyzed (or both) during the treatment of SE in whom the level of consciousness cannot be assessed adequately.

Subarachnoid Hemorrhage

Aneurysmal SAH has long been known to be associated with seizures. Studies have reported 4% to 9% rates of convulsive seizures after the initial bleeding,[20-23] often in the setting of a focal clot.[21,23,24] However, several more recent studies using cEEG suggest that these seizure rates underestimate the incidence of electrographic seizures after SAH, especially in comatose patients. In the Columbia series of 570 patients who underwent cEEG for altered mental status or suspicion of seizures, 19% of 108 SAH patients had seizures.[8] Most of these seizures were NCSzs, and 70% of the patients with seizures had NCSE. In a study of 11 patients with SAH and NCSE, the following clinical factors were associated with NCSE: advanced age, female sex, need for ventriculostomy, poor-grade SAH (Hunt-Hess grade III, IV, or V), thick cisternal blood clots, and structural lesions (ICH and stroke).[25] Because both convulsive seizures and NCSzs are associated with a poor outcome on multivariate analysis in patients with a diagnosis of SAH,[20,26] it may follow that seizures occurring after SAH are likely to worsen the brain injury (see the later section "Impact of Nonconvulsive Seizures in the Critically Ill"). However, the currently available data are insufficient to confirm a causal relationship.

Intracerebral Hemorrhage

ICH is associated with a 3% to 19% rate of in-hospital convulsive seizures.[10,24,27-30] In two recent studies using cEEG, 18% to 21% of patients with ICH were shown to have NCSzs.[7,10] cEEG may also predict outcome after ICH. Vespa and coworkers found that NCSzs were associated with an increased midline shift and a trend toward worse outcomes after controlling for hemorrhage size.[7] In a study of patients with ICH by Claassen and associates, NCSzs were associated with expansion of hemorrhage volume and a trend toward worse outcomes as well.[10] In addition, periodic epileptiform discharges (PEDs) were an independent predictor of poor outcome.

Ischemic Stroke

Population- and hospital-based studies have reported rates of acute clinical seizures after ischemic stroke ranging from 2% to 9%.[24,27,29,31-33] Again, more recent studies using cEEG have shown that this may be an underestimate. In the Columbia series, 11% of 56 patients with ischemic stroke undergoing cEEG had seizures; these seizures were purely nonconvulsive in 5 of these 6 patients.[8] In a recent study using cEEG, 6% of 46 patients with ischemic stroke demonstrated nonconvulsive seizure activity.[7] In the work of Jordan, who used cEEG in 57 consecutive patients admitted to the ICU with cerebral ischemia, 26% of the patients had EEG-defined NCSzs during the period of monitoring.[3] Several studies have shown that acute clinical seizures are associated with increased mortality in patients with ischemic stroke.[24,34,35] The relationship between NCSzs and outcome after stroke is currently unknown. However, in a rodent model of acute stroke, NCSzs were associated with increased infarct volume and a threefold increase in mortality.[36]

Traumatic Brain Injury

The incidence of convulsive seizures within the first week after TBI is 4% to 14%[37-39] and increases to 15% in patients with severe TBI.[37,39] Data regarding the incidence of NCSzs after TBI are relatively scant, but rates from 18% to 28% have been reported.[1,6,8] In 96 consecutive patients with moderate or severe TBI undergoing cEEG, Vespa found that 22% had seizures; more than half of the patients with seizures had NCSzs only, and many of these patients had therapeutic phenytoin serum levels.[40] In the Columbia series, 18% of the 51 patients with TBI monitored with cEEG had seizures, all of them had NCSzs, and 8% had NCSE.[8] The exact relationship between seizures and outcome is unclear, but some studies have shown that early posttraumatic seizures are an independent risk factor for poor outcome in adults[41] and children with severe TBI.[42] Whether NCSzs have a similar impact has not been studied properly.

FIGURE 54-1 Nonconvulsive seizures and status epilepticus, focal. **A,** This 49-year-old woman with a history of head trauma, seizures, and strokes was being evaluated for decreased mental status. During the recording, she had repetitive right-sided electrographic seizures beginning in the right frontal region (*highlighted*) and was in focal (also known as partial) nonconvulsive status epilepticus. **B,** Thirty seconds later, the discharge has become faster, thus demonstrating evolution in frequency and morphology and therefore unequivocally ictal. **C,** Four minutes later, the discharge continues and is becoming more widespread and slower, thus demonstrating evolution in location and further evolution in frequency and morphology. There were no associated movements.

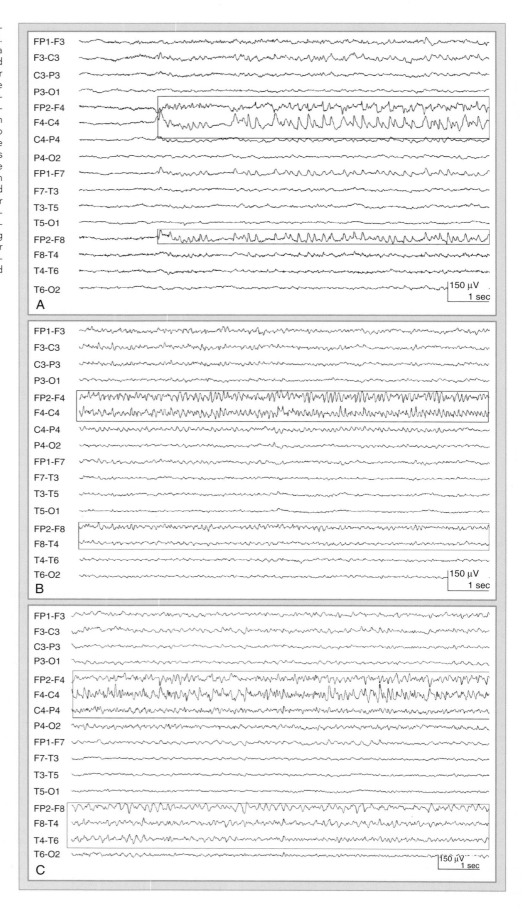

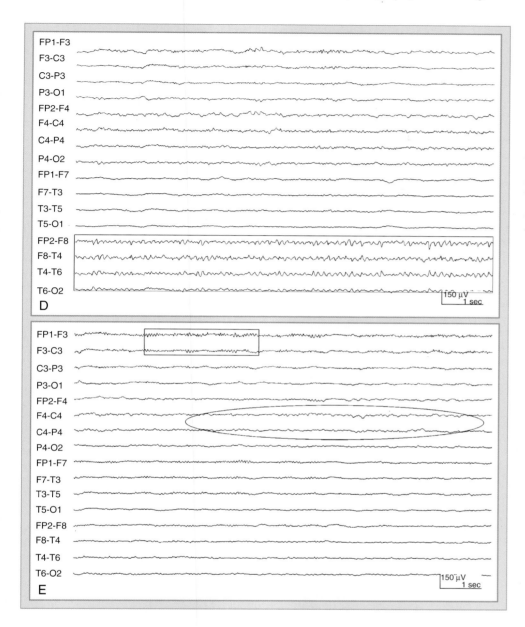

FIGURE 54-1, cont'd D, The discharge is now in the right temporal region only. The patient was given intravenous lorazepam. **E,** The discharge ceased after the administration of lorazepam. Beta activity (probably from the benzodiazepine) is present, but predominantly over the left hemisphere (*box*) (i.e., attenuated on the right—see *ellipse*—suggestive of cortical dysfunction on the right, as is commonly seen postictally); mild focal slowing (suggesting dysfunction, including subcortical white matter) can also be appreciated in the right parasagittal region (*ellipse*). (*From Hirsch LJ, Brenner RP. Atlas of EEG in Critical Care. London: Wiley-Blackwell, 2010.*)

Postoperative Patients

Neurosurgical procedures, especially those involving supratentorial lesions, are associated with a 4% to 17% risk for postoperative clinical seizures.[43-46] Patients with a presurgical history of epilepsy have a risk for postoperative seizures that has been reported to be as high as 34%.[46] Little is known about the rate of NCSzs in these patients. In the Columbia cEEG series, 3 of 13 patients monitored after neurosurgery (excluding patients with SAH) had seizures, all NCSzs, and 1 had NCSE.[8] Postoperative seizures can occur in any postoperative setting in which there is an acute neurological injury, a high risk for metabolic derangement, or neurotoxicity for any reason.

One particularly high-risk non-neurosurgical group is transplant patients. Seizures are common after pancreas, liver, lung, heart, kidney, and bone marrow transplantation[47-57] and often occur in the immediate postoperative period. Patients undergoing cardiac surgery are at risk for the development of acute neurological complications, including stroke or hypoxia,[58] that

may predispose them to seizures in the perioperative or postoperative period.[59] The incidence of NCSzs and NCSE in these patients has not been studied adequately.

Hypoxic-Ischemic Injury

In a series of comatose patients with NCSE, 42% of the patients had hypoxic/anoxic injury.[5] Rates of seizures have been reported to be as high as 35% after cardiac arrest.[60,61] Twenty percent of the patients with hypoxic-ischemic injury monitored in the Columbia series had seizures, most of which were NCSzs.[8] Aside from being a potential contributor to decreased mental status in these patients, the presence of seizures after cardiac arrest may have important prognostic implications (see the later section "Prognostication").[62] In addition, as hypothermia becomes more widely implemented for neuroprotection after cardiac arrest, cEEG may become an important tool for identifying NCSzs, especially during rewarming.[63]

TABLE 54-2 Criteria* for Definite Nonconvulsive Seizure

Any pattern lasting at least 10 seconds and satisfying any one of the following three primary criteria:

PRIMARY CRITERIA

Repetitive generalized or focal spikes, sharp waves, spike and wave complexes at ≥3/sec

Repetitive generalized or focal spikes, sharp waves, spike and wave or sharp and slow-wave complexes at <3/sec and the secondary criterion

Sequential rhythmic, periodic, or quasi-periodic waves at ≥1/sec and unequivocal evolution in frequency (gradually increasing or decreasing by at least 1/sec, e.g., 2-3/sec), morphology, or location (gradual spread into or out of a region involving at least two electrodes). Evolution in amplitude alone is not sufficient. Change in sharpness without other change in morphology is not enough to satisfy evolution in morphology

SECONDARY CRITERION

Significant improvement in the clinical state or appearance of previously absent normal electroencephalographic patterns (such as posterior-dominant "alpha" rhythm) temporally coupled to acute administration of a rapidly acting antiepileptic drug. Resolution of the "epileptiform" discharges leaving diffuse slowing without clinical improvement and without the appearance of previously absent normal electroencephalographic patterns would not satisfy the secondary criterion

*Satisfying these criteria is adequate for confirming nonconvulsive seizure activity. However, failing to meet these criteria does not rule out nonconvulsive seizure activity; clinical judgment and correlation are required in this situation.
Adapted from Chong DJ, Hirsch LJ: Which EEG patterns warrant treatment in the critically ill? Reviewing the evidence for treatment of periodic epileptiform discharges and related patterns. *J Clin Neurophysiol.* 2005;22:79, as modified from Young GB, Jordan KG, Doig GS. An assessment of nonconvulsive seizures in the intensive care unit using continuous EEG monitoring: an investigation of variables associated with mortality. *Neurology.* 1996;47:83.

Toxic-Metabolic Encephalopathy

Critically ill patients are susceptible to many toxic, metabolic, and electrolytic imbalances that may cause both changes in mental status and seizures. Such conditions include but are not limited to hypoglycemia and hyperglycemia, hyponatremia, hypocalcemia, drug intoxication or withdrawal, uremia, liver dysfunction, hypertensive encephalopathy, and sepsis.[16] In the Columbia series, 21% of the patients monitored with cEEG who had toxic-metabolic encephalopathy as their primary neurological diagnosis experienced NCSzs.[8] In other series, 5% to 10% of patients with acute NCSzs had metabolic derangements as the probable cause of their seizures.[5,64] In a recent study of 201 medical ICU patients without known brain injury who underwent cEEG, 22% had PEDs or seizures; sepsis and acute renal failure were significantly associated with electrographic seizures.[65]

Impact of Nonconvulsive Seizures in the Critically Ill

As evidenced by the preceding discussion, NCSzs are clearly common in critically ill patients, and this prompts the question of whether NCSzs require rapid identification and treatment and

whether this would have an impact on patient outcome. There is previous evidence that delay in diagnosis and the duration of NCSE are each independent predictors of a worse outcome, including higher mortality,[6,64] although mortality in patients with NCSE may be most influenced by the underlying cause.[66] In addition, although NCSE may be associated with a poor prognosis in the critically ill elderly,[67] aggressive treatment of NCSzs and NCSE itself may be associated with worse outcomes in this population.[68] Definitive proof that NCSzs worsen outcomes is lacking, however; to date, there has not been a single prospective controlled trial to determine whether treating NCSzs or NCSE improves neurological outcomes. Therefore, much of the justification for identifying and treating NCSzs in the critically ill comes from human and animal data demonstrating that seizures can lead to neuronal injury.

There is a large body of evidence that prolonged seizures, including NCSzs, can lead to neuronal damage in several animal models. Meldrum and colleagues found that paralyzed and artificially ventilated baboons exhibited hippocampal cell loss after treatment with a convulsant.[69] Despite careful control of factors such as oxygenation, temperature, and metabolic status, cell death occurred after 60 minutes of continuous electrographic seizures. Electrical- and chemoconvulsant-induced SE in rodents leads to cell loss, free radical production, inflammation, gliosis, and synaptic reorganization.[70] Pathologic changes can be seen in the absence of overt convulsions and can have profound long-term effects such as impaired performance on cognitive tasks[71] and the development of epilepsy.[72] There is also some evidence from animal models that even single or multiple brief seizures may lead to cell death and cognitive impairment.[73,74] SE in humans has likewise been associated with hippocampal cell loss in postmortem studies[75] and evidence of cell injury in hospitalized patients as demonstrated by elevated levels of serum neuron-specific enolase[76,77] (NSE). Although the sequelae of NCSzs and NCSE are not as well understood, evidence suggests that they can lead to neuronal damage in humans. In a study of NSE levels after seizures, DeGiorgio and associates showed that NSE levels were especially high after NCSzs and seizures of partial onset and that elevations were seen even in absence of acute brain injury.[77]

In addition to direct pathologic effects, seizures can place increased metabolic, excitotoxic, and oxidative stress on at-risk brain and lead to irreversible injury that may worsen the extent of the primary neurological insult. Microdialysis studies in patients with TBI have demonstrated that extracellular glutamate increases to excitotoxic levels after NCSzs.[78] Significant elevations in the ratio of lactate to pyruvate (suggesting neuronal stress and potential death), glycerol (suggesting membrane breakdown),[79] and intracranial pressure (ICP) are also seen.[80] As mentioned earlier, NCSzs in patients with ICH were associated with increased mass effect on serial imaging[7] and expansion of hematoma size.[10] NCSzs have been associated with increased infarct volumes after occlusion of the middle cerebral artery in rats,[36] treatment of which was shown to result in reduced infarct volumes.[81] In addition, even brief seizures can lead to hemodynamic changes, such as increased cerebral blood flow (CBF), which may lead to transient and potentially injurious elevations in ICP, even in the absence of tonic-clonic activity.[82,83] Hippocampal atrophy can be seen on long-term follow-up MRI ipsilateral to NCSz.[84]

Periodic Patterns on Continuous Electroencephalography—What Do They Mean?

There are several periodic patterns commonly seen in critically ill patients in which the relationship to seizures is unknown.[85] Although certain periodic discharges may be more closely related to systemic metabolic abnormalities, such as triphasic waves in patients with hepatic encephalopathy, others reflect injured tissue

TABLE 54-3 Studies Using Continuous Electroencephalographic Monitoring in Critically Ill Patients for Detection of Nonconvulsive Seizures

STUDY	STUDY POPULATION	TYPE OF EEG	DESIGN	N	PATIENTS WITH ANY SEIZURES	PATIENTS WHO HAD NONCONVULSIVE SEIZURES ONLY
Privitera et al.[4]	Patients with an altered level of consciousness or suspected subclinical seizures anywhere in the medical center	Routine EEG*	Prospective	198	37%	100% (32% had no subtle clinical signs)
Jordan[3]	Patients admitted to the neuro-ICU undergoing cEEG	cEEG	Retrospective	124	35%	74%
DeLorenzo et al.[19]	All patients with previous convulsive SE and an altered level of consciousness without clinical seizure activity	cEEG	Prospective	164	48%	100%
Vespa et al.[40]	All patients with moderate to severe traumatic brain injury admitted to the neuro-ICU	cEEG	Retrospective	94	22%	52%
Towne et al.[5]	ICU patients in coma without clinical seizure activity	Routine EEG	Retrospective	236	8%	100% (by definition)
Vespa et al.[7]	Patients admitted to neuro-ICU with stroke or intracerebral hemorrhage	cEEG	Prospective	109	19%	79%
Claassen et al.[8]	Patients of all ages with an unexplained decreased level of consciousness or suspected subclinical seizures	cEEG	Retrospective	570	19%	92%
Pandian et al.[9]	Neuro-ICU patients undergoing cEEG for diagnostic purposes or for titration of intravenous therapy for SE	cEEG	Retrospective	105	27%	68%
Jette et al.[11]	Patients <18 years old admitted to the ICU with an unexplained decreased level of consciousness or suspected subclinical seizures	cEEG	Retrospective	117	44%	75%
Claassen et al.[10]	Patients with intracerebral hemorrhage and an unexplained decreased level of consciousness or suspected subclinical seizures	cEEG	Retrospective	102	31%	58%
Oddo et al.[65]	Medical ICU patients without known brain injury undergoing cEEG with an unexplained decreased level of consciousness or suspected subclinical seizures	cEEG	Retrospective	201	10% (additional 17% with PEDs)	67%

*Routine EEG is 30 to 45 minutes of recording with or without video.
cEEG, continuous electroencephalography; NCSE, nonconvulsive status epilepticus; neuro-ICU, neurological-neurosurgical intensive care unit; PEDs, periodic epileptiform discharges without seizures; SE, status epilepticus.
Adapted with permission from Friedman D, Claassen J, Hirsch LJ. Continuous EEG monitoring in the intensive care unit. *Anesth Analg.* 2009;109:506.

at high risk for seizures, such as periodic lateralized epileptiform discharges (PLEDs, also known as lateralized periodic discharges[86]). See Figure 54-2 for an example of PLEDs evolving into a focal seizure. Furthermore, periodic patterns are sometimes definitively ictal, such as when they are associated with time-locked contralateral clonic jerking. Periodic discharges are typically thought to be interictal or on an interictal-ictal continuum.[85] However, the evidence that PLEDs are occasionally ictal include the following: positron emission tomography in patients with frequent PLEDs demonstrates increased regional glucose metabolism similar to that seen with focal seizures,[87]

single-photon emission computed tomography in patients with PLEDs demonstrates increased regional cerebral perfusion that normalizes when the PLEDs resolve,[88,89] and there are reports of PLEDs causing reversible confusion that resolves with antiepileptic drugs. In one series, seven patients older than 60 years experienced recurrent confusional episodes associated with PLEDs on EEG with interdischarge intervals as long as 4 seconds.[90] The clinical deficits resolved with a slowing of the EEG discharges, whether spontaneously or prompted by intravenous benzodiazepines. Carbamazepine appeared to be effective in preventing recurrences.

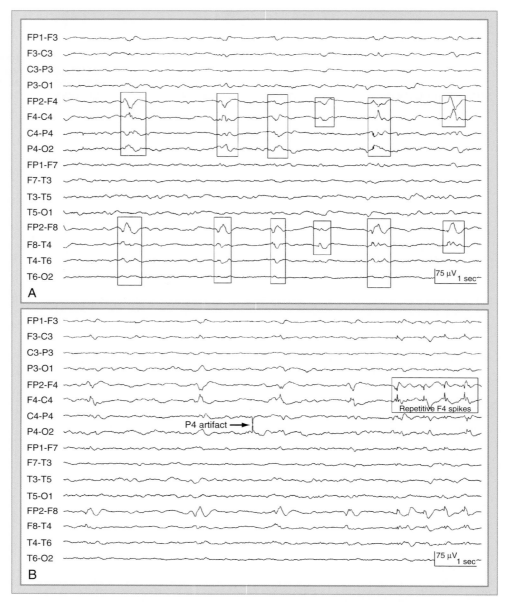

FIGURE 54-2 Periodic lateralized epileptiform discharges (PLEDs) evolving into focal seizure. **A,** First of four consecutive 10-second epochs from a 57-year-old woman after right "strokectomy" (resection of the necrotic area within a large infarct) and evacuation of right subdural hematoma. This sample shows blunt, approximately 0.5-Hz right-sided periodic discharges; these discharges still qualify as "PLEDs" even though they are not frankly "epileptiform." **B,** Ten seconds later, the discharges have changed morphologically, particularly toward the end of the sample, and now consist of faster repetitive spikes, maximal at electrode F4 (*box*). There is also an electrode artifact at P4 (*arrow;* note the lack of field, seen only in channels with P4).

A common practice used to distinguish ictal from nonictal EEG patterns in the critically ill is to see whether the periodic pattern is abolished by a trial of short-acting benzodiazepines. However, almost all periodic discharges, including the periodic triphasic waves seen in patients with metabolic encephalopathy, are attenuated by benzodiazepines.[91] Thus, unless clinical improvement accompanies the EEG change, the test is not helpful diagnostically. Unfortunately, improvement can take substantial time even if the activity represents NCSE and is aborted with benzodiazepines. It is important to recognize that lack of immediate clinical improvement does not exclude NCSE—it simply does not help determine its presence or absence. Our protocol for attempting to prove the presence of NCSE is shown

in Table 54-4. In a recent study of 91 ICU patients with SE diagnosed on EEG, 68 nonanoxic patients were treated with new or additional antiepileptic drugs after the diagnostic EEG. Thirty-eight (56%) had some improvement in level of consciousness that seemed to be due to treatment with the antiepileptic drugs. This improvement was never immediate but was often evident on the same day. The response was similar across medical or surgical ICUs and causes, regardless of whether patients had earlier clinical seizures. Improvement was significantly more likely in stuporous or confused patients (81%) than in comatose patients, but half (48%) of the comatose patients still improved. Patients with evidence of focal seizure onset improved more often (68%) than did those with generalized (50%) or myoclonic

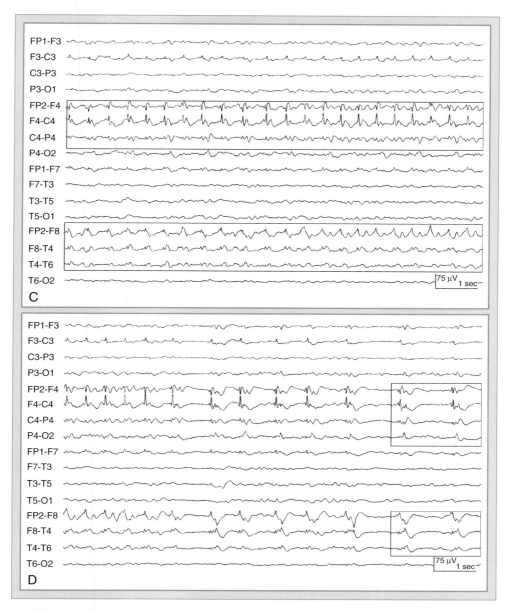

FIGURE 54-2, cont'd   C, Ten seconds later, the discharge becomes more widespread over the right hemisphere and is faster (now up to three per second) with slowly evolving morphology. **D,** The discharge is slowing and breaking up 10 seconds later, with a return to PLEDs in the last few seconds. *(From Hirsch LJ, Brenner RP.* Atlas of EEG in Critical Care. *London: Wiley-Blackwell, 2010.)*

seizures (25%) alone, but this did not reach statistical significance. Two thirds of these nonanoxic patients died. Although there is some evidence that the presence of periodic discharges is an independent risk factor for a worse prognosis in patients with ICH and SAH, it is unclear whether the presence of these discharges should change management. This is currently an area of active clinical research.

Another common pattern in encephalopathic ICU patients is ictal or quasi-ictal–appearing activity triggered by stimulation or arousal. The evoked activity is typically on the interictal-ictal continuum, and we have termed it *stimulus-induced rhythmic, periodic, or ictal discharges* (SIRPIDs).[92] There is usually no clinical correlate, as with most ICU seizures, but a small proportion of patients will have focal motor seizures consistently elicited by alerting stimuli.[93] This phenomenon of seizures or highly epileptiform patterns induced by alerting is most likely a result of

hyperexcitable cortex activated by the usual arousal pathways that involve the upper brainstem, thalamus, and widespread thalamocortical projections. The treatment and prognostic implications of SIRPIDs are currently unknown, but the relationship between ictal discharges and arousal raises the possibility that limiting unnecessary stimulation in patients with SIRPIDs may be beneficial.

CONTINUOUS ELECTROENCEPHALOGRAPHIC MONITORING WITH DEPTH ELECTRODES

Despite all the aforementioned potential applications, the use of conventional scalp electrode–derived EEG for continuous monitoring has significant limitations in the ICU setting.

TABLE 54-4 Benzodiazepine Trial for the Diagnosis of Nonconvulsive Status Epilepticus

Appropriate patients have rhythmic or periodic focal or generalized epileptiform discharges on EEG with an altered level of consciousness

Need to monitor EEG, pulse oximetry, blood pressure, ECG, respiratory rate by a dedicated nurse

Antiepileptic drug trial:

Sequential small doses of a rapidly acting short-duration benzodiazepine such as midazolam at 1 mg per dose

Between doses, repeated clinical and EEG assessment

Trial is stopped after any of the following:

1. Persistent resolution of the EEG pattern (and examination repeated)
2. Definite clinical improvement
3. Respiratory depression, hypotension, or other adverse effect
4. A maximum dose is reached (such as 0.2 mg/kg midazolam, although higher doses may be needed if the patient is taking benzodiazepines chronically)

The test is considered positive if there is resolution of the potentially ictal EEG pattern *and* either an improvement in the clinical state or the appearance of previously absent normal EEG patterns (e.g., posterior-dominant "alpha" rhythm). If EEG improves but patient does not, the result is equivocal.

ECG, electrocardiography; EEG, electroencephalography.

Adapted from Jirsch J, Hirsch LJ. Nonconvulsive seizures: developing a rational approach to the diagnosis and management in the critically ill population. *Clin Neurophysiol.* 2007;118:1660.

Interpretation of scalp EEG can be hampered by a poor signal-to-noise ratio, suboptimal long-term contact with the scalp, artifact from the numerous electrical devices used in ICU care, and other patient-related factors (such as movement artifact from standard clinical care). These confounding factors (most notably artifact) have largely precluded the development of practical bedside scalp EEG–driven alarm systems that could provide real-time information regarding ongoing or potentially reversible neurological injury. Early experience with the use of depth electrodes suggests that many of the limitations of EEG recordings derived from scalp electrodes can be overcome. We recently described our experience with recordings obtained from a small, intracortical eight-contact depth electrode (referred to as intracortical EEG) in a cohort of 16 ICU patients with acute brain injury requiring other invasive brain monitoring.[94] Depth electrode–specific EEG abnormalities were identified in 12 of 16 patients (75%), including electrographic seizures ($n = 10$) and PEDs without seizures ($n = 2$) (Fig. 54-3). The majority of seizures seen with the depth electrode were not seen with the scalp electrode: 6 of the 10 patients with electrographic seizures never had a scalp EEG recording correlate with the seizures seen intracranially; 2 showed an intermittent scalp correlate that could be considered potentially ictal, and 2 had intermittent delta rhythm only, without clear evolution and without a pattern that would traditionally be considered ictal. Significant nonepileptiform EEG changes were observed with the depth electrode only (not with the scalp electrode) in 2 patients who suffered secondary neurological complications during the monitoring period. In 1 patient with SAH and underlying vasospasm, widespread cerebral infarction develop after sepsis-associated hypoxia/hypotension, and in the other, hemorrhagic conversion of a large middle cerebral artery infarction developed. In both patients, dramatic changes in depth EEG tracings (marked attenuation or suppression-burst patterns) appeared before other devices detected any changes. These changes were not evident in simultaneous scalp EEG recordings (because of prominent muscle artifact on the scalp EEG or diminished signal amplitude). These depth EEG changes preceded the detection of concerning changes from other implanted neuromonitoring devices (by 2 to 6 hours) or changes in clinical examination (by >8 hours). These preliminary results indicate that the use of intracranial EEG can improve detection of abnormal brain electrical activity and provide early warning of secondary neurological complications. Intracortical EEG may thus facilitate the

development of EEG-based alarm systems and ultimately improve outcomes in patients with neurological injury.

MULTIMODALITY MONITORING

Invasive multimodality brain monitoring is increasingly being used to monitor comatose patients with severe brain injury.[95] Many different devices are available to measure and track either upstream effectors or downstream indicators of neuronal health, including neuronal activity, brain metabolism, brain tissue oxygenation, and perfusion.[96] Surface and depth EEG monitoring may become an integral part of multimodality monitoring, but few studies have investigated this potential to date.[78,80,94] Most investigators agree that focusing on a single parameter will not allow one to interpret changes adequately but that taking into account information from multiple devices may be helpful in detecting and defining clinical changes with reasonable sensitivity and specificity.

There are many promising applications for multimodality monitoring, including early detection of evolving brain injury, such as vasospasm and cerebral herniation. Multimodality monitoring may also help individualize treatment goals, such as adjusting blood pressure after ischemic stroke, ICH, or SAH. Multimodality monitoring could also give the clinician a more detailed look at brain function in patients who cannot be examined because of the need for pharmacologic paralysis or sedation. Finally, monitoring data could be used to help promote the metabolic health of brain tissue; for example, optimal body temperature, head position, and blood glucose levels could be studied more definitively. All these potential indications are areas for future research in the field and need to be prospectively evaluated before their use can be established. Currently, however, there are major practical limitations to multimodal monitoring capabilities in the neuro-ICU setting. In the future, as we gain a better understanding of the pathophysiology of secondary brain injury, we may be able to direct treatment toward a healthier profile of biochemical and electrical activity, thus preventing further damage after the primary injury.

Cerebral Microdialysis

Cerebral microdialysis monitors are increasingly being used as part of routine care in some neuro-ICUs. Many cerebral metabolites can be measured, but those that are now most commonly

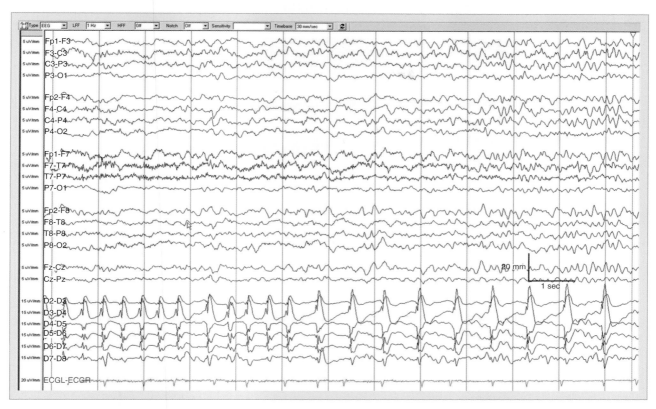

FIGURE 54-3 Cyclic seizures on an intracranial electroencephalographic recording from a woman in her seventies with a Hunt and Hess grade III subarachnoid hemorrhage and a left frontal mini–depth electrode (an eight-contact lead with 2.2 mm between electrode centers placed transcortically during the insertion of other invasive monitoring devices). She had no seizures for some time and then had a 5-hour period with cyclic seizures in the depth electrode only, each lasting about 1 minute and recurring every few minutes. A typical seizure is shown here. The bottom six channels show a clearly evolving seizure, with no hint of it seen on the scalp channels despite a high-quality recording with no missing electrodes. *(From Hirsch LJ, Brenner RP. Atlas of EEG in Critical Care. London: Wiley-Blackwell, 2010.)*

evaluated in the brain include glucose, lactate, pyruvate (energy metabolites), glutamate (an excitatory and potentially toxic amino acid known to be increased in patients with cerebral ischemia and seizures), and glycerol (a marker of cell membrane damage).[97-104] The principal microdialysis marker for neuronal stress is the lactate-pyruvate ratio (LPR). An LPR higher than 40 (normal, <30) is commonly seen in patients with permanent neuronal injury. Observing trends in individuals is probably more useful than interpreting absolute values.[105] Electrographic posttraumatic seizures have been shown to result in sustained elevations of ICP and LPR on microdialysis. Extracellular glucose is also reduced after TBI and may be related to a poor outcome.[106-108]

Detecting Other Changes in Brain Function

cEEG can reveal much more about the state of the brain aside from the presence or absence of seizures. There are distinct electrographic patterns associated with different states of arousal and with different levels of focal and global brain dysfunction, and because of the continuous nature of EEG monitoring, it is possible to assess changes on a second-by-second basis and observe trends.

DETECTION OF ISCHEMIA

It is well-known that EEG changes occur within seconds of a reduction in CBF, and this is the basis for intraoperative EEG monitoring of patients undergoing surgeries with a high risk for cerebral ischemia, such as carotid clamping during endarterectomy.[109-111] As CBF falls below 25 to 30 mL/100 g per minute, there is a progressive loss of higher frequencies and prominent slowing of background EEG activity. All EEG frequencies are suppressed when CBF falls below 8 to 10 mL/100 g per minute, a value low enough to cause irreversible cell death.[112,113] Therefore, cEEG can detect a window where intervention can potentially prevent permanent brain injury. This is becoming important inasmuch as thrombolytic and endovascular therapies have been shown to be effective in treating acute stroke and vasospasm, especially if the treatment is provided very early.[114,115] Recent advances in computing have allowed real-time application of quantitative EEG (qEEG) algorithms for using time-frequency data to measure changes in the background EEG rhythms and to set alarms leading to more detailed assessment for possible ischemia. See Figure 54-4 for an example.

In monitoring for cerebral ischemia, applications of qEEG include the detection of delayed cerebral ischemia (DCI) secondary to vasospasm after SAH and the detection of acute-onset cerebral ischemia. Vasospasm is common after aneurysmal SAH and causes symptomatic DCI in up to 36% of patients, which is associated with a 1.5- to 3-fold increase in mortality. Vasospasm typically occurs 3 to 12 days after the initial SAH and is diagnosed by a combination of serial clinical examinations, transcranial Doppler (TCD), and possibly CO_2 reactivity and invasive tissue oxygen monitoring, all typically with angiographic confirmation as needed.[116] TCD can detect abnormal cerebrovascular velocities only at one point in time (or rarely continuously for a short period), is typically performed every 24 hours, and has just moderate sensitivity and specificity for detecting symptomatic

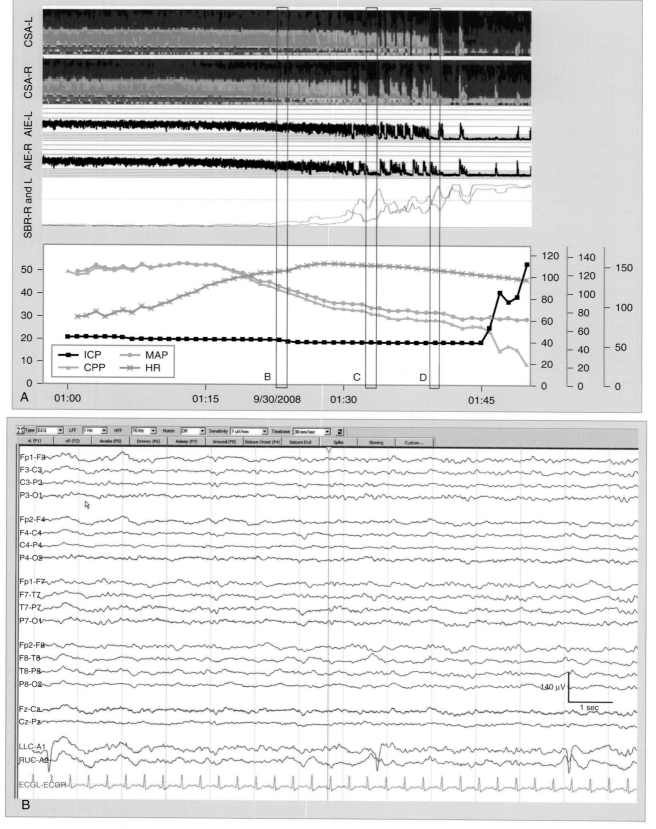

FIGURE 54-4 Quantitative EEG (qEEG) analysis during a drop in cerebral perfusion pressure (CPP). A 55-year-old-man was admitted with intraventricular hemorrhage and pneumonia. Refractory hypotension developed and resulted first in a drop in mean arterial pressure (MAP) and a delayed increase in intracranial pressure (ICP). qEEG analysis, with 1 hour shown here, demonstrates gradual attenuation of all frequencies in the compressed spectral array (CSA; *top two rows* of qEEG, with time on the x-axis and frequency on the y-axis), a bit more prominent and earlier on the right (**A**). Amplitude-integrated EEG (AIE) reveals a gradual decline in both the minimum and maximum amplitude per epoch, and the suppression-burst ratio (SBR) depicts the increasingly suppressed EEG background.

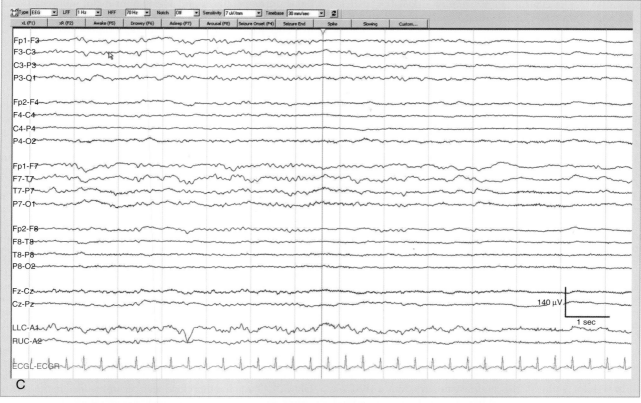

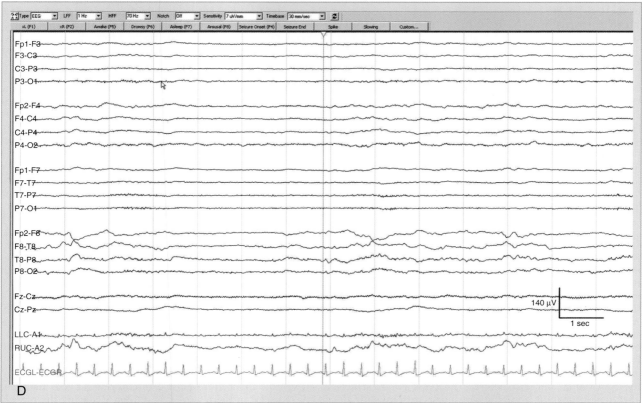

FIGURE 54-4, cont'd The raw EEG changes from diffuse background slowing and mild right hemisphere attenuation (**B**), to marked attenuation on the right (**C**), and then to a severely suppressed background (now more severe on the left; **D**) within approximately 1 hour. The EEGs in **B, C,** and **D** correspond to the times marked on the qEEG (**A**) with the same letters. *(Modified from Kurtz P, Hanafy KA, Claassen J. Continuous EEG monitoring: is it ready for prime time? Curr Opin Crit Care. 2009;15:99.)*

vasospasm.[117-119] The clinical examination of a comatose patient is also limited. Therefore, cEEG-based tools are well suited to detect DCI secondary to vasospasm in poor-grade SAH patients before it is apparent by current screening techniques. Several studies have demonstrated the feasibility of using qEEG for the early detection of DCI. An early report by Labar and colleagues using only two recording channels found that a reduction in total spectral power correlated with DCI and preceded clinical changes in 4 of 11 patients.[120] In a study of 32 patients with primarily good-grade SAH, Vespa and coworkers found that a reduction in the variability of relative alpha frequency (6 to 14 Hz, expressed as a percentage of total power between 1 and 20 Hz) was 100% sensitive and 50% specific for vasospasm as detected by TCD or angiography.[121] In the majority of patients, qEEG changes preceded the diagnosis of vasospasm by more than 2 days. In a study of 34 patients with poor-grade SAH (Hunt-Hess grade IV and V) monitored from postoperative days 2 to 14, Claassen and colleagues found that a reduction in the poststimulation ratio of alpha to delta frequency power of greater than 10% relative to baseline in six consecutive epochs of cEEG was 100% sensitive and 76% specific for DCI.[122] A reduction of greater than 50% in a single epoch was 89% sensitive and 84% specific. The authors examined cEEG epochs after routine stimulation of the ICU patient by caregivers and family to minimize the variability in EEG findings caused by levels of sedation or sleep-wake cycles.

Patients with acute ischemic stroke can also deteriorate after their initial event because of extension of the original infarct, a new infarct,[123] or reocclusion of a recanalized vessel[124] and thus may also benefit from cEEG for detection of new-onset ischemia. In a pilot study,[125] the brain symmetry index (BSI), a qEEG algorithm based on the difference in the mean spectral power for 1 to 25 Hz between the left and right hemispheres, was highly correlated with National Institutes of Health (NIH) stroke scale scores in patients with anterior circulation infarcts. The BSI was also found to correlate with changes on NIH stroke scale immediately after thrombolysis[126] and with outcome after stroke.[127,128] Other changes in the cEEG background pattern, such as regional attenuation without delta frequency (RAWOD), are useful to identify patients with massive acute ischemic strokes and can identify them earlier than computed tomography or magnetic resonance imaging can; these patients may benefit from early surveillance and intervention for cerebral edema, and the appearance of RAWOD on cEEG may assist in prognostication.[129]

MONITORING THE EFFICACY OF THERAPY

cEEG is often used to evaluate the response to interventions aimed at reducing neuronal activity to slow brain metabolism. It is commonly used to guide the treatment of refractory SE with intravenous infusions of anesthetic agents such as midazolam, propofol, or pentobarbital. cEEG may be helpful in adjusting infusion rates to maintain sufficient suppression, in preventing seizures while minimizing adverse drug effects, and in guiding withdrawal of anesthetics in these patients. Pharmacologic coma has been a tool for the treatment of refractory elevated ICP in head trauma; although it can help reduce ICP, it is also associated with a high risk for systemic complications such as hypotension, hepatic dysfunction, and renal failure.[130] cEEG is used to achieve the therapeutic goal of a suppression-burst pattern with the lowest dose of barbiturates possible in an attempt to limit adverse effects.[131] Finally, cEEG can provide information about the level of sedation in critically ill patients, especially in the setting of neuromuscular blockade. qEEG-based tools such as the bispectral index,[132] patient state index,[133] and Narcotrend[134] have been

in use intraoperatively and postoperatively for more than a decade to monitor the depth of sedation in neurologically normal patients. Unlike cEEG, these devices cannot detect seizures or ischemia reliably, and their performance has not been tested adequately in brain-injured patients.

PROGNOSTICATION

cEEG monitoring can provide prognostic information after brain injury that can guide treatment decisions for clinicians and family members alike. Prolonged monitoring can provide a continuous assessment of EEG reactivity, sleep architecture, seizures, and epileptiform discharges, all of which have been found to be factors in determining the prognosis in comatose patients.[135] Burst-suppression patterns after hypoxic-ischemic injury are almost always associated with a poor outcome and a lack of neurological recovery.[71] EEG patterns that are not affected by stimulation, such as alpha coma, are associated with an 88% likelihood of a persistent vegetative state or death after anoxia.[72] qEEG tools, such as amplitude-integrated EEG, can also be used to predict outcome after cardiac arrest, mostly by identifying very low-amplitude tracings or burst-suppression patterns.[136] It has also been shown that convulsive SE and NCSE after cardiac arrest are associated with less than a 25% chance of a good neurological outcome.[60,137] However, therapeutic hypothermia was not used in these studies investigating neurological outcomes in postanoxic patients. Therapeutic hypothermia has been shown in two recent, randomized controlled trials to improve neurological outcome in patients after out-of-hospital cardiac arrest secondary to ventricular fibrillation and without subsequent circulatory shock[138,139] and has therefore been recommended in this setting.[140] More recently, there is evidence suggesting that this benefit extends to patients in shock and is particularly notable when the duration of cardiac arrest is short (<30 minutes).[60,137,141] Thus, one cannot necessarily extrapolate findings from the older studies that did not use hypothermia to prognosticate after cardiac arrest. In fact, there are already case reports of patients with postanoxic coma who had refractory SE, myoclonic status, or generalized PEDs on EEG yet had excellent outcomes. Thus, the prognosis can no longer be presumed to be uniformly poor in these groups if therapeutic hypothermia is used; prognostic studies need to be repeated in the current era to evaluate this.[62,63,136,142]

EEG can provide useful prognostic information in other clinical settings. After convulsive SE, Jaitly and colleagues found that normalization of the EEG background was associated with an excellent outcome whereas patterns such as burst suppression and continued electrographic seizures were associated with mortality rates greater than 50%.[143] Many of the survivors with these patterns remained dependent. Periodic discharges also increased the risk for a poor outcome, but to a lesser degree. In a study of 116 patients with poor-grade SAH, absence of sleep architecture and the presence of PLEDs were independent risk factors for a poor outcome. All patients with absent EEG reactivity, generalized PEDs, bilaterally independent PLEDs, or NCSE had poor outcomes.[144] The percent alpha variability in the first 3 days after TBI has been shown to correlate with Glasgow Outcome Scale scores after 6 months, with a sensitivity of 87% and negative predictive value of 82%.[145,146]

FUTURE DIRECTIONS

Real-time application of cEEG monitoring is a goal that is potentially useful in the neuro-ICU setting. Reducing the raw cEEG traces to a few displayed variables with the use of improved qEEG algorithms will make it a practical tool that can be interpreted by nurses and intensivists. In addition, trend and critical value alarms can be used to alert the ICU staff to changes in neurological status. Computer algorithms have been used successfully to detect ongoing seizures in patients in epilepsy monitoring units. Because seizure patterns in the critically ill are different from those in ambulatory patients, new algorithms are being designed to detect seizures in this patient population. Refining techniques to help identify patterns of interest is an area of active research. Improvement is needed because many qEEG and data reduction tools are not sufficiently specific and are susceptible to contamination by artifact. Managing ICU-related artifact is the main impediment to developing accurate automated alarm systems that can be used at the bedside with acceptable sensitivity and specificity for the detection of seizure patterns, ischemia, and other changes. Although ICU staff can be trained to review raw trends and raw EEG traces for obvious artifacts and even pathologic patterns, an expert reviewer, typically a neurophysiologist, is usually still needed to verify the interpretation. It is necessary to standardize interpretation of the complex rhythmic and periodic EEG patterns seen in this population, an effort that is currently under way. It will then be possible to begin to study the relationship of these EEG patterns in the critically ill to ongoing brain injury for identification of exactly which patterns need to be treated and how aggressively. It may be necessary to individualize treatment by using multimodality monitoring to define the physiologic effects of a pattern in a given individual at a given time. Studies are also needed to determine whether using real-time monitoring with cEEG to detect ischemia can improve outcomes; the infrastructure for continuous expert interpretation (i.e., neurotelemetry, akin to cardiac telemetry) must be in place before this can be tested properly.

Finally, research is needed to determine whether conventional scalp EEG recording methods are sufficient for all patients. Recent studies with subdural electrodes in patients with severe TBI found episodes of cortical spreading depression and slow and prolonged peri-injury depolarizations lasting minutes near injured brain.[147] Similar types of cortical depolarizations have been observed in animal models of stroke, where they are associated with infarct enlargement because of N-methyl-D-aspartate receptor–mediated injury.[148] Recently, these events have also been demonstrated in patients with large middle cerebral artery strokes[149] and in patients with SAH,[150] in whom they have been associated with DCI. As described earlier, preliminary data suggest that depth electrodes inserted near injured cortex in severely brain-injured patients are able to detect seizures and changes in background activity not readily apparent with scalp electrodes.[94] Whether targeting these events for therapy can improve patient outcomes needs to be determined before more widespread application of these invasive recording techniques.

CONCLUSION

In summary, cEEG has become an important technique for assessing neurological status in critically ill patients admitted to neuro-ICUs. Its clearest utility at this point is to identify NCSzs, which are quite common and occur much more frequently than clinically recognizable seizures in this population. Dynamic monitoring of brain activity can help intensivists limit secondary injury in brain-injured patients and has the potential to detect neurological injury in at-risk patients at the moment that it occurs. Advances in cEEG analysis may soon make real-time bedside monitoring of brain activity and neurotelemetry a reality so that neurological status can be assessed and tracked as easily as cardiopulmonary status.

SUGGESTED READINGS

Bernard SA, Gray TW, Buist MD, et al. Treatment of comatose survivors of out-of-hospital cardiac arrest with induced hypothermia. *N Engl J Med.* 2002;346:557.

Chong DJ, Hirsch LJ. Which EEG patterns warrant treatment in the critically ill? Reviewing the evidence for treatment of periodic epileptiform discharges and related patterns. *J Clin Neurophysiol.* 2005;22:79.

Claassen J, Jette N, Chum F, et al. Electrographic seizures and periodic discharges after intracerebral hemorrhage. *Neurology.* 2007;69:1356.

Claassen J, Mayer SA, Kowalski RG, et al. Detection of electrographic seizures with continuous EEG monitoring in critically ill patients. *Neurology.* 2004;62:1743.

DeGiorgio CM, Heck CN, Rabinowicz AL, et al. Serum neuron-specific enolase in the major subtypes of status epilepticus. *Neurology.* 1999;52:746.

DeLorenzo RJ, Waterhouse EJ, Towne AR, et al. Persistent nonconvulsive status epilepticus after the control of convulsive status epilepticus. *Epilepsia.* 1998;39:833.

Dohmen C, Sakowitz OW, Fabricius M, et al. Spreading depolarizations occur in human ischemic stroke with high incidence. *Ann Neurol.* 2008;63:720.

Fabricius M, Fuhr S, Bhatia R, et al. Cortical spreading depression and peri-infarct depolarization in acutely injured human cerebral cortex. *Brain.* 2006;129:778.

Fountain NB, Waldman WA. Effects of benzodiazepines on triphasic waves: implications for nonconvulsive status epilepticus. *J Clin Neurophysiol.* 2001;18:345.

Hirsch LJ, Claassen J, Mayer SA, et al. Stimulus-induced rhythmic, periodic, or ictal discharges (SIRPIDs): a common EEG phenomenon in the critically ill. *Epilepsia.* 2004;45:109.

Hirsch LJ, Pang T, Claassen J, et al. Focal motor seizures induced by alerting stimuli in critically ill patients. *Epilepsia.* 2008;49:968.

Husain AM, Horn GJ, Jacobson MP. Non-convulsive status epilepticus: usefulness of clinical features in selecting patients for urgent EEG. *J Neurol Neurosurg Psychiatry.* 2003;74:189.

Jirsch J, Hirsch LJ. Nonconvulsive seizures: developing a rational approach to the diagnosis and management in the critically ill population. *Clin Neurophysiol.* 2007;118:1660.

Jordan KG. Emergency EEG and continuous EEG monitoring in acute ischemic stroke. *J Clin Neurophysiol.* 2004;21:341.

Oddo M, Carrera E, Claassen J, et al. Continuous electroencephalography in the medical intensive care unit. *Crit Care Med.* 2009;37:2051.

Oddo M, Schaller MD, Feihl F, et al. From evidence to clinical practice: effective implementation of therapeutic hypothermia to improve patient outcome after cardiac arrest. *Crit Care Med.* 2006;34:1865.

Towne AR, Waterhouse EJ, Boggs JG, et al. Prevalence of nonconvulsive status epilepticus in comatose patients. *Neurology.* 2000;54:340.

Vespa, P. Continuous EEG monitoring for the detection of seizures in traumatic brain injury, infarction, and intracerebral hemorrhage: "to detect and protect." *J Clin Neurophysiol.* 2005;22:99.

Vespa PM, Miller C, McArthur D, et al. Nonconvulsive electrographic seizures after traumatic brain injury result in a delayed, prolonged increase in intracranial pressure and metabolic crisis. *Crit Care Med.* 2007;35:2830.

Vespa PM, Nuwer MR, Juhasz C, et al. Early detection of vasospasm after acute subarachnoid hemorrhage using continuous EEG ICU monitoring. *Electroencephalogr Clin Neurophysiol.* 1997;103:607.

Vespa PM, Nuwer MR, Nenov V, et al. Increased incidence and impact of nonconvulsive and convulsive seizures after traumatic brain injury as detected by continuous electroencephalographic monitoring. *J Neurosurg.* 1999;91:750.

Vespa PM, O'Phelan K, Shah M, et al. Acute seizures after intracerebral hemorrhage: a factor in progressive midline shift and outcome. *Neurology.* 2003;60:1441.

Vespa P, Prins M, Ronne-Engstrom E, et al. Increase in extracellular glutamate caused by reduced cerebral perfusion pressure and seizures after human traumatic brain injury: a microdialysis study. *J Neurosurg.* 1998;89:971.

Waziri A, Arif H, Oddo M, et al. Early experience with a cortical depth electrode for ICU neurophysiological monitoring in patients with acute brain injury. *Epilepsia.* 2007;48(suppl 6):208.

Young GB, Jordan KG, Doig GS. An assessment of nonconvulsive seizures in the intensive care unit using continuous EEG monitoring: an investigation of variables associated with mortality. *Neurology.* 1996;47:83.

Full references can be found on Expert Consult @ www.expertconsult.com

CHAPTER 55

Neuroradiologic Evaluation for Epilepsy Surgery

Suzan Dyve ■ Leif Sørensen ■ Adam N. Mamelak ■
William W. Sutherling ■ Gregory D. Cascino

COMPUTED TOMOGRAPHY, MAGNETIC RESONANCE IMAGING, AND FUNCTIONAL IMAGING (DIFFUSION TENSOR IMAGING, POSITRON EMISSION TOMOGRAPHY, AND FUNCTIONAL MAGNETIC RESONANCE IMAGING)

Neuroimaging may point to the cause of epilepsy, aid in the planning of surgery, and serve as a guide during the neurosurgical procedure. The success of surgical resection for intractable epilepsy is highly dependent on presurgical delineation of the region responsible for generating the seizures. The aim of this chapter is to provide an overview of specific imaging modalities that can aid in providing the best surgical decision for epilepsy patients. The causes of epilepsy are varied, and each patient requires an individual approach. Seizures can occur in normal brain (hypoxia or hypoglycemia), in an apparently structurally normal brain (genetic, biochemical, microstructural), or in brains with a definite focal or general structural abnormality. Imaging can be classified broadly as anatomic or functional, and not all patients require use of the full repertoire that is available today. The decision to carry out epilepsy surgery depends on the surgeon's assessment of the potential benefit versus risk for each patient. Traditionally, therefore, epilepsy surgeons have made use of all modalities that can aid in decision making before and during surgery. In earlier neurosurgical and epilepsy-specific textbooks, chapters on imaging focused on computed tomography (CT) and magnetic resonance imaging (MRI). The rapid development and expansion of new methods in structural and functional imaging modalities present a challenge to keep up with and make use of. This chapter describes the more recent imaging techniques that have been adopted by neurosurgeons performing epilepsy surgery.

Anatomic imaging modalities include CT, MRI, and more recently, diffusion tensor imaging (DTI) based on water diffusion, an MRI technique that allows imaging of axonal white matter tracts. Functional imaging involves neurovascular coupling, where an increase in blood flow is associated with increased oxygen delivery, to satisfy the needs for increased oxygen and glucose consumption that occur in neurons with increased activity. Magnetic resonance spectroscopy (MRS) allows in vivo analysis of neurochemicals and their metabolites.

Some of these imaging tools require the injection of single-photon– or positron-emitting radioactive nuclides (single-photon emission computed tomography [SPECT] and positron emission tomography [PET]). Functional magnetic resonance imaging (fMRI) uses "blood oxygenation level–dependent" (BOLD) signals that arise when blood flow increases more than the oxygen consumption of active neurons. Magnetoencephalography (MEG) uses a relatively new "super-cooled" quantum interference device (SQUID) that registers changing magnetic fields with an extremely sensitive recording technique. Clinical uses for MEG include the detection and localization of epileptiform activity and localization of eloquent cortex for surgical planning.

Common to all these techniques is the potential for converting function to images on a screen.

Computed Tomography

CT is no longer the modality of choice, except in places with limited availability of MRI. Before the advent of MRI, CT had supplanted even earlier imaging methods. It was especially useful in detecting causes of focal epilepsy and revealing tumors, calcification, vascular anomalies, and atrophy. Its shortcomings include concern for ionizing radiation and problems caused by the presence of bone artifacts, especially (for epilepsy) in the temporal fossa. In addition, the spatial resolution of CT is on the order of millimeters lower than that of MRI. Nonetheless, CT still has a place in most centers as an acute screening method, for example, in the emergency department or in the event of postoperative complications.

Magnetic Resonance Imaging

Because of its high sensitivity and excellent tissue contrast, MRI should be the first step in screening an epilepsy patient because it detects underlying structural pathology in as many as 75% of patients with refractory focal seizures. MRI is the primary imaging modality when a patient experiences the first seizure or when the clinician suspects epilepsy. Most centers will have performed screening studies that usually include T1-weighted (with contrast enhancement if a space-occupying lesion is suspected), T2-weighted, and fluid-attenuated inversion recovery (FLAIR) sequences in the axial, sagittal, and coronal planes. These studies can be sufficient to reveal focal pathology. If focal pathology as shown by MRI is concordant with that noted on electroencephalography (EEG), a better surgical outcome is achieved, and identifying a focal lesion in patients with refractory epilepsy remains one of the most important factors in determining surgical outcomes.[1] However, if no focal lesion is seen and if EEG suggests a focal etiology, further MRI and other imaging studies should be performed.[2] In recent years, detection of lesions with MRI has improved by optimizing scan protocols with the use of FLAIR sequences, diffusion-weighted images, and volume acquisition with three-dimensional reconstruction.

MRI protocols specific for epilepsy patients can differ but often include variations of the following[3]:

1. Axial and sagittal T2-weighted imaging.
2. Coronal T2-weighted FLAIR, which dampens the signal of free water (cerebrospinal fluid) and thereby highlights areas of increased tissue water (gliosis and low-grade tumors).
3. Coronal T1-weighted FLAIR, which is extremely sensitive in defining gray and white matter and therefore useful in revealing migration anomalies (Fig. 55-1).
4. Axial T1-weighted three-dimensional spoiled gradient echo (SPGR), a thin-slice volume scan (1 to 2 mm, no gap) that can be reformatted in all planes. Images can be fused with other modalities in the neuronavigational system (DTI, fMRI,

3 T and 7 T versus 1.5 T

Some lesions, such as cortical dysplasia, can be difficult to detect, and there is ongoing interest in using new advances in MRI, such as high-field and multichannel technology. It remains to be tested whether multichannel 3- or 7-T imaging can provide additional useful information. Increasing field strength from 1.5 to 3 and 7 T for the clinical evaluation of epilepsy has required optimization of imaging protocols but has shown that increased field strength improves the SNR and may therefore prove useful in the detection of cortical dysplasia. However, some have found that 1.5 T appears to be more sensitive in cases of tissue loss and mesial temporal sclerosis.[8]

Diffusion Tensor Imaging

DTI, also known as "fiber tracking," is an MRI modality that has allowed three-dimensional study of white matter fiber bundles at visible resolution (millimeters). Previously, white fiber (axonal) tracts were mapped post mortem by using specialized preparations or chemical techniques. DTI provides imaging of major white matter bundles connecting functional groups of neurons (Fig. 55-3). Computer analysis can connect fiber bundles in close relation to a planned surgical field such as the motor cortex to motor areas in the brainstem. DTI can therefore aid in planning surgery by avoidance of not only eloquent cortex but also the white matter tracts that connect functional areas.

DTI visualizes the preferred movement of water molecules in the brain. Water molecules diffuse preferentially along white matter tracts (anisotropic movement). A diffusion-sensitizing magnetic field gradient is applied in multiple cartesian directions and yields representations of structures such as nerve fibers in three dimensions. The technique has the potential for elucidating the characteristics of tissue microstructure and therefore offers insight into the cause of the epilepsy and location, as well as serving as a guide during surgery.

Because white matter tract trajectories are complex, the use of DTI necessitates knowledge of the core or seed regions (voxels) of interest, specifically, where the tracts originate, where they pass through, and where they end. For example, when mapping the corticospinal tracts, the seed areas are the cortex in the motor area, the internal capsule, and the peduncles of the midbrain (Fig. 55-4). Placement of a seed area in the motor cortex is often preceded by fMRI to enable precise choice of the tracts of interest (Fig. 55-5).

In clinical practice, it is probably not necessary to study more than 20 prominent tracts in the cerebrum and brainstem. Regions of special interest to the epilepsy surgeon are tracts that connect areas of special functional importance and include the corticospinal tracts, corpus callosum, arcuate and uncinate fasciculi, and the inferior orbitofrontal tract, the latter including the optic tract and Meyer's loop. In recent years, papers and atlases have been published on white tract anatomy, placement of seed areas, and comparison of DTI with traditional white matter dissection.[9,10] Recent advances include intraoperative DTI, in which real-time images of white matter tracts are generated during neurosurgical procedures and shifting of tracts as a result of surgery can be depicted.[11] The role of DTI in neurosurgical practice is currently being defined.

Functional Brain Imaging

Magnetic Resonance Spectroscopy

MRS is a noninvasive functional neuroimaging tool that has been especially useful in studying hippocampal pathology. Hippocampal sclerosis is found by pathologic examination in 65% of

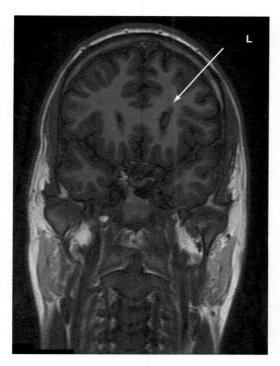

FIGURE 55-1 Coronal T1-weighted fluid-attenuated inversion recovery image showing a migration defect (*arrow*) adjacent to the anterior horn of the left lateral ventricle. (*Courtesy of Dr. Leif Sørensen, Århus University Hospital, Denmark.*)

functional PET [fPET] or 2-deoxy-2-[18F]fluorodeoxyglucose (FDG)-PET, and source localization from EEG and MEG) (Fig. 55-2). Functional or metabolic data can be coregistered to the three-dimensional anatomy to provide excellent separation and detail of gray/white matter boundaries.

5. Coronal T2*-weighted, gradient echo sequence, which is sensitive to paramagnetic substances such as blood and hemosiderin and useful in revealing cavernous angiomas.
6. Axial diffusion-weighted imaging (DWI), which can reveal infarct, abscess, or necrosis.

Recent imaging improvements include the following:

1. Arterial spin labeling (ASL), which measures cerebral blood flow (CBF) and is therefore similar in utility to SPECT but advantageous in that it is noninvasive and can be coregistered to structural MRI. A disadvantage is that ASL assesses CBF at the time of scanning and is therefore usually interictal. ASL has been found to be useful in lateralization and determining epileptic foci.[4]
2. Susceptibility-weighted imaging (SWI), which is extremely sensitive to iron in the brain, including the cortical layers, and can therefore reveal structures that were not previously identified on MRI. SWI is beginning to be used clinically and in the context of epilepsy and has proved helpful in visualizing small cavernous malformations and hemosiderin from old infarcts.[5] Improvements in the signal-to-noise ratio (SNR) are achieved with the use of phased-array surface coils with larger arrays. Phased-array coils are placed closer to the brain than earlier coil types and increase cortical signal. Each coil receives a signal from only a small area of cortex, thereby reducing noise. Increasing the number of arrays from 4 in the 1990s to 32 at 1.5 and 3 T at present, with up to 128 channels under development, will probably improve image quality in the future.[6]
3. Fetal MRI has enabled the diagnosis of cortical malformations and tuberous sclerosis in utero.[7]

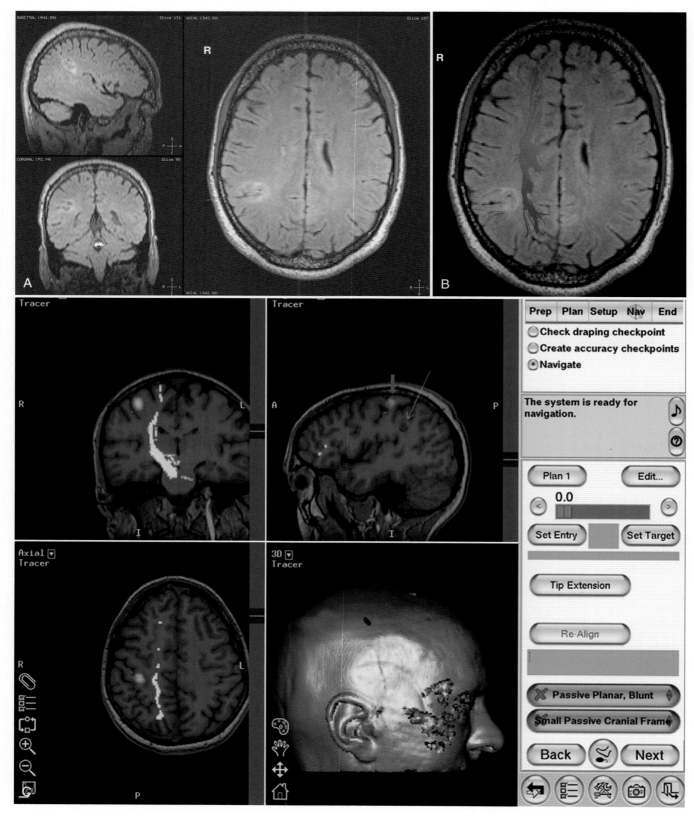

FIGURE 55-2 Cortical dysplasia in the right parietal region. **A,** T2-weighted fluid-attenuated inversion recovery (FLAIR) images in the sagittal, coronal, and axial planes. **B,** T2-weighted FLAIR image fused with T1-weighted three-dimensional spoiled gradient echo and diffusion tensor imaging (DTI). **C,** Images coregistered to the neuronavigational system (Medtronic Stealth Station) and fused with DTI and functional positron emission tomography (fPET). Lesion, *thin arrow*; fPET for the hand, *thick arrow*. *(Courtesy of J. Frandsen, K. Vang, and S. Dyve, Århus University Hospital, Denmark.)*

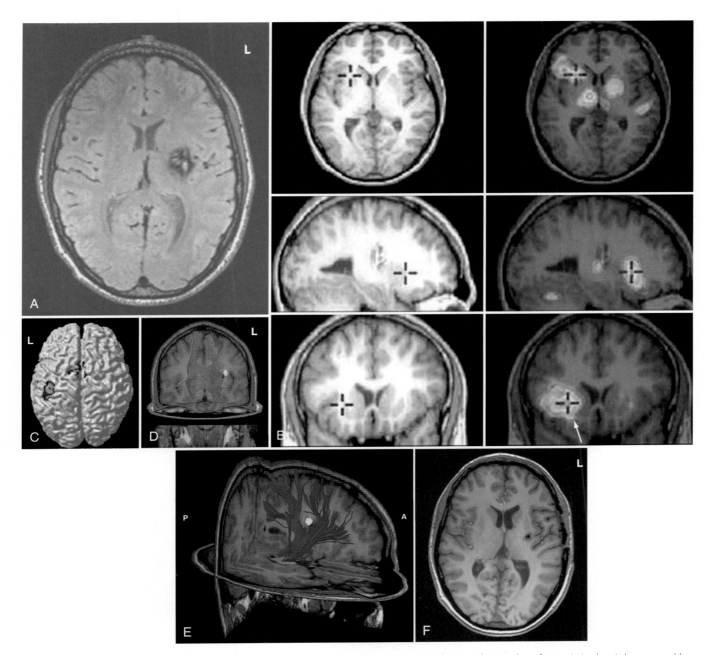

FIGURE 55-3 Cavernous angioma near the left internal capsule in a 23-year-old man with several episodes of paresis in the right arm and leg. Based on imaging studies and navigation, a path was chosen through the left frontal lobe, above Broca's language area, in front of the motor strip, and through the defect shown by tractography. Paralysis of the right arm and leg occurred postoperatively but resolved completely within 3 months. The patient had slight, permanent clumsiness in fine finger movement of his right hand. **A,** Axial T2-weighted fluid-attenuated inversion recovery image. **B,** Magnetic resonance imaging (MRI) and functional positron emission tomography (fPET) superimposed. fPET showed language activation in the left inferior frontal lobe (synonym production) (*arrow*). **C,** Preoperative superficial three-dimensional MRI reconstruction with fPET superimposed (right hand activation) in the left motor area to facilitate operative planning. **D,** Diffusion tensor imaging (DTI) in the corpus callosum (*pink*). The corticospinal tracts are *green* and the lesion is *white*. **E,** MRI with DTI showing disruption of the corticospinal tracts that was presumed to be due to a mass effect of the lesion and several episodes of hemorrhage. **F,** Postoperative 3-T MRI. *(Courtesy of S. Dyve, J. Frandsen, and A. Rodell, Århus University Hospital, Denmark.)*

patients with temporal lobe epilepsy and is characterized by loss of neurons, atrophy, and replacement gliosis.[12] It can be seen by visual inspection or volumetric analysis and can be defined by MRI in 70% of cases.[13] MRS allows in vivo analysis of neurochemicals and their metabolites. Attention has focused on proton [^{1}H] MRS, which has principally yielded data on *N*-acetylaspartate (NAA), choline, phosphocreatine, creatine, and lactate; MRS quantifies metabolites from brain regions that have underlying cellular abnormalities. NAA, which is an amino acid synthesized in mitochondria, is a neuronal and axonal marker that decreases with neuronal loss or dysfunction. Decreased levels of NAA can be interpreted as cell loss or neuronal damage. Total creatine, composed of phosphocreatine and its precursor creatine, is a marker of brain energy metabolism. Total choline is a marker for membrane synthesis or repair, inflammation, or demyelination and can reflect astrocytosis.

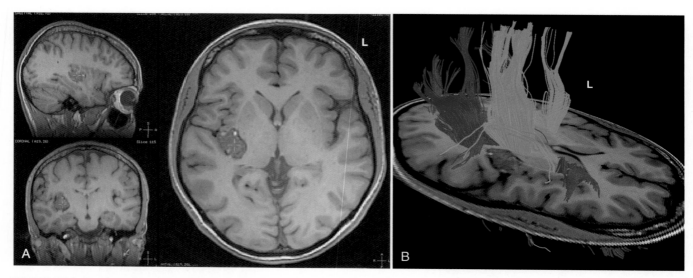

FIGURE 55-4 Cavernous angioma. **A,** T1-weighted magnetic resonance image showing cavernous angioma in proximity to the right posterior insula and internal capsule. **B,** Seed area placed in the internal capsule. *(Courtesy of J. Frandsen and S. Dyve, Århus University Hospital, Denmark.)*

Studies have shown that in comparison to controls, the temporal lobe ipsilateral to the seizure focus shows a reduction in NAA signal intensity and an increase in creatine and choline signal. Reduction of the ratio of NAA to choline, creatine, and phosphocreatine is a marker for neuronal loss and dysfunction. This method has shown promise for localizing epileptic foci with underlying pathology that is not visible with other imaging modalities. However, routine use of MRS for epilepsy is declining in many centers as a result of the increased application and improvement of other imaging modalities.

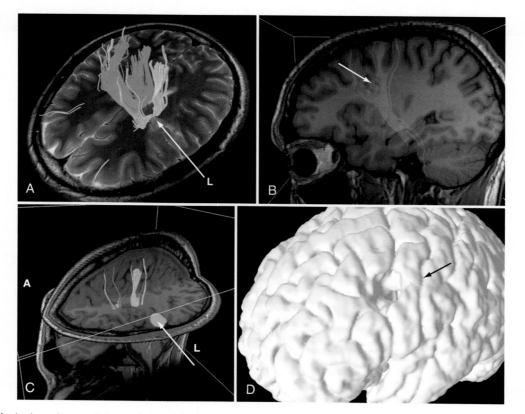

FIGURE 55-5 Meningioangiomatosis in proximity to the left motor area and corticospinal tract. **A,** T2-weighted magnetic resonance imaging (MRI) showing the corpus callosum *(green)* and a mesial defect in the corticospinal tracts *(arrow).* **B,** Sagittal T1-weighted MRI showing the mesial extent of the tumor with diffusion tensor imaging (DTI) superimposed *(arrow).* **C,** T1-weighted MRI, DTI, and functional positron emission tomography (motor movement of the tongue, *arrow).* **D,** Preoperative three-dimensional MRI surface reconstruction showing the planned surgical path. Central sulcus *(arrow).* Postoperative paresis of the tongue and lower part of the face resolved within 1 month. *(Courtesy of K. Vang, J. Frandsen, and S. Dyve, Århus University Hospital, Denmark.)*

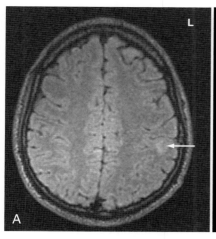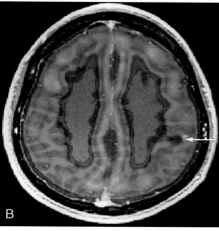

FIGURE 55-6 Low-grade ganglioglioma in the somatosensory area of the left parietal region. **A,** T2-weighted fluid-attenuated inversion recovery image of the tumor (*arrow*). **B,** Positron emission tomography ([^{15}O]H$_2$O) shows decreased blood flow in the area of the tumor (*arrow*). (*Courtesy of P. Borghammer, Århus University Hospital, Denmark.*)

Functional Mapping

Human brain mapping has produced new data that have added considerable information on the anatomy of specific cerebral functions. As already noted, there are two basic types of brain mapping methods for measuring brain function: first, techniques that detect electromagnetic activity (EEG and MEG) measure the electromagnetic fields generated by neural activity, and second, techniques that are based on hemodynamic or metabolic signals (PET and fMRI) measure signs of neural activity. These two methodologies differ, including their temporal and spatial resolution. fPET and fMRI produce data from most of the brain with a spatial resolution of a few millimeters and a temporal resolution of minutes (fPET) or seconds (fMRI). The electromagnetic techniques, in contrast, produce data with limited spatial resolution but with a temporal resolution of milliseconds. High temporal resolution is important to resolve rapidly changing patterns of brain activity that underlie cerebral function. However, traditionally, EEG and MEG have provided insufficient spatial detail to identify relationships between electrical events, structures, and functions, as visualized by MRI, PET, or fMRI. It is hoped that combining the two technologies will provide increasing information on processing in the human brain.[14] The rationale behind fPET and fMRI is to determine the spatial relationship between active eloquent brain areas and to identify the least traumatic neurosurgical approach. In the case of fPET, structural MRI images are required for coregistration.

Functional Magnetic Resonance Imaging

In simplified terms, fMRI is based on images of deoxyhemoglobin. Deoxygenated hemoglobin is found in the veins and capillaries and is seen in a magnetic field because of the presence of iron in the hemoglobin molecule. The presence of oxygen "neutralizes" the effect of the visible iron because it is bound to the iron in the hemoglobin molecule. There is therefore a loss of MRI signal in the absence of deoxyhemoglobin, and this loss of signal can be visualized in the veins and capillaries; in an animal breathing 100% oxygen, venous structure signal is lost. The oxygen content in blood therefore acts as a contrast agent: BOLD contrast. In activation studies, finger movement, for example, results in increased blood flow in the contralateral motor cortex and is visualized as signal loss because of an increase in the concentration of oxyhemoglobin.

Applications of fMRI include mapping of eloquent cortex, particularly sensorimotor function and language. Baseline studies are carried out, followed by presentation of relevant tasks to the patient. It is hoped that in the future fMRI will replace the Wada test for memory and language and mitigate the need for intraoperative cortical mapping in certain cases.[15] However, caution is necessary in comparing the localization of functions based on areas of brain activated, as with the use of fMRI, with areas inactivated by the Wada test or intraoperative stimulation mapping. There are also concerns of the accuracy of fMRI localization, which can be impaired by the low SNR (in comparison to fPET) and susceptibility to various artifacts, including movement during speech. Thus far, studies comparing fPET and fMRI in the same patient are rare.[16]

Positron Emission Tomography

PET records the accumulation of radioactively labeled compounds in regions of the brain. The radioactive compounds (tracers) follow the biochemical pathways of native molecules without altering the velocity of the reactions in these pathways. Although fMRI appears to be superseding fPET in terms of clinical use because of cost and availability, FDG-PET and fPET can assist in lateralization and localization of epileptogenic cortical areas (Fig. 55-6).

Functional Positron Emission Tomography

During functional activity, fPET shows significantly altered signals in comparison to a reference or baseline state. Functional activity results in altered signals in the region of interest, and fPET highlights the neuroanatomic correlates of changes in these processes by comparing the active state with the reference or baseline state. As in fMRI, activation typically involves sequential tasks contralateral to the lesion, such as thumb opposition, flexion-extension of the foot, or language tasks (Fig. 55-7). fPET is generally believed to be an accurate localization method that has demonstrated good correspondence with intraoperative cortical mapping methods and a high SNR. In fPET, uptake of radioactive water into the brain is proportional to blood flow during the first few minutes after the intravenous injection of [^{15}O]H$_2$O, and blood flow is assumed to change in proportion to functional activity.

The energy metabolism variable most commonly recorded with PET for epilepsy is uptake of the fluorine 18–labeled glucose analog FDG, which is trapped in brain tissue as FDG-6-phosphate in proportion to the glucose phosphorylation rate. The accumulated FDG-6-phosphate stays in the brain as a semipermanent index of the metabolic rate because it is neither further metabolized in the glycolytic pathway because of

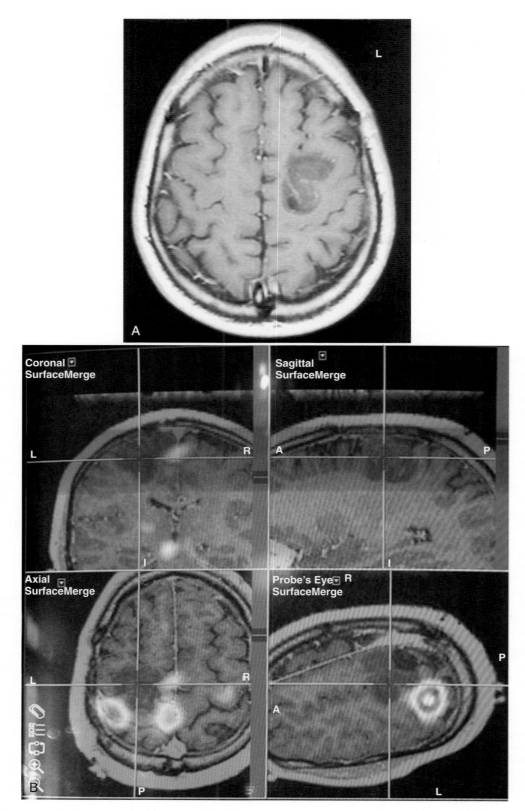

FIGURE 55-7 Dysembryoplastic neuroepithelial tumor in the left motor cortex. Limited resection was previously performed at another center. **A,** T1-weighted magnetic resonance imaging (MRI) with contrast enhancement. **B,** Functional positron emission imaging (fPET) of the hand and leg area merged with neuronavigation (Stealth, Medtronic) during resection.

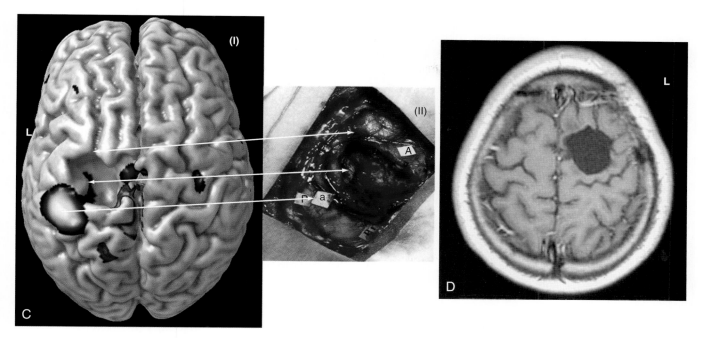

FIGURE 55-7, cont'd   C, (i) Preoperative three-dimensional MRI surface reconstruction with fPET (hand and leg) superimposed and the tumor "removed" was considered informative for the neurosurgeon and patient. (ii) Intraoperative comparison. *a,* fPET as shown by navigation; *p* and *p1,* intraoperative cortical mapping with movement of the anterior tibial muscle of the right leg and flexion of the fingers of the right hand (intubated, light anesthesia, and electromyographic electrodes placed in the relevant muscle groups); *A,* residual tumor, according to navigation, was close to the presumed supplementary motor area. **D,** T1-weighted MRI. Postoperative initial right-sided paralysis resolved within 3 months except for a slight decrease in fine finger movement. *(Courtesy of A. Rodell and S. Dyve, Århus University Hospital, Denmark.)*

incompatibility with the ensuing enzymes nor reconverted to FDG because brain tissue has negligible phosphatase activity.

FDG-PET has been found to be useful in nonlesional epilepsy by interictally locating areas of reduced glucose consumption (Fig. 55-8). This has been found to enhance the treatment of patients with cortical dysplasia.[17] Others have found that FDG-PET asymmetry such as left temporal lobe hypometabolism can predict verbal memory after temporal lobectomy.[18] Recent studies have indicated that FDG-PET can detect interictal hypometabolism in areas of cortical dysplasia in 81% of cases and has been found to be useful in identifying epileptogenic regions in patients with tuberous sclerosis.[19,20] PET remains of value in the diagnostic work-up of patients with epilepsy because of its simplicity, speed of performance, accuracy, and comfort in patients. There are usually no concerns for claustrophobic or overweight patients or those who have metal implants. Radioactivity is not commonly an issue because of its low concentration and the short half-life of positron-emitting isotopes.

In summary, functional brain-imaging techniques can support the presurgical diagnosis, especially in patients with nonlesional MRI findings or nonlateralizing or localizing scalp EEG recordings. Intraoperative cortical mapping is facilitated because

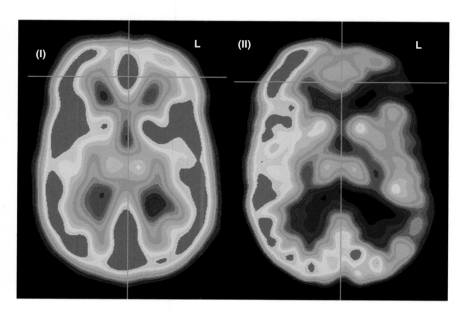

FIGURE 55-8 Fluorodeoxyglucose (FDG) and [^{15}O]H$_2$O positron emission tomography (PET) in a patient with seizures and no focus seen on magnetic resonance imaging. (i) Interictal [^{15}O]H$_2$O PET shows decreased blood flow in the left frontal region. (ii) Near ictal FDG-PET showing decreased FDG uptake in the left frontal area. *(Courtesy of A. Gjedde, Århus University Hospital, Denmark.)*

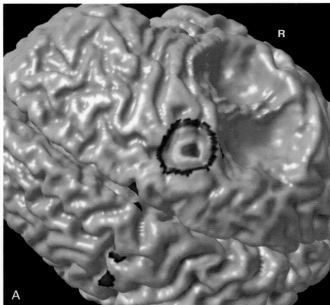

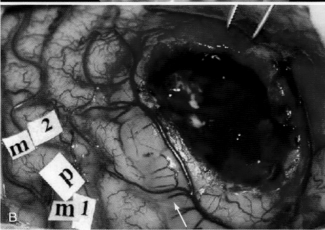

FIGURE 55-9 Large low-grade astrocytoma in the right hemisphere. **A,** Three-dimensional surface reconstruction from magnetic resonance imaging allowed informed consent for the patient and guidance for the neurosurgeon. **B,** m1 and m2, intraoperative cortical mapping showing the response of muscles in the left arm; p, positron emission tomography of the hand. (*Courtesy of S. Dyve and A. Rodell, Århus University Hospital, Denmark.*)

eloquent areas are mapped preoperatively and coregistered to the surgical navigational system. They aid in planning surgery and can serve as a basis for discussion with patients and families (Fig. 55-9).

MAGNETOENCEPHALOGRAPHY AND MAGNETIC SOURCE IMAGING IN THE PRESURGICAL EVALUATION FOR EPILEPSY

Fundamentals of Neuromagnetism

MEG measures the extracranial magnetic field activity arising from the electric currents produced in the brain. This activity arises largely from intracellular neuronal currents in the dendrites of tangentially oriented cortical pyramidal cells. MEG represents the magnetic signals corresponding to the brain's electrical activity recorded with standard EEG.[21-25] MEG is based on a fundamental principle of electromagnetism, namely, that for every electric current, there is a corresponding magnetic field. Applying the "right-hand rule" of electromagnetism, for every electric dipole, the corresponding magnetic field wraps around the dipole with the field flowing toward or away from the MEG detector in a counterclockwise fashion.[26] Much like its EEG counterpart, the majority of the magnetic signal produced by the brain arises from aligned groups of pyramidal cells in the six-layered cerebral cortex.[27] Because the detectors that measure the MEG signals are usually aligned perpendicular to the skull, MEG best detects the fields that arise from tangentially oriented current dipoles perpendicular to the cortical surface.[25,26,28,29]

The brain's magnetic fields are incredibly small, typically in the pico-tesla (10^{-12}) range. In contrast, the magnetic field activity of the earth itself is approximately 1 billion times (10^9) larger, ambient environmental sources such as room lighting and electric power lines are 10^5 to 10^6 times larger, and even those of the human heart are 10^2 times larger. SQUID detectors[2] must be used to measure these tiny magnetic fields (see elsewhere for further details[25,27]). These detectors are kept at very cold temperatures by bathing them in liquid helium in a magnetically shielded Dewar flask. Early MEG systems consisted of a single SQUID detector or small arrays of 3 to 7 detectors that were moved about the head to different positions during a recording session lasting several hours.[30] This would be equivalent to recording scalp EEG signals by moving a single EEG electrode from site to site on the scalp. Modern systems (Fig. 55-10A) consist of a whole-head helmet containing 36 to 240 or more detectors that simultaneously record MEG signals, again much the way that an EEG electrode montage records EEG signals from multiple brain sites simultaneously. These large sensor arrays allow recording of whole-brain activity, thereby providing excellent temporal and spatial resolution of brain activity.

As mentioned, the magnitude of the ambient environmental magnetic field is so large that it obliterates the ability to record MEG signals with even the most sensitive detectors. To overcome this obstacle, MEG is performed in a magnetically shielded room that essentially eliminates all environmental electric and magnetic fields. Unlike MRI unit shielding, which is designed to prevent magnetic fields from escaping the room, MEG shielding is designed to prevent magnetic activity from entering the room, thereby isolating the magnetic field to those generated by the patient alone. Similarly, the Dewar flask containing the MEG sensors and electronics is shielded. Because of the extremely specialized and sensitive equipment, the shielding requirements, and the need for cooling, MEG systems are extremely expensive to build and maintain, with typical costs exceeding $2 to $3 million. MEG studies are typically performed over a period of several hours or longer and require more analysis time than do MRI studies. MEG therefore has lower throughput than MRI, thus increasing the cost per study. This cost factor is a major limitation to the widespread availability of MEG in many epilepsy centers.

Magnetic Source Imaging

MEG signals are collected as traces of data much the way that EEG traces are collected. The majority of MEG data represent background brain activity and are of little clinical interest. However, MEG activity that is either provoked by a stimulus (evoked potential)[31-34] or arises from epileptiform spike activity is of primary interest. Identification of these evoked or spontaneous potentials is performed by off-line review of the individual MEG tracings. This requires manual review by an experienced technician or physician, or it can be done with automated spike detection algorithms.[35-37] Manual review with selection of spikes

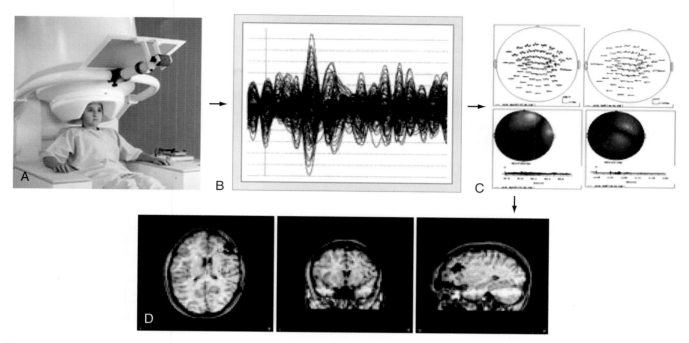

FIGURE 55-10 Generation of a magnetic source imaging (MSI) data set. **A,** A patient sits in the magnetoencephalography (MEG) unit with a whole-head array of "super-cooled" quantum interference device (SQUID) magnetometers enclosed in a helium-cooled casing. The casing contains an array of SQUID detectors and amplifying gradiometers to detect the MEG signals from each site on the scalp surface. **B,** After filtering, the raw MEG signals are collected as individual digital tracings and stored for off-line analysis. **C,** During off-line analysis, manual or automatic review of the data identifies individual interictal spikes or evoked potentials, and the tracings corresponding to each of these spikes are displayed on a traditional electroencephalogram-like spike map, with each tracing reflecting the amplitude and frequency of the signal recorded at each specific MEG sensor. Dipole source modeling is then applied. A computer algorithm finds a mathematical "solution" to the observed MEG pattern that represents the most likely location of the electric spike arising from a single source point in the brain. This is called the single equivalent dipole model. The topographic map for each dipole can be displayed, with *red* representing magnetic flux into the head and *blue* representing flux out of the head, and the electric dipole itself is oriented at right angles to the magnetic field by using the "right-hand rule" of electromagnetism. **D,** The individual dipoles, usually represented by *dots,* are then superimposed on a magnetic resonance image acquired after the MEG study and coregistered to the MEG detectors with fiducial markers. The result is a magnetic source imaging map of interictal spikes or evoked brain activity. Tight clustering of spikes in a single anatomic location seems to be most predictive of accurate localization of the ictal zone identified by intracranial electroencephalography.

is the most reliable and commonly used method. Automated detection programs often identify more artifactual spikes, so automatically detected spikes must be interpreted with some caution. Once a spike has been detected, the MEG tracings from all channels for the time period of that spike are displayed in the anatomic location of the sensor from which it was detected, thereby creating a "spike map." This map is then subjected to a process of dipole modeling in which various mathematical solutions are tested to identify the single best location for the current dipole that matches the pattern of MEG traces recorded around the brain. The most commonly used method is the "single equivalent dipole" (SED) model, in which it is assumed that any given pattern arises from a single brain area and that simultaneous spikes in distinct regions do not occur. More complex models involving other estimation methods, such as local minima, known anatomic features, and consideration of the skull as a multilayered structure with varying conductivities,[38-41] have been used more recently, although none have proved clearly superior in a clinical setting, and the SED model is the only Food and Drug Administration–approved algorithm for routine clinical use.

Once the MEG dipoles have been localized, they are superimposed on a brain MRI scan that has been coregistered to the MEG channels based on a set of fiducial markers to create a visual dipole map of the brain. This process is commonly referred to as magnetic source imaging (MSI) and represents the primary method by which MEG data are used in clinical and research settings. For most applications, the terms MEG and MSI are functionally interchangeable, although MSI is the preferred term for the complete process of data processing and display. An overview of this process is shown in Figure 55-10.

Magnetic fields are not significantly altered by passing in and out of the skull, whereas electric fields are "smeared" by conduction through the volume of the multilayered skull, analogous to the diffraction or bending of light going from air to water. Thus, localization with MSI is generally thought to be more spatially accurate and reliable than EEG source localization.[42] Recent investigations using more complex modeling methods are challenging this assumption, however.[43-45]

Uses of Magnetic Source Imaging

Early investigators saw that the clinical utility of MEG, for instance in comparison to EEG, would depend on the specific situation. Because MSI depends on the identification of event-specific spike activity, it is primarily useful for identifying the location of evoked brain activity or interictal epileptiform discharges. MSI has proved to be a highly reliable and reproducible method to identify and map the primary sensory cortex.[30,46-49] It can map the sensory homunculus with extreme precision and is superior to fMRI in this regard.[30,46,50-52] Similarly, MSI has been used to identify regions of receptive and expressive language.[53-57] These studies rely on the later component of the MEG signal in response to an evoked stimulus because the early component

(100 msec) represents activation of primary auditory cortex whereas the late component (150 to 700 msec) is specific to brain regions involved in language processing. Several language paradigms have been developed that primarily identify receptive language areas, and some groups have confirmed the results with intraoperative or intracranial EEG (ICEEG) language stimulation mapping. MSI has been proposed as an alternative to the intracarotid sodium amobarbital test for determining hemispheric language dominance.[57,58] Reliable reproduction of these methods has proved challenging, with significant patient-to-patient variability, although this method is promising. Because of the relative lack of availability of MSI and the inability to test for memory preservation, it is unlikely that MSI will supplant the intracarotid sodium amobarbital (Wada) test completely in the near future.

MSI has also been used as a method to identify brain regions involved in higher cortical functions such as visual and thought processing.[47,56] This application closely parallels work that has been carried out with fMRI- or EEG-based event-related potentials. Because MSI provides temporal resolution superior to that achieved with fMRI and measures neural activity rather than blood flow–related changes, it may be superior to fMRI for source localization. MSI has also been used in the study of psychiatric disorders.[59,60]

Epilepsy

Since its earliest introduction, a principal application of MSI has been to identify seizure foci.[33,61] In approximately 30% of patients, anticonvulsant medications cannot control their epilepsy, and about half of these patients are probably good candidates for seizure surgery. Focal excisional surgery has the highest chance of curing patients with intractable epilepsy, but it depends on accurate identification of the zone of seizure origin. The use of ICEEG monitoring with depth electrodes and subdural or epidural grid electrodes has resulted in a 36% increase in the number of patient who can benefit from seizure surgery. However, ICEEG monitoring is invasive, carries major surgical risks, and is time-consuming. The principal advantage of prolonged ICEEG monitoring is capture of stereotypic seizures on EEG and localization of the zone of origin with great precision. Although MSI can record true ictal events,[49,61-64] this is relatively rare because of the practical limitations of prolonged recording in an MEG unit. MSI does routinely capture interictal epileptiform discharges ("spikes"), which represent spontaneous brain irritability and often originate near the zone of seizure origin.[36,58,65-68] Thus, MSI has been used to identify the ictal zone indirectly and to help guide the placement of ICEEG electrodes for definitive identification of the ictal onset region.[36,45,51,58,65-68]

The accuracy of MEG localization has best been validated by studies comparing MEG spikes with simultaneously recorded ICEEG. These studies have demonstrated that a 2- to 4-cm^2 region (two to three EEG contacts on a standard grid) on the cortical surface must be activated to detect an MEG spike[69] and greater than a 6-cm^2 region for spikes in the basal temporal lobe.[70] Controlled studies with implanted dipoles have demonstrated that MEG-identified localizations were within about 1 to 2 cm of the true location, with greater errors for deeper sources.[71] For afterdischarge spikes recorded simultaneously on ICEEG with implanted subdural grids, MEG localization was within 12 mm[72] for lateral temporal spikes but up to 4 cm away for mesial temporal source spikes.[73] The large amount of tissue that must be activated on the medial temporal lobe indicates that few MSI spikes will reflect activation of the mesial temporal lobe or other deep structures, and therefore the MSI results are limited to regions that can be accurately sampled, namely, detection and localization of spikes close to the dorsolateral cortical surface. This does not mean that MEG has no predictive value for mesial

frontal or temporal lobe epilepsy but simply that the source localizations cannot be relied on to identify the ictal zone with the same confidence that can be applied in dorsolateral neocortical cases.

MESIAL TEMPORAL LOBE EPILEPSY

Mesial temporal lobe epilepsy originates from deep structures such as the amygdala and hippocampus, which are situated at least 3 to 4 cm below the cortical surface. Because of the intrinsic limitation of MEG for detecting such deep sources, MEG/MSI has not proved to be particularly useful for accurately identifying these deep sources.[74] However, correlative studies have implicated the orientation of the MEG dipoles as a potential predictor of outcome after temporal lobe surgery. In one study, correlation with ICEEG demonstrated that patients with vertically oriented anterior temporal dipoles tended to have mesial temporal seizure onsets whereas those with horizontally oriented dipoles had more basal or temporal polar origins.[65,75] Posterior vertically oriented dipoles were strongly correlated with lateral temporal lobe (neocortical) onset. This study suggests that dipole orientations are of greater value than actual dipole localization for temporal lobe epilepsy. Other studies have suggested that patients with more than 70% of the MEG spikes localized to the anterior temporal lobe are much more likely to become seizure free after lobectomy than are patients with spikes in the posterior temporal lobe.[76]

NEOCORTICAL EPILEPSY

The application of MSI to epilepsy has been best studied in patients with neocortical epilepsy. Because most neocortical epilepsy arises from sources on the surface or perisylvian area, their shallow location is ideal for detection by MEG. Several groups have reported their experiences and clinical outcomes with MEG for detection of neocortical seizure zones by comparing the findings with ictal localization by ICEEG or seizure outcome after resection (or both). For example, a study of 11 children with neocortical epilepsy demonstrated that the principal anatomic location of the MSI spikes correlated with the ictal onset zone determined by ICEEG grids in 10 of 11 children, with 9 of 11 experiencing a greater than 90% reduction in seizures after resection.[77] Similar studies have provided similar conclusions, namely, that presurgical MSI data generally correlate with the zone of seizure origin as determined by ICEEG or by seizure-free outcomes.[49,78-83] However, the majority of these studies have a sample size of 4 or fewer patients, are retrospective in nature, and do not define the exact role of MSI in the evaluation of a patient with epilepsy. It is not clear whether the MSI data altered the treatment plan, resulted in better localization, or had an impact on surgical resection. It is also not clear from the majority of these studies whether MSI supplies novel, nonredundant data or whether it truly has an effect on surgical decision making or outcome. In fact, a recent systematic review indicated that the currently available medical literature does not clearly support a causal relationship between the use of MSI and improved seizure-free outcomes in patients with intractable epilepsy.[45]

More recent, larger series have attempted to better define the exact role and utility of MSI in neocortical epilepsy. Mamelak and colleagues evaluated the correlation between MSI spike density and ICEEG ictal localization.[51] In 23 patients undergoing MSI and then ICEEG, ICEEG correctly identified the zone of seizure origin in 16 (70%). MSI demonstrated a pattern of densely clustered spikes, and the zone of seizure origin was localized to the same lobe as the MSI spikes in all cases. In contrast, when a dense clustering pattern was not observed, ICEEG failed to localize the zone of seizure origin. In 3 patients (8%) MEG provided novel localization information not available from other presurgical modalities that had a direct impact on the surgical outcome by altering electrode placement. These findings suggest that when MSI demonstrates tightly clustered dipoles, there is a high probability that ICEEG will correctly localize a zone of seizure origin and portend a subsequent good surgical outcome. In contrast, when MSI demonstrates diffuse spikes, the chances of discrete localization with ICEEG are low. In this regard, MSI may be useful for excluding poor surgical candidates and confirming good surgical candidates to yield better overall surgical results.

A similar study was performed in 22 children with normal MRI findings who underwent resective surgery.[84] In this series, 77% of the children had a good (Engel class IIA or better) outcome, but only 36% of them became seizure free. Analysis of this subgroup indicated that all seizure-free patients had a tight cluster of MSI dipoles in the resection area as determined by ICEEG. In contrast, freedom from seizures was not achieved in any patient who had bilateral MSI dipole clusters. When the MSI cluster was confined to fewer than five adjacent electrodes by ICEEG, all patients became seizure free, in contrast to the 7 patients in whom the MSI cluster extended beyond five electrodes. Other studies have confirmed that when 90% of the MSI spikes occur in one focal area, this overlaps the seizure zone and predicts a good outcome.[85,86] Taken as a whole, these studies suggest that MSI is valuable for predicting the ability of ICEEG to identify a resectable seizure focus but do not indicate that MSI can be used as a substitute for ICEEG to identify a seizure focus. Furthermore, these data indicate that if MSI spikes are diffusely distributed rather than tightly grouped, the seizure zone is far less likely to be correctly identified, and a seizure-free outcome after resection is much less likely.

Only recently have prospective, blinded, crossover, controlled clinical studies of MSI in epilepsy been conducted. Knowlton and associates evaluated 49 patients who completed both MSI and ICEEG studies in a prospective "intent-to-treat" design.[87] All patients were initially selected for ICEEG coverage by a consensus surgical conference, only after which the results of the MSI studies were made available. MSI data could be used only to supplement surgical coverage, but not alter it. Patients were then evaluated for seizure outcome, as well as the ability of MSI and ICEEG to localize the seizure focus. Based on their analysis, which included 55% of patients with neocortical epilepsy and 37% with medial temporal lobe epilepsy, they determined that MSI had a positive predictive value of 82% to 90% for seizure localization when compared with ICEEG localization. Of note, they included several epilepsy patients with completely negative ICEEG studies who still had successful surgery based on concordant data from other modalities. Thus, some of the patients underwent surgical resection based on concordant noninvasive data without identification of the ictal zone by ICEEG. These data do not indicate that MSI spike localization was accurate enough to be used for tailored neocortical resection, so MSI cannot be used in place of ICEEG for neocortical epilepsy. The general consensus remains that MSI is not sufficiently accurate at present to replace ICEEG for identification of the seizure focus.

A more recent study by Sutherling and coworkers evaluated 69 patients being evaluated for potential ICEEG studies in a prospective, blinded, basic "intent-to-treat" design.[88] Like the study by Knowlton and associates, a consensus surgical decision was made on the basis of preoperative data that excluded MSI. Once the surgical decision was made, the MSI data were disclosed to the conference attendees, and a new consensus decision was made. The subsequent analysis determined whether MSI changed the initial surgical decision and, if so, in what fashion. Additional features of this study versus the previous Knowlton study were the basic intention-to-treat approach and the ability to reduce or avoid ICEEG, as well as to add electrodes. MSI provided nonredundant information in 23 patients (33%). Incorporation of MSI

data into the surgical decision making resulted in the addition of electrodes in 9 patients (13%) and changed the surgical decision in 14 (20%). Sixteen patients (23%) were scheduled for ICEEG coverage that differed from that decided before the inclusion of MSI data. Twenty-six completed ICEEG and 30 completed resection or vagus nerve stimulator implantation, including 15 patients for whom MSI changed the decision. Additional electrodes placed in 4 patients covered the correct lobe in 3 and the sublobar ictal onset zone in 2. The addition of MSI data avoided contralateral electrodes in 2 patients. In 9 patients in whom MSI changed the decision and who had adequate postresection follow-up, it was determined that the MSI data contributed to improved outcomes in 3 patients. These data indicate that MSI can provide nonredundant, useful interictal localization information in approximately a third of patients undergoing work-up for neocortical epilepsy and that it affects outcome in approximately 26% of these patients without any increase in complications. This study shows the utility of MSI in the presurgical evaluation of the subset of patients with suspected neocortical epilepsy, principally by improving the yield of ICEEG. Like previous studies, it also indicated that MSI localizations cannot be used to perform tailored neocortical resections.

Landau-Kleffner Syndrome

Landau-Kleffner syndrome (LKS) is characterized by regression of language skills in children with previously normal development. LKS is caused by seizures arising from the perisylvian language cortex. Identification of LKS and treatment with either anticonvulsant agents or surgery can result in reversal of the symptoms. Because of the location of seizures arising from the perisylvian region, MSI has proved to be a very useful tool for identification of patients with LKS because it is better suited than EEG to identify interictal spikes arising from this location.[89,90] In light of this, MSI is recommended for the evaluation of all patients suspected of having LKS.

Conclusions Regarding the Use of Magnetic Source Imaging for the Presurgical Evaluation of Epilepsy

Based on the observations presented, we believe that MSI should be performed on all patients with suspected complex partial neocortical epilepsy for whom surgical resection is being considered, especially those without obvious structural lesions on MRI. Although MSI is not a mandatory test for the evaluation of mesial temporal lobe epilepsy or generalized epilepsies, MSI data can be used to help determine appropriate ICEEG coverage or to potentially avoid proceeding with ICEEG coverage altogether, but at present it should not be used to define a resection volume.

The Future of Magnetic Source Imaging

Unlike EEG, MRI, or even PET, MSI has not yet been proved to be an essential component of the presurgical evaluation of the majority of patients with intractable epilepsy. Certainly it has not been proved to be able to replace ICEEG, one of the main hopes for MSI when it was first developed. Even though multiple reports indicate the potential utility of MSI for the presurgical evaluation of epilepsy, the long-term future of routine MSI remains uncertain for several reasons. First, MSI is a very expensive technology that costs in the range of several million dollars, in addition to the need for considerable technical expertise with relatively low patient throughput. It is possible that improved EEG source and head modeling may be able to accomplish similar goals as MSI at a fraction of the cost.[91,92] Second, MSI, unlike long-term EEG or ICEEG, does not typically record seizures, but rather a limited sample of interictal spikes, which may correlate with the seizure focus but do not clearly define it. In the absence of true ictal recordings, MSI will remain predominantly a concordant rather than a definitive tool for seizure localization. Finally, for a technology to be of utility, it should provide information that is not available with other methods. Far less expensive and more widely available technologies such as ictal SPECT, PET, MRS, and MRI often provide concordant data that are as useful as those provided by MSI. Because MSI has excellent temporal resolution, it is likely to remain nonredundant for the foreseeable future. However, technology that provides novel information in about 33% of cases but is economically prohibitive may not remain a viable option in the long run unless more efficient use is made of this technology by referring a larger number of patients to a limited number of centers.

Summary

At present, MSI appears to be useful in about 30% to 50% of patients with neocortical epilepsy and has been demonstrated to affect seizure outcomes in about 5% to 10% of patients in studies to date. MSI provides significant predictive value to indicate whether neocortical resection based on ICEEG will be successful, but it cannot be used as a substitute for ICEEG ictal zone localization. It may be used to eliminate poor candidates for ICEEG, thereby avoiding surgery.

MSI is very useful for mapping the primary sensory cortex and for identification of language sites. The spatial resolution of MSI for these mapping tasks appears to be superior to that of fMRI. With further refinement, MSI may replace the intracarotid sodium amobarbital (Wada) test for determining hemispheric dominance. MSI will probably continue to enjoy increased use in human neurophysiology and psychology experiments involving higher cortical function. The high cost and limited availability of MSI units, especially when compared with the widespread availability of fMRI, may prove a decisive factor in determining which of these technologies becomes the standard for noninvasive brain mapping of cortical function.

ICTAL SINGLE-PHOTON EMISSION COMPUTED TOMOGRAPHY FOR DEFINITION OF THE SEIZURE ONSET ZONE

Partial or localization-related epilepsy is characterized by recurrent and unprovoked focal seizure activity and is the most common seizure disorder.[93-95] More than 90% of the incident cases of epilepsy in adults involve focal seizures. Individuals with partial epilepsy may experience focal sensory, focal motor (including temporal lobe automatisms), or secondarily generalized seizures. Approximately 30% to 40% of patients with newly diagnosed epilepsy will experience medically refractory seizures that are physically and socially disabling.[93] A minority of patients who fail to respond to the initial antiepileptic drug regimen will be rendered seizure free with "newer" medical treatments.[96-98] Epilepsy surgery is an effective and safe form of therapy for selected patients with intractable localization-related epilepsy.[93,94,99-104] Patients with mesiobasal limbic epilepsy and focal seizures related to foreign tissue lesional pathology may be favorable candidates for epilepsy surgery. Patients with these surgically remediable epileptic syndromes almost invariably experience a significant reduction in seizure tendency after focal cortical resection and excision of the pathologic findings underlying the epileptogenic zone.[94,99,100] The majority of these patients experience a significant reduction in seizure tendency after surgical ablation of the epileptic brain tissue.[99-108] The hallmark pathology of medial temporal lobe epilepsy is mesial temporal sclerosis.[106,108-110] The surgically excised hippocampus in these patients almost invariably shows focal cell loss and gliosis.[105,106,108-110] Patients with lesional epilepsy may have a primary brain tumor, vascular anomaly, or a malformation of cortical development (MCD).[102,103,106,107,110] The common surgical pathologies encountered in patients with lesional epilepsy include low-grade glial neoplasm, cavernous hemangioma, and focal cortical dysplasia.[102,103] Individuals with mesial temporal sclerosis and lesional pathology usually have abnormal findings on structural MRI, and the seizure types are classified as *substrate-directed partial epilepsy*.[94,102,110-112] MRI in these individuals may detect a specific intra-axial structural abnormality that may suggest the probable site of seizure onset and the surgical pathology.[112] MRI has a pivotal role in the selection and evaluation of patients for alternative forms of therapy.[99,102,105,108-110]

The rationale for presurgical evaluation is to identify the site of ictal onset and initial seizure propagation (i.e., the epileptogenic zone) and determine the probable pathologic findings underlying the epileptic brain tissue.[104,105] In patients with an MRI-identified foreign tissue lesion or unilateral mesial temporal sclerosis, the purpose of electroclinical correlation is essentially to confirm the epileptogenicity of the structural abnormality.[105,107,108,110] Demonstration of concordance between the pathologic substrate and the ictal onset zone indicates a highly favorable operative outcome in selected individuals. Approximately 80% of patients with unilateral mesial temporal sclerosis, a low-grade glial neoplasm, or a cavernous hemangioma are rendered seizure free after surgical treatment.[94,99,103,105-108,110] More than 90% of patients with these pathologic findings will experience an excellent surgical outcome (i.e., auras only or rare nondisabling seizures).[99] The operative outcome is distinctly less favorable in individuals with focal cortical dysplasia and other MCDs.[111] The most common operative strategy in patients with intractable partial epilepsy involves focal cortical resection of the epileptogenic zone with excision of the surgical pathology.[102,103] The goals of surgical treatment are to render the individual seizure free and allow the patient to become a participating and productive member of society.[93,94,101]

NON–SUBSTRATE-DIRECTED PARTIAL EPILEPSY

The seizure types in patients with localization-related seizure disorders and normal findings on MRI are classified as *non–substrate-directed partial epilepsy*.[112] The anatomic location of the epileptogenic zone in these individuals commonly involves the neocortex (i.e., extrahippocampal).[110,112] The most frequent site of seizure onset in patients with neocortical nonlesional partial epilepsy is the frontal lobe.[107,110] The surgical pathology in these patients includes gliosis, focal cell loss, MCD, or no histopathologic alteration.[110] MRI may rarely be indeterminate in selected lesional pathology, such as focal cortical dysplasia.[112] Only a minority of patients with neocortical, extratemporal seizures are rendered seizure free after surgical treatment.[107,110] An estimated 20% to 30% of these patients with extratemporal, mainly frontal lobe seizures will enter seizure remission after focal cortical resection.[110] An important reason for the unfavorable operative outcome in patients with non–substrate-directed partial epilepsy is the inherent difficulty in identifying the epileptogenic zone.[110] The potential limitations of interictal and ictal extracranial EEG and ICEEG monitoring in patients with partial seizures of extratemporal origin have been well defined.[110] The anatomic region of seizure onset may represent a continuum in these patients that lends itself to incomplete focal resection of the epileptogenic zone. A large resection increases the likelihood of rendering the patient seizure free, but it also increases the potential for operative morbidity.[110,112] Advances in peri-ictal imaging (see later) have assisted in the selection of operative candidates with non–substrate-directed partial epilepsy, altered the preoperative evaluation, and tailored the surgical excision.[113-118]

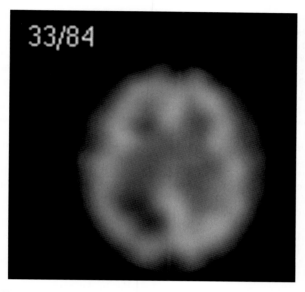

FIGURE 55-11 Interictal single-photon emission computed tomography in a patient with a remote right parietal lobe hemorrhage shows a region of hypoperfusion corresponding to the previous hematoma. (*Note:* The right side of the brain is on the *left* side of the figure.)

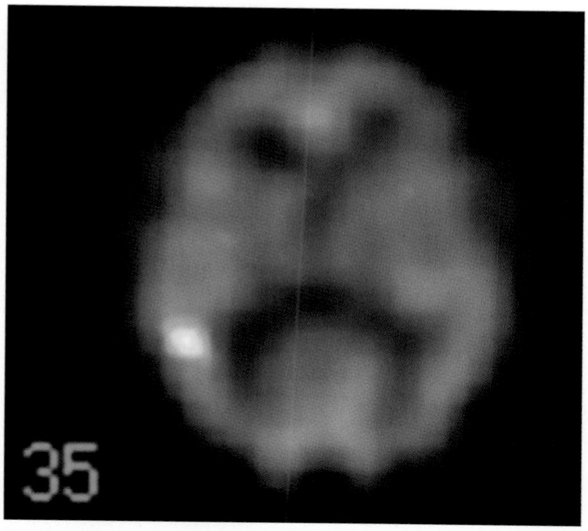

FIGURE 55-12 Peri-ictal single-photon emission computed tomography in this patient shows a region of hyperperfusion adjacent to the area of focal necrosis. (*Note:* The right side of the brain is on the *left* side of the figure.)

SINGLE-PHOTON EMISSION COMPUTED TOMOGRAPHY

SPECT is most appropriate for peri-ictal imaging in patients with partial epileptic syndromes being considered for epilepsy surgery.[113,117,119-129] There is a broad consensus that ictal SPECT studies are superior to interictal images (Fig. 55-11) in localization-related epilepsy.[117,119,120] SPECT studies involve CBF imaging with radiopharmaceuticals, principally either technetium 99m-hexamethylpropyleneamine oxime (^{99m}Tc-HMPAO) or ^{99m}Tc-bicisate, that have rapid first-pass brain extraction, with maximum uptake being achieved within 30 to 60 seconds of an intravenous injection.[113,119-121,126] These studies may produce a "photograph" of the peri-ictal cerebral perfusion pattern that was present soon after the injection (Fig. 55-12).[121] SPECT images can be acquired up to 4 hours after termination of the seizure so that the individual patient can recover from the ictus before being transported to the nuclear medicine laboratory. SPECT studies have an important clinical application in potential identification of epileptic brain tissue when the remainder of the noninvasive presurgical evaluation is unable to lateralize or localize the site of seizure onset.[121]

The initial blood flow SPECT studies in patients with intractable partial epilepsy involved interictal imaging, which variably detected focal *hypoperfusion* in the region of the epileptogenic zone (see Fig. 55-11).[114] Interictal SPECT images have proved to have low sensitivity and a relatively high false-positive rate in patients with temporal lobe epilepsy.[114] Interictal SPECT has also been shown to have a low diagnostic yield in patients with extratemporal seizures.[117] Ictal SPECT studies have been confirmed to be useful in patients with temporal lobe epilepsy for identification of a region of focal *hyperperfusion*.[117] The rationale for interictal SPECT at present is to serve as a reference baseline study for interpretation of the ictal SPECT images. The diagnostic yield of ictal SPECT has been established to be superior to that of interictal SPECT in patients being considered for surgical ablation procedures. The recent development of stabilized radiotracers that do not require mixing immediately before injection, such as ^{99m}Tc-bicisate, has made ictal SPECT more practical in patients with extratemporal seizures, which are often

not associated with an aura and may have a shorter seizure duration.[126] A potential limitation of ictal SPECT is that the spatial resolution of these studies is inferior to that of PET.[114]

SUBTRACTION ICTAL SINGLE-PHOTON EMISSION COMPUTED TOMOGRAPHY COREGISTERED TO MAGNETIC RESONANCE IMAGING

An imaging paradigm using computer-aided subtraction ictal SPECT coregistered to MRI (SISCOM) has been introduced in patients with intractable partial epilepsy.[113,121-129] SISCOM is a recent innovation in neuroimaging that may be useful in the evaluation of patients with non–substrate-directed partial epilepsy. The localized alteration in blood flow demonstrated with SISCOM may be intimately associated with the epileptogenic zone[121] (Figs. 55-13 and 55-14). Subtracting normalized and coregistered ictal and interictal SPECT images and then matching the resultant difference in images to high-resolution MRI for anatomic correlation has been shown to be a reliable indicator of localization of the epileptogenic zone in patients with localization-related epilepsy.[122-125] The technique used at the Mayo Clinic that was introduced by O'Brien and colleagues has compared favorably with traditional visual analysis of the interictal and ictal images.[121] SISCOM in a series of 51 patients had a higher rate of localization (88.2% versus 39.2%, $P < .0001$), had better interobserver agreement, and was a better predictor of surgical outcome than visual inspection of the interictal and ictal images.[121] The study demonstrated the inherent problems with visual interpretation of either peri-ictal or interictal SPECT studies alone.

The methodology used for SISCOM at the Mayo Clinic involves coregistering the interictal and the ictal SPECT study by matching the surface points on the cerebral binary images of the two procedures.[122,125,126] The normalized interictal image is subtracted from the normalized ictal image to derive the difference (subtraction) in CBF related to the partial seizure. Thresholding of the subtraction image to display only the pixels with intensities greater than 2 standard deviations (SD) above zero is

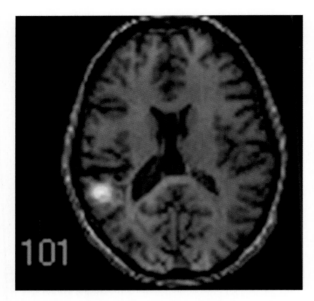

FIGURE 55-13 Subtracted peri-ictal single-photon emission computed tomography coregistered to structural magnetic resonance imaging (SISCOM) in the axial plane reveals a localized SISCOM focus.

performed. Finally, images with intensities greater than 2 SD are coregistered to the structural MRI scan. After the implantation of subdural electrodes for chronic ICEEG monitoring, the electrode positions can be segmented from a spiral CT scan and coregistered to the SISCOM image.[123] This allows determination of the relationship between the localized alteration in peri-ictal blood flow and the ictal onset zone.

The SISCOM region of alteration in blood flow is a surrogate for localization of the epileptogenic zone independent of the pathologic finding.[128] Clinical parameters that are significant in determining the diagnostic yield of SISCOM include the

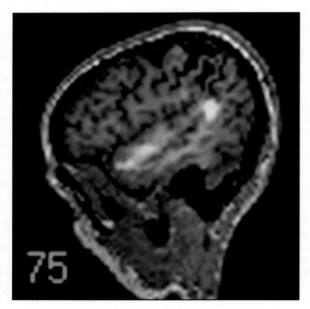

FIGURE 55-14 Subtracted peri-ictal single-photon emission computed tomography coregistered to structural magnetic resonance imaging (SISCOM) in the sagittal plane reveals a localized SISCOM focus in the right lateral temporal region reflecting seizure propagation.

duration of the seizure and the length of time from ictal onset to injection.[113,121] The seizure should be at least 5 to 10 seconds in duration, and the time after seizure onset should be less than 45 seconds.[121] The SISCOM findings also correlate with the operative outcome. Patients with a SISCOM alteration concordant with the epileptogenic zone are most likely to experience a significant re-education in seizure tendency if the focal cortical resection includes the region of change in peri-ictal blood flow.[121,128] Disadvantages of a SISCOM study include the need for hospitalization and long-term EEG monitoring, the use of radioisotopes for two imaging procedures, and the required presence of habitual seizure activity. Indications for SISCOM in patients undergoing presurgical evaluation include non–substrate-directed partial epilepsy and conflicting findings on noninvasive evaluation. SISCOM may be used to identify a "target" for the placement of ICEEG electrodes.[123] The presence of a SISCOM alteration may obviate the need for ICEEG recordings in selected patients. For example, patients with non–substrate-directed partial epilepsy of temporal lobe origin may not require chronic ICEEG monitoring if the extracranial ictal EEG pattern and peri-ictal SPECT studies are concordant. SISCOM also improves the diagnostic yield of postictal studies in patients with intractable partial epilepsy.[124]

The superiority of SISCOM in localizing the epileptogenic zone, particularly in extratemporal epilepsy, has previously been demonstrated.[128] The prognostic importance of the SISCOM *focus* in patients undergoing focal cortical resection for partial epilepsy of extratemporal origin has been evaluated.[128] O'Brien and colleagues in a previous series evaluated the operative outcomes of 36 patients with extratemporal epilepsy who underwent a SISCOM study before surgery.[128] The presence of a localizing SISCOM alteration concordant with the epileptogenic zone was a favorable predictor of an excellent surgical outcome ($P < .05$).[128] Eleven of 19 patients (57.9%) with a concordant SISCOM focus and 3 of 17 patients (17.6%) with a nonlocalizing or discordant SISCOM focus, respectively, were rendered seizure free or experienced only nondisabling seizures. Approximately three quarters of the patients with a localized SISCOM abnormality had normal structural MRI findings. In addition, this study demonstrated that the extent of resection of the SISCOM focus was also of prognostic importance ($P < .05$).[128] Failure to resect the neocortical region intimately associated with the localized change in blood flow concordant with the ictal onset zone was a predictor of an unfavorable operative outcome.[128]

CONCLUSION

The presurgical evaluation of patients with substrate-directed partial epilepsy is designed to determine the epileptogenicity of the alterations found on neuroimaging. The rationale for electrophysiologic studies is essentially *confirmatory* in patients with unilateral MRI-identified mesial temporal sclerosis or an isolated foreign tissue lesion. Video-EEG monitoring is performed in these individuals to confirm the diagnosis of a partial seizure disorder, establish the seizure type, and determine the disabling effect of the ictal behavior. Functional neuroimaging procedures may not be necessary in patients with medial temporal lobe epilepsy or lesional epilepsy in the presence of a structural MRI abnormality that is concordant with the remainder of the presurgical evaluation. Both MRS and PET have high diagnostic yield in patients with temporal lobe epilepsy. These techniques may be most useful in patients with indeterminate structural MRI studies, such as no intra-axial abnormality or bilateral hippocampal atrophy. In patients with non–substrate-directed partial epilepsy, there are significant concerns regarding localization of the epileptogenic zone. Chronic ICEEG monitoring may prove necessary in these patients, especially those with extratemporal epilepsy. Identification of a localized SISCOM focus may be a reliable indicator of the ictal onset zone. SISCOM may reveal a localized region of cerebral hyperperfusion or hypoperfusion in up to 80% of patients with intractable partial epilepsy. The SISCOM findings are also predictive of operative outcome. Ultimately, a decision regarding surgical treatment must be based on convergence of the neurodiagnostic evaluation. Electrophysiologic studies invariably need to be performed to localize the ictal onset zone in these patients. Resection of the SISCOM focus may be necessary to significantly reduce the seizure tendency in patients with a localized abnormality that is concordant with the epileptic brain tissue.

SUGGESTED READINGS

Assaf BA, Karkar KM, Laxer KD, et al. Magnetoencephalography source localization and surgical outcome in temporal lobe epilepsy. *Clin Neurophysiol.* 2004;115:2066.

Assaf BA, Karkar KM, Laxer KD, et al. Ictal magnetoencephalography in temporal and extratemporal lobe epilepsy. *Epilepsia.* 2003;44:1320.

Barkley GL. Controversies in neurophysiology. MEG is superior to EEG in localization of interictal epileptiform activity: Pro. *Clin Neurophysiol.* 2004;115:1001.

Barth DS. The neurophysiological basis of epileptiform magnetic fields and localization of neocortical sources. *J Clin Neurophysiol.* 1993;10:99.

Genow A, Hummel C, Scheler G, et al. Epilepsy surgery, resection volume and MSI localization in lesional frontal lobe epilepsy. *Neuroimage.* 2004;21:444.

Iwasaki M, Nakasato N, Shamoto H, et al. Surgical implications of neuromagnetic spike localization in temporal lobe epilepsy. *Epilepsia.* 2002;43:415.

Knake S, Halgren E, Shiraishi H, et al. The value of multichannel MEG and EEG in the presurgical evaluation of 70 epilepsy patients. *Epilepsy Res.* 2006;69:80.

Knowlton RC, Elgavish R, Howell J, et al. Magnetic source imaging versus intracranial electroencephalogram in epilepsy surgery: a prospective study. *Ann Neurol.* 2006;59:835.

Knowlton RC, Shih J. Magnetoencephalography in epilepsy. *Epilepsia.* 2004;45 (suppl 4):61.

Lau M, Yam D, Burneo JG. A systematic review on MEG and its use in the presurgical evaluation of localization-related epilepsy. *Epilepsy Res.* 2008;79:97.

Lee D, Sawrie SM, Simos PG, et al. Reliability of language mapping with magnetic source imaging in epilepsy surgery candidates. *Epilepsy Behav.* 2006;8:742.

Makela JP, Forss N, Jaaskelainen J, et al. Magnetoencephalography in neurosurgery. *Neurosurgery.* 2006;59:493.

Mamelak AN, Lopez N, Akhtari M, et al. Magnetoencephalography-directed surgery in patients with neocortical epilepsy. *J Neurosurg.* 2002;97:865.

Minassian B, Otsubo, H, Weiss, S, et al. Magnetoencephalographic localization in pediatric epilepsy surgery: comparison with invasive intracranial electroencephalography. *Ann Neurol.* 1999;46:627.

Morrell F, Whisler W, Smith M, et al. Landau-Kleffner syndrome: treatment with subpial intracortical transection. *Brain.* 1995;1:1529.

Nakamura A, Yamada T, Goto A, et al. Somatosensory homunculus as drawn by MEG. *Neuroimage.* 1998;7:377.

O'Brien TJ, So EL, Mullan BP, et al. Subtraction ictal SPECT co-registered to MRI improves clinical usefulness of SPECT in localizing the surgical seizure focus. *Neurology.* 1998:50:445.

Papanicolaou AC, Castillo EM, Billingsley-Marshall R, et al. A review of clinical applications of magnetoencephalography. *Int Rev Neurobiol.* 2005;68:223.

Papanicolaou AC, Simos PG, Castillo EM, et al. Magnetocephalography: a noninvasive alternative to the Wada procedure. *J Neurosurg.* 2004;100:867.

Ramachandran Nair R, Otsubo H, Shroff MM, et al. MEG predicts outcome following surgery for intractable epilepsy in children with normal or nonfocal MRI findings. *Epilepsia.* 2007;48:149.

Sato S, Balish M, Muratore R. Principles of magnetoencephalography. *J Clin Neurophysiol.* 1991;8:144.

Smith JR, King DW, Park YD, et al. A 10-year experience with magnetic source imaging in the guidance of epilepsy surgery. *Stereotact Funct Neurosurg.* 2003;80:14.

Sutherling WW, Crandall PH, Darcey TM, et al. The magnetic and electric fields agree with intracranial localizations of somatosensory cortex. *Neurology.* 1988;38:1705.

Sutherling W, Mamelak AN, Thyerlei D, et al. Influence of magnetic source imaging for planning intracranial EEG in epilepsy. *Neurology.* 2008;71:97.

Yoshinaga H, Ohtsuka Y, Watanabe Y, et al. Ictal MEG in two children with partial seizures. *Brain Dev.* 2004;26:403.

Full references can be found on Expert Consult @ www.expertconsult.com

CHAPTER 56

Evaluation of Patients for Epilepsy Surgery

Costas Michaelides ■ Garth Rees Cosgrove ■ Andrew J. Cole

Up to 40% of epilepsy patients have medication-resistant or medically intractable seizures.[1] As many as half of these patients may be candidates for curative or palliative epilepsy surgery. After successful epilepsy surgery, quality of life has been shown to improve significantly.[2] The degree of success of epilepsy surgery depends largely on careful presurgical evaluation for identification and selection of the most appropriate candidates. The evaluation usually takes place in centers with a dedicated multidisciplinary team of neurologists and neurosurgeons experienced in treating patients with epilepsy, supported by electroencephalographers, neuroradiologists, neuropsychologists, psychiatrists, and paramedical staff. The aim of this chapter is to review the key elements of the presurgical evaluation and to outline some of the principles used in the decision-making process for identification of appropriate candidates for epilepsy surgery.

INITIAL CONSIDERATIONS IN CHOOSING A CANDIDATE FOR PRESURGICAL EVALUATION

We apply three fundamental criteria to identify candidates for epilepsy surgery:

1. *The patient should have epilepsy that is refractory to standard medical treatment.* If the seizures can be controlled with medication that does not cause unacceptable side effects, epilepsy surgery is not necessary. Exceptions to this principle may occur in settings in which an obvious and accessible structural lesion is responsible for the epilepsy, especially when there are other reasons to pursue resection of the lesion, such as to reduce the risk for hemorrhage from a cavernous angioma or the need for tissue diagnosis of an apparent tumor. Operationally, intractability is typically defined as having persistent seizures after more than 2 years of working with a competent neurologist and failure of treatment (because of lack of efficacy, not lack of tolerability) with two or three major anticonvulsant drugs.
2. *The patient should have epilepsy that is disabling.* Importantly, determination of whether the epilepsy is disabling is, within reason, the province of the patient. Rare diurnal seizures may be disabling for some individuals, whereas frequent nocturnal seizures may be tolerable for others. Detailed inquiry into the impact of seizures on the individual is important in determining whether this criterion is satisfied.
3. *There must be a reasonable prospect that the patient's condition can be improved at an acceptable level of risk.* Satisfaction of this criterion is the responsibility of the epilepsy surgery team and ultimately the neurosurgeon before the decision to proceed to surgical resection.

In evaluating patients according to these three overarching criteria, it is important to note that intractable epilepsy is a progressive disorder that is medically, physically, and socially disabling.[3] Accidental injuries as a result of seizures, psychiatric morbidity, loss of independence attributable, in part, to the inability to drive, and chronic medication toxicity all have major impacts on the quality of life of affected individuals. Recognition of this situation has gradually led to earlier consideration of epilepsy surgery, although in many series the duration of refractory epilepsy before surgery still exceeds 10 to 15 years.[4]

Epilepsy surgery may be proposed as a curative treatment or as a palliative treatment. Curative procedures, aimed at focal epilepsy, are almost always resective and require clear and complete identification of the epileptogenic zone (EZ). The majority of epilepsy resections target the anterior temporal lobe, including the mesial structures, and are associated with a high rate of remission. By contrast, extratemporal foci, most commonly frontal, may present additional difficulties because the EZ may be difficult to fully delineate and may involve eloquent cortex. With high-resolution neuroimaging techniques and dedicated imaging protocols, extratemporal lesions such as small heterotopias, cavernous angiomas, and focal cortical dysplasias can be visualized in up to 50% of patients, thereby dramatically improving their chance for success after epilepsy surgery. Rates of long-term freedom from seizures after resection of extratemporal lesions have improved but may still be lower than those for temporal lobe resection.[5,6] In a recent meta-analysis, the median proportion of patients seizure free was 66% after temporal lobe resection, 46% after occipital or parietal resection, and 27% with frontal lobe resection.[7]

Palliative techniques include disconnection procedures and multiple subpial transections. Corpus callosotomy, typically performed as a two-stage procedure, may be helpful for patients with secondary generalized epilepsy syndromes and drop attacks.[8] The aim of this procedure is to primarily palliate patients with atonic seizures and improve their quality of life. This procedure may offer up to 35% freedom from the most disabling seizures.[7] Multiple subpial transections are thought to predominantly sever horizontal connections in the cortex while preserving columnar organization and efferent pathways.[9] This technique may be used in isolation for epileptic foci lying exclusively in eloquent cortex or as an adjunct along with partial resection to approach EZs that cannot be fully removed.

Evaluation of patients for consideration of epilepsy surgery includes a careful clinical history and physical examination, neuroimaging, and electroencephalographic (EEG) monitoring, often supplemented with detailed neuropsychological testing and psychiatric assessment when appropriate. The goal is to assess the concordance of multiple streams of data with respect to the probable EZ. Although the precise steps in the investigation vary somewhat from center to center, there is general consensus on the approach. Investigations are typically considered in phases. In general, phase I includes noninvasive recording, whereas phase II involves invasive intracranial EEG monitoring. Importantly, the investigation is an iterative process of hypothesis testing in which the results from each modality inform the interrogation of others. For example, identification of high-amplitude focal spikes on an EEG recording may prompt renewed scrutiny of magnetic resonance imaging (MRI) scans in the suspect area, thereby revealing a subtle developmental abnormality or vascular lesion (Fig. 56-1).

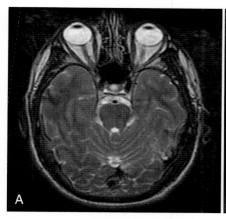
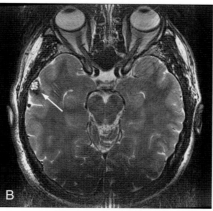

FIGURE 56-1 Cryptic cavernous angioma. Axial T2-weighted fast spin echo magnetic resonance images without (**A**) and with (**B**) phased-array surface coils. The initial scans (**A**) appeared unremarkable. Frequent interictal spikes at T4 led to rescanning with high-resolution phased-array surface coils. The resultant images (**B**) revealed a previously overlooked mulberry lesion (*arrow*) characteristic of a cavernous angioma. On review, subtle susceptibility artifact in the same region is apparent on the original scan.

PHASE I—NONINVASIVE INVESTIGATIONS

History and Physical Examination

Even in the age of modern neuroimaging, a thorough clinical history and physical examination may provide important clues regarding the etiology and location of the EZ. Specific auras such as experiential phenomena and somatomotor or somatosensory experiences may implicate specific areas of the brain. Symptoms at seizure onset, during progression, and after completion of the seizure can also offer lateralizing and localizing clues. For example, manual automatisms are frequently ipsilateral to the seizure focus, whereas ictal and postictal aphasia is typically associated with disease in the dominant hemisphere. Important features found on physical examination may include stigmata of a neurocutaneous syndrome such as tuberous sclerosis or neurofibromatosis; asymmetry of the size of the face, hand, or fingernails, which implies an insult to the contralateral hemisphere early in life; and of course focal findings on neurological examination. Although many patients may describe simple partial seizures, complex partial seizures, and secondarily generalized events as three different seizure types, from the perspective of localization they may each represent varying degrees of seizure propagation. Two or more fundamentally distinct semiologies, however, should alert one to the possibility of multifocal epilepsy.

Routine Electroencephalographic Recording

Although the value of routine outpatient EEG studies in the decision-making process for consideration of epilepsy surgery is limited in comparison to that of other tests such as prolonged video-EEG monitoring and neuroimaging, its usefulness in the diagnosis of epilepsy and elucidation of the underlying syndrome is invaluable.[10] Routine EEG findings are positive in 50% to 60% of patients with epilepsy, and the yield is increased by repeated or prolonged recordings that sample drowsiness and sleep. Even though focal slowing may signify an underlying structural abnormality, the major utility of routine EEG recordings is in the identification of interictal epileptiform discharges (IEDs) (sharp waves, spikes, or spike and wave complexes).[11] Routine EEG studies aim to answer certain key questions: (1) Are there any IEDs present, and if so, how frequent are they? (2) Are the IEDs diagnostic of an idiopathic generalized syndrome that would render the patient inappropriate for resective epilepsy surgery? (3) If not, are the IEDs confined to one hemisphere or are they bilateral? (4) If the IEDs are unilateral, are they confined to one area of the hemisphere, such as the temporal region, or are they

multifocal? The ideal surgical candidate would typically have a single population of well-localized IEDs, thus supporting the presence of only one EZ.

Continuous Video-Electroencephalographic Recording

Continuous computer-assisted video-EEG monitoring has become the mainstay of localization of the zone of epileptogenesis. The goals of video-EEG recording are threefold: (1) to further characterize the interictal EEG recording; (2) to detect, characterize, and quantify the patient's habitual seizures[12]; and (3) to acquire physiologic data regarding seizure localization that can be correlated and compared with anatomic data obtained from neuroimaging studies. These investigations typically occur over a 5- to 7-day inpatient hospital stay (for adults) but are obviously dependent on seizure frequency and last as long as required to capture a satisfactory number of seizures.[13,14] Characterizing the patient's seizures is crucial because it allows (1) correlation of the ictal behavior with the electrographic discharge, (2) establishment of whether a patient has more than one seizure type, and (3) lateralization (which hemisphere) and localization (which area of the hemisphere) of the onset of seizures and therefore identification of the EZ. Typically, activating procedures such as sleep deprivation are used in addition to reduction or cessation of antiepileptic drugs in an attempt to increase the likelihood of seizure occurrence. In patients with nonlesional mesial temporal epilepsy, statistical analysis indicates that five concordant seizures will yield a 95% chance that the patient's epilepsy is well lateralized (i.e., there is less than a 5% chance that five events would arise from the same side by chance alone).[15] In addition to lateralization and localization, video-EEG recording of clinical seizures allows assessment of the temporal relationship between behavioral and electrical seizure onset. Prolonged delay before the first appearance of ictal EEG discharge should raise suspicion that the scalp recording may represent propagated activity from a remote site of onset.

Imaging of the Epileptogenic Zone

Brain MRI is the neuroimaging modality of choice for the presurgical evaluation of patients for epilepsy surgery. Hippocampal sclerosis, the most common pathology associated with temporal lobe epilepsy, is diagnosed on MRI by identification of all or some of the elements of volume loss, increased T2 signal, and loss of normal internal architecture in the affected hippocampus. Although fluid-attenuated inversion recovery (FLAIR) imaging

FIGURE 56-2 Malformation of cortical development. Axial fluid-attenuated inversion recovery (**A**) and coronal T2-weighted fast spin echo (**B**) magnetic resonance images demonstrate subtle transmantle cortical dysplasia (*arrow*) in the right parasagittal convexity that corresponded to the patient's report of tingling in his left thigh at seizure onset. Note the subtle blurring of the gray-white junction, seen best in panel **B**.

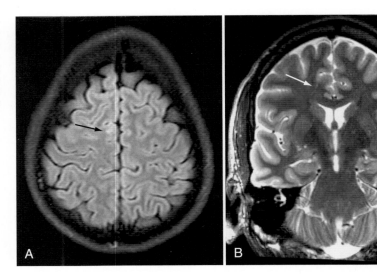

makes signal abnormalities most obvious, true T2-weighted fast spin echo (FSE) sequences provide optimal signal-to-noise ratios for the examination of volume and architecture. In some centers, quantitative image analysis techniques may be used to calculate the volume of the hippocampi to detect subtle asymmetries[16]; however, useful deployment of these tools is labor and resource intensive and requires a high level of technical skill and experience. In addition to hippocampal sclerosis, specific MRI epilepsy protocols involving T1-, T2-, and susceptibility-weighted sequences are used to identify congenital and acquired epileptogenic lesions, most commonly low-grade gliomas, dysembryoplastic neuroepithelial tumors, malformations of cortical development (MCDs), cavernous angiomas, and subtle posttraumatic encephalomalacia and ulegyria. Many MCDs are subtle and best appreciated by looking for blurring of the gray-white junction on high-resolution MRI (Fig. 56-2). Excellent anatomic definition of the gray-white junction is now possible with phased-array surface coils deployed in magnets with high field strength, now up to 7 T.[17]

Functional imaging with positron emission tomography (PET) and single-photon emission computed tomography (SPECT) offers information about ictal or interictal brain tissue metabolism. PET using [18F]fluorodeoxyglucose (FDG) typically shows regional hypometabolism around the EZ when the tracer is injected interictally. PET was therefore a very useful tool for lateralization in patients with temporal lobe epilepsy or for identification of extratemporal EZs, such as MCDs,[18] in the era before the development of high-resolution MRI scanning.[19] Recently, however, with the increasing anatomic definition offered by MRI, the number of patients with partial epilepsy and seemingly normal MRI findings has decreased. As a result, the value of PET in this respect has also decreased. Nevertheless, it remains a useful tool for verification of MRI and EEG findings and in patients with normal findings on MRI. Other tracers such as [11C]-flumazenil show comparable results to FDG, but with a more restricted distribution of hypometabolism, which may be advantageous, particularly with extratemporal EZs.[20]

SPECT images are generated by photons emitted after the intravenous injection of a radioactive isotope such as technetium 99m-hexamethylpropyleneamine oxime (99mTc-HMPAO). The isotope is taken up by brain tissue in proportion to blood flow. Therefore, when injected within the first few seconds of a partial seizure, it shows increased uptake in the area of highest blood flow. This *ictal* SPECT is then compared with a baseline *interictal* study from the same patient to detect the differences in regional perfusion. This allows identification of the area hyperperfused at the time of seizure onset. The main disadvantage of ictal SPECT

is that injection of the isotope has to be performed within the first few seconds after seizure onset, which is often impractical. The advantage, however, is that after injection, the window for scanning the patient is a few hours. SPECT can also be coregistered to MRI for better anatomic correlation of the EZ, and this can be used both for guidance of intracranial electrode placement and for subsequent surgical resection in a technique called subtraction ictal SPECT coregistered to MRI (SISCOM).[21]

Functional MRI (fMRI) images the blood oxygen level–dependent T2 signal (BOLD or T2*), a method whereby changes in metabolism and blood flow during an active process such as a simple motor or sensory task are detected. It has two roles in the identification of candidates for epilepsy surgery. fMRI is frequently used to map eloquent cortex during the surgical planning process. In this respect, fMRI aims to replace or limit the use of more invasive techniques such as the Wada test to identify language dominance and extraoperative or perioperative direct electrical brain stimulation to perform motor, sensory, and language mapping An emerging role for fMRI is in identification of the EZ. In this application, fMRI can be combined with simultaneous EEG recordings in an attempt to detect changes in blood flow and brain metabolism during an epileptic discharge.[22] With improving technology, this could be a useful tool in the future for identifying the EZ, particularly in patients with normal findings on MRI.

Magnetoencephalography (MEG) is also emerging as an adjunctive, noninvasive tool for identification of the EZ. This technique measures the magnetic fields produced by electric currents in the brain, in this case epileptiform discharges. The fields generated are very weak, and hence very sensitive devices are required to detect them. Furthermore, the MEG scanner needs to be in a magnetically shielded room to eliminate outside magnetic signals. For these reasons, the device remains expensive and available only in research centers. Its main advantage is that although both MEG and EEG signals are generated by the same neurophysiologic processes, the MEG signal is not distorted by the skull and scalp. One additional advantage is that MEG is a good tool for noninvasive localization of the central sulcus with the use of somatosensory evoked magnetic fields.[23] Overall, however, its value in surgical planning in relation to a seizure-free outcome has not yet been fully established.[24]

More recently, magnetic resonance spectroscopy (MRS) and diffusion tensor imaging (DTI) may offer additional clues to identification of the EZ in patients with MRI-negative partial epilepsy. MRS simultaneously detects and quantifies a number of brain metabolites and can therefore detect differences either between the two hippocampi, as in the case of hippocampal sclerosis, or between intralesional and perilesional tissue changes in MCD.[25] In patients with hippocampal sclerosis, the typical finding in the epileptogenic hippocampus is a reduction in *N*-acetylaspartate and an elevation in choline-related compounds and creatine plus phosphocreatine (total creatine); the contralateral hippocampus may be normal or show a lesser degree of abnormality.[26] Tractography, an important application of DTI, allows calculation of the direction of white matter tracts and may be helpful in determining the connections of the EZ to other brain areas, thus offering additional clues for identification of the EZ in patients with MRI-negative partial epilepsy.[27,28]

Neuropsychological Testing

Detailed neuropsychological testing is performed as part of the presurgical evaluation. Its goals are to identify epilepsy-related cognitive impairment, and it therefore complements EEG and neuroimaging in localization and lateralization of the EZ; prediction of potential postoperative deficits, particularly in memory domains, after resection of the EZ; and assessment of the patient's mental reserve capacity.[29] Comparison of the verbal and performance components of IQ testing may offer clear insight into the lateralization of dysfunctional cortex and hippocampus. Generally, a disparity of greater than 10 points between verbal IQ and performance IQ suggests significantly lateralized relative dysfunction in the dominant or nondominant hemisphere, respectively. The intracarotid sodium amobarbital procedure, also known as the Wada test, is used to determine which side of the brain is responsible for certain essential cognitive functions, namely, speech and memory. Further details related to the Wada test are provided in Chapter 57.

SURGICAL DECISION-MAKING AND PHASE II (INTRACRANIAL) INVESTIGATIONS

The information obtained from the clinical history and physical examination, EEG and video-EEG recording, neuroimaging, and neuropsychological testing is used to determine whether the EZ has been identified accurately. The degree of concordance of this information determines whether the region identified as the primary EZ is the only epileptic focus or whether other independent foci may exist. The information also determines whether resection of the candidate region is possible without significant risk for additional cognitive or neurological deficits. In an ideal scenario, a patient would have one type of seizure semiology, the seizure semiology would be typical for that of a particular area of the brain (such as the mesial temporal region), and the EEG/video-EEG recordings would identify IEDs and seizure onsets exclusively arising from that same region. Furthermore, there would be evidence of focal pathology in the implicated region on neuroimaging, for example, ipsilateral hippocampal sclerosis on MRI and anterior temporal hypometabolism on PET. Such complete concordance would then optimize the chance for postoperative freedom from seizures after complete resection of the identified EZ.

In clinical practice, however, the information obtained from phase I investigations is not always concordant, and therefore further intracranial electrode recordings are sometimes required (phase II recordings). Common problems that may lead to the need for intracranial electrode recordings are the following: (1) the seizure onsets are *lateralized* (i.e., onsets derived from one hemisphere) but not well *localized* (i.e., seizure onsets cannot be localized to one region within the hemisphere on scalp EEG recordings), (2) the seizures are localized but not clearly lateralized (e.g., both temporal regions appear to be involved at the onset), or (3) the seizures are neither lateralized nor localized (e.g., very diffuse scalp EEG onsets or scalp EEG onsets obscured

by muscle and motion artifact). Other examples include the presence of dual pathology (e.g., hippocampal sclerosis and an ipsilateral or contralateral lesion such as focal cortical dysplasia), where there is a need to establish a correlation between seizure onset and one or both of the lesions, or the presence of multiple cortical lesions such as in tuberous sclerosis, where there is a need to establish a correlation between seizure onset and one of these lesions. One other important application of intracranial electrodes is that they can be used for cortical mapping or stimulation to identify the central sulcus and eloquent cortex, respectively, and their relationship to the proposed area of resection.

Options for implanted electrodes include epidural, subdural (grids, strips, and foramen ovale [FO] electrodes), and intracerebral (depth) electrodes. These electrodes offer the advantage of recording in very close proximity to areas of the brain not readily sampled by scalp EEG studies, with both the scalp and skull being bypassed. Ictal electrocorticographic (ECoG) recordings can therefore define the exact area of seizure onset and reveal its propagation pathways, thus allowing accurate resection of the EZ and surrounding margin. The disadvantages are that implantation involves surgical risk and that the sampling area is relatively small, restricted to the tissue in immediate proximity to the recording electrodes.

Epidural Electrodes

Epidural electrodes are used infrequently and generally only for lateralization and approximate localization of the seizure onset.[30] These electrodes are placed through bur holes in the skull with the electrode contact resting on the dura to provide a high-amplitude EEG signal without muscle or movement artifact. Because they do not penetrate the dura, the risk for infection is minor. These electrodes record only from the lateral convexity of the cerebral hemispheres and are limited in their spatial resolution.

Subdural Electrodes

Three different kinds of subdurals electrodes are used: grid, strip, and FO electrodes. The strips are single columns of electrodes that can be placed mainly over the lateral convexity or over the frontal or temporal lobes,[31] but also in other less accessible regions such as the interhemispheric fissure. As with the other subdural electrodes, the strip is placed on the surface of the brain and records directly from the cortical surface. Although strip electrodes can be used for *lateralization* of seizure onset by being inserted through bur holes over, for example, the temporal lobes in each hemisphere, they are more commonly used for *localization* purposes in conjunction with grid electrodes, which offer additional coverage of adjacent areas of the cortical surface that abut the craniotomy site.

Grid electrodes are arrays of electrodes more than one column wide. Usually, rectangular grid arrays of 32 to 64 electrode contacts are used to maximize coverage over the craniotomy site. The site is determined from data gathered during the presurgical evaluation. Once placed, a grid is sutured to the dura to prevent motion. The grids are used to record from extratemporal regions and cannot be used to record from deeper cerebral structures such as the mesial temporal structures, which are often involved in medically refractory partial epilepsies. The main advantage of grid and strip electrodes is that they do not penetrate cerebral tissue and can record from a relatively wide area of the cortical surface. They can also be used for extraoperative cortical stimulation for mapping of specific areas of cortical function. Their disadvantages are that they have a small but significant rate of complications such as epidural and subdural bleeding, edema, or infection, often with an associated decrease in the level of consciousness and focal neurological signs.[32]

FO electrodes are intracranial electrodes introduced through the FO in the sphenoid bone, with the deepest contacts recording from the subdural space under the mesial temporal structures. FO electrodes frequently reveal striking epileptiform activity, including interictal epileptiform spikes and ictal discharges, which are not appreciated on associated scalp recordings (Fig. 56-3).

Implantation of FO electrodes is a minimally invasive procedure that in selected patients may provide significantly more information than scalp recordings and can preclude the need

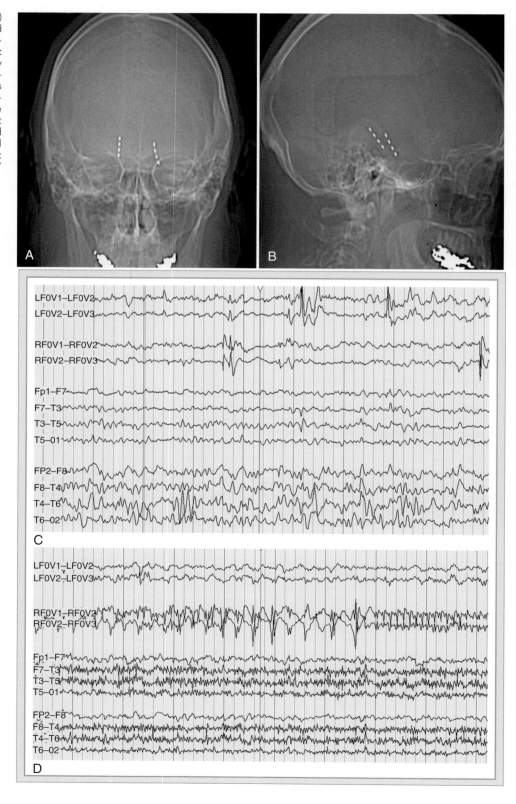

FIGURE 56-3 Foramen ovale (FO) electrodes. Anteroposterior (**A**) and lateral (**B**) skull radiographs demonstrate the position of four contact electrodes inserted percutaneously through the FO. Electroencephalography recorded with these electrodes demonstrates active bilateral independent interictal spikes from the FO electrode contacts that are not visualized in scalp channels recorded simultaneously (**C**) and a clear ictal onset from the right FO chain (**D**) that is not seen at the scalp until 47 seconds later (not shown).

for more invasive depth electrodes.[33] They have the additional advantage that they can be implanted "on the fly" in the course of a routine scalp investigation when required, without a lot of advanced planning. They are most useful in cases of suspected mesial temporal lobe epilepsy in which the phase I investigation failed to show unilateral seizure onsets. The advantage is that because the FO is a natural opening, implantation of FO electrodes does not involve disruption of the cranium or scalp. The disadvantage is that they record only from mesial temporal structures, *thus* offering biased information in cases in which the seizure onset is remote and therefore not captured by the FO electrodes but captured as it propagates through the mesial temporal structures. The complications related to FO implantation are relatively minor and transitory and include temporary facial pain and hypoesthesia in the trigeminal territory, temporomandibular joint dysfunction, and retromandibular hematoma.[34]

Intracerebral Depth Electrodes

Intracerebral or depth electrodes are flexible electrodes with multiple contact points that are placed stereotactically via bur holes into deep brain structures, usually the hippocampus, amygdala, and orbitofrontal and cingulate regions (Fig. 56-4).

Common methods for placement include the orthogonal, occipital, and parasagittal approaches.[35] Bilateral depth electrodes, like FO electrodes, are particularly useful for lateralization, especially in cases in which the scalp EEG recording is occluded by movement artifact at seizure onset. Unlike FO electrodes, however, multiple depth electrodes may be inserted and stereotactically targeted as clinically required. They are therefore better suited than FO electrodes for studying patients in whom the EZ may not be mesial temporal. They can also be used for localization in conjunction with ipsilateral subdural grids and strips, for example, in patients with suspected dual pathology in the same hemisphere involving a candidate neocortical region and the mesial temporal structures.[36] The indications for depth electrode placement are expanding as neuroimaging becomes more advanced and more subcortical lesions, such as MCDs, are identified. The major complications of depth electrodes include hemorrhage and infection, although the rates are relatively lower when only bur holes rather than a craniotomy are used.

After implantation of the intracranial electrodes, antiepileptic drug doses are decreased and eventually stopped to increase the likelihood of recording seizures. The use of MRI-compatible intracranial electrodes allows accurate visualization of the anatomic location of the electrodes. Specialized software systems that can combine the patient's segmented brain, postimplantation MRI scans, intracranial EEG findings, and results from cortical stimulation into one integrated environment of three-dimensional visualization have been developed to facilitate the planning of epilepsy surgery.[37]

Depending on the information obtained from the investigations described earlier, counseling is provided to each patient regarding the appropriateness of epilepsy surgery. Counseling also includes a psychosocial assessment to ensure that realistic goals and attitudes are engendered in the patient and family before surgery.

CONCLUSION

Success or failure of the surgical treatment of epilepsy depends in large part on proper identification and selection of patients. Recent advances, particularly in neuroimaging modalities, offer greater accuracy in localization of the EZ, thus improving the selection process even further. Given the increased assay sensitivity of modern imaging tools, however, clinical and neurophysiologic confirmation that a detected lesion is indeed the site of origin of the epileptic condition is critically important. Continued refinement of imaging and physiologic techniques should improve the results of surgical intervention for the treatment of epilepsy even further.

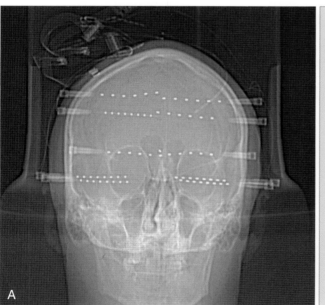
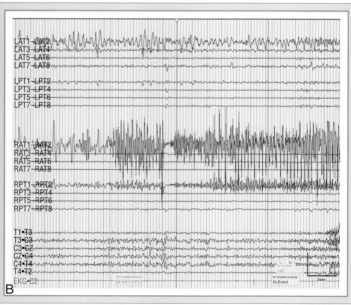

FIGURE 56-4 Intracerebral depth electrodes. **A,** An anteroposterior skull radiograph demonstrates the postioning of bilateral orthogonal depth electrodes. **B,** Electroencephalography (EEG) demonstrates an ictal onset from the deepest contact of the right anterior temporal chain and rapid involvement of the right posterior temporal chain. Simultaneous scalp EEG was unremarkable during the first 20 seconds of this event (lower six channels).

SUGGESTED REFERENCES

Alarcon G, Kissani N, Dad M, et al. Lateralizing and localizing values of ictal onset recorded on the scalp: evidence from simultaneous recordings with intracranial foramen ovale electrodes. *Epilepsia.* 2001;42:1426-1437.

Barnett GH, Burgess RC, Awad IA, et al. Epidural peg electrodes for the presurgical evaluation of intractable epilepsy. *Neurosurgery.* 1990;27:113-115.

Blatt DR, Roper SN, Friedman WA. Invasive monitoring of limbic epilepsy using stereotactic depth and subdural strip electrodes: surgical technique. *Surg Neurol.* 1997;48:74-79.

Blum D. Prevalence of bilateral partial seizure foci and implications for electroencephalographic telemetry monitoring and epilepsy surgery. *Electroencephalogr Clin Neurophysiol.* 1994;91:329-336.

Cascino GD. Surgical treatment for extratemporal epilepsy. *Curr Treat Options Neurol.* 2004;6:257-262.

Cascino GD. Surgical treatment for epilepsy. *Epilepsy Res.* 2004;60:179-186.

Cascino GD. Video-EEG monitoring in adults. *Epilepsia.* 2002;43(suppl 3):80-93.

Chen Q, Lui S, Li CX, et al. MRI-negative refractory partial epilepsy: role for diffusion tensor imaging in high field MRI. *Epilepsy Res.* 2008; doi:10.1016/j.eplepsyres.2008.03.009.

Chugani HT, Shields WD, Shewmon DA, et al. Infantile spasms: I. PET identifies focal cortical dysgenesis in cryptogenic cases for surgical treatment. *Ann Neurol.* 1990;27:406-413.

Cross JH, Connelly A, Jackson GD, et al. Proton magnetic resonance spectroscopy in children with temporal lobe epilepsy. *Ann Neurol.* 1996;39:107-113.

Engel J Jr, Kuhl DE, Phelps ME, et al. Comparative localization of epileptic foci in partial epilepsy by PCT and EEG. *Ann Neurol.* 1982;12:529-537.

Engel J Jr, Wiebe S, French J, et al. Practice parameter: temporal lobe and localized neocortical resections for epilepsy: report of the Quality Standards Subcommittee of the American Academy of Neurology, in association with the American Epilepsy Society and the American Association of Neurological Surgeons. *Neurology.* 2003;60:538-547.

Fitzsimons M, Browne G, Kirker J, et al. An international survey of long-term video/EEG services. *J Clin Neurophysiol.* 2000;17:59-67.

Fountas KN, Smith JR. Subdural electrode–associated complications: a 20-year experience. *Stereotact Funct Neurosurg.* 2007;85:264-272.

Gotman J, Benar CG, Dubeau F. Combining EEG and FMRI in epilepsy: methodological challenges and clinical results. *J Clin Neurophysiol.* 2004;21:229-240.

Helmstaedter C. Neuropsychological aspects of epilepsy surgery. *Epilepsy Behav.* 2004;5(suppl 1):S45-S55.

Jeha LE, Najm I, Bingaman W, et al. Surgical outcome and prognostic factors of frontal lobe epilepsy surgery. *Brain.* 2007;130:574-584.

Knake S, Triantafyllou C, Wald LL, et al. 3T phased array MRI improves the presurgical evaluation in focal epilepsies: a prospective study. *Neurology.* 2005;65:1026-1031.

Kwan P, Brodie MJ. Early identification of refractory epilepsy. *N Engl J Med.* 2000;342:314-319.

Lau M, Yam D, Burneo JG. A systematic review on MEG and its use in the presurgical evaluation of localization-related epilepsy. *Epilepsy Res.* 2008;79:97-104.

Morrell F, Whisler WW, Bleck TP. Multiple subpial transection: a new approach to the surgical treatment of focal epilepsy. *J Neurosurg.* 1989;70:231-239.

Rahimi SY, Park YD, Witcher MR, et al. Corpus callosotomy for treatment of pediatric epilepsy in the modern era. *Pediatr Neurosurg.* 2007;43:202-208.

Ryvlin P, Bouvard S, Le Bars D, et al. Clinical utility of flumazenil-PET versus [^{18}F]fluorodeoxyglucose-PET and MRI in refractory partial epilepsy. A prospective study in 100 patients. *Brain.* 1998;121:2067-2081.

Schuele SU, Luders HO. Intractable epilepsy: management and therapeutic alternatives. *Lancet Neurol.* 2008;7:514-524.

So EL. Integration of EEG, MRI, and SPECT in localizing the seizure focus for epilepsy surgery. *Epilepsia.* 2000;41(suppl 3):S48-S54.

Spencer SS, Spencer DD, Williamson PD, et al. Combined depth and subdural electrode investigation in uncontrolled epilepsy. *Neurology.* 1990;40:74-79.

Sutherling WW, Crandall PH, Darcey TM, et al. The magnetic and electric fields agree with intracranial localizations of somatosensory cortex. *Neurology.* 1988;38:1705-1714.

Tellez-Zenteno JF, Dhar R, Wiebe S. Long-term seizure outcomes following epilepsy surgery: a systematic review and meta-analysis. *Brain.* 2005;128:1188-1198.

Uijl SG, Leijten FS, Arends JB, et al. Decision-making in temporal lobe epilepsy surgery: the contribution of basic non-invasive tests. *Seizure.* 2008;17:364-373.

Van Paesschen W, Sisodiya S, Connelly A, et al. Quantitative hippocampal MRI and intractable temporal lobe epilepsy. *Neurology.* 1995;45:2233-2240.

Velasco TR, Sakamoto AC, Alexandre V Jr, et al. Foramen ovale electrodes can identify a focal seizure onset when surface EEG fails in mesial temporal lobe epilepsy. *Epilepsia.* 2006;47:1300-1307.

Velis D, Plouin P, Gotman J, et al for the ILAE DMC Subcommittee on Neurophysiology. Recommendations regarding the requirements and applications for long-term recordings in epilepsy. *Epilepsia.* 2007;48:379-384.

Wang Y, Agarwal R, Nguyen D, et al. Intracranial electrode visualization in invasive pre-surgical evaluation for epilepsy. *Conf Proc IEEE Eng Med Biol Soc.* 2005;1:952-955.

Widdess-Walsh P, Diehl B, Najm I. Neuroimaging of focal cortical dysplasia. *J Neuroimaging.* 2006;16:185-196.

Wiebe S, Blume WT, Girvin JP, et al. Effectiveness and Efficiency of Surgery for Temporal Lobe Epilepsy Study Group. A randomized, controlled trial of surgery for temporal-lobe epilepsy. *N Engl J Med.* 2001;345:311-318.

Woermann FG, McLean MA, Bartlett PA, et al. Quantitative short echo time proton magnetic resonance spectroscopic imaging study of malformations of cortical development causing epilepsy. *Brain.* 2001;124:427-436.

Wyler AR, Ojemann GA, Lettich E, et al. Subdural strip electrodes for localizing epileptogenic foci. *J Neurosurg.* 1984;60:1195-1200.

Full references can be found on Expert Consult @ www.expertconsult.com

PART 4

Intraoperative Mapping and Monitoring for Cortical Resections

CHAPTER 57

Motor, Sensory, and Language Mapping and Monitoring for Cortical Resections

Ben Waldau ■ Michael M. Haglund

Functional localization of eloquent regions of cortex is important for minimizing the morbidity associated with the removal of abnormal tissue. The techniques used for functional localization have been adapted from those that have been used for many years during epilepsy surgery for the removal of tumors and vascular malformations involving eloquent cortex and subcortical white matter. Because of our increased ability to identify functional and eloquent cortex, previously unresectable tumors and arteriovenous malformations are no longer inoperable.[1-4]

This chapter reviews the basics of functional mapping, including preoperative planning, the Wada test, intraoperative mapping techniques, language localization, and resection strategies. The major functional areas that can be defined during surgery are listed in Table 57-1.

PREOPERATIVE PLANNING

Magnetic resonance imaging (MRI) has been extremely helpful in predicting the relationship of motor cortex to a tumor by identifying a few constant MRI landmarks. On T2-weighted axial images near the convexity, a pair of mirror-image lines nearly perpendicular to the falx may be readily identified and represent the central sulcus.[5,6] Large lesions may compress the sulcus and distort the regional anatomy, but the landmark is usually identified by comparing the hemispheres on T1- and T2-weighted images. Although less sensitive, a midline sagittal image and a lateral parasagittal image may be viewed with respect to the marginal ramus of the cingulate sulcus and a perpendicular line drawn from the posterior roof of the insular triangle to identify the rolandic cortex.

The anterior suprasylvian region can have varying sulcus topography, and a classification based on anatomic landmarks has been published by Ebeling and coworkers.[7] Correlation has been shown between the structure of the frontal operculum as seen on MRI and the location of Broca's area, which allows preoperative prediction of this location.[8]

Patients with dense hemiparesis are not good candidates for mapping the motor pathways intraoperatively regardless of the stimulation used. Volitional movements of the face and extremities may be stimulated by cortical and subcortical mapping intraoperatively, but children younger than 5 to 7 years often have an electrically inexcitable cortex when a direct stimulating current is applied with a bipolar electrode.[9,10] Complex stimulating paradigms may still, however, bring out the excitability of pediatric motor cortex.[11] With the use of somatosensory evoked potentials (SSEPs), phase reversal over the central sulcus is available if direct stimulation mapping cannot be accomplished easily.[12-15] Insertion of a subdural electrode array under general anesthesia followed by extraoperative mapping may allow the mapping of motor, sensory, language, and ictal seizure onsets in children before early adolescence and in uncooperative adults. These techniques may be contraindicated in those with significant cerebral edema from malignant gliomas or metastatic tumors and may expose patients to a second craniotomy with its inherent risk of poor contact with the cortical surface as a result of blood or cerebrospinal fluid collecting underneath the electrodes. Delayed infection is also possible.[16]

FOUNDATIONS OF LANGUAGE MAPPING IN EPILEPSY SURGERY

Stimulation mapping during language measurement in awake adults has shown several features of the cortical organization of language that are not anticipated from the effect of brain lesions.[17]

Several of these features are of major importance in planning dominant hemisphere resections, including the high degree of localization of sites with repeated evoked errors in one language measure (and thus essential for function), but with broad variance across the patient population in terms of the exact locations of these sites. In a series of 117 patients undergoing intraoperative stimulation mapping in the left dominant perisylvian cortex during naming, Ojemann and colleagues found that most patients had essential sites with surface areas of 2 cm or less, with only 16% having an area of essential language sites as large as 6 cm.[18] It has been shown that if another language is acquired as a second language, more diffuse localization is seen than with the primary language (Haglund and Ojemann, unpublished observations). It has also been shown in sign language patients that localization of American sign language differs slightly from that of naming in hearing patients proficient in sign language.[19] The discrete localization is evident in both the frontal and temporoparietal sites and has been demonstrated with naming and word and sentence reading as language measures. Some sites have very sharp boundaries, whereas others have a surrounding area in which occasional

TABLE 57-1 Areas Identified by Functional Mapping

Motor pathways	Primary motor cortex, subcortical corona radiata, internal capsule, cerebral peduncle
Supplementary motor area	Motor cortex and descending motor pathways
Insula	Dominant: language localization and subcortical motor pathways Nondominant: subcortical motor pathways
Language localization	Dominant hemisphere: posterior frontal, perisylvian, temporal insula, subcortical arcuate fasciculus, inferior occipitofrontal fasciculus
Sensory pathways	Primary sensory cortex
Intractable seizures	Electrocorticography, grid mapping of ictal onsets

errors are evoked, thus suggesting a more graded transition from cortex unrelated to language to that essential for it.[20,21]

In most patients, several essential perisylvian areas are involved in language function. In a series of 117 patients, two thirds had two sites; in a quarter, three sites were present. Usually, there was one frontal site and one or more temporoparietal sites; however, in approximately 10% of patients there was no frontal language site, and around another 10% had no temporoparietal language site. Although a majority of patients have temporoparietal language sites, the critical issue here is the large variance between patients.

The considerable variance in language localization is illustrated in Figure 57-1. The percentage of essential language sites

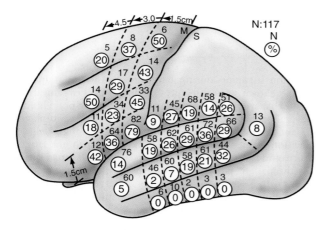

FIGURE 57-1 Localization of cortical sites essential for language (object naming) was assessed by stimulation mapping in the left, dominant hemispheres of 117 patients. Sites were related to language when stimulation at a current below the threshold for afterdischarge evoked repeated statistically significant errors in object naming. Small numbers above the *circles* indicate the number of patients who were tested at a site, and the number within the *circle* indicates the percentage of tested patients who were found to have a language site at this location. (*Adapted from Ojemann G, Ojemann J, Lettich E, et al. Cortical language localization in left, dominant hemisphere. An electrical stimulation mapping investigation in 117 patients. J Neurosurg. 1989;71:316.*)

in the entire series is shown in the circles and demonstrates a range in the temporoparietal region of 2% to 36% of patients with essential language sites in a single area. Note the 14% of essential language sites in the anterior superior temporal gyrus and 5% of such sites in the anterior middle temporal gyrus, in front of the central sulcus. In the posterior language area, no local area was crucial for language in more than about a third of the patients. This variation in language localization is substantially greater than the morphologic variability in the perisylvian cortex, although this is also substantial.[22,23] However, no cytoarchitectonic area seems to have a reliable relationship to language. It is the combination of discrete localization of essential language areas in the individual patient and the great variation in their location across the population that form the basis for using stimulation mapping rather than anatomic landmarks in planning resection near eloquent cortex.

Stimulation mapping in children has shown a lower frequency of sites of stimulation-induced errors than in the adult population.[24] This finding implies that new language areas may still arise with maturation in children during the age range of 4 through 16 years. In children younger than 10 years, language cortex is less likely to be identified by stimulation mapping than in older children. Wada testing seems to be more likely to be successful than stimulation mapping in this younger age group.[25] Extraoperative electrocortical stimulation mapping, however, is an established procedure for surgery near eloquent cortex in children.[26] Because awake craniotomy is less tolerable for children, implantation of subdural stimulation electrodes allows precise extraoperative mapping of cortical function without psychological trauma.

Anatomic knowledge of subcortical white matter tract connectivity in the temporal lobe is important for preventing postoperative deficits. The uncinate fasciculus connects the uncus, amygdala, and hippocampal gyrus to the orbital and frontopolar cortex.[27] No functional role has yet been attributed to the uncinate fasciculus, and resection of it is performed routinely in epilepsy surgery.

The inferior longitudinal fasciculus connects the anterior part of the temporal lobe to the occipital pole and has also been shown to play no role in language processing.[28] The inferior occipitofrontal fasciculus runs from the occipital lobe laterally to the lateral wall of the temporal horn of the lateral ventricle and then continues through the external capsule to the orbitofrontal and dorsolateral prefrontal cortices. Direct stimulation of this pathway induces semantic paraphasias,[29] so care should be taken to not disrupt this pathway during surgery. The superior longitudinal fasciculus is also called the arcuate fasciculus and connects Wernicke's area in the posterior and superior temporal cortex with Broca's area in the frontal lobe. Preservation of this pathway during surgery is mandatory because section of it produces phonemic paraphasias.[30] Finally, it is important to preserve the optical pathways to prevent the development of permanent postoperative hemianopia. Intraoperative stimulation mapping can elicit a transient shadow that can be used to identify the visual pathways.[31]

Assessment of the effects of stimulation on an array of language-related functions (naming, reading, recent verbal memory, orofacial mimicry, and speech sound identification) in a series of 14 patients provided the basis for a model of language organization in the lateral perisylvian cortex. This model included a perisylvian area involving the superior temporal and anterior parietal as well as the posterior frontal lobes important for speech production and perception, a surrounding zone of specialized sites, some of which are related to syntax, and an even more peripheral area related to recent verbal memory.[32,33] Significant interference with reading has been noted with stimulation of the lower part of the precentral and postcentral gyri; the dominant supramarginal, angular, and posterior part of the superior

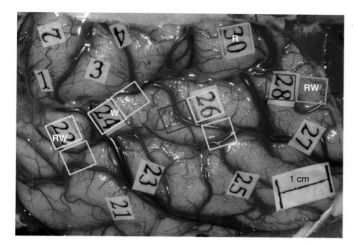

FIGURE 57-2 The human brain contains distinct as well as overlapping sites for visual naming, auditory naming, and sentence completion. This figure shows one example of intraoperative mapping results. *Blue boxes* represent visual naming sites; *yellow boxes*, auditory naming sites; and *white letters*, sites crucial for sentence completion (R, reading; W, word finding). *Green boxes* illustrate overlapping sites for visual naming, auditory naming, and sentence completion. *Light yellow boxes* mark sites that are shared by auditory naming and sentence completion only. Numbers 1 and 2 are placed on the face motor cortex and numbers 3 and 4 on the face sensory cortex.

temporal gyri; the dominant inferior and middle frontal gyri; and the posterior part of the dominant middle temporal gyrus.[34]

Positive language sites in bilingual patients may or may not colocalize. In an individual who acquired both languages during infancy, anomia was demonstrated for both languages when stimulation was performed at the same sites.[35] Four patients who acquired their second language during early school years (5 or 6 years of age) exhibited varying degrees of anomia in the second language.

Different tasks such as naming, reading, and responding may share the same cortical site, in which case they are referred to as multiuse sites.[36] Multimodality language mapping can generate an accurate map of eloquent language cortex in bilingual patients. Single-task sites are defined as sites where one task is disrupted across both languages with stimulation. Single-use sites are sites where one task is disrupted in only one language with stimulation. Cortical mapping of a bilingual patient has shown the presence of multiuse, single-task, and single-use sites, which underlines the necessity to test for both different languages and different language modalities if optimal postoperative functional outcomes are to be achieved.[37]

Many neurosurgical operating teams rely solely on visual naming tasks for the intraoperative testing of language function. Resection of auditory naming sites has, however, been shown to lead to postoperative word-finding difficulties.[38] Preservation of auditory naming and reading sites is critical for preserving language function, and intraoperative removal of these sites may account for up to 25% of the language deficits seen postoperatively.[39] Figure 57-2 illustrates that there are distinct as well as overlapping language sites that can be identified during intraoperative stimulation mapping for visual naming, auditory naming, reading, and word finding.

The extent of separation of language-related functions and the relationships of areas to one another constitute an active area of research in stimulation mapping techniques and single-unit microelectrode recordings.[40-43]

THE WADA TEST

In their original article in 1960, Juhn Wada and Theodore Rasmussen at the Montreal Neurological Institute described an invasive procedure for the lateralization of speech that has become to be known as the Wada test.[44] The procedure involves the injection of 150 to 200 mg of amobarbital (Amytal) sodium into the common carotid artery. An angiogram should be performed before the injection to rule out persistent trigeminal, otic, hypoglossal, or proatlantic arteries and avoid respiratory or circulatory problems as a result of shunting of the injection solution to the brainstem. The injection is made with the patient counting, the forearms up in the air, and the fingers either moving constantly or gripping an examiner's hands. As the injection is completed, the contralateral arm will become hemiplegic and flaccid. The patient is usually hesitant in counting on the dominant and nondominant side toward the end of the injection but then is quickly able to resume counting and naming objects while the contralateral hemiplegia still persists if the nondominant hemisphere is injected. In the case of injection into the dominant hemisphere, the patient is unable to continue counting or naming objects while the contralateral hemiplegia is complete. The patient is still able to follow commands, although on the side ipsilateral to the injection, which is tested to ensure that the aphasia is not due to confusion. At doses of 150 to 200 mg of Amytal Sodium, the contralateral hemiplegia typically lasts 1.5 to 5 minutes. Thirty to 90 seconds after the contralateral hemiplegia begins to resolve, the patient regains the ability to answer questions requiring yes and no answers. This is followed by a period of dysphasia that typically lasts for 1 to 3 minutes until normal speech is restored.

Although the Wada test has proved to be an important tool in the presurgical evaluation of epilepsy surgery patients for more than 50 years, it has lost some of its clinical significance over recent years with the advent of newer imaging techniques.[45] The majority of epilepsy centers no longer conduct a Wada test on every surgical candidate. In one multicenter study, 50% of respondents stated that they used the Wada test for less than 25% of their surgical epilepsy patients.[46] Functional MRI has largely replaced the Wada test for language lateralization in the preoperative evaluation of epilepsy patients to answer the question of whether language mapping should be performed during the resection. Therefore, the Wada test is now used mostly to screen for a patient's postoperative risk for memory deficits and amnesia. The indication for Wada testing in these cases may be limited to bilateral hippocampal pathology or epileptiform activity because one normal remaining hippocampus on fine-cut MRI scans after resection can usually sustain memory. The advent of MRI technology has further diminished the importance of Wada testing over the years since bilateral hippocampal anatomic abnormalities can now be studied with high-resolution coronal MRI.

Amnesia after unilateral anterior temporal lobe resection is a very rare occurrence.[47] Only about 20 patients have been reported in the literature.[48] In 3 of these patients, Wada testing had been performed before surgery and accurately predicted postoperative amnesia.[49-51] Therefore, surgical resection is often not performed on patients who fail the memory portion of the Wada test. However, one study involving 10 patients showed that all patients still retained memory after temporal lobe resections even if they failed the memory portion of the Wada test.[52] Other investigators have also demonstrated that a failed memory portion of the Wada test does not predict an amnestic syndrome,[53] and many epilepsy centers repeat the Wada test until the patient passes. Thus, use of the Wada test to evaluate for postoperative amnesia is also controversial. Noninvasive neuropsychological tests have been shown to be accurate predictors of postoperative neurocognitive and memory decline, so the Wada test does not always need to be used for this assessment as well.[54,55]

The Wada test is an invasive procedure with a reported complication rate of 0.5% to 10%.[56] Consequently, patients should be carefully selected on a case-by-case basis to determine the appropriateness of Wada testing. Many of the patients now undergoing Wada testing have disconcordant findings on video-electroencephalographic (EEG) recordings, high-resolution fine-cut hippocampal MRI, or neuropsychological testing. Furthermore, some clinicians have completely omitted Wada testing from their decision-making algorithms for epilepsy surgery.[57] Currently, the Wada test is used mostly to test for the ability to sustain memory in the setting of bilateral hippocampal pathology.

NONINVASIVE BRAIN MAPPING

Functional MRI, positron emission tomography (PET), and magnetoencephalography (MEG) are noninvasive tools used to search for the location of eloquent cortex.[58,59] Functional MRI is based on measurement of the real-time increase in deoxyhemoglobin in the venous structures associated with motor movement, sensory perception, or speech generation.[58]

The question is whether functional MRI as a noninvasive method can replace the Wada test in determining language lateralization. Although lesion and Wada studies have shown that only the left hemisphere is dominant in the majority of subjects, functional MRI typically demonstrates some degree of activity in the hemisphere contralateral to the Wada-dominant hemisphere in virtually all individuals. The language lateralization index is therefore used in functional MRI to determine hemispheric dominance. One method of calculating this index consists of defining an area of interest that has a known association with language function on MRI (Broca's area, for example) and subsequently performing a simple bilateral suprathreshold count in the region of interest.[60] Reproducibility of the language lateralization index has, however, been found to strongly vary between task analyses. Object naming has been found to be a more sensitive measure of speech localization than has number counting.[61] The language lateralization index showed significant correlation between sessions in the same individual for verb generation tasks, whereas no significant correlation was found for picture naming and only a weak correlation was seen in the antonym generation task.[62] Therefore, only the verb generation task allows a reliable calculation of the lateralization index across sessions. When the verb generation task was used to determine hemispheric dominance, functional MRI was concordant with invasive measures (Wada testing or cortical stimulation) in all but 1 of 23 patients in one study.[63] Correlation of the results for language lateralization between functional MRI and Wada testing was found to be highly significant in another study.[64] Thus, functional MRI based on the verb generation task has replaced Wada testing at many institutions in the United States for the determination of language dominance.

The inability of functional MRI to currently produce reliable results across all language tasks has raised concern about its general applicability to intraoperative surgical planning in eloquent cortex. Such concern is due to the fact that functional MRI has been shown to miss cortical sites that are found to be essential by intraoperative stimulation mapping.[65] To analyze its sensitivity and specificity with respect to direct cortical mapping, functional MRI data were registered in a frameless stereotactic neuronavigational device and correlated with the results of direct brain mapping. Although the specificity of functional MRI has been shown to be high for naming and verb generation tasks,[66] poor sensitivity was noted (only 22% in naming tasks and 36% in verb generation tasks).[65] A combined battery of language tasks may enhance the sensitivity of functional MRI in comparison to testing individual language tasks.[67] The results, however, have discouraged the use of functional MRI as a tool for making critical surgical decisions in the absence of direct brain mapping.

Functional MRI cannot replace stimulation mapping for positive language sites on the basis of the current state of technology.

Functional MRI has, however, been found to be a useful clinical tool for the prediction of selective motor cortex areas. Concordance between the contours of functional MRI and intraoperative electrical cortical mapping was found in 20 of 21 patients in one study that evaluated its reliability for the implantation of an epidural electrode for chronic motor cortex stimulation.[68]

Functional cortex can also be mapped with PET. Speech eloquent areas can be localized with 2-[18F]-2-deoxy-D-glucose (FDG) based on the higher consumption of glucose in eloquent areas during verb generation tasks. Although integration of functional PET data into frameless navigation systems for surgical planning is possible, its low reliability has precluded it from replacing direct stimulation mapping as well. In three of seven patients, preoperative PET findings were not supported by intraoperative mapping.[69]

In contrast to functional language areas, which vary in location between individuals, the primary motor cortex is always situated in the precentral gyrus. Pathology, however, can distort normal anatomy and make mapping procedures for cortical or subcortical motor structures essential to prevent a postoperative deficit.

In healthy individuals, MEG has been demonstrated to be capable of delineating the somatotopic organization of the motor cortex since its results were shown to correlate with anatomic landmarks.[70] Newer source reconstruction algorithms have increased its reliability in the clinical setting. In one patient with a perirolandic tumor, MEG correctly identified the hand motor area, which was subsequently confirmed by intraoperative cortical stimulation mapping.[71] Somatosensory mapping with MEG can be used to guide intraoperative mapping of motor cortex. One study found a consistent quantitative relationship in the distance between the mouth motor cortex identified by electrical stimulation and the lip somatosensory cortex delineated by MEG.[72] This relationship allows prediction of the location of the mouth motor cortex if the lip somatosensory cortex is detected by MEG. In one study including 15 patients, MEG depicted the central sulcus correctly in all patients and proved to be superior to functional MRI in localizing the somatosensory cortex.[73] MEG has also been shown to reliably map expressive and receptive language cortex.[74,75]

The pyramidal tract is the major output source of fibers arising from the motor cortex. Diffusion-weighted imaging (DWI) and diffusion tensor imaging (DTI) are noninvasive techniques that allow preoperative visualization of the pyramidal tract on MRI.[76] The disadvantage of preoperative tractographic imaging lies in the possibility of an intraoperative shift of brain tissue secondary to opening of the dura or the administration of mannitol and dexamethasone (Decadron). Intraoperative DWI has therefore been developed to acquire more reliable data. Early experience in a small number of patients has shown that the accuracy and image quality of intraoperative DWI with an MRI scanner of low magnetic field strength (0.3 T) are sufficient for possible incorporation into an intraoperative neuronavigation system.[77]

Bello and coworkers,[78] in contrast, were able to show that preoperatively performed motor and language DTI also allowed accurate intraoperative identification of eloquent fiber tracts through neuronavigation. They reported a sensitivity of 95% for detection of the corticospinal tract and 97% for language tracts, figures calculated by confirmation with intraoperative subcortical stimulation mapping. Another study consisting of nine patients found an average distance of 8.7 mm between positive stimulation sites and the preoperatively DTI-mapped fiber tracts and concluded that it can be used to define a safety margin around the tract.[79] Because DTI has only recently been added to intraoperative neuronavigational systems, further studies are needed to validate its reliability in the clinical setting.

PREOPERATIVE TESTING

To map language capabilities, the patient is tested before surgery with object naming. A baseline error rate of less than 25% is necessary for the intraoperative language mapping to reach statistical significance. Naming is used as the common test because of its involvement in many different types of language disturbances.[16,18,42] If the patient's inability to name objects is due to a mass effect, preoperative dexamethasone and mannitol may diminish the edema to the point where the patient's language ability returns sufficiently for intraoperative mapping.

Antiepileptic drug levels are checked on the evening before surgery and increased to the high therapeutic range. Patients undergoing electrocorticography have no significant change made in their medications before intraoperative recordings. Patients are kept in the high therapeutic range postoperatively and then adjusted back to their routine therapeutic levels.

INTRAOPERATIVE MAPPING

The patient is brought to the operating room and carefully positioned with a small shoulder roll so that the falx is approximately parallel to the floor. The neck is checked to make sure that it is in a neutral position, and a pillow can be placed between the head and the frame of the Mayfield head holder to provide comfort. Once the patient is positioned, an intravenous infusion of propofol (Diprivan) and remifentanil is begun to induce a deep hypnotic state,[80,81] and a Foley catheter is inserted. After the head is shaved and prepared, a local anesthetic (0.5% lidocaine with 1:100,000 to 1:200,000 units of epinephrine and 0.25% bupivacaine [Marcaine] with 1:100,000 to 1:200,000 units of epinephrine) is mixed in 1:1 fashion, and then 9.0 mL of this mixture is added to 1.0 mL of sodium bicarbonate solution. A field block is applied that initially extends anteriorly over the supraorbital nerves and in the region of the zygoma and the posterior auricular regions. The regional field block is completed with deep injections into the insertion of the temporalis muscle. If a 30-gauge needle is used, the patient can tolerate the injections well, but because propofol is not an analgesic, the patient is somewhat disinhibited during the scalp injection and the arms may have to be restrained. If the patient has become anxious or is overly sensitive to the injections, either the remifentanil can be increased or a small amount of intravenous fentanyl (25 to 50 μg) can be added. With the advent of hair-sparing incisions, the deep and field block portions of the injection are performed after the scalp opening.

Our preferred incision allows the anterior temporal lobe to be well exposed and the craniotomy to be as low as possible. A reverse–question mark incision may also be used, depending on the relationship of the lesion to eloquent cortex. The scalp flap and craniotomy are performed with the patient asleep. After the dura is exposed, peripheral tack-up sutures are placed and the skull clamp is positioned. The propofol drip is discontinued, and it usually takes 8 to 15 minutes (range, 5 to 55 minutes) for the patient to awaken and converse.

Stimulation mapping to localize the rolandic cortex is performed with a bipolar electrode with 5-mm spacing between the electrodes. A constant-current generator is used to produce a train of biphasic square-wave pulses with a frequency of 60 Hz and a 1-msec single-phase duration. The maximum train duration is 4 seconds. In an asleep patient, the current required to evoke motor responses may vary between 4 and 16 mA, but when the patient is awake, a lower current (2 to 5 mA) will usually suffice, especially in the face and hand motor-sensory cortex. The current is increased in 1- to 2-mA increments until the evoked responses are demonstrated. Alternatively, motor mapping may be performed with monopolar, anodal stimulation.[82] A train of 500 Hz (7 to 10 pulses) may be used for monopolar stimulation;

the current intensities applied are similar to those used for bipolar stimulation. Monopolar cortex stimulation was shown to be successful in generating compound muscle action potentials during intraoperative electrocortical stimulation of the primary motor cortex in 91% of 255 patients.[83] Bipolar cortical stimulation, however, has proved to be more sensitive than monopolar stimulation for mapping motor function in the premotor frontal cortex.[84] Both methods were found to be equally sensitive for mapping the primary motor cortex. Special electrodes have been designed that allow both monopolar and bipolar mapping.[85]

In an awake patient, the sensory cortex may be identified more easily at lower stimulation amplitudes. When motor and sensory responses are elicited, the cortical site is marked with a small numbered ticket. If a seizure is elicited by stimulation mapping, the cortex is irrigated with ice-cold Ringer's solution. The intraoperative risk for seizures induced by stimulation mapping has been found to be approximately 1.5%, and patients with symptomatic epilepsy do not have a higher risk than other patients for the intraoperative development of a seizure.[86]

When the operation is near the falx and identification of leg motor cortex is desired, a small strip electrode (four contacts spaced 1 cm apart) may be placed between the cortex and the falx to allow mapping of leg and foot motor cortex. The same current used to evoke motor responses on the cortical surface or slightly higher currents (1 mA) may be used in the white matter to identify the subcortical location of descending axons from the motor cortex.

Once the motor and sensory cortices have been identified in an awake patient, the electrocorticography equipment is attached to the skull clamp. If resection of the tumor includes an attempt to relieve the patient's seizure disorder, strip electrodes are inserted to record epileptiform activity. Usually, four strip electrodes are placed: anterior subtemporal, middle subtemporal, posterior subtemporal, and subfrontal. Single carbon-tipped electrodes are placed on the lateral cortical surface over the temporal lobe and the perisylvian region. Recording is then started, and with the assistance of the electroencephalographer, epileptic activity is identified or afterdischarge thresholds are determined. If the patient has intractable epilepsy, a tailored resection is then performed by identifying areas of interictal activity over the lateral or mesial cortical surfaces. Especially with temporal lobe lesions, our standard practice is to resect the lateral cortex and expose the ventricle to place strip electrodes along the hippocampus and subcortically along the parahippocampal gyrus for identification of the extent of resection needed to eliminate all interictal epileptiform activity.[18]

If preoperative planning did not call for identification of epileptic cortex, afterdischarge thresholds are determined. The choice of stimulating currents for language mapping depends on the selection of a current large enough to alter critical function but not so large that it will evoke seizure activity or long trains of afterdischarge activity. The long trains of afterdischarge activity may spread and thus confuse the localization being performed with stimulation. Usually, these requirements are met by setting the current 1 mA below the threshold for evoking single or small trains or afterdischarge activity. However, in cortex that involves adjacent or invasive tumor tissue, the afterdischarge thresholds may be significantly lower and several current levels for stimulation may be necessary for different cortical regions.[87] For example, in Figure 57-3, the afterdischarge threshold used in the posterior temporal region was 4 mA; in the anterior temporal lobe, which was undercut by the tumor, the afterdischarge threshold was just 3 mA; and it was 7 mA in the frontal region. Language sites were identified at sites 28, 41 , 44, 10, and 12. Afterdischarge thresholds vary considerably between patients and can range from 1.5 mA to greater than 10 mA.

To increase the confidence of the intraoperative mapping, stimulation should provide the information needed to know

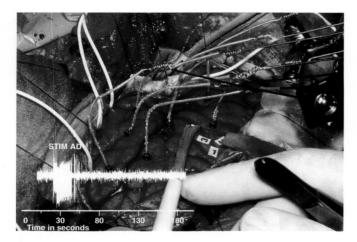

FIGURE 57-3 The choice of stimulating currents for language mapping depends on the selection of a current large enough to alter critical function but not so large that it will evoke seizure activity or long trains of afterdischarge activity. The long trains of afterdischarge activity may spread and thus confuse the localization being performed with stimulation. Usually, these requirements are met by setting the current 1 mA below the threshold for evoking single or small trains of afterdischarge activity. This figure illustrates afterdischarge activity elicited by stimulation; in this example, the current therefore needs to be adjusted to a lower level.

where language is localized and where it is not localized. Completely negative stimulation mapping does not always provide security that resection of the recorded sites will not cause a language deficit. In a series of 40 patients undergoing resection of temporal lobe tumors, two negative language maps resulted in language deficits in the postoperative period.[41] This finding has led to the concept that the region covered by stimulation mapping should include areas where language is likely to be found, as well as the area of planned resection.

Recently, however, Sanai and coworkers did not use the traditional approach of identifying positive language sites in every awake craniotomy and demonstrated that most gliomas could still be resected without causing language deficits.[88] Using a tailored approach to limit cortical exposure, 58% of 250 patients were found to have an intraoperative stimulation-induced speech arrest or anomia. Their 6-month functional outcome data, however, compared favorably with previous studies that relied on the identification of positive language sites. Only 4 of 243 surviving patients (1.6%) had a persistent language deficit 6 months after surgery, so the use of smaller, tailored craniotomies with testing for negative language sites seems to be a valid surgical strategy.

Cortical surface recordings of SSEPs can be helpful in localizing the sensorimotor cortex intraoperatively. SSEPs with approximately mirror-image waveforms can be recorded on either side of the central sulcus.[89] The precentral waveform is termed P20-N30 and the postcentral waveform P30-N20, corresponding to their polarity and average peak latency across subjects. In other words, stimulation of the median nerve on average leads to a negative wave (N) 20 msec later in recordings from the postcentral gyrus, followed by a positive wave (P) 30 msec after stimulation. The opposite order of waveforms is observed in the precentral gyrus. This phenomenon is called phase reversal. Intraoperative SSEP recordings enable the surgeon to identify the motor and somatosensory cortices under general anesthesia without the use of awake stimulation techniques. For localization of the hand motor area with SSEPs, the median nerve is typically stimulated intraoperatively. Trigeminal SSEPs with stimulating

electrodes in the chin, tongue, or palate can be used to identify face motor and sensory areas.[90]

Intraoperative infrared functional imaging has recently been developed as a means of measuring the increased neuronal heat production and capillary blood flow that are linked to greater neuronal firing.[91,92] This technique represents another modality to intraoperatively map motor, sensory, and language function.

As discussed earlier, the pyramidal tract is of crucial importance for avoidance of postoperative deterioration in motor function. The pyramidal tract can also be identified by intraoperative subcortical stimulation mapping. The subcortical stimulation settings are usually identical to the ones used for cortical mapping. Initially, the cortical motor region is identified and the same current is subsequently used to identify the descending motor pathways.[15] Multichannel electromyographic (EMG) recordings have been shown to be superior to mere visual observation in detecting motor responses elicited by stimulation of the internal capsule.[93] In 30% of 66 operations, motor responses during mapping were noted at least once on EMG recordings, although they were not apparent on visual inspection. Because lower electrical thresholds are required to elicit an EMG response during cortical mapping, it can be performed with lower currents, which potentially decreases the incidence of intraoperative seizures. This may be useful in patients who are susceptible to stimulation-induced seizures.

FUNDAMENTALS OF CORTICAL STIMULATION

The area of cortex inactivated by bipolar cortical stimulation has been studied in a number of ways. Bipolar stimulation pulses ensure that one electrode will not become the sole source of the direction of the current and produce a lesion. Imaging during bipolar stimulation in both human and monkey cortex has shown that the area activated is confined to the region around the recording electrodes[94] but that if afterdischarge activity is evoked, the spread is more diffuse.[95] Therefore, stimulation of motor movements should involve a very limited focal area of cortex to ensure accuracy of the functional maps. Stimulation at the afterdischarge threshold is sufficient to disrupt activity at that area of cortex. If language fails, the area is identified as an essential language site. Following Penfield's experience, object naming is the language measure primarily used with stimulation.[16,96] Naming seems to be adequate for localization of language, and naming deficits occur in all aphasic syndromes that result from pathologic lesions. Moreover, two studies investigating the relationship of changes in stimulation to language after resection cited naming as the only measure of language during stimulation that helped predict the effects of resection on a general aphasia battery measuring many language functions and significant clinical deficits.[16,97] However, with resections in the posterior temporal lobe and perisylvian area, other language functions may be assessed, such as auditory naming, reading, and memory, because these language functions have been noted to involve a somewhat wider cortical area than naming changes do.[18]

After the level of current for language mapping has been selected, 10 to 20 sites on the cortical surface in the area of the planned resection and the probable location of language are indicated by numbered tickets. The patient then begins a test that consists of repetitive measures of language function, usually naming pictures of common objects shown by a slide projector at a rate of one every 4 seconds. Stimulation at one of the numbered cortical sites is applied with a bipolar electrode at the onset of a randomly selected item in the language test, with contact being maintained until the correct response or the next item appears. At the point where the stimulation occurred, the number of the stimulation site and any errors are recorded. After one or two additional correct items, another site is stimulated. This process is continued until all the sites have been stimulated at least 3 times. No cortical site is stimulated twice in succession, and after each cortical stimulation, an image is shown on the computer screen and named by the patient to verify a return to baseline before further stimulation. When an essential language site is identified, further stimulation around that site may be done to determine how close the resection should approach that critical site. With this technique, stimulation mapping at 20 sites during naming requires approximately 20 minutes. The sites with repeated errors seem to be especially crucial for language. Errors can take a number of forms, although they are generally major errors with disruption of performance rather than just hesitations.

STRATEGIES FOR SURGICAL RESECTION

Localization of language is an important factor in planning for cortical resection.[98] In general, this is a concern only in the dominant hemisphere for language, and then usually in the perisylvian area. However, even in the anterior temporal lobe, a small percentage of essential language sites are identified within 3 cm of the temporal tip. The left hemisphere is commonly assumed to be dominant for language in right-handed patients, whereas in left-handed individuals, dominance is commonly established preoperatively with the intracarotid amobarbital perfusion test or functional MRI techniques, as discussed earlier in this chapter. In reality, the laterality of language may not be significantly different in left- and right-handed patients when those who are left-handed because of left hemisphere lesions are excluded.[99] The left hemisphere is most likely to be essential for language in either group, with a few patients demonstrating right or bilateral language in either group, although these unusual patterns seem to be slightly more common in left-handers with a strong family history. Overall, the left hemisphere alone is essential for language in about 85% of patients and the right in 6%, with language represented bilaterally in approximately 9%.[100] Within the dominant hemisphere, changes in language have been observed after lesions in a wide area. However, permanent deficits have generally been associated only with lesions in the perisylvian area; thus, localization of language in this area is particularly important. Changes in language are often evoked from the posterior superior frontal areas and often acutely follow resection there, but nearly all patients recover from the supplementary motor area syndrome.[101] The same situation seems to exist with regard to the basal temporal cortex.[14,102]

Two different approaches can be taken to minimize the risk for language deficits with cortical resection near the dominant hemisphere's perisylvian cortex. The traditional approach is to use anatomic landmarks that are thought to indicate areas not involved in language, for example, limiting temporal resection to the anterior 4 to 5 cm, anterior to the inferior aspect of rolandic cortex, or anterior to the vein of Labbé.[41,103] Sparing of the superior temporal gyrus has also been recommended. The pterion has been considered the safe posterior limit for inferior frontal resection. However, particularly in the temporal lobe, resections within these supposed safe limits are occasionally associated with postoperative aphasia,[97] and these landmarks provide no guidance for resection in the perisylvian areas, especially the posterior temporal and inferior parietal lobes. The alternative approach is to make a unique map for each individual and identify the essential language areas.

Functional cortex and subcortical white matter may be located within tumors or adjacent infiltrated brain regardless of the degree of tumor infiltration, swelling, apparent necrosis, and gross distortion by the mass. Direct stimulation mapping of the cortical and subcortical portions of tumors during resection has been shown to generate motor, sensory, or language dysfunction.[104]

Because of the bilateral representation of face motor function at the neocortical level, radical resection of tumors from the face motor cortex on the nondominant side may result in only transient contralateral facial weakness and apraxia, which resolves within 6 to 8 weeks after surgery.[105] Because language cortex is contiguous to the face motor area on the dominant side, resection of the face motor area is controversial in the dominant hemisphere but has been accomplished without major deficits (Friedman and Haglund, unpublished observations).

Verbal memory deficits may arise after temporal lobectomies in the dominant hemisphere. Ojemann and Dodrill found a significant correlation between a decline in postoperative verbal memory scores and the lateral, but not the medial extent of the temporal lobe resection.[106] Verbal memory scores measure the ability of a patient to recall a word after a short period of distraction. In their series of 14 adults undergoing left temporal lobectomy, the Wechsler verbal memory score was decreased an average of 22% at 1 month and 11% at 1 year. Thus, verbal memory is not only generated by medial temporal lobe structures such as the hippocampus but is also stored in the temporal cortex.

Functional intraoperative language mapping aims to limit the development of postoperative aphasias. Several investigators have examined the occurrence and time course of postoperative language dysfunctions after cortical mapping. A common theme of all studies is the finding that the majority of new postoperative aphasias improve or resolve over time. Ilmberger and colleagues found that in 32% of their 128 patients without preoperative deficits, a new aphasic disturbance developed within 21 days of microsurgical treatment of tumors in close proximity to or within language areas.[107] Seven months after treatment, only 10.9% of the 128 patients continued to demonstrate these postoperative language disturbances. Risk factors for the development of a postoperative aphasic disturbance included preoperative aphasia, intraoperative complications, language-positive sites within the tumor, and a nonfrontal lesion location. In patients without a preoperative deficit, normal but submaximal naming performance was found to be a strong predictor of early postoperative aphasia. The only risk factors that were identified for persistent postoperative language disturbances included age older than 40 years and preoperative aphasia.

Bello and coworkers identified language tracts through subcortical stimulation in 59% of 88 patients undergoing surgical removal of gliomas.[108] The identification of language tracts was associated with the development of a higher number of transient postoperative deficits (67.3% of patients), but permanent language deficits were ultimately noted in just 2.3% of their patients.

An important consideration when planning surgical resection of an intrinsic brain tumor is its proximity to positive language sites. Haglund and coworkers showed in a series of 40 patients with temporal lobe gliomas in the dominant hemisphere that the distance of the resection margin from the nearest language site is crucial for estimating the likelihood of a permanent postoperative language deficit.[41] In comparing the distance from the nearest language site to the resection margin, a clear association was found between the distance from the resection margin and the postoperative development of language deficits (Fig. 57-4). Patients with no postoperative deficit had an average distance between the nearest language site and the resection margin of 2.0 ± 0.43 cm; in contrast, the distance was 1.6 ± 0.2 cm in patients with deficits lasting 1 to 7 days, 0.71 ± 0.06 cm in those with deficits lasting 8 to 30 days, and 0.67 ± 0.05 cm in patients with permanent deficits. In the subgroup of patients with normal preoperative speech and comprehension, language sites identified by cortical stimulation and resection margins more than 1 cm away from the nearest language site resulted in normal language function by the end of the first postoperative week. Thus, resection of intrinsic brain tumors that follows a 1-cm safety margin from the nearest cortical language site is considered to be the best

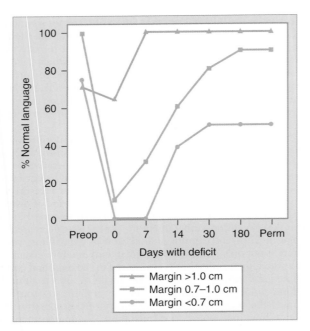

FIGURE 57-4 This graph illustrates the time course of postoperative object-naming language outcome based on the patient's preoperative status and the distance of the tumor resection margin from a language site. *(Data from Haglund MM, Berger MS, Shamseldin M, et al: Cortical localization of temporal lobe language sites in patients with gliomas. Neurosurgery. 1994;34:567.)*

surgical strategy for preventing the development of permanent postoperative aphasias while maximizing the extent of tumor resection.

Ojemann and Dodrill found that left anterior temporal resection within 2 cm of a site associated with repeated anomia or testing errors on naming tasks was linked to subtle increases in errors on the Wepman aphasia battery (administered 1 month postoperatively); no changes in the aphasia battery were evident when the resections avoided those sites, and changes in language were not induced with resections more than 2 cm away from such sites.[109] Moreover, there was no correlation between these postoperative aphasic errors and the size of the resection, preoperative language performance, or postoperative seizure control.

In a series of 294 patients, Keles and coworkers showed that subcortical stimulation to identify descending motor pathways could achieve an acceptable rate of permanent morbidity. Sixty patients (20.4%) had an additional postoperative motor deficit.[110,111] Of these patients, however, 76.7% regained their baseline function within 90 days of surgery, many of them returning to baseline in the first postoperative week.

Duffau and colleagues found that with subcortical stimulation mapping, 80% of their patients undergoing resection for low-grade gliomas experienced immediate postoperative neurological worsening.[112] However, 94% of these patients recovered to their preoperative status within 3 months, and 10% even improved. The same group also showed that postoperative morbidity and the extent of gross total resection in or near eloquent cortex at their institution significantly improved after the introduction of intraoperative stimulation mapping.[113] In a series of 115 patients who underwent intraoperative subcortical stimulation mapping, all but 2 (98%) had their language function return to baseline or better after resection of grade II gliomas in the left dominant hemisphere.[114]

FUNDAMENTALS OF SURGICAL RESECTION

With most of the cortical surface being buried within sulci, it is surprising that surface cortical stimulation can predict the effects of resections. It appears that the cortical language system has a major vertical organization and preferential location of essential areas in the crowns of gyri. Essential language areas in buried cortex, well away from those in the surface, do not seem to play a major role. Otherwise, surface stimulation would not reliably predict the effect of buried cortex resections. In fact, surface sites were identified by stimulation mapping in most patients (117 of 119), and this would not be the case if the language sites were randomly distributed. On a number of occasions, sulci that have been mapped for language have not shown independent sites, although occasionally a surface site extends a short distance into the sulcus.[13,26] The connections of essential language areas must also be somewhat vertically organized because surface stimulation predicts the effect of resections that remove white matter near the essential language areas. This relationship between surface stimulation effects and resection also seems to apply to frontal operculum stimulation, which can predict the results of resection of subinsular dominant hemisphere language sites (unpublished data).

There is a limited body of data on the stability of stimulation maps of language localization over time with or without an intervening brain lesion. On a few occasions, with repeated mapping after several months and without an intervening brain lesion, usually a comparison of extraoperative and intraoperative mapping shows that sites with or without changes in language function have had generally similar locations.[32] Remapping of language years after a static perisylvian brain injury (trauma or stroke) associated with partially recovered aphasia has shown language sites at the edge of the damaged cortex in locations where language sites are expected in nonaphasic patients. Repeated mapping for the development of aphasia in patients with recurrent brain tumors has shown disappearance of one of the localized essential language areas when the language deficit progressed, with other areas remaining stable (Haglund, Berger, and Ojemann, unpublished observations). None of these findings suggest any significant plasticity in adult language localization. In a series of nonaphasic patients with low-grade intrinsic tumors in the left temporal lobe, fewer language sites were found in the nonaphasic patients with left temporal epileptic foci, thus raising the possibility that the tumor had slowly destroyed some of the temporal lobe language sites without causing functional deficits. There was no evidence of an excess of extratemporal sites, as might be expected with reorganization.[41]

CONCLUSION

In many situations, intraoperative or extraoperative mapping can be used to identify eloquent areas for planning a safe resection. This includes the many patients in whom no intracranial ictal recordings are required and most adolescents and adults who can cooperate with an awake craniotomy that uses a local anesthetic technique. The major disadvantage of the intraoperative technique is the limited time available for language mapping. However, as we have indicated, multiple language functions at many sites can readily be assessed in 30 minutes or less, and all the information needed to plan a safe resection is usually provided. These intraoperative techniques have a number of advantages, including more flexibility in assessing essential areas of cortex and, once the essential areas have been identified, greater security in performing the resection. Intraoperative mapping also avoids the risks and cost of a second craniotomy for subdural grid placement and the risk for infection. For patients who can be managed with either technique, intraoperative stimulation mapping is the preferred method.

PART 5

Specific Operative Approaches

CHAPTER 60

Intracranial Monitoring

Kenneth P. Vives ■ Andy J. Redmond ■
Dennis D. Spencer

RATIONALE

Intracranial monitoring is one of an increasing number of tools available to neurosurgeons for the investigation of brain physiology and pathophysiology. The investigative process for neurological diseases always begins with the patient's history and physical examination to provide clues about the current state of brain function and dysfunction. For periodic disorders such as epilepsy, examination of the patient during the ictus and immediately after can provide further information about the areas of the brain involved. Neuroimaging with modalities such as computed tomography and magnetic resonance imaging (MRI) can further elucidate anatomic details of the pathology and its relationship to surrounding brain structures. Taken one step further, functional MRI can, in some patients, visualize areas of brain related to specific functions. Although these techniques are promising, the number of specific brain functions that can be mapped is limited. In many cases in which long-standing pathology exists and plasticity has allowed the relocation of function—perhaps in a more diffuse pattern—this type of imaging may not reveal the precise areas involved. Furthermore, the tasks that patients have to perform may be demanding, especially while confined in the MRI gantry. Such problems may be magnified in children and the neurologically impaired. Other imaging modalities, such as single-photon emission computed tomography (SPECT), can identify areas with abnormal blood flow, and positron emission tomography (PET) and magnetic resonance spectroscopy can identify areas of abnormal metabolism. These studies are somewhat lacking in anatomic resolution but can be enhanced by coregistration with anatomic MRI.

Scalp electroencephalograms (EEGs) may provide clues to regional localization of electrophysiologic disturbances; however, the anatomic resolution provided by such studies is inadequate to delineate the relationship of involved and uninvolved structures and allow safe operative intervention. The thick layers of the skin and skull protect the fragile structures of the central nervous system, but they the hinder electrophysiologic localization within the brain.

Thus, despite the technologic advances in functional and metabolic imaging and more sophisticated analysis of interictal abnormal electrophysiology with dipole modeling or magneto-encephalography, there are only two ways that the surgeon can be assured of localizing the epileptogenic substrate. The first is indirect and involves the use of MRI to identify anatomic abnormalities that are known to be highly epileptogenic, such as hippocampal atrophy in the setting of medial temporal lobe epilepsy or low-grade tumors. The second is the use of electrodes to directly record from suspected areas of the brain. The goal of such studies is twofold: to elucidate areas of brain pathology (i.e., epileptogenicity) and to localize brain functions for assessment of the potential risks and benefits of further intervention. Although the remainder of this chapter focuses primarily on intracranial monitoring for epilepsy, use of these devices for extraoperative brain mapping is also addressed.

HISTORY

The contribution of Otto von Guericke and later Ewald von Kleist and Pieter van Musschenbroek of Leyden in the late 1600s and early 1700s provided scientists with the means to generate and discharge static electricity. Although abundant hypotheses existed regarding the possible role of electricity in nerve and muscle conduction, Luigi Galvani was among the earliest scientists to demonstrate the role of, as he termed it, "animal electricity" in his experiments with frog leg preparations. Using electrostatic machines and static electricity generated from storms, he demonstrated contraction of muscle in response to the discharge of electricity and published these results in 1791. Galvani believed that these contractions resulted from the discharge of electricity from within the preparation; fortunately, not all agreed. Volta argued that intrinsic electricity was responsible, having been conducted into the tissue, possibly through the nerves. In the early 1800s, Hans Christian Oersted and J. S. C. Schweigger developed devices to measure small amounts of electricity (galvanometers). The development of such sensitive instruments allowed Richard Caton to record "feeble currents of the brain" directly from the cerebral cortex of animals in 1875.[1] Fifty-four years later, Hans Berger is credited with being the first to describe the human EEG. His initial measurements were performed on patients with skull defects or trephine holes and later on intact patients. In 1931, he recorded spike wave activity from the brain of a person with epilepsy. Similarly, in 1935, Frederic and Erna Gibbs recorded comparable spike wave patterns with a frequency of 3 Hz from the scalp of a woman suffering from petit mal seizures. In 1929, Sachs, Schwartz, and Kerr first recorded such activity from the surface of the human brain. Victor Horsely had been using direct cortical stimulation to guide resections for epilepsy, but it was Wilder Penfield and Herbert H. Jasper who began recording abnormal electrical activity directly from the surface of the brain at the time of such surgery. The first use of stereotactic depth electrodes for the treatment of intractable seizures dates to 1950, when E. A. Spiegel and H. T. Wycis recorded from and subsequently lesioned the lateral thalamus in an attempt to relieve seizures. These and other early studies emphasized the use of interictal recordings to guide resections. Talairach and Bancaud realized the limited ability of interictal activity to delineate the areas of paroxysmal ictal discharge,[2] and under this influence the American neurosurgeon Paul H. Crandall began chronic monitoring for the recording of spontaneous seizures in 1973.

INDICATIONS

Epilepsy

Patients being evaluated for intractable epilepsy undergo a fairly standard work-up, with some variability from center to center. Tertiary care centers, where patients with intractable seizures are referred for surgical evaluation, initially screen patients for appropriateness. In general, patients with focal epilepsy that is manifested as a consistent seizure type are likely to have an anatomic substrate for the symptomatic seizures. A second group of patients likely to benefit from surgery consists of those with multiple seizure types but with one type that is more frequent or more disabling. Last are patients with suspected diffuse or bihemispheric seizures that cause drop attacks on generalization. These patients may be candidates for monitoring before consideration of corpus callosotomy.

At Yale, we believe that the ictal onset best defines the volume of tissue that, when resected, will render the patient seizure free. The primary goal of intracranial monitoring of epilepsy patients for resection is to define this volume. It is worthwhile to note that not all institutions use these data in the same way. Some believe that interictal activity should play a major role in defining the resection and may use intraoperative interictal recordings to define the limits of resection.

In a typical phased epilepsy surgery evaluation, patients undergo detailed history taking and physical examination, followed by MRI and an outpatient EEG. This is usually followed by an inpatient continuous audiovisual EEG to further document interictal patterns on the EEG and to capture detailed semiologic (semiology, or the physical and experiential manifestation of a seizure) data, along with the ictal patterns on the EEG. During this time, patients may also undergo interictal and ictal SPECT and interictal PET. Neuropsychological examination may take place at this time as well. At the end of this period of monitoring, all the data are examined in detail to assess whether a specific area is responsible for the seizures. A decision tree is presented in Figures 60-1 and 60-2. Each part of the preoperative data set has its own characteristics that must be weighed in making the final decision with regard to concordance. Some data, by their very nature, point to only broad areas of brain dysfunction, whereas others may be very specific. Other pieces of data, such as an ictal scalp EEG, may be more regional at best and confer more weight to an MRI-detected structural abnormality, or the ictal EEG may indicate multifocality or generalization or be characterized only by muscle artifact.

Concordance of these data with an MRI abnormality is necessary to proceed to surgery without further monitoring. Several scenarios are likely. An initial determination of whether the patient has a lesion evident on MRI can be made. Patients with lesions can then be divided on the basis of whether their other data are concordant or nonconcordant. In general, patients with abnormal MRI findings and concordant data are good candidates for resection. In those with normal MRI findings, intracranial monitoring is necessary to delineate the areas of brain to be resected. The study may be designed as a focused study to cover the areas of brain identified by the initial data set as being potentially epileptogenic. In general, if the patient has one predominant seizure type, the ictal EEG may point to a particular area for invasive study. Some patients may have multiple areas of ictal onset but a common spread pattern, thus generating a single seizure type. Other patients may have a single area of ictal generation with a variable spread pattern that is manifested as multiple seizure types. Seizure onset in particular areas of the brain may be prone to rapid spread, thereby making the ictal EEG appear bilateral or diffuse.

These and many other factors need to be considered before deciding that a patient is or is not a candidate for further investigation. For example, a patient may have an ictal EEG that specifies one hemisphere, semiology on an audiovisual EEG that is consistently lobar (i.e., hemifield flashing lights from one occipital lobe), SPECT scans confirming regionally abnormal blood flow and metabolism, and neuropsychological testing that is abnormal but nonspecific. An invasive study should be designed to cover the posterior aspect of the hemisphere in question.

The other set of patients consists of those with evidence of a tumor, vascular malformation, or hippocampal sclerosis on MRI. Typically, these patients, in whom the other data are concordant, proceed to surgery without intracranial monitoring. Exceptions are individuals with evidence of brain developmental disorders on neuroimaging. These patients may have more diffuse brain abnormalities, and at our center, the threshold for invasive monitoring in these instances is low. In many cases in which a lesion is present and the other data are concordant, further study is warranted to ensure that the lesion is or is not responsible for the seizures. In other cases, patients may have multiple lesions, but all the data point to one particular lesion as being responsible for the seizures. Unless there are pressing reasons to address the other lesions (e.g., a patient with multiple cavernous malformations, one of which is larger and has evidence of hemorrhage, but the data point to a smaller lesion without evidence of hemorrhage), many of these patients can proceed directly to surgery.

A special case involves patients with lesions and evidence of hippocampal sclerosis. There is speculation in the literature about the relationship of these entities.[3-5] It is possible that an extrahippocampal lesion may cause seizures that spread through the hippocampus. Over time, this spread pattern could damage the hippocampus through excitotoxicity and render it an independent source of seizures. At our institution, in general, patients with hippocampal atrophy and dysfunction (temporal lobe–specific poor memory) in whom the other data are concordant for the temporal lobe undergo combined resection of the lesion and the hippocampus. The more medial the lesion, the more likely we are to assume true dual pathology and resect both. Patients without evidence of hippocampal dysfunction on neuropsychological studies and the intracarotid amobarbital (Amytal) procedure (IAP) undergo lesionectomy without hippocampectomy, regardless of the volume of the hippocampus, although a small proportion of these patients may need further resection. In the context of these cases, the IAP (Wada test) is also specifically used to ensure the ability of the contralateral hemisphere to encode memory when hippocampal resection is planned. Poor memory performance of the contralateral hemisphere on the IAP would largely be a contraindication to resection and would necessitate consideration of nonresective strategies for treatment of the patient's seizure disorder, such as investigational responsive electrical neurostimulation or multiple subpial transections, when applicable.

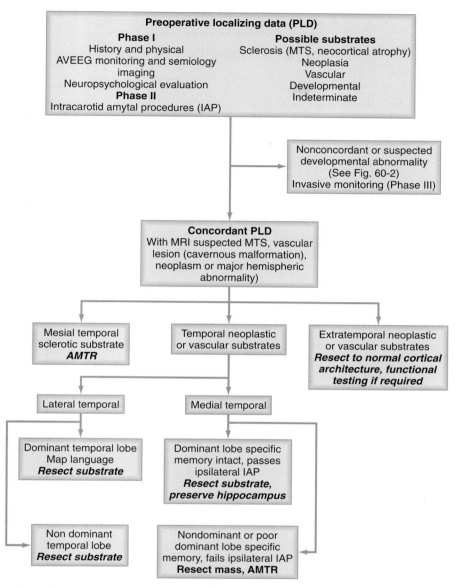

Preoperative localizing data (PLD)

Phase I	**Possible substrates**
History and physical	Sclerosis (MTS, neocortical atrophy)
AVEEG monitoring and semiology	Neoplasia
imaging	Vascular
Neuropsychological evaluation	Developmental
Phase II	Indeterminate
Intracarotid amytal procedures (IAP)	

Nonconcordant or suspected
developmental abnormality
(See Fig. 60-2)
Invasive monitoring (Phase III)

Concordant PLD
With MRI suspected MTS, vascular
lesion (cavernous malformation),
neoplasm or major hemispheric
abnormality)

Mesial temporal
sclerotic substrate
AMTR

Temporal neoplastic
or vascular substrates

Extratemporal neoplastic
or vascular substrates
***Resect to normal cortical
architecture, functional
testing if required***

Lateral temporal

Medial temporal

Dominant temporal lobe
Map language
Resect substrate

Dominant lobe specific
memory intact, passes
ipsilateral IAP
***Resect substrate,
preserve hippocampus***

Non dominant
temporal lobe
Resect substrate

Nondominant or poor
dominant lobe specific
memory, fails ipsilateral IAP
Resect mass, AMTR

FIGURE 60-1 Part 1 of a decision-making tree for the evaluation of patients with intractable epilepsy.

Brain Mapping

A separate indication for intracranial monitoring of patients without epilepsy is for extraoperative brain mapping (see Fig. 60-8). The goal is typically to map the areas of appreciable function in relation to a lesion (1) to provide data about the risks associated with surgical resection so that the clinician and patient can make a decision about the appropriateness of surgery and (2) to allow surgical planning to minimize those risks. In some instances, intraoperative monitoring may be the most efficient way to address these issues. Mapping of simple motor modalities can be accomplished at surgery through direct cortical stimulation. Similarly, sensory mapping can be performed via somatosensory evoked potentials. Intraoperative language mapping requires an awake patient who can participate at the time of surgery and demonstrate reversible deficits during cortical stimulation. Testing of higher cognitive function may be difficult during surgery because of the complexity of the tasks that must be performed. Beyond these straightforward tests, particular patients and particular types of mapping may make extraoperative mapping more desirable.

Some patients, such as children and adults who are unable to cooperate, may be unable to participate in an awake craniotomy. The claustrophobic nature of the drapes, even if they are transparent, can be overwhelming. No matter how good the anesthesia, the discomfort from craniotomy may also be a hindrance. Even preoperative language testing in children may be difficult because the patient is required to focus on the tests for a substantial period; the same can be said of neurologically impaired adults. Other brain modalities may be difficult to map intraoperatively. For example, a professional in the field of personal relations who has a lesion in the posterior fusiform gyrus near the facial recognition area may not desire resection if substantial impairment could result. Mapping this area requires multiple visual stimuli that would be difficult to accomplish intraoperatively.

HARDWARE

A variety of electrodes are available for use in electrophysiologic monitoring, and current research is focused on developing wireless implantable systems. A combination of depth electrodes and

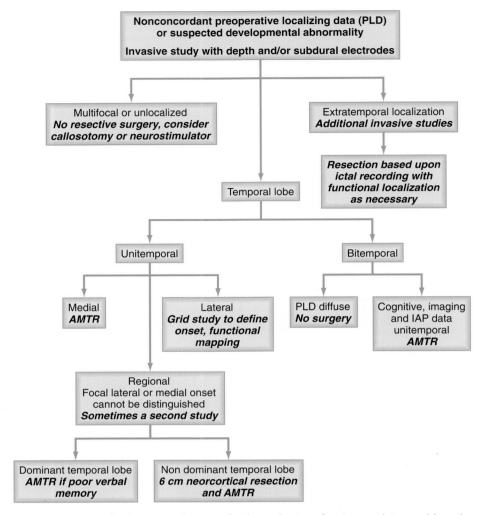

FIGURE 60-2 Part 2 of a decision-making tree for the evaluation of patients with intractable epilepsy.

subdural strip or grid electrodes are routinely used in most situations (Fig. 60-3). In certain situations in which the plane between the dura and brain surface is scarred and safe dissection is impossible, epidural peg electrodes can be used. Alternatively, a subdural electrode can be placed in the epidural space, but unless the dura has been denervated, these electrodes cannot be used for stimulation-based mapping. Some centers supplement scalp studies or intracranial studies with foramen ovale or sphenoidal electrodes. The construction, surgical technique, and use of each are discussed here.

Depth Electrodes

Depth electrodes are typically constructed with one or more contacts in a thin shaft with a blunt tip to minimize traumatic brain and vascular injury. Both rigid and flexible types exist. For insertion, the flexible electrodes are made rigid through a stylet that is fixed adjacent to the electrode or placed down the center and removed after insertion. An added advantage is that these electrodes can be tunneled subcutaneously, thereby reducing the risk for infection. The contacts themselves are usually made of platinum or platinum-iridium construction and spaced from 3 to 10 mm apart. For multicontact electrodes, individual insulated wires run up the inner cannula of the hollow electrode and lead to contacts that can be connected to a ribbon cable. Electrodes with multiple contacts can be used to record along the longitu-

dinal dimension of a structure, such as the hippocampus, or they may allow simultaneous recording of a deep structure and the cortical surface through which the electrode was inserted (Figs. 60-4 and 60-5).

Subdural Electrodes—Strips and Grids

Subdural electrodes are typically constructed from a flexible material that conforms to the surface anatomy of the brain. Usually, they have multiple contacts in one or more columns to allow simultaneous recording from different areas of the cortex. In general, two types are used: one that consists of a thin shaft or reed with multiple contacts (similar to depth electrodes) and one in which multiple disks are embedded in a thin sheet of Silastic. We find the second type to be more useful because of the enhanced ability to direct the electrodes to specific sites from a remote bur hole. The larger contact surface and the Silastic coating make cortical stimulation possible without dural pain. The wires from a single strip then exit together in a hollow Silastic tube. Newer constructs have multiple strips passing through a large Silastic tube that lead to contacts that can be connected to a ribbon cable. The contacts are constructed of stainless steel or platinum.

Most grids are similarly constructed, but they have columns of multiple contacts for a wider area of coverage (see Fig. 60-4). These grids terminate in multiple thin, hollow tubes with

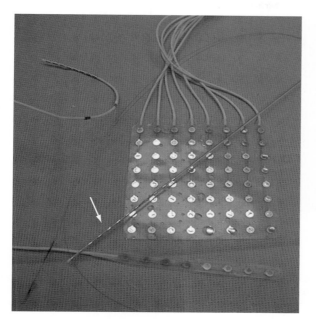

FIGURE 60-3 Intracranial monitoring hardware. The *arrow* points to a depth electrode.

contacts for connecting to ribbon cables. One special type is an L-shaped grid for recording from the medial surface of the hemisphere (Fig. 60-6). Once again, the contacts may be made of platinum or stainless steel. The platinum construction allows safe postoperative performance of MRI.[6]

Epidural Peg Electrodes

Recording of electrical activity from electrodes placed in the epidural space traces its history to Penfield and Jasper, who used epidural ball electrodes in a few difficult cases.[7] In comparison to scalp EEGs, epidural recordings have the advantage of providing an improved signal-to-noise ratio. The effect is created by reducing volume conduction and amplitude attenuation and by eliminating the myogenic and kinesigenic artifacts inherent with scalp EEGs.[8] Epidural recording has also been considered an alternative to subdural and intraparenchymal monitoring because of its semi-invasive nature and the presumed advantage of fewer infectious and hemorrhagic complications.

Epidural electrode designs have included ball electrodes,[7] screws,[8] and pegs.[9] Epidural screws and peg electrodes are widely applied in some epilepsy surgery centers. The screw is usually made of titanium and has a shaft to prevent overpenetration. Screw length varies to allow stable placement and to accommodate the varying thickness of the scalp and calvaria. The screw head is hexagonal to permit easy placement and removal of the

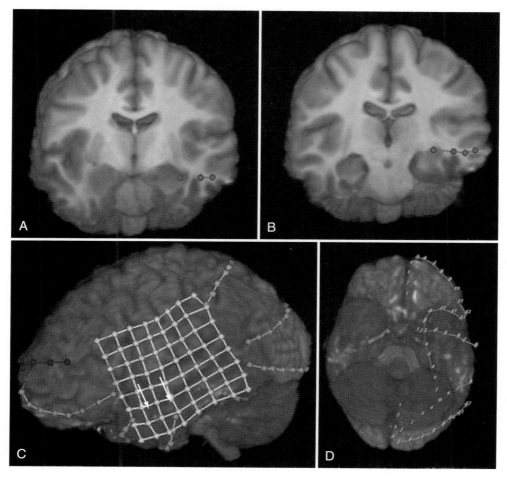

FIGURE 60-4 Reconstructions of electrode positions for a typical dominant frontotemporal study superimposed on preoperative magnetic resonance images. **A,** Anterior medial temporal depth electrode. **B,** Posterior medial temporal depth electrode. **C,** Electrode entrance sites (*arrows*) in the context of the rest of the study from a lateral view. **D,** Inferior view.

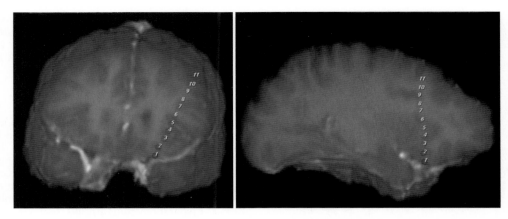

FIGURE 60-5 Coronal and sagittal reconstructions of an orbitofrontal depth electrode.

electrodes with a wrench. Right-angled EEG monitoring leads can be placed in the screw head.[8] Epidural peg electrodes are composed of mushroom-shaped Silastic elastomer, and the stalk tapers from a diameter of 4.7 mm to a diameter of 0.5 mm. At the base of the stalk, either stainless steel or platinum tips are used to conduct the electrical current. The tips are continuous with the Teflon-coated steel wire that is tunneled through the peg and exits through the cap. Strip arrays of epidural electrodes have also been described.[10]

Foramen Ovale and Sphenoidal Electrodes

Foramen ovale electrodes were first developed in 1985 as a semi-invasive EEG alternative to intracerebral depth electrodes for the evaluation of mesial temporal lobe epilepsy.[11] These electrodes generally consist of helical, wound, Teflon-coated silver wires that end in multicontact poles.[12] The construct is mounted on a thin stainless steel wire. The mechanical properties conferred to this construct allow appropriate flexibility to avoid puncturing the pia-arachnoid layer. The external diameter permits easy

passage through a specially constructed 18-gauge introducer cannula.[11]

Sphenoidal electrodes are used by many epilepsy centers as an adjunct to standard scalp EEG electrodes for the evaluation of temporal lobe epilepsy. These electrodes, in conjunction with scalp EEGs, can help determine whether the focus of the seizure is in the medial or lateral aspect of the temporal lobe. Sphenoidal electrodes were originally rigid, thus allowing only short-term monitoring, but they have evolved to a flexible design. Teflon-coated or multiple wires have silver or stainless steel tips, are flexible, and may be applied for EEG recordings for up to 3 weeks.[13]

Recording Equipment

After implantation, the leads are connected to an isolation box to prevent any inadvertent current from entering the patient. Impedances are checked with a small current in the vicinity of 10 nA.[14] The isolation box is then connected to a multichannel amplifier and a recording system. Typically, systems with at least 64-channel capabilities are used; however, more extensive studies necessitate more channels. An initial montage with sampling from the contacts of each implanted device is used. The information gained as the study continues usually dictates changes in the montage to focus on the relevant areas. Simultaneous video recordings provide the information necessary to correlate semiology with electrophysiologic data.

DESIGN OF STUDIES

Epilepsy Studies

In general terms, the preoperative localizing data dictate the areas to be studied. Localizing data from seizure semiology, scalp ictal EEGs, neuroimaging, and neuropsychological data are combined to establish which areas are suspected of being involved in seizure generation. If there is any doubt about the origin or spread of the seizure, one should have a low threshold for conducting bilateral hemispheric studies. Strip electrodes allow smaller craniotomies to be made than needed for grids and should be used generously over the convexities and sylvian fissure. Moreover, they allow accurate localization of language areas.

Several scenarios based on the type and multiplicity of lesions and the reliability or concordance of the preoperative data are typically encountered during the study design. Patients with lesions and discordant data generally require grid coverage over the lesion, as well as strip and depth electrode coverage of areas

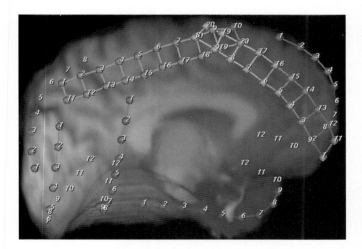

FIGURE 60-6 Reconstruction of two interhemispheric "L"-shaped grid placements for monitoring of the supplementary motor area and cingulate. The interhemispheric fissure is entered where the veins permit, and both strips are placed, one directed anteriorly and the other posteriorly. Frequently, both sides can be accessed from a unilateral approach by making an opening in the falx between the superior and inferior sagittal sinuses.

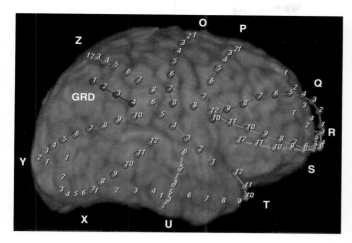

FIGURE 60-7 Reconstruction of a frontotemporal subdural strip study. This type of study is frequently used bilaterally as a survey study for patients with poorly lateralized PLD and frontotemporal semiology.

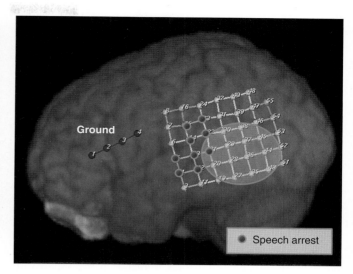

FIGURE 60-8 Reconstruction of grid placement for a patient with a temporo-occipital lesion for speech mapping before occipital lobectomy. The patient had previously undergone a subdural strip study localized to the temporo-occipital junction. The approximate location of the lesion is illustrated. This technique is frequently used in patients who will not tolerate an awake craniotomy.

as indicated by the other preoperative data. Patients with developmental abnormalities merit special consideration. In contrast to most other lesions, these malformative lesions may be inherently capable of seizure generation. Subdural grid coverage may not identify the seizure source if it is located in a malformed area of gray matter; therefore, depth electrode coverage of the lesion itself may be required. Other less accessible lesions may be suitable for depth electrodes, such as the medial hemisphere, orbitofrontal area, or the insula (see Figs. 60-4 and 60-5). Patients with multiple lesions typically require coverage over the lesions most likely to be responsible for seizure generation, as well as other potential epileptogenic regions demonstrated on preoperative studies. In patients with suspected bilateral medial temporal lobe seizures, bilateral hippocampal electrodes are used in combination with bilateral temporal lobe strip coverage (Fig. 60-7; also see Fig. 60-4A and B).

Patients without lesions but with concordant preoperative data undergo a focused study of the suspected area of the brain, as well as sampling of other areas. For patients with discordant preoperative data and negative MRI findings, a broad study is designed in which any localization data are used to direct the study. Many times, despite the paucity of imaging abnormalities and conflicting data, an invasive study may be useful. Usually, patients arrive at this stage because the seizure semiology is reproducible and may be distinct enough to define an area of seizure generation. This semiologic information can be used to at least help construct the study.

Two important facts must be kept in mind when designing and interpreting such studies. First, one cannot cover all possible epileptogenic locations with electrodes, and caution must be taken when interpreting electrical activity at the edge of grids or the end of strips. A source just beyond the area of coverage may appear to originate from the edge contacts. A clear voltage reversal between two adjacent electrodes is much better evidence of localization. Second, grids and strips record only from the surface of the brain. Gray matter in the sulci is also sampled from the surface, with problems similar to those encountered with scalp EEGs.

Brain Mapping Studies

Typically, these focused studies cover the areas of the lesion, as well as adjacent functional brain. In most locations, a subdural grid is well suited to such studies (Fig. 60-8). In other cases,

regional venous anatomy may dictate the use of custom-cut grids or subdural strips to avoid sacrificing a critical vein. For example, with lesions in the posterior fusiform gyrus, the location of the vein of Labbé may make grid placement difficult.

OPERATIVE CONSIDERATIONS

Preoperative Evaluation

Patients undergoing monitoring require routine preoperative management similar to that for any other patient undergoing craniotomy. Coagulation studies and particularly a bleeding time are necessary to screen for occult disorders of hemostasis. Many patients who require intracranial monitoring have also undergone an IAP, so the arterial and particularly the venous phase of the angiogram can be reviewed preoperatively to identify areas where the venous anatomy may limit the ability to place electrodes. For patients who have not undergone angiography and in whom the preoperative plan for electrodes requires defining the vascular anatomy, such as interhemispheric studies or studies around the vein of Labbé, a preoperative magnetic resonance venogram may be helpful. In patients who have seizures at particular times of the month, such as catamenial epilepsy, the study should be timed so that the monitoring precedes the patient's time of heightened seizure frequency by several days. In general, epilepsy patients need to be counseled carefully about the possibility of lengthy studies that require them to be confined to a single room for, in rare instances, weeks at a time. The electrodes and head dressing can be heavy and difficult to tolerate for some patients. Particularly with grid placement, we have found that the operation itself may cause a period of decreased seizure activity, which may prolong studies.

Placement of subdural strips or grids often requires the use of mild hyperventilation and administration of mannitol to provide adequate brain relaxation, thus necessitating general anesthesia. Depth electrodes may be inserted under local anesthesia with sedation; however, it is rare that such studies are performed without the simultaneous use of subdural strips.

Depth Electrodes

The insertion of depth electrodes is a stereotactic procedure in which either fixed frames or frameless devices are used. Identifying vascular structures via anatomic MRI is most useful when coregistered with magnetic resonance angiography and venography. The planned trajectory can be reviewed so that these structures can be avoided en route to the target. In contrast to biopsies, multiple contacts along the electrode trajectory need to be optimally positioned to obtain the maximal amount of information.

After preparation and draping, the area of skin through which the electrode is to be inserted is identified with stereotaxy. Alternatively, when planning a craniotomy for insertion of other subdural electrodes, if possible, the entrance site is designed so that it is close to a planned dural edge. This allows the electrode to be secured promptly and, in general, keeps it safely out of the way during the remainder of the procedure.

For longitudinal hippocampal placement, usually a small, vertical linear incision is made in the parasagittal occipital bone. Incisions for orthogonal temporal, frontal, or parietal study vary with location, but thoughtful consideration should be given to design of the skin incision so that it can be incorporated into a larger incision at the time of future resection. In patients with very thick bone, the trajectory of the depth electrode needs to be taken into account when creating a bur hole so that one can avoid having the trajectory blocked by the bone edge. After placement of the bur hole, the dura is coagulated and opened. If necessary, the entry point is replanned to avoid surface vessels. The electrode is then measured to ensure placement at the appropriate depth. After coagulation and incision of the pia-arachnoid, the electrode is inserted with the proper x, y, and z coordinates for framed stereotaxy or the appropriate visualized structure for frameless stereotaxy while feeling for areas of resistance as the electrode is passed. If unexpected resistance is met, the stereotaxy system is checked, the MRI trajectory is reviewed, and passage is reattempted. The stylet is then removed and the electrode is immediately secured to the dural edge, if possible. Frequently, this suture will be placed in the dura and looped loosely around the metal cannula, before its withdrawal. This allows the electrode to then be promptly secured with minimal manipulation. The electrode is tunneled under the skin with a cannula and trocar. A purse-string 4-0 nylon suture is placed at the site of exit from the skin and tied down, and then two separate 3-0 nylon sutures are used to secure the electrode to the skin. The ends of these electrodes are typically marked so that they can be identified postoperatively, with the head dressing on. After placement, the location of the electrode, along with its identifying mark, is recorded in the patient's chart. A hemostatic sponge is then placed in the bur hole and the skin closed. In many instances, a depth electrode must be inserted orthogonally through a grid that has been placed. In these cases, a small hole needs to be created in the grid to place the electrode. The electrode is sutured to the grid and tunneled out through the base of the flap.

When turning a large craniotomy flap, such as that needed for subdural grids, the brain may shift a number of millimeters. This shift occurs primarily at the cortical surface, not at the more medial structures such as the hippocampus, which typically makes the preoperative stereotaxy valid for the placement of depth electrodes. The one instance in which this does not apply is when the patient's head is positioned such that gravity is orthogonal to the direction of electrode placement, as in a patient with bitemporal craniotomies and the head in the neutral position. Cortical settling will occur in the direction of gravity (inferior and posterior) and possibly cause an error in this direction. Regardless, it is preferable to place depth electrodes before cortical settling.

Over the past 8 years we have been using frameless magnetic resonance stereotaxy almost exclusively for the insertion of depth electrodes. This system allows stereotactic placement when mul-tiple targets are planned in both hemispheres during grid placement. The absence of a frame prevents interference with the craniotomy and obviates the need to reset the x and y coordinates for each trajectory. However, placement of the Mayfield head holder and attachment of the stereotactic arm both require careful planning to allow access of the arm to both hemispheres, especially in the temporal regions.

Subdural Strips

Before preparation, the skin incision should be marked. Localization can be performed with simple craniometric measurement in conjunction with MRI, or stereotaxy can be used as an aid. Once again, the possible need to incorporate incisions into a future larger incision for resection should be considered. For example, in patients undergoing temporal lobe strip studies in which anteromedial temporal lobe resection may be required, we typically make the skin incision for insertion of the subdural strip in the same location as the upper limb of the temporal lobe craniotomy incision (see Fig. 60-7). After the skin incision, a small craniotomy is made, or a bony trough is created in the anteroposterior direction with multiple bur holes that are connected via a cutting bur. After removal of the bone, the dura is coagulated and opened. The strips are inserted with a pair of forceps while directing them toward the desired target with a steady stream of irrigation under the strip. This irrigation helps the strip slide smoothly over the surface of the brain and prevents trauma. If any resistance is felt, the strip is removed and reinserted. These areas of resistance may represent bridging cortical veins and thus should be avoided to prevent hemorrhage under the bone, to which the surgeon has no access through the same craniotomy. Finding the correct trajectory and depth of insertion for a given cortical location requires both patience and experience. After insertion, the intended location is recorded in the patient's chart, and the electrode is tunneled through the skin. A purse-string suture is placed around the site of exit, and the electrode is secured with a separate skin suture. Gelfoam is placed over the dural incision, and the skin is closed.

One particular technique of note is placement of a medial temporal subdural strip. Typically, a 12-contact strip is used, and the strip is inserted parallel to the sylvian fissure by gently pushing in a posterior to anterior direction, just below the sphenoid ridge. This strip will guide itself along the sphenoid and eventually place contacts close to the parahippocampal gyrus (see Fig. 60-4D).

Subdural Grids

Placement of large subdural grids requires a craniotomy flap of the same approximate size as the grid (see Fig. 60-4C). Once again, the skin flap should be designed so that if necessary, it can be incorporated into an incision for resection. The skin is incised in a U-shaped fashion and reflected. A periosteal graft may be harvested for use in dural closure after grid placement if desired. The bone flap is removed and the bone is cleaned thoroughly and sent to the bone bank for the duration of the study. Alternatively, an incision can be made in the abdomen and the bone inserted subcutaneously for safekeeping until the time of replacement, or it can be left in the craniotomy site but not secured tightly to the skull. After hemostasis, the dura is opened and removed in a circumferential fashion. This denervates the dura and decreases the frequency of postoperative headaches. A digital photograph of the brain is then taken. The grid is placed on the brain in the appropriate position and the multiple leads are tunneled subcutaneously and brought through the base of the skin flap, if possible. Purse-string sutures are placed around the exit of each site, and each electrode is secured to the skin with a separate suture. An additional photograph is taken with the grid, strip, and depth electrodes in place. These photographs often reveal gyral anatomy and electrode placement that cannot be achieved even with three-dimensional reconstructed MRI scans. The dura can then be closed with the previously harvested periosteal and dural grafts. Alternatively, we have been using a Gore-Tex dural substitute (Gore Preclude MVP Dura Substitute). Use of this particular product has drastically reduced scarring at the brain surface and facilitates dissection at the time of resection. An epidural drain is placed and tunneled through a distant separate stab incision. A "sleeper stitch" is placed around the drain exit site and wrapped around the drain. This stitch is used to secure the skin when the drain is removed the following morning. The skin is closed in two layers.

Epidural Peg Electrodes

Surgical placement of epidural peg or screw electrodes can be done with the patient under general or local anesthesia. The patient's head is placed in a favorable position for exposure of the desired brain area for electrographic examination, and multiple skin incisions of approximately 1.5 cm are made for placement of the epidural peg electrodes. For the placement of epidural screw electrodes, only 0.5-cm stab incisions are required. Small bur holes are made with a twist drill. When placing epidural screws, the electrodes are hand-tightened and then secured with a wrench. When placing epidural peg electrodes, electrodes with appropriate stalk length are selected and placed securely with a wrench until the cap of the peg can be covered by the edges of the galea, and the electrode wires are tunneled through the subcutaneous space. Usually, placement of epidural strips and grids requires a craniotomy.

Foramen Ovale and Sphenoidal Electrodes

Härtel's landmarks[15] are used to insert foramen ovale and sphenoidal electrodes. The introductory cannula is inserted 3 cm lateral to the oral commissure and passed to the foramen ovale via Kirschner's technique under fluoroscopic guidance. The cannula is guided along a line formed by the intersection of two orthogonal planes. The first plane is defined by the insertion point and the point on the lower eyelid corresponding to the medial border of the pupil. The second plane is defined by the insertion point and a spot 5 cm anterior to the external auditory meatus. Return of cerebrospinal fluid is visualized with removal of the inner cannula. The electrode is then placed through the cannula, usually without resistance, until its expected placement in the cistern. The cannula is then withdrawn, and the electrodes are fixed to the skin with gauze and adhesive tape. Removal of foramen ovale electrodes does not require anesthesia. Transient spasm or dysesthesias in the ipsilateral teeth may be elicited during withdrawal of the electrodes.

Sphenoidal electrodes are placed percutaneously under the zygomatic arch until they rest near the foramen ovale. The electrodes are directed toward the midportion of the foramen ovale. After insertion, the electrodes are taped securely to the skin and attached to a standard EEG jack.

POSTOPERATIVE CARE

The head is wrapped in a bulky dressing with a chin strap and the electrodes exiting from one or two sites. This type of dressing is necessary to prevent dislodgement of the electrodes during seizures and to contain any minor cerebrospinal fluid leaks. Patients who undergo grid placement usually receive a 1- to 3-day tapering course of methylprednisolone (Solu-Medrol). MRI and a high-resolution tomographic scan are performed the following morning to localize the electrodes. Before sending the patient for an MRI, care is taken to ensure that none of the electrodes form a loop. The electrode contacts are well visualized on computed tomographic scans; however, the signal artifact makes it difficult to delineate postoperative complications.[6] In addition, the superior resolution of MRI provides anatomic detail that is not possible to obtain with computed tomography. Therefore, we digitally fuse the MRI and computed tomographic images to create three-dimensional renderings of the electrodes and the brain (http://www.bioimagesuite.org/). This allows us to better understand the locations of the electrodes relative to the potential epileptogenic substrate. Interictal SPECT may be performed at this time for later substraction from an ictal injection.

Complications include small intraparenchymal hematomas associated with depth electrodes (2%), subdural electrodes mistakenly placed intraparenchymally (4%),[16] and placement of depth electrodes in the wrong position (2%).[17]

After the imaging studies are completed, the patient is taken to the epilepsy unit and connected to the monitoring equipment. The exiting electrodes and their connections must be tethered to the dressing. Wyler and colleagues found no difference in rates of meningitis in patient receiving continuous antibiotics after subdural strip placement versus those receiving only perioperative coverage[18]; thus, our patients routinely receive a 24-hour course of antibiotics and then no antibiotics during the remainder of the study unless other indications arise. Cerebrospinal fluid leaks may occur in up to 19% of patients,[19] so the head dressing is checked twice daily for evidence of leakage. A wet dressing is changed with sterile technique, and the source of the leak is sought and sutured. Patients usually experience low-grade fever and headache after the procedure. These fevers do not correlate with intracranial infection,[20] but care should be taken to evaluate patients with prolonged fever. Headache is especially troublesome and patients may require narcotics for 36 to 48 hours.

At the end of monitoring, the patient is returned to the operating room. Probes and strips are removed by gentle, steady traction without reopening the incision. Patients who have undergone grid placement are intubated and placed in pins, and the exiting leads from any grids and strips are tied into a bundle with umbilical tape that extends below the sterile field. After sterile preparation, the sutures are removed and the head is reprepared. The patient is draped and the incision is reopened. The leads are cut intradurally and then removed from the sterile field by pulling on the umbilical tape outside the field. The dura is reopened and the grid removed. Neocortical resections are performed at this time by using the acquired ictal data and functional mapping from grid stimulation. If ictal onset is localized to the medial temporal lobe or other sites that would require extensive additional bone work and brain retraction, the electrodes are removed, and the patient is brought back for resection in approximately 4 to 6 weeks. This avoids retraction of the mildly edematous brain caused by the electrode study. After any planned resection of tissue, the dura is closed, and the banked bone flap is reinserted and secured.

OUTCOME WITH INTRACRANIAL MONITORING

The outcome of resection in patients undergoing intracranial monitoring for epilepsy is linked to the selected population that undergoes such monitoring and interpretation of the data from such studies. We have outlined the general criteria used to select these patients for study, but the process is dynamic and changes over time. Patients with the best outcomes after surgical resection are those with hippocampal sclerosis or circumscribed lesions and concordant data. The majority of these patients do not require monitoring. Patients selected for invasive study are less likely to have excellent outcomes because of the nonconcordance of their preoperative data or the nonlesional extratemporal location.

Approximately 64% to 94% of patients are found to have sufficient localizing information to proceed to resection after intracranial study.[17,21-23] Thus, many more patients can be offered resection than those evaluated with scalp EEGs only.[24] An increasing percentage of patients being monitored are those with extratemporal epilepsy because MRI identifies most lesions and hippocampal atrophy.

After resection, 28% to 64% of patients are seizure free.[17,23,25] The range is so wide because series from different centers have substantially varied patient populations, experience, and indications for intracranial monitoring. In 21 patients with seizures localizing to the temporal lobe, Cascino and coworkers found that only 9 were seizure free after resection.[26] The largest number of patients with inferior outcomes had normal findings on MRI (without hippocampal atrophy), along with 3 patients who had hypothalamic masses and were thought to have gelastic seizures.

Epidural peg and screw electrodes have limited applications in the presurgical evaluation of epilepsy patients and have been used in addition to standard seizure monitoring techniques.[27,28] Their main advantages are the relative ease of placement and the probably decreased rates of major complications associated with subdural and intraparenchymal monitoring. Even though the signal-to-noise ratio of epidural monitoring is significantly improved over that of scalp EEG, it provides a lower density of coverage than possible with subdural or intraparenchymal monitoring and does not allow the definition of functional anatomy. The issues regarding the density of coverage may be overcome in part by the placement of epidural grid electrodes, which requires a craniotomy.

Surgical outcome regarding the preoperative use of epidural arrays was reported by Goldring and Gregorie, who reviewed 100 cases in which epidural electrode arrays were used to define the epileptic focus.[10] Sixty-four percent of the epileptic children and 62% of the epileptic adults had "good" outcomes. Kuzniecky and coauthors also reported greater than 90% improvement in seizures after resection based on the use of epidural grids and strips in 50 patients with predominantly temporal lobe epilepsy.[29] Epidural electrodes can identify epileptogenic foci in select patients with temporal lobe epilepsy and poorly localizing scalp EEG recordings.[30] Nevertheless, questions remain about whether surgical outcomes based on the use of epidural arrays are comparable to those of resections based on more invasive monitoring.

The efficacy of foramen ovale electrodes in identifying the mesolimbic temporal lobe as the epileptogenic substrate has been examined on a limited basis. However, in scenarios in which clinical, imaging, and scalp EEG data do not give clear temporal lateralizing information, there may be a safe and valuable adjunct.[20,31] With careful analysis, foramen ovale electrode recordings have been used to reliably identify the primary temporal source of seizures.[32] When candidates for amygdalohippocampectomy were studied preoperatively with foramen ovale electrodes, favorable outcomes were obtained by Wieser and associates[11]; similar outcomes were reported in that group (64% seizure free) and in the group studied with stereoelectroencephalography (59% seizure free). Similarly, Shih and colleagues demonstrated that 78% of patients with mesial temporal lobe epilepsy became seizure free after resection based on the use of foramen ovale electrodes.[31]

The advantages of foramen ovale electrodes are their semi-invasiveness, relative ease of placement, and elimination of the increased risk associated with the placement of depth electrodes and subdural grids and strips.[33] They may also be more cost-effective.[34] One drawback involves interpretation of the information generated without the appropriate context of having accurate electrographic information from other alternative epileptogenic sites. The most serious drawback may be the possibility of falsely localizing the seizure focus to the mesial temporal lobe and

missing the real epileptogenic focus, which may be in the neocortical temporal lobe or in an extratemporal location. Some centers with extensive experience in the technique emphasize the need to closely examine the seizure discharge pattern, as well as the scalp EEG, when interpreting the results recorded from foramen ovale electrodes. In light of the theoretical disadvantage of false localization, foramen ovale electrodes have not been used at our institution. We favor the techniques of intracranial depth electrodes and subdural grids and strips, which remain the "gold standard" in this field. Rather than replacing invasive monitoring, foramen ovale electrodes may have a more rational place as an adjunct, perhaps in the selection of patients for further invasive electrographic localization.

Early studies comparing sphenoidal electrodes with scalp EEG electrodes revealed that in patients suspected of having mesial temporal lobe epilepsy, the spike amplitude was largest with sphenoidal electrodes. It was believed that the proximity of these electrodes to the basal medial aspect of the temporal lobe increased their sensitivity for detecting mesial temporal discharges.[35] This notion of sphenoidal spikes' specificity for mesial temporal discharges has been questioned, however; Marks and coworkers found that the large sphenoidal spikes may be associated with extratemporal and extrahippocampal foci, thus raising questions regarding the specificity of sphenoidal electrodes.[36] Historically, many sphenoidal electrodes were passed blindly, which might have compromised the accuracy of the EEG recordings. When compared with the blind approach, Kanner and coauthors reported markedly improved sensitivity and specificity when sphenoidal electrodes were placed under fluoroscopic guidance.[37] Furthermore, when combined with scalp EEG, sphenoidal electrodes can be used to distinguish medial and neocortical epilepsy, with localization of medial temporal lobe ictal foci in 90% of patients.[38]

CONCLUSION

The use of intracranial monitoring to delineate brain function and dysfunction is largely dependent on the investigator's use of preoperative data to define a specific question that can be answered through the design and implementation of a study. Specific thought must be given not only to which areas are to be studied but also to which areas are to be omitted from the study. The recording and analysis of electrophysiologic data and data gained through stimulation studies can be used to determine the area of resection for epilepsy surgery, the anatomic relationship of a lesion to functional brain areas, or both. Electrophysiologic data constitute only a small amount of information that can be gained through these studies. A whole range of biosensors that in the future may detect changes in neurotransmitter levels, electrolyte disturbances, or metabolism can be envisioned to arm the neurosurgeon with more detailed information to allow safer, more successful resections.

SUGGESTED READINGS

Awad IA, Assirati JA Jr, Burgess R, et al. A new class of electrodes of 'intermediate invasiveness': preliminary experience with epidural pegs and foramen ovale electrodes in the mapping of seizure foci. *Neurol Res.* 1991;13:177-183.

Barnett GH, Burgess RC, Awad IA, et al. Epidural peg electrodes for the presurgical evaluation of intractable epilepsy. *Neurosurgery.* 1990;27:113-115.

Baumgartner C, Lindinger G, Lurger S, et al. Prolonged video EEG monitoring in differential diagnosis of seizures and in presurgical epilepsy diagnosis. *Wien Med Wochenschr.* 1998;148:2-8.

Behrens E, Zentner J, van Roost D, et al. Subdural and depth electrodes in the presurgical evaluation of epilepsy. *Acta Neurochir (Wien).* 1994;128:84-87.

Brazier MAB. *A History of the Electrical Activity of the Brain: The First Half-Century.* New York: Macmillan; 1961.

Carter DA, Lassiter AT, Brown JA. Cost-efficient localization of seizures of mesiotemporal onset with foramen-ovale electrodes. *Neurol Res.* 1998;20:153-160.

Cascino GD, Jack CR Jr, Parisi JE, et al. Operative strategy in patients with MRI-identified dual pathology and temporal lobe epilepsy. *Epilepsy Res.* 1993;14:175-182.

Cascino GD, Trenerry MR, Sharbrough FW, et al. Depth electrode studies in temporal lobe epilepsy: relation to quantitative magnetic resonance imaging and operative outcome. *Epilepsia*. 1995;36:230-235.

Cendes F, Cook MJ, Watson C, et al. Frequency and characteristics of dual pathology in patients with lesional epilepsy. *Neurology*. 1995;45:2058-2064.

Drury I, Schuh L, Ross D, et al. Ictal patterns in temporal lobe epilepsy recorded by epidural screw electrodes. *Electroencephalogr Clin Neurophysiol*. 1997;102: 167-174.

Goldring S, Gregorie EM. Surgical management of epilepsy using epidural recordings to localize the seizure focus. Review of 100 cases. *J Neurosurg*. 1984;60:457-466.

Härtel F. Über die intracranielle Injecktionbehandlung der Trigeminusneuralgie. *Med Klin*. 1914;10:582-584.

Kanner AM, Parra J, Gil-Nagel A, et al. The localizing yield of sphenoidal and anterior temporal electrodes in ictal recordings: a comparison study. *Epilepsia*. 2002;43:1189-1196.

Kanner AM, Ramirez L, Jones JC. The utility of placing sphenoidal electrodes under the foramen ovale with fluoroscopic guidance. *J Clin Neurophysiol*. 1995;12:72-81.

Kim OJ, Ahn JY, Lee BI. Analysis of electrical discharges made with the foramen ovale electrode recording technique in mesial temporal lobe epilepsy patients. *J Clin Neurophysiol*. 2004;21:391-398.

Kuzniecky R, Faught E, Morawetz R. Electroencephalographic correlations of extracranial and epidural electrodes in temporal lobe epilepsy. *Epilepsia*. 1991;32:335-340.

Kuzniecky R, Faught E, Morawetz R. Surgical treatment of epilepsy: initial results based upon epidural electroencephalographic recordings. *South Med J*. 1990;83: 637-639.

Li LM, Cendes F, Watson C, et al. Surgical treatment of patients with single and dual pathology: relevance of lesion and of hippocampal atrophy to seizure outcome. *Neurology*. 1997;48:437-444.

Marks DA, Katz A, Booke J, et al. Comparison and correlation of surface and sphenoidal electrodes with simultaneous intracranial recording: An interictal study. *Electroencephalogr Clin Neurophysiol*. 1992;82:23-29.

Nakase H, Tamura K, Kim YJ, et al. Long-term follow-up outcome after surgical treatment for lesional temporal lobe epilepsy. *Neurol Res*. 2007;29:588-593.

Pacia SV, Ebersole JS. Intracranial EEG substrates of scalp ictal patterns from temporal lobe foci. *Epilepsia*. 1997;38:642-654.

Penfield W, Jasper HH, eds. *Epilepsy and the Functional Anatomy of the Human Brain*. Boston: Little, Brown; 1954.

Rosenbaum TJ, Laxer KD, Vessely M, et al. Subdural electrodes for seizure focus localization. *Neurosurgery*. 1986;19:73-81.

Ross DA, Brunberg JA, Drury I, et al. Intracerebral depth electrode monitoring in partial epilepsy: the morbidity and efficacy of placement using magnetic resonance image–guided stereotactic surgery. *Neurosurgery*. 1996;39:327-333.

Ross DA, Henry TR, Dickinson LD. A percutaneous epidural screw electrode for intracranial electroencephalogram recordings. *Neurosurgery*. 1993;33:332-334.

Shih YH, Yiu CH, Huang CI. Role of foramen ovale electrodes in presurgical evaluation of intractable complex partial seizures. *Zhonghua Yi Xue Za Zhi (Taipei)*. 1997;60:155-160.

Silberbusch MA, Rothman MI, Bergey GK, et al. Subdural grid implantation for intracranial EEG recording: CT and MR appearance. *AJNR Am J Neuroradiol*. 1998;19:1089-1093.

Spencer SS. Depth electroencephalography in selection of refractory epilepsy for surgery. *Ann Neurol*. 1981;9:207-214.

Spencer SS, Spencer DD, eds. *Surgery for Epilepsy*. Boston: Blackwell Scientific; 1991.

Spencer SS, Spencer DD, Williamson PD, et al. Combined depth and subdural electrode investigation in uncontrolled epilepsy. *Neurology*. 1990;40:74-79.

Swartz BE, Rich JR, Dwan PS, et al. The safety and efficacy of chronically implanted subdural electrodes: a prospective study. *Surg Neurol*. 1996;46:87-93.

Talairach J, Bancaud J. Lesion, "irritative" zone and epileptogenic focus. *Confin Neurol*. 1966;27:91-94.

Velasco TR, Sakamoto AC, Alexandre V Jr, et al. Foramen ovale electrodes can identify a focal seizure onset when surface EEG fails in mesial temporal lobe epilepsy. *Epilepsia*. 2006;47:1300-1307.

Wieser HG, Elger CE, Stodieck SR. The 'foramen ovale electrode': a new recording method for the preoperative evaluation of patients suffering from mesio-basal temporal lobe epilepsy. *Electroencephalogr Clin Neurophysiol*. 1985;61:314-322.

Wieser HG, Siegel AM. Analysis of foramen ovale electrode–recorded seizures and correlation with outcome following amygdalohippocampectomy. *Epilepsia*. 1991;32:838-850.

Wilkus RJ, Thompson PM. Sphenoidal electrode positions and basal EEG during long term monitoring. *Epilepsia*. 1985;26:137-142.

Wyler AR, Ojemann GA, Lettich E, et al. Subdural strip electrodes for localizing epileptogenic foci. *J Neurosurg*. 1984;60:1195-1200.

Wyler AR, Walker G, Somes G. The morbidity of long-term seizure monitoring using subdural strip electrodes. *J Neurosurg*. 1991;74:734-737.

Full references can be found on Expert Consult @ www.expertconsult.com

CHAPTER 61

Surgery for Extratemporal Lobe Epilepsy

James W. Leiphart ■ Itzhak Fried

One of the most significant developments in the treatment of epilepsy has been the recognition of specific surgically remediable syndromes of epilepsy.[1] Foremost among these conditions has been the syndrome of mesial temporal lobe epilepsy, characterized by distinct patterns of semiology, electroencephalographic signature, imaging correlates, and histopathology.[2] The hallmark of this syndrome is hippocampal sclerosis, which underlies a hyperexcitable, recurrent, and pharmacologically resistant pattern of electrical activity. From the surgeon's standpoint, the significance of this syndrome is the feasibility of a uniform surgical approach to the disease.

In contrast, extratemporal epilepsy presents a more complex challenge for the surgeon. Because there is no analogue to the distinct pathology found in mesial temporal lobe epilepsy, there is no uniform resection plan for extratemporal epilepsy. A selection has to be made from a spectrum of resection plans such that the ablation is (1) sufficient and necessary to achieve seizure control and (2) functionally feasible (i.e., it should result in no neurological deficit or a deficit that is acceptable to the patient). This zone of planned resection may be delineated by using one or more of the following features: (1) concordance with the seizure semiology; (2) a focal abnormality on electroencephalography (EEG) or magnetoencephalography (MEG), or both; (3) a focal abnormality on magnetic resonance imaging (MRI); (4) a focal metabolic abnormality; (5) a focal abnormality in blood flow on single-photon emission tomography (SPECT); and (6) concordance with neurocognitive impairment. The existence of a focal MRI abnormality is probably the most useful diagnostic modality for planning a surgical approach for extratemporal epilepsy. The presence of such a focal structural abnormality immediately classifies a case as extratemporal *lesional* epilepsy, which usually correlates with a better surgical prognosis. Much of the challenge in surgery for extratemporal epilepsy is in the so-called nonlesional cases. In such cases, the resection plan cannot be based on an MRI abnormality, although pathologic studies of resected tissue may reveal a lesion not detected by MRI preoperatively. In this setting, the resection plan is based on findings from EEG (scalp or intracranial) and functional imaging techniques such as positron emission tomography (PET), MEG, SPECT, and magnetic resonance spectroscopy (MRS).

Although mesial temporal lobe epilepsy has become better defined as a clinicopathologic entity that can be treated with a standard surgical approach,[2,3] such is not the case for extratemporal lobe epilepsy syndromes. The semiology of extratemporal neocortical epilepsy is less well characterized, even when the seizure focus is localized to a single lobe (frontal, temporal, or parietal). Extratemporal lobe epilepsies also tend to spread rapidly, thus making localization based on their clinical characteristics difficult. In some cases, especially in patients with frontal lobe epilepsy, seizures cross to the contralateral side rapidly, which makes it difficult to even lateralize the site of seizure onset.

One of the reasons why temporal lobe epilepsy has proved especially amenable to surgical intervention is that resection of the anterior and anteromedial part of the temporal lobe can be performed with minimal loss of function. Careful neurocognitive, Wada, and functional imaging testing and electrical stimulation mapping in selected cases can minimize the possibility of language or memory impairment. Frequently, surgical resection can be tailored to the temporal tip and sclerotic hippocampus to limit the potential for cognitive deficit. Extratemporal lobe epilepsies commonly involve brain regions that subserve motor, sensory, language, or other critical neurological functions. Because of the risk for neurological injury, a standard resection strategy cannot be used. Instead, each resection must be tailored to the unique characteristics of each patient.

In contrast to temporal lobe epilepsy, which frequently has the consistent underlying pathology of hippocampal sclerosis, extratemporal lobe epilepsies have a wide variety of underlying pathologies ranging from tumors and other space-occupying lesions to developmental abnormalities and trauma. As might be expected, surgical outcomes differ for patients with different underlying pathologic conditions. In addition, there is a subset of patients with extratemporal epilepsy in whom no pathologic abnormalities are identified both preoperatively and in the resected tissue.

The presence of a lesion on preoperative imaging studies has a significant impact on the surgical prognosis. Seizure-free outcomes after lesional extratemporal epilepsy surgery are significantly better than those after nonlesional epilepsy surgery.[4] MRI scanners with higher magnet strength that can provide brain imaging with higher resolution offer promise for identifying anatomic abnormalities in more patients,[5,6] an especially promising area because many surgical specimens from "nonlesional" epilepsy surgery are found to have abnormalities on subsequent pathologic analysis.[7] New MRI and other imaging technologies that are being developed for the identification of epileptic foci are discussed later in the chapter in the section on patient evaluation.

Technologic advances have provided modern alternatives to resective surgery for medically intractable epilepsy, but none has supplanted surgical resection in efficacy. These alternatives include stimulation methods, such as vagal nerve stimulation or deep brain stimulation (DBS). The rate of significant seizure control with vagal nerve stimulation is approximately 30% to 50%.[8] DBS for severe intractable epilepsy is still largely experimental, and even more recent protocols using stimulation of the subthalamic nucleus (STN) or anterior thalamus have achieved only a modest rate of success.[9-11] Technologic advances have also made resective surgery safer. Advances in neurosurgical techniques and neuroanesthesia have made operative mortality a rare occurrence. Advances in functional imaging, stimulation brain mapping, and intraoperative image guidance help minimize the chance for neurological deficit. These considerations require that the surgical team have a good understanding of the different extratemporal seizure syndromes and the surgical risks and seizure control rates for each so that discussion among the surgical team members and with the patient can lead to an optimal decision.

This chapter discusses various important aspects of extratemporal lobe epilepsy surgery, including the characteristics, risks, and outcomes of epilepsies localized to each individual extratemporal lobe and the various pathologies underlying the extratemporal lobe epilepsies, along with their differences in postoperative seizure control outcomes. Also described are preoperative and intraoperative techniques used to (1) localize the seizure focus for resection and (2) establish the limitations of the resective area to avoid neurological deficit, with emphasis on more recent advances that have the potential to greatly facilitate the safety and efficacy of resective surgery for extratemporal lobe epilepsy.

GENERAL EPILEPSY SURGERY OUTCOMES

The earliest epilepsy surgeries performed in the late 1800s and early 1900s were targeted toward neocortical seizure foci.[12] Because of the limited utility of imaging and neurophysiologic modalities available to clinicians at that time, localization of the seizure focus was based primarily on anatomic features such as external signs of head trauma and underlying cortical encephalomalacia. Over time, improved imaging and electrophysiologic evaluation allowed delineation of medial temporal lobe epilepsy syndrome,[13,14] which is characterized by hippocampal sclerosis.[15,16] The work of several surgeons in developing and analyzing surgical approaches to this syndrome[17-21] has led to standardized approaches to epilepsy surgery for these patients. With these standardized approaches and distinct imaging characteristics of hippocampal sclerosis, many epilepsy surgery centers have proposed protocols that allow medial temporal lobe epilepsy surgery to be performed with a defined evaluation.[22] In addition, epilepsy surgery for medial temporal lobe epilepsy with hippocampal sclerosis is associated with a high seizure-free outcome rate on the order of 53% to 84%, a rate that has not been matched by extratemporal neocortical resections.[23-26] Probably for these and other reasons discussed later, modern series evaluating epilepsy surgery show that extratemporal lobe epilepsy surgery is much less common than temporal lobe epilepsy surgery.

The most recent multicenter source of information regarding current practice patterns of major epilepsy centers comes from a seven-center prospective observational study of resective epilepsy surgery. In this study, which included 355 patients at 1-year follow-up and 339 patients at 2-year follow-up, only 12% of the epilepsy surgery patients underwent extratemporal surgery.[27,28] In a review of 708 epilepsy surgeries at a major epilepsy surgery center in Germany, 429 of which were therapeutic, 35% of the therapeutic surgeries were extratemporal and consisted of frontal resection in 14%, parietal resection in 2%, occipital resection in 3%, multilobar resection in less than 1%, callosotomy in 8%, and hemispherectomy in 8%.[29] Based on these and other studies, it is clear that temporal lobe epilepsy surgery, especially medial temporal lobectomy, is much more common than extratemporal lobe epilepsy surgery. There are several probable reasons for this discrepancy, including a higher incidence of medial temporal lobe epilepsy that is intractable, better seizure-free rates with medial temporal lobe resection than with extratemporal resection, and frequently, more diffuse or obscure extratemporal seizure foci necessitating a more tailored approach for extratemporal resection and requiring additional evaluation for determination of the exact seizure location, often with surgically implanted electrodes.

Outcomes of extratemporal lobe epilepsy surgery are based mostly on retrospective case series reviews. Only one study has provided class I evidence for epilepsy surgery; however, this study looked only at medial temporal lobe resections but demonstrated a clear benefit of early surgery over maximal medical therapy for medically intractable epilepsy.[25] The multicenter epilepsy surgery study just mentioned was a prospective case series that grouped neocortical temporal with general extratemporal cases.[27,28] This study found that patients undergoing neocortical resection had a lower seizure-free rate than did patients undergoing medial temporal lobe resection at 1-year follow-up (56% for neocortical versus 77% for medial temporal resection) and 2-year follow-up (50% for neocortical versus 68% for medial temporal resection). These differences were statistically significant only at the 1-year follow-up. Interestingly, the seizure relapse rate for patients who were initially seizure free after surgery was lower with neocortical resection than with medial temporal lobe resection in both the 1-year (4% for neocortical versus 24% for medial temporal resection) and 2-year studies (19% for neocortical versus 25% for medial temporal resection), again only statistically significant at 1 year. A recent review of the adult and pediatric epilepsy surgery literature reported 1-year or greater freedom from seizures in 53% to 84% of patients undergoing medial temporal lobe resection, in 66% to 100% of patients with dual pathology, including medial temporal sclerosis and temporal neocortical involvement, and in 36% to 76% of patients undergoing neocortical resection.[23]

The American Academy of Neurology in association with the American Epilepsy Society and the American Association of Neurological Surgeons published a position paper that reviewed all the outcome studies for epilepsy surgery before the paper's publication in 2003.[30] The Quality Standards Subcommittee identified 33 studies reporting seizure-free outcomes after epilepsy surgery, but just 1 class I study was used (the one discussed earlier) and 32 class IV studies. Only 8 of these studies described outcomes after neocortical resection, including both temporal and extratemporal locations, and all were class IV studies. This group was able to conclude that the benefits of medial temporal lobe resection surgery for medically intractable disabling complex partial seizures are greater than the benefits with continued maximal medical therapy and that the risks related to surgery are at least comparable to the risks associated with antiepileptic drugs. However, they were not able to draw similar conclusions from the neocortical resection studies because of the low number of studies, lack of class I evidence, and great variability among the different neocortical epilepsies and their surgeries based on the lobe involved. This position paper simply states that further studies are needed to determine the benefits of surgery for treating neocortical epilepsies.

Many studies have supported the overall benefit of successful epilepsy surgery in several areas of patients' daily lives. These studies have not typically differentiated among patients according to the site of the resection, but it is likely that these quality-of-life studies are applicable to all patients who have successfully undergone epilepsy surgery, including surgery on the extratemporal lobe. The Multicenter Study of Epilepsy Surgery looked at some quality-of-life outcomes in their study patients. They found that quality of life was improved by 3 months after surgery regardless of seizure outcome but that scores at 1 and 2 years were statistically significantly lower in patients who were not seizure free than in those who were seizure free.[27] Others have found improved scores on quality-of-life measures after epilepsy surgery.[31] A study of pediatric epilepsy surgery also found that quality of life was improved to a greater degree in children rendered seizure free after surgery than in those who continued to have seizures.[32] Both anxiety and depression decreased significantly by 3 months after surgery, more in the seizure-free patients than in those who continued to have seizures, and scores remained improved at 1 and 2 years' follow-up.[33] Full-scale IQ has also shown improvements in long-term follow-up after temporal, parietotemporal, and frontal epilepsy surgery.[34] At 2 years after surgery, 75.5% of patients said that they would definitely undergo surgery again, 79.1% thought that they had a very strong or strong overall positive impact from the surgery, but in only 7% was employment status improved.[35] Other studies have shown no improvement in employment status for epilepsy surgery patients in comparison to epilepsy patients without surgical treatment despite a greater decline in the former group in both monthly seizure frequency and antiepileptic medication intake.[31] In a review of epilepsy surgery outcome papers, two studies evaluated multiple outcome factors in both temporal and extratemporal epilepsy surgery. Both studies found improvements in seizure outcome and decreased antiepileptic drug use, but only one of these studies found an improvement in social outcomes, and the one study that evaluated quality of life found no difference between surgical patients and controls.[24] This paper reported that in studies in which temporal lobe and extratemporal lobe resections were analyzed together, an average of 20% of patients were able to discontinue their antiepileptic drugs and an average of 41% were able to achieve monotherapy. Adverse outcomes associated with epilepsy surgery are relatively infrequent, with a series of 429 therapeutic epilepsy surgeries reporting no mortality, transient morbidity in 3%, and permanent morbidity in 2.3%.[29] Taken together, these results indicate a positive impact of epilepsy surgery on patients' lives that outweighs the risks.

LOBAR DISTRIBUTION OF EXTRATEMPORAL LOBE EPILEPSY

The distribution of lobes involved in various reported surgical series of extratemporal epilepsy may be skewed by the relative risk associated with ablative surgery and other factors that affect the decision for surgery, which differ for each lobe and may not represent the natural distribution of seizures in the general population of all patients with epilepsy. The surgical series are particularly instructive, however, in that they provide outcome data for cases in which relatively good localization has been achieved. The confidence in localization increases with invasive subdural or depth electrode monitoring, stimulation-induced replication of the seizure, and verification of seizure control postoperatively. Any or all of these criteria can be applied to the classification of surgical epilepsy patients but not nonsurgical patients.

Several case series have looked at epilepsy surgery in general or extratemporal epilepsy surgery in particular. These studies give an idea of the relative incidence of surgically remediable epilepsy in each of the lobes and the frequency of types of extratemporal epilepsy surgery. In adult epilepsy surgery series, extratemporal surgery represents 13% to 37% of operations.[36-38] Of the extratemporal resections, 60% to 84% were frontal, 4% to 20% were parietal, 3% to 20% were occipital, and 0% to 46% were multilobar.[36,38] Series combining adult and pediatric patients have reported extratemporal surgery in 12% to 44%.[27-29,36,38-41] Of these, 33% to 64% were frontal, 7% to 14% were parietal, 2% to 23% were occipital, 0% to 37% were multilobar, 0% to 34% involved corpus callosotomy, and 0% to 22% involved hemispherectomy.[29,36,38-44] The percentage of extratemporal epilepsy surgery cases in pediatric series varies from 32% to 83%.[36,38,45-52] The pediatric extratemporal epilepsy surgeries included frontal resection in 18% to 73%, parietal in 0% to 18%, occipital in 0% to 9%, multilobar in 0% to 72%, corpus callosotomy in 0% to 50%, and hemispherectomy in 0% to 52%.[36,38,45-52] Extratemporal resections, including corpus callosotomy and hemispherectomy, are more common in the pediatric population.

Parietal lobe epilepsy and occipital lobe epilepsy are rare in surgical series, a finding reported by several authors.[53,54] This very low incidence may be due to the relative resistance of these regions of the brain to the development of seizures, difficulty identifying these seizures because of the ambiguity of symptoms referable to seizures from these areas (especially in parietal lobe epilepsy), and the potential risk for permanent postoperative neurological deficit. The data also illustrate one of the characteristics of extratemporal lobe epilepsy that make it less amenable than

temporal lobe epilepsy to surgical therapy—a higher incidence of widespread pathology involving more than one lobe.

FRONTAL LOBE EPILEPSY

The frontal lobe is the largest lobe of the brain, and it encompasses several distinct anatomic-functional units, including the primary motor region; supplementary motor areas; language areas in the dominant frontal operculum; the frontal eye fields; part of the cingulate gyrus; a component of the limbic system; the orbitofrontal and ventromedial regions, which play a major role in the regulation of emotions; and the dorsolateral frontal region, which has major cognitive function, especially in executive functions and working memory. The regions responsible for clearly observable motor functions, the primary and supplementary motor areas, were the earliest to be classified anatomically[55,56] and the earliest targets for surgical treatment of epilepsy.[57-60] The clinical syndromes of primary and secondary motor cortex seizures are fairly well agreed on. Characterization of primary motor cortex seizures has remained essentially unaltered since the investigations of Penfield and Jasper[12]: focal clonic jerks without loss of consciousness if generalization does not occur. Supplementary motor cortex seizure morphology has been described by Ajmone-Marsan and Ralston[61] and later investigators and has been characterized by more complex motor semiology, including combined movements of the extremities and head version.

Seizures in other regions of the frontal lobe have shown significant variability, which has resulted in difficulty characterizing classic frontal lobe epilepsy syndromes.[62] Based on characterization of seizures in patients via depth electrode recording, Bancaud and Talairach[63] proposed that frontal lobe epilepsies be classified into (1) inferior frontal gyrus seizures in either the dominant or nondominant hemisphere with speech arrest, tonic or tonic-clonic contractions at the ipsilateral angle of the mouth, swallowing, salivation, gustatory hallucinations, vegetative signs, respiratory deficits, and possibly simple motor manifestations; (2) medial intermediate frontal seizures originating in the mesial frontal lobe, anterior to the supplementary motor cortex, superior to the cingulate gyrus, and posterior to the polar region, with frontal-type absence or complex motor seizures; (3) dorsolateral intermediate frontal seizures with contralateral deviation of the eyes followed by aversion of the head; (4) anterior cingulate gyrus seizures with intense fright, expressions of fear, and aggressive verbalizations and acts; (5) frontopolar seizures with dissociation from the environment, fixed eyes, immobility, flexion and turning of the head, falling, and tonic-clonic generalization; (6) orbitofrontal seizures with either olfactory illusions and hallucinations or vegetative symptoms, including cardiovascular, respiratory, or digestive system involvement; and (7) operculoinsular suprasylvian seizures with a variety of symptoms, including somatomotor involvement of the face and upper and lower limbs, disorders of verbal expression, contralateral oculocephalic deviation, dissociation from the environment, and postictal speech deficits. These syndromes are not universally accepted, with some authors expressing skepticism concerning the feasibility of anatomic localization by seizure semiology.[64]

Localization of a single resectable focus in patients with frontal lobe epilepsy is typically difficult because of the propensity for extensive epileptogenic zones with multiple pathways that allow rapid ictal spread within the frontal lobe and to other lobes and the contralateral side.[65] Even a determination of lateralization can be difficult.[66] In the absence of a distinct focal structural lesion, localization of frontal lobe epilepsy foci almost always requires intracranial ictal recording with either subdural electrodes[65] or depth electrodes.[63] The findings from these evaluations, combined with the variety of anatomic imaging modalities available, are the basis on which surgical resection plans are made.

with rTMS are minimal, with seizures occurring in 0% to 3.6% and the most common side effect being headaches, which occurred in 9.6%.[178,179] These various stimulation techniques under development would provide more options for patients with extratemporal lobe epilepsy who are not candidates for surgical resection.

PATHOLOGIC SUBSTRATES

The pathologic substrates underlying extratemporal lobe epilepsy syndromes are important in planning surgery and also influence the seizure control outcomes of patients. It is clear that the presence of a defined lesion with a pathologic substrate signifies a better prognosis and that the so-called nonlesional extratemporal epilepsy presents a more difficult challenge in epilepsy surgery. Focal abnormalities, such as tumors, vascular lesions, and some cortical abnormalities, may have relatively distinct borders that can be differentiated more easily from normal brain tissue intraoperatively. Such differentiation facilitates identification of the epileptogenic substrate and complete removal of the entire abnormality. Analysis of several extratemporal lobe epilepsy surgery series showed various categories of epileptogenic pathology.*

Neoplastic Lesions

Neoplasms frequently underlie epileptic foci. Based on frequency of occurrence in extratemporal epilepsy surgery series, these tumors, in order of their frequency, were dysembryoplastic neuroepithelial tumors, 2% to 36%; gangliogliomas, 2% to 35%; astrocytomas, 1% to 31%; oligodendrogliomas, 2% to 20%; glioneural hamartia, 14%; hamartomas, 1% to 13%; oligoastrocytomas, 2% to 12%; meningiomas, 6%; and ependymomas, 2%.† Some of the extratemporal lobe epilepsy series simply listed neoplastic causes in 2% to 70%.[41,45,48,75,81,87,89] In series that combined temporal lobe epilepsy and extratemporal epilepsy surgery, with the majority being temporal lobe surgery, the frequencies were slightly different, with gangliogliomas in 1% to 38%, astrocytomas in 2% to 31%, oligodendrogliomas in 1% to 15%, dysembryoplastic neuroepithelial tumors in 1% to 11%, hamartomas in 6%, xanthoastrocytomas in 3%, ependymomas in 3%, gangliocytomas in 2%, oligoastrocytomas in 1%, epidermoids in less than 1%, generically listed tumors in 2% to 33%, and gliomas in 5% to 7%.[36,39,46,69,182,183] Extratemporal series with adult patients only[53,77] differ in the underlying pathologies from extratemporal series with pediatric patients only[38,45,48,49,51,52] in that certain pathologies were found only in pediatric patients, such as gangliocytoma and hamartoma; some were more frequent in pediatric patients, such as dysembryoplastic neuroepithelial tumors; several were about equal in both groups, including astrocytoma, ganglioglioma, and oligodendroglioma; and only oligoastrocytoma was seen solely in adults.

Epileptogenic tumors may involve the limbic system[184] but are commonly seen in the temporal lobe and extratemporal locations. In general, epileptogenic tumors occur in young people, are slow growing, and involve the cortical gray matter. These tumors can be addressed best with an extended lesionectomy in an effort to remove the tumor and its margins in the surrounding brain. As long as the entire lesion with margins is removed, the seizure-free outcome after resection of neoplasms is likely to be good. Surgical outcome depends on the extent of resection. Partial resections of neoplasms usually yield a poor seizure outcome, and the best results are achieved with initial complete resection of the lesion and surrounding margins.[183] There are differing opinions in the literature regarding the benefit of resection of additional

contiguous tissue based on electrocorticography.[185,186] Reported seizure-free outcomes for extratemporal lobe epilepsy surgery vary by pathology, with gangliocytomas associated with a 100% seizure-free rate, oligoastrocytomas, 100%; dysembryoplastic neuroepithelial tumors, 75% to 100%; gangliogliomas, 67% to 100%; oligodendrogliomas, 50% to 100%; hamartomas, 0% to 100%; and astrocytomas, 0% to 100%.[49,51-53,77,81,86,88]

Vascular Lesions

The two vascular lesions classically associated with seizures are arteriovenous malformations (AVMs) and cavernous hemangiomas. Detection of cavernous hemangiomas as seizure foci has been improving since the development and refinement of MRI in the preoperative evaluation for epilepsy surgery. Venous angiomas have also been found in patients with epilepsy, but they are not always the cause of the seizures. Some associated underlying developmental abnormality may be the culprit, as illustrated in Case Study 61-1. The other vascular abnormality listed in some surgical epilepsy series is seen in connection with Sturge-Weber syndrome, a pathology more commonly found in pediatric patients. The vascular lesions reported in extratemporal lobe epilepsy series are Sturge-Weber syndrome in 1% to 30% of patients, AVMs in 2% to 10%, cavernous hemangiomas in 2% to 10%, and venous angiomas in 1% to 10%, with nonspecific vascular lesions being reported in 2% to 9%.* The combined temporal and extratemporal series report no venous angiomas and have lower frequencies of vascular lesions, with Sturge-Weber syndrome in 1% to 6%, cavernous hemangiomas in 4% to 5%, AVMs in 1% to 2%, and generically reported vascular lesions in 8%.[36,39,69,182] In comparing adult-only extratemporal series[53,77] with pediatric-only extratemporal series,[38,45,48,49,51,52] AVMs, cavernous hemangiomas, and venous angiomas were found only in the adult series, whereas Sturge-Weber syndrome was found predominantly in the pediatric series.

Seizure-free outcomes of extratemporal epilepsy surgery vary with the type of vascular lesion resected. Patients with cavernous hemangiomas and venous angiomas have a reported seizure-free rate of 100%, those with AVMs have a 67% to 100% seizure-free rate, and the rate in patients with Sturge-Weber syndrome is 0% to 100%.[45,51,53,77,81,86,88] Seizure outcomes after removal of cavernous hemangiomas appear to be comparable to those after resection of neoplasms. A paper looking only at cavernous hemangiomas found seizure-free outcome rates of 88% for frontal lobe, 78% for parietal lobe, 100% for occipital lobe, and 75% for multilobar resections.[187] We believe that removal of the margins of this lesion is important in achieving good seizure outcomes. This contrasts with a similar paper looking only at AVMs, which reported a lower seizure-free rate of 66%.[188]

Gliotic Lesions

Gliotic lesions, including posttraumatic, postischemic, and postinflammatory pathologies, are predominant in older surgical series that span several decades of operative experience, especially in series predating the use of computed tomography (CT) or MRI. Many of these lesions are related to perinatal or birth trauma or anoxia. Improvements in obstetric care have contributed to the decreasing incidence of these pathologies in modern epilepsy surgery series. Gliotic lesions remain a significant cause of epilepsy, however, particularly in the pediatric population. Seizures resulting from gliotic lesions can be difficult to control surgically.

Extratemporal lobe series report many types of epileptogenic lesions that would be gliotic in nature, including gliosis in 6% to 65%, scar or posttraumatic lesions in 2% to 40%,

---

*See references 29, 36, 40-44, 47, 50-54, 69, 77, 81, 86, 88, 89, 180, 181.
†See references 39, 42-44, 49-51, 53, 54, 74, 77, 78, 86, 88, 89, 94.

*See references 42-45, 50, 51, 53, 54, 74, 75, 77, 81, 86-89.

encephalomalacia in 2% to 25%, perinatal infarct or trauma in 15% to 19%, infarct in 1% to 18%, atrophy in 14%, necrosis in 10%, abnormal cysts including porencephalic cysts in 2% to 10%, gliomesodermal scar in 8%, postinfectious lesions in 2% to 7%, meningocerebral cicatrix in 5%, foreign body in 2%, and old hematoma in 2%.* Combined temporal and extratemporal series report only gliosis in 6% to 45%, infarct in 21%, perinatal infarct or trauma in 8%, and scar or posttraumatic lesions in 4% to 5%, but they do include hippocampal sclerosis in 5% to 23%, which is exclusively a temporal lobe pathology.[36,39,46,69,182] The pediatric-only series reported postinfarct cases, whereas the adult-only series did not; the adult-only series reported scar or posttraumatic cases only, whereas the pediatric series did not; but both groups reported many gliosis cases that may be from these causes but were not distinguished in the papers.[38,45,48,49,51-53,77] Surgery on these pathologies has mixed results, with seizure-free rates of 57% to 100% for infarct, 38% to 100% for scar or post-traumatic causes, 0% to 100% for gliosis, 0% to 71% for postinfectious causes, 58% to 67% for perinatal infarct or trauma, 0% for cysts including porencephalic cysts, and 0% for meningocerebral cicatrix.[45,49,51-53,77,86,88]

Developmental Lesions

Abnormalities in neuronal migration and development are increasingly being recognized as a cause of intractable epilepsy. With modern neuroimaging, some of these lesions can be identified and treated surgically. The most common developmental abnormality underlying seizures is cortical dysplasia. Other common developmental abnormalities include polymicrogyria and other cortical gyral malformations. Tuberous sclerosis and heterotopias have also been reported as lesions underlying epilepsy. Developmental lesions are seen more commonly in pediatric epilepsy patients and may involve extensive regions of cortex, sometimes more than one lobe.

Extratemporal lobe epilepsy surgery series report the following rates of developmental lesions: cortical dysplasia in 2% to 83%, neuronal migration disorders in 1% to 56%; cytoarchitectural abnormalities in 28%; macrogyria in 20%; cortical malformations in 3% to 17%,; tuberous sclerosis in 2% to 17%; hemimegencephaly in 7% to 10%; microgyria in 5% to 10%; heterotopia in 2% to 10%; ulegyric change in 6%; and ossification in 2% to 3%.[†] Many of these pathologies may overlap, given that they are dependent on the pathologist's interpretation and nomenclature for the abnormal developmental process.[7] The combined temporal and extratemporal series mention only cortical dysplasia (5% to 56%), neuronal migration disorder (15%), microgyria (5% to 14%), cortical malformation (6%), and tuberous sclerosis (1% to 6%) as developmental pathologies.[36,39,46,69,94,182] Cytoarchitectural abnormalities and microgyria were part of the adult-only series; cortical dysplasia, hemimegencephaly, macrogyria, neuronal migration disorders, and ulegyric changes were part of the pediatric-only series; and heterotopia and tuberous sclerosis were seen in both.[38,45,48,51,53,77]

This group of pathologies does not demonstrate as high seizure-free rates as the other categories, and this can be attributed to the diffuse nature of developmental pathologies, which do not have distinct borders and often have more widespread subtle abnormalities in neuronal migration and neuronal activity throughout the brain.[189] Seventy-five percent to 100% of patients with microgyria, 68% to 100% of patients with extratemporal cortical dysplasia, and 0% to 100% of those with tuberous sclerosis are seizure free postoperatively, all pathologies that can be more focal in manifestation, but only 50% of patients with macrogyria, 43% of patients with cytoarchitectural abnormalities,

0% to 43% of patients with hemimegencephaly, and 0% of those with nonspecific heterotopias become seizure free after epilepsy surgery in these surgical series.[45,51,53,77,86,88] These findings agree with reports of patients having better seizure control after surgery for focal cortical lesions than for developmental abnormalities such as cortical dysplasia.[50] In one epilepsy surgery series looking only at outcomes after resection of focal cortical dysplasia, there was a high seizure-free rate of 72%, whereas multilobar patients with more widespread disease had worse outcomes.[190] However, another paper summarizing studies of surgery for malformations of cortical development reported a 2-year seizure-free rate of only 38% for extratemporal focal cortical dysplasia and just 34% for all extratemporal malformations of cortical development.[191] The extent of resection for cortical dysplasia influences postoperative outcomes, with 80% of patients undergoing complete resection of the lesion being seizure free but only 20% with incomplete lesion resection being seizure free.[192] A small series of pediatric epilepsy surgeries for tuberous sclerosis demonstrated only a 33% seizure-free rate.[193]

These case studies demonstrate that epilepsy surgery for developmental lesions is not futile but does not carry a high chance for complete seizure control as with other epilepsy surgeries.

Inflammatory and Infectious Pathologies

Rasmussen's encephalitis is a highly epileptogenic process that progressively involves one entire hemisphere of the brain without spreading to the contralateral side. The etiology of the disorder is unknown, but it is a relatively frequent pathology in children with epilepsy who require epilepsy surgery. Given the involvement of an entire hemisphere, the surgery commonly used for this pathology is hemispherectomy or hemispherotomy. Other inflammatory processes that may cause seizures include encephalitis and inflammation from local infections. Although these processes may eventually burn out to produce postinfectious gliotic epileptic foci, they sometimes require earlier surgical intervention when the active process is still ongoing. Because of the active nature of the disease process, these pathologies can have the worst prognosis for seizure-free outcomes after epilepsy surgery.

The extratemporal epilepsy surgery series listed 2% to 17% with Rasmussen's encephalitis, 2% to 6% with other encephalitides, 1% to 5% with inflammation, one case of tuberculoma for a 1% incidence, and one case of cysticercosis for a 1% incidence.[41,43,45,50,54,75,86-88,94] The combined temporal and extratemporal series only reported encephalitis pathology in 1% to 17%.[36,182] In exclusively adult and exclusively pediatric extratemporal lobe epilepsy surgery series, inflammatory pathologies were reported just in the pediatric-only series and consisted of cases of inflammation and Rasmussen's encephalitis.[45] Seizure-free outcomes from inflammatory and infectious causes were poor overall, with 0% to 55% with Rasmussen's encephalitis being seizure free, 0% to 33% with encephalitis being seizure free, but complete seizure freedom for the patient with the tuberculoma.[45,86,88]

Normal Tissue

In general, surgical resections that yield tissue with no histopathologic abnormalities are a minority in epilepsy surgery. It may be that surgeons are less inclined to operate on normal-appearing substrates. Cryptogenic epilepsy surgical cases and cases producing normal resected tissue account for 2% to 43% of patients in extratemporal lobe epilepsy surgery series* and 1% to 15% of patients in combined temporal and extratemporal lobe epilepsy surgery series.[39,46,69,94,182] In these series, arachnoid cysts, which we consider "normal" anomalies, were reported as causes

---

*See references 38, 41-45, 48-51, 53, 54, 74, 75, 77, 78, 86-89, 94.
†See references 38, 42-45, 48, 50, 51, 53, 54, 74, 75, 77, 86-89, 94.

*See references 38, 41, 45, 50, 54, 74, 75, 77, 86, 88.

in 1% to 5% of epilepsy patients.[69,86] Cryptogenic and normal-tissue cases were seen in both the adult-only and the pediatric-only case series.[38,45,77] Seizure-free rates for cryptogenic patients and those with no abnormal substrate were 25% to 100%,[45,77,86,88] thus indicating that lack of cortical abnormality in an extratemporal epilepsy patient with good electrocorticographic localization of the focus should not deter the surgeon from attempting surgical intervention.

EVALUATIVE TECHNIQUES FOR EXTRATEMPORAL LOBE EPILEPSY

Preoperative Evaluation

Because extratemporal lobe epileptic foci in general are difficult to localize by semiology or scalp EEG, other ancillary techniques are required to obtain a concordant assessment of localization of the seizure focus for resection, particularly in the absence of a distinct structural abnormality on MRI. In many cases, invasive monitoring with intracranial electrodes is required. As part of the presurgical evaluation, three questions need to be answered: (1) is there a structural substrate for the disease? (2) are there physiologic markers for the zone that need to be removed? and (3) are there functional constraints to removal of the epileptogenic focus?

Video Electroencephalographic Monitoring

Modern imaging modalities often provide pivotal information for preoperative evaluation of patients for epilepsy surgery. EEG monitoring has therefore relinquished its role as the primary source of information on localization of the seizure focus in some cases. Despite the presence of a distinct lesion, it is nevertheless important to establish the relationship between a lesion seen on imaging and seizure onset. In some cases, the seizure focus is found to be distant from the lesion, and in rare cases, presumed epilepsy patients with space-occupying lesions were found to have nonepileptic seizures (i.e., pseudoseizures). At epilepsy centers, as many as 20% to 30% of patients admitted with a diagnosis of medically refractory seizures may actually have psychogenic nonepileptic seizures.[194] EEG monitoring is especially important in patients with multiple structural lesions such as tuberous sclerosis or familial multiple cavernous angiomas, each of which could be the causative substrate underlying the epileptic syndrome. In some epilepsy patients, no focal abnormality is found on imaging studies and EEG monitoring remains the primary modality for localization of the epileptic focus. In many of these patients, invasive monitoring is necessary for precise localization. Newer techniques allowing three-dimensional localization of interictal spikes make interictal scalp EEG potentially more useful for localization of the seizure focus than is the case currently.[195,196]

Interictal EEG is a good tool for differentiating an epileptic patient from a nonepileptic patient in that 50% of epilepsy patients will have interictal abnormalities on one EEG, which increases to 92% on four EEGs, as opposed to a 0.4% incidence of spikes in the normal population.[197] It has been argued that routine interictal EEG monitoring is frequently inadequate for accurate localization of the epileptogenic focus.[198] However, interictal spike frequency has been a predictor of postoperative seizure-free outcome in patients with temporal lobe epilepsy.[199] A study of interictal EEG for extratemporal epilepsy showed 100% concordance with subsequent surgical evaluation, including ictal and invasive recordings to localize the seizure focus to a specific lobe of origin.[44] Another study comparing ictal and interictal EEG showed that interictal EEG localized the seizure onset to the appropriate lobe 67% of the time, similar to the ictal EEG rate of 68%[200] and similar to rates in two other studies that showed ictal EEG localizing the seizure focus in 62% and 68% of patients.[201,202] These findings aside, most epilepsy surgery centers rely heavily on video EEG to capture ictal EEG activity for localization of the epileptic focus.

Invasive Electrode Monitoring

Invasive monitoring with surgically implanted electrodes is frequently necessary for more accurate localization of the epileptic focus than can be provided by scalp EEG, especially with extratemporal lobe epilepsy.[202] Depth electrodes have several contacts along their length and are surgically placed in specific locations within the brain parenchyma under frame-based or frameless stereotactic guidance. The use of multiplanar planning software has increased the accuracy of implantation of depth electrodes.[203] Depth electrodes allow investigation of mesial, basal, and deep structures. They are especially helpful in the evaluation of mesial temporal lobe epilepsy syndromes or when patterns of spread from an extratemporal focus may involve the mesial temporal lobe rapidly.[204] Examples would be distinguishing mesial temporal lobe epilepsy from orbitofrontal epilepsy or occipital lobe epilepsy because orbitofrontal and occipital seizures often spread rapidly to the temporal lobe.[91,205] The use of depth electrodes in patients with suspected extratemporal lobe epilepsy is supported by a study showing that 25% of these patients will be found to have mesial temporal foci rather than extratemporal foci.[206] Depth electrodes have a remarkably low complication rate, with a 2.4% infection rate, a 0.6% hemorrhage rate, no neurological deficits, and no deaths in one series in which there was an 85% rate of determining a surgically amenable seizure focus.[207] In addition, new technologies combining microdialysis catheters with depth electrodes[208] may make cerebral microdialysis clinically significant for the surgical evaluation of intractable epilepsy patients in the future.[209]

Subdural grid and strip electrodes are surgically placed in direct apposition to the cortex, either through bur holes or by craniotomy. Grid electrodes are especially useful in extratemporal lobe epilepsy because they provide sampling of cortical activity over the cerebral convexities and make recording from more extensive territories possible.[65] The advantage of subdural grids is that they enable detailed sampling of a cortical region in terms of seizure activity, along with functional mapping via electrical stimulation.[210] This coverage can be essential in defining the anatomic extent of the more diffuse epileptic foci that are seen frequently in extratemporal lobe epilepsy. For the best of both worlds, some surgical centers have been using both subdural and depth electrodes together to evaluate patients with intractable epilepsy.[211,212] Subdural electrodes alone appear to be preferable for the evaluation of frontal or multilobar seizure onset, whereas combined subdural and depth electrodes seem to be better for the evaluation of patients with dual pathology consisting of epileptic foci in both a neocortical region and the mesial temporal lobe.[204] Frameless stereotactic systems facilitate combined placement of subdural and depth electrodes in the same patient by eliminating the need for a stereotactic frame, which may obstruct the approach for the craniotomy.[213] The risk from limited subdural electrode studies is small, with one paper reporting a 0.85% rate of serious and minor complications in 350 patients,[214] but the risk can be significant when using larger grids, where the complication rate was reported to be as high as 26.3%, mostly without permanent deficits but with a 0.5% mortality rate.[215]

Invasive monitoring can also be performed in the epidural space with the use of grid or peg electrodes. Epidural peg electrodes are surgically implanted in small holes drilled into the skull such that they rest against the dura mater. They do not provide the same level of sensitivity or accuracy as depth and subdural electrodes, but they are useful in situations with significant subdural scarring in patients who have had previous surgery or trauma.

Imaging

The most important imaging modality in preoperative planning for extratemporal epilepsy surgery is MRI.[216] The advances in anatomic definition provided by modern MRI have contributed immensely to the identification of epileptic foci. The use of 3-T MRI and surface coils has made identification of a lesion underlying an epileptic focus 2.57 times more likely,[6,217] and new quantitative techniques have made lesion characterization more accurate in terms of the underlying histopathology.[218] Localized, well-circumscribed lesions on MRI, whether contrast-enhancing or signal abnormalities on T2-weighted or fluid-attenuated inversion recovery (FLAIR) images, delimit the target of resection, are associated with a higher occurrence of EEG focality,[219] and signify a greater possibility for postoperative seizure control. FLAIR imaging can be particularly useful and should be part of the routine epilepsy MRI protocol.[220,221] More diffuse lesions have a lower chance for postoperative seizure control,[50] and the absence of a lesion on MRI denotes a poorer prognosis for seizure control with surgery (44% seizure free in one study).[4,222,223] Three-dimensional reconstructions of CT and magnetic resonance angiographic images can now be fused with three-dimensional reconstructions of MRI in the frameless stereotactic system for more accurate representation of vascular structures in relation to cortical anatomy. Careful three-dimensional reconstructions of the cortical surface can reveal surface abnormalities associated with developmental lesions. Imaging of the brain with invasive monitors in place can also be fused with the preoperative MRI to provide exact localization and verification of electrode placement.[224]

Other imaging modalities have proved especially useful in the physiologic localization of epileptogenic regions in extratemporal lobe epilepsy. The first of these is fluorodeoxyglucose F 18 PET, which identifies areas of cortex with abnormal metabolic activity. Interictally epileptogenic zones tend to be hypometabolic relative to normal cortex.[225,226] PET has proved most useful in the evaluation of mesial temporal lobe epilepsy,[227] but it can also help delineate extratemporal epileptic foci and verify the likely epileptogenicity of structural lesions seen on MRI.[228] Another imaging modality for delineation of epileptic foci is SPECT. In SPECT scanning, a trace amount of radioisotope is injected intravenously, and areas of increased blood flow are revealed. When used in the ictal state and compared with the interictal state, it may show a significant seizure focus in which enhanced neuronal activity results in increased blood flow.[229,230] This technique has proved especially useful in tandem with coregistration to MRI (subtraction ictal SPECT coregistered to MRI [SISCOM]).[231-233] Hypoperfusion on interictal SPECT can verify the epileptogenicity of certain foci identified on MRI, such as areas of cortical dysplasia.[234] However, the disadvantage of ictal SPECT is that because of its inability to differentiate which region of activation occurred first, it can point to activated propagation pathways that do not need to be surgically removed to alleviate seizures.[227] Although ictal SPECT has proved useful in the localization of extratemporal epileptic foci,[228,235] interictal SPECT has not.[236]

Magnetic Source Imaging: Magnetoencephalography

Magnetic source imaging registered to MRI[237] has proved to be a particularly effective tool for epilepsy surgery, especially extratemporal epilepsy (see Case Studies 61-1 to 61-4). MEG uses superconducting quantum interference device magnetometers to detect the magnetic fields associated with intraneuronal electrical currents. The magnetic field, which can indicate the epileptic focus, is not attenuated or distorted by the overlying skull and scalp as in scalp EEG, thus increasing the accuracy of localization

without resorting to invasive EEG monitoring. MEG dipoles are registered to MRI by using fiducials, which allows structural localization in three dimensions. These images have proved useful in the localization of extratemporal lobe epileptic foci (see Case Study 61-1).[237-239] Magnetic source imaging is most useful for neocortical epilepsy[240] and correlates with intracranial recordings in the majority of cases.[241] MEG can be helpful in identifying a seizure focus when MRI appears normal, and clustering of the MEG signal in the subsequently resected region can predict effective postoperative seizure control.[242] In difficult cases requiring implantation of depth electrodes for evaluation of seizures, magnetic source imaging can be used to focus placement of the intracranial electrodes in a particular region suspected of epileptogenesis (see Case Study 61-3).

Another MRI modality showing promise in the localization of extratemporal seizure foci is MRS,[243,244] which depicts the relative distributions of various chemicals in selected areas of the brain. MRS has been explored extensively for mesial temporal lobe epilepsy but has also been used in studies of extratemporal lobe epilepsy.[245] Extratemporal epileptic foci have shown increased pH, decreased phosphomonoesters,[246] decreased N-acetylaspartate (NAA), and decreased NAA-to-creatine and NAA-to-choline ratios.[243,247-249] MRS is another imaging modality that can be used to localize extratemporal seizure foci in patients with negative MRI findings,[249] and with further development it may enjoy wider use by clinicians.

DTI, a technique used to evaluate white matter tract projections in the brain, has been investigated as a potential imaging modality for determining seizure foci in traditional MRI-negative epilepsy syndromes. DTI has shown changes in the brain that indicate neocortical seizure foci[5] but does not yet have the reliability to be used clinically for determination of seizure foci except in patients with tuberous sclerosis, in whom DTI was more accurate than structural MRI in localizing the epileptogenic cortex.[250]

fMRI is a maturing imaging technology that provides information on specific activation of cortical processing zones during motor, sensory, and cognitive functions. This modality is used as a preoperative tool to define the relationship of cortical functional anatomy and the epileptogenic zone.[72] fMRI is useful in the delineation of functional cortical anatomy for frontal lobe epilepsy resections that include motor and speech areas.[251] Although the clinical utility of fMRI activation outside the rolandic cortex is controversial,[252] it provides a noninvasive preliminary to intraoperative mapping that can avoid craniotomy in patients in whom the deficits would be unacceptable. It is useful in determining hemispheric language dominance and it correlates well with results obtained by the Wada test.[253,254] In addition to its role in defining functional cortical zones, fMRI is developing as a tool to localize interictal epileptiform discharges. Simultaneous EEG recording and event-related fMRI allow the linking of epileptiform activity with local hemodynamic changes in the brain.[255-260] On EEG-fMRI, a blood oxygen level–dependent (BOLD) effect corresponded to spiking in the temporal lobe in the majority of temporal lobe epilepsy patients, but there was also activation in other brain regions that was thought to represent activation of networks associated with the epileptic activity generated at the focus in the medial temporal lobe.[261] In addition, novel approaches involving quantitative methodologies in fMRI hold promise for localizing epileptiform neural activity in the future.[262]

Neuropsychological Testing

Careful neuropsychological testing can provide information concerning the impact of the epileptic focus on neurological function in the region of the focus.[263] Thus, it can be judiciously used as a confirmative tool in the presurgical evaluation. Preoperative neuropsychological testing is important to describe the current cognitive and behavioral functioning in the context of the seizure disorder and underlying neuropathology, to start interventions for cognitive and behavioral difficulties if present, and for postoperative prognosis, both for seizure-free outcome and for neuropsychological deficits.[263-265] This testing can be especially important in patients with frontal lobe epilepsy because specific abnormalities can become evident on testing, even though routine neurological examination appears normal. Frontal lobe epilepsy patients with either preoperative or postoperative deficits have difficulty with mental flexibility, planning, and fluency (verbal fluency from the left frontal lobe and nonverbal fluency from the right frontal lobe). Parietal lobe deficits are uncommon except in patients with extensive parietal lesions. Distortion in copying a complex figure representing distortion in conceptualization of spatial representation can be associated with parietal lobe lesions, right more than left, and somatosensory tests sometimes show differences in these patients. Occipital lobe lesions may be manifested as visual field deficits, and if significant, they may interfere with cognitive visual tests. Lateral occipital defects have profound cognitive effects on visual cognitive tasks only if they are bilateral, although unilateral occipitotemporal lesions may be accompanied by material-specific neurocognitive deficits, depending on the hemisphere involved. Some epilepsy surgery centers use neuropsychological testing to aid in localization and lateralization,[266] although neuropsychological findings alone are not reliable for the lateralization of seizure foci.[267]

The other important preoperative neuropsychological test commonly used is the intracarotid amobarbital procedure, or the Wada test.[268,269] The patient's language and memory functions are tested during injection of a barbiturate into one cerebral hemisphere to block function on that side, and the test is sometimes repeated with injection on the other side. A review of 1421 Wada tests suggested that the test has high reliability and validity for language lateralization but does not have as high reliability or validity for memory lateralization.[270] The memory component of the test is used to determine the safety of resection of medial temporal lobe tissue for the treatment of medial temporal lobe epilepsy. For extratemporal epilepsy, the memory part of the Wada test is less important. Establishing the side of language dominance is crucial, however, in planning frontal lobe and parietal lobe epilepsy surgery. Developments in fMRI hold promise in using this noninvasive modality to determine language hemispheric dominance,[271] thereby potentially obviating the need for the more invasive amobarbital procedure, which requires angiography and administration of amobarbital.

Intraoperative Evaluation

Intraoperative Mapping

It is often necessary to evaluate localization of functions such as language and movement in patients who are undergoing extratemporal lobe resection for seizures. Preoperative fMRI and other preoperative imaging modalities can be useful in providing a general impression of these functional regions in relation to the proposed site of resection.[272] fMRI is still under development, however, and thus most surgeons perform the "gold standard" intraoperative electrical stimulation mapping for proposed resections near regions of motor, sensory, or language cortex. In patients for whom EEG monitoring with grid electrodes is indicated for localizing the seizure focus, extraoperative mapping is performed on the ward.

For intraoperative language[18] or sensory[273] mapping, the patient needs to be fully conscious and able to cooperate. For motor mapping, patient cooperation is not required, and the procedure can be carried out under general, albeit light and nonparalytic anesthesia. In fact, there is some evidence that near a tumor, cortical stimulation motor mapping is inaccurate.[274] Evoked potential sensorimotor mapping can be performed with the patient under general anesthesia. To perform evoked potential sensorimotor mapping, the median nerve at the hand is stimulated with a small electrical current, and somatosensory evoked potentials are recorded from the cortical surface over the suspected rolandic cortex. Phase reversal of the N20 median nerve somatosensory evoked potential from one strip electrode lead to the next defines the central sulcus, with the precentral motor area being anterior and the postcentral sensory area being posterior. This process indirectly identifies the motor cortex and does not provide the detailed map offered by electrical stimulation mapping.

When patient cooperation is required, the operation is performed under local anesthesia, whereas intravenous sedation is used during periods of the procedure when the patient's cooperation is not required.[275] Awake craniotomy can be performed fairly routinely with few complications.[276] Agents such as propofol have greatly improved the ability to carry out such procedures with reasonable patient comfort. An alternative method, which we often use, is asleep-awake-asleep anesthesia,[277] in which the procedure is started with general anesthesia and intubation to enable the routine neurosurgical craniotomy protocol, including cranial fixation and image-guided surgery. Only at the stage of the procedure when mapping is required is the patient allowed to emerge from general anesthesia and subsequently extubated, with a small guide left in place through the vocal cords. After mapping, the patient can be reintubated and fully anesthetized. Electrical stimulation mapping or other patient testing can be carried out throughout the resection if the resection is close to functional processing zones. Intraoperative mapping can be especially important given the wide variability in the location of language areas.[18,278]

Intraoperative Electrocorticography

Extratemporal lobe epilepsy surgery requires extensive preoperative testing to localize and define the seizure focus as discussed earlier. Even with this significant preoperative evaluation, it is frequently necessary to perform intraoperative electrocorticography to define the seizure focus further and plan the extent of resection. To perform electrocorticography, grid electrodes of various sizes and configurations or individual electrodes are placed directly on the exposed cerebral cortex over suspected regions of epileptogenesis, and the electrical activity is recorded. Anesthesia is lightened as much as possible during electrocorticography so that epileptic activity is not suppressed. General anesthesia can suppress spike frequency[279]; however, propofol sedation[280] and dexmedetomidine sedation[281,282] can be used during electrocorticography. Spike activity is usually taken as an indication of an epileptogenic zone, but sometimes severe slowing of activity is also considered. After tissue resection, electrocorticography can be performed around the borders of the resection cavity to verify the elimination of pathologic electrical activity. The utility of electrocorticography in guiding extratemporal epilepsy surgery resection is controversial, with some clinicians arguing that it is not necessary in many situations[185] and others presenting some evidence that it may help increase the chance of postoperative freedom from seizures.[4,283-285]

Frameless Stereotaxy

The use of frameless stereotactic equipment in neurosurgery has become widespread in all areas, including epilepsy surgery,[286] and it is especially useful in extratemporal lobe epilepsy surgery. As discussed earlier, extratemporal lobe epilepsy has a better prognosis for postoperative seizure control if a structural lesion can be identified on imaging as the seizure focus. This improved prognosis depends on the ability to resect the lesion completely at the time of surgery. Complete resection can be especially difficult for some pathologic lesions underlying extratemporal lobe epilepsy, such as cortical dysplasia, because they frequently appear similar to normal brain tissue and do not have distinct borders. Frameless stereotactic systems can guide the surgeon directly to the lesion and help determine the borders of the lesion based on the imaging.[287]

Frameless stereotaxy is also useful in cases of nonlesional extratemporal lobe epilepsy. Many of the evaluation modalities described previously, such as MEG and SPECT, can be combined with the three-dimensional images to help guide surgery. CT or MRI with invasive electrodes in place can be fused with preoperative MRI to help localize the epileptogenic tissue more accurately during surgery.[288] fMRI can be added to suggest functional regions that may require extensive stimulation mapping. Frameless stereotaxy has proved very useful in other epilepsy surgeries as well, including corpus callosotomy[129] and the placement of intracranial electrodes.[213] The use of frameless stereotaxy in extratemporal lobe epilepsy holds considerable promise in improving the safety and efficacy of surgery.

New Modalities in Development

Novel intraoperative techniques are being developed that should prove useful in extratemporal lobe epilepsy surgery. One of these techniques is intraoperative MRI, which has been used in epilepsy surgery mainly for temporal lobe epilepsy,[289-291] although it is applicable to extratemporal lobe epilepsy as well. This technology has undergone considerable improvement in being compatible with the operating room environment. In its application to epilepsy surgery, it is especially helpful because it enables the use of various sequences intraoperatively, including FLAIR sequences, which are sensitive to the subtle tissue changes sometimes seen in epileptogenic lesions. With larger resections, especially those involving multiple lobes, brain shift poses difficulties for traditional image-guided navigation. Interventional MRI allows intraoperative evaluation of the extent of resection without the confounding effect of brain shift.

Intraoperative optical imaging of intrinsic signals (iOIS) is another technique under development that should prove useful during surgical resection of extratemporal epileptic foci.[292,293] The equipment is attached to the microscope and allows detection of cortical regions that are active during specific activities, such as hand movement and language. Intraoperative studies using this technique suggest that iOIS provides more detailed information about cortical function than stimulation mapping,[294] and functions localized by iOIS seem to correspond to localization by fMRI.[295] One study has shown that this procedure can be used to localize seizure foci intraoperatively as well.[296]

CONCLUSION

Extratemporal lobe epilepsies present a unique challenge to the neurosurgeon because of the frequent lack of obvious localized underlying pathology and common involvement of cortical regions with critical neurological functions. The key to successful extratemporal lobe epilepsy surgery is use of the specific preoperative and intraoperative technologies available to define a region where resection is necessary and sufficient to achieve seizure control with minimal neurological sequelae. Localization of a focal lesion responsible for the seizures is associated with the best seizure control outcome if the entire lesion can be resected. Even if not resectable, a localized epilepsy focus may now be a candidate for one of the newer stimulation technologies. Nonlesional extratemporal lobe epilepsies have a more modest prognosis for postoperative seizure control and usually require the use of additional modalities in planning the resection, including invasive electrode monitoring. Preoperative functional scans, intraoperative mapping techniques, and subpial transections, when indicated, minimize the risk for neurological deficit that could result from resection in an area necessary for a critical function. With the appropriate tools and careful multimodality evaluation at every stage, extratemporal lobe epilepsy surgery provides a reasonable chance of seizure control.

SUGGESTED READINGS

Asenbaum S, Baumgartner C. Nuclear medicine in the preoperative evaluation of epilepsy. *Nucl Med Commun.* 2001;22:835-840.

Berger MS, Ghatan S, Haglund MM, et al. Low-grade gliomas associated with intractable epilepsy: seizure outcome utilizing electrocorticography during tumor resection. *J Neurosurg.* 1993;79:62-69.

Cook SW, Nguyen ST, Hu B, et al. Cerebral hemispherectomy in pediatric patients with epilepsy: comparison of three techniques by pathological substrate in 115 patients. *J Neurosurg.* 2004;100:125-141.

Duchowny MS, Harvey AS, Sperling MR. Indications and criteria for surgical intervention. In: Engel J Jr, Pedley TA, eds. *Epilepsy: A Comprehensive Textbook.* Philadelphia: Lippincott-Raven; 1997:1677-1685.

Fried I. Magnetic resonance imaging and epilepsy: neurosurgical decision making. *Magn Reson Imaging.* 1995;13:1163-1170.

Fried I. Management of low-grade gliomas: results of resections without electrocorticography. *Clin Neurosurg.* 1995;42:453-463.

Fried I, Wilson CL, Maidment NT, et al. Cerebral microdialysis combined with single-neuron and electroencephalographic recording in neurosurgical patients. Technical note. *J Neurosurg.* 1999;91:697-705.

Hendler T, Pianka P, Sigal M, et al. Delineating gray and white matter involvement in brain lesions: three-dimensional alignment of functional magnetic resonance and diffusion-tensor imaging. *J Neurosurg.* 2003;99:1018-1027.

Hoh BL, Chapman PH, Loeffler JS, et al. Results of multimodality treatment for 141 patients with brain arteriovenous malformations and seizures: factors associated with seizure incidence and seizure outcomes. *Neurosurgery.* 2002;51:303-309; discussion 309-311.

Janjua FN, Eliashiv DS, Fried I. The added value of magnetic source imaging in a large series of medically refractory partial epilepsy patients that are candidates for epilepsy surgery. *Epilepsia.* 2003;44(suppl 9):251.

Jayakar P, Dunoyer C, Dean P, et al. Epilepsy surgery in patients with normal or nonfocal MRI scans: integrative strategies offer long-term seizure relief. *Epilepsia.* 2008;49:758-764.

Jobst BC, Velasco F, Lado F, et al. Brain stimulation for the treatment of epilepsy: What is the evidence in humans and animals [abstract 1W.27]. *Epilepsia.* 2008;49:176-177.

Jonas R, Nguyen S, Hu B, et al. Cerebral hemispherectomy: hospital course, seizure, developmental, language, and motor outcomes. *Neurology.* 2004;62:1712-1721.

Mamelak AN, Lopez N, Akhtari M, et al. Magnetoencephalography-directed surgery in patients with neocortical epilepsy. *J Neurosurg.* 2002;97:865-873.

McGonigal A, Bartolomei F, Regis J, et al. Stereoelectroencephalography in presurgical assessment of MRI-negative epilepsy. *Brain.* 2007;130:3169-3183.

O'Brien TJ, So EL, Mullan BP, et al. Subtraction peri-ictal SPECT is predictive of extratemporal epilepsy surgery outcome. *Neurology.* 2000;55:1668-1677.

Olivier A, Awad IA. Extratemporal resections. In: Engel J Jr, ed. *Surgical Treatment of the Epilepsies.* New York: Raven Press; 1993:489-500.

Spencer S, Huh L. Outcomes of epilepsy surgery in adults and children. *Lancet Neurol.* 2008;7:525-537.

Spencer SS, Berg AT, Vickrey BG, et al. Predicting long-term seizure outcome after resective epilepsy surgery: the multicenter study. *Neurology.* 2005;65:912-918.

Spencer SS, Schramm J, Wyler A, et al. Multiple subpial transection for intractable partial epilepsy: an international meta-analysis. *Epilepsia.* 2002;43:141-145.

Sporis D, Hajnsek S, Boban M, et al. Epilepsy due to malformations of cortical development—correlation of clinical, MRI and Tc-99mECD SPECT findings. *Coll Antropol.* 2008;32:345-350.

Téllez-Zenteno JF, Dhar R, Wiebe S. Long-term seizure outcomes following epilepsy surgery: a systematic review and meta-analysis. *Brain.* 2005;128:1188-1198.

Toczek MT, Morrell MJ, Risinger MW, et al. Intracranial ictal recordings in mesial frontal lobe epilepsy. *J Clin Neurophysiol.* 1997;14:499-506.

Williamson PD, Thadani VM, Darcey TM, et al. Occipital lobe epilepsy: clinical characteristics, seizure spread patterns, and results of surgery. *Ann Neurol.* 1992;31:3-13.

Full references can be found on Expert Consult @ www.expertconsult.com

CHAPTER 62

Standard Temporal Lobectomy

William Bingaman ■ Imad Najm

The term *standard temporal lobectomy* is commonly used in the medical literature but should be carefully interpreted because significant variations in the technique exist. The focus of this chapter is to describe current indications and technique for removal of both the lateral and mesial temporal lobe structures (corticoamygdalohippocampectomy). This technique is commonly used for medically intractable temporal lobe epilepsy (TLE) due to mesial temporal sclerosis. This procedure can also be used for other epileptic substrates (malformations of cortical development, cavernomas, neoplasms, and other focal epileptogenic lesions) involving the temporal lobe.

HISTORICAL BACKGROUND

The standard temporal lobectomy developed concurrently with the identification of the temporal lobe epilepsy syndrome and the emergence of electroencephalography (EEG) in the 1940s and 1950s. Much of the credit belongs to Penfield and Jasper at the Montreal Neurological Institute (MNI).[1] When Herbert Jasper joined the MNI in 1937, he brought the technique of EEG with him. By this time, Penfield and his partner William Cone had been performing surgery for epilepsy since Penfield arrived in 1928. As EEG became more established in the evaluation and diagnosis of focal epilepsy through the work of Jasper and Gibbs, the classification and study of temporal lobe epilepsies was under way. Through the close friendship of Jasper and Penfield, the MNI became a leader in the late 1930s in the surgical treatment of epilepsy. In 1941, Jasper and Kershman proposed a classification of epilepsy based on EEG waves.[2] In this report, they described the localization of psychomotor phenomena from within the deep regions of the temporal lobe. Despite increasing awareness of the role of the mesial temporal lobe in these seizures, the lack of understanding about the function of this tissue and the inability of the surgeon to "see" the lesion at the time of resection led to reluctance on Penfield's part to remove these structures.[1] In 1950, Penfield reported his success in anterolateral temporal resections.[3] In this series of 68 patients, 10 had partial removal of the uncus, and only 2 had hippocampal resections. EEG abnormalities were recorded from the temporal lobe in this group of patients, but an underlying substrate had not been identified. At the same time, Percival Bailey and Ernest Gibbs reported a series of 25 patients from the University of Illinois program who underwent temporal resection guided by EEG.[4] Similar to Penfield's series, these patients did not have hippocampal resections.

The second phase in the development of the modern surgical strategy to treat temporal lobe seizures took place in the 1950s as the role of the mesial temporal lobe structures in the pathogenesis of the epilepsy became better understood. This occurred as a number of scientists began to study the connections of the mesial temporal lobe to the rest of the brain and through the use of stimulation studies to reproduce seizure semiology in animals and humans.[5-8] In 1952, Penfield and Baldwin published a classic monograph describing their technique for anterolateral temporal lobectomy including the hippocampus and amygdala.[9] They reported that the most frequent pathologic abnormality in two of three of their cases was an atrophic lesion termed *incisural sclerosis*. Falconer in a report in 1953 recognized a connection with febrile seizures and introduced a modification allowing for en bloc resection of the hippocampus, which allowed the pathologists to study the tissue.[10] With the advent of neuroimaging, modifications to the technique reported by Penfield have been made to address specific pathology seen preoperatively. Despite these modifications, the operation developed and introduced by innovative neurosurgeons in the early 20th century remains one of the most successful operations for the treatment of epilepsy today.

IDENTIFICATION OF SURGICAL CANDIDATES: THE CONCEPT OF PHARMACORESISTANCE AND MEDICAL INTRACTABILITY

The indications for epilepsy surgery generally include the presence of focal epilepsy resistant to treatment with an adequate trial of anticonvulsant therapy. The precise definition of an adequate anticonvulsant trial is open to interpretation, but a study by Kwan and Brodie produced useful information regarding the efficacy of anticonvulsant therapy in newly diagnosed epilepsy.[11] This study suggests that after three medications fail to control seizures, further success is unlikely, and other options should be considered. Consider also the paper by Wiebe and associates, comparing temporal lobectomy to optimal medical therapy in a group of patients with temporal lobe epilepsy.[12] In this prospective randomized trial, surgical therapy in combination with medical therapy was far superior to ongoing medical therapy alone. These papers lend credence to the idea that patients with ongoing epilepsy despite a trial with a few anticonvulsants should be expeditiously evaluated for possible epilepsy surgery.

PREOPERATIVE EVALUATION

History and Neurological Examination

The preoperative evaluation for epilepsy surgery begins with a thorough history and physical examination by a trained and experienced epileptologist. Many clues to the possible etiology and the localization of the epileptogenic region can be elicited from the history (e.g., history of perinatal complications, childhood febrile convulsions, presence and type of auras) as well as the physical examination.

Video Electroencephalography Monitoring

The diagnosis and type of epilepsy should be confirmed through prolonged video-scalp EEG monitoring in a dedicated epilepsy monitoring unit (EMU).[13] Scalp EEG recording is a noninvasive monitoring technique that can sample extensive areas of the brain to give the best overview of the general distribution of interictal and ictal epileptic activities. It gives an excellent overview of the approximate location and extent of the epileptogenic area. Most epileptic patients with TLE (between 85% and 100%) show epileptiform discharges on their interictal scalp EEG recordings.[14,15] Both the localization and pathologic type of the epileptogenic lesion within the temporal lobe affect the scalp localization (and lateralization) of interictal and ictal EEG patterns. In addition, video recordings and analyses permit the characterization of the seizure semiology that may be helpful in the localization and lateralization of the ictal onset zone.

Semiology and Electroencephalography Patterns in Mesial Temporal Lobe Epilepsy Due to Hippocampal Sclerosis or Mesial Temporal Mass Lesions (Neoplasms or Cavernomas)

Hippocampal sclerosis is one of the most common pathologic substrates in patients with TLE. Patients with mesial TLE show a characteristic electroclinical syndrome that typically consists of a rising abdominal sensation aura that may be followed by mouth and hand automatisms and possible ictal contralateral hand dystonic posturing. The presence of postictal speech difficulties may help in lateralizing the seizure onset zone to the dominant hemisphere for language. Patients with TLE due to hippocampal sclerosis show slowing in the ipsilateral temporal electrodes and interictal epileptic sharp waves that are usually mapped to the anterior temporal lobe.[16] In addition, in less than 50% of these patients, sharp waves mapped to the contralateral anterior temporal lobe electrodes are found. Patients with mesial TLE due to amygdalohippocampal tumors or cavernomas are more likely to exhibit less localized sharp waves and less likely to have contralateral epileptiform abnormalities.

Ictal EEG patterns are typically mapped to the anterior temporal electrodes and consist of either relative attenuation of the background EEG activities or low-amplitude evolving alpha or theta patterns.

Semiology and Electroencephalography Patterns in Neocortical Temporal Lobe Epilepsy Due to Cortical Dysplasia or Temporal Mass Lesions (Neoplasms or Cavernomas)

Temporal neocortical epilepsies are increasingly recognized electroclinical entities in patients with pharmacoresistant epilepsy. The semiology of lateral neocortical temporal lobe seizures may be slightly different than that found in patients with mesial TLE because early motor phenomena are commonly seen. Interictal and ictal EEG patterns are characterized by a more lateral and posterior temporal distribution (T7/T8, P7/P8). The presence of a lateral temporal lesion (mainly tumor or cavernoma) may be associated with hippocampal sclerosis (so-called dual pathology) and warrants an invasive evaluation in most cases.

Imaging

Magnetic resonance imaging (MRI) of the brain, fluorodeoxyglucose (FDG) positron emission tomography (PET), ictal radionuclide blood flow studies (e.g., single-photon emission computed tomography [SPECT]), and functional MRI are the main neuroimaging tests that are used in the preoperative evaluation of patients with pharmacoresistant epilepsy that is suspected to arise from the temporal lobe. The typical MRI sequence involves thin-slice coronal T1-weighted imaging, fluid-attenuated inversion

recovery (FLAIR) coronal sequences, and T2-weighted coronal sequences. Typical findings of mesial temporal sclerosis include atrophy of the affected hippocampus and increased signal intensity on the FLAIR and T2 sequences. One must always carefully study the remainder of the temporal lobe because dual pathology occurs in about 10% to 30% of mesial temporal sclerosis cases.[17-19] Findings suggestive of dual pathology include blurring of the temporal pole gray-white interface or enlargement or distortion of the cortical ribbon. These are important findings that may influence the choice of surgical procedure.

The metabolism of the brain is studied with the use of interictal PET scanning. In this procedure, a radionuclide ([18]FDG) is injected, and computed tomography (CT) scanning is performed. This test gives the clinician a picture of how the brain takes up glucose. Originally designed for TLE, the test is said to be 70% specific when hypometabolism is seen in one of the temporal lobes.[20]

The localization of language is now possible by noninvasive functional MRI, which is slowly replacing the more invasive intracarotid sodium amobarbital testing. One possible advantage of the latter is the ability to test memory function at the same time, although recent reports suggest that cognitive functional MRI may offer an important, noninvasive, preoperative assessment of hippocampal memory function.[21-23]

Neuropsychological and Psychosocial Preoperative Evaluations

Neuropsychological testing and psychosocial and psychiatric evaluations are also completed during the initial work-up. Neuropsychological information is important because the temporal lobes play a role in emotion, language, and memory. In fact, patients with TLE are often aware of significant progressive memory and naming problems that lead them to pursue surgical intervention. Despite many years of experience in temporal lobe surgery, our understanding of function and prediction of neuropsychological deficits is still somewhat poor. During the preoperative evaluation of the TLE patient, it is important to gain a baseline measure of overall intellectual functioning as well as verbal and visual spatial memory scores. This is accomplished with standardized neuropsychological testing, which is then repeated 6 months after surgery. Preoperative and postoperative deficits in short-term memory and naming are common in patients with dominant (language-localized) TLE, and the risk for worsening must be discussed with the patient. This risk is dependent on baseline preoperative functioning and the individual substrate of the epilepsy (e.g., presence of mesial temporal sclerosis).[24-26]

When the preoperative evaluation is complete, the data should be discussed by the interdisciplinary team managing the patient. Ideally, this team consists of the epileptologist, neurosurgeon, neuropsychologist, psychiatrist, neuroradiologist, nurses and midlevel providers, EEG technicians, and social workers. At this time, the data are synthesized into a credible hypothesis regarding site of seizure origin, and a surgical strategy designed.

SURGICAL DECISION MAKING

For the TLE patient, decisions revolve around localizing the epilepsy to the lateral or mesial temporal lobe, the presence and nature of the epileptic lesion, and the presence of language or important short-term memory deficits. For the patient undergoing a standard temporal lobectomy, the epilepsy should be localized to the anteromesial temporal lobe, and ideally a well-defined lesion should be present (mesial temporal sclerosis, malformation of cortical development, neoplasm, cavernoma). The planned posterior extent of resection should not encroach on possible neocortical temporal lobe language areas. If the dominant temporal lobe is involved, a baseline memory or naming deficit in the presence of mesial temporal sclerosis would support the conclusion that the correct brain site was targeted, and the risk for causing further neurological deficits would be acceptably low.[27,28]

The anatomy of the temporal lobe deserves a brief discussion at this point. The temporal lobe has well-defined anterior, lateral, basal, and mesial surfaces. The posterior boundary is arbitrary, having no obvious anatomic demarcation separating it from the parietal area. The temporal lobe is made up of five gyri and their corresponding sulci. The lateral surface lies below the sylvian fissure and extends to the floor of the middle cranial fossa. The gyri from top to bottom include the superior temporal gyrus (T1), the middle temporal gyrus (T2), and the inferior temporal gyrus (T3), which often extends onto the basal surface. The basal surface includes the inferior temporal gyrus (T3), the fusiform gyrus, and the parahippocampal gyrus. The mesial surface includes the amygdala and the parahippocampal gyrus, including the uncus. The collateral sulcus separates the fusiform and parahippocampal gyri and serves as an important reference to locate the temporal horn of the ventricle. Within the temporal horn, important anatomic structures include the inferior choroidal point (anterior choroidal artery enters the choroid plexus here), the hippocampus occupying the mesiobasal portion of the ventricle, the fornix, the choroid plexus, the choroidal fissure, and the amygdala in the anterior-superior-medial portion of the ventricle. The reader is referred to an excellent series of articles describing in detail the temporal lobe anatomy.[29]

Functional anatomy in the temporal lobe includes comprehensive language cortex in the dominant temporal lobe, visual field fibers (Meyer's loop) subserving the contralateral upper quadrantic visual field information, and potential important memory and naming centers. The anatomy of language cortex in the temporal lobe can be quite variable.[30,31] Cortical stimulation testing can be performed to further identify and protect lateral language cortex when posterior temporal lobe resections are anticipated on the dominant side. This can be done either intraoperatively with the patient awake or extraoperatively with implanted electrodes. After the language cortex has been identified, the temporal resection can be tailored to the patient's individual anatomy. The standard temporal lobectomy is designed to avoid temporal lobe cortical language sites by limiting the resection of the superior temporal gyrus to 3 to 4.5 cm from the anterior temporal pole. There is some controversy as to whether even this practice is safe, and some centers advocate leaving the entire superior temporal gyrus in place. This is based on language-stimulation data suggesting the presence of language sites in the anterior 3 cm of the superior temporal gyrus in a small percentage of patients.[30] Of course, these sites were not resected, and thus it is difficult to know whether they were essential language sites. Other "nonessential" language sites in the temporal lobe have been demonstrated through cortical stimulation followed by resection.[32] These sites were located in the basal temporal lobe by direct cortical stimulation but left no permanent language deficit after they were resected. Insufficient data, however, are available from the limited numbers of patients reported to conclude with certainty that no patient will develop a permanent language deficit after resection of a basal temporal language site.

Visual field fibers are also located in the temporal lobe as they extend forward from the lateral geniculate body before turning posterior on their way to calcarine cortex. These fibers are located unpredictably in the roof of the temporal horn, and standard temporal lobe resections cause injury to this fiber tract in as many as 50% of cases.[33] This leads to the "pie in the sky" visual field deficit with loss of peripheral vision in the opposite upper quadrant. In most cases, the visual field defect noted with careful perimetry testing is not clinically significant.

Finally, other important anatomic structures the surgeon should be familiar with include the sylvian fissure and associated structures (sylvian vein, middle cerebral arterial cascade, and underlying insula), the vein of Labbé, and the region of the tentorial incisura, including the brainstem, posterior cerebral artery, basal vein of Rosenthal, and third and fourth cranial nerves. Familiarity with these anatomic structures is critical to avoid a potentially devastating injury during resection of the mesial temporal lobe structures.

SURGICAL TECHNIQUE

When the decision has been made to perform a standard temporal lobectomy, the technique varies little from patient to patient. The word *standard* implies a reproducible operation from patient to patient and even surgeon to surgeon. It is best used to treat the "standard" syndrome of mesial TLE consisting of reproducible EEG, MRI, and seizure semiology elements. The targets of this operation are the mesial temporal lobe structures that are "sclerotic": the parahippocampus, hippocampus, and amygdala. The exact posterior extent of resection of the hippocampus to improve outcomes is unknown, but at least one prospective trial correlated improved outcome with more aggressive resection of the hippocampus.[34]

The procedure does vary slightly for the language-nondominant and language-dominant sides. On the dominant side, the surgeon limits resection of the superior temporal gyrus to avoid a possible postoperative language deficit. This usually translates into a resection of 3 to 4.5 cm measured along the superior temporal gyrus from the anterior aspect of the middle fossa. On the nondominant side, the posterior extent of resection can be farther from the temporal pole, although it is usually limited by the vein of Labbé about 4.5 to 6 cm posterior to the temporal pole. One must be careful with resections extending posteriorly beyond these measurements because there is increased risk for injuring the geniculocalcarine tract with resultant homonymous hemianopsia.

Preoperatively, the patient is given antibiotics within 1 hour before incision. A general anesthetic is administered, and bladder and arterial cannulations are performed. Intravenous access is maintained throughout the case with peripheral catheters. Before incision, hyperventilation therapy and intravenous mannitol can be used to relax the brain and minimize retraction during surgery. The patient is positioned supine on the operating table with the head rigidly fixated by a head clamp attached directly to the operating table. Stereotactic navigation is optional and is not routinely used at our institution. The position of the head is important because optimal positioning allows the surgeon to access the mesial structures with less retraction on the temporal lobe. Optimal positioning includes placing an ipsilateral shoulder roll to minimize torsion on the neck and then turning the head 30 degrees from the midline so that the operative side is up. The head is slightly extended to bring the sylvian fissure to a perpendicular plane to the operating approach. Finally, dropping the vertex down toward the floor allows the surgeon easier access to the mesial structures and allows less retraction on the temporal lobe.

Once positioned, the hair in the frontotemporal region is clipped, and a "reverse question mark" incision is made from just above the zygoma, extending back in the temporal region to the posterior part of the pinna and then curving anteriorly just above the insertion of the temporalis muscle. A larger skin flap is not necessary and may lead to increased risk for cosmetic deformity. The skin incision is carried out staying in the plane above the temporalis fascia. I (W.B.) prefer to split the fascia of the temporalis muscle and then elevate the muscle using a T incision based on the zygoma, with most of the muscle bulk reflected anteriorly.[35] This approach is done with a scalpel to minimize shrinking of the muscle fibers and facilitates an easier reattachment of the muscle at the end of the procedure. One should also be careful to leave enough muscle cuff attached to the temporal bone to allow secure suturing of the muscle at closure. Despite all these efforts, a significant cosmetic deformity may occur from wasting of the temporalis muscle, and this should be discussed with the patient before surgery. At this stage, exposure of the temporal bone from the root of the zygoma to the anatomic "keyhole" should be visualized. The anterior aspect of the temporalis muscle is undermined with electrocautery in case the bone in the region of the sphenoid wing needs to be rongeured away to allow additional exposure of the temporal pole. In most cases, this additional removal of bone is unnecessary and further increases the chances of a cosmetic deformity after surgery.

The craniotomy should facilitate exposure of the lateral aspect of the temporal lobe from the base of the middle fossa to the sylvian fissure. In our practice, the frontal lobe is not exposed during this procedure, but other epilepsy surgeons do routinely expose the posterior-inferior aspect of the frontal lobe during this operation. The anterior aspect of the bone removal should extend to the sphenoid wing, and the spine of the sphenoid bone is removed with a fine rongeur. The craniotomy can be performed with two bur holes, respectively located at the base of the zygoma and the keyhole. The bone is then removed with high-speed drilling, and the final break across the sphenoid is performed after removing the outer cortex with the drill or fine rongeur. All bone edges should be waxed as necessary to stem bleeding, and any exposed air cells along the temporal base are sealed. Restricting the craniotomy to the bone below the temporalis muscle cuff allows placement of the titanium fixation plates entirely below the muscle, which prevents the patient from feeling them through the scalp after surgery.

At this point, the dura is inspected, and bleeding is controlled. The dural opening should be created to maintain some blood flow into the dural flap. This is best accomplished by reflecting the flap anteriorly and inferiorly so that the middle meningeal branches are maintained. The dural flap is reflected, and the temporal lobe is visualized. The sylvian fissure is recognizable along the superior limit of the temporal lobe, and the floor of the middle fossa should be visualized with minimal retraction of the inferior temporal gyrus. Additionally, as the surgeon looks anteriorly along the sylvian fissure, the anterior extent of the temporal pole should be visualized within 1 to 2 cm of the anterior bony edge of the craniotomy. If not, additional bone is removed as discussed earlier. Also at this stage, brain swelling should be assessed and changes in the anesthetic technique made if necessary. Head elevation can be a useful maneuver to reduce intracranial swelling.

The posterior limit of resection along the superior temporal gyrus is now measured with a Penfield dissector placed so that the curve of the instrument follows the curve of the temporal pole and the tip of the instrument contacts the dura of the anterior middle cranial fossa. The appropriate distance is chosen based on the side of surgery and the location of important draining veins and arterial branches supplying the posterior temporal lobe. The lateral cortical resection is designed to allow access to the deeper mesial structures; therefore, preservation of the veins and arteries supplying the posterior temporal cortex is extremely important. It is possible to achieve the goals of surgery with a small lateral resection but is difficult to reverse neurological deficits associated with a larger resection that damages the blood supply to brain tissue that is not resected. It is wise to attempt to preserve all draining veins that connect to the sylvian venous system or to the vein of Labbé. Smaller veins draining to the anterobasal dura of the middle fossa (temporal tip veins) can be ligated. Assessment of the venous drainage pattern of the frontotemporal region should be performed before the start of the lateral resection because the sylvian venous system is often vari-

able. Care should be exercised as one dissects along the anterior-superior temporal gyrus and temporal pole to avoid injury to the outflow of the sylvian vein where it enters the sphenoparietal sinus. If significant variations in the venous pattern exist, modifications of the lateral resection should be attempted to minimize disruption to these veins. In the worst-case scenario, the operation can be converted to a selective transcortical or transsulcal amygdalohippocampectomy (when removal of the mesial temporal structures is the goal of the operation).

After the posterior line of resection is marked, dissection begins along the superior temporal gyrus a few millimeters inferior to the sylvian fissure. This is done with bipolar coagulation and sharp dissection of the pia mater followed by subpial aspiration of the cortical tissue. This allows exposure of the temporal pia of the sylvian fissure and the underlying insula and middle cerebral artery. The cortex should be aspirated down to the level of the inferior circular sulcus of the insula, where the pia ends and the temporal white matter begins. This marks the depth of the initial lateral resection to avoid injury to deeper structures. This dissection should extend anteriorly along the pia of the superior temporal pole until the dura of the anterior aspect of the middle fossa is reached. The posterior extent continues to the premeasured point determined by the side of surgery (3 to 4.5 cm left, 5.5 to 6 cm right). The posterior line of resection extends from just below the sylvian fissure at the superior temporal gyrus angling posteriorly along the middle and inferior temporal gyrus so that slightly more inferior temporal gyrus is removed than superior temporal gyrus. The pia along the superior and inferior temporal sulci is coagulated and divided during this phase of the procedure. The cortical tissue is aspirated down to the depth determined by exposure of the inferior circular sulcus. The basal temporal lobe is divided along the line of the posterior cut as the fusiform gyrus is aspirated to expose the collateral sulcus. This can sometimes be confusing, and it is important to retain orientation during this stage so as not to injure the deeper midline structures. This can be avoided by ensuring that the dura of the middle cranial fossa is still beneath the pia being dissected and also by gently retracting the basal temporal tissue and looking for the edge of the tentorium. If the edge of the tentorium is encountered, it is likely that the collateral sulcus has already been divided. The collateral sulcus is an important landmark because it facilitates controlled entry into the inferior horn of the lateral ventricle. This entry point is designed to be on the inferior-lateral aspect of the temporal horn to avoid potential injury to the optic radiations. The ventricle is identified by gently aspirating the white matter just distal to the end of the collateral sulcus, and cottonoid patties can be placed to keep the ventricle open and protect the choroid plexus. The lateral aspect of the ventricle can then be opened and the white matter of the anterior temporal lobe divided in a line connecting the lateral opening of the ventricle and the inferior circular sulcus of the insula. As the dissection progresses, the intraventricular surfaces of the amygdala and hippocampus become apparent. The final disconnection of the lateral temporal lobe occurs as a cut through the lateral ventricular sulcus (collateral eminence) is made and the basal temporal pia divided just deep to the collateral sulcus. This pia is then divided anteriorly to the prior cut made from above and ending at the temporal pole. With this, the lateral temporal lobe is free and can be removed after inspecting to ensure all draining veins to the dura have been coagulated and divided.

The next stage of the operation can be performed with loupe magnification or the operating microscope. The operating microscope has the advantage of magnification and illumination and is recommended. The anatomy in this region is complex, and careful removal of the parahippocampus, hippocampus, and amygdala requires a thorough understanding of the relationships existing among the structures in the perimesencephalic cistern, the hippocampal sulcus, and the choroidal fissure and point. These relationships are better visualized with the operating microscope. At this point, the mesial resection can be thought of in two stages, with either stage proceeding first. These consist of the amygdalar-uncal removal and the hippocampal-parahippocampal removal. These stages are performed using the subpial aspiration technique, the one exception being division of the superior aspect of the amygdala in a line connecting the choroidal point and the middle cerebral artery visualized through the pia of the anterior sylvian fissure. It is important to stay below this line to avoid injury to the globus pallidus and the cisternal segment of the anterior choroidal artery (injury to this vessel is a significant source of hemiplegia and hemianopsia after temporal lobectomy).

The amygdala removal begins with identification of the choroidal point. This is located at the anterior extent of the choroidal plexus where the anterior choroidal artery enters the temporal horn of the lateral ventricle. Once identified, this demarcates the posterior-superior point of resection of the amygdala, as mentioned previously. The surgeon extends an imaginary line across the gray matter of the amygdala from the choroidal point to the middle cerebral artery visualized through the pia of the anterior sylvian fissure. In my experience, this is often difficult to visualize, and the line is extended horizontally from the roof of the temporal horn so that resection in a plane above the roof does not occur. Remember that the goal is to avoid resecting the superior amygdala, which blends imperceptibly into the globus pallidus, and to avoid exposure of the anterior choroidal artery in the cistern. After the superior line of resection is begun, it is carried down to the pia overlying the brainstem, third nerve, and interpeduncular fossa. The remaining dissection should be subpial and will remove temporal polar tissue, lower portion of the amygdala, and uncus. The posterior limit of this stage involves subpial aspiration of the uncus where it joins the head of the hippocampus. During division and removal of this tissue, the free edge of the hippocampal sulcus becomes visible as it arises from the perimesencephalic cistern. When this stage is complete, the anterior free edge of the tentorium, the third nerve, and the anterior aspect of the posterior cerebral artery should be seen.

The hippocampal removal begins with gentle aspiration of the parahippocampal tissue just deep to the remnant of the collateral sulcus. This tissue is removed in subpial fashion and can be carried as far medially as the edge of the tentorium and posteriorly curving deep below the hippocampus to the region of the hippocampal tail. This allows for gentle retraction of the hippocampus down toward the floor of the middle cranial fossa and reduces the need for retraction on the roof of the ventricle as the choroidal fissure is explored. After the parahippocampal tissue is removed, the lateral ventricle sulcus in the posterior aspect of the ventricle is further divided to allow easier access to the tail region of the hippocampus. This step effectively disconnects the overlying temporal cortex from the hippocampus and allows safer removal of the posterior aspect of the hippocampus. During the hippocampal removal, retraction on the roof of the ventricle and on the remaining posterior temporal lobe is undesirable and should be minimized by using the steps described earlier and by changing the position of the microscope to enhance the view of the tissues. Excessive retraction on the roof of the ventricle can lead to a retraction hemiparesis or injury to the optic tract, and similar retraction on the dominant posterior temporal lobe can lead to a postoperative language deficit. After the parahippocampus is removed, the choroidal fissure is exposed by gently retracting the choroid plexus superiorly with the use of a cottonoid patty or Telfa sponge cut to size. The fornix of the hippocampus and dentate gyrus are identified and gently aspirated, which exposes the underlying hippocampal sulcus. This is an extremely important landmark because it contains the arterial and venous supply to the hippocampus. It is much more robust in the head and anterior body region of the hippocampus and becomes more inconsistent in the posterior hippocampal regions. It should be exposed by aspiration of the fornix, dentate gyrus, and uncal tissue so that the entire width is visualized. The anterior extent is a free edge around which the parahippocampus curls to become the uncus. As this tissue is aspirated, the free edge is apparent. The deep origin of the sulcus is the pia overlying the brainstem, and care is necessary to avoid injury. The hippocampal arteries arise directly from the lateral aspect of the posterior cerebral artery, and direct visualization of the course of the hippocampal arteries should be obtained before coagulating and dividing them. This reduces the chances of ligating a traversing vessel that arises from the posterior cerebral artery and crosses the hippocampal sulcus before reentering the perimesencephalic cistern to irrigate the posterior thalamus and brainstem. To reiterate, only those vessels terminating in the hippocampus should be divided. After the arteries are coagulated, divide them so as to leave an arterial tail that is easily reached and coagulated. This avoids a scenario in which the divided stump retracts into the perimesencephalic cistern and causes subarachnoid hemorrhage. After the hippocampal sulcus is divided, the hippocampus and any remaining parahippocampus can be gently peeled off the underlying pia and removed to be sent to pathology for study. The mesial resection is then assessed and any remaining accessible posterior hippocampus removed. The posterior cut across the tail of the hippocampus ideally should allow for 3 to 4 cm of hippocampus to be removed.

When the resection is complete, hemostasis is achieved by time, irrigation, and the judicious use of hemostatic materials. Bipolar coagulation of bleeding points in the mesial temporal or sylvian fissure region is best avoided to prevent injury to underlying structures. Similar bleeding points in the residual amygdala tissue are also best treated with application of hemostatic agents, irrigation, and time. The cavity is then filled in with saline and the dura closed in watertight fashion. The craniotomy flap is attached with titanium fixation and the muscle sewn together and reapproximated to the residual cuff. The skin is then closed in anatomic layers over a subgaleal drain to reduce postoperative swelling.

OUTCOMES

After the surgery is completed, time must pass before determining outcome. Long-term seizure-free outcomes after temporal lobectomy, especially when performed for mesial temporal sclerosis, are often stated to be the best of all surgical procedures for medically resistant epilepsy. A number of long-term studies following patients for 5 to 10 years after surgery describe an initial seizure-free rate reaching 80%, which then noticeably declines over time to a 5-year seizure-free rate of about 50%.[36-40] Factors predicting an unfavorable outcome may include the presence of epileptic activity on the 6-month postoperative EEG, frequent preoperative seizures, generalized motor seizures, bilateral MRI abnormalities, and increased epilepsy duration.[36,41-43] Interestingly, in the report by Jeha in 2006, the presence of a normal MRI preoperatively did not lead to a worse outcome after surgery.[36] This is in disagreement with other studies suggesting a worse outcome in the face of a normal preoperative MRI and would suggest that patients with well-localized nonlesional TLE should be considered for temporal lobectomy.[40,44] Another important factor in the postoperative management of these patients is the "running-down" phenomenon described to occur in as many as one third of patients experiencing postoperative seizures after temporal lobectomy.[43,45-47] In a recent study, the presence of rare postoperative seizures 6 months after surgery was observed in a group of patients who subsequently were documented to have long-term seizure freedom in 74% of cases.[43] The authors hypothesized that the epileptogenic zone (EZ) in these patients was considerably reduced but not completely removed.

The running-down theory implies that this greatly reduced EZ gradually loses the power to generate seizures or that the anticonvulsant medications are able to control them.

Outcome analysis is extremely important in this group of patients because questions regarding return to employment, driving, and cessation of medication hinge on the success of surgery. Concrete information regarding potential risks and benefits of anticonvulsant withdrawal are necessary to allow these patients to reintegrate into society safely without medications. The National Library of Medicine has indexed more than 4400 articles that focus on epilepsy surgery, and 75% of these were published after 1990.[48] As Wiebe points out, the quality of these studies is reflected by the fact that only seven randomized controlled trials have been performed, and four of these involved the efficacy of vagus nerve stimulation.[49-52] Two others compared different surgical procedures to treat temporal lobe epilepsy without medical controls, and the final study compared temporal lobectomy with medical treatment.[12,34] Importantly, the results of the randomized trial by Wiebe in which 58% of surgically treated patients remained free of seizures appear comparable to the results of the systematic review of class IV nonrandomized studies involving 1952 patients.[53] In this large review, overall 66% of patients remained seizure free after surgery.

SURGICAL COMPLICATIONS

The rate of significant complications after temporal lobectomy is fortunately quite low. In general, the neurosurgical risks that need to be discussed with the patient include the general risks of craniotomy and the more specific risks of manipulating the temporal lobe. General complications include infection (wound, craniotomy, meningitis, urine), hemorrhage (wound, epidural, subdural, intracerebral), red blood cell transfusion related to acute blood loss anemia, deep venous thrombosis, anesthetic complications, and death. The incidence of mortality after temporal lobectomy is approaching zero as experience and technology improves.[12,53,54]

Complications specific to the temporal lobe include visual field loss, naming and language deficits (dominant temporal lobe), memory deficits, cranial nerve palsies, hemiparesis or plegia, and psychiatric morbidity (depression, anxiety). Common postoperative conditions (not complications) include headache, wound swelling, jaw discomfort, retro-orbital pain, and cosmetic deformity. These conditions largely resolve over 2 to 3 months, although preoperative headaches and temporomandibular joint dysfunction can predispose the patient to a longer recovery period after surgery.

Visual field loss after temporal lobectomy is related to injury of the geniculocalcarine fibers as they make their way from the lateral geniculate body to the occipital cortex. The most common pattern of injury results in a contralateral superior quadrantanopsia ("pie in the sky") from damage to Meyer's loop as it courses forward in the roof of the temporal horn of the lateral ventricle. Its variable course and lack of anatomic distinction at surgery make it a difficult structure to protect. The incidence of superior quadrantanopsia reported on retrospective studies is variable, but likely a realistic estimate is 35% to 50% after standard temporal lobectomy.[33,55,56] Contralateral homonymous hemianopsia is much less common and usually results when larger temporal lobe resections are performed and damage to the geniculocalcarine tract occurs at the posterior aspect of the inferior temporal horn (trigone region). The optic tract can also be injured in the prethalamic region by dissections that stray too far superiorly at the level of the amygdala and anterior hippocampus. Finally, a contralateral hemianopsia may accompany a hemiparesis when damage to the anterior choroidal artery occurs in its cisternal segment. This artery is an important structure to protect during removal of the mesial structures. Respecting the anatomic land-

marks during removal of the amygdala and hippocampus is the best way to avoid this potentially devastating complication. Hemiparesis may also result from manipulation or retraction injury of the ipsilateral cerebral peduncle. This type of postoperative deficit generally improves with time and is best avoided by limiting retraction during surgery on the roof of the temporal horn.

Other neurological complications encountered include horizontal and vertical diplopias resulting from irritation to the third and fourth cranial nerves, respectively. These usually resolve over a few months and may need to be treated with ocular patching therapy. Fourth cranial nerve dysfunction is likely the less frequent cause of diplopia, although because it is difficult to diagnose, it may be underrecognized. The patient typically complains of double vision, especially when descending stairs or looking down. The nerve is vulnerable during temporal lobectomy because it travels under the medial edge of the tentorium, and injury is best avoided by limiting pressure or coagulation in this region.

Postoperative aphasias can occur after dominant temporal lobe resections. These are generally characterized by perseveration, naming difficulties, paraphasias, and word substitutions. Fortunately, these are usually transient and peak 24 to 48 hours after surgery before resolution. Although the exact cause is unknown, this language disturbance can be quite severe when it occurs. Potential mechanisms include retraction and ischemic infarction of comprehensive language cortex and resection of anterior and basal temporal lobe language sites that ultimately are not essential language sites.[32] Management of this complication should include postoperative MRI with stroke protocol, corticosteroid therapy, and speech therapy services. The patient and family should be reassured that language function will improve when the MRI does not demonstrate a posterior temporal lobe infarction. Strategies to avoid injury to the posterior temporal neocortex during surgery include minimizing retraction during removal of the posterior hippocampus and protecting the arterial and venous structures serving this area.

COGNITIVE OUTCOME AND QUALITY OF LIFE

Complaints centered on cognitive function are common in the temporal lobe epilepsy patient. Many patients have significant neuropsychological deficits before surgery thought to be related to damage to the mesial temporal lobe structures involved in memory as well as the effects of anticonvulsant therapy on normal cortical tissue. Preoperative and postoperative cognitive assessment is important to help counsel the patient on existing deficits and to predict and document the effects of temporal lobectomy on memory function. Preoperative risk factors for worsening memory function after surgery include dominant TLE, lack of hippocampal sclerosis, normal baseline neuropsychological function, and later age of onset of the epilepsy.[27,28,57] Additionally, postoperative memory function and quality of life appear to be positively related to seizure freedom after surgery.[24]

Memory assessment includes the use of standardized neuropsychological testing, intracarotid sodium amobarbital testing (Wada's test), and more recently functional MRI.[21-23] Additionally, detailed patient questioning regarding their own observations about memory and cognitive functioning are important because little correlation may exist between neuropsychological testing results and how the patient functions in day-to-day life. Although dominant temporal lobe surgery predisposes the patient to a decline in verbal memory and short-term memory functioning, the risks associated with nondominant temporal lobe surgery are less predictable. Visual spatial memory can be quantified during testing, and although removal of the nondominant hippocampus usually results in no apparent clinical deficits, impaired performance may be observed on postoperative retesting.

Considerable interest has focused on quality of life and psychiatric comorbidities associated with TLE. Depression and anxiety appear to be the most common psychiatric disturbances encountered before surgery, and depression is the most common encountered after surgery.[58,59] Patients undergoing temporal lobectomy generally experience improved quality of life compared with medically treated patients.[12,60-62] Measuring an individual's improvement in day-to-day functions and well-being is important, and health-related quality-of-life (HRQOL) measurements are being used with increasing frequency in patients with medically intractable epilepsy. In a recent study by von Lehe and colleagues, HRQOL scores correlated positively with seizure control, and the authors suggested that to obtain better quality of life after epilepsy surgery, seizures must be controlled.[63] In a randomized controlled trial for temporal lobectomy, the average quality of life measures at 6 months and 1 year were significantly higher in those treated with surgery.[12] In this study, there were no differences in the rates of psychiatric comorbidities between the two groups.

CONCLUSION

Temporal lobectomy is well established as a safe and effective treatment option for medically intractable TLE. Although some of the terminology is inexact, and the details of the surgical technique vary somewhat across centers, the reported results are very similar for patients with the same underlying epileptic substrate. The preoperative work-up and patient selection process can be complicated and should be carried out at a center experienced in the surgical treatment of epilepsy. Overall, patients with medically resistant TLE are better managed with epilepsy surgery rather than continued medical treatment. These patients should be referred for surgical evaluation promptly.

SUGGESTED READINGS

Helmstaedter C. Neuropsychological aspects of epilepsy surgery. *Epilepsy Behav.* 2004;5:S45-S55.

Jeha L, Najm I, Bingaman W, et al. Predictors of outcome after temporal lobectomy for the treatment of intractable epilepsy. *Neurology.* 2006;66:1938-1940.

Kwan P, Brodie MJ. Early identification of refractory epilepsy. *N Engl J Med.* 2000;342:314-319.

Nogueira de Almeida A, Teixeira MJ, Feindel WH. From lateral to mesial: the quest for a surgical cure for temporal lobe epilepsy. *Epilepsia.* 2008;49:98-107.

Seidenberg M, Hermann B, Wyler A, et al. Neuropsychological outcome following anterior temporal lobectomy in patients with and without the syndrome of mesial temporal lobe epilepsy. *Neuropsychology.* 1998;12:303-316.

Spencer SS. The relative contributions of MRI, SPECT, and PET imaging in epilepsy. *Epilepsia.* 1994;35:S72-S89.

Tanriverdi T, Olivier A, Poulin N, et al. Long-term seizure outcome after mesial temporal lobe epilepsy surgery: corticalamygdalohippocampectomy versus selective amygdalohippocampectomy. *J Neurosurg.* 2008;108:517-524.

Wen HT, Rhoton AL, De Oliveira E, et al. Microsurgical anatomy of the temporal lobe. Part 1: mesial temporal lobe anatomy and its vascular relationships as applied to amygdalohippocampectomy. *Neurosurgery.* 1999;45:549-591.

Wiebe S, Blume WT, Girvin JP, et al. A randomized, controlled trial of surgery for temporal lobe epilepsy. *N Engl J Med.* 2001;345:311-318.

Wyler AR, Hermann BP, Somes G. Extent of medial temporal lobe resection on outcome from anterior temporal lobectomy: a randomized prospective study. *Neurosurgery.* 1995;37:982-991.

Full references can be found on Expert Consult @ www.expertconsult.com

CHAPTER 63

Selective Amygdalohippocampectomy

Kim J. Burchiel ■ Andrew C. Zacest ■ David Spencer

HISTORICAL CONSIDERATIONS

Over the course of the past century, two main factors have driven the surgical approach to epilepsy. First, an appreciation of the central role of the mesial basal temporal structures in many cases of human epilepsy has been gained from clinical observation and neuropathologic, electrophysiologic, and radiologic studies.[1] Second and in parallel has been accumulating evidence from numerous surgical series demonstrating that temporal lobe resection, in particular, resection of mesial temporal structures, leads to an 80% to 90% rate of freedom from seizures in patients with medically intractable temporal lobe epilepsy.[1-7]

A number of surgical techniques have evolved in the process. The standard temporal resection procedure has been en bloc anterior temporal lobectomy (ATL) involving anterior neocortical resection of up to 4.5 to 6.5 cm, depending on whether the dominant temporal lobe is being operated on, and mesial temporal resection encompassing the amygdala and at least 3 cm of hippocampus. This approach was originally advocated by Falconer and colleagues in 1955[8] and is still used today.

Selective surgical approaches to the amygdala and hippocampus evolved as evidence increasingly indicated a critical role for these structures in epileptogenesis, and methods were sought to minimize collateral surgical injury to important temporal neocortical structures. Niemeyer was the first to describe selective transcortical transventricular amygdalohippocampectomy (STTAH) in 1958.[9] A direct approach to the mesial temporal structures via the middle temporal gyrus was used, an approach that Olivier would later refine with the assistance of frameless stereotaxy.[1]

Other surgeons have approached the mesial temporal structures via less direct paths. Weiser, Yasargil, and their coworkers reported a transsylvian approach to the medial temporal structures that had the theoretical advantage of complete avoidance of neocortical injury; however, the approach was technically more demanding and placed critical vascular structures at risk.[10,11] Hori and associates described a subtemporal selective approach and reported fewer neuropsychological sequelae as an advantage.[12,13]

With the recent confirmation that temporal lobectomy is superior to the best medical therapy for patients with intractable temporal lobe epilepsy,[7] focus has now shifted toward understanding what is the best surgical approach to achieve this end. Selective amygdalohippocampectomy (SAH) represents an approach to the mesiobasal temporal structures that is as effective as ATL in selected patients, has the potential to minimize neocortical injury and its neurological sequelae, and is an approach that may be used by most neurosurgeons.

SURGICAL RATIONALE FOR SELECTIVE AMYGDALOHIPPOCAMPECTOMY

The surgical rationale for performing SAH is to limit surgical resection to brain structures that must be removed to eliminate seizures while minimizing the risk for injury to important collateral structures. For example, in the case of well-defined mesial temporal sclerosis, these objectives can be met with a more selective approach than the traditional ATL.

Seizure outcome after epilepsy surgery has been noted to depend largely on diagnostic and clinical variables that have an impact on patient selection.[3,6] The efficacy of selective approaches versus traditional en bloc ATL with mesial resection for seizure control has been examined in a number of noncontrolled series and found to be comparable in most,[3,5] but not all reports,[2] and this variability may reflect differences in the types of patients selected for surgery. Indeed, even in studies that have claimed the highest rates of freedom from seizures with the selective approach,[1] it is evident that strict attention to preoperative selection is important.

In the absence of surgical complications such as stroke or infection, neuropsychological complications, particularly memory loss, are the major potential morbidity after all temporal resections. It is argued that these complications must arise from resection of functioning normal tissue and are therefore less likely to occur in patients undergoing more selective resection. Although confounding variables such as the dominance of the resected side, the absence of ipsilateral hippocampal sclerosis, the focality of the epileptic source, the presence of intact memory, and methodologic differences in neuropsychological testing make direct comparisons difficult, there is accumulating evidence that individually tailored or selective approaches may have a more favorable cognitive outcome than standard resections[3,5,14,15]; however, not all studies have shown such results.

Although SAH has been performed via the transsylvian and subtemporal routes, the rationale for the frameless stereotaxy transcortical approach described in this chapter is that it is the most direct and simplest approach that results in minimal disruption of nontargeted tissue and avoids the arachnoid dissection and vessel manipulation or excessive retraction inherent with other selective approaches.

PREOPERATIVE EVALUATION AND DECISION MAKING

Preoperative evaluation is concerned primarily with selecting patients who have surgically remediable epilepsy and a favorable risk-to-benefit ratio for surgery.

Patients under consideration for epilepsy surgery have medically refractory epilepsy. Although the definition of medical intractability may vary, data from Kwan and Brodie and from others suggest that these patients can be identified early, perhaps after as few as two failed trials of antiepileptic drugs.[16]

Confidence in localization of the surgical epileptic focus depends on concordance of the seizure history and semiology, electrophysiologic monitoring (interictal and ictal), neuroimaging, and in some cases, metabolic imaging, positron emission tomography, or single-photon emission computed tomography. In select cases in which lateralization of the temporal focus is not clear, semi-invasive or invasive electroencephalographic methods

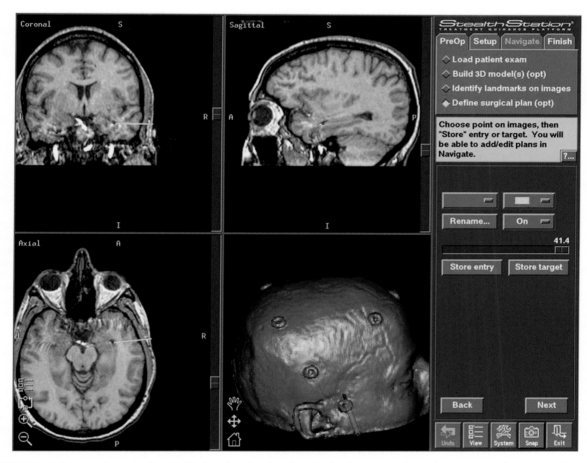

FIGURE 63-1 Image from the Stealth Workstation showing the plan for the entry point and trajectory to the temporal horn.

such as foramen ovale depth electrodes or surface grid electrodes may be used.

Neuropsychological assessment, including quantitative measures of visuospatial and verbal memory, is performed on all preoperative patients. A Wada test to assess hemispheric language dominance and lateralized memory deficits is considered mandatory at some centers and applied more selectively at others. Psychiatric assessment may also be sought in patients with a past history of depression.

Clinically significant postoperative memory loss is more likely in patients with left (dominant) temporal lobe epilepsy, intact preoperative verbal memory, normal magnetic resonance imaging (MRI) results, bilateral hippocampal abnormalities, and later age at seizure onset.[3,17] Assessment of these factors guides preoperative counseling regarding the risk for postoperative memory deficits. These risks are tempered by the hazards associated with not operating (some patients with medically treated refractory temporal lobe epilepsy have accelerated memory loss) and by the knowledge that some cognitive skills can stabilize or improve after successful surgery.

The patients being considered for surgery are presented at a multidisciplinary epilepsy conference, where the results of all investigations performed to date are discussed. A management plan is then agreed on, and any additional diagnostic studies needed are requested. Patients who are deemed appropriate candidates for surgery are then seen in the neurosurgery clinic. The treating surgeon describes the aims, risks, and benefits of surgical resection. Risks include persistent seizures; infection; hematoma; neurovascular injury causing stroke, loss of memory function, and loss of language function; wound complications; death; and other complications. Care is taken to ensure that the patient and family understand all the relevant issues and their questions are answered.

SELECTIVE TRANSCORTICAL TRANSVENTRICULAR AMYGDALOHIPPOCAMPECTOMY— OPERATIVE PROCEDURE AND AVOIDANCE OF COMPLICATIONS

All patients undergo preoperative stereotactic brain MRI with fiducial scalp markers in place. Images are transferred to a Stealth Workstation (Medtronic, Minneapolis, MN), and the surgical entry point and trajectory are planned so that the most direct route is taken to the ipsilateral temporal horn from the middle temporal gyrus, approximately 3 cm from the tip of the temporal lobe (Fig. 63-1).

The patient undergoes routine general anesthesia and endotracheal intubation with insertion of a urinary catheter and administration of antibiotics. Mannitol is not used routinely. The patient is positioned supine with the head rotated 90 degrees to the opposite side, parallel to the floor with the head held in a three-pin fixateur. Attention to level positioning of the head is important to achieve a true lateral trajectory. Fiducials are registered and the planned cortical entry point marked on the scalp along with the intended bone flap and scalp incision (Fig. 63-2). The scalp is then prepared, draped, and infiltrated with 1% lidocaine and a 0.25% bupivacaine mixture with epinephrine.

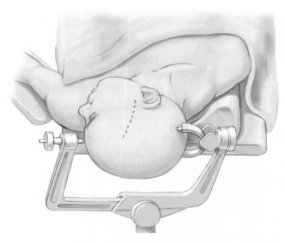

FIGURE 63-2 Operative drawing showing patient positioning and the proposed incision.

The linear scalp incision is opened, the temporalis fascia sharply incised, and the longitudinal fibers of the temporalis dissected from the periosteum and retracted laterally. The neuronavigation system is then used to direct the position of the temporal craniotomy, which invariably reaches the floor of the middle cranial fossa. After the dura is exposed and the surface vessels controlled with diathermy, the dura is opened and reflected inferiorly (Fig. 63-3).

The neuronavigation system is used to estimate the distance from the tip of the temporal lobe, which is confirmed manually, and to select the cortical entry site on a portion of the middle temporal gyrus that is free of significant cortical vessels. For the dominant temporal lobe, we select an entry point no farther than 3.5 cm from the temporal tip and plan for a cortical incision 1.5 to 2 cm in length (Fig. 63-4). With the use of bipolar cautery, the cortical surface is opened and an endopial dissection is performed toward the temporal horn guided at all times by the image guidance system (Fig. 63-5).

Once the temporal horn is entered, two self-retaining brain retractors are placed to optimize visualization of the intraventricular anatomy (Fig. 63-6). The following structures

should be identified to aid navigation: the medial prominence of the hippocampus; the collateral eminence, which overlies the collateral sulcus separating the parahippocampal and occipitotemporal gyri; and the choroid plexus.

Resection of the mesial temporal lobe structures is commenced by entering the parahippocampal gyrus located ventral to the hippocampus (Fig. 63-7). The resection begins at the pial surface of the most ventrolateral portion of the gyrus and then progresses medially toward the uncus. After this part of the resection is complete, it possible to visualize the edge of the tentorium and the contents of the basal cisterns and be sufficiently oriented to perform the amygdalectomy safely. The navigation system is used throughout the procedure. The mesial pial border must be strictly preserved to avoid injury to the posterior cerebral artery and third nerve. These structures can be visualized through the preserved pial membrane.

After the anterior portion of the parahippocampal gyrus and the amygdala have been removed, attention is directed toward the hippocampus (Fig. 63-8). Here, identification of the choroid plexus and choroidal fissure guides the resection by defining the superomedial limit of resection. The hippocampus is dissected first from this border starting anteriorly from the posterior limit of the amygdalectomy and extending posteriorly to the level of the tectal plate. Again, frameless stereotaxy is used to ensure the completeness of resection from the uncus to the posterior of the hippocampus. At the posterior limit of the planned resection the hippocampal tail is removed and the lateral margin of the hippocampus is then dissected down the pia of the middle cranial fossa to completely isolate the structure. The body of the hippocampus can then be removed piecemeal via a suction technique on either side of the hippocampal sulcus. While removing the hippocampus and separating it from the hippocampal sulcus, it may be necessary to coagulate small hippocampal vessels, but great care should be taken to preserve small branches of the anterior choroidal artery and posterior cerebral artery in this vicinity.

The resection cavity is then inspected and hemostasis is achieved (Fig. 63-9). The brain retractors are removed and the dura is closed in watertight fashion. The bone flap is secured with miniplates, the temporalis muscle is reapproximated, and the scalp is closed in layers with absorbable suture.

The patient is awakened from anesthesia, checked neurologically, and transferred to the neurosurgical intensive care unit. Postoperative computed tomography is performed, and all anti-

FIGURE 63-3 A and **B,** Operative drawings showing the scalp retracted and the site and size of the stereotactically guided temporal craniotomy and durotomy.

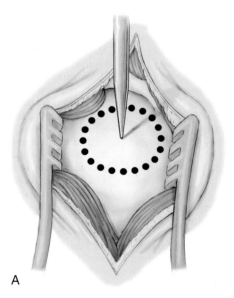
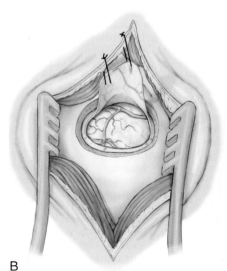

A   B

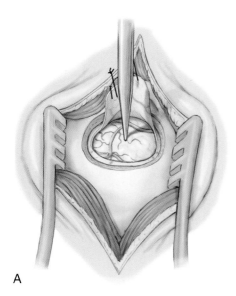

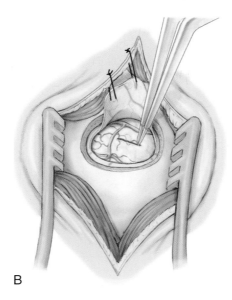

A

B

convulsant medications are continued. The patient is observed in the hospital for 4 to 5 days until discharge.

Potential complications of STTAH include inadvertent vascular injury, hematoma, infection, quadrant visual field deficit, psychiatric disorders (delirium, depression, and anxiety), brainstem injury, and neuropsychological sequelae. Particular attention must be paid to the technical details of this procedure to reduce the risk for complications. Strict attention to patient positioning to allow a perpendicular transcortical trajectory to the temporal horn of the lateral ventricle will greatly facilitate navigation. Careful identification of the choroidal fissure and the entry point of the anterior choroidal artery and meticulous preservation of the medial pial boundary will minimize the likelihood of serious vascular and brainstem injury. Adequate resection of the amygdala and hippocampus will depend largely on accurate

intraoperative navigation and direct visualization to verify the anterior and posterior limits of resection.

OUTCOME

There are no randomized controlled trials comparing SAH with ATL. Hence, the existing nonrandomized comparative studies suffer from potential selection bias, and many compare groups of patients who are not comparable with each other.[3,5,18] Nonetheless, the overwhelming finding from these studies is therapeutic equivalence; both SAH and ATL lead to high rates of freedom from seizures in carefully selected patients. Many studies restricted SAH to a highly selected group of patients with hippocampal sclerosis as the sole pathology. Others have reported excellent outcomes with SAH in patients with lesions identified

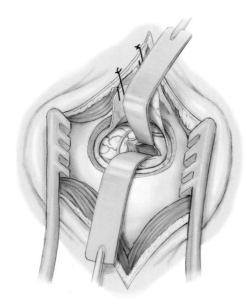

FIGURE 63-5 A subpial dissection to the temporal horn of the lateral ventricle has been made with the use of neuronavigation, and the exposure is maintained by retractors.

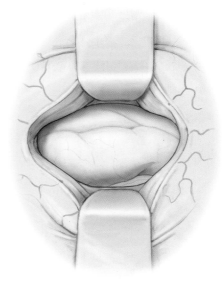

FIGURE 63-6 The temporal horn of the lateral ventricle has been opened and the temporal neocortex retracted. The ventricular structures visible include the lateral sulcus, which is the junction of the hippocampus and the lateral wall of the ventricle.

FIGURE 63-7 A, The parahippocampal gyrus is entered with suction to commence resection of the amygdala until (**B**) the medial pia of the anterior aspect of the uncus is located, exposing the floor of the middle fossa, tentorial edge, and suprasellar cistern.

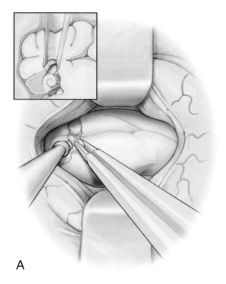
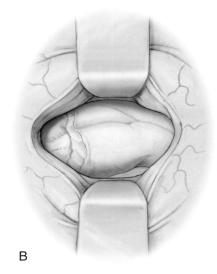

A   B

on preoperative imaging studies, as well as those with normal MRI studies.[19] It is clear, however, that surgical outcomes suffer if the patient selection process deviates from the strict criteria that are used to identify patients with unilateral mesial temporal lobe epilepsy who may benefit from conventional temporal lobe resection surgery.[20] Although there is little dispute that patients with unilateral hippocampal sclerosis are excellent candidates for SAH, the characteristics of other patients who might benefit from this procedure have yet to be fully defined.[3,5,12,13,17,21-23]

Neuropsychological outcomes in most,[3,5,12,13,17,21-23] but not all[24-26] studies favor SAH over ATL. Nonetheless, this remains a subject of controversy. Many test measures examining postoperative neurological function are similar between the two surgical groups; however, several studies have reported superior outcomes with SAH in terms of verbal memory, attention, and some composite measures of neuropsychological outcome.[3,5] However, it is clear from large, well-conducted trials that patients undergoing left (dominant) SAH are not immune to substantial verbal memory impairment and that the more selective procedure is not

a panacea.[17,21] Careful preoperative neuropsychological assessment and counseling remain critical.

A large, randomized, controlled comparison of transsylvian and transcortical SAH demonstrated no differences in seizure-free outcomes or most neuropsychological measures between the two surgical groups. However one performance measure (verbal fluency) was superior in the transcortical group.[2] Hori and colleagues have argued that cognitive sequelae are minimized by a subtemporal approach,[12,13] but this remains to be demonstrated convincingly.

CONCLUSION

In summary, SAH represents a more direct and less invasive surgical approach to the critical mesiobasal structures that have been implicated as sites of seizure onset in patients with temporal lobe epilepsy. Technical advances and accumulating clinical evidence support SAH as an acceptable alternative to ATL in carefully selected patients. There is evidence to support comparable

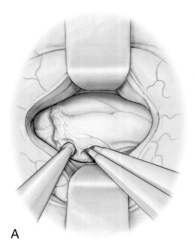
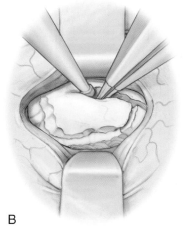
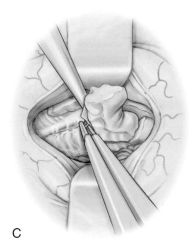

A   B   C

FIGURE 63-8 A-C, Once the amygdalectomy is performed, the choroidal fissure is identified and followed posteriorly to the tail of the hippocampus as the superomedial margin of resection. The hippocampal tail is then cut level with the tectal plate. Lateral dissection of the hippocampus is next accomplished while leaving the hippocampus on its vascular pedicle, the hippocampal sulcus. As the hippocampus proper is dissected, the sulcal vessels must be carefully identified, dissected, and coagulated.

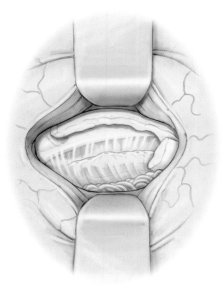

FIGURE 63-9 The empty resection cavity within intact pial margin. The underlying midbrain, posterior cerebral artery, and third nerve can be visualized through the pia.

efficacy for the two approaches in this select patient group, and the SAH procedure may produce fewer neuropsychological sequelae in some patients.

SUGGESTED READINGS

Abosch A, Bernasconi N, Boling W, et al. Factors predictive of suboptimal seizure control following selective amygdalohippocampectomy. *J Neurosurg.* 2002;97: 1142.

Arruda F, Cendes F, Andermann F, et al. Mesial atrophy and outcome after amygdalohippocampectomy or temporal lobe removal. *Ann Neurol.* 1996;40:446.

Bate H, Eldridge P, Varma T, et al. The seizure outcome after amygdalohippocampectomy and temporal lobectomy. *Eur J Neurol.* 2007;14:90.

Clusmann H, Schramm J, Kral T, et al. Prognostic factors and outcome after different types of resection for temporal lobe epilepsy. *J Neurosurg.* 2002;97:1131.

Falconer MA, Meyer A, Hill D, et al. Treatment of temporal-lobe epilepsy by temporal lobectomy; a survey of findings and results. *Lancet.* 1955;268:827.

Gleissner U, Helmstaedter C, Schramm J, et al. Memory outcome after selective amygdalohippocampectomy in patients with temporal lobe epilepsy: one-year follow-up. *Epilepsia.* 2004;45:960.

Gleissner U, Helmstaedter C, Schramm J, et al. Memory outcome after selective amygdalohippocampectomy: a study in 140 patients with temporal lobe epilepsy. *Epilepsia.* 2002;43:87.

Goldstein LH, Polkey CE. Short-term cognitive changes after unilateral temporal lobectomy or unilateral amygdalo-hippocampectomy for the relief of temporal lobe epilepsy. *J Neurol Neurosurg Psychiatry.* 1993;56:135.

Hori T, Yamane F, Ochiai T, et al. Selective subtemporal amygdalohippocampectomy for refractory temporal lobe epilepsy: operative and neuropsychological outcomes. *J Neurosurg.* 2007;106:134.

Hori T, Yamane F, Ochiai T, et al. Subtemporal amygdalohippocampectomy prevents verbal memory impairment in the language-dominant hemisphere. *Stereotact Funct Neurosurg.* 2003;80:18.

Jones-Gotman M, Zatorre RJ, Olivier A, et al. Learning and retention of words and designs following excision from medial or lateral temporal-lobe structures. *Neuropsychologia.* 1997;35:963.

Kwan P, Brodie MJ. Early identification of refractory epilepsy. *N Engl J Med.* 2000;342:314.

Lacruz ME, Alarcon G, Akanuma N, et al. Neuropsychological effects associated with temporal lobectomy and amygdalohippocampectomy depending on Wada test failure. *J Neurol Neurosurg Psychiatry.* 2004;75:600.

Mittal S, Montes JL, Farmer JP, et al. Long-term outcome after surgical treatment of temporal lobe epilepsy in children. *J Neurosurg.* 2005;103:401.

Morino M, Uda T, Naito K, et al. Comparison of neuropsychological outcomes after selective amygdalohippocampectomy versus anterior temporal lobectomy. *Epilepsy Behav.* 2006;9:95.

Niemeyer P. The transventricular amygdalohippocampectomy in temporal lobe epilepsy. In: Baldwin M, Bailey P, ed. *Temporal Lobe Epilepsy.* Springfield, IL: Charles C Thomas; 1958:461.

Olivier A. Transcortical selective amygdalohippocampectomy in temporal lobe epilepsy. *Can J Neurol Sci.* 2000;27(suppl 1):S68.

Paglioli E, Palmini A, Portuguez M, et al. Seizure and memory outcome following temporal lobe surgery: selective compared with nonselective approaches for hippocampal sclerosis. *J Neurosurg.* 2006;104:70.

Pauli E, Pickel S, Schulemann H, et al. Neuropsychologic findings depending on the type of the resection in temporal lobe epilepsy. *Adv Neurol.* 1999;81:371.

Radhakrishnan K, So EL, Silbert PL, et al. Predictors of outcome of anterior temporal lobectomy for intractable epilepsy: a multivariate study. *Neurology.* 1998;51:465.

Wiebe S, Blume WT, Girvin JP, et al. A randomized, controlled trial of surgery for temporal-lobe epilepsy. *N Engl J Med.* 2001;345:311.

Wieser HG. Selective amygdalohippocampectomy: indications and follow-up. *Can J Neurol Sci.* 1991;18:617.

Wieser HG, Ortega M, Friedman A, et al. Long-term seizure outcomes following amygdalohippocampectomy. *J Neurosurg.* 2003;98:751.

Wieser HG, Siegel AM, Yasargil GM. The Zurich amygdalo-hippocampectomy series: a short up-date. *Acta Neurochir Suppl.* 1990;50:122.

Wolf HK, Campos MG, Zentner J, et al. Surgical pathology of temporal lobe epilepsy. Experience with 216 cases. *J Neuropathol Exp Neurol.* 1993;52:499.

Yasargil MG, Teddy PJ, Roth P. Selective amygdalo-hippocampectomy. Operative anatomy and surgical technique. *Adv Tech Stand Neurosurg.* 1985;12:93.

Full references can be found on Expert Consult @ www.expertconsult.com

CHAPTER 64

Tailored Resections for Epilepsy

David W. Roberts

Although the first operations performed for the treatment of medically intractable epilepsy were obviously directed by the specific findings in individual patients[1,2] and by the large formative experience of Penfield and Jasper in using electrocorticography (ECoG) to guide temporal resection,[3] the majority of surgical interventions that have been performed since have been fairly standardized procedures. The recognition of certain epilepsy syndromes and their associated pathologies has enabled widespread application of such procedures as anterior temporal lobe resection, selective amygdalohippocampectomy, and hemispherectomy with remarkable success.[4] There are certain settings, however, in which the surgical procedure may be improved in terms of seizure outcome or safety, or both, through tailoring of the surgical procedure to the specific patient. Indeed, in many instances such an approach is the only one possible.

In this review, the concept of tailored resection for epilepsy is presented as an alternative to more standardized procedures, particularly with respect to the temporal lobe, and as an approach to frontal lobe, parietal lobe, and multilobar epilepsy. A description of the surgical technique and results is presented.

THE BASIS FOR TAILORED RESECTION

Temporal Lobe Resection

The role of tailored resection is least agreed on for epilepsy involving the temporal lobe. There are standardized approaches to temporal lobe epilepsy surgery that vary slightly according to side with respect to language dominance and inclusion of mesial structures, and reasonably good seizure outcomes overall have long been reported with these standardized approaches. The 1991 survey of epilepsy surgery centers compiled by Engel for the Second Palm Desert International Conference on the Surgical Treatment of the Epilepsies, held in Indian Wells, California, in February 1992, found seizure-free outcomes in 67.9% of patients undergoing anterior temporal resection.[4] Recognition of variability among patients with respect to both the epileptogenic zone and language cortex, however, has led a number of surgical epilepsy teams to advocate tailoring the resection.

Distinguishing between mesial temporal sclerosis and temporal neocortical epilepsy represents one of the first rationales for implementation of this strategy. It was the ability to diagnose seizure onset localized to the hippocampus or amygdala that made selective amygdalohippocampectomy a viable treatment in the first place. Intracranial recording, usually with depth electrodes, made possible the successful selective procedures reported from Zurich[5,6]; alternatively, neuroimaging showing localized lesions limited to medial structures similarly sufficed. Conversely, neurophysiologic or radiographic data indicating a pathologic process confined to neocortical tissue justified a surgical procedure that spared the amygdala and hippocampus. These strategies are widely implemented today with the use of advanced magnetic resonance imaging (MRI) data or invasive monitoring, or both. Surgical planning and decision making in these instances generally occur outside the operating room, before the actual resective procedure.

Intraoperative "tailoring" of the resection procedure with the assistance of ECoG and functional mapping data obtained at the time of surgery is widely performed today. Intraoperative recordings, with rare exception, necessarily rely on interictal epileptiform discharges, or spikes, rather than ictal onset, which can be diagnosed only with extraoperative studies. The relationship of such interictal spikes to the epileptogenic zone or the area whose resection will result in a seizure-free outcome is not as clear as that for ictal-onset data. Animal models using either penicillin or alumina foci have demonstrated tight correlations between spikes and the epileptogenic zone.[7,8] However, human clinical investigations have shown varying degrees of correlation. Using preresection and postresection intraoperative ECoG in a series of 29 patients undergoing standard temporal resection for mesial temporal sclerosis, Schwartz and colleagues investigated the predictive value of corticography for seizure outcome and found no correlation.[9] Sugano and associates, in contrast, reported an analysis of 35 temporal lobe epilepsy patients who had undergone either lesionectomy or resection of a lesion plus tissue with residual spike activity (most often the hippocampus) and noted 3-year seizure-free rates of 76.9% and 90.9%, respectively.[10] This relationship plus the enhanced ability of ECoG recording to accurately define an epileptogenic zone whose resection will lead to cessation of seizures is one of the two major rationales for tailoring resections.

The other rationale for individualization of temporal lobe seizure surgery relates to the known variability in the spatial representation of normal temporal lobe functions, particularly those related to language. Conventional teaching for untailored temporal lobe resection surgery advocates removing no more than the most anterior 4.5 cm of the middle temporal gyrus in the language-dominant hemisphere and preferably sparing the superior temporal gyrus entirely. With extensive experience in mapping language during epilepsy resections, however, Ojemann and coworkers have clearly documented the high variability of cortical language representation, with some critical language sites observed within anterior temporal lobe regions that would be removed during a standardized resection procedure.[11-13] On this basis, cortical mapping has been strongly advocated.[14] Those who argue against this position would note that others have reported the absence of new language deficits after standard resection.[15]

Extratemporal Neocortical Resection

The strategy of resecting identified epileptogenic cortex while preserving normal function similarly applies to surgery on the frontal, parietal, and occipital lobes. Individualized investigation is generally required, given the absence of analogous epileptic syndromes and standardized surgeries, with the possible exception of some epilepsy cases associated with well-defined lesions. Although recognition of structural pathology on imaging studies may guide the approach, appreciation of the extent of the surrounding resection and the proximity of eloquent cortex usually benefits from extraoperative or intraoperative recording with or without functional mapping. MRI-negative or nonlesional epilepsy necessitates such an approach.

Frontal lobe epilepsy resection requires preservation of primary motor cortex and, on the language-dominant side, speech cortex. Although variability in the primary motor areas has been noted, it is considerably less variable than the critical language sites. Under image guidance, planned surgical approaches well anterior to the precentral gyrus may be performed in accordance with the structural anatomy; incorporation of tractography or functional MRI (fMRI) data provides only further reassurance. Resections that are planned closer to eloquent brain regions, however, are facilitated by intraoperative mapping and monitoring. Language preservation with frontal resection requires sparing of Broca's area in the posterior inferior frontal gyrus, but recent intraoperative studies have documented more extensive and variable frontal lobe language representation as well.[16,17]

Parietal resections must preserve primary sensory cortex and, on the language-dominant side, perisylvian language areas. Optic radiations, generally deep to the epileptogenic cortex, are at risk with larger resections but are not generally mapped intraoperatively. When operating within the occipital lobe, the primary visual cortex must be preserved. Although the accumulated surgical experience in posterior brain regions is much more limited than that in the temporal and frontal lobes, surgical interventions in these posterior regions are being carried out with increasing frequency and encouraging results.[18-23]

Multilobar Resection

Multilobar resection for the treatment of medically intractable epilepsy has understandably been used far less frequently than well-recognized interventions such as anterior temporal lobe resection or single-lobe cortical resection. The extent of surgery, its potential morbidity, associated functional consequences, and not least, the lower seizure control efficacy rate underlie the smaller surgical numbers, and the published experience with multilobar surgery is limited. Engel's 1991 survey described comparative seizure control outcomes, with multilobar resection achieving seizure-free outcomes in 45.2% of patients and improvement in an additional 35.5%; anterior temporal lobe resection and lesionectomy, in contrast, achieved seizure-free outcomes in 67.9% and 66.6% of patients, respectively.[4] Patients undergoing these different procedures, however, are distinctly different patient populations, and it would be a misinterpretation of that previous experience to deny multilobar epilepsy patients consideration of possible surgical intervention. Since the time of Engel's survey, developments in both evaluation—neuroimaging as well as intracranial investigation—and surgical technique have improved the risk-benefit ratio for these patients.[24-27]

METHODOLOGY AND TECHNIQUE

Preoperative Evaluation

Surgical evaluation of an epilepsy patient today requires the multidisciplinary team approach of a dedicated epilepsy service. In addition to a general and epilepsy-focused history and physical examination, routine evaluation will include scalp electroencephalography (EEG) and epilepsy-protocol MRI; in those in whom surgery appears to be a reasonable preliminary consideration, further neuroimaging with positron emission tomography or single-photon emission computed tomography (SPECT), or both, inpatient video-EEG monitoring, ictal SPECT, and neuropsychological testing generally follows. Not all patients require all of these studies. In patients with MRI-negative epilepsy, subtraction SPECT (ictal minus the coregistered baseline) has often proved invaluable in directing subsequent intracranial investigative studies.[28,29] Review and consideration of all this information

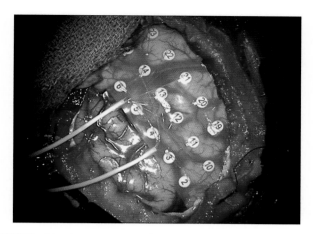

FIGURE 64-1 Intraoperative electrocorticography is being performed in this patient with complex partial epilepsy and a right temporal cavernous angioma. A 4 × 8 subdural grid has been placed over the right temporal lobe convexity (anterior is *top left;* superior is *bottom left*).

by a multidisciplinary epilepsy team in a regular working conference subsequently ensue. At this point, patients without surgically treatable epilepsy, those who require additional medical management, and those with straightforward conditions such as medial temporal lobe epilepsy or structural lesions confined to a single lobe will have been identified. More challenging patients, such as those with discordant data, apparent multifocal or bilateral disease, MRI-negative epilepsy, or a more extensive pathophysiologic substrate, require further evaluation.

Intraoperative Mapping and Electrocorticography

When used, intraoperative ECoG may be performed with either awake or general anesthesia; in either instance, attention to anesthetic considerations is critically important. Wide exposure of the suspected cortical region is essential. After visual inspection of the cortical surface, electrodes of a variety of types may be used. A combination of grids and strips can be used to obtain the desired number of contacts, regularity of spacing, and access to less exposed surfaces such as the inferior temporal or orbitofrontal cortex. Large 4 × 8 or 8 × 8 subdural grids with 1-cm spacing of contacts may be placed easily over the convexity (Fig. 64-1); smaller subdural grids and strips (most typically 1 × 8) may supplement the larger grids. In lesional cases, image guidance may be helpful in directing manual placement of these electrode arrays. Intraoperatively placed depth electrodes may be used, particularly electrodes placed into the medial temporal lobe structures, but this has become less common. Once placed, ample recording is performed, and in collaboration with electrocorticographers in the operating room, the epileptogenic zone that would ideally be resected is defined. After the initial recording, mapping (see the next paragraph), and subsequent resection, further ECoG is often performed, although the significance of postresection spikes and the appropriate surgical response are debated. Advocates of this technique cite reports of better outcomes associated with absence of residual epileptiform activity,[30-32] although resection in pursuit of residual spike activity is controversial and not universally advised.[9]

Intraoperative mapping, most commonly for language, motor, or sensory function (or any combination of these functions), typically follows the initial ECoG. For the primary sensorimotor cortex, mapping has a long and successful history. Integration of

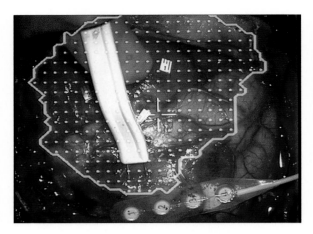

FIGURE 64-2 Functional mapping of language in the left temporal lobe with a handheld bipolar stimulator. Numbered tags identify previously tested sites. The *green* outline, superimposed on the surgical field with the heads-up display of a neuronavigation system, represents the boundary of an underlying lesion.

preoperative MRI or ideally fMRI data through the use of image guidance methods greatly facilitates this activity. Placement of a subdural strip perpendicular to the presumed central sulcus is a method that can be used to obtain somatosensory evoked potentials and assist in localization of the precentral and postcentral gyri. Direct motor mapping may be performed with either a handheld stimulator or a 1 × 4 subdural strip, with appropriate electromyographic recording increasing the sensitivity. Once the motor cortex has been identified, an extremely useful practice involves placing a subdural strip electrode over that area, delivering repeated electrical stimuli, and monitoring motor evoked responses to examine the integrity of the corticospinal tract during the resection.[33-35]

Language mapping requires an awake craniotomy, and with an experienced team, this approach can be used routinely in an efficient and safe manner. Numerous descriptions of awake craniotomy techniques have been published.[13,16] A handheld bipolar stimulator consisting of 1-mm electrodes with a separation of 5 mm is used to apply a 5-second, 60-Hz, biphasic square-wave constant-current or constant-voltage stimulus at sequential sites across the exposed cortex of interest, beginning with low-stimulation parameters and gradually increasing the stimulation intensity until either language is disrupted or the maximal subthreshold for afterdischarges is reached (Fig. 64-2). Adjacent electrodes monitor the cortex for afterdischarges, and cold irrigation or intravenous propofol is available as needed to manage stimulation-induced seizures. Broca's area is most easily identified, with arrest of speech during counting being readily elicited; speech interference by a direct motor response must be excluded. Beyond Broca's area, naming is assessed by using pictures of objects presented on an appropriately positioned computer screen during application of the stimulus. The cortex is investigated in this manner at approximately 1-cm intervals, with each site typically tested three times. Numbered labels are used to identify sites that have been tested, and intraoperative photographs can be used to document the results of the functional mapping procedure. Subsequent resections are generally kept a minimum of 1 cm from positive language sites, although this conventional dictum does not take into account sulcal patterns that may warrant its modification.

Extraoperative Intracranial Investigation

Localization of the area of seizure onset, as well as cortical function, can also be achieved extraoperatively with implanted electrode arrays. Although this strategy necessitates an additional operative procedure, there are also advantages related to intraoperative recording. ECoG data recorded outside the operating room are obtained in a setting that more closely resembles the patient's normal environment, and these recordings can be obtained for periods of days or even weeks. Actual seizure onset may be recorded rather than relying on interictal spike activity as its surrogate. Repeated seizures can be captured, and when a consistent pattern is observed across all events, it is likely that these data accurately reflect the patient's usual pattern of epilepsy. With respect to mapping normal function, the extraoperative setting enables more extensive and repeated testing without the constraints of anesthetic requirements or operative time. Extraoperative methods are most valuable in a patient in whom the actual region of seizure onset has not been confidently defined. Bilateral, multilobar subdural strip and depth electrode placement, for example, may identify seizure onset in patients who would otherwise be deemed unsuitable for surgical resection. Particularly in patients with MRI-negative epilepsy, placing multiple electrode types and large grid arrays over the general regions of interest may be the only effective strategy for identifying a resectable seizure focus. The utility and low morbidity associated with subdural grid electrodes have been well documented.[36]

Intracranial Electrode Implantation Procedure

The actual array that may provide the most information in any given case is individualized. Relatively restricted, superficial cortical lesions may require subdural grid coverage only. If there is a question of involvement of the hippocampus or other deep structures or if some coverage of the opposite hemisphere is also desired, the addition of depth electrodes can be helpful. The craniotomy exposure required for grid placement readily accommodates multiple subdural grids, as well as placement of subdural strip electrodes. Determination of an individual electrode implantation plan is optimally a multidisciplinary process.

Implantation is generally performed with the patient under general anesthesia, and in most instances, use of an image guidance system is helpful in ensuring accurate electrode placement. After induction of general anesthesia, the patient is positioned with the head secured in three-point pin fixation, the head is coregistered with the neuronavigation system by using scalp fiducials and preoperative MRI, and the scalp is shaved, prepared, marked, and draped in conventional manner. Incisions are planned in anticipation of having sufficient exposure for subsequent resection. Attention to preparing a wide field, with planning of electrode exit sites, is essential. During this preparation the patient is administered prophylactic antibiotics, and if the array will entail a more difficult exposure requiring retraction, such as for an interhemispheric array, mannitol is also administered. If the array involves depth electrodes in a region apart from the subdural grid array, they are usually placed (whether by frame-based or frameless stereotactic methodology) before the craniotomy. If depth electrodes will be placed in the same region as the subdural grid, they are most easily placed via a frameless methodology, and in that instance accuracy is best ensured by implantation of the depth electrodes through the craniotomy exposure but before grid placement.

The craniotomy is performed with standard neurosurgical technique. There are two schools of thought regarding management of the bone flap. Many centers in the past have replaced the bone flap at the close of the implantation, in the same manner as for any craniotomy. Alternatively, in an attempt to reduce the risk for subsequent infection by bacterial colonization along the electrode leads and at the same time to simplify the procedure, the bone flap may be left out during the interval while the patient is monitored, with replacement at the time of the subsequent procedure for electrode removal and resection. We keep the bone flap sterile in a freezer and have not experienced significant morbidity or other difficulties related to using this approach. Particular attention to hemostasis during the opening as well as throughout the procedure reduces the risk for development of a symptomatic epidural or subdural hematoma; the postoperative appearance of some blood in the region of the electrodes has been specifically reported but is without clinical significance.[37]

If placement of depth electrodes in the craniotomy site is planned, they are inserted immediately after opening the dura. We have placed them through cut openings in an already placed subdural grid, as well as before grid placement, with a right-angle bend at the pial surface held in place by the overlying grid, and found the latter preferable. Subdural grid placement is planned preoperatively so that it covers the suspected areas of seizure involvement, in addition to any relevant areas of potential functional eloquence. More difficult electrode placements are performed first to minimize displacement of others, and more easily displaced electrodes, including subdural strip electrodes, are placed last. Besides these electrodes, a four-contact subdural electrode is placed away from the cortex of interest, with the contacts facing the dura, to serve as a reference electrode during recording.

All electrode leads are brought through separate exit sites with the use of temporarily placed, large-bore catheter sheaths; typical tunneling distances are several centimeters. Electrodes are secured to the scalp at their exit sites with a single suture, which also serves to tighten the track and prevent leakage of cerebrospinal fluid. The dura is reapproximated around the electrode leads, but no attempt is made to render the closure watertight at the level of the dural openings. With hemostasis ensured, the galea is then reapproximated and the scalp closed with running nylon or Prolene suture. Bacitracin ointment, Xeroform, and sterile dressings are applied. Most importantly, the electrodes are individually and securely labeled in the recognition that a mislabeled electrode is far worse than none.

Postoperatively, a fine-resolution CT scan of the head is obtained before the patient goes to the epilepsy monitoring unit, and this study is then fused with the patient's preoperative MRI for optimal understanding of the final electrode positions (Fig. 64-3). The patient is now monitored until (ideally) at least three typical seizures have been recorded, during which time prophylactic antibiotics are administered, although this is a recognized controversial precaution. Use of anticonvulsants is weaned if necessary. Recording is usually performed for 2 days up to 4 weeks, with an average time of 7 days. Functional mapping, unless not required, is performed during this interval. The data are reviewed by the multidisciplinary team, and surgical recommendations are developed and discussed with the patient and family.

Resective Procedure

With a treatment plan in place, the extraoperatively investigated patient is returned to the operating room and generally reregistered with an image guidance system using either the remaining scalp fiducials or natural landmarks. In addition, the intracranial electrodes in place may be used to guide the resection. With the patient and head positioned, the sutures securing the exiting electrode leads are cut, and then the previous incision line and adjacent scalp are prepared and draped so that the exit sites are left outside the sterile field. The incision is now reopened, the electrode leads divided at the level of the dura, and the now divided distal electrode leads withdrawn from the exposed surgical field from under the drapes. The dura is reopened, and the exposed cortex and subdural electrodes are inspected for any evidence of displacement. Electrodes away from the area to be resected are removed, and if image guidance is not reliably available, the locations of the contacts of the subdural grid overlying

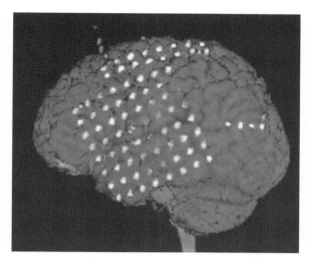

FIGURE 64-3 This composite graphic using coregistered preoperative magnetic resonance imaging (for surface anatomy) and postoperative computed tomography (for electrodes) shows the electrode contacts of two contiguous 4 × 8 subdural grid electrodes overlying the left frontal and temporal lobes. This array was used both for electrocorticographic localization of seizure onset and for functional mapping.

the margins of the planned resection are marked on the cortical surface with bipolar cautery.

The actual resection is performed under the operating microscope with standard microsurgical technique. If there is any question of functional cortex being at risk, functional mapping or monitoring, or both, may be performed at the time of resection. Should recordings implicate cortex whose functionality precludes resection, that cortex is generally preserved; alternatively, multiple subpial transections in this portion of the cortex may be combined with resection elsewhere. With large resections, care must be taken to preserve large arteries and veins within the resection margins that may be associated with brain tissue outside the planned resection. On completion of the resection, the dura is closed over Gelfilm, and the bone flap is secured in place with a standard plating system. The remainder of the closure follows standard technique. The patient is mobilized immediately after the procedure, and attention is directed at ensuring appropriate anticonvulsant levels. Discharge follows in 1 to 3 days.

SEIZURE OUTCOMES

No prospective, randomized clinical studies have compared the results of tailored resection with other surgeries, and the dominating influence of patient selection as a confounding variable limits comparison of historical outcomes. Nevertheless, a number of series have reported seizure outcome data that may further our understanding of the capabilities of resective surgery.

For anterior temporal lobe resection, with or without tailoring, Engel's survey had found seizure-free outcomes in 67.9% of patients.[4] A recent series of 434 consecutive temporal resections selectively using ECoG for tailoring in patients without medial temporal sclerosis has been reported by Elsharkawy and colleagues, who achieved Engel class I seizure outcomes at 2 years in 72.3% of patients.[38]

The report of Sugano and colleagues already alluded to involved 35 patients with temporal lesions who underwent lesionectomy alone or lesionectomy plus resection of additional tissue shown to generate spike activity on postresection ECoG; seizure-free outcomes were achieved in 90.9% of the latter group (versus 76.9% with lesionectomy alone).[10]

Kanner and colleagues analyzed their results of tailored anterior temporal resection and assessed outcome with respect to the extent of resection based on postoperative MRI. Through the use of intraoperative recording, they were frequently able to spare the amygdala or hippocampus, or both, and yet achieve seizure-free outcomes in 21 of 24 patients, with rare seizures in the remaining 3.[3,32]

It should also be noted, however, that untailored temporal resections continue to produce good results. Cukiert and coauthors reported a series of untailored corticoamygdalohippocampectomy procedures in 100 patients with mesial temporal sclerosis, with 89 patients becoming seizure free or experiencing simple partial seizures only; the other 11 patients all experienced greater than a 90% reduction in seizure frequency.[39] Also to be noted is the report of Schwartz and associates, who in a series of 29 patients undergoing untailored temporal resection with ECoG performed before and after resection, found no correlation between seizure outcomes and the presence or absence of residual epileptiform activity on the postresection recording.[9]

For lesional epilepsy surgery, Engel's survey reported that 66.6% of patients became seizure free.[4] There are two clinical series of lesionectomy alone without resection of surrounding cortex. In the extended (4-year) follow-up series of Cascino and coworkers, 13 of 23 (56.5%) lesional patients achieved seizure-free outcomes, and 17 patients (73.9%) experienced greater than a 90% reduction in seizure frequency.[40] In Giulioni and colleagues' series of 15 children, 13 (86.6%) became seizure free.[41] Comparing the results of lesionectomy alone with resection tailored by ECoG, Jooma and coauthors reported a study of 16 lesional epilepsy patients treated by lesionectomy and 14 patients whose resection was guided by intraoperative ECoG. Seizure-free outcomes were achieved in just 3 patients (18.8%) in the lesionectomy-alone group but in 62.5% of the tailored resection patients.[42] In a similar comparison, Sugano and associates' previously cited study showed improvement in seizure-free outcomes from 76.9% for lesionectomy alone to 90.9% for tailored resection.[10]

Extratemporal resections in Engel's series led to seizure-free outcomes in 45.1% of patients.[4] In more recent surgical series, Engel class I outcomes have been reported in 49.5% to 60% of patients operated on for frontal lobe epilepsy[43-45] and in 39.5% to 90% of patients with parietal or occipital lobe epilepsy.[18,46-48] With respect to larger, multilobar resections, Engel's survey found seizure-free outcomes in 45.2% of patients.[4] More recent series have reported seizure-free outcomes in 30% to 47% of patients.[24,25,49]

For the present purposes it is useful to distinguish whether patients included in the series had lesional or nonlesional epilepsy. In nearly every series in which it has been examined, the presence of a discrete MRI-detectable lesion has been associated with a better outcome.[43,45,50] In patients with no structural abnormality found on neuroimaging, reliance on intracranial recording and mapping, with subsequent formulation of a tailored resection plan, is essential. In addition to determining an epileptogenic region for resection, individualized intracranial monitoring can serve to enable sparing of suspected but then exonerated uninvolved structures. With such a strategy, seizure-free outcome rates have been reported to be in the range of 29% to 41%, with a considerable additional percentage of patients becoming almost seizure free.[45,50] Although generally not as favorable as results seen with lesional epilepsy, these surgical outcomes are best compared with the results of nonoperative treatment, the only actual alternative.

CONCLUSION

Tailored surgical resections are performed with the objectives of identifying the seizure focus and eloquent brain regions of individual patients and thus optimizing each patient's chance of achieving a seizure-free outcome without new neurological deficits. The surgical literature does not unambiguously confirm the superiority of this approach over standard resection techniques, but existing data do provide strong support for the tailored resection strategy. It may improve outcomes in patients with known structural pathology, and in those with normal MRI findings, it may be the only viable surgical option.

SUGGESTED READINGS

Binder DK, Podlogar M, Clusmann H, et al. Surgical treatment of parietal lobe epilepsy. *J Neurosurg*. 2009;110;1170.

Cascino GD, Hulihan JF, Sharbrough FW, et al. Parietal lobe lesional epilepsy: electroclinical correlation and operative outcome. *Epilepsia*. 1993;34:522.

Cascino GD, Kelly PJ, Sharbrough FW, et al. Long-term follow-up of stereotactic lesionectomy in partial epilepsy: predictive factors and electroencephalographic results. *Epilepsia*. 1992;33:639.

Elsharkawy AE, Alabbasi AH, Pannek H, et al. Long-term outcome after temporal lobe epilepsy surgery in 434 consecutive adult patients. *J Neurosurg*. 2009;110:1135.

Hata D, Isu T, Nakanishi M, et al. Intraoperative electrocorticography and successful focus resection in a case of Sturge-Weber syndrome. *Seizure*. 1998;7:505.

Hermann BP, Wyler AR, Somes G. Language function following anterior temporal lobectomy. *J Neurosurg*. 1991;74:560.

Jeha LE, Najm I, Bingaman W, et al. Surgical outcome and prognostic factors of frontal lobe epilepsy surgery. *Brain*. 2007;130:574.

Jooma R, Yeh HS, Privitera MD, et al. Lesionectomy versus electrophysiologically guided resection for temporal lobe tumors manifesting with complex partial seizures. *J Neurosurg*. 1995;83:231.

Kanner AM, Kaydanova Y, deToledo-Morrell L, et al. Tailored anterior temporal lobectomy. Relation between extent of resection of mesial structures and postsurgical seizure outcome. *Arch Neurol*. 1995;52:173.

Kasowski HJ, Stoffman MR, Spencer SS, et al. Surgical management of parietal lobe epilepsy. *Adv Neurol*. 2003;93:347.

Leiphart JW, Peacock WJ, Mathern GW. Lobar and multilobar resections for medically intractable pediatric epilepsy. *Pediatr Neurosurg*. 2001;34:311.

Mosewich RK, So EL, O'Brien TJ, et al. Factors predictive of the outcome of frontal lobe epilepsy surgery. *Epilepsia*. 2000;41:843.

Ojemann G, Ojemann J, Lettich E, et al. Cortical language localization in left, dominant hemisphere. An electrical stimulation mapping investigation in 117 patients. *J Neurosurg*. 1989;71:316.

Olivier A, Boling W Jr. Surgery of parietal and occipital lobe epilepsy. *Adv Neurol*. 2000;84:533.

Salanova V, Andermann F, Rasmussen T, et al. Parietal lobe epilepsy. Clinical manifestations and outcome in 82 patients treated surgically between 1929 and 1988. *Brain*. 1995;118:607.

Schwartz TH, Bazil CW, Walczak TS, et al. The predictive value of intraoperative electrocorticography in resections for limbic epilepsy associated with mesial temporal sclerosis. *Neurosurgery*. 1997;40:302.

Sugano H, Shimizu H, Sunaga S. Efficacy of intraoperative electrocorticography for assessing seizure outcomes in intractable epilepsy patients with temporal-lobe-mass lesions. *Seizure*. 2007;16:120.

Van Gompel JJ, Worrell GA, Bell ML, et al. Intracranial electroencephalography with subdural grid electrodes: techniques, complications, and outcomes. *Neurosurgery*. 2008;63:498.

Wennberg R, Quesney F, Olivier A, et al. Electrocorticography and outcome in frontal lobe epilepsy. *Electroencephalogr Clin Neurophysiol*. 1998;106:357.

Wieser HG, Yasargil MG. Selective amygdalohippocampectomy as a surgical treatment of mesiobasal limbic epilepsy. *Surg Neurol*. 1982;17:445.

Full references can be found on Expert Consult at @ www.expertconsult.com

CHAPTER 65

Topectomy and Multiple Subpial Transection

Patrick J. Connolly ▪ Atsushi Umemura ▪ Gordon H. Baltuch ▪ Richard W. Byrne

TOPECTOMY

The prevalence of epilepsy is approximately 1%. In the majority of cases, it can be effectively treated medically with antiepileptic drugs, but 30% to 40% of all new epilepsy patients will ultimately become refractory to treatment.[1] Some investigators report that ongoing medication trials can be a satisfactory approach to managing refractory epilepsy.[2] However, it is important to consider surgery for such patients.[3]

In the Montreal Neurological Institute series covering the period from 1929 to 1980, the anatomic distribution of surgical resection in 2177 patients was as follows: temporal, 56%; frontal, 18%; central, 7%; parietal, 6%; occipital, 1%; and multilobar, 11%.[4]

"Topectomy" generally indicates resection of focal cerebral cortex from the frontal, parietal, or occipital lobe. Outside the temporal lobe, localization of the seizure origin is much more difficult, seizure outcome is less favorable, and surgery in some brain sites is associated with higher risk for major morbidity than with temporal lobe resection.[5] Although temporal lobe resection is much more common in modern epilepsy practice, topectomy is the foundation of modern epilepsy surgery.[6] In 1886, Sir Victor Horsley performed what would now be considered lesionectomies with excellent results. Before the invention of electroencephalography (EEG) in 1928, epilepsy surgery was exploratory and based on clinical localization pioneered by Jackson and identification of visibly abnormal tissue. EEG removed this requirement and decreased negative explorations considerably through the 1950s and 1960s.[7] Magnetic resonance imaging (MRI) now provides a priori knowledge of structural cortical abnormalities. Table 65-1 shows types of procedures for epilepsy.

A fundamental concept underlying focal cortical resection is that the epileptic focus contains electrically abnormal neurons that are the source of seizures. Hence, if this epileptogenic focus can be accurately identified and resected, the seizure will cease. Epileptogenicity is assumed to derive from physiologic events that occur within the cell body and dendrites of neurons rather than axons.[8] Therefore, resection of only epileptogenic gray matter (cerebral cortex) rather than white matter should in theory be sufficient to eliminate seizures. Recent work suggests that epilepsy may arise as a result of abnormalities of a distributed cellular network.[9] Therefore, intrinsic cellular abnormalities may not be required to create an epileptic condition. The most characteristic and ubiquitous pathologic changes are the presence of gliosis, loss of neurons, and dendritic abnormalities.[10,11] This chapter reviews the principles and methods of surgical localization and cortical resection in patients who may be candidates for topectomy or multiple subpial transection (MST).

Patient Selection

In general, surgical treatment of epilepsy should be considered when (1) the seizures have not been controlled by adequate attempts at treatment with maximally tolerable doses of correct anticonvulsant medications; (2) the seizures interfere with psychological and intellectual development, employment, or social performance; (3) all potentially epileptogenic areas have matured, the seizure tendency (pattern and frequency) is stable, and there is no tendency toward spontaneous regression; and (4) the patient must be strongly motivated to cope with an exhaustive diagnostic regimen and a lengthy operative procedure, possibly under local anesthesia.[12-14] Chronic psychosis is a contraindication to surgical treatment, but epilepsy-related acute psychosis is not. Mental retardation is not a contraindication.[15,16]

The length of time that patients have seizures before being referred for surgery has become shorter as referring physicians recognize that superior surgical results may be obtained when the period of uncontrolled seizures is shortened, particularly in children.[17] Currently, adequate, but unsuccessful antiepileptic drug therapy for 1 to 5 years may be a sufficiently long trial period to warrant referral for consideration of epilepsy surgery.[16] In exceptional cases, urgent cortical resection may be considered for the relief of status epilepticus.[18,19]

Table 65-2 is a representative list of neurological diagnoses that may be considered for surgery involving focal cortical resection.[20] Topectomy can be considered when the seizure arises from a focal and functionally silent area of the brain, which usually means that the focus is not in the speech or motor cortex. Additionally, neuropsychological testing is performed to identify any functional deficits that may be related to the epileptic cortical region.[21] Multiple widespread or bilateral foci are generally contraindications to resective surgery. A series of diagnostic studies, including EEG, are necessary to confirm the site of seizure onset. In eloquent brain regions, MST may be considered.

Presurgical Evaluation

The optimal surgery for epilepsy is resection of just enough neuronal tissue to eliminate the patient's seizures without causing unacceptable neurological deficits. Presurgical evaluation enables the surgeon to determine the volume of cortex involved in seizure initiation and propagation and whether it can be safely resected. As stated by Rasmussen, epileptogenic lesions outside the temporal lobe are considerably more varied in extent and geographic configuration than the more common temporal lobe epileptogenic lesions.[22] A variety of diagnostic tests are used for this purpose, but there is no consensus on how much information is actually needed before a particular surgical intervention can be recommended.[23]

The initial preoperative evaluation process includes careful examination of clinical seizure characteristics, ictal and interictal scalp EEG, neuroimaging, and neuropsychological testing. The results of this testing should provide considerable lateralizing and localizing information. Video-EEG monitoring is the "gold standard" of the evaluation. When noninvasive tests do not show the source of seizures clearly, invasive testing is considered. Localization of the seizure focus is difficult in patients with extratemporal epilepsy, and invasive EEG is almost always required.[5]

TABLE 65-1 General Categories of Epilepsy Surgery

Resection
  Hemispherectomy: resection of the cerebral hemisphere
  Lobectomy: resection of one cerebral lobe
  Topectomy: resection of a focal area of cerebral cortex
Disconnection
  Corpus callosotomy: disconnection of two hemispheres
  Multiple subpial transection: disconnection of a focal area of
    cerebral cortex
  Hemispherectomy: disconnection of a cerebral hemisphere
Stimulation
  Vagal nerve stimulation
  Anterior thalamic stimulation
  Responsive neurostimulation

Noninvasive Evaluation

Symptomatic Localization

The initial symptoms and signs often have localizing value. A detailed history may elucidate auras, partial seizures, the presence and timing of secondary generalization, preservation or loss of consciousness, postictal dysphasia, or Todd's palsy. Extratemporal epilepsy is more frequently manifested as convulsive phenomena than is temporal lobe epilepsy.

In frontal lobe epilepsy, clinical localization of the seizure origin is difficult because the ictal behavioral manifestations in patients with frontal lobe epilepsy are largely due to spread of seizures to neighboring or distant functionally connected brain regions.[24] Rasmussen characterized six distinct convulsion patterns, some of which he believed indicated a frontal lobe focus:[25,26]

1. Loss of consciousness and then generalized tonic-clonic convulsion
2. Loss of consciousness, head and eyes turning opposite, and generalized convulsion—anterior third of the frontal lobe
3. Head and eyes turning opposite, preserved consciousness, contralateral attacks, loss of consciousness, and generalized convulsions—lateral intermediate frontal region
4. Posturing movements of the body with tonic elevation of the contralateral arm, downward extension of the ipsilateral arm, and turning of the head away from the side of the lesion—mesial aspect of the intermediate frontal region
5. Vague sensation in the head or body often followed by a brief arrest of activity, confused thinking, staring, followed by a generalized convulsive seizure
6. Automatisms similar to those seen with temporal lobe epilepsy.

TABLE 65-2 Representative Conditions Treatable
  by Topectomy

Tuberous sclerosis
Sturge-Weber syndrome
Neurofibromatosis type 1
Dysembryoplastic neuroepithelial tumors
Migrational disorders
Focal cortical dysplasia
Closed/open-lipped schizencephaly
Polymicrogyria
Lissencephaly
Hamartoma
Subcortical/periventricular heterotopia

In parietal lobe seizure, most patients have attacks consisting of unilateral motor or sensory phenomena with additional features such as dizziness, cephalic sensation, contraversion, perceptual illusions, informed visual hallucinations, mental confusion, epigastric sensation, dysphasia, or automatisms.[26,27]

In central epilepsies, the attacks are somatomotor or somatosensory. The attacks sometimes remain localized, but in most patients a certain portion of the attacks progress to generalized convulsive seizures. Epilepsia partialis continua is particularly common.[26,27]

In occipital lobe seizure, visual symptoms such as transient blindness or visual hallucinations are usually characterized by flashes of lights, colored balls, and other geometric patterns. These symptoms have a strong relationship with seizure activity.[26]

However, some initial seizure symptoms may not reflect the region of seizure origin because many cortical regions are clinically silent. Seizures originating in these regions produce signs and symptoms only after spreading outside the epileptogenic region.[27]

Extracranial Electroencephalography

Scalp EEG often provides important information about the location and size of the epileptogenic area. An interictal epileptiform abnormality consisting of spikes, spike and slow wave complexes, sharp waves, and sharp and slow wave complexes repeated on several occasions may be particularly informative.[28] Activation procedures such as withdrawal of medication, hyperventilation, or drug-induced sleep may enhance abnormalities or even provoke a seizure.[13]

In addition, long-term video-EEG monitoring is generally performed in an epilepsy monitoring unit to correlate clinical seizure activity with the accompanying electrical abnormalities with the intent of identifying the seizure origin electrographically.[5] The specific ictal symptomatology can help greatly in some cases in which localization of the focus is problematic. The EEG pattern of seizure onset is most frequently rhythmic, fast, spike-like discharges, often building in amplitude.[9]

Neuroimaging

MRI is the imaging modality of choice in patients with intractable partial epilepsy. Computed tomography (CT) is also helpful because it demonstrates intracranial calcifications more clearly than MRI does. MRI provides visualization of focal dysplastic cortical lesions in many patients previously assigned a diagnosis of cryptogenic neocortical epilepsy.[5,29] An MRI-identified lesion may prove to be the cause of the seizure disorder. These abnormalities are then correlated with the results of electrophysiologic studies to accurately identify the source of the patient's seizures.[30] MRI is also useful in the diagnosis of structural and developmental epileptogenic pathologies. The most common findings in this category are ischemic lesions or developmental abnormalities, specifically, neuronal migration disorders.[31] Structural lesions include ischemic infarctions (prenatal, perinatal, or postnatal), Sturge-Weber syndrome, Rasmussen's encephalitis, and others. Progressive unilateral cortical atrophy is demonstrated in patients with Rasmussen's encephalitis. Unilateral megalencephaly is one characteristic example of a developmental pathology associated with seizures. The most common neuronal migration disorders are lissencephaly and diffuse pachygyria. The complete absence of gyri and sulci in lissencephaly and the development of a few thick, wide gyri separated by shallow sulci in diffuse pachygyria are clearly identifiable on MRI.[31]

Ictal perfusion single-photon emission computed tomography (SPECT) may demonstrate increased blood flow at the site of seizure onset.[15,32-34] The tracer isotope (usually technetium

99m–labeled hexamethyl-propyleneamine-oxime [HMPAO]) is administered immediately after seizure onset, and the scan should be performed within several hours. There are some reports of localized hyperperfusion in ictal studies of patients with frontal, parietal, or occipital epilepsy.[15,16] Interictal SPECT has been of only limited value; it occasionally shows local reduced blood flow.[33] Timing demands and other technical issues associated with SPECT scanning present barriers to its use. There is some evidence that functional anatomic correlation is more reliable with a technique called *SISCOM,* an acronym for *subtraction ictal single-photon tomography coregistered to MRI.*[35]

Interictal positron emission tomography (PET) with a tracer for glucose metabolism (^{18}F-fluorodeoxyglucose) has regularly demonstrated hypometabolism in the epileptic focus of temporal lobe epilepsy.[15,36] However, PET is less reliable in identifying extratemporal, nonlesional foci.[29]

Neuropsychological Testing

Neuropsychological examinations contain a personality inventory and tests of memory, language function, and intelligence. These tests are useful in localization and lateralization of speech, memory, spatial, cognitive, and cerebral dominance functions. They also evaluate mental states such as mental retardation.[29,37] These traditional roles of neuropsychological evaluation are now augmented by the discipline's ability to predict cognitive and behavioral outcomes after surgery.[22] Additionally, neuropsychology can have therapeutic benefit as well,[38] and it can be combined with advanced imaging techniques to make highly specific predictions about cognitive function after epilepsy resection.[39]

Invasive Evaluation

The Wada Test

The Wada test (intracarotid amobarbital [Amytal] test) is performed to identify the dominant hemisphere for language functions and to determine the degree to which memory functions are subserved by each hemisphere.[40] In the series from the Montreal Neurological Institute, in right-handers, 96% had speech lateralized to the left cerebral hemisphere and 4% to the right hemisphere. In left-handed or ambidextrous individuals 70% had speech on the left, 15% had it on the right, and 15% had some representation of speech in each hemisphere. Therefore, the Wada test is necessary in all left-handed and ambidextrous patients and in right-handed patients with some ambiguous evidence of lateralization from psychological tests, x-ray films, EEG studies, or the seizure pattern.[13] Unusual language lateralization can be seen in patients who sustain left hemisphere injury in early life or have early onset of intractable epilepsy.[15] Recently, work has been done to supplant the invasive Wada test with functional MRI (fMRI).[41,42] Although fMRI has some cost and risk advantage,[43] the diagnostic accuracy of the technique is insufficient to completely supplant the WADA test at this time.

Invasive Electroencephalography

When an epileptogenic focus is not clearly lateralized, invasive EEG monitoring is necessary for cortical resection. In extratemporal epilepsy, subdural strip electrodes are used primarily to lateralize an epileptogenic focus (Fig. 65-1), and large subdural grids are used to define the limits of a focus that has already been lateralized but not sufficiently localized (Fig. 65-2). It is important to cover as much of the suspected area as possible for accurate lateralization and localization.[29,44] In our center, we routinely identify electrode locations in image space by coregistering postoperative MRI and CT images.[45] If the electrodes are properly

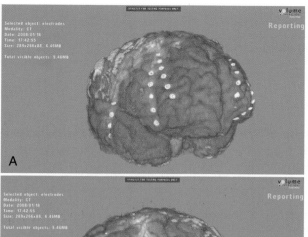

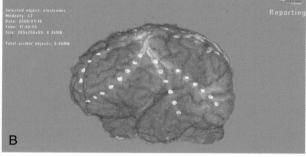

FIGURE 65-1 **A,** Fused postoperative MRI and CT demonstrate three subdural strip electrodes over the surface of the right frontal and temporal lobes. **B,** The same data set shows the left frontal and temporal electrodes. The data processing was performed with the Dextroscope virtual reality system (Volume Interactions, Ltd., Singapore).

indexed in the image, an electroradiographic record of the eloquent and epileptogenic regions can be obtained and used as a navigational tool during resection.

Subdural strip electrodes are placed through a bur hole and passed blindly into the subdural space. Multiple electrodes may be inserted through one bur hole to cover wide regions of the brain. In patients with bifrontal discharges, strip electrodes are placed over the medial and lateral surfaces of the posterior frontal lobe from bur holes at the coronal suture, just off the midline (see Fig. 65-1).[15]

Subdural grid electrodes are placed with a craniotomy (see Fig. 65-2). They are used not only for determining the site of seizure onset over the convexity of one hemisphere but also for extraoperative functional mapping (motor, sensory, speech, and so on) by stimulation of each electrode. The maximal extent of

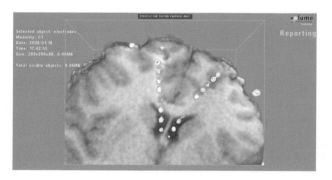

FIGURE 65-2 Cingular depth electrodes from the same patient as in Figure 65-1. The patient had intractable frontal lobe epilepsy. The goal was to determine from which side the seizures arose.

an epileptogenic focus and areas of cortical function are determined with these evaluation methods.[4] With invasive EEG methods, the electrode leads are brought out through the scalp and the patient is monitored for many days. The most common complications are infection and leakage of cerebrospinal fluid, especially with a large subdural grid.[42]

Surgical Topectomy Procedure

General Principles from Anatomic Considerations

The extent of cortical resection is based on the results of presurgical evaluation and findings on intraoperative recording and stimulation. Resection of essential cortex such as the language and precentral arm or leg motor cortex should be absolutely avoided in adults because of the resultant hemiparesis or aphasia. Therefore, it is particularly important to identify language and motor cortical sites before proceeding with resection surgery.

Anatomically, the frontal lobe Broca speech area is identified in the opercular, inferior frontal gyrus (usually the posterior 2.5 cm of this gyrus). It is difficult to identify Wernicke's area by anatomic criteria. The parietal speech area is identified 1 to 4 cm above the sylvian fissure and 2 to 4 cm behind the postcentral sulcus. The temporal speech areas usually extend posteriorly behind the level of the postcentral sulcus and 2 to 3 cm from the adjacent convolution above, behind Heschl's gyri. Lack of defining anatomic features for Wernicke's area renders language mapping essential for cortical dominant hemisphere resections.[13,14,46]

Large frontal resections in the nondominant hemisphere can be carried out in front of the precentral gyrus. Identification of the precentral and postcentral gyri is best accomplished by stimulation under anesthesia without neuromuscular blockade.[4,27] It can also be done more coarsely by identifying the somatosensory evoked potential (SSEP) phase reversal over the central sulcus.[47] Resection of precentral arm or leg motor cortex is permitted only if significant contralateral paresis is already present.[15,47] The lower precentral face area can be resected. The resulting contralateral facial paresis improves but may not return to normal.[27]

Resection of the postcentral sensory arm or leg area causes a profound proprioceptive deficit and is rarely indicated, although improvement over a period of several months is possible.[27,47] Conversely, the lower 2.5 to 3 cm of the postcentral face area can be resected without significant deficit as long as the resection does not extend into the underlying white matter.[27] In the nondominant hemisphere, the entire parietal cortex posterior to the postcentral gyrus can be removed without inducing a sensorimotor deficit.[27,47,48] Resection in the parietal operculum may produce contralateral lower quadrantic hemianopia if resections are carried beyond the depths of the sulci into the white matter.[47] In the dominant hemisphere, parietal lobe resections should be limited to the superior parietal lobule. Language functions are subserved by cortex of the inferior parietal lobule, and a disabling Gerstmann syndrome can also result from extensive parietal lobe resection.[27]

Large resections of occipital cortex produce a contralateral homonymous hemianopia. Therefore, if vision is intact preoperatively, the calcarine cortex and optic radiations are spared as much as possible. Because cortex essential for reading is often more widespread than that for naming, excision within 2 cm of Wernicke's area may cause a persisting dyslexia.[47]

The vascular territory of each crucial artery or vein should be studied to assess the consequences of occlusion of the vessel during surgery. This approach is essential to minimize morbidity, especially with surgery on the motor and speech areas. Any ascending vein to the superior sagittal sinus draining from the central or postcentral sulci should be left intact to avoid significant morbidity.[4,27]

Preoperative Care and Anesthesia

It is our practice to reduce the doses of antiepileptic medications the week before surgery so that the epileptogenic cortex is as active as possible during surgery.[13] Some epilepsy centers do not use this strategy, particularly in situations in which they will be carrying out awake craniotomies. When resecting noneloquent cortical areas, general anesthesia can be used.[27] However, when intraoperative electrocorticography (ECoG) is required, the use of drugs that depress cortical electrical activity, such as benzodiazepines and barbiturates, should be avoided. In addition, when functional mapping of speech and sensory areas is performed, the patient should be conscious and cooperative during the procedure. In this situation, local and total intravenous anesthesia with analgesic drugs (fentanyl and droperidol or propofol) should be used.[14,49] Local anesthesia alone has the disadvantages of taking more time to create a complete block and limiting the range of head positions that can be used. Furthermore, it cannot be used with uncooperative patients and young children. Constant supervision by a specially trained anesthesia team is essential.[4,27]

Intraoperative Electrocorticography

Sufficient brain exposure via craniotomy is essential during ECoG. ECoG is performed to further delineate the extent of the epileptogenic zone. The intention is to identify regions with primary epileptic neurons by identifying brain sites that have interictal ECoG spikes. In our experience, there is a clear relationship among the site of interictal discharges, the site of ictal onset, and the tissue that must be removed to control seizures. This ECoG hallmark is used to determine what part of the brain should be resected.[4,15,50]

ECoG also provides prognostic information by indicating areas with residual discharges after cortical resection. Patients with no interictal discharges on postresection recordings are more likely to be free of seizures than those with persisting discharges.[4,51,51] For "standard" temporal lobectomy surgery, the value of ECoG is not as clear.[52]

Cortical Stimulation (Functional Mapping)

The purpose of intraoperative cortical stimulation is to localize eloquent cortex such as the motor cortex, sensory cortex, or language area in the dominant hemisphere. Functional mapping is necessary when cortical resections are carried out near eloquent brain areas. Identification of motor cortex is useful for any resection in the posterior frontal or parietal lobes. Identification of language cortex is necessary for any dominant-hemisphere resection in the perisylvian cortex and posterior superior frontal lobe.

The location of the central sulcus is determined by electrical stimulation of the precentral and postcentral gyri after preliminary identification by monitoring for the SSEP phase reversal.[48] The suspected site of the motor and sensory cortex is stimulated and mapped with a motor response detected by the anesthetist, measurement by electromyographic electrodes, or a report of sensory change by the patient.[15,47,51] In practice, the best way to identify the postcentral gyrus is to induce sensory responses in the tongue area located at the bottom of the postcentral gyrus.[27,53]

The frontal, parietal, and temporal language areas in the dominant hemisphere are stimulated while the patient carries out simple verbal tasks such as naming objects shown on picture cards. A language critical area is identified if the patient is unable to speak (speech arrest) when the site is being stimulated or if the patient can speak but is unable to name objects.[14,15,47,51] Although failure to produce speech arrest or anomia does not always exclude the presence of language critical sites in the stimulated cortex, intraoperative mapping is nevertheless the most reliable

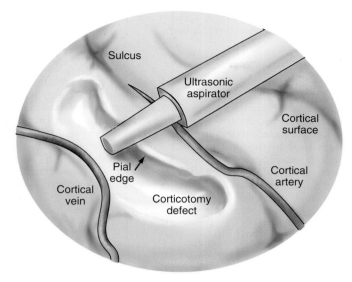

FIGURE 65-3 Simple cartoon illustrating basic microsurgical principles. 1. Open the pia with bipolar cautery and microscissors. 2. For cortical resection, it is not necessary to remove tissue deeper than the bottom of the sulcus. 3. The cortical veins and arteries are preserved when traversing a sulcus. 4. Use the arachnoid flap to retract veins and arteries. 5. Use an ultrasonic aspirator on low power to resect to the pia of the parallel sulcus.

method currently available for indentifying these language critical sites.

Surgical Technique

Unlike temporal lobectomy, there are no anatomically standard operations for extratemporal cortical resection.

A craniotomy is performed to expose the epileptic focus that will be resected. The extent of neocortical resection is based on the gross pathology and the results of ECoG and functional mapping. In general, effort is made to resect all areas with interictal discharges. Essential motor and language areas should be preserved (preferably with a 2- or 1-cm margin), regardless of involvement in the epileptic focus.[15] Special attention is also given to the vascular supply of the area to be resected.[47] The extent of the resection is individually tailored to each case.

A subpial dissection technique is used for cortical resection (Fig. 65-3).[9,14,15,16,47,54] This procedure was used by Horsley (1909) and has remained the technical basis of surgery for epilepsy to this day. The pial surface is coagulated and incised in a relatively avascular area. Gyral resection is then carried out in a subpial fashion. An ultrasonic aspirator at a low suction/vibration setting is extremely useful for focal resections in a subpial plane. Meticulous, slow removal of epileptogenic gray matter is carried to the bottom of the sulcus without damaging vessels within the pia that might supply other nonresected tissue. Hemostasis is achieved principally with topical agents such as Gelfoam or Surgicel and minimal use of electrocautery. With the topectomy procedure, unnecessary resection of the underlying white matter is avoided to preserve the integrity of projection, association, and commissural fibers.

Appropriate antiepileptic medication and dexamethasone are administered after cortical resection.

Surgical Outcome

Extratemporal nonlesional resection is associated with worse seizure control rates and a higher incidence of major postopera-

TABLE 65-3 Outcome of Seizures

	ATL (%)	ETR (%)
Seizure free	2429 (67.9)	363 (45.1)
Improved	860 (24.0)	283 (35.2)
Not improved	290 (8.1)	159 (19.8)
Total	**3579 (100)**	**805 (100)**

ATL, anterior temporal lobectomy; ETR, extratemporal resection.
From Engel J, Ness PCV, Rasmussen TB, et al. Outcome with respect to epileptic seizures. In: Engel J, ed. *Surgical Treatment of the Epilepsies*, 2nd ed. New York: Raven Press; 1993:609-621.

tive morbidity than is lesional or temporal lobe resection surgery. Table 65-3 presents the seizure outcome reported by Engel and colleagues in 1993.[55] Extratemporal surgery results in seizure-free rates of 45% and improvement in 35%. More recent work is highlighted in Table 65-4.

With localized resective surgery, less than 5% of patients have some postoperative neurological deficit as a result of unintended vascular compromise or other accidental damage to essential neural tissue. Most of these deficits are transient and resolve within months, however. Postoperative bleeding and infection are uncommon. Seizures in the acute postoperative period may portend a poor prognosis, and most patients will continue to require pharmacologic treatment.

Conclusion

Extratemporal epilepsy encompasses a broad range of diagnoses and is associated with greater difficulty in identifying a discrete seizure focus. There is no "standard" operation to treat these disorders; the surgical procedure must be customized to each individual patient. This variability and the comparatively poor seizure control results after surgery support the contention that extra–temporal lobe epilepsy is a much more complex and variable disorder than temporal lobe epilepsy. Extratemporal epilepsy surgery requires a more extensive and invasive preoperative diagnostic evaluation, and the probability of an excellent outcome is lower with this type of epilepsy surgery than with temporal lobe epilepsy. Nevertheless, topectomy can decrease and sometimes eliminate disabling epilepsy at a reasonable neuropsychological cost. Topectomy should be considered for carefully selected patients who have the highest probability of benefiting from the procedure and unattractive management alternatives.

TABLE 65-4 Comparison of Recent Work with the Engel Report

STUDY	YEAR	CENTRAL THEME	ENGEL CLASS 1 (%)
Elsharkawy et al.[56]	2008	Extratemporal	54.5
Kral et al.[57]	2007	Focal cortical dysplasia	76
Bauman et al.[58]	2005	Multistage	60
Tellez-Zenteno et al.[59]	2005	Meta-analysis	27F/46PO
Chapman et al.[60]	2005	Normal MRI	37

MULTIPLE SUBPIAL TRANSECTION

From the inception of epilepsy surgery, it has been clear that resective surgery for medically intractable seizure foci can be done in noneloquent areas with acceptably low rates of morbidity and a reasonable chance for seizure control in carefully selected patients. Resection of seizure foci in eloquent cortex, however, results in unacceptable deficits. The surgical procedure MST addresses this difficult problem by capitalizing on the difference between the vertical and horizontal organization of the cortical structures of the brain.[61] The master organizational principle in the cerebral cortex is the functional vertical column, with its vertical orientation of incoming and outgoing fibers and blood supply.[62-64] At the same time, seizures in part spread horizontally through the gray matter. MST involves disconnecting the gray matter columns that lie in eloquent cortex. This technique can inhibit synchronization and spread of the seizure focus with minimal injury to the cortex. In this section we review the history of the development of MST, patient selection, surgical indications, technique, results, pitfalls, and areas for further exploration. New horizons for the application of MST, including hippocampal transection for mesial temporal epilepsy, are also reviewed.

History

In the 1930s, two treatments emerged for patients with chronic epilepsy that brought hope for better seizure control. The anticonvulsant effects of phenytoin were discovered in 1938, and it was effective in controlling the seizures of patients with chronic epilepsy.[65] At the same time, Wilder Penfield at the Montreal Neurological Institute expanded the use of surgical resection of seizure foci, primarily in the temporal lobe, for "psychomotor seizures."[66] News of Penfield's success spread, and in 1951, Percival Bailey and Fred Gibbs at the University of Illinois Neuropsychological Institute reported their results of temporal lobectomy for psychomotor seizures guided by EEG findings.[67] One class of patients who would not benefit from standard surgical therapy consisted of those with a seizure focus in eloquent cortex because excision of this seizure focus would lead to unacceptable deficits.

Several discoveries in neuroscience in the 1950s and 1960s, along with his own work, led Frank Morrell to believe that nonresective surgical therapy might be safe and effective. The first discovery, by Mountcastle, was that gray matter in the neocortex was organized in vertical functional columns with afferent and efferent connecting fiber tracts oriented perpendicular to the surface of the cortex.[62,63] Although some horizontal interconnections between neurons exist, experiments by Sperry and colleagues demonstrated that if these horizontal connections are interrupted in the cat visual cortex, the function of that cortex is largely preserved.[68-70] In these experiments, they placed mica plates in gray matter perpendicular to the cortical surface, thus severing the horizontal fibers in the cortex but preserving the vertical fibers. Visual testing showed preservation of function. Experiments by Morrell demonstrated the role of these horizontal fibers in the synchronization and spread of an epileptic discharge.[71,72] He found that in the monkey, he could inhibit the seizure focus but preserve motor function when he transected through a penicillin-induced seizure focus in the motor cortex.[61] These findings led to a long-term collaboration in the surgical treatment of seizure foci in eloquent cortex between the neurologist Morrell and the neurosurgeon Walter Whisler, who had worked at the Illinois Neuropsychological Institute with Gibbs. By 1999, Morrell and Whisler had used MST to treat more than 120 patients at Rush Epilepsy Center in Chicago, where they developed and perfected the technique. Since the report of their

original series,[61] many other epilepsy centers have duplicated that success and reported their findings.[73-99]

Patient Selection

The great majority of surgical epilepsy cases can be treated by standard resective techniques such as temporal lobectomy with amygdalohippocampectomy and extratemporal resection in noneloquent cortex. Subpial transection is reserved for patients in whom the seizure activity originates in eloquent cortex. MST has been used to treat patients with epileptogenic lesions of the speech, motor, or primary sensory cortex. Although MST has been used for Rasmussen's encephalitis, it is of questionable benefit for progressive disease states when the underlying disease cannot be controlled.[100,101]

MST can be used for the treatment of carefully selected cases of

1. Epilepsia partialis continua
2. Focal sensory, somatosensory, or visual cortex seizures
3. Persistent epileptogenic activity in eloquent areas adjacent to a previous resection
4. Landau-Kleffner syndrome
5. Rasmussen's encephalitis[102]
6. Status epilepticus[100,103]

Operative Procedure

In most cases, subdural grid recording and mapping have been done, and general anesthesia with methohexital is used. Methohexital has been shown to induce epileptic activity, with some evidence that it preferentially induces epileptiform activity within the primary seizure focus.[104-106] If intraoperative mapping is planned, lighter doses of methohexital are used, along with intravenous sedation and generous use of local anesthetic. Patients are positioned so that the planned operative exposure is superior in the field and the head is in three-point fixation. A standard frontotemporal craniotomy with an exposure large enough to allow ECoG is carried out. ECoG is performed with a grid, and additional strip electrodes are placed as needed. In many patients in whom MST is being considered, the seizure focus lies in both eloquent and noneloquent cortex. In these cases, surgical resection is performed in the noneloquent cortex to within 1.5 cm of eloquent cortex, as delineated by intraoperative or subdural grid stimulation mapping with standard techniques.[107,108] If repeat ECoG does not show significant resolution of the interictal activity and the primary residual focus lies within eloquent cortex, MST is performed on the crown of the involved gyri at 5-mm intervals through the gray matter. Transections are made in parallel rows in the direction perpendicular to the long axis of the gyrus (Fig. 65-4). If significant resolution of the seizure focus is noted on ECoG, no further transection is done. If no significant resolution is noted and a clearly focal area is active despite transection of the crown of the gyrus in that area, transection is sometimes carried out vertically into the gray matter within the depth of the sulcus. This is illustrated in a cadaver in Figure 65-5. This transection is performed along the same plane as transection of the crown. If the primary seizure focus is truly in the MST area, these maneuvers usually stop or significantly reduce the intraictal epileptic discharges. If they do not, it is possible that the preoperative evaluation and ECoG have not shown the primary seizure focus, which may be projecting abnormal electrical activity from a distance.

In the less common scenario, the seizure focus is located entirely in eloquent cortex. In such cases, MST is the only surgical option. The procedure is done as described earlier, the only exception being that no cortical resection is performed. All intraoperative decision making relies on ECoG, grid mapping, and

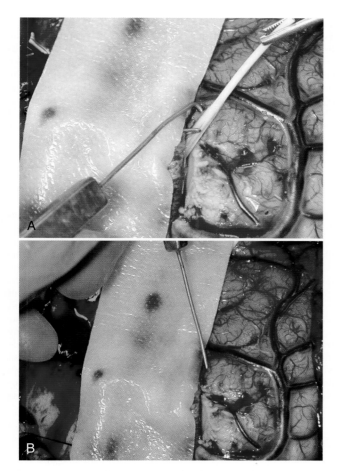

FIGURE 65-4 **A,** The transection hook enters through the hole. **B,** The hook is advanced stepwise across the gyrus, with the tip of the hook visible beneath the pia. The transector is then withdrawn along the same path.

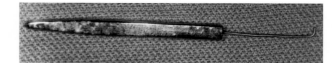

FIGURE 65-6 The transector has three parts. The rectangular handle is connected to a malleable wire with a 4-mm tip. The tip is angled 105 degrees to prevent snagging of vessels.

the preoperative evaluation. Evidence of a true focal-onset seizure focus with spread through the surrounding cortex must be differentiated from mere cortical "spiking," which is not appropriate for treatment with MST. This requires an experienced epileptologist familiar with the interpretation of ECoG.

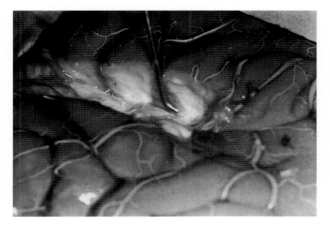

FIGURE 65-5 On a cadaver specimen in the coronal plane, the transector is seen advancing into the depth of a sulcus. The tip is reversed and pointed away from the sulcus to lessen the possibility of vessel injury.

Transections

Transections are performed with a specially designed fine, malleable wire that is bent into a 4-mm blunt hook at the tip (Fig. 65-6). The hook of the subpial transector (Whisler-Morrell Subpial Transector, Redman Neurotechnologists, Lake Zurich, IL) measures 4 mm in length to match the average depth of gray matter in the neocortex.[63] This hook is bent at an obtuse angle of 105 degrees relative to the main shaft of the wire. The wire is connected to a rectangular handle with the tip of the hook aligned with the flat sides of the handle. This is important because it prevents the hook from going into the cortex at any angle other than perpendicular. If the hook is advanced through the cortex at an angle off the perpendicular, extensive undercutting of the cortex will result, with corresponding deficits. The transection hook shank can be bent to any shape necessary for use in technically difficult locations. This is useful in the intrahemispheric motor and visual cortices and in the posterior temporal lobe when the sylvian fissure is opened to allow access to the depths of the fissure.

The area to be transected is carefully inspected. The gyral and microgyral patterns are noted. The course of the vascular supply and bypassing vessels is traced. After ECoG, transections are usually begun in the most dependent area because subarachnoid bleeding may occur. If a large amount of subarachnoid blood accumulates, a small opening can be made in the pia to let the blood escape. Each transection is begun by opening a hole in an avascular area of the pia. This is done at the edge of a sulcus with a 20-gauge needle. As the transector hook enters the gray matter through this opening, it is important to keep the hook vertically oriented to avoid undercutting and advancing the tip too deep and thus injuring white matter. The hook is advanced in stepwise fashion in a straight line across the crown of the gyrus in a direction perpendicular to the long axis of the gyrus. The hook is then withdrawn along the same path, with the tip of the hook visible just below the pia.[109-111] As the hook is withdrawn from the pial puncture site, a small amount of blood sometimes escapes. This is easily controlled with a small piece of Gelfoam and gentle pressure. The next transection line is made parallel to and 5 mm from the first. Because the hook is 4 mm long, it can be used to estimate the distance to the next transection line. The transections are thus done along the gyrus in the area of the seizure focus. Great care must be taken to note the course of the major blood vessels, particularly around the sylvian and intrahemispheric fissures. When transection must be performed in the depths of a sulcus or fissure, the hook is inserted upside down, with the tip pointed away from the pial surface. This lessens the likelihood of damaging a vessel in the sulcus or fissure. The obtuse angle of the hook also helps lessen the likelihood of injury to vessels. In cases of perisylvian-onset epilepsy, it is often useful to open the sylvian fissure to record from the depths of the fissure and transect under direct vision. In some cases, transection at 5-mm intervals is not possible because of microgyral patterns or a large confluence of vessels that may cover the area to be transected (Fig. 65-7).

An alternative approach to transection was proposed by Wyler and colleagues in which the transection device is inserted with

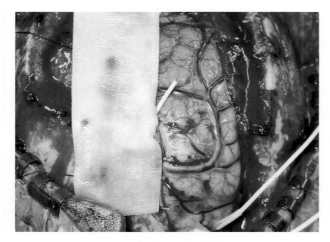

FIGURE 65-7 After transections are completed, fine lines can be seen beneath the pia at 5-mm intervals. Petechial bleeding is easily controlled with Gelfoam and gentle pressure.

the point projected downward into the cortex.[74] Other authors have described alterations of the technique.[86,87]

A recent publication by Shimizu and coauthors reported hippocampal transection in patients with temporal lobe epilepsy.[97] Shimizu and associates stated that the primary indication for this procedure was normal hippocampal cases in which there is a high risk for memory loss with hippocampal resection. In their technique, the ventricle is accessed from above via a corticotomy in the superior temporal gyrus. Hippocampal ECoG is followed by transections in the hippocampus in a coronal plane to varying depths by a specially designed transection device. The amygdala is resected if ECoG shows epileptic discharges. They reported that active epileptic discharges usually disappear after transection. If further discharges are noted, they may resect the basal temporal region. In their series, they reported the results of this procedure in 21 patients with normal preoperative MRI findings. In the 17 patients who had at least 1 year of follow-up, 14 were free of seizures. Postoperative neuropsychological testing (Rey auditory verbal learning test, Benton Visual Retention Test, and Wechsler Adult Intelligence Scale–Revised) was reported to be unchanged from preoperative testing in all patients by 6 months after surgery. The confounding variables of having performed a corticotomy on the superior temporal gyrus, transgression of the temporal stem, resection of the amygdala, and in some cases, resection of basal cortex make it difficult to determine that the efficacy of the procedure is entirely due to transection of the hippocampus. Regardless, the reported stability of memory testing makes this procedure intriguing. Long-term follow-up in these patients will be required to determine the potential usefulness of this procedure.

Pathology

When tissue that has been treated with the MST method has been removed and analyzed, the acute pathologic changes are consistent with microscopic focal injury along the transection line (Fig. 65-8). On the transection line, microscopic hemorrhage, edema, and mild cell injury are seen. When the transection lines are done properly and perpendicular to the gyral surface, the columns of cell bodies and their vertical afferent and efferent fibers are preserved. In the study by Pierre-Louis and colleagues,[112] the majority of transections were entirely in gray matter and were perpendicular to the gyral surface. Limiting transections to surface gray matter may explain the kainic acid–induced animal models of epilepsy, which show evidence that MST suppresses epileptic activity in the transected cortex but does not stop subcortical spread of epilepsy. Kaufmann and associates described more variable results with transections deviating from the perpendicular and at varying depths.[113]

Radiology and Functional Imaging

The acute changes as a result of MST seen on CT and MRI include small subcortical hemorrhages and edema, along with loss of definition of the gray-white junction. On MRI, the transections themselves can often be seen acutely. At 6 months, MRI shows clear, fine transections in gray matter. If subcortical hemorrhage occurs, microcystic changes and focal gyral atrophy may be seen.

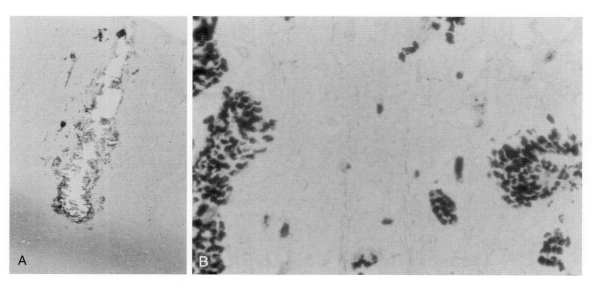

FIGURE 65-8 The pathology of multiple subpial transection is illustrated with hematoxylin-eosin staining. The transection shown reaches down to the white matter but remains within gray matter. Edema and mild inflammatory changes are noted on higher power. Intervening vertical cell columns are preserved.

TABLE 65-5 Postsurgical Outcomes

SURGICAL PROCEDURE	N	ENGEL'S CLASSIFICATION*				NEUROLOGICAL COMPLICATIONS	
		Class I (%)	Class II (%)	Class III (%)	Class IV (%)	Transient (%)	Permanent (%)
MST only, partial seizures	16	6 (37.5)	4 (25)	2 (12.5)	4 (25)	1 (6)	3 (19)
MST only, LKS	16	9 (57.7)	2 (12.5)	2 (12.5)	3 (18)	2 (12.5)	—
MST/resection	68	33 (48.5)	7 (10)	16 (23.5)	12 (18)	7 (10)	4 (6)
Total	**100**	**48**	**13**	**20**	**19**	**10**	**7**

*Classes I to III indicate significant worthwhile improvement; class IV indicates no significant improvement.
LKS, Landau-Kleffner syndrome; MST, multiple subpial transection.
From Morrell F, Kanner A, Whisler W. Multiple subpial transection. In: Stefan H, Andermann F, eds. *Plasticity in Epilepsy*. New York: Lippincott-Raven; 1998.

Hashizume and Tanaka demonstrated the effects of MST on an experimental seizure focus.[114] In a kainic acid rat seizure model, they found that MST suppressed the spread of seizure activity to the ipsilateral hemisphere and reduced the frequency of seizures but did not eliminate them. They tested glucose metabolism in the transected cortex and found that it was not altered, thus suggesting that function of the cortex was preserved.

Leonhardt and coworkers reported PET findings after MST.[115] In one patient who had undergone MST in the central sensorimotor cortex, they found that PET activation during a hand motor task was maintained in the transected cortex. They also found that there was more widespread activation in motor association cortex bilaterally, thus suggesting active recruitment of cortex after MST.

Complications

In our series of more than 100 patients and in published series by others, no deaths have been reported (Table 65-5). In the early postoperative period, most patients who undergo MST in eloquent cortex have subtle, transient deficits corresponding to the area transected. These deficits are most pronounced in the first week after surgery. As the edema and microhemorrhage resolve, most patients return to their baseline function within 2 to 4 weeks. In many patients undergoing careful, detailed examination, deficits in fine motor control or speech can be detected. Moo and coworkers reported a prospective evaluation of motor recovery after MST.[116] fMRI was performed before and after transection and then repeated 6 weeks postoperatively. Findings included an initial loss of dexterity corresponding to an initial loss of focal fMRI activation. The focal fMRI activation and the dexterity had returned by 6 weeks.

In the series reported by Morrell, there was a 5% incidence of permanent, disabling complications corresponding to the area transected. In two patients, motor deficits arose after retraction and transection of the intrahemispheric leg motor cortex. Two cases of permanent postoperative dysphasia occurred after transection of speech areas. One case of hemiparesis occurred after a basal ganglia hemorrhage distant from the site of transection. Eight patients had deficits corresponding to the area transected that lasted longer than the expected 2 to 4 months, but they eventually resolved over a period of several months. One was related to speech, and seven were related to sensory or motor function. Seven other complications occurred that were clearly related to the resection or craniotomy. Permanent visual field loss and permanent sensory loss were clearly related to the surgical resection. A transient sixth nerve palsy was attributed to temporal lobe resection. A single case of meningitis, orchitis, and phlebitis was associated with the craniotomy procedure but resolved with appropriate treatment. The final permanent complication rate was 7% as reported by Morrell. A later publication by Smith and Byrne on 84 patients with MST, with or without additional resection, reported a complication rate of 17%.[100]

Complication rates similar to ours have been reported in other series (Table 65-6). A period of transient dysfunction has also been commonly noted. Higher complication rates can be expected if the interval of transection is narrowed to 4 mm or less.[76] Although perpendicular transection through cortex causes little damage to the surrounding neurons, as the pathologic studies indicate, it does cause some damage.[112,113] As the interval is narrowed, one would expect a higher percentage of neurons in the cortex to be injured. This would also be expected if the depths of the sulci in the cortical area were transected. This maneuver is not routinely done at our center but is performed routinely by some surgeons.

In a multicenter meta-analysis reported by Spencer and coworkers, the complication rate for MST without resection was 19% and that for MST with resection was 23% in a series of 211 patients.[117] These results are similar to those reported by Smith and Byrne and reflect the nature of operating in eloquent cortex in patients with severe medically intractable epilepsy.[100] Results from other series are listed in Table 65-6.

Seizure Outcome

To evaluate the effects of MST on seizure outcome, it is useful to examine MST procedures in the following categories:

1. MST for focal-onset epilepsy in which MST is the only procedure done.
2. MST for focal-onset epilepsy in which cortical resection of noneloquent cortex is also performed. In such cases, preoperative evaluation showed seizure activity in eloquent and noneloquent cortex, and the cortical resection had no significant effect on ECoG findings. MST was then performed on adjacent eloquent cortex.

Seizure outcome after MST is analyzed in this fashion because the cortical resection done in the majority of cases introduces a confounding variable: one cannot be certain whether MST or the resection had the effect on seizure outcome or on morbidity. In these cases, one can be certain only that MST had an effect on intraoperative ECoG. The group that underwent MST as the only surgical intervention gives the clearest indication of the effect of MST on seizure outcome because there are fewer confounding variables and the pathology is more uniform in this group. In 16 patients who underwent MST alone for focal-onset seizures in eloquent cortex with at least 2 years of follow-up, 6

TABLE 65-6 Postsurgical Outcome after Multiple Subpial Transection at Epilepsy Centers

| AUTHOR | N | SIGNIFICANT IMPROVEMENT | | NO WORTHWHILE IMPROVEMENT | | NEUROLOGICAL COMPLICATIONS | |
		MST Only	MST/Resection	MST Only	MST/Resection	n	Type (n)
Shimizu et al.[80]	12	12	—	0	0	0	—
Devinsky et al.[77]	3	0	0	0	0	2	Mild speech deficits (2)
Sawhney et al.[78]	21	8	12	1	0	0	—
Lui et al.*	50	32	—	18	—	0	—
Wyler et al.[74]	6	6	—	0	—	1	Mild motor deficits (4)
							Mild speech deficits (2)
Hufnagel et al.[79]	22	4	15	2	1	7	Overt speech deficits (2)
							Mild dysnomia (7)
							Moderate dysphasia (1)
Pacia et al.[73]	21	3	18	0	1	9	Loss of proprioception in the hand (1)
							Permanent (7)
							Transient (8)
Rush Epilepsy Center	100	25	56	7	12	17	Sensorimotor (13)
Schramm et al.[87]	20	9	—	11	—	0	—
Shimizu et al.[98]	17	—	17	—	—	0	—
Spencer et al.[117]	211						
Simple partial	85	14	47	5	19	10	Aphasia, memory, hemiparesis
Complex partial	113	17	71	4	21	37	Aphasia, memory, hemiparesis

MST, multiple subpial transection.
*In this study it was not clear whether MST alone or MST plus resection was performed.
From Morrell F, Kanner A, Whisler W. Multiple subpial transection. In: Stefan H, Andermann F, eds. *Plasticity in Epilepsy*. New York: Lippincott-Raven; 1998.

were made seizure free (see Table 65-5). An additional 6 patients had only rare seizures or had a 90% or greater reduction in seizures. Four patients had no worthwhile benefit. Overall, 75% of patients in this category had a worthwhile Engel's class I to III seizure outcome. Because all of these patients would have been rejected for standard resective surgery, their outcomes should be compared with best medical therapy. Other groups have reported similar results (see Table 65-6). In Wyler and coworkers' series of 6 patients with uniform pathology in the sensorimotor cortex, all 6 had a significant reduction in their seizures.[74] There was only one permanent mild motor deficit. Schramm and colleagues reported on a series of 20 patients who underwent MST without resection.[87] Forty-five percent of the patients at the 1-year follow-up had a worthwhile outcome (Engel's class I to III). They reported that lesional epilepsy and large areas of epileptic discharge predicted a worse outcome. Mulligan and coauthors reported a 42% rate of significant improvement in seizure frequency in a series of 12 patients.[86] Spencer and associates reported an international meta-analysis on 212 patients who underwent MST at six epilepsy centers.[117] In cases of MST alone without resection, they reported rates of excellent outcome with regard to seizure control of 71% for generalized epilepsy, 62% for complex partial epilepsy, and 63% for simple partial seizures.

The next category of patients underwent a combination of MST and resection. This was the most common type of case in the series of Morrell and Whisler.[61] It is rare for a seizure focus to lie entirely in eloquent cortex. A total of 82% of patients in this category were seizure free or had a significant reduction in their seizures (Engel's class I to III; see Table 65-5). Although the majority of patients exhibited worthwhile improvement, the initial report by Morrell of 52% being free of seizures was not sustained later in the series.[61] The meta-analysis reported by Spencer and coauthors showed similar results for patients who underwent resection plus MST, with excellent outcomes (>95%

reduction) reported in 87% of patients with generalized seizures, 68% of patients with complex partial seizures, and 68% of patients with simple partial epilepsy.[117] These collective data support the efficacy of MST, both as a stand-alone procedure for highly localized cases in eloquent cortex and for cases in which the epileptogenic zone overlaps eloquent cortex. The expected outcome of MST, however, is more likely to be improvement than cure. Results from other series are listed in Table 65-6.

The question of long-term efficacy has been raised. Orbach and coworkers reported an 18.5% seizure recurrence rate in a series of patients who underwent MST and had at least 5 years of follow-up.[118] In a series of 20 patients who underwent pure MST, Schramm and coauthors reported that outcomes changed over time.[87] Five patients improved during the long-term follow-up period, whereas 7 worsened. This phenomenon has also been described in patients who have undergone resective epilepsy surgery.

Conclusion

The initial experience with MST was reported in 1989.[61] In that group of patients with intractable seizures, 11 of 20 were free of seizures after a follow-up of at least 5 years. Subsequent cases in which MST was performed without resection proved the independent efficacy of the procedure. Since then, MST has proved helpful in patients with intractable epilepsy and foci in unresectable cortex. Similar results at other centers have confirmed its efficacy and safety if done properly on well-selected patients. The exact mechanism of action of MST is being delineated with functional testing. Other centers attempting MST have added different techniques and new protocols.[73,74,76] As we learn more about MST and about the nature of epileptogenic cortex, the technique will be further refined and will probably result in improved outcomes in patients with unresectable seizure foci.

SUGGESTED READINGS

Abson Kraemer DL. Diagnostic techniques in surgical management of epilepsy: strip electrodes, grids and depth electrodes. In: Schmidek HH, Roberts DW, eds. *Schmidek & Sweet Operative Neurosurgical Techniques: Indications, Methods, and Results*. 4th ed. Philadelphia: WB Saunders; 2000:1359-1374.

Barkovich AJ, Rowley HA, Andermann F. MR in partial epilepsy: value of high-resolution volumetric techniques. *AJNR Am J Neuroradiol*. 1995;16:339-343.

Bauman JA, Feoli E, Romanelli P, et al. Multistage epilepsy surgery: safety, efficacy and utility of a novel approach in pediatric extratemporal epilepsy. *Neurosurgery*. 2005;56:318-334.

Chapman K, Wyllie E, Najm I, et al. Seizure outcome after epilepsy surgery in patients with normal preoperative MRI. *J Neurol Neurosurg Psychiatry*. 2005;76:710-713.

Cohen-Gadol AA, Stoffman MR, Spencer DD. Emerging surgical and radiotherapeutic techniques for treating epilepsy. *Curr Opin Neurol*. 2003;16:213-219.

Devinsky O, Perrine K, Vazquez B, et al. Multiple subpial transections in the language cortex. *Brain*. 1994;117:255-265.

Faught E. Collective data supports efficacy of multiple subpial transection. *Epilepsy Curr*. 2002;2:108.

Hashizume K, Tanaka T. Multiple subpial transection in kainic acid–induced focal cortical seizure. *Epilepsy Res*. 1998;32:389-399.

Hufnagel A, Zenter J, Fernandez G, et al. Multiple subpial transection for control of epileptic seizures: effectiveness and safety. *Epilepsia*. 1997;38:678-688.

Kaufmann W, Kraus G, Uematsu S, et al. Treatment of epilepsy with multiple subpial transections: an acute histological analysis in human subjects. *Epilepsia*. 1996;37:342-352.

Leonhardt G, Spiekermann G, Muller S, et al. Cortical reorganization following multiple subpial transection in human brain—a study with positron emission tomography. *Neurosci Lett*. 2000;292:63-65.

Morrell F, Whisler WW, Bleck T. Multiple subpial transection: a new approach to the surgical treatment of focal epilepsy. *J Neurosurg*. 1989;70:231-239.

Mulligan LP, Spencer DD, Spencer SS. Multiple subpial transections: the Yale experience. *Epilepsia*. 2001;42:226-229.

Ojemann GA. Surgical treatment of epilepsy. In: Wilkins RH, Rengachary SS, eds. *Neurosurgery*. 2nd ed. New York: McGraw-Hill; 1996:4173-4183.

Ojemann GA. Awake operations with mapping in epilepsy. In: Schmidek HH, Sweet WH, eds. *Operative Neurosurgical Techniques*. 3rd ed. Philadelphia: WB Saunders; 1995:1317-1322.

Olivier A, Awad IA. Extratemporal resections. In: Engel J, ed. *Surgical Treatment of the Epilepsies*. 2nd ed. New York: Raven Press; 1993:489-500.

Pierre-Louis SJC, Smith MC, Morrell F, et al. Anatomical effects of multiple subpial transection. *Epilepsia*. 1993;34(suppl):104.

Rasmussen T. Surgery of frontal lobe epilepsy. *Adv Neurol*. 1975;8:197-205.

Schramm J, Aliashkevich AF, Grunwald T. Multiple subpial transections: outcome and complications in 20 patients who did not undergo resection. *J Neurosurg*. 2002;97:39-47.

Shimizu H, Kawai K, Sunaga S, et al. Hippocampal transection for treatment of left temporal lobe epilepsy with preservation of verbal memory. *J Clin Neurosci*. 2006;13:322-328.

Shimizu H, Kawai K, Sunaga S, et al. [Surgical treatment for temporal lobe epilepsy with preservation of postoperative memory function.] *Rinsho Shinkeigaku*. 2004;44:868-870.

Smith MC, Byrne R. Multiple subpial transection in neocortical epilepsy: part I. *Adv Neurol*. 2000;84:621-634.

Spencer SS, Schramm J, Wyler A, et al. Multiple subpial transection for intractable partial epilepsy: an international meta-analysis. *Epilepsia*. 2002;43:141-145.

Sperry RW, Miner N, Myers RE. Visual pattern perception following subpial slicing and tantalum wire implantation in visual cortex. *J Comp Physiol Psychol*. 1955;48:50-58.

Tanaka T, Hashizume K, Sawamura A, et al. Basic science and epilepsy: experimental epilepsy surgery. *Stereotact Funct Neurosurg*. 2001;77:239-244.

Wada J, Rasmussen T. Intracranial injection of Amytal for the localization of cerebral speech dominance. *J Neurosurg*. 1960;17:266-282.

Whisler WW. Multiple subpial transection. In: Kaye A, Black P, eds. *Operative Neurosurgery*. London, United Kingdom: Churchill Livingstone; 1997.

Whisler WW. Multiple subpial transection. In: Rengachary SS, ed. *Neurosurgical Operative Atlas*. Vol 6. Park Ridge, IL: American Association of Neurological Surgeons; 1997:125-129.

Wyler AR, Wilkus RJ, Retard SW, et al. Multiple subpial transection for partial seizures in sensorimotor cortex. *Neurosurgery*. 1995;37:1122-1128.

Full references can be found on Expert Consult @ www.expertconsult.com

CHAPTER 66

Hemispheric Disconnection Procedures

Johannes Schramm

DEFINITION

Hemispheric disconnection procedures are a group of surgical interventions for chronic epilepsy that are used as alternatives to anatomic hemispherectomy. The common denominator of these procedures is disconnection of the cortical layer of one hemisphere from the contralateral hemisphere and from the deeper structures of the basal ganglia. The term *hemispherotomy* is frequently used as an alternative expression for the same group of operations. Although the terms *hemispheric deafferentation* and *hemispherotomy* imply that the hemispheric tissue is not removed, other techniques such as *hemicorticectomy* or *hemidecortication* also disconnect the cortex from the deeper structures but do so by removing the cortex. Preferably, *hemispheric deafferentation* should be reserved for techniques in which no or very little resection of cortical brain tissue is included.

DEVELOPMENT

The first *anatomic hemispherectomy* was done for glioma surgery by Dandy in 1928,[1] and Krynauw performed the first resection for drug-resistant epilepsy in 1950.[2] A change from *anatomic hemispherectomy*, frequently used in the 1950s and 1960s and in which one whole hemisphere was removed (with or without the basal ganglia block), to the less invasive disconnection techniques has taken place since the early 1990s. An important step in the evolution from large resection to large disconnection occurred with development of the technique of *functional hemispherectomy*, introduced by Rasmussen.[3] It included removal of two larger brain segments (temporal lobe and central suprasylvian tissue block), combined with callosotomy and disconnection of the frontal, parietal, and occipital lobes. Although the hemisphere as such is no longer totally removed, the effect of this surgery is functionally equivalent to total hemispherectomy. For the aims of epilepsy surgery, it is not important whether parts of the hemisphere are removed or just disconnected because to achieve a seizure-free outcome, it is sufficient to disconnect the ictogenic cortical part of the hemisphere from its connections to the other hemisphere and the long tracts to the basal ganglia. It makes sense to limit use of the term *functional hemispherectomy* to Rasmussen's and Mathern's techniques.[4] The latter consists of a large central peri-insular resection, including the basal ganglia block and the temporal lobe, combined with disconnection of the frontal, parietal, and occipital lobes.

After a period of increased use of anatomic hemispherectomy in the 1960s and 1970s, a high rate of late complications was described, such as superficial cerebral hemosiderosis (SCH), occlusion of the foramen of Monro and aqueduct, development of hydrocephalus and its complications,[5-8] and even fatal outcomes.[3,9,10] In 27 anatomic hemispherectomies performed in Montreal between 1952 and 1968 with long-term follow-up, hydrocephalus developed in 52% of patients, 33% from SCH and 19% from other causes. Three of nine patients with SCH died of hydrocephalus.[11] SCH is thought to be caused by recurrent minor intracranial bleeding in the large cavity as a result of the resection surgery. Such bleeding may occur after minor head trauma or intermittent rises in intracranial pressure from physiologic events such as sneezing.

Less Resection—More Disconnection

Because of the considerable mortality from these complications, the use of anatomic hemispherectomy decreased until the 1970s, when Rasmussen described an alternative technique based on the observation that in patients with multilobectomies, these complications did not occur. Because the frontal lobe and the parieto-occipital lobe are left in situ, a lower incidence of hydrocephalus and hemosiderosis was expected and later confirmed. Rasmussen demonstrated in his patient series that seizure-free outcome rates after anatomic and functional hemispherectomies were very similar, 83% and 85%, respectively, but the rate of complications from increased intracranial pressure was reduced from 35% to 7%. A lower rate of SCH has been reported for functional hemispherectomy techniques after a follow-up of 20 years.[3,10,12] Another approach to avoid these complications was the technique by Adams, who occluded the foramen of Monro, excised the choroidal plexus, and obliterated the subdural space by folding down the dura toward the midline and over the residual basal ganglia.[13] The *hemidecortication* and *hemicorticectomy* techniques[14-16] approached the problem of these complications by preserving nearly all of the ventricular system and leaving the cerebrospinal fluid (CSF) space uncontaminated.

It also makes sense to consider hemidecortication and hemicorticectomy separately from disconnection procedures (e.g., transsylvian/transventricular keyhole procedure,[17] Delalande's vertical parasagittal hemispherotomy, and perisylvian window techniques[18,19]), which usually include very little brain resection. Differentiation between mostly disconnective procedures and functional hemispherectomies[3,4] or decortications, including larger resections, is useful because the latter procedures appear to have a different set of characteristics and disadvantages.

The modern transition to nearly exclusively disconnective techniques started in 1992 after a brief description of two quite different approaches developed independently by Schramm, Delalande, and their colleagues.[20,21] This was followed in the mid-1990s by the first patient series treated via perisylvian techniques.[17,19] Closely related to Villemure's technique is a variation of a perisylvian resective approach by Shimizu and Maehara.[18] Among the disconnective procedures, the technique by Delalande and associates (vertical parasagittal hemispherotomy)[22] and the transsylvian transventricular keyhole procedures[23] include minimal tissue removal and mostly consist of disconnections. The change to less resective procedures during the past 15 years is being made in many centers, and a number of reports have confirmed the initial results indicating that disconnection procedures are associated with shorter operative time, less blood loss, fewer intraoperative complications, and possibly a lower rate of hydrocephalus.

INDICATIONS, PATIENT SELECTION, AND TIMING

Because anatomic hemispherectomy, functional hemispherectomy, hemispherotomy, and hemispheric deafferentation are similarly effective, all are established and very successful methods used to treat drug-resistant epilepsy resulting from diffuse damage to one hemisphere. Such damage is usually associated with hemiparesis, hemianopia, and frequently, delayed cognitive development. The indications, selection of patients, and timing are similar for all variants of these procedures.

Causes

The diagnoses typical in these patients may be grouped into inborn, perinatal, or acquired conditions (Table 66-1) and include Sturge-Weber syndrome (SWS), developmental defects (multilobar cortical dysplasia, polymicrogyria, lissencephaly, hemimegalencephaly [HME]), cystic defects from intrauterine or perinatal infarction or hemorrhage, and hemiplegia-hemiconvulsion-epilepsy syndrome (HHE) (Fig. 66-1). Rasmussen's encephalitis leads to hemiatrophy, which may also be posttraumatic, postencephalitic, or of unknown origin. The epilepsy syndromes associated with these lesions may include several seizure types occurring with different frequencies. Patients can have up to hundreds of seizures per day or suffer from focal status epilepticus (i.e., epilepsia partialis continua, typical of Rasmussen's encephalitis).

Hemimegalencephaly

Patients with HME usually have an enlarged hemisphere displaying different features of abnormal architecture. Parts of the ventricle may be enlarged, whereas others may be compressed by abnormal brain tissue. There may be pachygyria, polymicrogyria, grossly enlarged gyri, and areas of ectopic gray matter around the ventricle in the white matter (Fig. 66-E1).

(Figure 66-E1 can be found on Expert Consult @ www.expertconsult.com)

The cause is commonly a neuronal migration disorder. HME is often associated with seizures that are frequent and intractable. The hemiparesis can be mild or pronounced, and a marked degree of mental retardation is usually present.

Sturge-Weber Syndrome

SWS is a rare congenital disorder with a variable natural history. Its characteristic feature is leptomeningeal angiomatosis, and in a proportion of cases it may be associated with a facial nevus, the latter variant occasionally described as encephalotrigeminal angiomatosis. The clinical syndrome is characterized by a progressive neurological disorder consisting of epilepsy, cortical calcifications, cerebral atrophy, and if the epilepsy is untreatable, frequently the development of mental retardation. Seizures usually develop by the end of the first year, may respond to medical treatment initially, but often become resistant to drugs. The cerebral manifestations generally involve the occipital or parietal cortex, or both, but the entire cortex or large parts of it may be involved; however, the pathologic changes remain restricted to one hemisphere. Epilepsy surgery should be considered for patients with refractory seizures, but one has to differentiate between the need for hemispheric deafferentation and a multilobar or more restricted resection. Hemianopia may be present from the beginning or may develop together with hemiparesis during progression of the epileptic encephalopathy, which is associated with cognitive decline and mental retardation. Children with widespread hemispheric involvement are classic candidates for hemispheric deafferentation. The results from three multicenter series have been reported.[24-26] Seizure-free rates after hemispherotomy were reported to be 100% in 8, 6, and 5 patients.[24,25,27] In three larger series, rates of 80% to 82% were reported in 12, 28, and 70 patients.[22,26,28]

Rasmussen's Encephalitis

The origin of Rasmussen's encephalitis is unknown. The clinical syndrome is characterized by intractable epilepsy and progressive hemiparesis inexorably resulting in hemiplegia, mental decline, and hemispheric atrophy. The median age at onset in a multicenter study of 16 patients was 4.2 years with a range of 2 to 11 years.[28] Most of the brain damage occurs during the first 8 to 12 months.[29] Progression to hemiplegia or aphasia (or to both) and finally cognitive decline occur invariably. The seizure disorder may begin with generalized seizures, but focal seizures are most frequent and epilepsia partialis continua develops in a large proportion of patients. A characteristic histologic finding is a perivascular infiltrate of T lymphocytes, which is associated with destruction of neurons.[30] Seventy-seven percent of 83 patients in that study were seizure free after hemispheric surgery. Once the diagnosis is suspected, the atrophic process may be staged by serial magnetic resonance imaging (MRI).[31] A difficult decision on when to operate will arise. These patients are classic candidates for hemispheric deafferentation.

Indications

The decision to perform hemispherotomy is straightforward for unihemispheric lesions that are either inborn or occurred around the time of birth and became manifested during infancy or early childhood as frequent and intractable seizures. Hemispherotomy is also indicated for small infants with so-called catastrophic epilepsy, or very severe epilepsy manifested early after birth, usually from severe hemispheric damage or an inborn malformation in which lengthy drug treatment is known to be unsuccessful. The procedure is less frequently performed in adults, generally after long-standing drug-resistant epilepsy.

Why is it possible to have a useful life after such a procedure? The disconnection is performed on a mostly nonfunctional or partly destroyed hemisphere, where language and motor function either have been or will be transferred to the other hemisphere, as is the rule if the damage occurred intrauterinely or perinatally. These patients already have spastic hemiparesis, and although the procedure always results in loss of fine motor control of the hand and occasionally deterioration of gait, the majority of patients are able to walk and even use their arm and hand to a certain degree. Hemispherotomy is associated with a 70% to 80% probability of

TABLE 66-1 Etiology of Seizures	
Infarct, ischemia, porencephaly	54
Cortical dysplasia, migration disorders	10
Hemimegalencephaly	12
Sturge-Weber syndrome	6
Rasmussen's encephalitis	15
Hemiatrophy, unclear etiology	7
Postencephalitic, HHE, or other	6
Total	**110**

HHE, hemiplegia-hemiconvulsion-epilepsy syndrome.

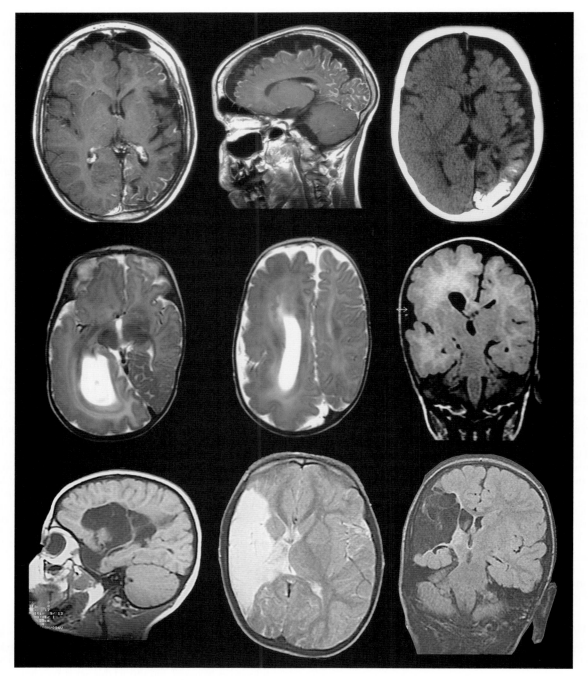

FIGURE 66-1 Magnetic resonance images and computed tomography scans from three typical causes. *Upper row,* Sturge-Weber syndrome. *Middle row,* Hemimegalencephaly. *Bottom row,* Perinatal porencephalic cyst, most likely of ischemic origin. *(Copyright J. Schramm, with permission.)*

being seizure free in most series and up to 90% with some causes. Frequently, improvement in cognition and behavioral problems is seen.

Timing

Children with holohemispheric malformations or HME with unilateral severe and continuous seizures may be operated on very early (in our group at 4 months), even without demonstrating classic hemiparesis because it may be difficult to detect early in life and would surely become evident later. If hemiparesis is

well established or severe, little motor function will be lost. The timing of surgery in children with a progressive disease such as Rasmussen's encephalitis is more difficult to determine. Progressive worsening of epilepsy with deteriorating cognitive deficits and increasing hemiparesis may also be found in patients with SWS or HME or after encephalitis. Particularly problematic is the timing of surgery in children older than 7 or 8 years if the language-dominant hemisphere is affected by progressive disease. Some language function may still develop after surgery, even in children between 4 and 7 years of age. Nonetheless, it should not be forgotten that Rasmussen's encephalitis invariably leads to severe atrophy of the affected hemisphere together with complete hemiplegia and loss of language function. It is not infrequent in many institutions to elect to proceed to surgery at a time when the relentless series of severe epileptic seizures has not caused irreversible damage to the unaffected hemisphere. This outcome may be minimized by accepting earlier surgery and earlier motor loss from surgery and not waiting until the disease process has destroyed the hemisphere. Performing surgery earlier for children with Rasmussen's encephalitis also increases the chance that the healthy hemisphere may compensate better for the loss of motor (or speech) function from the affected hemisphere.

Another argument in support of hemispheric disconnection is the deleterious effects of frequent seizures on cognition and behavior, as well as other neurological functions. These seizures may be clinically apparent or subclinical. This complex of frequent seizures and neurological decline is sometimes called *epileptic encephalopathy*, and abolishing it constitutes a legitimate aim for this extensive type of epilepsy surgery. Instead of giving the epileptic encephalopathy a chance to further impair the developmental and cognitive potential of the infant, this approach is particularly applicable when the cause of the epilepsy has been recognized as being untreatable early in the clinical course (such as hemispheric cortical malformations) and when repeated trials of antiepileptic drugs appear useless.

Contraindications

Hemispheric deafferentation is contraindicated if the presurgical evaluation cannot demonstrate that all typical ictal activity originates from the affected hemisphere. A relative contraindication may be seen in patients with independently arising seizures from the so-called healthy hemisphere. Occasional isolated contralateral seizure episodes may be acceptable because they do not automatically result from an independent seizure focus. Bilateral epileptogenic activity may be seen on the electroencephalogram in as many as 75% of patients, but it may be secondary and originate from the diseased hemisphere. Because bilateral involvement may represent an independent seizure focus and not just activity conducted from the diseased hemisphere, it is associated with a somewhat reduced probability of a seizure-free outcome after surgery. Nonetheless, high rates of freedom from seizures[32] can still be achieved,[33] as demonstrated in a large series in which 77% of patients with suspected bilateral disease were found to either be seizure free or have only "minor events."[34]

Occasionally, the presence of incomplete hemianopia may be considered a contraindication, especially in older children. However, it has been our experience that patients who have grown up with hemianopia adjust well to this deficit. Mental retardation is no longer considered a contraindication in our institution and others.[35]

PRESURGICAL EVALUATION

The mainstays of the presurgical evaluation are high-quality MRI and video electroencephalographic monitoring of seizures. In most patients, this plus the clinical history is sufficient to establish the indications for surgery. If possible, neuropsychological testing is also performed to be able to quantify any changes that occur after surgery. An intracarotid amobarbital test (Wada test) will frequently be necessary to demonstrate which hemisphere is language dominant and to exclude the presence of dissociated sensory and motor speech areas. With late-onset disease or other progressive disease types in which there are doubts about the hemispheric transfer of language functions, this test will be particularly important. In patients with contralateral ictogenic activity, the Wada test may be helpful for differentiating between ictal activity conducted from the diseased hemisphere and ictal activity arising from an autonomous focus in the "healthy" hemisphere.

If the contralateral ictal activity disappears when amobarbital is injected into the affected hemisphere, it is safe to assume that the contralateral activity is a conducted phenomen on and will not adversely affect the prognosis. If Rasmussen's encephalitis is suspected, it may be necessary to perform a brain biopsy to confirm the diagnosis. The use of implanted electrodes is rarely necessary to establish the indication for surgery. Intradural recordings may occasionally be used to identify the few patients in whom the hemispheric damage seems to be confined to several but not all lobes of the brain for the purpose of identifying those in whom multilobectomy would be sufficient rather than complete hemispheric deafferentation.

GOALS OF SURGERY

Hemispheric deafferentation has three goals: (1) cessation of seizures, (2) relief of the epileptic encephalopathy and neurologic deterioration, and (3) better cognitive development and improvement of behavioral disturbances. Achievement of these goals will lead to better psychosocial development and improved quality of life. Although the second and third goals are very ambitious and cannot be attained in all cases, in some situations this objective is realized when the seizures are eliminated. Elimination of seizures is achieved by completely disconnecting the epileptogenic area, which in these cases refers to all cortex of the affected hemisphere. Disconnecting the cortex is functionally equivalent to anatomic removal. When total cortical disconnection is performed, the results are comparable to those obtained with anatomic hemispherectomy.

SIDE EFFECTS AND COMPLICATIONS

Distinction must be made between expected side effects and unexpected complications. Patients or parents need to be informed about the unavoidable *side effects* of hemispheric deafferentation: complete hemianopia and loss of some motor function, such as fine pincer movement of the thumb and index finger. The impact of postoperative loss of motor function is influenced by the patient's preoperative condition. Adverse effects are more severe when the disease develops late and the hemiparesis is mild. In the case of incomplete transfer from the affected dominant hemisphere, severe aphasia may be unavoidable after surgery. Typical *risks* that patients or parents need to be informed about include lack of success with regard to seizures, need for shunting of CSF, need for transfusions, superficial wound infection or meningitis, or both, and rarely, death.

SURGICAL TECHNIQUES

The various forms of hemispheric deafferentation surgery currently in use all evolved from Rasmussen's functional hemispherectomy technique. The principle behind this surgery is to forgo anatomic removal of brain tissue by instead disconnecting brain regions. One of the early variations of Rasmussen's method was developed by Mathern's group in Los Angeles.[4] This procedure involved performing a large resection of the operculum, insula, underlying basal ganglia, and temporal lobe to achieve a functional hemispherectomy. An intermediate step short of a pure deafferentation procedure involves perisylvian techniques in which only restricted parts of the opercula (Fig. 66-E2D), corona radiata, or temporal lobe are resected. This is usually combined with disconnection of the frontal and parieto-occipital lobes and callosotomy, which is performed from within the ventricular system.[17,18,36] The latest versions of these evolving procedures are two disconnection operations that involve little or no brain removal and extensive disconnections: transsylvian keyhole hemispheric deafferentation[21,23] and central vertical hemispherotomy (Fig. 66-2).[20,22]

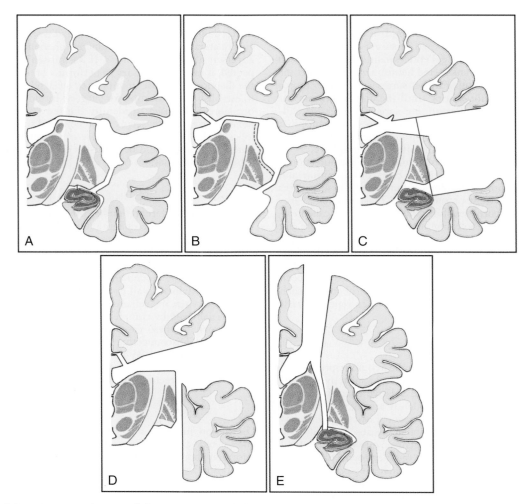

FIGURE 66-2 Schematic coronal views of the perisylvian and disconnection techniques. **A,** Step 1 of the transsylvian/transsulcal keyhole approach to the ventricle.[23] **B,** Step 2 of the transsylvian/transventricular keyhole approach: facultative temporomesial resection, removal of the insular cortex, and paramedian callosotomy. **C,** Peri-insular window technique.[36] **D,** Japanese variant of the peri-insular window technique.[18] **E,** Vertical parasagittal hemispherotomy.[22] *(Modified from Schramm J. Hemispherectomy techniques.* Neurosurg Clin N Am. *2001;37:113.)*

Hemispheric Deafferentation Techniques

Transsylvian Keyhole Technique

This technique requires limited exposure of the brain and uses disconnection steps almost exclusively. A lateral transsylvian/transventricular approach is performed through a keyhole opening. A 4 × 4 or 4 × 5 cm craniotomy is performed superior to the sylvian fissure to gain access to the underlying insula, which has an average length of 49 to 57 mm,[38] and to the corpus callosum, which has a maximal length of 7.5 cm in adults (Fig. 66-3).

This approach is characterized by four main features:

1. *Transsylvian exposure of the circular sulcus* (or sulcus limitans) of the insular cortex via a small craniotomy through a linear or curvilinear incision (see Fig. 66-E2A to C).
2. *Temporomesial disconnection* via a transventricular approach through the temporal stem (Fig. 66-4A). A pure disconnection is possible from the choroidal point anteromesially to the lateral mass of the bulging amygdaloid body to the arachnoid covering the mesial aspect of the uncus. Alternatively, the uncus and amygdala may be removed by suction. The hippocampus may be left in place as long as the mesiotemporal disconnection is carried backward along the choroidal fissure

to the trigone, but some hippocampus may be harvested for histologic examination.

3. *Complete opening of the* entire *lateral ventricle* through a transcortical incision from the insular cistern along the circular sulcus into the ventricle from the temporal horn to the tip of the anterior horn (Fig. 66-5; also see Fig. 66-4).
4. *Mesial disconnection* in the frontal and parieto-occipital area and *callosotomy.* This fourth step may be subdivided into two parts: frontobasal and posteromediobasal lobar disconnection and paramesial callosal disconnection via an intraventricular approach (see Fig. 66-4C, red lines).

Orientation during this fourth step is made easier by disconnecting the frontobasal cortex and white matter along a line drawn from the ascending middle cerebral artery through the tip of the frontal horn. The disconnection then continues by following the anterior cerebral artery in the A1 and A2 segment around the anterior knee of the corpus callosum. The next step is paramesial callosotomy. While working from within the ventricle, the pericallosal artery is followed by disconnecting callosal fibers in the white matter in a paramedian plane (Fig. 66-E3). Posteriorly, the inferior rim of the falx and the anterior rim of the tentorium are used as guiding structures all the way around to the trigone area until one reaches the temporomesial discon-

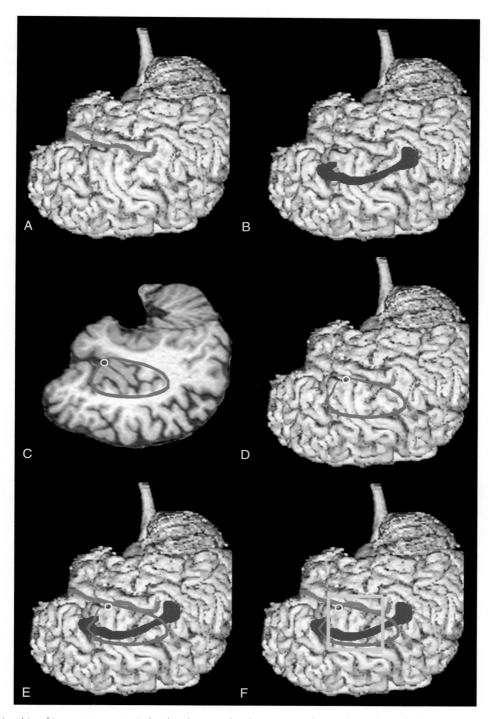

FIGURE 66-3 Relationship of important anatomic landmarks to each other projected onto the surface of a brain reconstructed from magnetic resonance images. The pictures are arranged from the surgeon's perspective. The reformatted images are taken from an unaffected hemisphere. **A,** The *red line* shows the sylvian fissure. **B,** The shape and position of the corpus callosum are shown in *blue* as projected onto the surface. **C,** The circular sulcus, which represents the border of the insular cistern, is portrayed in *green*. The *white ring* delineates the position of the ascending M1 just in front of the limen insulae. **D,** Outline of the circular sulcus projected onto the lateral surface of the hemisphere. **E,** Relationship of the position of the corpus callosum, circular sulcus, and sylvian fissure projected onto the surface. **F,** Outline of a 4 × 4-cm craniotomy, shown in *yellow*, superimposed on the sylvian fissure, the outline of the circular sulcus, and the shape of the corpus callosum. *(Based in part on a figure from Schramm J, Kral T, Clusmann H. Transsylvian keyhole functional hemispherectomy. Neurosurgery. 2001;49:891.)*

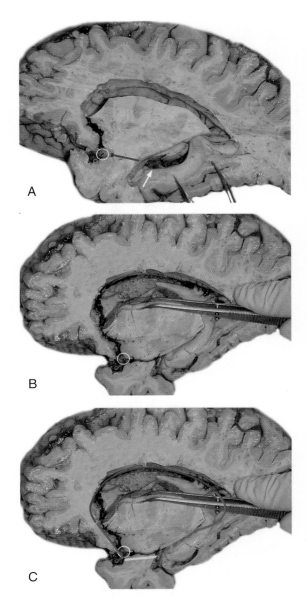

FIGURE 66-4 Demonstration of mesial disconnection lines for the technique of transsylvian/transventricular hemispheric deafferentation. **A,** In a formalin-fixed brain, a parasagittal cut exposes the lateral ventricle and the temporal horn simultaneously. The *white circle* marks the position of the ascending M1 division of the middle cerebral artery. One *blue line* above M1 marks the frontobasal disconnection leading from the tip of the frontal horn to the base of the frontal lobe. The other *line* marks the transection of the temporal stem and disconnection of the amygdaloid body leading from the choroidal point to the arachnoid parallel to the ascending M1 down to the uncus. The *arrow* marks the choroidal point, which corresponds to the end of the choroidal fissure (i.e., the terminal end of the attachment of the choroid plexus). Anterior to this point, the entorhinal cortex is located between the head of the hippocampus and the amygdaloid body. **B,** Paramesial transection of the callosal fibers within the lateral ventricle is shown by the *line* as a prolongation of the frontobasal disconnection. **C,** The different types of disconnection lines shown in one picture: the *blue line* is the paramedian callosal transection, the *anterior red line* represents the frontobasal disconnection, the *yellow line* represents the temporomesial disconnection anterior to the choroidal point, the *posterior red line* shows the occipitotemporomesial disconnection through the trigonal area, and the *dotted red line* shows the temporomesial disconnection along the choroidal fissure, used if one chooses not to resect the hippocampus. The *green oval* shows resection of the hippocampus, which is frequently done to obtain a good specimen. *(Copyright J. Schramm, with permission.)*

nection in the temporal horn (Fig. 66-E4). Details of this procedure have been described previously.[23,39,40]

A reduction in blood loss, reduced need for blood transfusion, and a decrease in operative time have been demonstrated with this procedure, as well as with related peri-insular hemispherotomy techniques, albeit to a lesser extent.[4,18,41] This procedure is suitable for patients with hemispheric atrophy and is particularly quick and well suited for patients with porencephalic cysts or with very marked atrophy of the insula–basal ganglia complex (Figs. 66-E5 and 66-E6). This technique may be used in patients with hemispheric cortical dysplasia, lissencephaly, and HME, but with extensive HME, it is advisable to combine it with opercular resection or temporal lobe resection to gain space for postoperative swelling and better transinsular exposure of the ventricles. The use of neuronavigation is advisable to correctly place the craniotomy so that the upper border is at the level of the corpus callosum and the lower border is 0.5 cm below the sylvian fissure. The ascending M1 segment should be visualized at the anterior border (see Fig. 66-3).

The disadvantages of this technique include its limitations in patients with HME, unless it is combined with a suprasylvian window (as in 7 of 9 of our own patients) (Figs. 66-6 and 66-E7). A certain risk for incomplete disconnection exists, which may either be true incomplete disconnection or occur as a result of a too anteriorly placed disconnection line frontobasally (i.e., not parallel to the M1, A1 segment but anterior to it). Hydrocephalus can develop postoperatively, as is the case with all transventricular disconnection procedures (hydrocephalus occurred in 4 of 56 of our patients and was treated with two shunts and two ventriculocisternostomies, equivalent to a shunt rate of 3.6%). Shunt rates of 8%, 16%, 19%, and 23% were seen with related procedures,[22,42-44] but even higher rates are reported for the older techniques. The pros and cons of this and related approaches have recently been discussed.[41,45-47]

Vertical Parasagittal Hemispherotomy

This technique differs from the perisylvian and transsylvian approaches in two main aspects as described in detail by Delalande and coauthors[22] and may descriptively be called a *dorsal transcortical subinsular hemispherotomy:*

1. Much less brain resection and more disconnection
2. Use of a vertical approach through a parasagittal craniotomy

The approach is characterized by five features:

1. A parasagittal frontal craniotomy approximately 3 × 5 cm, one third anterior and two thirds posterior to the coronal suture
2. Transcortical access to the lateral ventricle via limited cortical resection to enable access to the foramen of Monro and the posterior thalamic region
3. Paramedian callosotomy, including transection of the posterior column of the fornix
4. Lateral transection between the thalamus and the striatum starting in the lateral ventricle and reaching down to the temporal horn
5. After completion of the anterior callosotomy, resection of the posterior part of the gyrus rectus and extension of the transection line laterally so that the head of the caput caudatum meets the substriatal transection line lateral to the thalamus

To date, reports of this procedure have been confined to one center,[48] but the series consists of 83 children and has a seizure-free outcome rate of 74%. The transfusion rate was just 8%, and the shunt rate was 16%. The insular cortex is automatically disconnected. Shunt implantation was most often required in a large subgroup of patients with HME, thus demonstrating that the

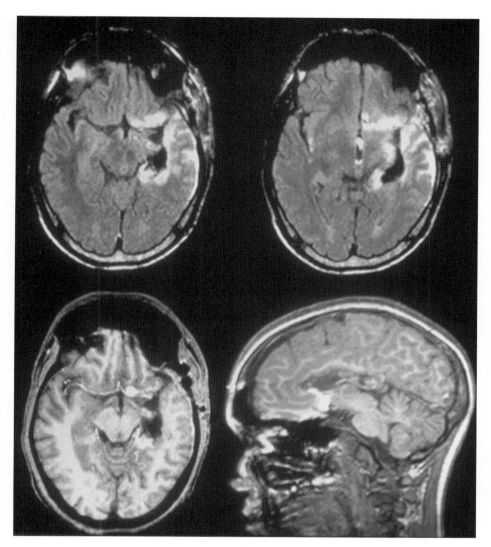

FIGURE 66-5 Early postoperative magnetic resonance images of transsylvian keyhole hemispheric deafferentation with resection of the insular cortex show an ideal position of the frontobasal disconnection along the course of A1 and M1. *(Reproduced from Schramm J. Hemispherectomy techniques. Neurosurg Clin N Am. 2001;37:113.)*

underlying pathologic condition influences the rate of this complication. The advantages of this procedure include a low level of blood loss that necessitated transfusion in just 8% of cases. Data on operative time are not available. Another advantage is preservation of superficially located large vessels, including the middle cerebral artery. A possible disadvantage is the long distance that must be traversed between the cortical surface to the temporal horn and the frontal lobe base.

Combined Resection-Deafferentation Techniques

The *peri-insular hemispherotomy techniques* combine moderate to limited resection of brain tissue with disconnections. The group consists of hemispheric deafferentation through Schramm's peri-insular transcortical approach,[17,21] Villemure's peri-insular hemispherotomy,[19] and the Japanese peri-insular modification.[18] These three procedures involve a certain degree of brain resection, disconnection from the contralateral hemisphere via transventricular-paramedian callosotomy, transection of the long tract fibers around the insula, and disconnection of the frontal and

parieto-occipital lobes (see Fig. 66-2). These techniques may be considered progressive variants of Rasmussen's functional hemispherectomy because they involve removal of either a peri-insular tissue block or the temporal lobe. The new features common to all these procedures are the transventricular approach to the callosal fibers, transventricular disconnection of the frontal and parieto-occipital lobes, and a more limited craniotomy and exposure. When compared with the older anatomic resections, the incidence of hydrocephalus and severe intraoperative complications is decreased. Operative times are shorter and blood loss is less than with the anatomic hemispherectomy techniques, but possibly higher than with the two deafferentation procedures described by Schramm and Delalande.

In the perisylvian window technique, the frontoparietal and temporal opercula are resected (see Fig. 66-E2D), including parts of the corona radiata above the basal ganglia block, to create a large opening in the lateral ventricle and the temporal horn. Parts of the insular cortex are removed during this approach.[19,49] In the Japanese modification, the insular cortex is partly removed and the inferior portion is disconnected when the dissection is directed downward to the mesiotemporal lobe at the bottom of

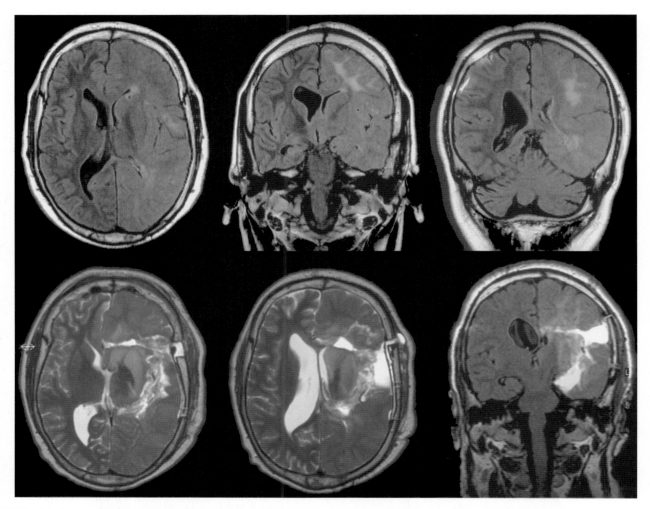

FIGURE 66-6 Preoperative (*upper row*) and postoperative (*lower row*) magnetic resonance images from a 29-year-old with hemimegalencephaly. The small opercular window and the limited temporomesial resection, as well as the disconnection lines reaching the midline anteriorly, posteriorly, and superiorly, are shown clearly. (*Copyright J. Schramm, with permission.*)

the peri-insular window.[18] The temporomesial structures are resected. In the peri-insular transcortical disconnection procedure,[17] the opercula are not resected, but the ventricle is opened through a disconnection line from the surface into the lateral ventricles through the opercular tissue. The insular cortex is left behind, but this procedure could be combined with a temporal lobectomy.

It remains unclear whether removal of the insular cortex is necessary. Residual insular cortex may be a source of persistent postoperative seizures, but not all surgical techniques include systematic removal or disconnection of the insular cortex. Some surgeons make an intraoperative decision based on electrocorticography and remove the cortex if abnormal spiking is present.[50] In a large multicenter case collection ($N > 300$)[28] and in an older series,[6] no correlation was found between the amount of residual insular cortex after surgery and the degree of seizure control. In a recent study of 28 patients, the presence of residual insular cortex was positively correlated with persistent seizures.[51] However, this study was based on a small sample size. For several years our policy has been to routinely remove the insular cortex by subpial suction during the transsylvian keyhole approach (see Figs. 66-6 and 66-E7).

Alternative Classic Techniques

Four techniques based on extensive resection are described briefly for comparison purposes. *Anatomic hemispherectomy* involves a large hemicraniotomy, clipping of the anterior and middle cerebral arteries and parasagittal veins, and stepwise or en bloc removal of the hemisphere. Peacock and colleagues combined anatomic hemispherectomy with routine implantation of a shunt into the cavity after a 5-day period of subdural drainage after the operation.[52] The *Oxford modification* is based on anatomic hemispherectomy but is supplemented by a muscle plug in the foramen of Monro and by folding down the convexity dura onto the falx and the basal ganglia and into the temporal cavity.[1] This technique does not prevent problems resulting from the large exposure and long duration of surgery, such as blood loss, but it seems to lead to a lower rate of hydrocephalus. *Hemidecortication* or *hemicorticectomy* procedures rely on the principle that all seizures originate from the cortex and thus only the ictogenic cortex needs to be removed.[14-16] Opening of the ventricle is avoided except at the temporal tip, where one has to enter to remove the hippocampus. No callosotomy is required, but extensive brain exposure is necessary. This technique is associated with a number of possible untoward effects linked to the large exposure, including severe hypotension, blood loss, and prolonged operative times. The technique also risks damaging the arachnoid granulations at the midline, which may result in impairment of CSF resorption. Hydrocephalus rates of 20% and 32% have been reported.[53,54] There is also a risk of the surgeon becoming spatially disoriented, particularly in the setting of holohemispheric dysplasia or HME.

POSTOPERATIVE MANAGEMENT

All patients spend the first night in intensive care, but small infants and those with HME may be kept in intensive care somewhat longer. The usual blood and neurological parameters are recorded, output is monitored, and if necessary, blood components are replaced. Any postoperative seizures need to be compared carefully for similarities to or differences in preoperative seizure types. Typically, mild to moderate increases in temperature are observed that last for a few days up to 10 days, and they are thought to be caused by contamination of CSF by material entering the ventricles during surgery. Anticonvulsive medications in the postoperative period remain the same as preoperatively. More than five acute postoperative seizures (in the first 10 days) have been shown to be associated with worse seizure control at 0.5 and 1 year after surgery.[55] Early physiotherapy is mandatory, and if necessary, transfer to a rehabilitation center is arranged. Early postoperative MRI using the blood along the disconnection slit as contrast medium is useful to prove the completeness of disconnection (see Fig. 66-4).

CHOICE OF PROCEDURE

Provided that the various types of procedures are performed completely and correctly, the chance for freedom from seizures should be similar. Regardless of procedure type, it is safer to remove or disconnect the insular cortex. In a setting in which seizure-free outcome rates are comparable for different procedures, safety considerations and differences in complication risk profiles play a dominant role in surgical decision making. There is considerable published evidence demonstrating that seizure outcomes are comparable for disconnective procedures and functional or anatomic hemispherectomy. Functional hemispherectomy techniques are associated with reduced risk for late complications and a somewhat lower rate of intraoperative complications than anatomic hemispherectomy is. For these reasons we prefer to use functional hemispherectomy techniques. There is increasing evidence that the perisylvian hemispherotomy method and associated disconnection techniques (transsylvian keyhole and vertical parasagittal hemispherotomies) are associated with an even lower rate of complications, shorter operative time, and less blood loss than the older methods. It is critically important, however, that surgeons be comfortable and knowledgable about the technique that they elect to use.

The choice of appropriate surgical procedure for HME is more difficult. Because of the malformed anatomy and distorted anatomic structures, it is possible for the surgeon to become spatially disoriented (Fig. 66-E8). Abnormal vascularization patterns are frequently encountered, particularly large atypical veins within the white matter. It is advisable to create a larger craniotomy that is at least large enough to expose the entire insular cistern through an opercular resection. For HHE, a deafferentation procedure should be used that provides full exposure and visualization of the opened ventricular system, such as the hemispheric window technique (see Fig. 66-5).

OUTCOME

Seizure-free rates range from mid 50% to mid 80%. They were 61.1% for anatomic hemispherectomy and 63.2% for functional hemispherectomy in a 1997 review from 13 centers for cases done between 1980 and 1990.[56] More recent series report seizure outcome rates ranging from 75% to 80%.[27,41,47,51,57-59] For some causes, seizure-free rates may be better. Patients with SWS tend to have better outcomes,[26] as do those with Rasmussen's encephalitis. Patients with cortical dysplasia do less well, and the poorest outcomes are reported in the setting of HME,[34,60-62] although some series describe more favorable outcomes.[57] Interpretation of outcome data per center needs to be done carefully because cause influences outcome and the composition of the patient groups varies considerably from center to center. A high proportion of HME and cortical dysplasia cases will lead to overall lower seizure-free rates. Early outcome must be differentiated from late follow-up results. Long-term stable good seizure control outcomes have been reported from some centers at follow-up periods as long as 15 years,[22,63] but in another large patient cohort, seizure-free rates of 78% at 6 months dropped to 70% at 2 years and just 58% at 5 years.[64]

In view of all the factors influencing outcome, it is difficult to ascertain with certainty whether one of the older more resective techniques, one of the newer perisylvian techniques, or the primarily disconnective procedures lead to consistently better results. It is safe to assume that in principle all techniques should achieve similar seizure-free rates, although in Holthausen and colleagues' review of 328 cases from 12 centers, differences in seizure-free outcome between operative techniques were described, with hemispherotomy techniques showing better results (85.7% class I) than Rasmussen's technique (66.1% class I) or the hemicorticectomy-hemidecortication techniques (60.7% class I).[28] The high number of 12 contributing centers and the variable mixture of causes do not allow one to conclude that hemispherotomies are truly associated with better outcomes. In the University of California, Los Angeles, series, seizure control was not statistically different for the various techniques used in 115 cases.[4] In the Bonn series, the transsylvian keyhole technique and Rasmussen's technique both had greater than 80% class I outcomes.

There is incontrovertible evidence, however, that the cause of the seizure disorder influences outcome. Many series describe poorer seizure-free rates for congenital malformative diseases, with HME cases showing even poorer outcome than other migration disorders (polymicrogyria, cortical dysplasias). Patients with dysplasia and HME do less well with all the surgical techniques used.[28,40] Surgery for HME carries a higher risk of bleeding, a higher shunt rate, a higher rate of incomplete disconnection, and the lowest success rates among the causes typical for this procedure. Acute postoperative seizures were seen in 22.6% of 114 patients and were associated with a worse short-term seizure outcome.[55] The significance of contralateral spikes over the good hemisphere remained unclear in Holthausen and associates' large case collection.[28] Seizure-free rates of 80% to 100% have been reported for SWS.[22,24,25,27,28,58] Results for Rasmussen's encephalitis have been reported at 77% in a large series of 83 patients.[28]

Cognition and Behavior

Patients with a typical cause and indication for hemispheric deafferentation often have low intelligence or mental retardation. This may be combined in a smaller subgroup with behavioral problems such as aggression or temper tantrums.[12] Hemispheric surgery in this pediatric patient population does not result in a decline in health-related quality of life.[65] The postoperative pattern of cognition and behavioral changes observed in patients is influenced by whether the patient is seizure free after surgery and the nature of the underlying pathologic process. Seizure-free patients tend to do better and dysplasia patients tend to do worse.[65-67] The necessity of continuing antiepileptic drug use appears to have a negative impact on quality of life in the pediatric population, although having undergone a hemispherotomy procedure predicted fewer epilepsy-related limitations.[65] In an unpublished analysis of 46 of our own cases, over half the patients were reported by parents to have improved behavior, whereas only 7% of patients had a deterioration in behavior. IQ may improve in a proportion of cases but may decline in a smaller subgroup.[3] Schooling is frequently improved, but this depends highly on preoperative IQ levels.

Complications

Incomplete disconnections can be unintentional and unrecognized in the operating room and are usually listed as a postoperative complication. They can occur not only with the pure disconnection technique but also with Rasmussen's technique.[52] Incomplete disconnection has been described as a cause of persisting seizures in up to 30% of patients[18,28,42-44,52,68-70] and may be classified as a complication. Other complications may develop intraoperatively, in the postoperative period, and late.

Typical examples of *intraoperative complications* are marked blood loss, electrolyte disturbances, and coagulation disorders resulting from excessive blood loss or blood replacement therapy. Hypovolemia with bradycardia, hypothermia, and in extreme situations, even cardiac arrest may occur. *Early postoperative complications* include electrolyte disturbances, diabetes insipidus, and swelling of the contralateral healthy hemisphere. Transient rises in temperature for a few days and even to up 10 days are typical and must be differentiated from true bacterial meningitis. Subdural hygroma or acute hematomas (epidural and subdural) may occur. Expected losses in motor function, speech, or visual fields are accepted and expected side effects, not complications. Death in the postoperative period in historical series was observed in 4% to 6% of cases, is reduced to around 2% with functional hemisperectomy techniques, and in modern series is reported to be between 1% and 2%.[22,28,41,69,71-73] Classic bone flap infections do seem to appear a bit more frequently with larger craniotomies and types of procedures requiring longer operative time.[13,74] Hydrocephalus may develop in the early postoperative period, as well as later. SCH has not yet been reported with the modern perisylvian or disconnection techniques, but the observation period for these more modern techniques is still less than 20 years, so no definite judgement is possible at this time. A certain incidence of hydrocephalus appears to be unavoidable, as with all procedures that involve opening the ventricular system. Shunt rates between 8% and 23% have been described.[13,22,42-44,74] Recently, some forms of hydrocephalus have been treated effectively by cisternostomy, so shunt rates may be a bit lower than hydrocephalus rates. Shunt rates after functional hemisperectomy or disconnection procedures tend to increase with removal of a larger volume of brain tissue.[48,51] The underlying cause also influences the rate at which shunts are required, with the highest frequency observed in patients with HME.[18,22,48]

Late complications include bone flap infections and hydrocephalus requiring shunting. Late reappearance of seizures has been observed with variable frequency, rarely in some groups[22] and more frequently in other series.[4,64] Late death may also occur because of persistent or reappearing seizures.

CONCLUSION

Surgery for unihemispheric drug-resistant epilepsy has evolved considerably over the past 15 years. The key element in this change was to replace resective steps with disconnective steps, which culminated in nearly exclusive disconnective surgery. These techniques are successful and less demanding on the patient because of decreased operative time and less blood loss. Outcomes are influenced more by the cause of the seizure disorder and less by the specific technique used. Hemispherotomies and hemispheric deafferentations continue to be some of the most successful types of epilepsy surgery.

SUGGESTED READINGS

Adams CB. Hemispherectomy—a modification. *J Neurol Neurosurg Psychiatry.* 1983;46:617.

Bien CG, Urbach H, Deckert M, et al. Diagnosis and staging of Rasmussen's encephalitis by serial MRI and histopathology. *Neurology.* 2002;58:250.

Carson BS, Javedan SP, Freeman JM, et al. Hemispherectomy: a hemidecortication approach and review of 52 cases. *J Neurosurg.* 1996;84:903.

Cook SW, Nguyen ST, Hu B, et al. Cerebral hemispherectomy in pediatric patients with epilepsy: comparison of three techniques by pathological substrate in 115 patients. *J Neurosurg.* 2004;100:125.

Delalande O, Bulteau C, Dellatolas G, et al. Vertical parasagittal hemispherotomy: surgical procedures and clinical long-term outcomes in a population of 83 children. *Neurosurgery.* 2007;60:ONS19.

Ellenbogen RG, Cline MJ. Hemispherectomy: historical perspective and current surgical overview. In: Miller JW, Silbergeld DL, eds. *Epilepsy Surgery: Principles and Controversies.* New York: Taylor & Francis; 2006:563.

Gonzalez-Martinez JA, Gupta A, Kotagal P, et al. Hemispherectomy for catastrophic epilepsy in infants. *Epilepsia.* 2005;46:1518.

Griffiths SY, Sherman EM, Slick DJ, et al. Postsurgical health-related quality of life (HRQOL) in children following hemispherectomy for intractable epilepsy. *Epilepsia.* 2007;48:564.

Holthausen H, May T, Adams C. Seizures post hemispherectomy. In: Tuxhorn I, Holthausen H, Boenigk H, eds. *Paediatric Epilepsy Syndromes and their Surgical Treatment.* London: John Libbey; 1997.

Jonas R, Nguyen S, Hu B, et al. Cerebral hemispherectomy: hospital course, seizure, developmental, language, and motor outcomes. *Neurology.* 2004;62:1712.

Kestle J, Connolly M, Cochrane D. Pediatric peri-insular hemispherotomy. *Pediatr Neurosurg.* 2000;32:44.

Kossoff EH, Vining EP, Pyzik PL, et al. The postoperative course and management of 106 hemidecortications. *Pediatr Neurosurg.* 2002;37:298.

Peacock WJ, Wehby-Grant MC, Shields WD, et al. Hemispherectomy for intractable seizures in children: a report of 58 cases. *Childs Nerv Syst.* 1996;12:376.

Pulsifer MB, Brandt J, Salorio CF, et al. The cognitive outcome of hemispherectomy in 71 children. *Epilepsia.* 2004;45:243.

Rasmussen T. Hemispherectomy for seizures revisited. *Can J Neurol Sci.* 1983;10:71.

Schramm J. Hemispherectomy techniques. *Neurosurg Clin N Am.* 2002;13:113.

Schramm J, Behrens E, Entzian W. Hemispherical deafferentation: an alternative to functional hemispherectomy. *Neurosurgery.* 1995;36:509.

Schramm J, Kral T, Clusmann H. Transsylvian keyhole functional hemispherectomy. *Neurosurgery.* 2001;49:891.

Shimizu H, Maehara T. Modification of peri-insular hemispherotomy and surgical results. *Neurosurgery.* 2000;47:367.

Smith JR, Lee MR. Functional hemispherectomy. In: *American Association of Neurological Surgeons. Neurosurgery Operative Atlas,* 2nd ed. Vol 5. 1996:155.

Tinuper P, Andermann F, Villemure JG, et al. Functional hemispherectomy for treatment of epilepsy associated with hemiplegia: rationale, indications, results, and comparison with callosotomy. *Ann Neurol.* 1988;24:27.

Villemure JG, Daniel RT. Peri-insular hemispherotomy in paediatric epilepsy. *Childs Nerv Syst.* 2006;22:967.

Villemure JG, Mascott CR. Peri-insular hemispherotomy: surgical principles and anatomy. *Neurosurgery.* 1995;37:975.

Wilson PJ. Cerebral hemispherectomy for infantile hemiplegia. A report of 50 cases. *Brain.* 1970;93:147.

Winston KR, Welch K, Adler JR, et al. Cerebral hemicorticectomy for epilepsy. *J Neurosurg.* 1992;77:889.

Full references can be found on Expert Consult @ www.expertconsult.com

CHAPTER 67

Vagus Nerve Stimulation for Intractable Epilepsy

James E. Baumgartner ■ Gretchen K. Von Allmen

Since receiving Food and Drug Administration (FDA) approval in 1997, vagus nerve stimulation (VNS) delivered via the implantable Neurocybernetic Prosthesis (NCP) from Cyberonics, Inc. (Houston, Tex) has become an established method for treating patients with medically refractory seizures. The NCP delivers intermittent afferent electrical stimulation to the left cervical vagus nerve trunk, which secondarily transmits impulses that exert widespread effects on neuronal excitability throughout the central nervous system.[1] More than 46,000 NCP devices have been implanted to treat epilepsy worldwide. Since introduction of the original model 100 generator, the device has been made progressively smaller and easier to implant and program (Figs. 67-1 and 67-2).

BRIEF HISTORY

Experimental use of VNS to treat epilepsy can be traced to the 1880s.[2] In 1938, Bailey and Bremmer demonstrated desynchronization of orbital cortex activity with the use of VNS in a cat model.[3] Zanchetti and colleagues showed that intermittent VNS reduced or eliminated interictal epileptic events that were chemically induced in the frontal cortex of cats.[4] In 1980, Radna and MacLean found that VNS caused changes in single-unit activity within the basal limbic structures of squirrel monkeys.[5] Based on these experiments, Zabara in 1985 proposed that if VNS could desynchronize electroencephalographic activity, it might be effective in attenuating epileptic seizures.[6] Subsequent animal work by Zabara[7] and others[8-10] supported Zabara's hypothesis and allowed clinical trials to be performed in humans.

In 1987, a company—Cyberonics, Inc. (Houston, Tex)—was founded to develop VNS therapy in humans. In 1988, the first epileptic patient to undergo implantation of a VNS therapy device became seizure free.[11] Five acute-phase clinical studies analyzing the safety and effectiveness of VNS therapy followed[12-16] and culminated in FDA approval of VNS therapy "for use as an adjunctive therapy in reducing the frequency of seizures in adults and adolescents over 12 years of age with partial onset seizures that are refractory to antiepileptic medications."[17]

Cyberonics, Inc., created a long-term outcome registry that compiled information on patients receiving VNS therapy. The registry opened on November 7, 1997, and closed on April 1, 2003. Participation was voluntary and data were provided by participating physicians. Data were not available for all patients at all time intervals. Median reductions in seizure activity were 46% (n = 4448) at 3 months, 57% (n = 2696) at 1 year, and 63% (n = 1114) after 2 years of VNS therapy.[18] Overall, studies report that in responding patients, the effectiveness of VNS steadily improves over the first 3 to 12 months of stimulation. Many subsequent long-term studies have been published supporting the efficacy, durability, and cost-effectiveness of VNS therapy for epilepsy.[19-33] In addition to refractory partial-onset seizures, VNS is used, off-label, to treat children younger than 12 years with generalized epilepsy and as an adjunct to other surgical procedures (when they are insufficient to control seizure activity).[34-37]

PATIENT SELECTION

Before considering VNS therapy, patients with medically refractory epilepsy should undergo evaluation at a comprehensive epilepsy center. The evaluation usually includes a complete history and physical examination, video electroencephalographic monitoring to obtain ictal and interictal data, neuropsychological testing, and anatomic and functional neuroimaging. Antiepileptic medications are optimized by an epileptologist, and surgery is considered only after failure of two or more adequate antiepileptic drug trials and the completion of a phase I evaluation. VNS is generally considered palliative because it is rarely curative. Surgical resection of the epileptogenic zone, when indicated, typically achieves higher rates of seizure control. Therefore, VNS is usually offered to those who are not candidates for potentially more effective resective surgical procedures or for patients who refuse resective surgery. In addition, with current clinical data, it is not possible to predict which patients will achieve a favorable response to VNS therapy or in what way VNS therapy will affect their seizure control. VNS therapy, when effective, can cause decreases in seizure duration, frequency, or intensity and may make it feasible to decrease the amount of antiepileptic medications needed to achieve adequate seizure control.

Once identified as candidates for the device, patients should be counseled about the potential risks and benefits of VNS therapy, as well as the risks and benefits of other therapeutic options, including resective or other surgeries, further medication trials, and a ketogenic diet (in the case of eligible children). It is also important to describe the long-term outcome and seizure control data that are available, including the possible length of time needed to achieve full efficacy of the device. This approach will result in more realistic expectations and better compliance.

ANATOMIC CONSIDERATIONS

The majority of vagal nerve fibers are general somatic and special visceral afferents projecting to the brain, along with efferent projections to the larynx and parasympathetic projections to the heart, lungs, and gastrointestinal tract. The VNS electrode is applied to the midcervical portion of the vagal nerve, which is relatively free of branches. The upper cervical vagal nerve gives off branches to the pharynx, carotid sinus, and superior and inferior cardiac branches leading to the cardiac plexus. Studies in dogs suggest that the right vagal nerve preferentially innervates the sinoatrial node of the heart whereas the left vagal nerve projects to the atrioventricular node. Accordingly, the NCP electrode is usually applied to the left vagal nerve to avoid stimulation-related asystole or bradycardia.[38] A small series of right-sided VNS implants in children, which included Holter monitoring of patients after surgery, failed to demonstrate any changes in heart rate with stimulation.[39]

The recurrent laryngeal nerve travels with the main vagal nerve trunk and then branches caudally at the aortic arch before ascending in the tracheoesophageal groove. As a result, changes

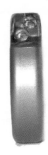
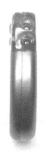
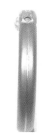

Model 100
Thickness: 0.52" (13.2 mm)
Volume: 31 cc

Model 101
0.41" (10.3 mm)
26 cc

Model 102/102R
0.27" (6.9 mm)
14/16 cc

Model 103/104
0.27" (6.9 mm)
8 cc/10 cc

FIGURE 67-1 Side views of vagal nerve stimulation generators showing a progressive decrease in size over time, from the original model 100 generator (1994) to the current model 103/104 generator (2007).

in the character and quality of voice are common during nerve stimulation in the early period after NCP implantation. The voice changes usually resolve within weeks of surgery.

Other nerves in the region of the vagal nerve can be affected at surgery. The phrenic nerve lies deep to the carotid sheath, and unilateral paralysis of the left hemidiaphragm has been reported during periods of VNS. Hypoglossal and facial nerve fibers are found well above the midcervical trunk, but injuries to both have been reported after VNS implantation. The sympathetic trunk runs deep to the common carotid artery and provides fibers that ascend with the internal carotid artery. There is a report of Horner's syndrome developing after VNS implantation, presumably caused by injury to the sympathetic plexus or the fibers along the internal carotid.[40]

NEUROCYBERNETIC PROSTHESIS

The NCP has two implantable components: a generator and a stimulating electrode (Figs. 67-3 to 67-6; also see Figs. 67-1 and 67-2). The generator consists of an epoxy resin header with a receptacle for the connector pin or pins from the electrode and a titanium module containing a lithium battery and the generator. The electrode is secured to the connector pin receptacle with a set screw or screws tightened with a hexagonal torque wrench included with the generator packaging. The generator contains an antenna that receives radiofrequency signals from the pro-

gramming telemetry wand and transfers them to a microprocessor that regulates the electrical output of the pulse generator. The generator delivers a charge-balanced waveform characterized by five programmable parameters: output current, signal frequency, pulse width, signal-on time, and signal-off time. Higher stimulation frequencies and longer signal-on times result in a shorter duration of battery service life. The NCP electrode is insulated with a silicone elastomer and can be implanted safely in patients with latex allergies. One end of the lead has a connector pin or pins that insert directly into the generator (see Figs. 67-3 and 67-4); the other end has an electrode array consisting of three discrete helical coils that are placed around the vagal nerve (see Figs. 67-5 and 67-6). The middle and distal coils are the positive and negative electrodes, respectively, and the most proximal coil serves as an anchoring tether to prevent excessive force from being transmitted to the electrodes when patients turn their neck. Each electrode helix contains three loops. Embedded inside the middle turn is a platinum coil that is welded to the lead wire. Suture tails extending from either end of the helix allow manipulation of the coils without injuring the platinum contacts. A silicone electrode collar is included with the electrode and is used to anchor the electrode to the soft tissue of the neck, proximal to the helical coils. The portion of the electrode between the electrode collar and the inferior helix creates a "strain release loop" that further protects the vagal nerve from unwanted traction. A handheld NCP magnet performs several functions. When passed over the chest wall overlying the generator, it triggers stimulation superimposed on the baseline output. This on-demand stimulation can be performed by a patient or caregiver at the onset of an aura and can sometimes diminish or abort an impending seizure. In addition, if the NCP appears to be malfunctioning or if the patient wishes to terminate stimulation for any other reason, the system can be turned off by placing the magnet over the generator site continuously.

The NCP has undergone a series of revisions since introduction of the model 100 (see Fig. 67-1). The original model 100 and the second-generation model 101 were used with a bipolar helical lead. The third- and fourth-generation models (102 and 103) incorporated a monopolar lead. Generators 102R and 104 have bipolar lead acceptors, so revision of models 100 and 101 (with bipolar electrodes) can be performed without replacing the electrodes (see Figs. 67-3 and 67-4). The original programming hardware included a programming wand attached to a laptop computer. The laptop has been replaced with a personal digital assistant (PDA) and a similar programming wand (Fig. 67-7). Typically, we turn the generator on at low stimulation settings in the operating room at the time of implantation. The device is turned up sequentially over a period of several weeks until the

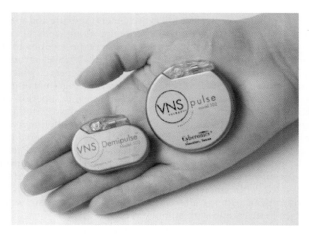

FIGURE 67-2 A model 103 generator (*left*) next to a model 102 generator (*right*) demonstrating decreased size.

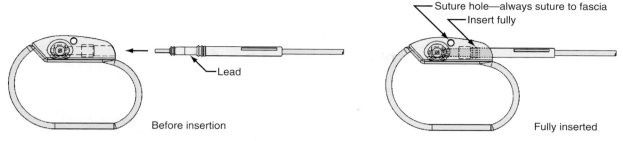

FIGURE 67-3 Diagram demonstrating connection of a monopolar electrode to a monopolar vagal nerve stimulation generator.

desired stimulation parameters are reached, and then adjustments can be made every few months as needed.

With the early generators and diagnostic software, it was difficult to estimate time until the end of service of the battery. This is important because replacement of the generator before the battery stops working allows the stimulation parameters to continue unchanged without an interruption in VNS therapy. Replacement of the generator after the battery's end of service requires that the stimulation parameters be set at minimal settings and be slowly increased as though the VNS were newly implanted. With the new PDA software, an estimate of remaining battery lifetime is possible, thereby allowing improved planning for replacement of the generator before the end of service of the battery.

OPERATIVE PROCEDURE

General Considerations

Although implantation of the NCP system can be performed by any surgeon familiar with the anatomy and exposure of the carotid sheath, neurosurgeons active in comprehensive epilepsy programs are ideal NCP implanters. As discussed earlier, VNS therapy should be considered only for refractory epilepsy patients who have undergone evaluation through a comprehensive epilepsy program and who are not candidates for resective epilepsy surgery.

The operation is typically performed with the patient under general anesthesia. Patients receive prophylactic intravenous antibiotics preoperatively and for 24 hours postoperatively. Patients are admitted for 23 hours and observed for vocal cord dysfunction, dysphagia, respiratory compromise, or seizures induced by anesthesia. It is our practice to turn the generator on while the patient is under general anesthesia and to turn the device up on the day after surgery, before discharge.

Operative Technique

After endotracheal intubation, the operating table is rotated 90 degrees clockwise from the anesthesia setup to expose the left side of the neck and chest to the surgeon. The patient's head is supported on a horseshoe headrest, and a small roll is placed between the patient's shoulder blades. The neck is slightly extended. After the preparation has been completed, attention is directed to the patient's neck. At the midbody of the sterno-cleidomastoid (SCM), a horizontal incision measuring 2 to 3 cm in length is created sharply. Dissection is continued sharply through the platysma and then bluntly along the medial border of the SCM to the carotid sheath. Soft tissues are retracted with vein retractors. At the level of the thyroid cartilage, the carotid sheath is opened bluntly and the vagal nerve is found deep to the internal jugular vein and lateral to the common carotid artery. The vagal nerve is exposed by blunt dissection and mobilized over a length of approximately 4 cm. The nerve is then gently retracted superiorly with a vessel loop. The inferior two electrode helices are placed around the nerve. The nerve is then gently retracted inferiorly with the vessel loop, and the superior helix is placed around the nerve. The vessel loop is divided at the level of the skin and gently withdrawn while applying gentle digital compression of the helical electrodes and vagal nerve to prevent displacement of the electrode. Next, the strain release electrode loop is created by anchoring the electrode to the mesial border of the SCM with an electrode collar, with roughly 6 cm of electrode between the inferior helix and the electrode collar.

Attention is then directed to the chest wall overlying the lateral border of the pectoralis major (PM). An incision overlying and running parallel to the PM and measuring between 2 and 1.5 cm (models 103 and 104) to 6 cm (models 100 to 102) is created sharply. Dissection is then continued through soft tissue to the lateral border of the PM. A plane is developed between the PM and pectoralis minor with a blunt technique. Once a pocket large enough to accommodate the generator has been created between the two muscles, a NCP tunneling device is used

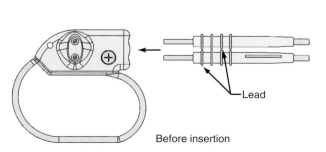
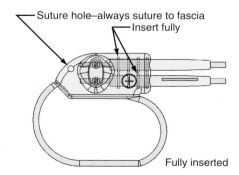

FIGURE 67-4 Diagram demonstrating connection of a bipolar electrode to a bipolar vagal nerve stimulation generator. Note that the positive lead is inserted into the inferior pin site. The positive electrode pin has a white mark.

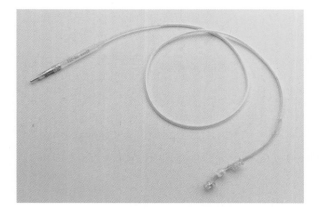

FIGURE 67-5 Monopolar vagal nerve stimulation electrode.

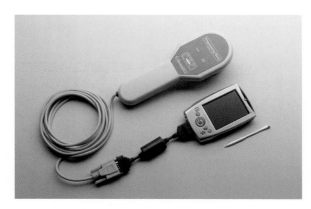

FIGURE 67-7 Vagal nerve stimulation programming wand and personal digital assistant–type programming computer.

to create a track from the chest wall pocket to the neck incision (Fig. 67-8). Tunneling can be performed in either direction (chest to neck or neck to chest). Care must be taken to avoid injuring the soft tissues of the neck with the tunneling device. The tunneling device has a bullet tip that screws onto the end of the metal shaft of the tunneling device and holds a clear hollow sheath around the tunneler. Once the track has been created, the bullet tip is removed and the shaft withdrawn from the clear sheath. The free end of the electrode is then placed inside the sheath and drawn, with the sheath, from the neck incision to the chest wall incision. The electrode is then removed from the sheath. The generator is next brought into the field and attached to the electrode with the set screw or screws and torque wrench. The generator is then introduced into the chest wall pocket while keeping the electrode deep to the generator. An anchoring stitch can be passed through the generator header and pectoralis to secure the generator to the chest wall. The platysma and subcutaneous structures of the neck, as well as the pectoralis fascia and soft tissues of the chest, are closed in layers. Next, the programming wand is introduced into the operative field within a sterile drape. Electrodiagnostic testing is performed by the neurologist with the PDA. The draped programming wand is held over the generator during this process. Anesthesia personnel are alerted before performing the lead test portion of the electrodiagnostics and asked to carefully monitor the patient's vital signs during this test. Rarely, profound bradycardia/asystole necessitating the use of atropine has been reported during the lead test. If the diagnostic parameters are unsatisfactory, the neck wound is reopened to confirm or adjust electrode placement, and the chest wall wound is reopened to confirm good contact between the electrode and generator. The diagnostics are repeated until satisfac-

tory data are obtained. The NCP is then programmed by the neurologist to the initial stimulating parameters with the PDA. Closure of the neck and chest wall incisions is completed with Dermabond.

Generator Revision

As discussed earlier, it is desirable to replace the generator before the end of battery service. The patient is returned to the operating room where general endotracheal anesthesia is induced and antibiotics are administered. The operating table is rotated clockwise away from the anesthesiologist, and the neck and chest are prepared, including both the chest wall and neck incisions. The chest wall incision is reopened, and dissection is carried down to the generator capsule with Bovie cautery at low-coagulation settings. Care is taken to avoid damaging the electrode, the generator is removed, and the electrode or electrodes are disconnected from the generator after the set screws have been loosened. If a monopolar electrode is present, the appropriate single-channel generator is brought into the field and attached to the electrode with the torque screwdriver. If a bipolar electrode is present, the appropriate bipolar generator is brought into the field. The positive electrode has a white mark proximal to the actual connector and is introduced into the inferior lead channel closest to the titanium portion of the generator. The set screws are tightened for both connectors with the torque screw driver. The generator is then placed into the chest wall pocket and the incision is closed in layers. The programming wand in a sterile drape is then introduced into the operative field and used for diagnostics and programming. The chest wound is closed in layers and the skin closed with Dermabond.

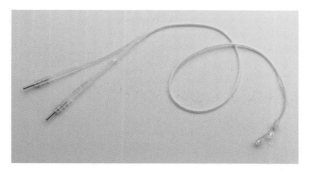

FIGURE 67-6 Bipolar vagal nerve stimulation electrode.

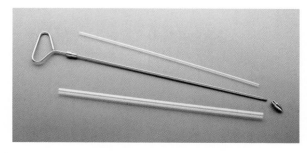

FIGURE 67-8 Disassembled vagal nerve stimulation tunneling device, with the screw on the bullet head and clear electrode sheaths.

Lead Revision

If preoperative or intraoperative electrodiagnostics suggest lead failure, the neck incision is reopened and blunt dissection is used to follow the electrode to the helical coils. Typically, the electrodes and vagal nerve are engulfed in a dense field of fibrosis. The electrodes can, however, be safely removed from around the nerve.[41]

AVOIDANCE AND MANAGEMENT OF COMPLICATIONS

Infection

In a meta-analysis of 454 patients enrolled in five controlled clinical trials, the most frequent surgical complication was generator or lead implant site infection. The overall infection rate was 2.86%, but most were successfully treated with antibiotic therapy alone. Only 1.1% required explantation of the device for infection.[16] Smyth and coauthors reported a higher rate of deep infection of 3.5% that required removal of the device in children.[42]

Vocal Cord Abnormalities

Transient vocal cord paralysis was reported in 0.7% of patients in the meta-analysis.[16] Because no preoperative or postoperative vocal cord examination was performed, this is probably an underestimate of postimplant vocal cord dysfunction. Happily, most clinically significant cases are self-limited. Smyth and associates reported one case of vocal cord paralysis and one case of fatal aspiration pneumonia in a series of 74 children after VNS implantation.[42] A prospective study in which 13 patients underwent preimplantation and postimplantation laryngeal electromyography, videolaryngoscopy, measurement of maximal phonation time, determination of the Voice Handicap Index, and Consensus Auditory-Perceptual Evaluation of Voice was published in 2006. Six of the patients had significant abnormalities in vocal fold mobility 2 weeks after surgery. Five patients had significant electromyographic abnormalities before implantation, and all 5 experienced vocal cord paresis 3 months after implantation. The data suggest that patients with preexisting vocal cord abnormalities are at greater risk for long-term vocal cord paresis after VNS implantation than those with normal preimplant vocal cord function.[43] It is our practice to refer patients with hypotonia for preoperative ear, nose, and throat evaluation to assess their vocal cord function. If vocal cord dysfunction is detected, VNS therapy is not offered to the affected patient.

Bradycardia/Asystole

Ventricular asystole occurring intraoperatively during the lead test portion of VNS electrodiagnostic testing has been observed rarely in adult patients. The estimated incidence is 1 in 800 to 1000 patients. The asystole is treated with atropine and the VNS is turned off. Some affected patients are able to tolerate VNS at very low settings initially, which are slowly turned up to therapeutic levels.[44,45]

Sleep-Related Breathing Disorder

Some children evaluated after VNS implantation are found to have decreased respiratory airflow during sleep. In one patient, obstructive sleep apnea on polysomnography had been reported to have developed but resolved with cessation of VNS stimulation.[46] This can be managed with positive pressure treatment or by varying VNS stimulation parameters. Patients with known sleep apnea should be monitored carefully after VNS implantation. If the sleep apnea worsens, positive pressure treatment or adjustment of the VNS stimulation should be pursued.

Magnetic Resonance Protocol for Patients with Vagus Nerve Stimulation Implants

Recent FDA warnings have caused many clinicians to avoid magnetic resonance imaging (MRI) in patients with VNS implants. We have developed a protocol that has been used without adverse event to image patients with VNS and that satisfies the medicolegal concerns of our hospital administration. The patient is informed of the FDA concerns, and consent for MRI with VNS is obtained. The device is turned off, and imaging is performed on a 1.5-T GE Excite MRI machine. Only the patient's brain is imaged, and the scan is performed with a GE quad head coil. Once the scan has been completed, the VNS is reprogrammed to the same settings programmed before the scan. We are working to extend this protocol to 3.0-T MRI machines.

CONCLUSION

VNS is a safe and effective method for treating some patients with medically refractory epilepsy. Off-label uses of VNS have expanded from children younger than 12 years to patients with tuberous sclerosis complex, patients who have failed resective surgery, and others. Two recent reports suggest that the earlier in the course of refractory epilepsy that the VNS is implanted, the better the outcome. Indications for VNS use are likely to continue to expand and the frequency of VNS use to increase for the foreseeable future.

SUGGESTED READINGS

Ali II, Pirzada NA, Kanjwal Y, et al. Complete heart block with ventricular asystole during left vagus nerve stimulation for epilepsy. *Epilepsy Behav*. 2004;5:768-771.

Amar AP, Apuzzo MI, Liu CY. Vagus nerve stimulation therapy after failed cranial surgery for intractable epilepsy: results from the Vagus Nerve Stimulation Therapy Outcome Registry. *Neurosurgery*. 2004;55:1086-1093.

A randomized controlled trial of chronic vagal nerve stimulation for treatment of medically intractable seizures. The Vagus Nerve Stimulation Study Group. *Neurology*. 1995;45:224-230.

DeGiorgio CM, Amar AP, Apuzzo MLJ. Vagus nerve stimulation: surgical anatomy, technique and operative complications. In: Schacter S, Schmidt D, eds. *Vagal Nerve Stimulation*. London: Dunitz; 2001:31-50.

Handforth A, Degiorgio CM, Schachter SC, et al. Vagus nerve stimulation therapy for partial onset seizures: a randomized active control trial. *Neurology*. 1998;51:48-55.

Helmers SL, Griesemer DA, Dean JC, et al. Observations on the use of vagal nerve stimulation earlier in the course of pharmacoresistant epilepsy: patients with seizures for six years or less. *Neurologist*. 2002;9:160-164.

Hsieh T, Chen M, McAfee A, et al. Sleep-related breathing disorder in children with vagal nerve stimulators. *Pediatr Neurol*. 2008;38:99-103.

MacLachlan RS. Suppression of interictal spikes and seizures by stimulation of the vagus nerve. *Epilepsia*. 1993;34:918-923.

Morris GL, Mueller WM. Vagus nerve stimulation study group E01-E05: long-term treatment with vagus nerve stimulation in patients with refractory epilepsy. *Neurology*. 1999;53:1731-1735.

Penry JK, Dean JC, Prevention of intractable partial seizures by intermittent vagal nerve stimulation in humans: preliminary results. *Epilepsia*. 1990;31(suppl 2):S40-S43.

Renfro JB, Wheless JB. Earlier use of adjunctive vagus nerve stimulation for refractory epilepsy. *Neurology*. 2002;59(suppl 4):S26-S30.

Shaw GY, Sechtem P, Searl J, et al. Predictors of laryngeal complications in patients implanted with the Cyberonics vagal nerve stimulator. *Ann Otol Rhinol Laryngol*. 2006;115:260-267.

Smyth MD, Tubbs RS, Bebin EM, et al. Complications of chronic vagus nerve stimulation for epilepsy in children. *J Neurosurg*. 2003;99:500-503.

Tatum WO, Moore DB, Stecker MM, et al. Ventricular asystole during vagal nerve stimulation for epilepsy in humans. *Neurology*. 1999;52:1267.

Uthman BM, Reichl AM, Dean JC, et al. Effectiveness of vagal nerve stimulation in epilepsy patients: a 12-year observation. *Neurology*. 2004;63:1124-1126.

Uthman BM, Wilder BJ, Hammond EJ, et al. Efficacy and safety of vagus nerve stimulation in patients with complex partial seizures. *Epilepsia*. 1990;31(suppl 2):S44-S50.

Uthman BM, Wilder BJ, Penry JK, et al. Treatment of epilepsy by stimulation of the vagus nerve. *Neurology*. 1993;43:1338-1345.

Zabara J. Inhibition of experimental seizures in canines by repetitive vagal nerve stimulation. *Epilepsia*. 1992;33:1005-1012.

Full references can be found on Expert Consult @ www.expertconsult.com

CHAPTER 68

Radiosurgical Treatment of Epilepsy

Isaac Yang ■ Edward F. Chang ■ Nicholas M. Barbaro ■
Jean Régis ■ Marc Lévêque ■ Fabrice Bartolomei ■ Patrick Chauvel

RADIOSURGICAL THERAPY FOR TEMPORAL LOBE EPILEPSY

Radiosurgery is the precise application of focused radiation under stereotactic guidance to a targeted volume area within the brain identified on magnetic resonance imaging (MRI).[1] Conceptualized by Lars Leksell for use in functional neurosurgery, radiosurgical treatment of neurological disorders has progressively widened its utility[2-34] and is now also a treatment modality option for several neoplastic[35-84] and vascular indications.[62,85-118] Unlike standard-dose fractionated radiotherapy, radiosurgery allows the neurosurgeon to deliver effective, precise, and accurate doses of radiation to a smaller volume without affecting large portions of normal parenchyma, thereby allowing a powerful radiobiologic effect on the chosen targeted volume.[1,119-121]

Epilepsy is one of the most common serious neurological diseases and has a prevalence of 0.5% to 1.0% in the U.S. population.[122,123] Approximately, 20% of patients with epilepsy have seizures that are medically refractory (i.e., failing to respond to medications). Despite modern advances in new antiepileptic medications, the percentage of patients with medically refractory epilepsy has not significantly improved. Patients with medically refractory seizures may be referred for possible surgical management, and approximately half of them are found to be suitable candidates for open surgical resection of a seizure focus.[124] Focal partial epilepsies such as temporal lobe epilepsy are typically responsive to open surgical resection and are increasingly being treated with "structural" treatment modalities.[117,125]

The most common type of open surgery performed for temporal lobe epilepsy is anterior temporal lobectomy, which is resection of a portion of the temporal lobe.[123,125-127] With modern advances in surgical and anesthetic techniques, microsurgical resection of mesial temporal lobe structures can be performed with low morbidity and even lower mortality.[121] Open invasive surgical procedures, however, have inherent risks, including damage to the brain (either directly or indirectly by injury to important blood vessels), bleeding (which can require reoperation), blood loss (which can require transfusion), infection, and general anesthetic risks.[128-131] In addition, significant postoperative pain can result from surgical incisions and scars. Several clinical studies evaluating the morbidity and mortality associated with open microsurgery for temporal lobe epilepsy have reported that approximately 5% to 23% of patients undergoing open microsurgery experience a symptomatic neurological deficit postoperatively.[126,128,129,132,133] Furthermore, open surgical procedures require several days of care in the hospital, typically including one night in the intensive care unit, which contributes to the economic costs of open microsurgical treatment.[117] There is also a significant population of patients with medically intractable epilepsy who are unsuitable for conventional open microsurgery.[117] These patients may have their epileptic focus in regions that are difficult to access or in eloquent functional regions of the brain where surgical resection could result in irreversible language, motor, or visual impairment.[117,118]

Radiosurgery is now being evaluated as an alternative treatment modality to open resective microsurgery for intractable temporal lobe epilepsy. High-dose radiation is toxic to all living cells, but the highly focused nature of radiosurgery allows stereotactic guidance and sparing of adjacent tissues from the damaging effects of radiation. Although performed in a hospital setting, radiosurgery is relatively noninvasive, with frame-based radiosurgery using just frame pins that penetrate only the skin to firmly fix the stereotactic frame to the skull. Typically, patients can return to full activity within 1 to 2 days after treatment. Currently, radiosurgery is under investigations as a treatment modality for epilepsy associated with vascular malformations, hypothalamic hamartomas, and medial temporal lobe epilepsy (MTLE) associated with mesial temporal sclerosis (MTS).*

Preclinical Evidence

Preclinical studies investigating focused high-dose radiosurgery in animal models of epilepsy have demonstrated the potential utility of radiosurgical treatment applied to nonhuman epilepsy models. Early animal experiments indicated the efficacy of focused irradiation in a feline model of epilepsy in reducing seizure activity.[117,134,135] At doses between 10 and 20 Gy (1 Gy is equivalent to 1 J of energy per kilogram of tissue), cats with epileptic foci treated with an implanted cobalt radiation source had reduced seizure activity. Histologic analysis of these radiosurgically treated animal specimens revealed "neuronal reafferentation" as a proposed potential mechanism for amelioration of seizures with focused irradiation.[134,135]

Recently, Sun and colleagues reported that radiosurgery successfully reduced seizure activity and raised seizure thresholds in a nonhuman epilepsy model.[118] In this preclinical investigation, a linear accelerator (LINAC) was used to deliver radiosurgery doses of 10 or 40 Gy at the 90% isodose line. These investigators reported that seizure thresholds in these radiosurgically treated rats were significantly increased and that the length of afterdischarges was significantly decreased in the group treated with 40 Gy. These antiepileptic effects were observed 1 week after radiosurgical treatment, and the antiseizure effects persisted at the 3-month follow-up period.[118]

In animal studies from the University of Virginia, the effects of radiosurgery on a chronic spontaneous epilepsy model in rodents were reported.[153] In this preclinical investigation, hippocampal electrodes were implanted to produce a rodent temporal lobe epilepsy model. Ten weeks later, Gamma Knife radiosurgery (GKRS) with radiation doses between 10 and 40 Gy was applied as the therapeutic modality. Although the group receiving the lowest dose (10 Gy) showed no improvement in seizure activity, the 20-Gy group did exhibit a gradual and progressive reduction in seizures 2 to 6 months after radiosurgery. Also reported in this animal study, the 40-Gy group displayed a more dramatic and earlier reduction in seizures by the second month of follow-up. On histologic analysis of temporal lobe regions treated by radiosurgery in this rodent study, no necrosis in the tissue specimens was reported. Synaptically driven

---

*See references 1, 30, 86, 91, 93, 96, 101, 118, 120, 121, 134-152.

neuronal firing was reported to be intact in these radiosurgically treated rodent brain slices, thus suggesting that functional neuronal death was not responsible for the identified reduction in seizures.[153]

Recent preclinical experiments from the University of Pittsburgh were designed to estimate the radiation dose in radiosurgery that was needed to reduce seizure activity in a rat kainic acid–induced epilepsy model.[144] In this animal investigation, rats underwent stereotactic injection of kainic acid into the hippocampus to induce seizures. Ten days after the injections, the focal epileptic injection site was treated by GKRS at a dose range of 20 to 100 Gy. Even animals treated with the lowest dose of 20 Gy in this study were reported to demonstrate a progressive reduction in the number of daily seizures during each week of observation after radiosurgery. Furthermore, 3 weeks after radiosurgery, all treated rats in this study at each radiosurgery dose—20, 40, 60, and 100 Gy—showed a statistically significant reduction in seizure activity. The authors reported that histologic evaluation revealed radiation-induced necrosis only at the highest 100-Gy radiosurgery dose. However, injection of kainic acid induces a loss of CA3 neurons in all animals, and for this reason, interpretation of the histologic findings, especially for radiation-induced necrosis, is extremely difficult and problematic in this kainic acid–based epilepsy model. Small areas of kainic acid–induced necrosis were, however, reported in 2 of 20 control animals and in 14 of 37 radiosurgically treated animals, but only in the animals treated with 100 Gy of radiosurgery did the observed histologic necrosis match the collimator size.[144]

A second preclinical study using the same kainic acid–induced epilepsy model was undertaken to further evaluate the histopathologic and behavioral effects of "subnecrotic" radiosurgery doses.[154] Stereotactic hippocampal kainic acid injections were subsequently followed by GKRS at doses of either 30 or 60 Gy. A statistically significant reduction in seizures was reported in all radiosurgically treated animals, and this antiepileptic effect was observed earlier in the animals treated with the higher radiosurgery dose (weeks 5 to 9 versus weeks 7 to 9). Furthermore, in this preclinical investigation, no animals treated with radiosurgery were reported to demonstrate a deficit in new memory attainment tasks on water maze testing in comparison to control animals only injected with kainic acid, but both groups showed "cognitive" impairment when compared with rats that did not receive any kainic acid injection or radiosurgical treatment. For the histopathologic analysis in this study, two blinded observers evaluated the specimens from all animals at 13 weeks after radiosurgery. Typical changes with kainic acid injections were seen in all injected animals. Furthermore, in 25 of 46 injected animals, unilateral hippocampal atrophy was also observed. Again as noted earlier, histopathologic assessment is difficult given the use of kainic acid, but radiation-induced necrosis matching the target volume of radiation was not reported in any of the animals treated with radiosurgery.[154] These preclinical animal findings suggest that reduction of seizure activity after radiosurgery does not require necrosis or concomitant functional loss of treated neurons.[154]

With the suggestion that necrosis is not necessary for reduction of seizures, the radiosurgery group in Prague reported on their preclinical characterization of a "subnecrotic" dose of radiosurgery in a rat model.[155,156] This preclinical investigation evaluated radiosurgery doses of 25, 50, 75, or 100 Gy delivered bilaterally to the rat hippocampus and then assessed the rats with cognitive tests, MRI, and histopathologic examinations at 1, 3, 6, and 12 months after radiosurgery. A progressive time- and dose-dependent response curve was observed in cognitive memory function, edema on MRI, and necrotic histopathology. All animals radiosurgically treated with the 100-Gy dose died by 6 months after radiation therapy, and all histopathology specimens from these rats had radiation-induced necrotic lesions. All animals

treated with 75 Gy displayed cognitive memory functional impairments, edema on MRI, and radiation-induced necrotic lesions, whereas only one of the animals treated with the 50-Gy radiosurgery dose had observable edema and necrosis. Animals treated with radiosurgery doses of 25 and 50 Gy were not reported to demonstrate any functional or structural impairments after radiosurgery.[155] This observation of a potential subnecrotic radiosurgery dose that could improve seizure activity prompted a second follow-up preclinical study in which a 35-Gy radiosurgery dose was used with a long-term follow-up period of 16 months.[156] In this study, 6 months after radiosurgical treatment, edema was observed on MRI, and this edema was most pronounced at 9 months after radiosurgery. After 16 months, two of six treated animals were reported to have radiation-induced necrotic cavities after treatment with a 35-Gy dose of radiosurgery. The four treated animals without frankly necrotic cavities had other notable histopathologic findings such as severe atrophy of the corpus callosum, loss of thickness of the somatosensory cortex, and damage to the stratum oriens hippocampi.[156] These preclinical animal studies suggest that the full radiobiologic and histopathologic effect of radiosurgery may be manifested only several months after radiosurgery.

These preclinical studies reported amelioration of seizures, as well as histologic neuronal changes associated with radiosurgical treatment in different animal epilepsy models. These animal studies suggested that the antiepileptic efficacy of radiosurgery is dose dependent.[121,144,153,154] Most of these studies suggest that a radiosurgery dose of approximately 25 Gy is required to induce a therapeutic antiepileptic effect and that the full histologic and other toxicity may require several months to fully develop.[117,118,144,153-156] Animal models, however, may be poor predictors of radiation effects for translation to human biologic responses.

Clinical Evidence

The first application of radiosurgery for epilepsy surgery is attributed to Talairach in the 1950s, who implanted radioactive yttrium in patients with temporal lobe epilepsy without a lesion.[117,118,121] Further clinical experiences with GKRS and LINAC-based radiosurgery for the treatment of arteriovenous malformations and low-grade tumors also reported the incidental antiseizure effects of radiosurgery.* Although it is not clear whether lesion resolution itself may contribute to the reduction in seizure activity, these clinical reports of improvement in seizures with radiosurgery provided the impetus for investigating radiosurgery as a potentially effective treatment of medically intractable epilepsy.

Medial Temporal Lobe Epilepsy

MTLE associated with MTS is perhaps the most well defined epilepsy syndrome responsive to structural intervention. MTS is an idiopathic process associated with extensive loss of neurons and an increase in astrocytes in the mesial temporal structures, which include the amygdala and hippocampus in the temporal lobe. When temporal lobe epilepsy is due to underlying MTS, improvements in seizures with open microsurgical structural resections can be expected in between 65% and 90% of patients.[117,123,125,127,157-162] This form of temporal lobe epilepsy is particularly amenable to structural interventions such as radiosurgery because 80% to 90% of these patients show detectable changes on MRI.[120,159]

Radiosurgery has also been explored as an alternative to open microsurgery for MTS-associated MTLE. In a small series of patients with MTLE treated with GKRS, Régis and coauthors

---

*See references 86, 91, 96, 101, 121, 138, 142, 143, 151, 152.

reported clinical and effective amelioration of seizures with minimal morbidity.[145,146] A recent, prospective, multicenter European study evaluating GKRS for MTS showed comparable efficacy rates (65%) for reduction of seizures by conventional microsurgery and radiosurgery after 2 years of follow-up.[121] Using a marginal dose of 24 Gy, Régis and colleagues reported that radiosurgery can be used as an alternative to conventional open microsurgery to effectively treat MTLE associated with MTS and improve quality of life with comparable rates of morbidity and mortality.[121] In the United States, a multicenter pilot trial is currently being conducted, and the initial results show that 85% of patients treated with 24 Gy (to the 50% isodose line) delivered to the medial temporal lobe, including the amygdala, anterior hippocampus, and nearby cortex, are seizure free at 2 years of follow-up with minimal morbidity (Barbaro and coworkers, unpublished). This study group is also planning a follow-up, phase III multicenter trial to compare open microsurgery with radiosurgery for patients with clinically and radiographically defined MTS-associated MTLE.

Although radiosurgery has proved effective and safe in improving MTLE-associated seizures, the beneficial effects of radiosurgery are not demonstrated immediately. Typically, patients with MTLE treated by radiosurgery can achieve improvement in seizures between 9 and 12 months and dramatic improvement in seizures between 18 and 24 months after treatment. A transient increase in partial seizures (auras) has been reported at approximately the same time that the complex seizures decrease.[121] Most patients require a temporary course of corticosteroids to treat the delayed radiation-induced edema associated with the initial radiosurgical effect, commonly 10 to 15 months after treatment (Fig. 68-1) (Barbaro, personal observation).[121]

One of the difficulties in applying radiosurgery broadly as an application for intractable MTLE is the definition of the radiosurgical target (Fig. 68-2). Because the MTS associated with MTLE is not clearly defined anatomically, the precise boundaries and structures for radiosurgical treatment are yet not well characterized. Hence, standardization among different academic and community treatment centers has not been implemented and is difficult to achieve thus far, and consensus on treatment targets remains elusive. Successful radiosurgical treatment, however, is correlated with the targets treated with radiosurgery. For example, in recent reports, Régis and colleagues radiosurgically targeted the mesial temporal lobe structures in their series, whereas Kawai and associates restricted their treatment to the amygdala or hippocampus structures, and each series reported varying rates of successful amelioration of MTLE.[121,140,145,146] Although target definition may vary among different neurosurgeons, radiosurgery for MTS-associated

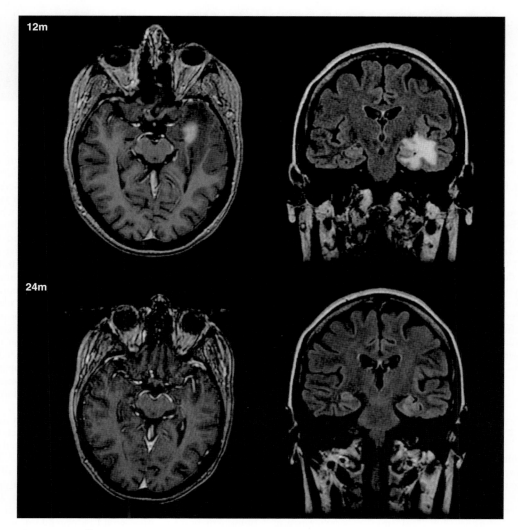

FIGURE 68-1 Changes on magnetic resonance imaging at 12 months and 24 months after radiosurgery.

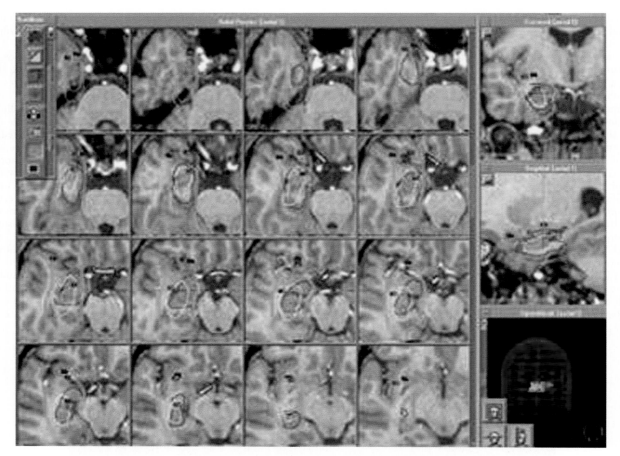

FIGURE 68-2 Treatment planning session for Gamma Knife radiosurgery.

MTLE remains an attractive therapeutic option because of its effectiveness, low morbidity and mortality, and the consistent manifestations of this disease with identifiable imaging characteristics on MRI. Moreover, conventional open microsurgical temporal lobectomy is still possible if the initial radiosurgical treatment is ineffective after sufficient time has elapsed for the delayed radiosurgical antiepileptic effect.[121]

Furthermore, recent dose studies have also suggested that a lower dose of 20 Gy at the margins may be less effective than higher marginal doses in reducing seizure activity. Cmelak and coauthors reported unsuccessful reduction of seizures with a 15-Gy marginal radiosurgery dose.[163] Similarly, Kawai and coworkers reported two cases of radiosurgery with an unsuccessful antiepileptic effect at a marginal radiosurgery dose of 18 Gy.[140] Finally, Srikijvilaikul and colleagues from the Cleveland Clinic also reported their series of ineffective radiosurgical treatment for seizure control with a 20-Gy marginal dose.[164]

Histologic Evaluation after Radiosurgical Treatment of Medial Temporal Lobe Epilepsy

Histologic examination of radiosurgically treated human mesial temporal tissue for MTLE has been limited because of the efficacy of radiosurgery for MTS-associated MTLE. However, histologic analysis of radiation-treated tissues has been reported in patients who underwent resection as a result of ineffective seizure control after radiosurgery.[140,163,164] Using a subtherapeutic dose, Cmelak and coauthors reported no radiation-induced histopathologic changes in tissues treated with radiosurgery at 15 Gy.[163] In another series in which two patients were treated with 18 Gy, one patient was noted to have a necrotic focus with some prominent vascular changes consisting of vessel wall thickening and fibrinoid and hyaline degeneration, whereas the other patient treated with this subtherapeutic dose showed no necrosis or vascular histopathologic changes.[140] When treated with a higher, yet subtherapeutic dose of 20 Gy, all five patients from a series reported from the Cleveland Clinic demonstrated histopathologic necrosis, perivascular sclerosis, and macrophage infiltration on resection and evaluation.[164] These reports suggest that in the clinical use of radiosurgery, significant identifiable histologic changes may be observed only with radiosurgical doses of 20 Gy or greater. These radiobiologic and histologic markers such as necrosis and vascular changes may be required for an effective antiseizure effect to become manifested. Thus, a dose that produces some tissue necrosis and histopathologic effects without inducing an excessive biologic response (e.g., edema), such as 24 Gy, may be the optimal effective dose for the radiosurgical treatment of MTLE.[121,145,146]

Currently, the radiobiology of radiosurgery in the setting of MTS-associated MTLE is not yet completely understood. Although some preclinical studies have suggested an antiepileptic effect of radiation with subnecrotic doses,[154] human clinical studies have suggested that a certain amount of tissue necrosis and histopathologic changes may be required to produce significant amelioration of MTS-associated seizures. The importance of this issue on biologic effect is that radiosurgical treatment of eloquent brain regions would be possible if an effective subnecrotic dose could be found.

CHAPTER 69

Deep Brain Stimulation for Epilepsy

Robert S. Fisher ■ Brian Litt ■ William C. Stacey

Epilepsy is a highly prevalent, serious neurological and sometimes neurosurgical disorder that affects approximately 1% of the world's population. In the majority of people, epilepsy can be controlled adequately with antiepileptic medications, but some continue to experience breakthrough seizures or unacceptable side effects of medications. For this highly needy population, new treatment strategies are required. Deep brain stimulation (DBS) is one such new modality of treatment and at the time of this writing is just on the verge of probable admission into the mainstream of epilepsy therapies. Although palliative, DBS has the advantage of tissue preservation and also the potential ability to favorably influence multifocal epilepsy.

Electrical stimulation of the nervous system has a very long history. Legend holds that a freed slave of Emperor Tiberius in 15 AD accidentally stepped on a torpedo electric fish. After recovering from the shock, he noted improvement in his gout. A local physician consequently recommended torpedo fish treatment of pain.[1,2] From early times, electrical stimulation therapies were prone to adoption by charlatans. The "grand electrical machine of Francis Lowndes" produced static electricity with impressive effects on the subject's hairstyle and purported benefits for a wide list of maladies.[3] In the 1700s, a Leyden jar, an early form of a battery, was used to generate sparks claimed to be beneficial for paralysis, blindness, warts, toothache, St. Vitus' chorea, and death by drowning. A theatrical high point of DBS was accomplished by Dr. José Delgado, who stopped a charging bull with handheld radio control of brain electrodes implanted in the animal's internal capsule and basal ganglia.

The first legitimate scientific use of electrical brain stimulation in a live patient was probably performed by Dr. Roberts Bartholow.[2] The patient had an infected scalp ulcer and osteomyelitis. Débridement led to exposure of the brain. During the procedure, Dr. Bartholow stimulated the exposed cortex with a sporadic current source and noted muscle contractions. Intraoperative electrical brain stimulation came into mainstream medicine through the efforts of the neurosurgeon Wilder Penfield and the neurologist Herbert Jasper at the Montréal Neurological Institute in the 1940s and 1950s. Their use of stimulation was diagnostic rather than explicitly therapeutic, and the information gained from electrical stimulation mapping was used to aid tailored resections of the brain for lesions and seizures.

Many innovators used depth wires to record deep in the brain in the late 1940s and early 1950s, but therapeutic stimulation via implanted wires was probably first performed by Heath in the early 1950s, with stimulation of the posterior frontal/septal region being used to alleviate pain and psychosis. In a 1963 article, R. G. Heath refers to work begun in 1952 with electrodes implanted into the centromedian nucleus, septal region, and mesencephalic tegmentum in a patient with psychomotor epilepsy.[4] Stimulation was set at 100 Hz, 3 to 5 mA for 15 minutes and could be triggered by the patient. A variety of subjective symptoms were produced by stimulation, some of which were sufficiently positive that patients would initiate stimulation up to 300 times per hour. At one point the patient's acute psychotic symptoms were interrupted with septal stimulation.

CEREBELLAR STIMULATION

Irving Cooper, working from Valhalla, New York, pioneered the use of DBS as chronic therapy for epilepsy.[5] His first therapeutic target of DBS for epilepsy was the cerebellum based on previous animal work. Sherrington showed in 1897 that the cerebellar cortex provoked inhibitory activity in various structures. In 1941, Moruzzi demonstrated that motor twitches in cats from strychnine on the cortex could be attenuated by cerebellar stimulation.[6] In 1955, Cooke and Snider demonstrated that 60-Hz stimulation of the cerebellar cortex could modify seizures provoked by electrical stimulation of the cat cerebral cortex.[7] Cooper and colleagues used a silicon mesh with four to eight pairs of bipolar platinum electrodes applied to the midline cerebellum or neocerebellum to stimulate the cerebellar cortex chronically in patients.[8] Electrodes were stimulated through a subcutaneous antenna on the chest by inductive coupling through the skin. Their 1973 article reported cerebellar stimulation in seven patients with intractable seizures, three with "psychomotor seizures," three with "grand mal" seizures, two with petit mal seizures, and one with focal seizures involving the left side of the face, arm, and leg. Six of the seven were said to improve over a period of 8 months, and "virtually complete control of seizures" was achieved in four of them.

The original article by Cooper and coworkers in 1973 stimulated a small series of cerebellar implantation in people with epilepsy. As summarized by Krauss and Fisher, 11 uncontrolled studies showed benefit of cerebellar stimulation.[9] Two blinded controlled studies, one by Wright and colleagures[10] and the other by Van Buren and associates,[11] were, however, negative. The Wright study was performed in 12 patients with treatment lasting 6 months. The Van Buren study included 5 patients. Neither showed efficacy over sham stimulation. Even though these two controlled studies were criticized methodologically and totaled just 17 patients, they served to place cerebellar stimulation for epilepsy on the back burner for many years. Certain practitioners, notably the neurosurgeon Ross Davis, continued arguments that cerebellar stimulation could be effective in selected people with epilepsy.[12-16] At a mean follow-up of 17 years, 19 patients with cerebellar stimulators were contacted by Davis, and 53% indicated that that they were seizure free and 32% had reduced seizures.[12] Generalized tonic-clonic seizures appeared to show the best response.

Velasco and colleagues performed a small double-blind, randomized trial of bilateral stimulation of the superomedial surface of the cerebellum in five patients with refractory motor seizures.[17] The parameters of the stimulation consisted of 10 pulses per second, 4 minutes on and 4 minutes off adjusted to a current density of 2 microcoulombs (μC) per square centimeter per pulse. Statistical analysis indicated a beneficial effect of stimulation. The three patients who completed the protocol for 2 years showed a reduction in generalized tonic-clonic seizures to a mean of 24% of baseline levels. Definitive documentation of the efficacy of cerebellar stimulation will probably be provided only by a large, controlled clinical trial.

FIGURE 69-1 Sites in the brain (and vagus nerve) that have been subjected to deep brain stimulation to treat seizures. CM, centromedian thalamus. Except for *direct focus* and *vagus*, black lines indicate the approximate areus superficial to the deep brain stimulation sites.

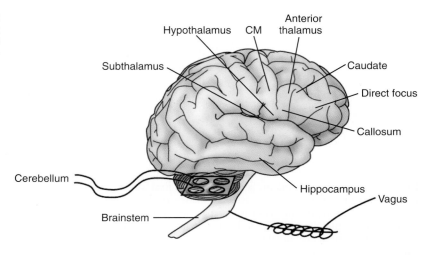

STIMULATION SITES FOR TREATING EPILEPSY

Figure 69-1 illustrates various regions of the nervous system that have been stimulated in humans to treat seizures. Direct cortical stimulation is discussed separately in this text. Exemplary studies at the different sites are tabulated in Table 69-1. No attempt is made to list all DBS studies in the literature. Only stimulation of the peripheral vagus nerve is licensed in the United States for epilepsy therapy. Vagus nerve stimulation is not discussed in this chapter.

The literature on DBS for neurological disorders is difficult to interpret. Reports usually consist of small, uncontrolled studies. Particularly in the early phases of DBS, descriptions of seizure types, specific seizure frequencies, and concurrent therapies were lacking. Most articles reported various degrees of improvement in seizure frequency after stimulation, but it remains unclear how much of this was due to stimulation. An important alternative explanation would involve either a placebo effect or regression to the mean, by which patients would return to their baseline seizure frequency after entering a clinical trial at a particularly bad point in their disorder. Early studies were done without the benefit of magnetic resonance imaging (MRI) to accurately localize placement of the stimulating electrodes. Stimulation parameters often varied widely among patients in a particular series. The actual number of patients treated is difficult to estimate because authors frequently published different reports with overlapping patients. Nevertheless, we briefly review each of the brain sites (other than direct stimulation of the cortex) stimulated to treat seizures. Cerebellar simulation was discussed earlier in its historical context.

Brainstem

The brainstem is the source of the reticular activating system classically described by Moruzzi and Magoun.[6] Activation of the reticular activating system would be expected to result in electroencephalographic (EEG) desynchronization and make the formation of seizures, which consist of highly synchronous rhythms, more difficult. Only two studies have evaluated brainstem stimulation for epilepsy in patients. In these studies,[19,20] the locus caeruleus was stimulated in a total of three patients. Benefit was reported in the form of a reduction in seizures and prolongation of auras, but the benefit was mild and sustained for only a few days.

Posterior Hypothalamus

The mammillary bodies of the posterior hypothalamus are on the classic circuit of Papez, which links hippocampal outflow to the mammillary bodies and anterior thalamus, to the cingulate, and then back to the entorhinal cortex and hippocampus. Interruption of the mammillothalamic tract prevents pentylenetetrazol-induced seizures in guinea pigs.[55] Stimulation of the mammillary nuclei at high frequency with depth electrodes similarly increases the pentylenetetrazol seizure threshold in rats.[56] Activation of the histamine system mediated by the mammillary nucleus was hypothesized to be involved in the mechanism of action of mammillary body DBS.[57] With these experimental data as background, van Rijckevorsel and colleagues in Brussels implanted DBS electrodes in three patients with refractory epilepsy.[21] They observed paroxysmal epileptiform discharges in the mammillary bodies. Although potentially beneficial for seizures, stimulation and further implantations were not continued because of the potential risk for hemorrhage.

Corpus Callosum

Marino Junior and Gronich in São Paulo implanted DBS electrodes in 10 patients with disabling convulsive disorders.[22] Preliminary evaluation suggested that such implantation was better tolerated than corpus callosotomy and possibly beneficial against the seizures.

Caudate

A long history of animal experimentation suggests the possible utility of DBS in the caudate for controlling seizures. The caudate has been shown to exert inhibitory control over propagation of seizures. In 1982, Oakley and Ojemann showed that caudate stimulation attenuated seizures produced by placing alumina cream on the cortex of monkeys.[58] After continuous caudate stimulation, five of the six monkeys exhibited a rebound in increased seizure activity. Psatta showed that caudate stimulation at 5 Hz, 0.3 msec, 1- to 5-V pulses for 1 to 3 seconds reduced interictal spiking in freely moving cats made epileptic by cobalt on the neocortex.[59] La Grutta and Sabatino placed bipolar stimulating electrodes bilaterally in the caudate of cats, followed by hippocampal injection of penicillin. Hippocampal spiking decreased by 55% with stimulation.[60]

TABLE 69-1 Studies of Stimulation Sites

SITE	ILLUSTRATIVE AUTHOR, YEAR	N	FINDING
Cerebellum	Cooper and Upton,[18] 1978	?	Original DBS for epilepsy
	Davis,[12] 2000	19	Follow-up of patients, 53% seizure free
	Velasco et al.,[17] 2005	5	Double-blind study. Statistically significant reduction in tonic-clonic seizures in 3 of 5 patients
Locus caeruleus	Faber and Vladyka,[19] 1983	1	Stimulation of the right locus caeruleus in a 24-year-old woman with "petit mal" and "grand mal" seizures reduced EEG discharges but had clinical benefit for only a few days
	Feinstein et al.,[20] 1989	2	Stimulation reduced seizures and lengthened auras
Mammillary bodies	Van Rijckevorsel et al.,[21] 2005	3	Patients with epilepsy underwent implantation of electrodes in the mammillary bodies. Anecdotal report of seizure benefit, but potential concern for hemorrhage
Corpus callosum	Marino Junior and Gronich,[22] 1989	10	Patients with epilepsy had electrodes implanted in the anterior callosum as an alternative to callosotomy. Well tolerated, but efficacy not analyzed
Caudate	Sramka et al.,[23] 1976	6	Patients with caudate stimulation either became seizure free over a 6-day period or improved
	Sramka and Chkhenkeli,[24] 1990	74	Epilepsy patients with caudate stimulation
	Chkhenkeli and Chkhenkeli,[25] 1997	38	Stimulation (4-6 Hz) of the caudate head, with a reduction in mesial temporal and neocortical seizures
	Chkhenkeli et al.,[26] 2004	21	Ventral caudate head stimulation at 4-8 Hz reduced seizures to 10%-30% of baseline
Centromedian thalamus	Velasco et al.,[27] 1987	5	Original CM stimulation, performed for 2 hr/day in patients with generalized or multifocal seizures. At 3 mo, saw a 60%-100% reduction in partial and 80%-100% reduction in generalized seizures
	Fisher et al.,[28] 1992	7	Randomized crossover design showed a nonsignificant 30% reduction in seizures
	Velasco et al.,[29] 1993	23	Patients with mixed seizure types: reduced seizures in GTC but not CP or LGS patients
	Velasco et al.,[30] 1995	5	GTC almost disappeared and absence seizures improved, but not CPS
	Velasco et al.,[31] 2000	13	Improved GTC and absence seizures. Partial benefit for LGS. No help for CPS or focal EEG spikes
	Velasco et al.,[32] 2001	49	Summary of patients stimulated for 0.5-15 yr. Highly significant decrease in GTC, absence, tonic, atonic, but not CPS
	Velasco et al.,[33] 2006	13	Patients with LGS; 80% reduction in seizures
Hippocampus	Sramka et al.,[23] 1976	26	This article was primarily about caudate stimulation, but a few underwent beneficial direct hippocampal stimulation
	Velasco et al.,[34] 2000	16	Patients with CP and SGTC. In 7 patients, seizures were abolished after 6 days
	Velasco et al.,[35] 2000	10	Patients with temporal seizures. Seizures were abolished in 7 patients after 5-6 days
	Velasco et al.,[36] 2001	?	Patients with LGS. Seizures as a percentage of baseline: total, 25%; GTC, 10%; atypical absence seizures, 25%; CPS, 60%
	Vonck et al.,[37] 2002	3	Patients with CPS. All had >50% reduction
	Vonck et al.,[38] 2005	7	Patients with bilateral hippocampal electrodes. More than half improved >50%
	Osorio et al.,[39] 2005	4	Electrodes were implanted bilaterally into the amygdala-hippocampal region. A seizure-detection algorithm trigger stimulation. Seizures were reduced by 56%
	Tellez-Zenteno et al.,[40] 2006	4	Left hippocampal stimulation tested with a double-blind crossover design. Seizure frequency was reduced by 15%, but not significant
	Velasco et al.,[41] 2007	9	Patients monitored for 18 mo to 7 yr. Those with normal MRI findings had a >95% reduction in seizures; those with MTS, reduction of 50%-70%
	Boon et al.,[42] 2007	12	With hippocampal stimulation, 1 became seizure free, 1 with 90% reduction, 5 with 50% reduction, 2 with 30%-49% reduction, 1 with no help
Subthalamic nucleus	Chabardes et al.,[43] 2002	5	3 of the 5 patients had a 67%-80% reduction in seizures
	Benabid et al.,[44] 2003	5	Seizures decreased in the 5 patients by 84%, 71%, 35%, 80%, and 0%
	Neme et al.,[45] 2004	4	Patients with partial epilepsy; 2 showed reduction of 42% to 75%. No benefit occurred in the other 2
	Handforth et al.,[46] 2006	2	Patients with partial seizures; reduced by 33%-50% during the time of stimulation
	Vesper et al.,[47] 2007	1	A patient with progressive myoclonic epilepsy had seizures improved by 50%
Anterior nucleus	Cooper et al.,[8,18,48] 1970s	?	Several series with improvement. Amount of improvement was not quantifiable
	Sussman et al.,[49] 1988	4	Seizures reduced to 23% of baseline
	Hodaie et al.,[50] 2002	5	Seizures reduced to a mean 47% of baseline. Benefit occurred mainly after implantation, before turning on the stimulator
	Kerrigan et al.,[51] 2004	5	Seizures reduced to 33% of baseline. Particular benefits for seizures that could produce falls
	Lee et al.,[52] 2006	6	Seizures reduced to 44% of baseline
	Lim et al.,[53] 2007	4	Seizures reduced to 49% of baseline
	Osorio et al.,[54] 2007	4	Seizures reduced to 25% of baseline
	Fisher et al.,[54a] 2010	110	Seizures reduced to 40.5% of baseline in stimulated group vs. 14.5% in control group (p-38)

CM, centromedian nucleus of the thalamus; CP, complex partial seizure; DBS, deep brain stimulation; EEG, electroencephalogram; GTC, generalized tonic-clonic seizure; LGS, Lennox-Gastaut syndrome; MRI, magnetic resonance imaging; MTS, mesial temporal sclerosis; SGTC, secondarily generalized tonic-clonic seizure.

Clinical application of caudate stimulation was first performed by Sramka and associates. In a study of various DBS sites for epilepsy, six patients underwent unilateral or bilateral caudate stimulation. Over a period of 4 to 6 days of treatment, two were said to be without seizures and four improved.[23] Further studies by Sramka and the Chkhenkelis of low-frequency (4 to 8 Hz) stimulation of the head of the caudate reduced the frequency of mesial temporal neocortical seizures, often to 10% to 30% of baseline levels.[24-26]

Centromedian Thalamus

The centromedian thalamus (CM) is part of the so-called non-specific thalamic activating system that interacts with diffuse regions of the cortex and, in the case of the CM, also with the basal ganglia and brainstem. In 1987, the Velasco brothers and colleagues implanted electrodes in five patients with multifocal or primary generalized refractory seizures.[27] Stimulation parameters were bipolar square pulses 0.1 msec in duration, 60 to 100 Hz, and 0.8 to 2.0 mA in trains of 1 minute every 5 minutes, alternating on the right and left side for 2 hours daily. The stimulator wires were external. Generalized tonic-clonic seizures were reduced 80% to 100% and complex partial seizures 60% to 100%. One patient with myoclonic seizures had the seizures abolished completely with stimulation.

Fisher and associates tested this protocol in a double-blind, randomized crossover trial in seven patients.[28] Stimulation was on or off for 3 months, then off in all patients for a 3-month "wash-out," and then off or on as the opposite treatment of the first 3 months for an additional 3 months. Patients could not tell whether the stimulator was on or off. Overall seizure frequency improved 30% but the difference was not statistically significant. The patient with the greatest improvement could not be analyzed because the family did not wish the stimulator settings to be changed from the apparently beneficial effects in the first 3 months (stimulator on). The degree of carryover effect from stimulation in the first cycle could not be estimated but may have influenced the frequency of seizures during the control months. Subsequently, Velasco and colleagues implanted deep brain stimulators into the centromedian nucleus in 50 to 100 patients.[30-33,61,62] Further experience suggested that generalized tonic-clonic seizures improved the most and atypical absence seizures in part, but complex partial seizures and focal EEG spiking improved little. Patients with the otherwise highly intractable Lennox-Gastaut syndrome had up to an 80% reduction in seizures. The only controlled study of CM stimulation has been that of Fisher and associates,[28] and no definitive large randomized trial has been performed.

Hippocampus

Most brain regions subjected to DBS for seizures are synaptically connected to but remote from the seizure focus or foci. Hippocampal stimulation provides an exception to this rule in that the hippocampus is often the primary site of the seizure focus. Direct hippocampal stimulation in humans to treat epilepsy was again pioneered by the Velasco brothers. In 2000, Velasco and colleagues published a study of 16 patients with complex partial and secondarily generalized tonic-clonic seizures.[34] Hippocampal stimulation was delivered at high frequency, low amplitude continuously with 130 pulses per second, 450-μsec pulse duration, and an amplitude of 200 to 400 μA. In 7 patients, seizures were abolished after 6 days of stimulation. Long-term follow-up by Velasco and associates of 9 patients for 18 months to 7 years showed that the reduction in seizures was greater than 95% with hippocampal stimulation, provided that the baseline MRI findings were normal, versus a 50% to 70% reduction in the presence of mesial temporal sclerosis.[41]

Vonck, Boon, and colleagues extended the findings of Velasco for hippocampal stimulation.[37,38] In an initial study of 3 patients with complex partial seizures, all had greater than 50% improvement in their seizures. In a later study of 7 patients implanted with bilateral hippocampal electrodes, seizures were reduced by half or better. Boon and coworkers evaluated 10 patients with long-term hippocampal stimulation: 1 became seizure free, 1 had a 90% reduction, 5 had at least a 50% reduction, 2 had a 30% to 49% reduction, and 1 was not helped.[42] A paradigm of seizure detection and hippocampal stimulation in response was used by Osorio and colleagues in 4 patients.[39] With this paradigm, seizures were reduced by 56%. A small, randomized crossover trial involving 4 patients was performed by Tellez-Zenteno and associates.[40] Left hippocampal stimulation at 190 Hz was on for a month and off for a month or in the reverse order. Seizure frequency decreased a median of 15%, which was not statistically significant. No large, randomized trial of hippocampal stimulation has been completed as of the time of this writing, but such a trial is under development.

Subthalamic Nucleus

The subthalamic nucleus (STN) is a target for the treatment of certain movement disorders.[63] In 1998, Vercueil, Benabid, and colleagues demonstrated that high-frequency stimulation of the STN suppressed absence seizures in a genetic absence seizure strain of rats.[64] In the clinic of Benabid, this was carried forward to patients.[43] DBS electrodes were inserted bilaterally into the STN of five patients. Stimulation was mostly continuous at 130 pulses per second, a duration of 90 μsec, and an amplitude 1.5 to 5.2 V. Mean reductions in seizure frequency for each patient were 81%, 42%, 68%, 67%, and 0%. Neme and colleagues implanted electrodes in the STN in four patients with partial epilepsy.[45] Two of the patients had a reduction in seizures in the range of 42% to 75%. No benefit occurred in the other two. Handforth and coworkers showed a 33% to 50% reduction during the time of STN stimulation in two patients with partial seizures.[46] Vesper reported 50% improvement with STN stimulation in a patient with progressive myoclonic epilepsy.[47]

Anterior Nucleus of the Thalamus

The anterior nucleus of the thalamus (AN) was an original target of Cooper in his early studies of DBS for epilepsy. His rationale for implanting in this particular nucleus was not clearly expressed in his publications, except that it was considered to be part of the nonspecific thalamus. The AN can influence EEG activity in regions of the frontal cortex. Cooper, Upton, and associates published several case series reporting the beneficial effects of AN stimulation on seizures,[65-68] but the results were not quantifiable from the publications. In 1988, a group from the Medical College of Pennsylvania published two abstracts on 5 patients who underwent AN stimulation.[49] Seizures were reduced to 23% of baseline. A pilot study was then initiated by Fisher and colleagues to develop parameters and methodology for a controlled trial of AN stimulation.[28] The results in the 10 patients in the pilot study were published in two separate reports. The group from Toronto reported on 5 of the patients.[50] Seizures were reduced to a mean of 47% of baseline. Interestingly, benefit appeared to occur mainly after implantation, before turning on the stimulator. The second cohort of 5 different patients in the pilot trial was reported from the Barrow Neurological Institute and the University of Pennsylvania.[51] Seizures were reduced to 33% of baseline. There appeared to be particular benefit against seizures of a type that could produce falls and injuries. In South Korea, Lee and associates showed seizures to be reduced to 44% of baseline with AN stimulation in 6 patients.[52] Lim and colleagues in Taiwan showed a reduction to 49% of baseline in 4 patients.[53] Osorio and

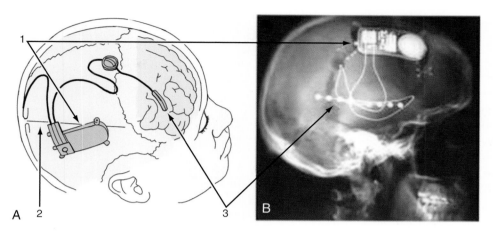

FIGURE 69-4 The NeuroPace responsive neurostimulator (RNS, Mountain View, CA). **A,** Schematic, and **B,** radiograph of the RNS. The stimulator (1) is implanted in a recessed skull window and connected to depth (2) or subdural strip (3) electrodes (or both). *(From Stacey WC, Litt B: Technology insight: neuroengineering and epilepsy: designing devices for seizure control. Nat Clin Pract Neurol. 2008;4:190. **A,** © NeuroPace, Inc., Mountain View, CA. **B,** Nursing Spectrum Nurse Wire © 2004.)*

Their proximal contacts are secured to the implanted device after being tunneled under the scalp. The neurostimulator contains the battery and microprocessor, which is programmable through a telemetric wand.[118] It has the capability of sensing four channels of electrocorticography (ECoG), performing analog-to-digital conversion of the signals, extracting three quantitative features from these data, detecting seizures, recording them in memory, and triggering programmable electrical stimulation in response to detection of events. The detection and stimulation parameters are individually adjustable via multiple settings so that it can be tuned to individual patients. The processor uses custom algorithms to determine when to stimulate and is capable of producing a wide variety of stimuli that can be used in attempts to stop seizures.

The key to developing the RNS device was crafting and testing algorithms that could be performed on board the device, thereby allowing the patient to be "unplugged" from higher powered acquisition and processing machines while being monitored for seizure activity. This fully contained monitoring and therapeutic solution therefore works during "real life" rather than only in the hospital and has real potential to improve the patient's quality of life. Early work demonstrated that computationally feasible algorithms could be reliably implemented in such a device.[119] Shortly thereafter, a pilot study demonstrated that seizures could be controlled by responsive stimulation in one patient.[120] These results were presented at the annual meeting of the American Epilepsy Society (AES) in 2002, along with work demonstrating further refinement in parameter optimization and tuning[121] and the establishment of a clinical trial for the RNS.[122] Since that time, the AES meeting has served as the venue for periodic updates in the status of this trial.[123-126] This device successfully completed its pivotal clinical trial in 2009 and showed significant improvement in seizure control during the blinded phase. The device is currently seeking FDA approval. One clear benefit of the closed-loop approach is the versatility of having recorded feedback: it effectively provides ambulatory ECoG data and allows tuning of the system in patient-specific training sessions.[123] Although the trial is still under way, the preliminary results are promising and the device has a favorable safety record.[126] Examples of early success in terminating seizures with both the RNS and the system described by Osorio and coworkers are shown in Figure 69-5.[39]

Closed-Loop Device Considerations for the Future

With current technology, an implantable closed-loop device can perform a significant amount of onboard processing and recording and can upload data via telemetry. The RNS has these capabilities, but there is much room for improvement in that processing speed and storage capacity have greatly increased since its creation. For instance, the RNS device can store only a limited number of discrete short segments of ECoG and needs to download them externally to avoid overwriting them.[127] This is only one of several features of the device that can be enhanced as a result of recent advances in hardware and consequently improve clinical results with closed-loop control. Onboard data storage is rapidly dropping in cost and becoming increasingly compact. Available flash memory will allow longer recording times and more feedback data. Battery technology continues to improve and will increase the longevity of the devices. Early devices have significant memory, processing, and battery limitations, thus forming strong motivation for using simple algorithms in a device,[119] but these limitations become less stringent with every passing year. Thus, there may be a greater selection of algorithms available in future devices. Perhaps the most important improvements, however, have yet to be discovered. As described in the following section, there is a growing community of researchers trying to determine which electrographic biomarkers of epilepsy can be used as feedback and how best to intervene to prevent seizures.

This chapter has focused on electrical stimulation to abort seizures, but there are many other methods that can also be incorporated into the next-generation implantable antiseizure devices.[128] One promising method is being developed by two independent groups and uses a Peltier device to induce focal cooling of the brain cortex to stop seizures.[129-132] No clinical trials in humans have yet been attempted, but Peltier devices are becoming small enough to be considered for human implantation. Transcranial magnetic stimulation has had mixed success[133-136] but is not feasible as an implantable device. Another method with tremendous therapeutic potential is local drug delivery.[137-141] This method uses known antiepileptic medications, stored in a reservoir, and injects them automatically at specific times into the seizure focus. The technology for these systems already exists on

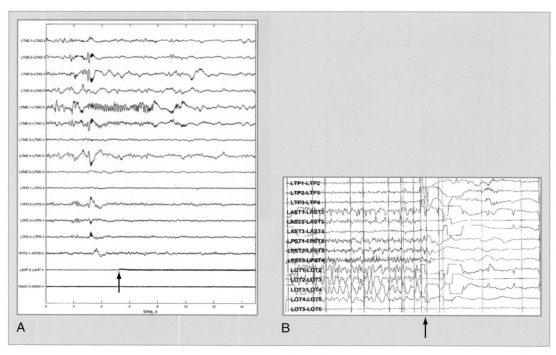

FIGURE 69-5 Examples of responsive antiseizure stimuli. **A,** An applied stimulus (*arrow*) after detection of an event prevents the event from lasting its typical length.[39] **B,** An event detected in the Responsive Neurostimulator device is halted by an abortive stimulus (*arrow*). (© NeuroPace Inc., Mountain View, CA. *Used with permission.*)

both the macroscopic and microscopic scale. It can be used both for open-loop infusion and as a responsive rescue medication and has the added benefit of proven efficacy in stopping seizures. Future nanotechnologies, such as light-triggered ion channel modulation, may provide even more opportunities for closed-loop seizure control devices.[142] Other technologies, such as adapting the vagus nerve stimulator (Cyberonics, Inc., Houston) with closed-loop control, are also being explored.[143]

MAPPING EPILEPTIC NETWORKS

The addition of recording elements with onboard or telemetrically retrieved storage will provide a wealth of information about epilepsy. Acutely, this technology allows real-time monitoring during surgical implantation, thereby aiding in lead placement. It can then be used for early training of the system to set the initial parameters, followed by iterative tuning throughout the life of the device. This information will provide patient-specific information about the network dynamics that are creating the seizures, data that may prove invaluable in understanding how to control seizures in an individual and the systemic nature of seizures.

SEIZURE DETECTION AND PREDICTION

Automated methods to detect seizures allow the RNS device to administer stimuli after initiation of the seizure.[144-146] Further refinement of seizure detection technology is needed to improve both sensitivity and specificity. Impending signs of seizures may be evident on intracranial EEG traces before the emergence of traditional EEG seizure patterns.[147,148] Study of these preictal changes, known as seizure prediction, attempts to find early biomarkers of seizure generation. In the past decade several methods have been tried, including the use of nonlinear mathematics, hidden Markov models, and statistics.[149-153] A related problem is refining the data processing within a device by using machine

learning algorithms, neural networks, or other methods that use classifiers and feature extraction to help maximize the system's accuracy in an automated fashion.[154-156] To date, these methods have had mixed results, but researchers are optimistic that automated analysis will be able to predict seizures before they occur in some patients.[128]

BIOMARKERS OF EPILEPSY: HIGH-FREQUENCY OSCILLATIONS

High-frequency oscillations of EEG potentials may signal impending seizures.[157-160] High-frequency discharges, called ripples or fast ripples, tend to localize to epileptic tissue, and changes in their temporal and spatial characteristics may predict seizures before they occur, both temporally and spatially. Additionally, studies of intracranial EEG signals sampled at higher frequencies than typically used in clinical machines have found that there is abnormal activity well above 70 Hz long before seizures occur.[147] While clinical research further evaluates the characteristics of this activity, basic science research is striving to understand its physiologic mechanisms.[161-166] These findings may indicate that fast activity can be used as a biomarker for seizures, and future technologies may discover ways to use such activity as an early feedback for advanced closed-loop devices.

CONCLUSION

DBS is a promising therapy for intractable seizures. The mechanisms by which DBS might help are unknown. In simple systems, high-frequency stimulation results in release of potassium into the extracellular space and depolarization block of neurons. In more complex systems, stimulation appears to have mixed inhibitory and excitatory effects that ultimately modify the properties of disordered neural networks.

The first site to be stimulated for epilepsy therapeutics was the cerebellum. Uncontrolled case series were positive, but two small controlled trials were negative, and interest in DBS for treating epilepsy declined. Attention to DBS redeveloped with the success of vagus nerve stimulation for epilepsy and STN and GPi stimulation for movement disorders. Since then, small uncontrolled case series of DBS for epilepsy have been attempted in several sites, including the locus caeruleus, mammillary bodies, corpus callosum, head of the caudate nucleus, CM, AN, STN, hippocampus, and direct stimulation of the cortex. Stimulation can occur on a scheduled basis or can be programmed to be responsive to epileptiform EEG patterns. Interpretation of these trials, however, is difficult in the absence of control groups. Typical reductions in seizure frequency in the range of 30% to 90% are reported, but it is impossible to be certain that these reductions are due to the stimulation. A multicenter, randomized clinical trial of bilateral stimulation of the anterior thalamic nucleus[54a] showed a 40.5% median reduction in seizures compared with 14.5% in the control group (p = 0.038). Adverse events were typical of those see for implanted brain electrodes. At time of this writing, deep brain stimulation for partial and secondarily generalized seizures in adults now is approved in Europe and several other countries, but not yet in the United States. A multicenter, randomized trial of responsive neurostimulation similarly showed efficacy for stimulation; however, results are not yet published.

Adverse events from DBS are common, but most are minor; serious, lasting complications are rare. Hemorrhage caused by implantation occurs in 1% to 2% of patients, but the hemorrhage is not always significantly symptomatic. A small proportion of implanted patients have infections or mechanical problems such as lead migration or fracture. The impact of stimulating various structures, such as the hippocampus, on cognitive function remains an open but important question. Long-term generation of epilepsy by a "kindling" effect of stimulation has not yet been convincingly documented.

Closed-loop devices using feedback technologies are becoming more important to the field of epilepsy. In recent years, momentum has been building to follow in the successful footsteps of analogous cardiac devices to treat arrhythmias, but there is need for caution in fostering expectations of rapid success in this area. The spatial and temporal circuits generating seizures are far more complex than those generating cardiac arrhythmias. Nonetheless, slow, steady, and impressive progress is being made.

Open-loop (scheduled) stimulation and closed-loop (responsive) stimulation are complementary rather than competitive. Open-loop stimulation does not require detection of the onset of a seizure, nor knowledge of the precise geography of a seizure focus. Closed-loop stimulation specifically addresses a patient's particular seizure pattern at a particular time and place. This may prove more effective in circumstances in which the seizure focus or foci can be localized. The true benefits and risks associated with either variety of DBS for epilepsy will be shown only by large, randomized, double-blind clinical trials. At the time of this writing, one such trial of AN stimulation has been completed, and another of responsive neurostimulation to the cortex or hippocampus is just being.

SUGGESTED READINGS

Benabid AL, Vercucil L, Benazzouz A, et al. Deep brain stimulation: what does it offer? *Adv Neurol*. 2003;91:293.

Beric A, Kelly PJ, Rezai A, et al. Complications of deep brain stimulation surgery. *Stereotact Funct Neurosurg*. 2001;77:73.

Boon P, Vonck K, De Herdt V, et al. Deep brain stimulation in patients with refractory temporal lobe epilepsy. *Epilepsia*. 2007;48:1551.

Chkhenkeli SA, Sramka M, Lortkipanidze GS, et al. Electrophysiological effects and clinical results of direct brain stimulation for intractable epilepsy. *Clin Neurol Neurosurg*. 2004;106:318.

Cooper IS, Amin I, Gilman S. The effect of chronic cerebellar stimulation upon epilepsy in man. *Trans Am Neurol Assoc*. 1973;98:192.

Dostrovsky JO, Lozano AM. Mechanisms of deep brain stimulation. *Mov Disord*. 2002;17(suppl 3):S63.

Gildenberg PL. Evolution of neuromodulation. *Stereotact Funct Neurosurg*. 2005;83:71.

Graves NM, Fisher RS. Neurostimulation for epilepsy, including a pilot study of anterior nucleus stimulation. *Clin Neurosurg*. 2005;52:127.

Handforth A, DeSalles AA, Krahl SE. Deep brain stimulation of the subthalamic nucleus as adjunct treatment for refractory epilepsy. *Epilepsia*. 2006;47:1239.

Krauss GL, Fisher RS. Cerebellar and thalamic stimulation for epilepsy. *Adv Neurol*. 1993;63:231.

Lehnertz K, Mormann F, Osterhage H, et al. State-of-the-art of seizure prediction. *J Clin Neurophysiol*. 2007;24:147.

Litt B, Echauz J. Prediction of epileptic seizures. *Lancet Neurol*. 2002;1:22.

McIntyre CC, Savasta M, Walter BL, et al. How does deep brain stimulation work? Present understanding and future questions. *J Clin Neurophysiol*. 2004;21:40.

Osorio I, Frei MG, Sunderam S, et al. Automated seizure abatement in humans using electrical stimulation. *Ann Neurol*. 2005;57:258.

Osorio I, Overman J, Giftakis J, et al. High frequency thalamic stimulation for inoperable mesial temporal epilepsy. *Epilepsia*. 2007;48:1561.

Peters TE, Bhavaraju NC, Frei MG, et al. Network system for automated seizure detection and contingent delivery of therapy. *J Clin Neurophysiol*. 2001;18:545.

Sramka M, Fritz G, Galanda M, et al. Some observations in treatment stimulation of epilepsy. *Acta Neurochir (Wien)*. 1976;23(suppl):257.

Velasco AL, Velasco F, Velasco M, et al. Electrical stimulation of the hippocampal epileptic foci for seizure control: a double-blind, long-term follow-up study. *Epilepsia*. 2007;48:1895.

Velasco F, Velasco AL, Velasco M, et al. Deep brain stimulation for treatment of the epilepsies: the centromedian thalamic target. *Acta Neurochir Suppl*. 2007;97:337.

Velasco M, Velasco F, Velasco AL. Centromedian-thalamic and hippocampal electrical stimulation for the control of intractable epileptic seizures. *J Clin Neurophysiol*. 2001;18:495.

Velasco M, Velasco F, Velasco AL, et al. Subacute electrical stimulation of the hippocampus blocks intractable temporal lobe seizures and paroxysmal EEG activities. *Epilepsia*. 2000;41:158.

Vonck K, Boon P, Claeys P, et al. Long-term deep brain stimulation for refractory temporal lobe epilepsy. *Epilepsia*. 2005;46(suppl 5):98.

Worrell G, Wharen, R, Goodman R, et al. Safety and evidence for efficacy of an implantable responsive neurostimulator (RNS) for the treatment of medically intractable partial onset epilepsy in adults. *Epilepsia*. 2005;46:226.

Wright GD, McLellan DL, Brice JG. A double-blind trial of chronic cerebellar stimulation in twelve patients with severe epilepsy. *J Neurol Neurosurg Psychiatry*. 1984;47:769.

Full references can be found on Expert Consult @ www.expertconsult.com

CHAPTER 70

Epilepsy Surgery: Outcome and Complications

Anthony L. Petraglia ■ Christian B. Kaufman ■ Webster H. Pilcher

The past 25 years has witnessed the evolution of epilepsy monitoring and surgery into a mature neuroscience subspecialty.[1,2] The proliferation of multidisciplinary epilepsy centers has increased our capacity to provide multidisciplinary evaluations of patients with intractable epilepsy, thereby leading to greater numbers of patients being offered surgical treatment (Table 70-1). A robust clinical literature has documented both improvements in surgical approaches and a set of measures of surgical outcomes that has stimulated changes in our approach to these patients. In addition, the emergence of a nosologic context of "surgically remediable syndromes" has been spurred by advances in brain imaging and studies of the neurobiologic underpinnings of epileptogenesis.

Traditional en bloc resective approaches, which predominated during the first 60 years of epilepsy surgery, have been supplemented by more focused, minimalistic approaches, including selective amygdalohippocampectomy (SAH), multiple subpial transection (MST), keyhole deafferentation hemispherotomy, radiosurgery, and neuromodulatory approaches such as deep brain stimulation (DBS), vagal nerve stimulation (VNS), and the NeuroPace device (Table 70-2).

Advances in our understanding of the intractable epilepsies have facilitated a discrete taxonomy of "surgically remediable syndromes" (Table 70-3).[1] Each syndrome and each new treatment approach engender a new data set with regard to (1) seizure, neurobehavioral, and psychosocial outcomes; (2) complications (surgical, neurological, neuropsychological, and psychobehavioral); (3) "health outcomes" expressed in terms of alterations in quality of life (QOL); and (4) "cost-effectiveness" in comparison to alternative therapeutic interventions.

EPIDEMIOLOGY AND HEALTH CARE COSTS OF INTRACTABLE EPILEPSY

Epilepsy is a relatively common disorder, with more than 2 million Americans (1.3%) afflicted and approximately 1 in 10 Americans having a minimum of one seizure over the course of a lifetime.[3] Up to a third of all individuals with epilepsy are refractory to medical therapy.[4] Medically intractable epilepsy is costly. Estimates of the lifetime cost of intractable epilepsy incorporate both *direct cost* (cost of medical care) and *indirect cost* (i.e., productivity, lost earnings). In a 2000 study, patients with medically intractable epilepsy in the United States were found to account for 42% of the estimated $1.7 billion in annual direct medical costs for epilepsy and 86% of the $10.8 billion in indirect costs.[5] Beyond these estimates, the burden of epilepsy incorporates additional, unmeasurable indirect costs that encompass pain, suffering, and reduction in the QOL of epileptic patients and their caretakers.[6,7]

ADVANCES IN OUTCOME ASSESSMENT OF EPILEPSY SURGERY

Seizure frequency, previously considered the "gold standard" of outcome measures, is an inadequate measure of surgical outcome for many reasons. Persistent epileptic seizures are often associated with significant psychosocial, psychiatric, and neuropsychological impairments, as well as medication toxicity and excess mortality rates (Fig. 70-1).[8] These disabilities may persist despite relief of seizures after "successful" surgery. Therefore, contemporary studies of postoperative outcome emphasize neuropsychological and psychosocial functions and "health outcomes" commensurate with the World Health Organization's definition of health as "… a state of complete physical, mental and social well-being …".[3,8]

Classification of Seizure Outcomes

Studies have demonstrated that "health-related quality of life" (HRQOL) and psychosocial measures may not improve significantly with as much as a 70% reduction in seizure frequency after surgery.[9] In recognition of the benefits of postoperative freedom or near freedom from seizures, contemporary seizure outcome classification schemes have emphasized patterns of seizure reduction that are likely to have an impact on QOL.[10-12] The Engel classification scheme (Table 70-4) provides four categories of seizure outcome: I, seizure free; II, "rare" seizures (two to three per year): III, "worthwhile improvement" (>90% reduction); and IV, "no worthwhile improvement" (<90% reduction).[8,11] That a class IV ("no worthwhile improvement") outcome may be associated with a 70% reduction in frequency is emphasized by HRQOL studies showing that epilepsy-specific measures are affected even by a few seizures per year.

Neuropsychological Outcomes

Neuropsychological assessment is useful both during the surgical patient selection process and as a tool to assess outcomes after surgery. The aim of the evaluation is to establish a profile of the patient's strengths and weaknesses in multiple domains on a variety of standardized tests and questionnaires (Table 70-5) in relation to normative values derived from the general population.[13]

Of particular concern in temporal lobe surgery are losses of memory function, including the rare but disabling syndrome of global amnesia, as well as the more common material-specific memory losses affecting short-term verbal memory in the language-dominant hemisphere and visual-spatial memory in non–dominant-hemisphere, temporal lobe operations. The Wada test, which was originally developed to determine hemispheric lateralization of language function,[14] was subsequently adapted by Milner and colleagues[15] to provide a measure of the risk for loss of memory function postoperatively. The Wada test has been used for many years to identify patients at risk for global memory loss,[16] and in fact, such losses are uncommon since the Wada test was universally adopted. However, reports of favorable memory outcomes in patients who failed the Wada test preoperatively ("false positives") have called into question the reliability of this procedure in some patients.[17] The Wada test has also been useful in identifying lateralized temporal lobe dysfunction, which may correlate with the side of seizure onset,[18,19] the likelihood of a favorable seizure outcome, and more recently, prediction of the

TABLE 70-1 Worldwide Surgical Procedures for Temporal Lobe Epilepsy

PROCEDURE	BEFORE 1986*	1986-1990†
ATLX	2336	4862
SAH	—	568
Neocortical resection	825	1073
Lesionectomy	—	440

ATLX, anterior temporal lobectomy; SAH, selective amygdalohippocampectomy.
*Total of 139 centers.
†Total of 2107 centers.
From Engel J. Surgery for seizures. *N Engl J Med.* 1996;334:647-652.

TABLE 70-2 Surgical Approaches for Epilepsy

Resective surgery
    Temporal lobe resections: "standard," selective
       amygdalohippocampectomy (SAH)
    Extratemporal resections
    Lesional resections
    Anatomic or functional hemispherectomy
Radiosurgery
Disconnection surgery
    Corpus callosotomy
    Keyhole hemispherotomies
    Multiple subpial transection (MST)
Neuroaugmentive surgery
    Vagal nerve stimulation (VNS)
    Deep brain stimulation (DBS)

TABLE 70-3 Surgically Remediable Syndromes

Temporal lobe epilepsy (TLE)	Idiopathic
	Mesial temporal sclerosis/mesial temporal lobe epilepsy
	Lesional (tumor, vascular malformation, developmental, ischemic, traumatic)
Extratemporal epilepsy	Idiopathic
	Lesional (tumor, vascular malformation, developmental, ischemic, traumatic)
Catastrophic epilepsy	Lesional
	Hemimegalencephaly
	Diffuse cortical dysplasias
	Sturge-Weber syndrome
	Rasmussen's encephalitis
	Porencephalic cysts
Secondarily generalized epilepsies	Lennox-Gastaut syndrome

TABLE 70-4 Engel's Outcome Classification

I. Free of disabling seizures
    Auras
    ≥2 years seizure free
    Generalized tonic-clonic seizures with drug withdrawal
II. Rare disabling seizures (≤2 per year) cusert ≥2 years
    Nocturnal seizures only
III. Worthwhile improvement
    ≥2 years
IV. No worthwhile improvement (≤90%)

From Engel J. Surgery for seizures. *N Engl J Med.* 1996;334:647-652.

TABLE 70-5 Neuropsychological Assessment of Epileptic Patients

FUNCTIONS	TESTS
Sensory functions	Halstead-Reitan examination
Motor functions: dexterity, coordination, speed, flexibility	Purdue Pegboard, Grooved Pegboard, Thurstone's Uni- and Bimanual Coordination Test
Perceptual-motor functions	Beery Visuo-Motor Integration Test, Block Design, Rey-Osterrieth Complex Figure
Psychomotor development and intelligence	Griffith or Bayley Developmental Scales, Wechsler Intelligence Scales for Adults or Children (WISC, WAIS), Stanford-Binet
Attention	Concentration Endurance Test, Auditory Continuous Performance Test
Memory and Learning	
General	Wechsler Memory Scales for Children and Adults
Verbal: word lists, story recall	California Verbal Learning Test (CVLT)
Visual: faces, patterns	Rey-Osterrieth Complex Figure
Expressive: sentence construction	Boston Naming Test, Token Test
Receptive: comprehension	Peabody Picture Vocabulary Test (PPVT)
Written: reading, spelling	Wide Range Individual Achievement Test (WIAT)
Numerical operations	WIAT, Woodcock-Johnson Achievement Battery
Executive functions	Tower of London, Wisconsin Card Sorting Test, Fluency Tests
Personality	Rorschach, Thematic Apperception Test for Children or Adults, SCL-90R
Affective state	Beck Depression Inventory, Hamilton Anxiety Scale
Social adjustment	Vineland Adaptive Behavior Scales, Achenbach Child Behavior Check List (CBCL)
Quality of life	Quality of Life in Epilepsy questionnaires (e.g., QOLIE-31, QOLIE-AD-48)

TLE AS A CHRONIC ILLNESS

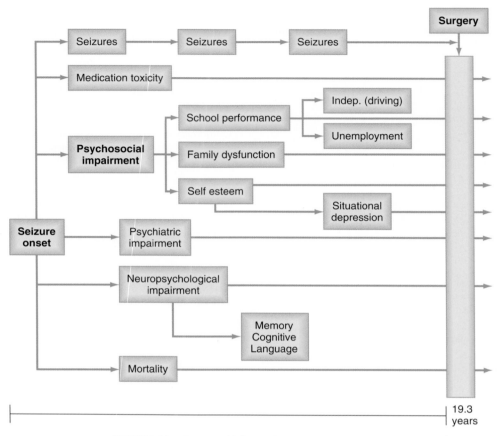

FIGURE 70-1 Temporal lobe epilepsy as a chronic illness.

risk for material-specific memory loss (particularly verbal memory loss) after surgery.[20,21] Nonetheless, the Wada test is invasive and requires a degree of patient cooperation, which may be suboptimal in young children and mentally retarded patients. Wada test results may be difficult to interpret in patients with bilateral language representation, excessive agitation, insufficient hemispheric inactivation by amobarbital (Amytal), or other procedural factors.[13,22] Functional neuroimaging modalities (i.e., functional magnetic resonance imaging [fMRI], [18F]fluorodeoxyglucose positron emission tomography [FDG-PET], and [99mTc]-hexamethylpropyleneamine oxime single-photon emission computed tomography [HMPAO-SPECT]) are increasingly being used as noninvasive tools for localization of epileptogenic cortex and assessment of focal functional deficits in patients with intractable epilepsy.[23-26] [18F]FDG-PET, by imaging the rate of cerebral glucose metabolism, reflects neuronal losses and focal functional deficits in epileptic patients and serves as a predictor of postoperative seizure outcomes. In 70% to 90% of patients with temporal lobe epilepsy (TLE), interictal [18F]FDG-PET detects unilateral temporal hypometabolism or asymmetric bitemporal hypometabolism. This reflects neuronal loss in the damaged temporal lobe, correlates with clinical and neurophysiologic findings,[24-26] and has been associated with favorable postsurgical seizure control in several studies.[25,27,28] Patients with left mesial temporal lobe epilepsy (MTLE) and regional left hemispheric hypometabolism tend to have impairments in verbal memory and word fluency.[29] Although the laterality of hypometabolism as determined by [18F]FDG-PET is related to memory deficits

measured by the Wada test,[30-33] the location or spatial pattern of the metabolic changes that can predict impairment in Wada memory performance has not been characterized. If future studies can demonstrate a strong correlation between Wada memory scores and metabolism on [18F]FDG-PET, presurgical [18F]FDG-PET could play a role in predicting memory laterality during the presurgical evaluation.

fMRI represents neuronal activity indirectly via hemodynamic changes in the brain. The size of the cortical area activated and the number of involved neurons directly influence the magnitude of the changes in regional cerebral blood flow.[34] Studies comparing fMRI and Wada test results in the same patient have shown a high correlation (from 80% to 100%) between the two procedures when the studies were aimed at either investigating language lateralization[35-38] or assessing memory asymmetries.[39-41]

Even though it is likely that functional neuroimaging will ultimately supplant the Wada test, more studies are required to confirm the reliability of data obtained in the context of presurgical evaluation of epilepsy.

Health-Related Quality of Life

Over the past decade, epilepsy-specific HRQOL instruments have been developed to assess the impact of epilepsy surgery on the "health" and "quality of life" of patients afflicted with intractable epilepsy. These instruments incorporate "generic" measures of health status previously validated in studies of health outcomes in other disease states, as well as "epilepsy-specific" measures of

in whom global amnesia occurred only after the hippocampus was removed.[145] This is further supported by reports of global amnesia after SAH.[149] Contemporary series report rare postoperative global memory deficits at a frequency of less than 1%,[49,143,150,151] whereas a less profound postoperative "severe amnesia" may be more common.[152]

MATERIAL-SPECIFIC MEMORY DEFICITS

Reported "material-specific" memory deficits include loss of short-term verbal and nonverbal memory postoperatively. In particular, short-term verbal memory loss is common after dominant temporal lobe resections, with significant decrements in verbal memory being reported in 25% to 50% of operated patients.[153] Verbal memory loss may accompany resections in the nondominant hemisphere, although at a much lower frequency.[153] Nonverbal memory deficits are less commonly identified, even after non–dominant-hemisphere resections,[154] although some authors report that these losses may be obscured by "practice effects."[153] In the Graduate Hospital series, evidence of significant short-term verbal memory loss was identified in many patients after dominant-hemisphere temporal lobe resections, with a trend toward improvement after nondominant temporal lobe resections.[12] In a recent 10-year series of 321 TLE patients undergoing a variety of surgical approaches for the treatment of nonlesional and lesional TLE, verbal memory declined in 34%, improved in 19%, and remained stable in 46% of patients.[121] Weak preoperative performance on measures of verbal memory, young age at surgery, and operations on the nondominant side were associated with stability or improvement in verbal memory. Short-term nonverbal memory measures exhibited similar rates of improvement and deterioration. Weak preoperative performance on measures of nonverbal memory and dominant-side operations were associated with improvement, whereas advanced performance preoperatively and older age were associated with deterioration.[121]

The high frequency at which verbal memory impairment occurs after dominant-hemisphere temporal lobe surgery has stimulated interest in predicting which patients are at risk for postoperative deficits.[8] Recent studies have documented significantly greater risk for verbal memory loss in two categories of patients: (1) those with intact memory function and a normal hippocampus ipsilateral to the seizure focus ("functional adequacy" hypothesis) and (2) those with ipsilateral hippocampal atrophy but impaired memory function, presumably related to poor function within the hemisphere contralateral to the seizure focus to be resected ("functional reserve" hypothesis).[8,155] Patients with dominant-hemisphere TLE and a reversed Wada memory asymmetry score (i.e., better memory performance in the epileptogenic temporal lobe, with poor right temporal lobe performance) have been shown to have a greater risk for memory morbidity after left-sided resection, as well as poorer seizure outcome postoperatively.[156] Patients with dominant-hemisphere hippocampal atrophy who undergo contralateral, non–dominant-hemisphere resections are also at risk for verbal memory deficits.[157] Preoperative MRI studies of hippocampal volumes and left hippocampal MRS profiles (creatine/NAA ratio) also help predict the risk to verbal memory performance after surgery.[62]

In a recent study, a multivariate risk factor model for predicting postoperative decline in verbal memory was developed in which five risk factors were independently associated with outcome, including (1) dominant-hemisphere resection, (2) MRI findings other than exclusively ipsilateral MTS, (3) intact preoperative delayed recall verbal memory, (4) relatively poorer preoperative immediate recall verbal memory, and (5) intact ipsilateral memory performance on the Wada test.[8,158] With this model, individual patients can be assessed with respect to their risk for deficits in verbal memory function after surgery.

STANDARD ANTERIOR TEMPORAL LOBECTOMY VERSUS SELECTIVE AMYGDALOHIPPOCAMPECTOMY: MEMORY OUTCOME

In patients thought to be at risk for global or material-specific memory deficits postoperatively, various management strategies have been proposed to reduce these losses,[8] including memory mapping in the temporal neocortex with restriction of neocortical resection, SAH, or simple denial of surgery to these patients.[159] With reports of global amnesia occurring in patients undergoing SAH,[149] it was thought that it may be advantageous to perform selective mesial resection from the standpoint of preservation of material-specific memory, particularly short-term verbal memory function. Although some early outcome studies in small series of patients suggested a possible advantage of SAH over standard anterior temporal lobectomy from the standpoint of postoperative memory outcome,[88,160] this has not been supported by other studies, and there have been reports to the contrary.[161]

In a recent review of 140 patients undergoing either right or left SAH, a decline in verbal learning and memory occurred after 32% of the right-sided and 51% of the left-sided resections.[54] The left SAH patients were particularly at risk when preoperative testing revealed intact verbal memory function, late onset of epilepsy, and the absence of MTS on MRI. Collateral damage to adjacent temporolateral tissue during the transsylvian dissection may exacerbate the deficits caused by hippocampal resection.[54,162] The role of deafferentation of the temporal circuitry during resection of the parahippocampal gyrus, amygdala, and hippocampus also needs to be considered. This is supported by PET evidence of worsening hypometabolism of the remaining temporal lobe neocortex after SAH.[163]

POSTOPERATIVE LANGUAGE DYSFUNCTION

After dominant-hemisphere temporal lobe resection, a syndrome of transitory postoperative dysnomia or even aphasia is observed in as many as 30% of operated patients.[164] In most cases, the dysnomia or aphasia gradually disappears over a period of a few weeks. This occurs even when resections are guided by intraoperative or extraoperative language mapping.[126,127] The cause of this transitory phenomenon is unclear, but it is more common when resections are carried to within 1 to 2 cm of essential language sites as determined by mapping procedures.[8,159,165] Other explanations for this phenomenon include resection of inferior temporal lobe "inessential" language sites,[166] brain retraction and associated "neuroparalytic edema,"[167,168] or deafferentation of white matter pathways. Some authors have suggested that such word-finding deficits represent an acute postoperative exacerbation of the preoperative deficits common in patients with TLE and that they last no longer than 1 year.[169]

Although some investigations of naming have not revealed enduring deficits at 6 and 18 months postoperatively,[170-172] others have suggested that significant, persistent word-finding difficulties do occur commonly after standard or anteromesial temporal lobe resection.[164,173,174] Such deficits have been reported to be associated with early risk factors for the development of seizures[173] and with the pathologic state of the resected hippocampus.[175] In one study, 7% of patients undergoing standard dominant-hemisphere resections exhibited persistent postoperative dysnomia.[174] Ojemann described enduring language deficits after resections within 1 to 2 cm of identified language sites.[176]

The aforementioned findings stimulated interest in the value of intraoperative mapping and tailoring of the lateral neocortical resection. Ojemann and colleagues suggested that up to 17% of patients undergoing left temporal resections 4.0 to 4.5 cm from the temporal tip (a "standard" temporal lobe resection) without mapping would experience postoperative deficits.[8,177]

Some centers now restrict cortical resections to 3 cm of the middle and inferior gyrus without mapping and have reported minimal postoperative language deficits.[103] A general trend toward restricted lateral cortical resection in the temporal lobe has resulted in language mapping being less commonly used. It has not been studied whether such restricted resection may engender deficits not seen in patients undergoing mapping.

Persistent, severe dysphasia has been reported in 1% to 2% of patients undergoing dominant-hemisphere temporal resections, even with language mapping.[116,143,178,179] Such adverse postoperative outcomes occur as a result of resection of essential language cortex or manipulation or thrombosis of the middle cerebral or anterior choroidal artery.[180]

Neurobehavioral and Psychosocial Outcomes

PSYCHIATRIC OUTCOME

Psychiatric morbidity has been reported to occur in 15% to 50% of patients with epilepsy in the literature.[181,182] There is a high prevalence of psychopathology, including depression, in candidates for temporal lobe resection both preoperatively and postoperatively.[183,184] One study reported postoperative improvement or resolution of long-standing depressive symptoms in 47% of patients undergoing temporal lobe resections, thus suggesting that preoperative depression is not a contraindication to surgery.[185] In the same study, depression occurred de novo in 10% of operated patients. Improvement in depression postoperatively is more likely in patients who are rendered seizure free.[186,187] Preoperative assessment of the risk for chronic depressive symptoms postoperatively may be achieved by using measures of emotional adjustment, such as the Washington Psychosocial Seizure Inventory.[187] The early postoperative period is characterized by the dynamic expression of varying psychopathologic conditions. In one study, half of the patients with no psychopathology preoperatively exhibited symptoms of anxiety, depression, and emotional lability 6 weeks postoperatively.[188] Other reports have documented new psychiatric problems in 31% of patients and resolution of psychiatric diagnoses in 15% of patients in the 6 months after surgery.[183] One study reported that 10% of 121 patients with TLE who underwent epilepsy surgery required postoperative psychiatric hospitalization.[189] The de novo appearance of hypomania requiring psychiatric hospitalization,[190] psychogenic seizures (particularly in females undergoing nondominant temporal lobe surgery),[183,191] and neurotic or psychotic symptoms[192] postoperatively demonstrates the necessity for comprehensive psychosocial and psychiatric assessments both preoperatively and postoperatively. In the context of a thorough preoperative evaluation, a history of psychotic symptoms does not represent an absolute contraindication to surgical intervention, although an exacerbation of symptoms may occur postoperatively.[8]

PSYCHOSOCIAL OUTCOME

It is increasingly being recognized that the syndrome of intractable TLE embraces comorbid conditions beyond the encumbrance of frequent, intractable seizures. Such comorbidity includes psychosocial, psychiatric, and neuropsychological impairment, medication toxicity, and excess mortality rates.[8] These impairments develop as a result of frequent, disabling seizures during critical stages of personal development and may not resolve immediately after surgery.

Patients are aware of epilepsy-associated disabilities and hope for their resolution after surgery. In a study of 69 preoperative patients, their aims for epilepsy surgery beyond freedom from seizures included desire for work, ability to drive, independence, socializing, and freedom from AEDs.[9] The psychosocial

outcomes of successful surgery were assessed in a 5-year follow-up study of the long-term changes in 61 surgical and 23 medically managed TLE patients.[193] In this study, 68% of the surgery group exhibited improved psychosocial status, as opposed to 5% of the medically managed group. Individuals who underwent surgery were found to be more likely to drive, live independently, work full-time, and be financially independent. Remaining seizure free was not a prerequisite for improvement in psychosocial measures in this study, although other investigations have documented diminished psychosocial adjustment in patients with recurrent seizures.[194]

Health-Related Quality of Life

A clear relationship has been documented between psychosocial status and quality of seizure control in medically managed epileptics.[195] Similarly, in postoperative patients, seizure-free patients score more favorably than those with either auras or recurrent seizures on a variety of measures.[45] In the only randomized, controlled trial of epilepsy surgery versus best medical management to date, patients who underwent surgery were documented to have improvement in both seizure outcomes and HRQOL.[2] The surgical group consistently scored higher than the medical group as early as 3 months after surgery and continuing to 12 months on both the QOLIE-89 and measures of school or job performance. Another study showed better HRQOL in postoperative seizure-free patients than in those with persistent auras and persistent seizures.[42] In another study of patients 2 years postoperatively, both seizure-free patients and those with a 90% reduction in frequency experienced significant improvement in HRQOL.[89] When compared with the health status of patients with other chronic diseases, postoperative patients with persistent seizures scored worse than did those with heart disease, hypertension, or diabetes. When patients were seizure free postoperatively, they scored better than patients with these non-neurological illnesses.[196] In a study reviewing nonsurgical and surgical patients evaluated preoperatively and 1 and 2 years postoperatively, significant improvement was identified on 10 of the 17 scales of the QOLIE-89 in patients who were entirely seizure free.[197] Significantly more improvement was noted at 2-year follow-up than at 1-year follow-up. In addition, patients with persistent auras were not significantly improved when compared with patients with persistent seizures.[197]

In a large prospective surgical series of 396 patients in which the QOLIE-89 was administered before surgery and up to 5 years after surgery, the most substantial improvement in HRQOL occurred immediately after surgery in all patients, but additional improvements over time were seen in the seizure-free group.[198] The effect, in this study, seemed to stabilize at 2 years after surgery and was related to the duration of freedom from seizures. Another method of determining well-being is to assess patients' perceived effect of surgery or their satisfaction with the results. A recent study found that of 396 patients, 80% would make the same decision (to have surgery) if given the choice again, and 91% to 92% reported a strong or very strong positive impact of surgery (influenced by freedom from seizures and gainful employment).[199]

Cost-Effectiveness of Surgical Treatment

Wiebe and coworkers used decision-analysis modeling and an intention-to-treat approach to compare medical and surgical treatment of intractable TLE in a Canadian population of 200 patients treated either surgically or medically over a 35-year period.[48] In their model, surgery required a larger initial expenditure; however, by 8 years after surgery, the cost savings engendered by the 57 seizure-free patients made surgical management less expensive than medical management across the entire cohort of surgical patients. Thus, surgical therapy was more cost-effective than medical management in this population.

In a decision-analysis model of surgical versus best medical management of intractable TLE, Langfitt used Rochester, New York, cost data to address the relative cost-effectiveness of different treatments.[8,47] This investigation used public health clinical research methods that express the cost-effectiveness of treatment as a "marginal cost-effectiveness ratio" (MCER), which represents the dollar cost per QALY added to treated patients' lives postoperatively. Each postoperative outcome state was assigned a quality adjustment on the basis of the ESI-55 scores achieved by 42 patients undergoing evaluation for surgery. With a state of total health adjusted to 1.0, patients with intractable seizures preoperatively were adjusted to 0.62; postoperative states were adjusted as follows: no seizures, 0.89; auras only, 0.80; and recurrent complex partial seizures, 0.72. In this model, a patient rendered seizure free after surgery would improve from 0.62 to 0.89 on the adjustment scale, and if this patient lived for 40 years in this state of health, the patient would accrue an additional 10 QALYs. The calculated MCER was $15,581 per QALY, which compares quite favorably with the cost of other health care interventions. Another study reported a cost-effectiveness ratio of $27,200 per QALY.[200] By comparison, the calculated MCER for lifetime tuberculosis screening for a 20-year-old African American was $324,537 per QALY.[47] The MCER calculated for stenting versus balloon angioplasty for symptomatic, single-vessel coronary artery disease was $29,893 per QALY.[47] In addition, the calculated MCER for asymptomatic intracranial aneurysm repair was $28,441 per QALY.[47]

A recent study sought to determine whether health care costs change when seizures become controlled after surgery.[201] Total costs for seizure-free patients had declined 32% by 2 years after surgery because of less use of AEDs and inpatient care. Costs did not change in patients with persisting seizures, regardless of whether they underwent surgery. In the 18 to 24 months after evaluation, epilepsy-related costs were $2068 to $2094 in patients with persisting seizures versus $582 in seizure-free patients. They concluded that costs remain stable for more than 2 years after evaluation in patients with TLE whose seizures persist but that patients who become seizure free after surgery use substantially less health care than before surgery. Further cost reductions in seizure-free patients can be expected as AEDs are successfully eliminated.

Complications of Temporal Lobe Resection

In a review of the accumulated worldwide experience on temporal lobe resective surgery before 1993,[49] significant/impairing complications were uncommon and included *death*,[51,124,143,202-204] *infection*,[49,143,167] *hemiparesis* from manipulation or thrombosis of the middle cerebral artery or anterior choroidal vasculature or from direct brainstem injury or resection,[203,205-209] *visual field deficits* from resection of Meyer's loop fibers in the roof of the temporal horn,[209-211] *hemianopia*[179,211,212] as a result of excessive tissue resection or infarction, postoperative *hematoma* formation,[124,143,202] and rare *third cranial nerve*[203,206] and *seventh cranial nerve*[213] palsies. There was a trend toward reduced mortality and morbidity over time in a large, single-center series and in a worldwide survey of 2282 operations performed between 1928 and 1973.[124]

In a contemporary, single-center study of 329 temporal lobe neurosurgical interventions (in 321 consecutive patients), 28 complications were reported (8.5%), including no mortalities, meningitis (1.5%), subdural hematoma (0.6%), deep venous thrombosis (1.2%) and neurological complications (5.2%).[121] In another single-center study of 215 patients undergoing temporal lobe surgery between 1984 and 1999, complications included mild hemiparesis, hemianopia, transient cranial nerve palsies, and transient language difficulties.[214]

In a multicenter study at six different centers in Sweden, the complications in 449 operated patients were reviewed.[56] In 247 temporal lobe resections, one mortality occurred in a 62-year-old woman who experienced a postoperative hematoma. Hemiparesis occurred in 5 patients, in 1 patient after neocortical resection and in 4 patients after resections involving the hippocampus. These complications were thought to be due to anterior choroidal artery infarction and manipulation of "perforating vessels." Other complications included hemianopia (0.4%) and cranial nerve injury (0.9%). A clear correlation between age and severity of complications was noted. Few complications occurred in those younger than 35 years. "Manipulation hemiplegia" was originally described by Penfield and colleagues[208] and may be caused by manipulation/injury to the anterior choroidal artery or the middle cerebral artery in the sylvian fissure. The resultant hemiparesis was thought to be more likely in older patients with atherosclerosis and hypertension and was one of the main complications of temporal lobe surgery in those older than 35 years. In a Norwegian epilepsy surgery series,[215,216] "large" complications occurred in 1 of 64 patients younger than 19 years and in 7 of 61 adult patients, thus confirming an increased risk for postoperative complications in older patients. Additional support is provided by another study of 215 operations performed between 1983 and 1999 in which permanent complications occurred in only 3 of 215 patients, and these patients were older than 30 years.[214]

Recent reports of unusual complications after temporal lobe resection include four cases of cerebellar hemorrhage believed to be related to postoperative epidural suction drains[217] and diplopia associated with transient trochlear nerve palsy in three patients.[218]

MORTALITY AFTER TEMPORAL LOBE RESECTION

The annual death rate attributable to epilepsy, which reflects accidents, suicide, and sudden unexpected death due to epilepsy (SUDEP), is higher in patients with chronic epilepsy than in the general population.[8] Studies of the impact of postoperative freedom from seizures have revealed that successful temporal lobe surgery lowers but does not normalize the overall mortality associated with chronic epilepsy.[219] In the Graduate Hospital series, all late mortalities (four) occurred in patients with recurrent seizures, including three with SUDEP and one suicide.[12] In another study, late mortality was studied and occurred in 2% of seizure-free patients and in 11.9% of patients with recurrent seizures.[214]

Lesional Temporal Lobe Epilepsy

Lesions of various types are identified in 15% to 30% of patients with intractable TLE.[8,220,221] These lesions may be neoplastic (astrocytoma, ganglioglioma, pleomorphic xanthoastrocytoma, dysembryoplastic neuroepithelial tumor), vascular (cavernous hemangioma, arteriovenous malformation [AVM], angioma), dysgenetic (microdysgenesis, focal or diffuse dysplasia, Sturge-Weber syndrome, tuberous sclerosis), or traumatic/ischemic. In a review of 167 patients with temporal or extratemporal lesions, 15% had hippocampal sclerosis or "dual pathology."[68] In further investigations of dual pathology, significant hippocampal neuron loss was identified in patients with lesions located adjacent to the hippocampus and in those with a history of "early injury."[222,223]

In patients with mesial temporal lobe lesions and intractable epilepsy, studies of lesional resection alone, without resection of mesial structures ("lesionectomy"), have produced disappointing results, with 22%,[224] 19%,[225] and 43%[226] of patients rendered seizure free in small series.[8] In those with laterally located lesions, seizure outcome is improved when complete lesion resection is achieved.[117] When lesional removal is performed along with standard mesial resection, seizure outcomes were improved, with 85%,[226] 91%,[227] and 92%[228] of patients being rendered seizure free in various series. Other authors have recommended gross total resection of the lesion along with an additional 5 to 10 mm of adjacent epileptogenic tissue ("lesionectomy plus") and sparing of mesial structures in the case of lateral lesions without dual pathology (i.e., normal hippocampus) and have reported favorable seizure outcomes with this approach.[8,121,229] In patients with temporal lobe lesions and dual pathology, resection of mesial structures along with the lesion has been recommended.[230]

The value of ECoG in guiding decisions regarding the extent of extralesional tissue resection is controversial[231] and has been addressed in reports of patients with TLE and various tumors[57,111,225,228] and AVMs[227]; these reports suggest an advantage conferred by resection of epileptogenic tissue, including mesial structures, along with lesional resection. Despite a possible advantage from the standpoint of seizure control, hippocampal resection in lesional cases may cause significant neuropsychological morbidity when hippocampal sclerosis is absent on MRI, particularly in dominant-hemisphere resections. In cases in which the hippocampus is not invaded by tumor, the approach of "lesionectomy plus" may confer less morbidity in dominant-hemisphere resections while maintaining favorable seizure outcomes.[229] Excision of a presumed epileptogenic region without lesional resection tends to result in poor outcomes.[231]

Extratemporal Epilepsy

The protean clinical manifestations of the extratemporal epilepsies result from the varied pathogenetic features of these disorders and the eloquent brain regions that are affected by seizures arising in the broad expanse of the frontal, parietal, and occipital lobes.[8] Extratemporal epilepsy patients undergo surgery less commonly than do patients with TLE.[1] The epileptogenic regions are often large and ill defined, thus mandating larger resections, and surgical approaches include lobar and multilobar, central and tailored resections, topectomy, and MST. Extratemporal resections are often combined with callosotomy or MST to improve efficacy. In a series of 2177 patients older than 51 years at the Montreal Neurological Institute, operations included temporal (56%), frontal (18%), central/rolandic (7%), parietal (6%), occipital (1%) and multilobar resections, as well as hemispherectomy (11%).[49,232]

Seizure Outcomes

The outcomes of extratemporal resections have historically been less favorable than those achieved with temporal lobe surgery, with approximately 45% being seizure free after surgery.[1] Improved imaging, patient selection, mapping, and surgical methods have resulted in improved outcomes in contemporary reports. In a study of 60 patients with extratemporal epilepsy, structural abnormalities were present in 83% of the patients.[233] Surgical resection of the frontal, parietal, and occipital lobes was performed. Preoperative mapping with grids and strips was performed in 50%, and the remainder underwent intraoperative mapping with ECoG. At 4 years' follow-up, 61% of the patients with focal lesions were seizure free versus 20% of the patients without histopathologic abnormalities. In a review of patients undergoing frontal lobe resections with adjunctive MST and callosotomy when appropriate, 72% were Engel class I or II postoperatively.[234] In another study of patients undergoing frontal lobe surgery, 24 underwent intracranial monitoring and 80% were Engel class I or II postoperatively (64% seizure free).[235] In this series, patients without lesions had better outcomes than those with lesions. In a review of frontal lobe epilepsies, 72% of lesional and 40% of nonlesional patients had an excellent outcome (Engel class I, II) after frontal lobe resection, with seizure-free

rates of 44% and 24%, respectively.[236] In a report of seizure outcomes in 37 patients with intractable frontal tumoral epilepsy, 67% of patients were Engel class I or II with 35% being seizure free.[237]

Complications of Extratemporal Resection

Complications of extratemporal resections include those related to invasive monitoring with grids, surgical complications of resection or MST, and neurological sequelae of intentional resection of or inadvertent injury to regions of eloquent cortex.[8] The complications in one study included three wound infections and three neurological deficits that resolved slowly.[233] In frontal lobe resections in Broca's area, within the posterior 2.5 cm of the opercula, the inferior frontal gyrus is usually spared,[232] and language sites identified by stimulation mapping techniques within the middle frontal gyrus may contribute, if resected, to transient or long-standing expressive aphasias.[177] Resection of the supplementary motor cortex may produce a transient syndrome consisting of postoperative mutism, contralateral neglect or hemiparesis, and diminished spontaneous movement, which usually resolves spontaneously over a period of weeks.[238,239] The cognitive effects of frontal resections are usually well tolerated.[240] Preservation of draining veins and arterial supply to the central area is a key consideration.[49] Partial resection of the non–dominant-hemisphere facial motor cortex is usually well tolerated; however, complete removal may produce long-standing perioral weakness.[115,241,242] The superior resection margin should be located no closer than 2 to 3 mm below the lowest elicited thumb response. Rasmussen described successful removal of the dominant-hemisphere facial motor cortex, provided that the vascular supply to the central area is meticulously preserved.[8,241,242] Large parietal resections behind the rolandic cortex can be accomplished with reported hemiparesis rates as low as 0.5%.[242] When resections are extended into the parietal operculum, visual field defects may occur if the resections are carried deep into the white matter.[203,242] A non–dominant-hemisphere parietal syndrome develops in some patients after large parietal resections, and in the dominant hemisphere, care must be taken to preserve Wernicke's area. In the occipital lobe, complete resection produces the expected contralateral hemianopia, and excision in the dominant hemisphere to within 2 cm of Wernicke's area may result in dyslexia.[242]

Extratemporal Lesional Epilepsy

Lesional resection alone has provided favorable results in extratemporal sites, with 9 of 14 patients (64%) being seizure free in one study[224] and 17 of 18 patients (94%) being seizure free in another study.[243] A meta-analysis of lesional epilepsy in all sites showed that 44% of the patients were seizure free after simple excision and 67% were seizure free after "seizure surgery."[244] Lesionectomy with removal of hemosiderin-stained brain resulted in freedom from seizures in 73% of patients with occult vascular malformations.[245]

Cortical dysplasias are associated with a unique pattern of intrinsic epileptogenicity, and intraoperative ECoG is thought by some authors to provide useful information for guiding resection and ensuring optimal seizure outcomes.[246,247] In a large series of patients undergoing surgery for focal epilepsy secondary to cortical dysplasia, 49% were seizure free.[248] Fifty-eight percent of those undergoing complete resection and 27% of those with incomplete resection were seizure free. Other reports suggest universal freedom from seizures in 100% of patients with Taylor's balloon cell–type cortical dysplasia after complete lesionectomy without ECoG mapping.[249] Other neuronal migration abnormalities, such as "double cortex," do not benefit from resective surgery.[250]

Hypothalamic Hamartomas

"Intrahypothalamic" hypothalamic hamartomas (HH) may be associated with intractable partial, gelastic, and generalized seizures,[251] as well as retardation and behavioral disorders, whereas precocious puberty predominates in the "parahypothalamic" subset.[252] Although several reports have documented successful surgical removal of these lesions and relief of seizures with transcallosal or modified subfrontal approaches,[253] such intrahypothalamic surgery raises concern regarding complications of the approach, as opposed to direct intrahypothalamic resection of these lesions. A recent study reported the results of transcallosal surgical resection of HH in 26 patients with refractory epilepsy in a prospective outcome study.[254] Fourteen (54%) patients were completely seizure free, and 9 (35%) had at least a 90% improvement in total seizure frequency. They also reported postoperative improvement in behavior and cognition. The likelihood of a seizure-free outcome seemed to correlate with younger age, shorter lifetime duration of epilepsy, smaller preoperative HH volume, and 100% HH resection. Another recent study looked at 37 patients with HH and symptomatic epilepsy who underwent transcortical transventricular endoscopic resection.[255] Eighteen patients (48.6%) were seizure free. Seizures were reduced more than 90% in 26 patients (70.3%) and by 50% to 90% in 8 patients (21.6%). Additionally, the mean postoperative hospital stay may be shorter in endoscopic patients than in patients who undergo transcallosal resection.

Cerebellar Seizures

The classic teaching that epileptic seizures do not arise from the cerebellar cortex has been challenged by several reports of focal motor seizures with secondary generalization in which the seizure focus appeared to be within the cerebellum.[8,256] Five of eight patients achieved freedom from seizures after resection of their cerebellar lesions.

Catastrophic Epilepsy

"Catastrophic epilepsies" are those in which panhemispheric syndromes are associated with intractable seizures. Such syndromes include Rasmussen's encephalitis, developmental syndromes (i.e., hemimegalencephaly, tuberous sclerosis, hamartomas, Sturge-Weber syndrome), and congenital hemiplegia/porencephaly.[257]

Hemispherectomy

Although the original surgical approach of anatomic, complete, en bloc hemispherectomy with sparing of the basal ganglia, hypothalamus, and diencephalon[114,242,258] was successful from the standpoint of seizure control, the immediate and delayed complications were daunting.[49] In particular, these procedures created a large area of denuded, unsupported subcortical tissue and significant volumes of intracranial dead space that led to repeated microhemorrhage and subdural membrane formation, referred to as "superficial cerebral hemosiderosis."[8] Late complications in the postoperative course occur in as many as 38% of patients[259] and include hydrocephalus,[260] increased intracranial pressure, neurological demise, or even death.[261] An alternative approach to hemispheric decortication (i.e., removal lobe by lobe) was reviewed in a large pediatric series.[257] The study reported that 26 of 48 patients were seizure free with a reduced rate of delayed complications.[257] Nevertheless, perioperative mortality occurred in 3 patients, and intraoperative blood loss and coagulopathy complicated the clinical course, particularly in children without brain atrophy or with hemimegalencephaly. In another version of "cerebral hemicorticectomy," the entire cortical surface is "degloved" to the level of the white matter. In one study this

resulted in 8 of 11 patients being seizure free, 1 patient with hydrocephalus, and no mortalities or delayed complications.[262]

With the introduction by Rasmussen of the technique of modified or "functional hemispherectomy," in which a generous central and temporal resection is juxtaposed with deafferentation of the frontal and occipital lobes, postoperative complications were significantly reduced.[115,242] With deafferentation rather than removal of the frontal and occipital lobes, the volume of intracranial dead space is reduced.[8] In a 7-year follow-up study of 14 patients, no hemosiderosis or hydrocephalus occurred, and 10 of the 14 patients were seizure free.

Over the last 15 years, the approach of hemispheric deafferentation as a preferred alternative to resection has been advanced by several authors, all of whom perform increasingly limited resections in concert with hemispheric deafferentation. During this period, "peri-insular hemispherotomy" was introduced, in which a smaller craniotomy and a much reduced peri-insular (opercular frontal, parietal, temporal) resection are combined with deafferentation of the frontal, parietal, occipital, and temporal lobes.[263] This study reported favorable seizure outcomes (9 of 11 patients seizure free and 1 of 11 improved 95%). In addition, the study documented reduced operative time, as well as a decrease in perioperative and delayed complications. Hemispherectomy in children has been found in recent studies to result in freedom from seizures in 43% to 79% of patients.[264-273]

The "transsylvian keyhole functional hemispherectomy" advanced by Schramm and colleagues[274,275] represents a true "minimalist" approach to hemispheric deafferentation.[8] A linear scalp incision and a 4- by 4-cm craniotomy provide the limited exposure required for a transsylvian approach to the circular sulcus, through which access to the entire ventricular system is gained.[8] Transventricular hemispheric deafferentation and amygdalohippocampectomy resulted in significantly decreased blood loss and a reduced mean operating time when compared with a Rasmussen-type functional hemispherectomy. Of the 20 patients reviewed, 88% were seizure free, and 6% had improvement in their seizures. This approach is facilitated in patients with hemispheric atrophy and not recommended in those with hemimegalencephaly.[8] In a modification of this technique, another study evaluated 34 patients undergoing "transopercular hemispherotomy," after which 67% of patients were seizure free.[276]

DISCONNECTION SURGERY

Multiple Subpial Transection

MST was developed by Morrell and colleagues to permit the treatment of partial epilepsies in which the seizure focus resides exclusively or partially within eloquent cortical regions.[277] In a review of the Rush Presbyterian experience with 100 patients, seizure outcomes were stratified according to MST performed alone (32 patients) or in conjunction with cortical resection (68 patients).[277] Class I and II outcomes were achieved, respectively, in 38% and 25% of patients with partial seizures undergoing MST alone, in 58% and 13% of patients with Landau-Kleffner syndrome treated by MST alone, and in 49% and 10% of patients when MST was performed in conjunction with resection procedures. In another review of 20 MST procedures performed without resection, less favorable outcomes were reported.[278] Yet another study of 12 patients undergoing MST with or without resection revealed less favorable outcomes, including Engel class II (1), III (2), and IV (9).[279] A study of long-term outcome reported a late increase in seizure frequency in 19% of patients treated by MST with or without resection.[280] A meta-analysis of an aggregate international experience consisting of 211 patients at six centers revealed that 53 underwent MST alone and 158 underwent MST plus resection.[281] An "excellent outcome," defined as greater than a 95% reduction in seizures, was achieved with MST plus resection in 87% of patients with generalized seizures and in 68% with complex partial seizures; with MST alone, 71% of patients with generalized seizures and 62% of patients with complex partial seizures had excellent outcomes.

As an increasing number of patients have undergone MST, we have been able to evaluate the neurological deficits resulting from this procedure. MST has been associated with a reduction in verbal fluency but preservation of spoken and written language abilities.[277] In this same study, 41 of 45 patients undergoing MST in Wernicke's area had preserved receptive function, including comprehension of spoken and written words. One patient suffered a deep hemorrhage causing a speech deficit. In 44 transections in the hand motor cortex, strength was preserved, and activities of daily living could be performed with the affected hand.[277] Of 7 transections in the leg area, which were described as technically difficult, 2 patients suffered footdrop because of subcortical venous hemorrhage. Overall, neurological complications were observed in 17% and permanent deficits were identified in 7%. No mortalities occurred. Two cases of "remarkable" intraoperative brain swelling and edema have been described, with a large intracerebral hematoma discovered in 1 patient.[278]

Corpus Callosotomy

The procedure of subtotal or staged total corpus callosotomy has been recommended less frequently since widespread introduction of the vagal nerve stimulator.[8] Nevertheless, an abundant literature attests to the utility of callosotomy as palliative treatment in patients with multiple or poorly lateralized (and unresectable) epileptogenic foci, secondarily generalized tonic-clonic seizures, and injurious drop attacks because of tonic or atonic seizures with resultant falls and injury.[282-286] Early studies revealed increased focal seizures in 25% of patients undergoing callosotomy.[285] It has been reported that 70% of patients will achieve elimination of seizures or at least a greater than 80% reduction in their frequency.[284,285,287]

In a recent series of 23 patients with intractable generalized seizures, patients underwent partial division (17) or total division (6) of the corpus callosum.[288] Forty-one percent of the patients were completely seizure free or nearly free of the seizure types targeted for treatment. Forty-five percent of the patients experienced a greater than 50% reduction in seizure frequency. Simple partial motor seizures developed in 4 patients postoperatively. In addition, mentally retarded patients tended to have poorer outcomes. Fifty-seven percent of patients experienced a transient disconnection syndrome that resolved. One patient suffered a clinically silent right frontal infarction related to venous thrombosis. The average hospital stay was 7.7 days.

Callosotomy is particularly effective for drop attacks. In a study of 52 patients with drop attacks (tonic or atonic seizures), 42 (81%) exhibited complete cessation of drop attacks, with greater success occurring in those undergoing total callosal section.[289] Two adult patients suffered a marked disconnection syndrome that gradually remitted, and 14 patients experienced transient akinetic states that resolved in several weeks. In another study of 20 patients monitored for 3 years, 10 exhibited a marked improvement in QOL, and 10 had greater than a 50% reduction in their seizures.[290] In another cohort of 17 patients, 9 had greater than an 80% reduction in targeted seizures, and overall, 88% of the parents reported satisfaction with the surgical outcome because of improved alertness and responsiveness.[291]

The surgical and functional complications attributable to corpus callosotomy are well described in the literature, with a larger number of complications noted in earlier series.[49,228] The main complications reported are acute disconnection syndromes, more common with total callosotomy, and the rare "split brain" syndrome. Subtotal (70% to 80%) callosotomy has been recommended as an initial procedure to minimize this complication. Surgical complications such as hemorrhage and infarction are related more to obtaining access to the interhemispheric fissure. With modern advances in microsurgical approaches and careful patient selection, corpus callosotomy is a safe procedure and a technique that is currently underused.

NEUROMODULATORY SURGERY

Vagus Nerve Stimulation

Since Food and Drug Administration approval in 1997 of VNS as palliative treatment of patients older than 12 years with intractable partial seizures, tens of thousands of patients have undergone implantation of a left vagus nerve stimulator.[292,293] In prospective clinical trials, a median partial seizure reduction of 34% after 3 months and 45% at 12 months was achieved in patient groups both younger and older than 50 years. Twenty percent of patients at 12 months had 75% or greater reductions in seizures, thus demonstrating improved seizure control over time.[292,293] At 3 months, generalized seizures were reduced by 46%. Improvements in mood have also been reported.[294] Although it has been observed that figural memory worsens when VNS is active during memory tasks,[295] no change in cognitive functions has been noted.[296] In patients with greater than 50% improvement in seizure frequency, QOL measures were improved.[296,297] In a long-term study looking at the effectiveness of VNS in epilepsy patients, seizure frequency was reduced by 26% 1 year after implantation, by 30% 5 years after surgery, and by 52% 12 years after implantation.[298] A more recent study suggested that VNS could be a safe and effective alternative therapy in children with drug-resistant epilepsy who are not candidates for epilepsy surgery.[299] In this study, after a mean follow-up of 31 months, 38% of the patients had a reduction in seizure frequency of greater than 90%.

Reported side effects include voice alteration, hoarseness, throat or neck pain, headache, cough, and dyspnea.[300] Adverse events in adults include infection requiring antibiotics or removal of the device (or both) and transient paralysis of the left vocal cord with hoarseness and aspiration.[301] There is an extraordinary report of self-inflicted vocal cord paralysis in 2 developmentally disabled patients by manipulation and rotation of the pulse generator within the subclavicular pocket.[302] Such a report mandates that patients be observed for manipulation of the device. In a review of adverse events in 24 children implanted with the vagal nerve stimulator, 15 events occurred in 11 patients, including lead fractures, wound erythema, requested removal of the device, abscess, malfunction, gastrostomy, recurrent psychosis, and diminished speech volume.[300] Removal of electrodes from the vagus nerve can be difficult. One paper reported resolution of a deep wound infection with antibiotics alone, thus suggesting that removal of the device might not always be necessary.[303] No increase in sudden unexpected, unexplained death with the vagal nerve stimulator was identified when implanted patients were compared with appropriate cohort populations.[304]

Deep Brain Stimulation

In the past, brain stimulation in the cerebellum, the caudate nucleus, and the anterior, centromedian, and ventralis intermedius thalamic nuclei has been performed in an attempt to modulate cortical excitability.[305,306] Small controlled trials in 14 patients who underwent cerebellar stimulation showed that 2 were improved and 12 were unchanged.[307] In another study, 4- to 6-Hz stimulation of the ventral caudate nucleus led to a reduction in neocortical and mesial temporal epileptic discharges and electrical spread of seizures, but clinical seizure data were not assessed. Caudate nucleus stimulation for epilepsy has not yet been tested in controlled studies. A small placebo-controlled study of stimulation of the centromedian nucleus showed no significant benefit.[308] An initial report of patients undergoing DBS in the subthalamic nucleus described a greater than 80% reduction in daytime seizures.[305] In another study, 5 patients with various seizure types underwent stimulation through bilateral electrodes in the anterior thalamus.[309] They reported a significant decrease in seizure frequency, with a mean 54% reduction (mean follow-up of 15 months). Two of the patients had a 75% or greater reduction in seizures. The observed benefits, however, did not differ between stimulation-on and stimulation-off periods, thus suggesting that either a placebo or carryover effect was present. Currently, a multicenter prospective randomized trial of scheduled chronic anterior thalamic stimulation in patients with medically intractable localization-related epilepsy is under way. Electrical stimulation of the hippocampus has also been reported in an attempt to block temporal lobe seizures.[310] In another small series, 3 patients with complex partial seizures had DBS electrodes implanted in the amygdala-hippocampal region.[311] Over a mean follow-up of 5 months, all patients had a greater than 50% reduction in seizure frequency. In 2 patients, AEDs could be reduced. Complications with DBS for epilepsy, such as hemorrhage and infection, have been reported in about 5% of patients,[312] although the hemorrhage is often not clinically significant.

There is growing interest in methods of neurostimulation that are modulated by input from sensing devices. A small pilot study reported that responsive stimulation controlled with an external computer system terminated some spontaneous seizures in eight patients, four with bilateral anterior thalamic stimulation and four with focal cortical stimulation.[313] In this study, analysis of electrographic seizure severity in stimulated versus nonstimulated events was used to rule out non–stimulation-associated effects and suggested both an immediate effect and a possible cumulative antiepileptic effect of high-frequency stimulation. A multi-institutional clinical study is also under way in patients with medically intractable partial onset seizures treated with a cranially implanted responsive neurostimulator (RNS). The RNS pulse generator continuously analyzes the patient's ECoG tracings and automatically triggers electrical stimulation when specific ECoG characteristics programmed by the clinician are detected. An initial single-center experience in a feasibility study of this device described a 45% decrease in seizures in seven of eight patients with a mean follow-up of 9 months.[314]

STEREOTACTIC RADIOSURGERY

Radiosurgery for Hypothalamic Hamartomas

HH may be associated with an epileptic encephalopathy marked by medically intractable gelastic and other seizures and behavioral and cognitive decline. Recent reports of successful treatment of HH with Gamma Knife surgery (GKS) have offered an attractive alternative to open surgery.[315-318] In a multicenter study of 10 patients undergoing GKS in seven centers, 4 patients were seizure free (Engel class I), 1 had rare nocturnal seizures, 1 had rare partial seizures, and 2 were improved.[316] A European, multicenter, prospective trial of GKS for HH has enrolled 60 patients, 27 of whom have exceeded 3 years of follow-up.[319] Ten of the 27 patients (37%) were seizure free (Engel class I). This study emphasized a temporal evolution of changes in seizure frequency during the postradiation period: a slight improvement in seizure frequency within the first 2 months, followed by

transient worsening, with a subsequent reduction and ultimate remission in favorable cases. Behavioral improvements, in addition to EEG normalization, occurred in a more linear fashion. Minimal side effects were reported. Patients treated with doses exceeding 17 Gy to the margins of the HH seemed to have greater rates of seizure remission than did those receiving less than 13 Gy.

Radiosurgery for Supratentorial Tumors

Given the diverse pathologic features and locations of central nervous system tumors associated with intractable epilepsy, the effects of GKS on tumor progression and seizure outcome are not well studied. One study divided 24 patients into two groups distinguished by the amount of radiation directed to surrounding tissue.[320] Outcome was assessed at a mean of approximately 2 years after GKS as "excellent" (Engel class I or II) or not. Patients in the high-dose group achieved a 66% improvement rate as compared with 42% in the low-dose group, with all patients exhibiting adequate tumor control. This report suggested that higher GKS doses to the epileptogenic region surrounding the tumor may improve seizure outcomes.

Radiosurgery for Arteriovenous Malformations

The potential efficacy of GKS in the treatment of symptomatic localization-related epilepsies has best been demonstrated in the treatment of AVMs. One large series reported that seizures remitted after GKS in 69% of patients with AVM and epilepsy.[321] Subsequent studies of both proton beam treatment and GKS showed a combined rate of seizure remission of 73% to 80%.[322-324] A recent large case series emphasized that the incidence of seizure remission is better with smaller AVMs.[324] However, another study noted that seizures remitted independent of radiologic remission of the AVM, thus suggesting that the effects of irradiation near the lesion, rather than improvement of the AVM itself, may be important in control of seizures after GKS.[321]

Radiosurgery for Cavernous Malformations

It is difficult to draw conclusions about seizure outcome after radiosurgery for cavernomas given the limited studies in the literature. In general, seizure remission appears to be lower than that encountered in patients after treatment of AVMs. The effect of dose to adjacent brain tissue around the margin of the cavernous malformation, thought to be important in the case of tumors and possibly AVMs, has not been systematically studied with regard to seizure control for patients with cavernomas. Excess morbidity in terms of postoperative hemorrhage and edema remains a concern. An early study suggested that GKS did not appreciably alter the natural course of cavernous malformations while exposing patients to radiation-induced complications that exceeded by seven times those expected with the same dose for AVMs.[325] A more recent retrospective comparison concluded that traditional open resection resulted in better seizure control and a lower risk for hemorrhage than GKS did.[326] A retrospective multicenter trial reported on 49 patients with cavernomas treated by GKS.[327] All patients had epilepsy that was medically intractable and were monitored for more than 12 months after treatment. The mean marginal dose was 19.2 Gy. Twenty-six patients (53%) became seizure free (Engel class I), 10 patients (20%) had a substantial decrease in the number of seizures (Engle class II), and 13 patients (26%) had little or no improvement. The average time to seizure remission was 4 months, and severe radiation-induced edema developed in 7 patients, but they recovered fully.

Radiosurgery for Mesial Temporal Lobe Epilepsy

The rationale for treatment of MTLE with GKS is less compelling than in the disorders discussed previously because MTLE is amenable to open surgery.[328] All of the studies in the literature differ in their treatment protocols and results, with most failing to achieve complete remission from seizures.[329-334] An earlier study had demonstrated that 6 of 7 patients (86%) studied over a 2-year follow-up period were seizure free after radiosurgery.[329] A more recent trial reported that 13 of 21 patients (62%) were seizure free (Engel class I) after radiosurgery for MTLE.[334] The variability in outcome of GKS therapy for MTLE may reflect differing approaches to the dose and target volume more than the anatomic target of the mesial temporal lobe structures.[328] Taken together, these studies suggest that low-dose protocols are less successful than higher-dose protocols. No significant clinical or neuroimaging changes occur until approximately 9 to 12 months after treatment, and the most dramatic drop in the seizure rate occurs between 12 and 18 months, coincident with the development and resolution of maximal MRI changes. Reported morbidities include visual field deficits, headache, nausea, vomiting, and depression.

Beyond seizure control, studies have begun to evaluate secondary outcome measures such as cognition and QOL. Three reports of neuropsychological outcome after GKS for MTLE are available.[332-334] One prospective, multicenter trial reported no mean neurocognitive changes through a 2-year follow-up period.[334] Similarly, one small series reported no group mean changes at 6 months of follow-up, although some individuals showed a decline in at least one cognitive domain.[332] Another small series reported on three participants with a 27-month follow-up who underwent dominant-hemisphere low-dose GKS.[333] No long-term consistent changes in neurocognitive measures were found, although each patient showed a decline in a measure of verbal memory. They concluded that the neurocognitive changes after GKS appear to be similar to those after anterior temporal lobectomy.

Overall, although GKS for MTLE is promising, the optimal treatment protocol has not yet been determined and the relative benefits in terms of seizure resolution and avoidance of complications have yet to be clearly demarcated from those of open surgery. A National Institutes of Health–sponsored multicenter pilot study on the safety of GKS for MTLE has recently been completed.[328] In this study, patients who would normally qualify for anterior temporal lobectomy for unilateral MTLE were randomized to either a 20- or 24-Gy dose. A total of 30 subjects were enrolled and monitored for 3 years; the preliminary results are promising, with safety well within that expected after routine GKS and favorable efficacy and neuropsychological profiles.

SUGGESTED READINGS

Bien CG, Kurthen M, Baron K, et al. Long-term seizure outcome and antiepileptic drug treatment in surgically treated temporal lobe epilepsy patients: a controlled study. *Epilepsia.* 2001;42:1416-1421.

Clusmann H, Schramm J, Kral T, et al. Prognostic factors and outcome after different types of resection for temporal lobe epilepsy. *J Neurosurg.* 2002; 97:1131-1141.

Engel J. Surgery for seizures. *N Engl J Med.* 1996;334:647-652.

Feindel A, Rasmussen T. Temporal lobectomy with amygdalectomy and minimal hippocampal resection: review of 100 cases. *Can J Neurol Sci.* 1991;18:603-605.

Fontaine D, Capelle L, Duffau H. Somatotopy of the supplementary motor area: evidence from correlation of the extent of surgical resection with the clinical patterns of deficit. *Neurosurgery.* 2002;50:297-305.

Gleissner U, Helmstaedter C, Schramm J, et al. Memory outcome after selective amygdalohippocampectomy: a study in 140 patients with temporal lobe epilepsy. *Epilepsia.* 2002;43:87-95.

Langfitt JT. Cost-effectiveness of anterotemporal lobectomy for medically-intractable complex partial epilepsy. *Epilepsia.* 1997;38:154-163.

Langfitt JT, Holloway RG, McDermott MP, et al. Health care costs decline after successful epilepsy surgery. *Neurology.* 2007;68:1290-1298.

Milner B. Psychological defects produced by temporal lobe excision. *Res Publ Assoc Res Nerv Ment Dis.* 1958;36:244-257.

Ng Y, Rekate HL, Prenger EC, et al. Transcallosal resection of hypothalamic hamartoma for intractable epilepsy. *Epilepsia.* 2006;47:1192-1202.

Ojemann G, Ojemann J, Lettich E, et al. Cortical language localization in left dominant hemisphere. *J Neurosurg.* 1989;71:316-326.

Ojemann G. Surgical therapy for medically intractable epilepsy. *J Neurosurg.* 1987;66:489-499.

Olivier A. Extratemporal resections in the surgical treatment of epilepsy. In: Spencer SS, Spencer DD, eds. *Surgery for Epilepsy.* Boston: Blackwell Scientific; 1991.

Quigg M, Barbaro NM. Stereotactic radiosurgery for treatment of epilepsy. *Arch Neurol.* 2008;65:177-183.

Salanova V, Markand O, Worth R. Temporal lobe epilepsy surgery: outcome, complications and late mortality rate in 215 patients. *Epilepsia.* 2002;43:170-174.

Schachter SC, Wheless JW. The evolving place of vagus nerve stimulation therapy. *Neurology.* 2002;59(6 suppl 4):S1-S2.

Schramm J, Aliashkevich A, Grunwald T. Multiple subpial transections: outcome and complications in 20 patients who did not undergo resection. *J Neurosurg.* 2002;97:39-47.

Schramm J, Kral T, Clusmann H. Transsylvian keyhole functional hemispherectomy. *Neurosurgery.* 2001;49:891-901.

Schwartz TH, Bazil CW, Walczak TS, et al. The predictive value of intraoperative electrocorticography in resections for limbic epilepsy associated with mesial temporal sclerosis. *Neurosurgery.* 1997;40:302-311.

Spencer SS, Huh L. Outcomes of epilepsy surgery in adults and children. *Lancet Neurol.* 2008;7:525-537.

Sperling M, O'Connor, M, Saykin, A, et al. Temporal lobectomy for refractory epilepsy. *JAMA.* 1996;276:470-475.

Stroup E, Langfitt J, Berg M, et al. Predicting verbal memory decline following anterior temporal lobectomy. *Neurology.* 2003;60:1266-1273.

Wiebe A, Blume W, Girvin, J, et al. A randomized, controlled trial of surgery for temporal-lobe epilepsy. *N Engl J Med.* 2001;345:311-318.

Wieser HG, Siegel G, Yasargil G. The Zurich Amygdalohoppocampectomy series: a cohort up-date. *Acta Neurochir Suppl.* 1990;50:122-127.

Wyler AR, Hermann BP, Somes G. Extent of medial temporal resection on outcome from anterior temporal lobectomy: a randomized prospective study. *Neurosurgery.* 1995;37:982-991.

Full references can be found on Expert Consult @ www.expertconsult.com

Functional Neurosurgery

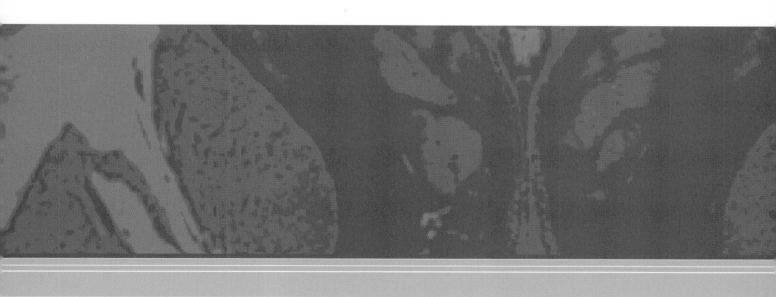

PART 1

Overview

CHAPTER 71

Introduction

Andres M. Lozano ■ Ron L. Alterman

As we complete work on this edition of Youmans, the field of stereotactic and functional neurosurgery is experiencing an unprecedented period of renaissance and growth. Advances in neuroscience and functional neuroimaging, improved understanding of the pathophysiologies of movement and neuropsychiatric disorders, innovations in medical devices, and an expanding armamentarium of minimally invasive, neuromodulatory, and biologic modifying techniques are all driving a strong innovation pipeline of novel concepts and clinical applications. Disorders that were long ago in the realm of neurosurgeons but had largely escaped our grasp are being repatriated, and disorders that were once considered to be well outside neurosurgery's purview are now within our sights.

Neurosurgeons were at the forefront of treatment of Parkinson's disease in the 1950s and 1960s but gave way to neurologists when the introduction of levodopa seemed to provide a lifelong cure. Similarly, psychiatric disorders were treated with neurosurgery in the 1930s, 1940s, and 1950s until the introduction of chlorpromazine and the indiscriminate use of frontal lobotomy by some practitioners (many of whom were not neurosurgeons) created a public backlash that forced all but a few neurosurgeons to abandon further development of this field. In the 1980s and 1990s, armed with better science and technology and the understanding that the limits of contemporary medical therapy had been reached, neurosurgeons revisited the treatment of Parkinson's disease, tremor, and dystonia to the enormous benefit of thousands. Likewise, as we now learn the limits of even the most sophisticated medical therapies for psychiatric illness, interest in surgical intervention for obsessive-compulsive disorder, depression, and addiction is on the rise.

In the chapters that follow, today's leaders in stereotactic and functional neurosurgery provide an up-to-date and comprehensive view of our rapidly developing field. The interested reader will find that we are continuing to make significant inroads in the treatment of movement disorders as we begin our exploration of the treatment of psychiatric illnesses, epilepsy, and pain. It will also be clear that deep brain stimulation will soon be accompanied by techniques such as intraparenchymal drug infusions, gene therapy, and brain-machine interfaces to alter the course of biologic processes, modulate aberrant neurological activity, or harness brain power for various purposes. In short, we are just beginning to learn how to work with our patients' brains to improve their lives. The possibilities are limitless.

PART 2

Basic Science of Movement Disorders

CHAPTER 72

Anatomy and Synaptic Connectivity of the Basal Ganglia

Yoland Smith

Our knowledge of the functional anatomy of the basal ganglia has increased greatly over the past decades as a result of tremendous developments in the field. The use of sensitive tracing methods combined with high-resolution immunocytochemical methods has revealed complex features of the microcircuitry and macrocircuitry of the basal ganglia. The results of these studies led us to reconsider various aspects of the pathophysiology of basal ganglia disorders and the potential role of the basal ganglia in motor and nonmotor functions. In-depth knowledge of the basal ganglia circuitry is a prerequisite for a deeper understanding of the neural systems and functional network changes that underlie the beneficial effects of surgical therapies for movement disorders. This chapter provides an overview of the functional anatomy of the primate basal ganglia with an emphasis on recent findings that led us to reconsider the complex functions of the basal ganglia in normal and diseased states. Because of space constraints, this review does not aim at covering the whole literature on basal ganglia anatomy. Readers are referred to previous comprehensive reviews and compendiums for a survey of the early literature and a more general overview of this field.[1-41]

FUNCTIONAL CIRCUITRY OF THE BASAL GANGLIA

The basal ganglia structures comprise the caudate nucleus and putamen, which make up the dorsal striatum and the nucleus accumbens and olfactory tubercle that form the ventral striatum. In rodents, the dorsal striatum is made up of a single mass of gray matter called the caudate-putamen complex. Other basal ganglia nuclei include the pallidum, which in primates consists of two parts, the internal and external segments of the globus pallidus, commonly referred to as GPi and GPe, respectively. In rodents, the homologue of the GPi is the entopeduncular nucleus and that of the GPe is the globus pallidus. The complex made up of the putamen and globus pallidus is called the lenticular nucleus. The subthalamic nucleus (STN), a small almond-shaped nucleus located laterally just below the thalamus at the junction between the diencephalon and midbrain, is another key basal ganglia structure often referred to as the "pacemaker" or "driving force" of the basal ganglia.[10,20,21,30,31] The fact that the STN is the prime target of surgical therapy for Parkinson's disease (PD) heavily supports its critical role in regulating basal ganglia function in normal and pathologic conditions.[42-52] Finally, another major component of the basal ganglia network is the substantia nigra,

located at the basis of the mesencephalon. The substantia nigra is divided into two major subnuclei; the substantia nigra pars compacta (SNc) consists of dopaminergic neurons, whereas the substantia nigra pars reticulata (SNr) is made up of GABAergic projection neurons. Other neighboring cellular groups related to the dopaminergic SNc include the ventral tegmental area (VTA) along the midline and the more caudal retrorubral field (RRF) lying along the ventrolateral edge of the upper brainstem. The basic circuit of the basal ganglia involves information originating from the entire cortical mantle and thalamus sent to the striatum, known as the main entrance of the basal ganglia. Once this information has been processed, it is sent to frontal cortical regions or the brainstem via functionally segregated basal ganglia thalamocortical channels of information that flow through the GPi and SNr, commonly known as the basal ganglia output nuclei (Fig. 72-1).

THE STRIATUM: AN ENTRANCE TO THE BASAL GANGLIA CIRCUITRY

The striatum consists of dorsal and ventral components based on their respective location along the dorsoventral extent of the telencephalon. These striatal regions are functionally different and process segregated information from the cerebral cortex; the main cortical input to the dorsal striatum originates from associative and sensorimotor areas, whereas the ventral striatum is predominantly innervated by limbic cortical regions.[1]

The striatal neuropil is further compartmentalized into two distinct territories called the patch (or striosomes) and the extrastriosomal matrix. These two striatal compartments receive distinct afferent projections and display a significant degree of neurochemical heterogeneity.[2,53] Despite a pretty clear understanding of the anatomic organization of these compartments, their functional significance long remained poorly understood. However, there is recent evidence that imbalanced activity between the patch and matrix compartments may underlie some aspects of repetitive motor behavior known as stereotypies.[54-57] The preferential recruitment of patch (or striosome) neurons after chronic exposure to psychostimulants probably represents a neural end point of the transmission from action-outcome associative behavior to conditioned habitual responding.[57] The differential regulation of the Ras/Rap/extracellular signal–related kinase (ERK) mitogen-activated protein (MAP) kinase signal transduction cascades between the striosomal and extrastriosomal

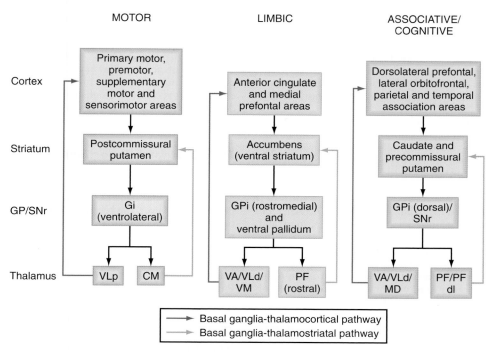

FIGURE 72-1 Segregated basal ganglia–thalamocortical and basal ganglia–thalamostriatal functional loops. Each functional modality is processed and travels through segregated regions of the basal ganglia and thalamic nuclei (ventral anterior/ventral lateral [VA/VL] and centromedian/parafascicular [CM/PF]) involved in motor, limbic, and associative/cognitive functions. GPi, globus pallidus pars interna; MD, mediodorsal nucleus; PFdl, dorsolateral extension of the PF; SNr, substantia nigra pars reticulata; VLd, dorsal VL; VLp, posterior VL; VM, ventromedial nucleus.

matrix compartments predicts the severity of the motor side effects induced by chronic dopaminergic antiparkinsonian therapy,[58] and preferential loss of striatal patch projection neurons occurs in X-linked progressive dystonia-parkinsonism.[59,60] Differential changes in $GABA_A$ receptor subunit expression between the patch and matrix compartments may underlie the variation in clinical symptomatology related to changes in mood in patients with Huntington's disease.[61]

Cellular Organization of the Striatum

The striatum is largely made up of the so-called GABAergic medium spiny projection neurons, which can be divided into two major phenotypes based on their peptide and relative dopamine receptor expression (see later). There are about 2.8×10^6 medium spiny neurons in the rat striatum, which accounts for 95% to 97% of the total striatal neuronal population.[62] These neurons have a small to medium-sized cell body from which emerge smooth proximal dendrites that give rise to a profuse and heavily spiny distal dendritic tree. Two main subtypes of striatal projection neurons have been identified: the "direct pathway" neurons preferentially express D_1 dopamine receptors, substance P, and dynorphin and project directly to the GPi and SNr, whereas "indirect pathway" neurons express preferentially D_2 dopamine receptors and enkephalin and project mainly to the GPe. Although both neuronal populations look morphologically similar, a recent rodent study has indicated that the dendritic length of D_1 projection neurons is significantly greater than that of D_2 neurons, an anatomic feature correlated with increased excitability of D_2 neurons in adult mice.[63-66]

The abundance and plasticity of dendritic spines are other important morphologic criteria that could contribute to the physiologic role of medium spiny neurons. On average, single striatal projection neurons of either pathway are covered by about

5000 spines distributed quite homogeneously at about 1 spine/μm of distal dendritic length across species.[67-70] The fact that in PD there is severe loss of striatal spines suggests an important regulatory role of dopamine and glutamate in striatal spine plasticity in normal and pathologic conditions.[67-70] Although recent data from transgenic mice indicate that the loss of striatal spines in dopamine-depleted animals is specific to D_2-containing neurons of the indirect pathway,[68] these findings could not be confirmed in 1-methyl-4-phenyl-1,2,3,6-tetrahydropyridine (MPTP)-treated monkeys and humans with parkinsons, both of whom display more homogeneous spine loss between direct and indirect pathway striatofugal neurons.[33,70]

Medium spiny neurons give rise to a rich plexus of intrinsic axonal arborization within the vicinity of the parent cell bodies and contact neighboring projection neurons.[71] Although this local connectivity has long been considered the main substrate for lateral inhibition in the striatum,[71] electrophysiologic data have demonstrated that these connections are sparse and distal and consequently are poorly influential on the activity of striatal projection neurons.[72,73] However, these connections are specifically organized and unidirectional between pairs of D_1- or D_2-containing neurons or from D_2- to D_1-positive projection neurons,[74] with connections from D_1- to D_2-positive neurons being rare. The strength of these intrinsic connections is significantly reduced in dopamine-depleted parkinsonian conditions.[74]

The striatum also comprises four main populations of interneurons that represent about 2% to 3% of the total striatal neuronal population in rats, whereas in monkeys they account for as much as 23% of all striatal neurons.[15,16,75,76] The *cholinergic interneurons*, which probably correspond to the "tonically active" neurons physiologically identified in the rat and monkey striatum,[76-79] display a significant degree of colocalization with calretinin in primates.[80] These neurons receive strong synaptic input from GABAergic axon collaterals of substance P–containing striatofugal neurons in rats[81] and play a key role in reward-related learning and motivated behavior.[77,78,82-89] In rats, they are connected to one another through GABAergic interneurons, thus providing a mechanism for their widespread recurrent inhibition via nicotinic excitation.[90] The cholinergic interneurons are key mediators of dopamine-dependent striatal plasticity and learning.[24,91-95]

The *GABA/parvalbumin interneurons* are known as the "fast-spiking interneurons." They form axosomatic synapses on projection neurons, are electrotonically coupled through gap junctions, and control spike timing in projection neurons, thereby providing the substrate for fast-forward intrastriatal inhibition of projection neurons in response to cortical activation (but see the article by Berke[96]).[15,16,76]

The *GABA/nitric oxide synthase/neuropeptide Y/somatostatin interneurons* are categorized physiologically as "persistent and low-threshold spike" neurons.[15,16,76] These cells induce large inhibitory currents in projection neurons and release nitric oxide to modulate plasticity at glutamatergic synapses.[16] In addition, because somatostatin actions entrain projection neurons into the rhythms generated by some interneurons, they are capable of modifying the processing and output of the striatum.[97]

The *medium-sized GABA/calretinin interneurons* represent the largest population of striatal interneurons in humans,[80] display physiologic characteristics similar to the persistent and low-threshold spike neurons, and exert powerful monosynaptic inhibition of medium spiny projection neurons.[76]

Extrinsic Connectivity of the Striatum

Corticostriatal Projections

The cerebral cortex is the main source of glutamatergic input to the striatum. The corticostriatal pathway originates from all cortical areas and displays a highly topographic pattern of distribution in the striatum that imposes functionally segregated maps on it (see Fig. 72-1).[98] The anatomic organization of the corticostriatal system has been extensively studied in rats and monkeys and more recently in humans via functional imaging approaches.[99-119] These findings led to a basic scheme of functional connectivity between the cerebral cortex and striatum. The somatosensory, motor, and premotor cortices innervate the postcommissural region of the putamen somatotopically in a band-like pattern; the associative cortical areas from the frontal, parietal, and temporal lobes project to the caudate nucleus and the precommissural putamen; and the limbic cortices, the amygdala, and the hippocampus terminate preferentially in the ventral striatum (see Fig. 72-1).[1,98] Functionally related associative or sensorimotor cortical inputs from areas connected through corticocortical projections either overlap or remain segregated in the striatum.[116-119]

In rats, corticostriatal neurons are divided into two distinct subsets: the superficial "intratelencephalic neurons," which project solely to the striatum and the cerebral cortex, preferentially target "direct pathway" neurons, whereas the deep "pyramidal tract" neurons, which send their main axonal projections to the brainstem and spinal cord with collaterals to the striatum, preferentially target "indirect pathway" neurons.[120,121] However, the physiologic significance of these anatomic observations remains unclear because electrophysiologic data suggest that intratelencephalic neurons are the main source of functional excitatory input to both populations of striatal projection neurons.[122] There is also significant controversy regarding the existence of pyramidal tract corticostriatal neurons in primates.[123-125]

The dendritic spines of medium spiny neurons and GABA/parvalbumin-containing (PV) interneurons are the main targets of corticostriatal afferents,[126-127] thereby laying the foundation for feedforward inhibition of striatal projection neurons in response to corticostriatal input.[15,16,126-128] The cortical drive of feedforward inhibition from GABA/PV interneurons contributes to the imbalance of activity between the two populations of striatal projection neurons in the rat model of PD.[129] However, this concept has recently been challenged by electrophysiologic evidence of the lack of correlation between cortical information flowing to GABA/PV neurons versus projection neurons.[96]

Thalamostriatal Projections

The thalamus is another major source of glutamatergic projections to the striatum, but very little is known about the functional integration of the thalamostriatal pathways in the basal ganglia network. However, the recent evidence that deep brain stimulation (DBS) of the caudal intralaminar nuclei, the main sources of thalamostriatal projections, alleviates some symptoms of PD and Tourette's syndrome (see later) has generated significant interest in the thalamostriatal systems. Two major sources of thalamostriatal projections have been recognized: those from the caudal intralaminar nuclei and those from other thalamic nuclei.

Thalamostriatal Projections from the Caudal Intralaminar Nuclei

The intralaminar thalamic nuclei are a major source of excitatory afferents to the striatum. In primates, the centromedian (CM) and parafascicular (PF) nuclei give rise to projections that largely terminate in different functional regions of the striatum. The medial part of the CM nucleus projects to the sensorimotor postcommissural sensorimotor putamen, whereas the PF nucleus predominantly innervates the associative caudate nucleus and the limbic ventral striatum.[14,37] The dorsolateral PF nucleus selectively projects to the precommissural putamen. CM/PF neurons send only sparse projections to the cerebral cortex.[130] At the synaptic level, CM and PF input preferentially targets the dendrites of striatal projection neurons.[131-133] CM neurons also innervate striatal interneurons immunoreactive for choline acetyltransferase, parvalbumin, and somatostatin, but not calretinin.[134] In line with these electron microscopic data, projections from the CM/PF complex tightly regulate the electrophysiologic activity and release of neurotransmitters from cholinergic interneurons[135-137] and are required for the sensory responses of the "tonically active neurons "(probably cholinergic) that are acquired through sensorimotor learning in monkeys.[138-140]

Thalamostriatal Projections from Other Thalamic Nuclei

The CM/PF complex is not the only source of thalamostriatal projections. Albeit sparse, most thalamic nuclei also contribute to a topographically and functionally organized striatal innervation.[14,37,141-145] However, the synaptology of striatal projections from the CM/PF nuclei is strikingly different from that of other thalamic nuclei; that is, CM/PF terminals form synapses predominantly with the dendritic shafts of medium spiny neurons and interneurons, whereas projections from other thalamic nuclei, including the rostral intralaminar, midline, and relay thalamic nuclei, almost exclusively target dendritic spines.[14,37,144,145] The degree of axon collateralization to the striatum and cortex of projections from the CM/PF complex versus other thalamic nuclei is significantly different. In contrast to CM/PF projections, which are directed mainly toward the striatum with minimal innervation of the frontal cortical areas, the relay and rostral intralaminar nuclei project predominantly to the cerebral cortex with modest striatal innervation.[14,37,131,133,144,146] In general, thalamostriatal projections from single CM/PF neurons are much more focused and give rise to a significantly larger number of terminals than do individual corticostriatal axons.[37,125,130] The functional significance of such differences in the pattern of striatal innervation between CM/PF and cortical input remains poorly understood.

Vesicular Glutamate Transporters as Specific Markers of Thalamostriatal versus Corticostriatal Projections

The vesicular glutamate transporters 1 and 2 (vGluT1 and vGluT2) are selective markers of the corticostriatal and thalamostriatal glutamatergic terminals, respectively.[14,37,145,147] More than 95% of vGluT1 terminals contact spine heads, whereas only 50% to 60% of vGluT2 terminals do so in monkeys, a pattern that does not change in parkinsonism.[145] In rats, there is a significant difference in the microcircuitry of vGluT2 terminals between the patch and matrix striatal compartments such that most axodendritic vGluT2 synapses are found in the matrix, consistent with the idea that the CM/PF complex is the main source of this synaptic input.[14,37,133]

Functional Roles of the Thalamostriatal Systems

The role or roles of the thalamostriatal systems probably differ between projections that arise from the CM/PF nuclei and those arising from other thalamic nuclei. In nonhuman primates, CM/PF neurons most likely supply striatal neurons with information that has attentional value in that they act as detectors of behaviorally significant events occurring on the contralateral side.[138,139] In line with these data, changes in CM/PF activity are induced in response to attention-demanding reaction time tasks in humans.[148] Electrical stimulation of the CM nucleus induces complex excitatory and inhibitory electrophysiologic responses in striatal projection neurons and cholinergic interneurons.[135-137] In contrast, stimulation of rostral intralaminar nuclei results in complex alterations in cognitive processing, most likely through regulation of cortical and striatal activity.[149,150] The function of other thalamostriatal systems is unknown, but they probably act as a positive reinforcer of specific populations of striatal neurons involved in performing a selected cortically driven behavior.[14,37,151]

Centromedian/Parafascicular Degeneration in Parkinson's Disease

Postmortem studies of patients' brains affected with progressive supranuclear palsy, Huntington's disease, or PD revealed as much as a 50% loss of cells in the CM/PF nuclei.[152,153] In patients with PD, the parvalbumin neurons are affected mainly in the PF nucleus, whereas the nonparvalbumin/noncalbindin neurons are specifically targeted in the CM nucleus.[153] Asymmetric changes in the shape of the thalamus between patients with PD and healthy controls were recently reported.[154] It is not clear whether these thalamic pathologies are also induced in animal models of parkinsonism. In rodents, some studies showed significant loss of PF thalamostriatal neurons in 6-hydroxydopamine–treated rats and MPTP-treated mice, whereas others did not find any cell loss in the PF nucleus under similar conditions.[14,37] In nonhuman primates, a significant reduction in the relative abundance of vGluT2-positive terminals forming axodendritic synapses in the putamen of MPTP-treated monkeys was reported, thus suggesting a possible loss of CM-striatal neurons in this animal model.[145]

The Mesostriatal Dopaminergic Systems

Three main groups of dopaminergic neurons are found in the ventral midbrain: the A8 (RRF), A9 (SNc), and A10 (VTA) regions. Each of these subnuclei consists of predominantly dopaminergic neurons among which are interspersed small populations of GABAergic interneurons, except in the VTA, which has a significant population of GABAergic projection neurons.[9] Various neuropeptides, including neurotensin and cholecystokinin, have been identified in subsets of dopaminergic neurons in the medial SNc and VTA.[155-158] Ventral tier SNc (SNc-v) neurons are more significantly enriched with dopamine transporter than other ventral midbrain dopaminergic neurons,[159] which may account for the preferential vulnerability of SNc-v neurons in response to MPTP.[160,161] In addition, the calcium-binding protein calbindin D28k (CB) is strongly expressed in neurons of the VTA and RRF, as well as in dorsal tier neurons of the SNc (SNc-d), but it is not found in SNc-v neurons.[9,162] A neuroprotective role of CB in SNc-d and VTA neurons in PD has been suggested, whereas the absence of CB may contribute to the selective vulnerability of SNc-v neurons in parkinsonism.[163-165] The pattern of nigrostriatal degeneration at both the striatal and nigral levels is, indeed, correlated with the expression level of CB. At the striatal level, the sensorimotor postcommissural putamen, the most sensitive striatal region to dopaminergic denervation in PD (see later), is devoid of CB-containing neurons.[166] In the substantia nigra, the more sensitive SNc-v neurons express a low level of CB immunoreactivity, whereas the relatively spared SNc-d and VTA neurons are enriched in CB.[159,167] Finally, SNc neurons targeted by a strong CB-containing innervation from the striatum are more resistant than nigral neurons in CB-poor pockets called nigrosomes.[164] Together, these findings highlight the potential neuroprotective role of CB in the pathogenesis of PD.

Based on various tract-tracing studies in monkeys, the following pattern emerged for organization of the nigrostriatal dopaminergic system in primates: (1) the sensorimotor striatum (i.e., postcommissural putamen) receives its main dopaminergic innervation from neuronal columns in the SNc-v, (2) the limbic striatum (i.e., nucleus accumbens) is the main recipient of dopaminergic projections from VTA and SNc-d neurons, and (3) the associative striatum (i.e., caudate nucleus and precommissural putamen) is preferentially innervated by dopaminergic neurons in the densocellular part of the SNc-v.[9,33] In rats, the pattern appears to be slightly different in that SNc-d neurons project predominantly to the dorsal striatum.[168]

Single-cell filling studies have identified two main types of nigrostriatal axons: thin, varicose and widespread fibers that arise from neurons in the SNc-d, VTA, and RRF and preferentially terminate in the matrix striatal compartment, as well as thick varicose fibers that arise from the SNc-v and terminate mostly in the patch striatal compartment.[169] A recent study using a more sensitive viral tracing method challenged this concept of dual nigrostriatal fiber systems and instead suggested a much more extensive axonal arborization of individual SNc dopaminergic neurons that do not display any preferential innervation of the patch or matrix compartments.[170]

It is well established that the pattern of progressive dopaminergic cell loss in PD is not homogeneous but rather displays a complex topographic and regional organization. In PD patients and MPTP-treated monkeys, two main features of nigrostriatal denervation have been well characterized: (1) the dopaminergic projections to the sensorimotor striatum (postcommissural plus dorsolateral precommissural putamen) are affected before those to the associative (caudate nucleus) and limbic (nucleus accumbens) striatal regions,[171,172] and (2) VTA projections to the ventral striatum display a much lower degree of degeneration than do other midbrain dopaminergic cell groups.[173,174] A preferential dopaminergic denervation of patch over matrix has also been suggested in MPTP-treated monkeys, but these data remain controversial and may be dependent on the animal species used and the method of MPTP administration.[165,175]

Dopamine has long been known to be a critical neuromodulator of basal ganglia neuronal activity through both presynaptic and postsynaptic mechanisms. Five dopamine receptor subtypes are expressed in striatal projection neurons and interneurons, thus providing multiple targets through which dopamine can mediate its effects. The dopamine-mediated regulation of glutamatergic and cholinergic transmission is severely affected in parkinsonism, thereby contributing to the abnormal changes in basal ganglia network activity described in PD. The morphology and plasticity of dendritic spines are also tightly regulated by dopamine/glutamate interactions, and this provides a substrate for integration and processing of extrinsic information to the basal ganglia circuitry.[6,9,33,70]

Other important modulatory systems that are not discussed in this review include the serotoninergic system from the raphe nuclei and the noradrenergic ascending projections from the locus coeruleus. Although not as well studied as the dopaminergic system, there is evidence that these two neurotransmitters regulate physiologic activity in various basal ganglia nuclei and possibly contribute to midbrain dopaminergic neuron loss and the development of nonmotor deficits and motor side effects from long-term dopaminergic therapy in patients with PD.[176-183]

Intrastriatal Dopamine Neurons: A Potential Compensatory Mechanism in Parkinson's Disease

Dopaminergic interneurons have been described in the striatum of dopamine-depleted rats and monkeys and in the caudate nucleus and putamen of humans with PD.[184-188] These aspiny neurons are small and coexpress various markers of dopaminergic neurons—glutamic acid decarboxylase and, in a small subset, calretinin.[184,187] They receive scarce synaptic input and show up preferentially in the precommissural putamen and caudate nucleus in MPTP-treated monkeys.[187] Their density significantly increases after dopamine depletion and the administration of glial-derived neurotrophic factor in the striatum,[189] thus suggesting a potential compensatory role for dopaminergic interneurons in PD.

Extrastriatal Dopaminergic Systems

Although the striatum is well recognized as the main target of midbrain dopaminergic neurons, there is significant evidence that extrastriatal dopamine acting directly at the level of the globus pallidus, STN, and SNr also plays an important role in regulating basal ganglia function in normal and pathologic conditions.[9,33] In addition, the existence of a dopaminergic afferent system to the ventral motor thalamus has recently been suggested.[189-192] Although the exact origin of this system remains controversial, it could play a critical role in regulating the activity of thalamocortical neurons in basal ganglia–receiving nuclei, thereby contributing to the fine-tuning of information flow through the basal ganglia–thalamocortical loops in normal and parkinsonian conditions. Because of space limitations, this topic cannot be discussed extensively in this chapter, but readers are referred to recent publications and reviews that discuss the anatomic and physiologic evidence for these projections.[9,33]

THE DIRECT AND INDIRECT PATHWAYS OF THE BASAL GANGLIA

Although overly simplistic, the direct and indirect pathway model of the basal ganglia has driven the field of basic and clinical basal ganglia research for the past decades. Obviously, since its introduction, this model has been challenged, revised, and

updated as a result of gain in new knowledge of the basal ganglia circuitry, but it remains the most reliable working model of normal and abnormal physiology of the basal ganglia. The "direct pathway" refers to the monosynaptic connection between the striatum and the basal ganglia output nuclei, the GPi and the SNr, whereas the "indirect pathway" refers to the polysynaptic pathway linking the striatum and GPi/SNr via the GPe and STN.[193-195] GABAergic striatal neurons give rise to either of these pathways, but they can be segregated into two populations by their peptide content (substance P—direct; enkephalin—indirect) and their preferential expression of dopamine receptor subtypes (D_1—direct; D_2—indirect).[195] A balance between the activity of the two pathways is essential for normal functioning of the basal ganglia. In PD, the loss of striatal dopamine results in increased activity of indirect striatofugal neurons and decreased output from direct striatofugal neurons. Because of the polarity of connections in the direct/indirect pathways, this results in increased GABAergic basal ganglia outflow to the thalamus, which in turn may reduce cortical excitability and decrease motor behavior (Fig. 72-2).

This traditional scheme of the basal ganglia circuitry has been challenged over the past decades because of some anatomic and molecular data suggesting that the two pathways may not be as segregated as previously thought. On the one hand, single-cell

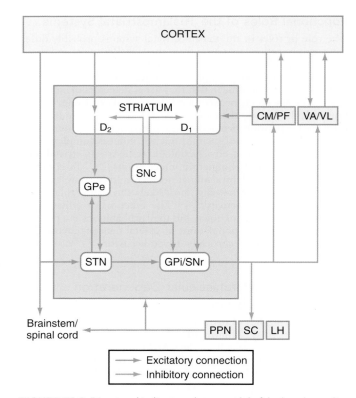

FIGURE 72-2 Direct and indirect pathway model of the basal ganglia. The *blue box* indicates tightly interconnected basal ganglia nuclei that receive extrinsic input from the cortical, thalamic, and brainstem regions. The extrastriatal substantia nigra pars compacta (SNc) dopaminergic projections to the globus pallidus pars externa (GPe), subthalamic nucleus (STN), and globus pallidus pars interna/substantia nigra pars reticulata (GPi/SNr) have been omitted from this diagram. The connections between the basal ganglia and the pedunculopontine nucleus/superior colliculus/lateral habenula (PPN/SC/LH) are depicted in more detail in Figure 72-4. CM, centromedian nucleus of the thalamus; D_1 and D_2, dopamine D_1-type and D_2-type receptors; PF, parafascicular nucleus of the thalamus; VA/VL, ventral anterior and ventrolateral nuclei of the thalamus.

filling studies have demonstrated that most striatofugal neurons of the direct pathway give off collaterals to the GPe.[8,196-198] Although the functional significance of these collateralized projections still remains poorly understood, they surely deserve consideration in the interpretation of functional changes in basal ganglia circuitry in normal and diseased states.

Another challenge to the model comes from molecular studies showing that D_1 and D_2 receptor mRNA may not be as segregated as originally thought.[199-205] Significant controversy about dopamine receptor segregation was also raised in immunocytochemical studies; some reports have shown that D_1 and D_2 receptor protein immunoreactivity was largely segregated in two distinct populations of striatal spines,[121,206] whereas others demonstrated a high level of D_1 and D_2 receptor immunoreactivity at the single-cell level in the rat striatum.[207,208]

More recently, bacterial artificial chromosome (BAC) transgenic mice have been developed.[209,210] These BAC-D_1 and BAC-D_2 mice display complete segregation of D_1 and D_2 receptor mRNA, even when measured with the highly sensitive single-cell mRNA amplification method, an approach that revealed significant D_1/D_2 colocalization in normal rats.[25,68,200,201,205] Whether this strict segregation of the two dopamine receptor subtypes underlies distinct functional dopamine-mediated physiologic effects or different mechanisms of synaptic plasticity between normal animals and these transgenic mice remains to be established. Another important fact to keep in mind while interpreting dopamine-mediated effects in individual striatofugal neurons is the possible coexpression of other D_1 or D_2 receptor family subtypes (i.e., D_3, D_4, and D_5 receptors) in the two main populations of striatofugal neurons.[211-216] To our knowledge, the relative expression level of D_3, D_4, and D_5 receptors in striatofugal neurons of BAC-D_1/enhanced green fluorescent protein (EGFP) or BAC-D_2/EGFP transgenic mice remains unknown. We believe

that such information is absolutely essential to clearly determine the chemical phenotype of striatofugal neurons in these animals and ensure that the functional data gathered from these mice can be translated to normal brains.

THE HYPERDIRECT CORTICOSUBTHALAMIC SYSTEM: ANATOMIC AND FUNCTIONAL SIGNIFICANCE

The STN is another major entry station for delivery of extrinsic cortical information to the basal ganglia circuitry. Information flowing along the corticosubthalamic tract is transmitted to the SNr and GPi at a faster pace than information transmitted along the direct and indirect corticostriatofugal systems.[217] Basal ganglia output neurons do indeed respond with a fast excitation to electrical stimulation of the motor cortices. Excitotoxic STN lesions abolish these responses. In monkeys, the corticosubthalamic projection originates mainly from the motor cortices. Input from M1 flows along the dorsolateral sector of the nucleus, whereas projections from the supplementary motor area, premotor cortices, and the cingulate motor cortex overlap in the dorsomedial STN. There is a reversed somatotopy between the dorsolateral "M1 domain" and the dorsomedial "supplementary motor area/premotor cortices/cingulate motor cortex domain."[217-219] The ventrolateral half of the STN receives some input from the frontal and supplementary eye field areas, whereas the medial tip of the STN is involved in the processing of limbic-related information (Fig. 72-3). However, the exact sources and pattern of termination of cortical input to the ventral sectors of the STN have been less studied and remain poorly characterized.

An important role for the hyperdirect corticosubthalamic projection in the selection of motor programs has been

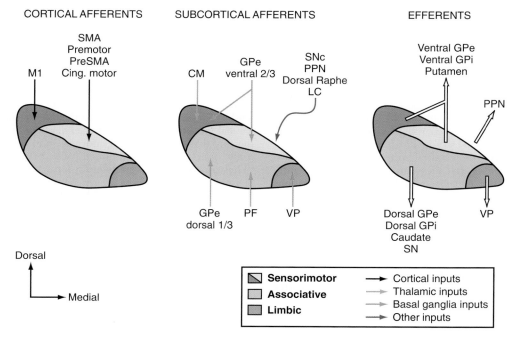

FIGURE 72-3 Afferent and efferent connections of functional subregions of the subthalamic nucleus. The sensorimotor region is further subdivided according to the source of primary motor versus premotor, supplementary, and cingulate motor cortical input. Cing. mot., cingulate motor area of the cortex; CM, centromedian nucleus of the thalamus; GPe, globus pallidus pars externa; GPi, globus pallidus pars interna; LC, locus caeruleus; M1, primary motor area of the cortex; PF, parafascicular nucleus of the thalamus; PPN, pedunculopontine nucleus; Premotor, premotor area of the cortex; SMA, supplementary motor area of the cortex; SN, substantia nigra; SNc, substantia nigra pars compacta; VP, ventral pallidum.

proposed. According to this hypothesis, the cortical information flowing along the hyperdirect pathway is transmitted to a large and diffuse pool of GPi neurons in a nonspecific manner, thereby exciting a large population of basal ganglia output neurons not related to the selected motor act (i.e., the "surround neurons"). In contrast, the corollary signal transmitted along the corticostriatal system is much more focused and influences a restricted pool of GPi neurons (i.e., the "center neurons"). Via these projections, the cortical input flowing through the striatum and the STN generates a "center-surround" motor act selection model in the GPi that allows proper movements to be performed.[217]

Although this model generated significant interest, caution must be exercised in its interpretation in light of the anatomic and physiologic observations gathered from monkeys. First, the anatomic relationships between the STN and both pallidal segments are highly specific and topographic, with functionally related neurons in the GPe, GPi, and STN being connected,[220,221] which is contrary to the assumption made by the model that the STN provides a diffuse projection to the GPi. Second, a majority of STN neurons increase their activity around the time of movement onset or after the movement during active step tracking movements in monkeys,[222] thereby reducing the likelihood that the corticosubthalamic projection is involved in the preparation for movements as suggested by the center-surround hypothesis. However, recent reports have indicated that most STN neurons are active before self-paced movements in the parkinsonian human.[223] Thus, the relative importance of the hyperdirect corticosubthalamic system in the basal ganglia circuitry remains a matter of debate that should be addressed in future studies.

Although the functional anatomy of the corticosubthalamic system largely relies on the processing of motor-related input from primary and secondary motor cortices, there is also evidence, gathered largely from rodent studies, that this system may be involved in processing limbic and cognitive information. The recent work of Baunez, Robbins, and colleagues led to the suggestion that the corticosubthalamic projection from the prefrontal cortex to the medial STN plays a role in preparatory processes, attention, perseveration, and other important cognitive or limbic functions in rats.[224-233] However, the sources of nonmotor cortical afferents to the STN remain poorly characterized in nonhuman primates. In contrast, the recent use of diffusion-weighted magnetic resonance imaging methods has revealed connections between high-order associative areas of the frontal lobe and the STN in humans.[234] It is also important to note that cognitive effects are sometimes induced by bilateral STN-DBS in PD patients.[235-242] Although direct connections with the cerebral cortex remain to be established, it is worth noting that the ventromedial STN is tightly linked with the caudate nucleus and related associative regions of the GPe and GPi, thus providing another substrate for STN stimulation–mediated effects on complex cognitive functions.[220,221,243,244] The caudal intralaminar nuclei and the brainstem pedunculopontine nucleus (PPN) are two additional sources of glutamatergic input to the STN that may contribute to the increased firing activity of STN neurons in parkinsonian conditions (see Fig. 72-3).[221] In turn, the STN sends glutamatergic projections back to the cerebral cortex and PPN.[221,243-245]

The exact origin of corticosubthalamic neurons remains unknown. Although early data suggested that cortico-STN axons may be collaterals of the descending pyramidal tract in rats[246] and cats,[247] the recent filling of single pyramidal tract neurons in M1 led to the anterograde labeling of only a few scarcely distributed fibers in the monkey STN,[125] thus suggesting that this projection may have a more complex origin than previously thought in primates.

THE PEDUNCULOPONTINE NUCLEUS AS AN INTEGRATIVE COMPONENT OF THE BASAL GANGLIA

Cellular Organization and Connectivity of the Pedunclulopontine Nucleus

The PPN is made up of a chemically heterogeneous group of neurons in the upper brainstem that lies around the superior cerebellar peduncle. It is surrounded laterally by fibers of the medial lemniscus, medially by the decussation of the superior cerebellar peduncle, dorsally by the RRF, rostrally by the dorsomedial sector of the caudalmost tip of the substantia nigra, and caudally by the cuneiform nuclei. Two major neuronal groups have been identified: the PPN pars compacta (PPNc), which consists of densely packed cholinergic neurons in the caudolateral half of the nucleus, and the PPN pars diffusa (PPNd), which is more medially located and consists of sparsely distributed noncholinergic neurons along the dorsoventral extent of the superior cerebellar peduncle. In humans, the PPN comprises about 10,000 to 15,000 cholinergic neurons,[248,249] which make up more than 90% of the PPNc.[250] In nonhuman primates, the 40% of cholinergic neurons in the PPN express glutamate immunoreactivity.[251] GABAergic, dopaminergic, noradrenergic, and various peptidergic neurons have also been identified within the boundaries of the PPN.[252-257]

It has long been known that the PPN is tightly linked with the basal ganglia. It receives major projections from the GPi and SNr (see later) and more modest input from the STN. Additional input to the PPN originates from the spinal cord, raphe nuclei, locus coeruleus, deep cerebellar nuclei, superior colliculus, and SNc.[255-257] In turn, the PPN sends ascending projections to all basal ganglia nuclei, but most particularly to the SNc and the STN.[258,259] Both glutamate and acetylcholine are used as neurotransmitters by these projections. In addition to feedback projections to the basal ganglia, the PPN is also an important source of descending projections to the pontine, medullary, and spinal structures. Through these connections, the PPN can thus be considered a possible relay station where information from the basal ganglia could bypass the thalamocortical loop and be transmitted directly to the reticular formation and spinal cord (see later).

The PPN also sends massive cholinergic and noncholinergic projections to the thalamus. This ascending PPN-thalamus system is critical for mediation of cortical desynchronization during waking and rapid eye movement sleep. Both cholinergic and glutamatergic PPN input to thalamostriatal neurons in the caudal intralaminar thalamic nuclei has been shown,[260] thus suggesting that the PPN sends information to the basal ganglia not only directly but also indirectly via thalamostriatal neurons. Therefore, the PPN is strategically located to modulate neuronal activity in functional basal ganglia–thalamocortical and basal ganglia–thalamostriatal loops.[253,257,260]

Recent studies using diffusion tensor imaging have confirmed and extended our knowledge of PPN connectivity in humans. Despite the obvious limitations of this approach in differentiating afferent from efferent fiber pathways and the likelihood that small fiber tracts may not be detected with tractography, diffusion tensor imaging surely deserves strong interest because of its noninvasive nature and possible use in tracing neural connections in the human brain.[261-264]

The Pedunculopontine Nucleus as a Target for Functional Deep Brain Stimulation in Movement Disorders

There is experimental evidence that the PPN plays a role in the initiation and modulation of gait and other stereotyped movements in animals.[255,265-267] Bilateral lesions of the PPN in normal monkeys induce bradykinesia.[267-269] Postmortem studies have revealed as much as a 50% loss of cholinergic neurons in the PPN of parkinsonian patients.[270,271] Blockade of GABA$_A$ receptors or low-frequency stimulation in the PPN reverses akinesia in MPTP-treated parkinsonian monkeys.[272-274] This series of experimental data led to the hypothesis that DBS in the PPN area may be a suitable antiparkinsonian strategy for patients who suffer from gait freezing and poor balance, two late-onset symptoms of PD that are resistant to dopamine therapy.[255,275-281] Although such procedures have been successfully applied to some patients,[275-281] the exact brainstem site of stimulation remains controversial.[282-283] Some authors have argued that the peripeduncular nucleus, a cell group located rostral and lateral to the PPN, has been the main target of DBS performed thus far in some PD patients.[280-284]

BASAL GANGLIA OUTPUT TO THE THALAMUS AND BRAINSTEM

The GPi and SNr are the two main output stations of the basal ganglia. They integrate functionally segregated striatal input and send this information through massive GABAergic projections that profusely innervate thalamic, brainstem, and reticular targets. These projections, which often originate from collaterals of the same axons, are specific and functionally compartmentalized in their respective targets (Fig. 72-4). In the following account, the anatomic organization of GPi and SNr outflow is discussed, and the relevance of these projections in the transmission and processing of basal ganglia information through cortical and subcortical loops in normal and pathologic conditions is examined.

Efferent Projections of the Globus Pallidus Pars Interna

Two major types of projection neurons have been identified in the primate GPi: type I neurons send collateralized axonal

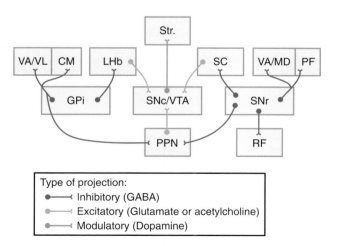

FIGURE 72-4 Main output projections of the globus pallidus pars interna (GPi) and substantia nigra pars reticulata (SNr). This diagram also illustrates some of the subcortical input to the substantia nigra pars compacta (SNc)/ventral tegmental area (VTA) dopaminergic neurons that have been considered as sources of reward- or sensory-related influences on midbrain dopaminergic neurons. CM, centromedian nucleus; GABA, γ-aminobutyric acid; LHb, lateral habenular nucleus; MD, mediodorsal nucleus; PF, parafascicular nucleus; PPN, pedunculopontine nucleus; RF, reticular formation; SC, superior colliculus; Str, striatum; VA, ventral anterior nucleus; VL, ventral lateral nucleus.

projections to the thalamus and PPN, whereas type II neurons, located along the border of the GPi, project to the lateral habenula with rare collaterals to the anterior thalamic nuclei (see later).[285] Each of these projection systems is discussed in more detail.

The Pallidothalamic Projection

The pallidothalamic projection travels via the ansa lenticularis and lenticular fasciculus to reach the ventral anterior/ventral lateral (VA/VL) nuclei,[1,286,287] where it terminates in a topographic fashion. The exact origin of fibers that make up the two major pallidal outflow tracts remains controversial. On one hand, some studies have demonstrated that pallidothalamic fibers from the caudal sensorimotor portion of the GPi travel medially through the lenticular fasciculus to reach the thalamus whereas fibers coursing in the ansa lenticularis originate mostly from cells in the rostral GPi.[288] This scheme is much simpler than that proposed in other studies in which it is suggested that fibers coursing through the ansa lenticularis frequently follow lengthy courses through the caudorostral extent of the GPi to reach the thalamus.[285,289] This discrepancy may be the result of a significant degree of neuronal heterogeneity in the primate GPi.[285] Such delineation is critical for effective surgical treatment of various movement disorders.[288]

Efferent projections from the sensorimotor GPi remain largely segregated from associative and limbic GPi outflow. In squirrel monkeys, the sensorimotor GPi output is directed toward the posterior VL (VLp) nucleus, whereas the associative and limbic GPi regions preferentially innervate the parvocellular VA (VApc) and the dorsal VL (VLd) nuclei. The ventromedial nucleus receives input from the limbic GPi only.[98,286,287]

The pallidal-, nigral-, and cerebellar-receiving territories are largely segregated in the primate thalamus, but they slightly overlap in rodents.[290-292] In contrast to previous belief, pallidothalamic outflow to the cerebral cortex is not restricted to the supplementary and premotor cortices but also gains access to the primary motor cortex, as does information flowing along the cerebellothalamic tract.[1,3-5,293-295] However, the sources of GPi or cerebellar projections to specific motor cortical areas are quantitatively different and largely segregated such that GPi outflow to thalamocortical neurons that innervate the supplementary and presupplementary motor areas is more massive than projections from the dentate nucleus to these areas.[293] In the VL nucleus, the differential level of CB expression can be used as a landmark between GPi and cerebellar termination sites.[286] About 10% to 20% of pallidothalamic neurons in the monkey GPi project to the contralateral VA/VL nuclei.[296]

Most pallidal neurons in the sensorimotor portion of the GPi that project to the VA/VL nuclei send axon collaterals to the CM nucleus (see Figs. 72-1 and 72-4), where they form synapses with thalamostriatal neurons projecting back to the sensorimotor territory of the striatum (i.e., the postcommissural putamen). Similarly, associative GPi outflow innervates the dorsolateral extension of the PF (PFdl) nucleus, which projects back to the precommissural associative region of the putamen, whereas the limbic GPi innervates the rostrodorsal PF nucleus, which preferentially innervates the nucleus accumbens. The CM/PF complex is therefore integrated into series of closed and open basal ganglia–thalamostriatal loops that run in parallel with the basal ganglia–thalamocortical system (see Fig. 72-1).[14,37,297]

The Pallidotegmental Projection

The main target of descending pallidotegmental fibers is the PPN. In monkeys, more than 80% of GPi neurons projecting to the PPN send axon collaterals to the VA/VL nuclei (Fig. 72-4). Because the PPN sends significant descending projections to lower brainstem regions and the spinal cord,[253-256] the pallidotegmental projection may be a route by which cortical information processed in the basal ganglia can bypass the thalamocortical system to directly reach lower motor and autonomic centers. In contrast to the thalamus, where motor, associative, and limbic information is largely segregated, there is significantly more overlap between projections from different functional regions of the GPi in the PPN,[298] thus suggesting a higher degree of functional convergence at the level of individual PPN neurons than in the thalamus. The medial pars diffusa of the PPN is the main site of termination of basal ganglia input from the GPi and SNr, which suggests that some of these PPN neurons may send projections back to the basal ganglia, thereby forming additional subcortical loops integrated within the basal ganglia circuitry.[255,257,259,298]

The Pallidohabenular Projection

As mentioned earlier, the pallidohabenular projection arises from a distinct population of neurons located along the borders of the GPi in nonhuman primates.[1,285] Although originally seen as a rather minor projection, recent studies using sensitive tracing methods have demonstrated that the pallidohabenular projection is functionally organized and more massive than previously thought.[284] In primates, the sensorimotor GPi preferentially innervates the centrolateral part of the lateral habenular nucleus, whereas the limbic and associative GPi regions project massively to the medial part of the nucleus (Smith and colleagues, unpublished data). Although the pallidohabenular projection is mainly GABAergic like other GPi output systems, cholinergic neurons also contribute to this projection in rats.[299,300] In light of its close connections with various subcortical limbic regions, the lateral habenula is considered to be a functional interface between the limbic system and the basal ganglia.[301-307]

The lateral habenula is a major source of GABAergic inhibitory projections to midbrain dopaminergic neurons,[301,308] although the anatomic and functional organization of this system has been studied mainly in rodents and remains to be carefully examined in primates (see Fig. 72-4). Recent studies have suggested that the pallidohabenular neurons convey reward-related signals to the lateral habenula, which then influences the striatum and other basal ganglia nuclei through regulation of the dopaminergic and serotoninergic systems (see Fig. 72-4).[306] The lateral habenula also plays important roles in learning, memory, and attention.[309,310] Because of its close relationships with the different monoaminergic systems, the lateral habenula is thought to be a potential target site for DBS in patients with severe depression.[311]

Efferent Projections of the Substantia Nigra Reticulata

The Nigrothalamic Projection

SNr and GPi input to the ventral thalamus is largely segregated from each other and from cerebellar afferents in primates.[290] In monkeys, nigrothalamic cells form the largest population of nigrofugal neurons. Input from the medial part of the SNr terminates mostly in the medial magnocellular division of the VA (VAmc) and mediodorsal (MDmc) nuclei, which in turn innervate anterior regions of the frontal lobe, including the principal sulcus and the orbital cortex.[1,11,312-317]

Neurons in the lateral part of the SNr preferentially project to the lateral posterior region of the VAmc nucleus and to different parts of the MD nucleus, mostly related to posterior regions of the frontal lobe, including the frontal eye field areas of the premotor cortex (see Fig. 72-4). SNr outflow also gains

access to thalamocortical neurons that project to the area TE in the inferotemporal cortex, thereby providing a substrate whereby the basal ganglia can influence higher order aspects of visual processing.[316] Dysfunction in this system may therefore contribute to alterations in visual perception, including visual hallucinations in some basal ganglia disorders.

In rats, functionally segregated striatal neurons project to different lamellae of SNr neurons, which in turn send the information to different thalamic nuclei. The dendrites of individual SNr neurons largely conform to the geometry of striatonigral projections, which strongly supports the concept of a parallel architecture of striatonigral circuits.[318-320] SNr neurons also project to the rostral and caudal intralaminar thalamic nuclei. In monkeys, SNr projections terminate in the PF nucleus, where they form GABAergic synapses with thalamostriatal neurons that project to the caudate nucleus.[14,37,297]

The Nigrotegmental Projection

The nigrotegmental projection has not been studied in detail in primates, but in rats it displays a dorsoventral topography and terminates preferentially on noncholinergic neurons in the medial two thirds of the PPNd.[321,322] In monkeys, the cells that give rise to the nigrotegmental projection are found throughout the mediolateral extent of the SNr, and most send axon collaterals to the VA thalamic nucleus (see Fig. 72-4).[1,312]

The Nigrocollicular Projection

The nigrocollicular projection is massive and terminates in the intermediate layer of the superior colliculus, where nigral terminals form distinctive clusters that innervate neurons projecting to the spinal cord, medulla, and periabducens area (Fig. 72-4). This projection is critical for control of saccadic eye movements and orients the eyes toward a stimulus in response to auditory or visual stimuli.[18,32,323-325] This is consistent with the fact that the SNr-receiving neurons of the intermediate layer of the superior colliculus are targeted by visual input from the cortex and project to brainstem regions that control eye movement. In turn, the superior colliculus sends a projection to dopaminergic neurons in the SNc in rats and primates.[326-331] This projection is considered a prime source of sensory-related events to dopaminergic nigrostriatal neurons, thereby suggesting that the phasic responses of midbrain dopaminergic neurons in complex tasks may be related to "sensory prediction errors" instead of "reward prediction errors" (see Fig. 72-4).[332-340]

The Nigroreticular Projection

The SNr also sends projections to the medullary reticular formation. In rats, this projection arises from a population of neurons in the dorsolateral SNr and terminates in the parvicellular reticular formation. Identified nigroreticular neurons receive GABAergic input from the striatum and the globus pallidus. This projection probably plays a role in orofacial movements because the part of the SNr receiving neurons of the reticular formation is directly connected with orofacial motor nuclei.[341-343]

CONCLUSION

Our understanding of the functional anatomy of the basal ganglia has grown substantially over the past decades, which has led to significant changes in our current view of basal ganglia functioning under normal and pathologic conditions. Although the exact role of the basal ganglia remains highly speculative, there is a general consensus that these brain regions are endowed with highly complex integrative properties of information that extends far beyond the sensorimotor domain. The close interconnections between basal ganglia nuclei and associative or limbic cortical areas provide a solid substrate through which integration and processing of nonmotor information can be performed. The complex nonmotor symptomatology of basal ganglia diseases is another indication that functional changes in cortical and subcortical basal ganglia–related networks may encompass multifarious motor and nonmotor deficits, which in many cases also include complex neuropsychiatric symptoms. The recent finding that STN-DBS in patients with PD may result in complex neuropsychiatric and cognitive changes is more evidence of basal ganglia regulation of nonmotor functional modalities. The continued development of sensitive neuroanatomic tracing methods and brain imaging techniques should provide the necessary tools to deepen our understanding of the neuronal microcircuits and macrocircuits that should be targeted to further improve the outcome of therapies for basal ganglia disorders.

Acknowledgment

I wish to thank Adriana Galvan for her help in the preparation of figures and various members of my laboratory who have contributed to the original publication of some of the data discussed in this chapter. Thanks are also due to the various funding agencies that have contributed to support of the research from my laboratory that was discussed in this review, including the National Institute of Neurological Disorders and Stroke and the National Parkinson Foundation and Tourette Syndrome Association. I am also grateful for the continued support from the Yerkes National Primate Center National Institues of Health–based grant.

SUGGESTED READINGS

Benabid AL, Chabardes S, Mitrofanis J, et al. Deep brain stimulation of the subthalamic nucleus for the treatment of Parkinson's disease. *Lancet Neurol.* 2009;8:67-81.

Fornai F, di Poggio AB, Pellegrini A, et al. Noradrenaline in Parkinson's disease: from disease progression to current therapeutics. *Curr Med Chem.* 2007;14:2330-2334.

Graybiel AM. Habits, rituals, and the evaluative brain. *Annu Rev Neurosci.* 2008;31:359-387.

Haber SN, Calzavara R. The cortico-basal ganglia integrative network: the role of the thalamus. *Brain Res Bull.* 2009;78:69-74.

Kimura M, Minamimoto T, Matsumoto N, et al. Monitoring and switching of cortico-basal ganglia loop functions by the thalamo-striatal system. *Neurosci Res.* 2004;48:355-360.

Matsumoto M, Hikosaka O. Representation of negative motivational value in the primate lateral habenula. *Nat Neurosci.* 2009;12:77-84.

Matsumoto M, Hikosaka O. Lateral habenula as a source of negative reward signals in dopamine neurons. *Nature.* 2007;447:1111-1115.

May PJ, McHaffie JG, Stanford TR, et al. Tectonigral projections in the primate: a pathway for pre-attentive sensory input to midbrain dopaminergic neurons. *Eur J Neurosci.* 2009;29:575-587.

Mazloom M, Smith Y. Synaptic microcircuitry of tyrosine hydroxylase-containing neurons and terminals in the striatum of 1-methyl-4-phenyl-1,2,3,6-tetrahydropyridine–treated monkeys. *J Comp Neurol.* 2006;495:453-469.

McHaffie JG, Stanford TR, Stein BE, et al. Subcortical loops through the basal ganglia. *Trends Neurosci.* 2005;28:401-407.

Mena-Segovia J, Winn P, Bolam JP. Cholinergic modulation of midbrain dopaminergic systems. *Brain Res Rev.* 2008;58:265-271.

Middleton FA, Strick PL. Anatomical evidence for cerebellar and basal ganglia involvement in higher cognitive function. *Science.* 1994;266:458-461.

Nambu A, Tokuno H, Takada M. Functional significance of the cortico-subthalamo-pallidal 'hyperdirect' pathway. *Neurosci Res.* 2002;43:111-117.

Pahapill PA, Lozano AM. The pedunculopontine nucleus and Parkinson's disease. *Brain.* 2000;123:1767-1783.

Parent A, Hazrati LN. Functional anatomy of the basal ganglia. I. The cortico-basal ganglia-thalamo-cortical loop. *Brain Res Rev.* 1995;20:91-127.

Redgrave P, Gurney K, Reynolds J. What is reinforced by phasic dopamine signals? *Brain Res Rev.* 2008;58:322-339.

Rommelfanger KS, Weinshenker D. Norepinephrine: the redheaded stepchild of Parkinson's disease. *Biochem Pharmacol.* 2007;74:177-190.

Sanchez-Gonzalez MA, Garcia-Cabezas MA, Rico B, et al. The primate thalamus is a key target for brain dopamine. *J Neurosci.* 2005;25:6076-6083.

Schultz W. Multiple dopamine functions at different time courses. *Annu Rev Neurosci.* 2007;30:259-288.

Smith Y, Kieval JZ. Anatomy of the dopamine system in the basal ganglia. *Trends Neurosci.* 2000;23:S28-S33.

Smith Y, Raju D, Nanda B, et al. The thalamostriatal systems: anatomical and functional organization in normal and parkinsonian states. *Brain Res Bull.* 2009;78:60-68.

Stefani A, Lozano AM, Peppe A, et al. Bilateral deep brain stimulation of the pedunculopontine and subthalamic nuclei in severe Parkinson's disease. *Brain.* 2007;130:1596-1607.

Surmeier DJ, Ding J, Day M, et al. D1 and D2 dopamine-receptor modulation of striatal glutamatergic signaling in striatal medium spiny neurons. *Trends Neurosci.* 2007;30:228-235.

Villalba RM, Lee H, Smith Y. Dopaminergic denervation and spine loss in the striatum of MPTP-treated monkeys. *Exp Neurol.* 2009;215:220-227.

Wichmann T, Delong MR. Deep brain stimulation for neurologic and neuropsychiatric disorders. *Neuron.* 2006;52:197-204.

Full references can be found on Expert Consult @ www.expertconsult.com

CHAPTER 73

Rationale for Surgical Interventions in Movement Disorders

Thomas Wichmann ■ Mahlon R. DeLong

Neuroscience research has led to major insights into the structure and function of the basal ganglia and the pathophysiologic basis of basal ganglia disorders such as Parkinson's disease (PD).[1-4] Several factors have contributed to progress in this field, specifically, the availability of effective animal models, improved methods of physiologic and pharmacologic investigation, and the development of powerful brain imaging methods for studies of patients and animal models of these disorders.

When functional neurosurgical procedures were first introduced in the 1940s and 1950s, they were carried out largely on an empirical basis. Over time, the rationale for performing focal neurosurgical interventions has become clearer. Researchers and clinicians have refined patient selection criteria and better defined neurosurgical targets, thereby increasing the success rate, effectiveness, and safety of these interventions. This chapter examines the anatomic and physiologic foundations underlying current neurosurgical strategies, reviews the pathophysiology of several common disorders that are treated surgically, and discusses the mechanism of action of both ablative procedures and deep brain stimulation (DBS).

OVERVIEW OF ANATOMY AND FUNCTION OF THE BASAL GANGLIA

PD and other movement disorders are increasingly being recognized as "circuit disorders" that involve not only the basal ganglia but also related nodes in the thalamus and the cerebral cortex. This chapter focuses on a description of these larger cortical-subcortical circuits. The anatomic organization of the basal ganglia is discussed in detail in Chapter 74.

Anatomic and physiologic studies have demonstrated that the basal ganglia are components of a family of parallel reentrant brain circuits in which cortical information is sent to the basal ganglia, processed, sent to the thalamus, and then returned to the cerebral cortex.[5-9] The different circuits are segregated but share anatomic features, thus supporting the view that the basal ganglia and cortex interact in a modular fashion in which similar processing steps are carried out in each module even though the different modules are engaged in different functions. Depending on the presumed function of the cortical region that is involved in these different circuits, the circuits are commonly designated as "motor," "oculomotor," "prefrontal," and "limbic" (Fig. 73-1). As shown in Figure 73-1, dysfunction within the individual circuits may be associated with specific disease states.

Movement disorders prominently affect the "motor" circuit, which takes origin in the frontal cortical precentral and postcentral sensorimotor areas, including the primary motor cortex (M1), the supplementary motor area (SMA), the premotor cortex (PMC), the cingulate motor area (CMA), and interconnected sensory cortical areas, and involves specific "motor" portions in each of the basal ganglia structures and thalamus. Similar to the other transbasal ganglia circuits, the motor circuit is at least partially closed, with thalamocortical projections terminating in the same frontal cortical regions from which the circuit origi-

nates. The anatomy of the motor circuit is shown in greater detail in Figure 73-2A.

The basal ganglia are composed of the neostriatum (caudate nucleus and putamen), the ventral striatum, the external and internal segments of the globus pallidus (GPe and GPi, respectively), the subthalamic nucleus (STN), and the substantia nigra pars reticulata and pars compacta (SNr and SNc, respectively).

The striatum and STN are the main entry points for cortical input, whereas the GPi and SNr provide basal ganglia output to the thalamus. The corticostriatal projections are topographically organized.[5-7,10,11] Movement-related cortical input terminates in the postcommissural putamen, and nonmotor projections terminate in other areas of the striatum. Thus, prefrontal cortical areas project to the caudate nucleus and the precommissural putamen, and projections from limbic cortices, amygdala, and hippocampus terminate preferentially in the ventral striatum. The cortical-subthalamic projections are also topographically arranged.[12,13] Afferents from M1 reach the dorsolateral STN, whereas afferents from the PMC and SMA innervate mainly the mediodorsal third of the nucleus.[14]

The striatum is linked to the basal ganglia output structures, GPi and SNr, via two distinct pathways, the so-called direct and indirect pathways (Fig. 73-2).[1,5,7] The direct pathway arises from sets of striatal medium spiny neurons (MSNs) that project monosynaptically to neurons in the GPi and SNr. These neurons also contain the neuropeptides substance P and dynorphin and preferentially express dopamine D_1-like receptors. It is thought that MSNs in the direct pathway receive a larger share of the thalamostriatal pathway than do neurons in the indirect pathway. The indirect pathway arises from a set of striatal MSNs that project to the GPe.[15,16] The striatal neurons that give rise to the indirect pathway preferentially express enkephalin and dopamine D_2-like receptors.[17,18] Although most authors emphasize the separation of these pathways, single-cell labeling of striatal MSNs has shown that at least some send collaterals to both segments of the globus pallidus (thus participating anatomically in both the direct and indirect pathways).[19,20]

Similar to the corticostriatal projections, the direct and indirect pathways are topographically organized. For instance, populations of GPe neurons within the sensorimotor, associative, or limbic territory are reciprocally connected with populations of neurons in the same functional territories of the STN, and neurons in each of these regions, in turn, innervate the same functional territory of the GPi.[15,16]

In terms of basal ganglia output, the caudolateral "motor" territory of the GPi projects almost exclusively to the posterior part of the ventrolateral (VL) nucleus, which sends projections toward the SMA,[21,22] M1, and PMC.[23] The outflow from pallidal motor areas directed at M1, PMC, and SMA appears to arise from separate populations of pallidothalamic neurons.[23] These findings indicate that the larger "motor circuit" is composed of segregated subcircuits centered on the individual cortical motor areas.[24,25] The more rostromedial associative areas of the GPi project preferentially to the parvocellular part of the ventral anterior (VA) and the dorsal VL nucleus (VLc in macaques),[26,27]

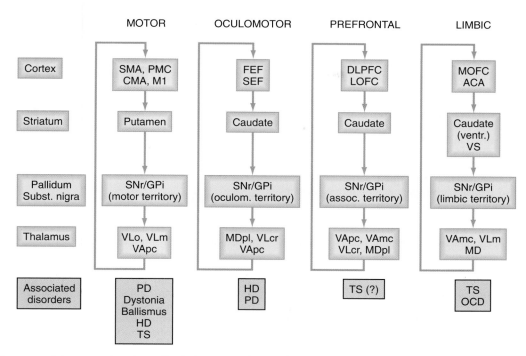

FIGURE 73-1 Anatomy of the cortex–basal ganglia–thalamocortical circuits. ACA, anterior cingulate area; CMA, cingulate motor area; DLPFC, dorsolateral prefrontal cortex; FEF, frontal eye fields; GPi, globus pallidus interna; HD, Huntington's disease; LOFC, lateral orbitofrontal cortex; M1, primary motor cortex; MDpl, mediodorsal nucleus of the thalamus, pars lateralis; MOFC, medial orbitofrontal cortex; OCD, obsessive-compulsive disorder; PD, Parkinson's disease; PMC, premotor cortex; SMA, supplementary motor area; SEF, supplementary eye field; SNr, substantia nigra pars reticulata; TS, Tourette's syndrome; VApc, ventral anterior nucleus of the thalamus, pars parvocellularis; VAmc, ventral anterior nucleus of the thalamus, pars magnocellularis; VLm, ventrolateral nucleus of the thalamus, pars medialis; VLo, ventrolateral nucleus of the thalamus, pars oralis; VLcr, ventrolateral nucleus of the thalamus, pars caudalis, rostral division; VS, ventral striatum. *(From Wichmann T, Delong MR. Deep brain stimulation for neurologic and neuropsychiatric disorders. Neuron. 2006;52:197.)*

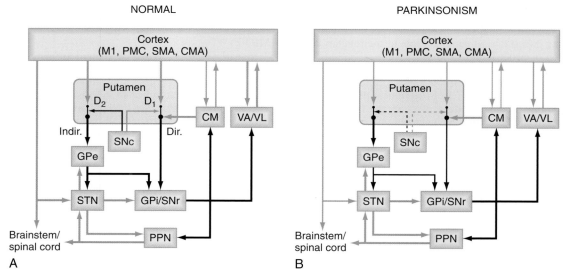

FIGURE 73-2 Parkinsonism-related changes in overall activity in the basal ganglia–thalamocortical motor circuit. *Black arrows* indicate inhibitory connections; *blue arrows* indicate excitatory connections. The thickness of the *arrows* corresponds to their presumed activity. CM, centromedian nucleus; Dir., direct pathway; D_1, D_2, dopamine receptor subtypes; Indir., indirect pathway; PPN, pedunculopontine nucleus; SNc, substantia nigra pars compacta; STN, subthalamic nucleus. For other abbreviations, see the legend to Figure 73-1. *(From Galvan A, Wichmann T. Pathophysiology of parkinsonism. Clin Neurophysiol. 2008;119:1459.)*

specifically to thalamic areas preferentially connected to the prefrontal cortex.[28,29]

Collaterals from the pallidofugal and nigrofugal projections also reach the intralaminar nuclei of the thalamus, the centromedian (CM) and parafascicular (PF) nuclei. These projections are part of a system of segregated basal ganglia–thalamostriatal feedback projections.[27,30] In primates, the CM nucleus receives input from motor areas in the GPi and projects to the motor portions of the putamen and STN, whereas PF input and output are related to the associative and limbic territories of the basal ganglia.[31,32] CM terminations are found mostly along the shafts of striatal direct pathway MSNs,[33,34] separate from the sites of termination of cortical input and of dopaminergic synapses.[30,35-41] Basal ganglia output also reaches the pedunculopontine nucleus (PPN),[42,43] which in turn gives rise to ascending projections to the basal ganglia, thalamus, and basal forebrain and to descending projections to the pons, medulla, and spinal cord.[44,45]

Electrophysiologic and metabolic mapping studies in animals and functional imaging data in humans support the view that the anatomically and physiologically defined basal ganglia "motor" areas are indeed involved in movement.[25,46-48] The model of the basal ganglia–thalamocortical motor circuit shown in Figure 73-2 is often used as the basis for speculations regarding the function of the basal ganglia in movement. The model poses that activation of MSNs that give rise to the direct pathway reduces inhibitory basal ganglia output from targeted neurons with subsequent disinhibition of related thalamocortical neurons.[5,49,50] The net effect of this process is increased activity in appropriate cortical neurons that results in facilitation of the movement. By contrast, activation of MSNs that give rise to the indirect pathway would lead to increased (inhibitory) basal ganglia output on thalamocortical neurons and to suppression of movement. The balance between direct and indirect pathway activity may regulate the overall amount of movement, whereas specific activation patterns (for instance, a center-surround type of activation involving the direct and indirect pathways) may limit the extent or duration of ongoing movements.

Other views of basal ganglia function are currently evolving.[51-55] Thus, synaptic processing and modification of synaptic strength in the striatum, or alteration of the level of interneuronal synchrony, may give the basal ganglia a role in the regulation of habit formation or procedural learning.[51-53,55]

In models of basal ganglia function, the modulatory effects of dopamine on striatal transmission are highly important. Dopamine is released in the striatum from terminals of projections from the SNc and modulates the activity of the basal ganglia output neurons in the GPi and SNr by facilitating corticostriatal transmission on the direct pathway and inhibiting corticostriatal transmission on MSNs that give rise to the indirect pathway. These opposing actions are probably mediated by the two different sets of dopamine receptors (D_1-like and D_2-like receptors) that are differentially expressed in these pathways.[56-59] Through the different effects of activation of the direct and indirect pathways, the net effect of striatal dopamine release appears to be reduction of basal ganglia output to the thalamus and other targets. Evidence indicates that dopamine also acts directly on receptors in the STN and pallidum to influence discharge patterns and rates in these structures.

Dopamine receptor activation may not only act to modulate the activity of the direct and indirect pathways but might also have a role in the proposed learning functions of the basal ganglia. Activation of dopamine receptors on MSNs has been shown to be involved in the induction of long-term potentiation and depression at glutamatergic (presumably corticostriatal) synapses.[60-64] Recent research has elucidated complex interactions between dopaminergic transmission and transmission involving adenosine, glutamate receptors, and endocannabinoid receptors in this process.[61,63-66]

In summary, the basal ganglia, thalamus, and cortex are linked by a number of segregated circuits that partition these structures into "motor," "oculomotor," "limbic," and "associative" functional territories. This provides the substrate whereby these subcortical structures may participate in the full range of behavior and whereby dysfunction within these disparate circuits may result in a wide spectrum of motor and nonmotor behavioral abnormalities. As will be discussed in some detail, it is now apparent that the various clinical disorders of movement with their signature clinical features may be viewed as *circuit disorders* and that they can be addressed by specific manipulations of the individual loops at several different nodes.

PARKINSONISM

The cardinal features of PD—the triad of akinesia/bradykinesia, tremor at rest, and muscular rigidity—result from decreased dopaminergic transmission in the motor portions of the basal ganglia, in particular, the putamen, as a result of progressive loss of dopaminergic neurons in the SNc. Dopaminergic replacement therapies are highly effective in reversing these features of the disorder. These dopamine-responsive features are often accompanied by other issues that are poorly or entirely unresponsive to dopaminergic medications, such as depression, autonomic dysfunction, sleep disorders, cognitive impairment, and gait/balance problems. Although some of these problems may result, in part, from decreased dopamine within the nonmotor portions of the basal ganglia, widespread progressive pathologic changes in the brainstem, thalamus, and eventually the cerebral cortex appear to play a major role.[67]

Pathophysiology of Parkinsonism

The following paragraphs are focused on the motor aspects of PD that result from dopamine deficiency. Study of these changes has been facilitated by the development of animal models of dopamine depletion in which changes in the basal ganglia, thalamus, and cerebral cortex can be conveniently studied, including the 6-hydroxydopamine (6-OHDA)-treated rat and primates treated with 1-methyl-4-phenyl-1,2,3,6-tetrahydropyridine (MPTP).[68,69]

In early studies of MPTP-treated primates, alterations in activity of the striatopallidal pathways were strongly emphasized. Such changes were suggested by studies of metabolic activity in the basal ganglia that indicated increased synaptic activity in the GPe and GPi.[70,71] Possible interpretations of this finding were that the activity of the striatal-GPe connection and the STN-GPi pathway is increased in parkinsonism or that the STN projections to both pallidal segments were overactive. Subsequent microelectrode recording studies in MPTP-treated primates showed a reduction in neuronal discharge in the GPe and increased firing in the STN, GPi, and SNr in comparison to normal controls,[72-75] as well as high neuronal discharge rates in the GPi in PD patients undergoing functional neurosurgical procedures.[76-78] These changes may be related to one another in that striatal dopamine depletion may lead to increased activity of striatal neurons in the indirect pathway and result in inhibition of the GPe and subsequent disinhibition of the STN and GPi/SNr (Fig 73-2B). A role of local dopamine loss in the extrastriatal structures (specifically in the STN, GPi, and SNr) may play a role as well, specifically with regard to the emergence of abnormal firing patterns in these nuclei (see later).

Other structures and feedback loops, such as those involving the PPN and CM, may contribute to the abnormalities in discharge that are found in the basal ganglia output nuclei. A series of studies have demonstrated that brainstem areas such as the PPN may also be involved in the development of parkinsonian signs. Lesioning of the PPN in normal monkeys was shown to lead to akinesia.[79,80] At the cortical level, positron emission tomography (PET) studies in parkinsonian patients have consistently shown reduced activation of motor and premotor areas.[46,81]

The notion that rate changes in the basal ganglia underlie the development of parkinsonism (the so-called rate model, depicted in Fig. 73-2) is generally supported by studies that have shown that inactivation of the sensorimotor portions of the STN or GPi increases metabolic activity in the cortical motor areas and improves bradykinesia and tremor in parkinsonian subjects. Thus, lesions of the STN, GPi, or SNr in MPTP-treated primates reverse some or all signs of parkinsonism, presumably by reducing basal ganglia output,[19,82,83] and GPi or STN lesions are highly effective antiparkinsonian treatments in patients with PD.[84-90] However, the "rate model" has largely been rejected because several crucial observations contradict a purely rate-based view of basal ganglia–processing abnormalities. For instance, lesions of the VA/VL nuclei of the thalamus (which completely removes thalamic output) do not lead to parkinsonism and are, in fact, beneficial in the treatment of tremor and rigidity.[91,92] Similarly, lesions of the GPi in the setting of parkinsonism improve the cardinal features of PD without producing dyskinesias or other obvious detrimental effects. In fact, they are highly effective in reducing drug-induced dyskinesias.[86,87,93]

Because of these discrepancies, the rate model has given way to the view that abnormalities in basal ganglia activity other than rate changes are more relevant to the pathophysiology of parkinsonism. Among the most discussed changes in discharge patterns in the basal ganglia of parkinsonian subjects (Fig. 73-3) is the development of oscillatory phenomena.[94,95] Abnormal oscillations have been identified in the activity of single neurons in the GPi, SNr, and STN in animals and patients and, more recently, in recordings of local field potentials (LFPs) in patients, and these oscillations may reflect the activity of more extensive networks of connections. The LFP recordings were made by using implanted DBS macroelectrodes as recording probes during the time immediately after the implantation surgery. Recordings in the STN and other basal ganglia areas with this method have demonstrated the presence of LFP oscillations in the 10- to 25-Hz (beta) range in the STN, GPi, and cortex in unmedicated PD patients. The studies have also shown that beta-range oscillations give way to oscillations in the 60- to 80-Hz (gamma) range when the patients are treated with levodopa or when the STN is stimulated at high frequencies.[95,96] The prominence of beta-band activity is apparent throughout the basal ganglia–thalamocortical circuitry. For example, the desynchronization of electroencephalography (EEG) oscillations that normally precedes movement

was shown to be abnormally small in parkinsonian patients, perhaps interfering with the initiation of movement.[97-99]

Another parkinsonism-related abnormality in spontaneous discharge is the emergence of abnormal synchrony between neurons. Under physiologic conditions, basal ganglia activity is highly specific in its relation to movement parameters and body part and appears to be segregated even at the cellular level, where neighboring neurons are rarely found to fire in synchrony.[100] In parkinsonism, this level of segregation is lost, and the discharge of neighboring neurons is often found to be correlated and abnormally synchronized.[95,101]

Finally, the proportion of cells in the STN, GPi, and SNr that discharge in bursts (oscillatory or nonoscillatory) is greatly increased in parkinsonism.[73,95,101-103] Oscillatory burst discharge patterns are also seen in conjunction with tremor, which may reflect tremor-related proprioceptive input or more active participation of basal ganglia in the generation of tremor.

Although spontaneous basal ganglia firing has been extensively studied in MPTP-treated monkeys, much less is known about the way information processing is altered in the basal ganglia. Studies of changes in neuronal firing patterns preceding or following active movements are difficult to perform and interpret in akinetic or bradykinetic animals. However, studies of neuronal responses to passive limb manipulation have been carried out and showed that such responses in the STN, GPi, and thalamus occur more often, are more pronounced, and have widened receptive fields after treatment with MPTP.[72,73,101,104]

The importance of specific electrophysiologic features in basal ganglia, thalamic, or cortical activity for development of the behavioral signs of parkinsonism remains unclear. Although burst-like, synchronized oscillatory activity in the basal ganglia–thalamocortical circuits is associated with parkinsonism,[105] direct links between oscillatory activity and specific parkinsonian deficits have not been established. In fact, recent studies in monkeys that underwent a gradual MPTP treatment protocol in which parkinsonism was slowly induced have cast doubt on the notion that synchronous oscillatory firing contributes strongly to (early) parkinsonism.[106] In these single-neuron recording studies, synchrony and oscillations in neuronal spiking activity were detected only after the development of bradykinesia and akinesia. Similarly, recent rodent experiments have suggested that abnormal oscillations in the basal ganglia do not result simply from (acute) lack of dopaminergic stimulation but may rather be due to the chronic absence of dopamine.[107] Such "late" changes could be related to anatomic alterations secondary to dopamine depletion, such as loss of the dendritic spines of MSNs,[108-110] which has been

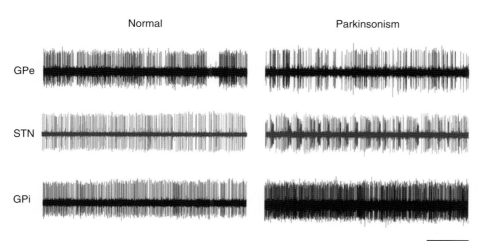

FIGURE 73-3 Changes in the activity of single cells in the globus pallidus externa (GPe), globus pallidus interna (GPi), or subthalamic nucleus (STN) of 1-methyl-4 phenyl-1,2,3,6-tetrahydropyridine (MPTP)-treated monkeys. Shown are examples of separate neurons recorded by standard methods for extracellular electrophysiologic recording in normal and parkinsonian animals. Each data segment is 5 seconds in duration. *(From Galvan A, Wichmann T. Pathophysiology of parkinsonism. Clin Neurophysiol. 2008;119:1459.)*

Normal   Parkinsonism

GPe

STN

GPi

1 sec

described as homeostatic pruning in response to altered glutamatergic transmission in the striatum.[108,109]

Rationale for Treating Parkinsonism by Surgical Interventions

Arguably, the most important lesson from the aforementioned anatomic and functional studies is the insight that parkinsonism, like other diseases of basal ganglia origin, is not just a basal ganglia disorder but should be viewed as a circuit disorder. This insight is the primary rationale to carry out focal neurosurgical procedures in patients with parkinsonism, where disruption of basal ganglia–thalamocortical activity at almost any level of the motor circuit has been shown to constitute effective treatment of the disease. Although the earliest loss of dopamine occurs in the putamen, the receptive portion of the basal ganglia, neurosurgical interventions generally target motor areas of the STN and GPi. Given the focal nature of the procedures, basal ganglia areas in which motor functions are represented in a small volume of tissue are preferred, thus rendering the ventral posterolateral GPi or the dorsal and central STN ideal targets for such interventions.

Two general types of procedures are used to surgically treat patients with parkinsonism: lesioning and DBS. Unilateral lesioning of the sensorimotor territory of the GPi results in significant contralateral antiparkinsonian effects and significantly reduces drug-induced involuntary movements and motor fluctuations. For DBS, a stimulation electrode is introduced into the same targets in the GPi and STN, and high-frequency stimulation is applied by way of an implanted, externally programmable pulse generator. DBS alleviates parkinsonian motor signs and reduces the severity of "off" periods and the dyskinesias, dystonia, and motor fluctuations that result from long-term drug administration.[111-113]

The mechanism of action of these interventions remains unclear. The therapeutic benefits of GPi and STN lesions suggest that a total lack of basal ganglia output is more tolerable in PD patients than disruptive abnormal output on the brainstem and thalamocortical systems. Although it was initially believed that DBS, like lesioning, functionally inactivates the target because both procedures lead to almost identical outcomes, considerable evidence now suggests more complex mechanisms of action of DBS. The electrophysiologic effects of GPi or STN DBS appear to depend on the distance of the stimulated elements from the electrode and may differ between the elements themselves. Stimulation in the STN has been demonstrated to evoke complex excitatory effects in the GPi, one of the primary recipients of STN efferents,[114] and may alter the oscillatory resonance characteristics of the STN-GPi network.[115] Modeling studies have shown that STN DBS may inhibit the somata of STN cells through activation of local release of γ-aminobutyric acid from GPe afferents while simultaneously directly activating STN axons[116] and thereby activating synaptically innervated GPi cells. Anterograde activation of efferents plus retrograde activation of afferents by DBS is likely to secondarily alter firing patterns in the associated corticosubthalamic and thalamocortical circuitry. Recent modeling studies have suggested that this may strongly affect (normalize) thalamic bursting activity.[117] STN DBS has also been shown to normalize intracortical inhibitory mechanisms in studies of the effects of transcranial magnetic stimulation,[118] and functional imaging studies have shown that pallidotomy or DBS of the STN or GPi acts to restore relatively normal levels in the frontal motor areas.[87,119,120]

DBS at other nodes along the basal ganglia–thalamocortical motor circuitry has also been shown to be useful. For instance, parkinsonian tremor is effectively treated by thalamic DBS at the border between the thalamic nucleus ventralis oralis and nucleus ventralis intermedius.[121,122] Stimulation of the PPN may also be beneficial.[123-126]

The finding that ablation and DBS are effective only when they are carried out within the sensorimotor territories of the nodes of the motor circuit strongly supports the concept that in PD, the motor circuit has been commandeered by abnormal firing patterns and more normal function can be achieved by elimination or modification of the abnormal basal ganglia output.

DYSTONIA

In patients with dystonia, normal movements are profoundly disrupted by co-contraction of agonist and antagonist muscles and by excessive activation of inappropriate musculature (overflow), thereby leading to abnormal postures and involuntary movements. The earliest manifestation of dystonia is often an "action dystonia" that occurs only with attempted voluntary movement. In adults, dystonia most commonly occurs in a focal manner, such as cervical dystonia, blepharospasm, or spasmodic dysphonia. In children, generalized forms of dystonia are more common.

Dystonia may arise from a variety of disease processes, and many of these processes involve the basal ganglia. Dystonia is categorized as "primary" if no clear cause is identified and as "secondary" if an underlying structural or biochemical defect is present. One of the main forms of generalized dystonia, idiopathic torsion dystonia, is caused by a genetic defect in the *DYT1* gene on chromosome 9.[127,128] Secondary dystonia may occur in the setting of PD, after exposure to drugs (tardive dystonia), as a sequela of focal damage to the striatum (particularly the putamen) or the thalamus, or even after peripheral injuries. The onset of dystonia is typically delayed for weeks or months after the inciting lesion.

Pathophysiology of Dystonia

The pathophysiology of dystonia is far less clear than that of PD and potentially varies substantially between different forms of dystonia. Research in this field is hampered by the fact that no fully convincing mouse or primate model of dystonia exists[129] and, of course, by the fact that clear pathologic changes do not appear to be present in most cases of dystonia.

There is some evidence that a disturbance in the dopamine system may be involved in *DYT1* dystonia[130] and other forms of dystonia. For instance, dystonia may develop acutely in normal individuals treated with dopamine receptor blocking agents or appear after long-term treatment with these drugs (tardive dystonia). In PD, dystonia usually develops in patients who have been exposed to dopaminergic drugs, but it may also occur as an early sign of the disease itself, independent of medications. Dystonia is also present in a group of patients with familial dystonia and parkinsonian features who respond dramatically to treatment with low-dose levodopa (dopamine-responsive dystonia [DRD]).[131,132] Most of these patients suffer from a genetic defect in dopamine synthesis caused by reduced activity of guanosine triphosphate cyclohydrolase,[133-135] the rate-limiting enzyme in the biosynthesis of a cofactor of the dopamine-synthesizing enzyme tyrosine hydroxylase, tetrahydrobiopterin.

When dystonia results from lesions affecting the striatum or its dopaminergic supply,[136] these lesions may affect the affinity or number of dopamine receptors in the nonlesioned portion of the striatum or may lead to reorganization of striatal topography, which eventually results in altered activity in the basal ganglia output structures. Metabolic studies in primates have suggested that dystonia may be associated with a reduction of activity along the putamen-GPe connection and increased inhibition of the STN and GPi by GPe efferents.[137,138] Other PET and single-cell recording studies in human patients with dystonia have emphasized changes in activity in the direct pathway instead (see later).

Involvement of the direct and indirect pathways in the pathophysiology of dystonia is also supported by pharmacologic studies. For instance, it has been shown that D_2-like receptor antagonists may induce dystonia, presumably by increasing striatal outflow to the GPe via the indirect pathway, whereas D_1-like receptor antagonists may be beneficial in this regard, presumably by reducing striatal outflow to the GPi along the direct pathway.[139,140] These data suggest that a relative increase in activity along the direct pathway (versus that along the indirect pathway) contributes to dystonia. Single-cell recording studies in human patients undergoing functional neurosurgical procedures are in partial agreement with this concept. These studies have demonstrated that discharge rates in the GPe and GPi are lower than expected,[141-146] although such changes in firing rate were not found by Hutchison and colleagues.[147]

Similar to parkinsonism, oscillatory activity in the basal ganglia may also be involved in the pathophysiology of dystonia. Low-frequency coherence between the discharge of neurons in the basal ganglia[142] or thalamus[146,148] and the electromyographic activity of dystonic muscles has been demonstrated. LFP recordings from DBS electrodes implanted in the GPi have shown increased power in the 4- to 10-Hz band[149,150] and high correlation with simultaneously recorded electromyographic activity.[149,151]

True to the concept that dystonia is a circuit disorder similar to PD, there is substantial evidence for altered cortical functioning in dystonia, specifically from imaging and electrophysiologic studies that have used transcranial magnetic stimulation and other methods. These studies are strongly suggestive of abnormal plasticity in dystonia. For instance, PET studies in dystonic patients have demonstrated widespread changes in activity of the prefrontal areas,[152-155] specifically, changes involving the SMA, anterior cingulate, and dorsolateral prefrontal motor areas.[152,153,155] In focal dystonia, abnormal somatotopic maps were demonstrated in M1,[156,157] with increased intracortical excitability in the motor areas[158] and a decreased Bereitschaftspotential/contingent negative variation.[159-162] Patients with writer's cramp were also shown to have an abnormally small degree of beta-band EEG desynchronization.[163]

Sensory abnormalities may also play a role in dystonia. There is convincing evidence of reduced corticocortical inhibition in the sensory system[164-167] and increased and improperly modulated precentral sensory evoked potentials (N30).[168-174] In addition, single-cell recording and imaging studies have suggested altered somatotopic representation at the cortical,[175-177] putamen,[178] and thalamic levels,[148,179] although such changes were not seen in recent GPi recording studies.[143,180]

Rationale for Treating Dystonia by Surgical Interventions

Despite the lack of an overarching pathophysiologic model of dystonia, the disease has been treated for decades by inducing pallidal or thalamic lesions and, more recently, by DBS. Specifically, GPi DBS is currently used in many cases of advanced intractable dystonia. This procedure is highly effective in cases of generalized dystonia[181-183] but less so for secondary dystonia.[184] Other emerging indications for GPi DBS are cervical and tardive dystonia.[182,185,186] Recent case reports suggest that STN DBS may also be effective.[20,187]

As is the case with ablative or DBS surgeries for PD, selection of the surgical target for treatment of dystonia is primarily driven by our knowledge of the functional anatomy of the basal ganglia. The effects of surgical interventions for dystonia remain unclear. It has been shown that GPi DBS, administered to motor portions of the GPi, modulates activity in the basal ganglia–thalamocortical motor circuit. PET activation studies have shown that GPi DBS reverses the overactivity of the motor cortical areas present in dystonia,[188] and electrophysiologic studies have demonstrated that GPi DBS enhances motor cortex excitability through modulation of thalamocortical projections.[189] In distinction to the use of neurosurgical treatments in PD, the clinical benefits of DBS or pallidotomy in dystonia are usually delayed, often by weeks or months,[190] thus suggesting that anatomic or functional remodeling of neuronal interactions, reflecting abnormal plasticity within the basal ganglia–thalamocortical circuitry, may be necessary for the beneficial effects to occur.

TOURETTE'S SYNDROME

Tourette's syndrome is a familial disorder characterized by the presence of motor and vocal tics. In many cases, comorbid psychiatric symptoms such as obsessive-compulsive disorder, attention-deficit/hyperactivity disorder, or depression are also present and may dominate the clinical findings. The symptoms typically peak in the early teens and decline thereafter. Imaging studies have suggested that Tourette's syndrome may involve abnormalities in the limbic and motor circuitry, although information about the specific alteration in neuronal activity that may underlie the symptoms of Tourette's syndrome is lacking.

Rationale for Treating Tourette's Syndrome by Surgical Interventions

In the small group of patients in whom incapacitating tics persist despite conventional treatments, surgical procedures may be useful.[191] Given the paucity of knowledge regarding the pathophysiology of the disease, target selection and other aspects of these procedures remain entirely empirical. Several targets are currently being explored, including the medial thalamus CM/PF nuclei,[192-194] the motor and limbic portions of the GPi,[192] and the anterior limb of the internal capsule.[195] In small open-label studies, these procedures are reported to substantially reduce vocal and motor tics.

CONCLUSION

Movement disorders of the basal ganglia are now recognized as circuit disorders that result from disturbances arising within the basal ganglia, which then affect the function of the entire associated basal ganglia–thalamocortical network of connections. Surgical procedures are increasingly being used to treat conditions such as PD, dystonia, and Tourette's syndrome. The choice of targets for lesioning or stimulation procedures is now strongly influenced by our knowledge of the anatomy of the basal ganglia–thalamocortical circuits. The clear therapeutic effects of these procedures, directed at multiple nodes of the circuit, provide further support for the notion that both hypokinetic and hyperkinetic disorders such as PD and dystonia result from specific disturbances within the motor circuit. The effectiveness of ablative procedures and stimulation in treating both hypokinetic and hyperkinetic disorders argues against specific effects of these procedures on pathophysiologic processes. Instead, it is more likely that these interventions either remove, in the case of ablative procedures, or override and replace, in the case of DBS, the abnormal signals directed to the thalamus, cortex, and brainstem, thus allowing the otherwise relatively intact systems to function more normally.

SUGGESTED READINGS

Albin RL, Young AB, Penney JB. The functional anatomy of basal ganglia disorders. *Trends Neurosci.* 1989;12:366.
Alexander GE, DeLong MR, Strick PL. Parallel organization of functionally segregated circuits linking basal ganglia and cortex. *Annu Rev Neurosci.* 1986;9:357.

Braak H, Del Tredici K, Rub U, et al. Staging of brain pathology related to sporadic Parkinson's disease. *Neurobiol Aging*. 2003;24:197.

Breakefield XO, Blood AJ, Li Y, et al. The pathophysiological basis of dystonias. *Nat Rev Neurosci*. 2008;9:222.

Brown P. Oscillatory nature of human basal ganglia activity: relationship to the pathophysiology of Parkinson's disease. *Mov Disord*. 2003;18:357.

Butefisch CM, Boroojerdi B, Chen R, et al. Task-dependent intracortical inhibition is impaired in focal hand dystonia. *Mov Disord*. 2005;20:545.

Ceballos-Baumann AO, Brooks DJ. Basal ganglia function and dysfunction revealed by PET activation studies. *Adv Neurol*. 1997;74:127.

Coubes P, Cif L, El Fertit H, et al. Electrical stimulation of the globus pallidus internus in patients with primary generalized dystonia: long-term results. *J Neurosurg*. 2004;101:189.

DeLong MR. Primate models of movement disorders of basal ganglia origin. *Trends Neurosci*. 1990;13:281.

Doyon J. Motor sequence learning and movement disorders. *Curr Opin Neurol*. 2008;21:478.

Eidelberg D, Moeller JR, Ishikawa T, et al. The metabolic topography of idiopathic torsion dystonia. *Brain*. 1995;118:1473.

Gerfen CR, Engber TM, Mahan LC, et al. D1 and D2 dopamine receptor–regulated gene expression of striatonigral and striatopallidal neurons. *Science*. 1990;250:1429.

Grafton ST, Turner RS, Desmurget M, et al. Normalizing motor-related brain activity: subthalamic nucleus stimulation in Parkinson disease. *Neurology*. 2006;66:1192.

Graybiel AM. Habits, rituals, and the evaluative brain. *Annu Rev Neurosci*. 2008;31:359.

Hammond C, Bergman H, Brown P. Pathological synchronization in Parkinson's disease: networks, models and treatments. *Trends Neurosci*. 2007;30:357.

Hashimoto T, Elder CM, Okun MS, et al. Stimulation of the subthalamic nucleus changes the firing pattern of pallidal neurons. *J Neurosci*. 2003;23:1916.

McIntyre CC, Savasta M, Walter BL, et al. How does deep brain stimulation work? Present understanding and future questions. *J Clin Neurophysiol*. 2004;21:40.

Mena-Segovia J, Bolam JP, Magill PJ. Pedunculopontine nucleus and basal ganglia: distant relatives or part of the same family? *Trends Neurosci*. 2004;27:585.

Middleton FA, Strick PL. Basal ganglia and cerebellar loops: motor and cognitive circuits. *Brain Res Brain Res Rev*. 2000;31:236.

Mink JW. Neurobiology of basal ganglia and Tourette syndrome: basal ganglia circuits and thalamocortical outputs. *Adv Neurol*. 2006;99:89.

Smith Y, Raju DV, Pare JF, et al. The thalamostriatal system: a highly specific network of the basal ganglia circuitry. *Trends Neurosci*. 2004;27:520.

Temel Y, Visser-Vandewalle V. Surgery in Tourette syndrome. *Mov Disord*. 2004;19:3.

Turner RS, Grafton ST, Votaw JR, et al. Motor subcircuits mediating the control of movement velocity: a PET study. *J Neurophysiol*. 1998;80:2162.

Full references can be found on Expert Consult @ www.expertconsult.com.

CHAPTER 74

Neuropathology of Movement Disorders

Kurt A. Jellinger

Movement disorders, can be divided into four major groups according to clinical phenomenology (Table 74-1); only the first two are discussed in this chapter. Most rigid-kinetic and hyperkinetic forms have their origin in dysfunction of the dorsal basal ganglia (BG), which work in tandem with the cortex via complex information circuits of the brain, although virtually the entire nervous system is engaged in motor control. Recent progress has provided insight into the anatomy, functional organization, and pathophysiologic significance of BG in specific types of movement disorders, as well as the role of different neuron subpopulations in mediating different aspects of motor control.[1-9]

FUNCTIONAL ANATOMY OF BASAL GANGLIA

The interconnections of the nuclei of the BG are shown schematically in Figure 74-1. The three main transmitter systems involved in the integration of BG function are glutamate, γ-aminobutyric acid (GABA), and dopamine (DA).[10] Normal movement is controlled by cortico-BG-thalamocortical circuits, in which the striatum receives glutamatergic input from the cerebral cortex. It sends GABAergic output to the substantia nigra reticulata (SNr) and globus pallidus (pars) interna (GPi), which release projections to specific thalamic nuclei and, to a lesser extent, to the deep layers of the superior colliculus and mesencephalic reticular formation. The respective thalamic nuclei have an excitatory glutamatergic input to specific regions of the cerebral cortex involved in motor function. In this major circuit, the GABAergic output of the substantia nigra compacta (SNc) and GPi diminishes the glutamatergic projections from the thalamus back to the cortex. Projections of the globus pallidus (pars) externa (GPe), the dopaminergic SNc, and the subthalamic nucleus (STN) remain primarily within the realm of the BG, and these nuclei modulate the main flow of information through the BG. The functional specialization of the striatum is closely related to its chemical heterogeneity along the dorsoventral and mediolateral axes.[11] The topography of cortico-BG projections has led to a model of their function based on parallel and segregated pathways operating through discrete functional channels that are represented in specific regions of each BG structure, whereas others have suggested a more complicated pattern of BG connections that indicate potential complex interactions between these channels.

CORTICOBASAL GANGLIA–THALAMOCORTICAL CIRCUITS

The BG are tightly linked to the frontal cortex and are thought to be involved not only in motor control but also in learning processes, behavior motivation, and planning.[9,12] A bidirectional pattern of cortico-BG communication is differentially patterned across bands and during changes in movement.[13] These circuits involve, in a sequential manner, specific parts of the prefrontal cortex, striatum, pallidonigral complex, medial and ventral thalamus, and the frontal or prefrontal cortical area. Five such BG-thalamocortical circuits have tentatively been defined: the motor and oculomotor circuits and the dorsolateral prefrontal, lateral orbitofrontal, and anterior cingulate or limbic circuits involving different parts of the striatum, the pallidonigral complex, and the medial and ventral thalamus.

A nigrostriatal circuit in which the SNc receives a GABAergic inhibitory projection from the striatum feeds back to the striatum with a modulating dopaminergic input. DA causes excitation of striatal neurons that project to the GPi and SNr (by D_1 receptors) and releases the inhibition of thalamic nuclei to maintain normal speed and tone of movements. DA also inhibits neurons that project to the GPe or STN (by D_2 receptors) to keep check on the normal negative effect on motor speed and tone associated with high output from the STN. The GPe receives GABAergic input from the striatum and sends glutamatergic projections to the STN, which in turn sends glutamatergic projections to the SNr and GPi to inhibit glutamatergic excitation of the cortex. The STN-GPe system is considered a central pacemaker of the BG, with heavy implications for their function and dysfunction. By inhibiting BG output neurons in the GPi and SNr, the thalamocortical system can be disinhibited, thereby resulting in higher output at the cortical level.

Activity of the BG output structures is controlled by two opposing striatal pathways, direct and indirect. The *direct pathway* includes projections from the glutamatergic cortex to the medium spiny neurons (MSNs), which contain GABA, substance P (SP), and dynorphin and express the D_1 receptor projecting to GABAergic neurons in the GPi and SNr. Activation of striatal MSNs leads to inhibition of the tonically active pallidal and nigral neurons and consequently to inhibition of the BG target structures in the thalamus and midbrain. This pathway facilitates thalamocortical activity and thereby motor and behavioral output. It can be thought of as the "go" pathway.

The *indirect pathway* includes projections from the glutamatergic cortex to the striatal MSNs (containing enkephalin [ENK] and GABA and expressing the DA D_2 receptor) along with sequential striatal projections to the GPe, GABAergic GPe projections to the STN, and glutamatergic STN projections to the GPi and SNr. Activation of striatal neurons in this pathway leads to inhibition of the tonically active neurons in the GPe, thereby inducing decreased inhibition (disinhibition) of the STNs and their thalamic and mesencephalic targets and causing suppression of motor and behavioral output. It is the "stop" pathway. Experimental evidence indicates that the STN is a critical component of complex networks controlling not only motor function but also emotion, cognition, and corticothalamic excitability.[1,5]

Balance between these two pathways at the level of the pallidum and substantia nigra (SN) appears to be crucial for normal functioning of the BG-thalamocortical circuits, and in pathologic situations (in particular in movement disorders), this equilibrium is disrupted. The circuits subserving abnormal movements in primates and humans with specific lesions may be different from those governing normal movements in intact subjects. This core model has helped explain some of the pathophysiologic mechanisms for the major movement disorders, in which there is either increased inhibition of the thalamocortical pathway, which results in hypokinetic disorders, or decreased inhibition of thalamacortical output, which results in hyperkinetic disorders. DA has opposite effects on the two pathways. The direct pathway has D_1 receptors, and when DA binds to them, this pathway is activated.

TABLE 74-1 Clinical Classification of Movement Disorders

Akinetic-rigid forms
   Parkinsonism: Parkinson's disease, parkinsonian syndromes
   Stiff man syndrome
Hyperkinetic forms
   Chorea syndromes
   Tremor syndromes
   Dystonias
   Myoclonus
   Ballism
   Tics
Atactic movement disorders (not discussed here)
   Cerebellar ataxias
   Spinocerebellar degeneration
Motor neuron disorders (not discussed here)
   Motor neuron disease
   Spinal muscular atrophy and related disorders

The indirect pathway has D_2 receptors, and when DA binds to them, this pathway is inhibited. Therefore, the overall effect of DA is to decrease GPi activity, thereby promoting movement. In contrast, DA depletion, as in Parkinson's disease (PD), leads to higher neuron activity in the output structures and consequently to inhibition of their thalamic and midbrain targets, with reduced activity in "direct" cortical-putamen-GPi projections. This model provides a reasonable explanation for the origin of the akinetic features in PD and the response to drugs and surgery.[14] However, the concept of direct and indirect pathways is likely to be far too simplistic and will probably be modified as more complex organization emerges. Recent studies have led to refinement of the model and the development of a novel hypothesis for better understanding how DA regulates the BG and contributes to BG pathophysiology in PD. Although the striatum remains the main functional target of DA, it is now appreciated that there is dopaminergic involvement of the globus pallidus (GP), STN, and SN. The differential distribution of D_1 and D_2 receptors on neurons in the direct and indirect striatopallidal pathway has been re-emphasized, and cholinergic interneurons are recognized as an intermediary mediator of DA-mediated communication between the two pathways.[15] Recently, two "hyperdirect" pathways were reported. One is a direct excitatory connection from the cortex to the STN, which has an excitatory connection to the GPi. Activity in this pathway will increase GPi activity and reduce thalamic and cortical activity.[16] A new dopaminergic-thalamic system has also been uncovered that sets the stage for direct DA action on thalamocortical activity.[17] Its degeneration in the monkey model of PD provides further evidence for a critical

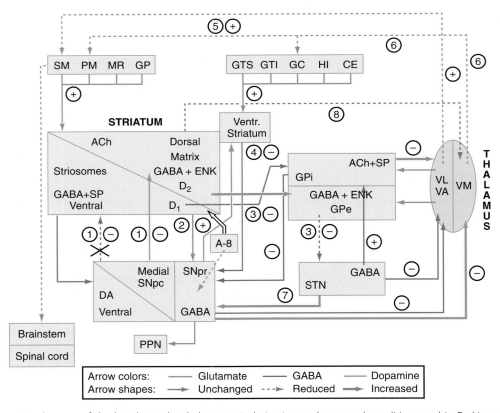

FIGURE 74-1 Schematic diagram of the basal ganglia–thalamocortical circuitry under normal conditions and in Parkinson's disease. Several pathways are shown: 1, nigrostriatal dopaminergic pathway; 2, striatonigral pathway; 3, "indirect" loop; 4, "direct" loop; 5, motor or complex loop; 6, thalamocortical pathway; 7, pallidosubthalamic pathway. *Cortex:* CE, entorhinal cortex; GC, gyrus cinguli; GP, postcentral gyrus; GTI, gyrus temporalis inferior; GTS, gyrus temporalis superior; HI, hippocampus; MR, motor cortex; PM, premotor field; SM, supplementary motor field. *Basal ganglia:* A-8, retrorubral field; ACh, acetylcholine; DA, dopamine; ENK, enkephalin; GABA, δ-aminobutyric acid; GPi/GPe internal/external globus pallidus; PPN, pedunculopontine nucleus; SNpc, substantia nigra zona compacta; SNpr, substantia nigra reticulata; SP, substance P; STN, subthalamic nucleus; VA, ventral anterior; VL, vental lateral; VM, ventral medial; +, excitatory; –, inhibitory.

extrastriatal site whereby DA depletion could induce pathologic changes in neuronal activity and behavior.[15] Another ultra-short DA pathway from SNc to SNr regulates the intensity and pattern of these BG outputs by dendritically released DA that excites SNr GABA neurons via D1-5 receptor activation enhancing active TRPC3 channels.[17a] Parallel processing and integrative networks probably work together rather than in conflict to allow coordinated behavior and motor control to be maintained, as well as to be modified and changed according to the appropriate external and internal stimuli, which are key deficits in BG disorders.[8] A model for altered neural network dynamics related to movement disorders in PD has recently been presented.[18]

CLASSIFICATION OF MOVEMENT DISORDERS

Most movement disorders related to BG dysfunction are neurodegenerative diseases that are morphologically characterized by neuronal degeneration and loss accompanied by astrocytosis in various, often disparate parts of the central nervous system (CNS). According to recent genetic and molecular-biologic data, movement disorders can be classified into several groups (Table 74-2).[16] They may or may not be associated with cytoskeletal abnormalities, which represent important histologic signposts pointing to the diagnosis (Table 74-3). For some of these disorders, consensus criteria for their clinical and neuropathologic diagnoses have been established.[19-25]

Movement disorders are classified into *synucleinopathies*, a heterogeneous group of neurodegenerative disorders caused by misfolded α-synuclein (α-Syn) protein that forms amyloid-like filamentous inclusions in many brain areas. They include Lewy body (LB) disorders—sporadic and rare familial forms of PD (brainstem type of LB disease [LBD]), dementia with Lewy bodies (DLB), and pure autonomic failure (PAF)—multisystem atrophy (MSA), and Hallervorden-Spatz disease, renamed neurodegeneration with brain iron accumulation type I (NBIA-I) or pathothenate kinase–associated neurodegeneration (PKAN). Other major groups are *tauopathies*, all of which feature neurofibrillary pathology (progressive supranuclear palsy [PSP], corticobasal degeneration [CBD], and so on); *polyglutamine* (*CAG*) *disorders*, such as Huntington's disease (HD) and related disorders; the recently described *TDP-43 proteinopathies*, such as frontotemporal lobe dementia with ubiquitin (Ub) inclusions (FTLD-U); and other *neurodegenerative movement disorders* without hitherto detected genetic or specific disease markers (Table 74-4). Movement disorders have additional importance in differentiating Creutzfeld-Jakob disease from Alzheimer's dementia (AD) and DLB.[26]

SYNUCLEINOPATHIES

α-Syn is a partially unfolded, 140–amino acid presynaptic protein with potential for self-oligomerization and fibrillary aggregation under pathologic conditions. Its gene, located on chromosome 4, is mutated in rare familial forms of PD.[27] For its molecular basis, functions, aggregation modes, interaction with DA metabolites, and relevant animal models, see other sources.[28-31] α-Syn assembles into special oligomers and is potentially prone to misfold,[32] which may lead to neuronal death,[33] but other modes of toxicity have also been proposed.[34] The lysosomal protease cathepsin D influences α-Syn processing, aggregation, and toxicity in vivo.[35] α-Syn was demonstrated to be a major component of LBs, Lewy-related dystrophic neurites (LNs), and astroglia in PD and DLB[36,37] and neuronal and glial inclusions in MSA.[38] Given the fundamental nature of the α-Syn–containing lesions, these and other disorders are referred to as *synucleinopathies*.[39] The reliability of assessment of α-Syn pathology and its dysfunction in LBD

TABLE 74-2 Morphologic and Biochemical Classification of Degenerative Diseases with Movement Disorders

α-SYNUCLEINOPATHIES

Invariable Forms (Consistent α-Synuclein Deposition)

Parkinson's disease (brainstem type of Lewy body disease)
  Sporadic
  Familial with α-synuclein mutation
  Familial with other mutations
  Incidental Lewy body disease (subclinical Parkinson's disease)
  Pure autonomic failure
  Lewy body dysphagia
Dementia with Lewy bodies; diffuse Lewy body disease
Multiple system atrophy (MSA)
  Striatonigral degeneration (MSA-P)
  Olivopontocerebellar atrophy (MSA-C)
Hallervorden-Spatz disease (pantothenate kinase–associated neurodegeneration)

Variable Forms (Inconsistent α-Synuclein Deposition)

Parkinson's disease with parkin- and LRRK2-linked mutations
Alzheimer's disease (and other tauopathies)

TAUOPATHIES

Progressive supranuclear palsy (PSP) (4-repeat tau doublet + exon 19)
Corticobasal degeneration (CBD) (same)
Amyotrophic lateral sclerosis/parkinsonism-dementia complex (ALS-PDC) of Guam (3+4-repeat triplet)
Postencephalitic parkinsonism (3+4-repeat triplet)
Chromosome 17–linked familial dementia (frontotemporal dementia and parkinsonism [FTDP-17]) (tau doublet)
Pallidopontonigral degeneration (PPND) (4-repeat tau)
Multiple system tauopathy with presenile dementia (MSTD)
Pick's disease (3-repeat tau doublet without exon 10)
Hallervorden-Spatz disease (with tangles)
Advanced Alzheimer's disease with subcortical neurofibrillary tangles

TDP-43 PROTEINOPATHIES

Frontotemporal lobe degeneration with ubiquitin inclusions (FTDLD-U)
Amyotrophic lateral sclerosis (ALS)
Dementia with Lewy bodies
Amyotrophic lateral sclerosis/parkinsonism-dementia complex (ALS-PDC) of Guam

POLYGLUTAMINE REPEAT (CAG) DISORDERS

Huntington's disease—rigid type (CAG triplet repeat)
Choreoacanthocytosis (neuroacanthocytosis)
Machado-Joseph disease (SCA3) + spinocerebellar ataxia (SCA) type 2
Dentatorubral-pallidoluysian atrophy (DRLPA)
X-linked dystonia parkinsonism (Lubag)

OTHER HEREDITARY DEGENERATIVE DISORDERS

Hereditary striatal degeneration
Pallidal degeneration and related variants
Hallervorden-Spatz disease (without α-synucleinopathy)
Wilson's disease, Menkes' disease
Neuronal intranuclear inclusion (NIID) and basophilic inclusion (BIBD) disease
Inherited dystonias

TABLE 74-3 Ultrastructure, Immunohistochemistry, Biochemistry, and Distribution of Neuroglial Inclusions

TYPE OF INCLUSIONS	ULTRASTRUCTURE	IMMUNOHISTOCHEMISTRY									BIOCHEMISTRY	LESION PATTERN
		AS	PHF	pNF	pTau	Ub	ChrA	αBCrys	APP	αβTub		
AD-NFT	22-nm PHF + 18-nm SF	−	+++	+++	+/+++	+/+++	−	−	+	−	PHF-tau (60-, 64-, 68-kD 3-4-repeat triplet)	Hippocampus, cortex, amygdala
PEP-NFT	22-nm PHF	−	++	++	+/++	+	−	+	+	−	PHF-tau triplet	Brainstem, basal ganglia
PSP-NFT	12- to 18-nm SF + 10-nm PHF	−	±	+/+++	+++	+	−	−	+	−	64-, 68-kD tau 4-repeat doublet	Basal ganglia, brainstem, cortex
PSP, balloned cells	?	−	−	++	+	+	−	+	−	−	Same	Same
PSP, threads	12- to 18-nm SF	−	±	++	+	±/+	−	+	−	+	Same	Same
Lewy bodies, subcortical	7- to 20-nm SF (mean, 10 nm)	+++	±	+++*	±†	+++	−	+	−	+	AS + pNF + ubiquitin	Brainstem, forebrain, nucleus basalis, olfactory bulbs, autonomic ganglia
"Pale" (pre-Lewy) bodies	10-nm SF	++	?	+	−	++	?	?	?	?	Same	Same
Lewy bodies, cortical	10-, 12- to 18-nm SF	+++	+	+‡	−/±	++	+	?	+	?	AS + 68-kD NF fragment	Cortex, amygdala, limbic cortex
CBD inclusions (NFT-like)	22- to 24-nm TR + 22- to 24-nm SF	+/−	+	+/++	++§	±/−	−	−	?	?	64- to 69-kD 4-repeat tau doublet	Cortex
CBD, balloned cells	12- to 15-nm SF + 26-nm SF	−	−	+	±	−/+	−	++	−	?	Same	Basal ganglia, brainstem
MSA, neuronal inclusions (NCI)	18- to 28-nm fibrils + 10-nm filament	++	−	±	−	+++	−	?	?	+	AS	Cortex, basal ganglia
MSA, oligodendroglial inclusions (GCI)	15- to 30-nm tubules	+++	+	−	++	++	−	−	?	++	AS + ubiquitin	White matter, cortex, basal ganglia, pons
Pick bodies	10- to 16-nm SF + 22- to 24-nm TR	−	++	+++	++	++	++	+	+	−	60- to 64-kD 3-repeat tau doublet	Hippocampus, neocortex, pons
Pick balloned cells	Same	−	+	+++‡	++	++	+	+	?	−	Same	same
Astrocytic inclusions PSP, CBD, PiD	15- to 22-nm SF	−	−	+	++	±/+	−	−	?	?	64-, 69-kD tau doublet/triplet	Cortex, basal ganglia, brainstem, white matter
Oligodendroglia "coiled bodies," PSP, CBD, AD	13- to 15-nm SF (PSP), 15- to 20-nm SF (CBD) + 26-nm TR	−	−	−	+	−	−	−	?	?	Tau doublet or triplet	White matter, cortex

*Not persistent after phosphatase treatment.
†Also contains microtubule-associated protein 5 (MAP 5).
‡Persistent after phosphatase treatment.
§Different from AD and PSP.

AD, Alzheimer's disease; APP, amyloid precursor protein; AS, α-synuclein; αBCrys, αB-crystallin; CBD, corticobasal degeneration; ChrA, chromogranin A; GCI, α-Syn–immunoreactive oligodendroglial cytoplasmic inclusions; MND, motor neuron disease; MSA, multiple system atrophy; NCI, neuronal cytoplasmic inclusions; NF, neurofilaments; NFT, neurofibrillary tangles; PEP, postencephalitic parkinsonism; PHF, paired helical filaments; PiD, Pick's disease; pNF, phosphorylated neurofilament epitopes; PSP, progressive supranuclear palsy; SF, straight filaments; pTau, phosphorylated tau protein; TR, twisted ribbons; αβTub, tubuline; Ub, ubiquitin.

has been reviewed.[29,31,40-44] α-Syn phosphorylated at serine 129 has a central role in both familial and nonfamilial forms of PD in dysregulating the DA synthesis pathway.[45] Recently, elevated levels of soluble α-Syn oligomers have been detected in postmortem brains of patients with DLB.[46]

Akinetic-Rigid Movement Disorders—Parkinsonism

This group includes various forms of parkinsonism, tauopathies, and other hereditary degenerative disorders causing atypical parkinsonian syndromes.[47] *Parkinsonism* describes the presence of extrayramidal movement disturbances manifested by a combination of rigidity and bradykinesia with or without resting tremor and postural instability. It has many causes (Table 74-5), with frequent clinical misclassification even if strict diagnostic criteria are used.

Lewy Body–Associated Disorders

The prominent cytoskeletal lesions in this group are α-Syn–positive LBs, cytoplasmic inclusions occurring in many regions of the CNS and autonomic nervous system.[48,49] They are the morphologic hallmarks of PD and DLB but are also found in a variety of neurodegenerative disorders, for example, in 7% to 71% of sporadic and familial forms of AD[50,51] and in 2% to 61% of aged individuals with or without dementia.[52-55] The variation in the estimated prevalence of LB pathology in the older population depends mainly on case selection and the methods used for detecting LBs.[53] α-Syn pathology has been encountered in autonomic nuclei, plexuses, and nerves[49] and more recently in cutaneous nerves[56] as an essential or coincidental feature.

Lewy Bodies

There are two types of LBs: the classic brainstem and the cortical type. Classic LBs are spherical cytoplasmic intraneuronal inclusions 8 to 30 μm in diameter with a hyaline eosinophilic core, concentric lamellar bands, and a narrow pale-stained halo. Although most LBs are single, some neurons contain multiple or polymorphic inclusions. In some brain regions, such as the dorsal motor nucleus of the vagus (DMX), similar inclusions within neuronal processes are intraneuritic LBs. They can be detected in routine histopathologic preparations and should be distinguished from LNs, which are not visible on routine histology. Ultrastructurally, classic LBs are non–membrane-bound, granulofilamentous structures composed of radially arranged, 7- to 20-nm intermediate filaments associated with electron-dense granule material and vesicular structures, with the core showing densely packed filaments and dense granular material and the periphery having radially arranged 10-nm filaments. Cortical LBs—eosinophilic, rounded, angular, or reniform structures without a halo—are more difficult to detect by routine histology. Ultrastructurally, they are poorly organized, granulofibrillary structures with a felt-like arrangement composed of 7- to 27-nm–wide filaments, mostly devoid of a central core.[57] They are found in small nonpyramidal neurons in the lower cortical layers, with densest accumulation in the insular cortex, amygdala, and parahippocampal and cingulate gyri. Similar lesions—rounded areas of granular, pale-staining eosinophilic material displacing neuromelanin (NM) in brainstem neurons—are referred to as "pale bodies" and have been considered precursors of LBs.[58]

Both classic and cortical LBs share immunocytochemical and biochemical characteristics, the major components being α-Syn, Ub, and phosphorylated neurofilaments associated with many other substances, including parkin and synphilin-1 isoforms.[22,25,59,60] LBs, the morphologic hallmark of PD and DLB,

have a distinct central parkin- and Ub-positive domain with α-Syn in the periphery,[61] but it is incorporated into LBs and dystrophic neurites before ubiquitination.[62,63] Colocalization of α-Syn and parkin within LBs suggests that parkin plays a role in ubiquitination and posttranslational modification of α-Syn.[64] The latter results in changes in protein size, structure, or charge[28] (e.g., phosphorylation and nitration, both enhancing fibrillation and formation of LBs[65,66]). A functional Ub–3-ligase complex consisting of early-onset familial PD associated with parkin, PINK-1, and DJ-1 mutations promotes the degradation of unfolded or misfolded proteins and may be a pathogenetic mechanism for PD.[67,68] Full-length leucine-rich repeat kinase 2 (LRRK2) is not a major component of the LBs and tau inclusions in AD. Proteomic analysis of cortical LBs has revealed 296 proteins related to multiple or unknown functions.[69] In brainstem LBD, 90 proteins were identified that differ from those in Pick bodies, thus suggesting a complex formation process.[70] Classic LBs show an initial intraneuronal appearance of dust-like particles related to NM or lipofuscin that are cross-linked to α-Syn, with homogeneous deposition of α-Syn and Ub in the center. Septin 4 (SEPT4), a polymerizing guanosine triphosphate–binding protein that serves as a scaffold for diverse molecules, has been found to colocalize with α-Syn in LBs. Because it serves as a substrate for parkin, it may play a central role in the etiopathogenesis of PD.[71] In the MPTP model of parkinsonism, no Lewy pathology was seen in old monkeys.[72]

Cortical LBs show diffuse α-Syn and Ub labeling, whereas subcortical LBs have a distinct, central Ub-positive domain with α-Syn occurring primarily in the periphery and ubiquitination being the later event. The developmental stages of cortical LBs include granular accumulation of α-Syn in the neuronal cytoplasm initially, stepwise accumulation of dense filaments, spreading to dendrites, later deformation of LBs, and final degradation by astroglial processes.[73] Extraneuronal LBs are related to death and disappearance of the involved neurons.

LBs are associated with coarse, dystrophic neurites—LNs—and also contain α-Syn and Ub as inclusions in axonal processes, which according to recent three-dimentional studies may evolve into LBs.[74] They occur in many regions of the CNS and peripheral and autonomic nervous systems; absence of tyrosine hydrolase (TH) immunoreactivity suggests that many of these neuritic processes are not derived from dopaminergic neurons.

Although not all LBs contain Ub, 7% to 10% have only α-Syn, which is more widespread than Ub staining, thus making specific antibodies against α-Syn the best markers for diseases with LBs and other synucleinopathies and for differentiating LBs and LNs from negative neurofibrillary tangles (NFTs), Pick bodies, and other protein inclusions.[75] Despite the presence of high Aβ affinity binding sites on α-Syn filaments, no discernible interaction of [³H]–Pittsburgh Compound B (PIB) was detected on amygdala sections from patients with PD that contained frequent α-Syn–immunoreactive LBs and LNs, thus indicating that LB pathology is unlikely to contribute significantly to the retention of PIB in positron emission tomography (PET) studies.[76]

Intranuclear inclusions, referred to as Marinesco bodies, are found at higher frequency in elderly individuals in the pigmented neurons of the SN and locus caeruleus (LC) that contain LBs than in those without such inclusions, and their frequency appears to have an inverse relationship with striatal concentrations of DA transporter (DAT) and TH.[77]

LEWY BODIES AND NEURONAL CELL DEATH

The biologic significance of these insoluble proteinaceous cytoplasmic inclusions, the mechanism of LB formation, and their impact on neurodegeneration await further elucidation. LBs, which are the sequelae of frustraneous proteolytic degradation of abnormal cytoskeletal elements, may represent—similar to other

TABLE 74-4 Summarized Diagnostic Criteria for Some Neurodegenerative Movement Disorders

NEUROPATHOLOGIC FEATURES	PARKINSON'S DISEASE (LEWY BODY TYPE)	LEWY BODY DISEASE (DIFFUSE)	PROGRESSIVE SUPRANUCLEAR PALSY*		
			Typical	**Atypical**	**Combined**
Lewy bodies, Lewy neurites	Brainstem, nucleus basalis of Meynert, amygdala, cerebral cortex, autonomic ganglia, olfactory bulbs	Cerebral cortex (cingulate gyrus, hippocampus), brainstem nuclei	None or rare	Rare	Rare
Neurofibrillary tangles and/or neuropil threads	Absent or age-related numbers, except when AD coexists, none in brainstem	Only in Lewy body type of AD	High density in at least 3 of the following areas: basal ganglia/brainstem, subthalamic nucleus, substantia nigra, pons; and low to high density in at least 3 of the following areas: striatum, oculomotor complex, basis pontis, medulla, dentate nucleus	Similar distribution as in typical PSP, except that the severity or distribution of the abnormalities deviates from the typical pattern	Similar distribution as in typical PSP, but coexisting with other neurological disorders
Neuronal loss and astrogliosis	Severe in substantia nigra, zona compacta, locus caeruleus, many brainstem areas	Variable in substantia nigra or other brainstem area	Variable in affected areas	Variable in affected areas	Variable in affected areas
Atrophy	Only if AD coexists	Only if AD coexists	Brainstem	None	Only if another neurological disorder with atrophy coexists
Ballooned and achromatic neurons	None	None	Rare	Rare	Only if another neurological disorder coexists
Pick argyrophilic inclusions (Pick bodies)	None	None	None	None	As above
Basophilic inclusions	None	None	None	None	As above
Neuronal inclusions, α-synuclein positive	None	None	None	None	None
Oligodendroglial, inclusions, α-synuclein positive	None	None	None	None	None
Oligodendroglial inclusions, tau positive	None	None	In affected areas	None	None
Astroglial inclusions, tau positive	None	None	In affected areas	In affected areas	None

*The presence of Lewy bodies, oligodendroglial argyrophilic inclusions, changes diagnostic of Alzheimer's disease (neuritic plaques), prion P–positive amyloid plaques, and larger or numerous infarcts exclude the diagnosis of any of these disorders, except combined progressive supranuclear palsy.
AD, Alzheimer's disease; FTDP-17, frontotemporal dementia and parkinsonism; PSP, progressive supranuclear palsy.

POSTENCEPHALITIC PARKINSONISM	CORTICOBASAL DEGENERATION	FTDP-17	MULTIPLE SYSTEM ATROPHY	NEURONAL INTERMEDIATE FILAMENT INCLUSION DISEASE	HUNTINGTON'S DISEASE
None	None		Rare	None	Lewy neurite–like bodies in cerebral cortex
Similar severity and distribution as in typical or atypical PSP, with minimal involvement of the oculomotor complex, nucleus IV, pontine basis, and inferior olives	Numerous in substantia nigra	Neuronal pretangles, neuronal tangles, and globose tangles	None or extremely rare	None	None or extremely rare
Severe in substantia nigra, less in other brainstem nuclei	Severe in substantia nigra and atrophic areas in basal ganglia or dentatorubrothalamic tract	Severe in substantia nigra, cortex, hippocampus (resembles hippocampal sclerosis)	Severe in striatum, substantia nigra, cerebellum, inferior olives, pontine nuclei (spinal cord)	Severe in frontal and temporal lobe, striatum	Severe in neostriatum (caudate > putamen), less in pallidum, nucleus accumbens
None	Parietal or frontoparietal areas, circumscribed or lobar	Frontal, temporal, parietal lobes; substantia nigra	Striatum, pontine basis, inferior olives	Frontal, temporal cortex, putamen	Striatum, caudate nucleus > putamen; cerebral cortex (layers III and V)
None	In affected areas	In affected areas	None	Occasional	None
None	None	In rare mutation form	None	Hyaline conglomerate inclusions	None
None	In substantia nigra	None	None		None
None	None	None	Isocortex, parahippocampus, hippocampus	None	None
None	None	None	In affected and other areas	None	None
In affected areas	In affected areas	In affected areas (white matter)	None	Occasional	None
None	In affected areas (white matter!)	In affected areas (midbrain)	None	Occasional	None

TABLE 74-5 Causes of Parkinsonism

COMMON CAUSES OF PARKINSONISM

Idiopathic Parkinson's disease

Drug-induced parkinsonism

Multiple system atrophy

Dementia with Lewy bodies

Progressive supranuclear palsy (Steele-Richardson-Olszewski
    syndrome)

UNCOMMON NEURODEGENERATIVE CAUSES OF PARKINSONISM

Vascular pseudoparkinsonism

Corticobasal degeneration

Alzheimer's disease, Pick's disease

Frontotemporal lobe degeneration (FTDP-17)

Wilson's disease

Neuroacanthocytosis

Huntington's disease

Multisystem degeneration

Dentatorubral-pallidoluysian atrophy

Lubag (X-linked dystonia-parkinsonism)

Dopa-responsive dystonia

Pallidal degenerations

Neuronal inclusion body and neurofilament inclusion body disease

SECONDARY CAUSES OF PARKINSONISM

Space-occupying lesions

Hydrocephalus (normal pressure)

Drugs (especially dopamine receptor blocker)

Toxin-induced disease (manganese, carbon monoxide, carbon
    disulfide, MPTP, rotenon)

Boxer's encephalopathy (dementia pugilistica)

Infections and postinfectious diseases—HIV encephalopathy,
    Creutzfeldt-Jakob disease, neurosyphilis, Japanese B encephalitis

Anoxic brain injury

Metabolic disorders (e.g., Wilson's disease)

Basal ganglia calcification (Fahr's syndrome, hypoparathyroidism)

HIV, human immunodeficiency virus;
MPTP, 1-methyl-4-phenyl-1,2,3,6-tetrahydropyridine.

inclusions such as NFTs in AD or Pick bodies—end products or reactions to unknown neuronal degenerative processes.[78] Inhibition of complex I (reduced nicotinamide adenine dinucleotide ubiquitinone oxidoreductase) may be a central cause of sporadic PD, and derangement of complex I causes aggregation of α-Syn, which contributes to the impairment in protein handling and detoxification,[79] whereas mitochondrial accumulated α-Syn may interact with complex I and interfere with its functions.[80] Complex I deficiency in PD brain is not confined to the SN but has also been demonstrated in the frontal cortex.[81]

Involvement of the Ub-proteasome system (UPS) and the autophagy-liposome pathway (ALP) suggests that LBs are structural manifestations of a cytoprotective process. Inhibition of proteasomal function or generation of misfolded proteins exceeding the degradative capacity of the UPS causes the formation of aggresomes, which are cytotoxic inclusions formed in the centrosome, or a cytoprotective response to sequester and degrade excess levels of potentially cytotoxic proteins.[61,82,83] Aggresomal proteins such as β-tubulin and others have been demonstrated in LBs.[84,85] There is no correlation between the density of LB formation and cell loss,[86] and the comparatively low number of

neurons containing LBs in any brain region would not be expected to result from altered synaptic function. Oligomerization of α-Syn at the initial stage of LB development is well documented,[87] and accumulation of α-Syn oligomeres coincides with behavioral and pathologic changes, thus indicating that these oligomeres may initiate protein aggregation, disrupt cellular function, and eventually lead to neuronal death.[88] Accumulation of small α-Syn aggregates at presynaptic terminals has been linked to synaptic pathology in LBD,[89] a finding suggesting that PD is caused by presynaptic accumulation of α-Syn aggregates and resultant synaptic degeneration and that loss of dopaminergic neurons is rather an epiphenomenon after the loss of synapses. LRRK2 expression is found widely in the human brain and may be associated with early-age α-Syn pathology in the brainstem in PD.[90] Fragmentation of the Golgi apparatus, seen in 5% of PD nigral neurons with LBs and 3% of those without LBs and in 19% of neurons containing pale bodies, suggests that the cytotoxicity of α-Syn aggregates is reduced by the process of LB formation,[91] whereas SN neurons showing DNA fragmentation have no somal LBs. LBs bear similarities to some intermediate filament inclusions, such as Mallory bodies, Rosenthal fibers, and others, which have been proposed as a structural manifestation of a cytoprotective response designed to confine and eliminate damaged cellular elements.[91,92a] Nevertheless, significant intracellular protein aggregation, such as LB formation, is a pathologic process reflecting changes in the cellular environment that may contribute to dysfunction of the involved cells. Recent studies have shown the development of LBs in grafted neurons in individuals with PD, thus suggesting host-to-graft disease propagation.[93,94] In the SN, the proportion of LB-bearing neurons appears to be stable, with 3.6% of neurons involved on average. This suggests that destruction of LBs may be equal to their production, and with the hypothesis that neuronal death is related to LBs, their life span was estimated to be around 6.2 months (15.9 months for any type of α-Syn inclusion).[95] Thus, neuronal loss of 71%, necessary for the manifestation of motor symptoms, would be reached after about 20 years, which is in line with standard progression of the disease.[95]

Deposition of tau can be demonstrated in a proportion of LBs and is greatest in neurons vulnerable to both LB and NFT formation, such as in the LC, nucleus basalis of Meynert (NBM), and amygdala.[96,97] Tau phosphorylation at Ser396 has been observed in synaptic-enriched fractions of the frontal cortex in patients with PD and DLB and in advanced stages of AD with and without amygdala LBs.[98] Aβ inhibits the proteasome and enhances amyloid and tau accumulation.[99] This suggests that α-Syn and tau may be related to several pathologic processes (bystander effect), which may explain the frequent overlap between synucleinopathies and tauopathies.[100-102] Interactions between Aβ, α-Syn, and tau may be a molecular mechanism in the overlapping pathology of AD and PD/DLB.[103,104]

Sporadic Parkinson's Disease

PD or the brainstem type of LBD, the most common neurodegenerative disorder in patients with advanced age, is manifested clinically by bradykinesia, rigidity, tremor at rest, postural imbalance, and various nonmotor features.[105] Subtle cognitive dysfunction and depression are often present early in the disease,[105] whereas dementia is common in later stages.[106] PD is characterized by progressive degeneration of the dopaminergic nigrostriatal system and other cortical and subcortical networks associated with widespread α-Syn pathology, and the resultant striatal DA deficiency and multiple other biochemical deficits produce a heterogeneous clinical phenotype.[107] Accepted clinical criteria for the diagnosis of possible and probable PD[108-110] have high sensitivity but a specificity of just 75% for identifying and differentiating PD from other LBDs.[111] For the diagnosis of definite PD, histopathologic confirmation is required. Although LBs are not specific to PD and occur in a variety of conditions as secondary pathology, a positive diagnosis of PD can usually be made by inspecting two unilateral sections from the midportion of the SN and finding LBs. If no LBs are found, two further sections should be examined. If LBs are not seen in either the SN or LC, the diagnosis of PD of the LB type can be excluded. In case of cell loss in the SN and LC in the absence of LBs or other α-Syn–positive inclusions, an alternative cause of parkinsonism should be pursued.[22,25] Several clinicopathologic studies have shown that LBD accounts for 73% to 83% of cases of parkinsonism, including 42% to 63% of cases of PD, whereas other degenerative disorders masquerading as PD, such as DLB, MSA, or PSP, account for 9% to 33%.[59] Awareness of the high rate of misdiagnosis and refinements in the clinical diagnostic criteria for PD seem to have improved the accuracy of diagnosis.[109] Although data on the lesion pattern of α-Syn pathology and the multisystem degeneration in PD have provided insight into its course and the pathophysiology of its clinical subtypes, the cause and pathogenesis of PD remain unclear.[112,113]

NEUROPATHOLOGY OF PARKINSON'S DISEASE

The brain is usually grossly unremarkable or may show mild cortical atrophy, enlargement of the ventricles, and pallor of the SN and LC. Histopathologic examination reveals widespread α-Syn–immunoreactive deposits in neurons (LBs) and dystrophic neurites throughout the CNS. Recent studies have demonstrated α-Syn–positive deposits in presynaptic terminals of the cerebral cortex.[89] Although PD is generally considered a disease of the CNS, LBs may also be found in sympathetic and parasympathetic neurons in PD patients, including the heart[83,114] and the enteric nervous system.[49] These findings have been related to gut dysmobility and cardiac disorders in many PD patients. For the distribution of LBs in PD, see other sources.[25,59]

Glial pathology is present in PD, with argyrophilic, α-Syn–positive, tau-negative inclusions in both oligodendroglia and astrocytes, including Bergmann glia.[115-117] Ultrastructurally, they are composed of approximately 23- to 40-nm filamentous structures.[118]

There is variable neuronal loss in the midbrain and other subcortical nuclei, in particular the SNc, LC, and NBM: severe depletion of melanized neurons (45% to 66%) and dopaminergic neurons immunoreactive for TH (60% to 85%) in the A9 group of the SNc, particularly in the ventrolateral tier (area A, 91% to 97%) projecting to the striatum, followed by the medioventral, dorsal, and lateral areas. The susceptibility of dopaminergic neurons, among others, depends on their distribution within compartments of the SN defined by calbindin (CAB) immunoreactivity. The CAB-rich matrix is separated from the CAB-poor zones of nigrosomes, which show greater cell loss in the caudal and mediolateral region (98%) than in the adjacent matrix. From there it spreads to other nigrosomes and finally to the matrix along a caudorostral, lateromedial, and ventrodorsal progression.[119] This temporospatial disorder corresponds to a somatotopic pattern of dopaminergic terminal loss that is more severe in the dorsal and caudal putamen than in the caudate nucleus (CN). The degree of A9 SNc cell loss and the resulting reduction of TH and DAT immunoreactivity in the putamen followed by the CN and nucleus accumbens show close correlation with the duration and severity of motor dysfunction.[120,121] DAT immunoreactivity in the striatum is inversely correlated with the total α-Syn burden in the SN, but not with the LB count; nigral TH immunoreactivity does not correlate with α-Syn immunopositivity.[122] These data support the concept of synaptic dysfunction and impairment of axonal transport by pathologic α-Syn aggregation.

A close relationship between decreased TH-negative neurons, LBs, and neuronal loss has been shown for the SN.[123] The

reduced intensity of DAT mRNA in the remaining SNc neurons is associated with decreased α-Syn mRNA expression in the SN and cortex with loss of the vesicular monoamine transporter VMAT2 (a dopaminergic neuronal marker) in the striatum, orbitofrontal cortex, and amygdala, but not in the SN in the early stages of PD,[124] whereas α-Syn inclusions and neuritic changes in the neostriatum increase with progression of PD.[125] Akinesia and rigidity are linked to neuronal loss, but the percentage of LB-bearing and α-Syn–positive neurons in the SN is not correlated with disease duration and is apparently stable over time, with 39% of the neurons being involved on average. Such stability suggests that during the course of disease the destruction of LBs is equal to their production and that they are destroyed with the afflicted neurons.

The A10 group of dopaminergic neurons—ventral tegmental area, nucleus parabrachialis, and nucleus parabrachialis pigmentosus—projecting to the striatal matrix,[126] thalamus,[127] and cortical and limbic areas (mesocorticolimbic system) show less severe involvement (40% to 50% cell loss), whereas the periretrorubral A8 region, which contains only a few dopaminergic but CAB-rich neurons, and the central periventricular gray matter show little or no degeneration.[128] Others have reported greater cell loss in the LC (area A6) than in the SN in both PD and AD patients.[129] These changes differ from the age-related lesions in the dorsal tier of the SNc, which is involved only in the late stages of PD.[130,131] Morphometric studies have shown a 35% to 41% reduction in pigmented SN cells, with severe loss of DAT-immunoreactive neurons in older persons[132] and an increase in the volume of these cells.[133] Some studies have estimated the loss to be 4.3% per decade,[133] whereas others have reported almost 10% per decade.[134] Recent morphometric stereologic studies of the human SN have revealed a significant loss of pigmented (−28.3%) and TH+ (−36.2%) neurons in older controls versus younger individuals, with hypertrophy of cells in older controls being interpeted as a compensatory mechanism to allow normal motor function despite neuronal loss. Patients with PD had a massive loss of SN neurons with significant atrophy of the remaining cells (20% of controls), but most of the patients examined were in the end stage of the disease.[135]

Degeneration of the nigrostriatal system causes dopaminergic denervation in the striatum progressing from the ventrorostral to the posterior putamen and CN. These changes are preceded by a preclinical phase ranging from 4.6 years for the anterior putamen to 6.6 years for the posterior putamen,[136] with an annual decline of striatal DA intake of 8% to 10% and of DAT between 5.7% and 6.4% or 10% to 13%. Higher striatonigral dopaminergic neuron loss is suggested in early-onset than in late-onset PD.[137] There is marked loss of DA (−89%) in the CN and more severe loss in the putamen (−98.4%), whereas DA loss in the GPi (−89%) and GPe (−51%) is not related to the pattern of putaminal DA loss.[138] Reduction of striatal DA by 57% to 80%[139] and DAT loss of 56% cause motor symptoms. Therefore, about 50% of dopaminergic striatal innervation appears to be sufficient for normal motor function.[140] Striate DA release was reduced by 60% in PD patients, whereas frontal DA release was within the normal range, thus indicating that it remained preserved even in severe stages of disease.[141] Sprouting of DA terminals and decreased DAT, which prevent the appearance of parkinsonian symptoms until about 60% loss of SN neurons takes place, also contribute to altered DA release and increased DA turnover and predispose to the occurrence of motor complications and dyskinesias as the disease progresses.[142]

SN cell degeneration is preceded by loss of neurofilament proteins; neuronal TH immunoreactivity; TH, DAT, and neurofilament mRNA; TH and DAT proteins; and cytochrome *c* oxidase—findings indicative of functional neuronal damage.[143] Neuronal loss is accompanied by extracellular release of NM with uptake into macrophages, rare neuronophagia or phagocytosis of neurons by macrophages, astroglial reaction, and an increase in major histocompatibility complex class II–positive microglia, which may release proinflammatory cytokines and other substances that mediate immune reactions.[144,145] Microglial reaction, together with the 35% to 80% pigmented neuronal loss reported in normal aging human SN, indicates the presence of a pathologic process that may be additive with specific age-related changes.[146] Activated microglia may also be a source of trophic factors that upregulate neurotrophins in response to signals received from failing nigral neurons and may protect against reactive oxygen species and glutamate.[147] Demonstration of microglial activation and corresponding dopaminergic terminal loss in the affected nigrostriatal pathology in early PD (and DLB) by PET and in the rat SN suggests that neuroinflammatory reaction contributes to the progressive degenerative process.[145,148-150]

Development of Lewy Body–Related Pathology

A hypothetic staging of brain pathology related to sporadic PD with ascending progression has been proposed.[151-153] LB pathology may begin in the lower brainstem and involve the DMIX/DMX, intermediate reticular zone, and anterior olfactory nucleus, with the NBM and midbrain regions being preserved (stage 1), and then extend to the caudal raphe nuclei, gigantocellular reticular nucleus, and ceruleus-subceruleus complex (stage 2). These initial stages are considered asymptomatic or presymptomatic and may explain the early nonmotor (autonomic and olfactory) symptoms that precede the somatomotor dysfunctions.[154,155] In stage 3, the LC, the central nucleus of the amygdala, the nuclei of the basal forebrain, and the posterolateral and posteromedial SNc are the focus of cytoskeletal changes and neuronal depletion, whereas the allocortex and isocortex are preserved. In stage 4, the anteromedial temporal limbic and neocortex and amygdala are additionally affected. Stages 3 and 4 have been correlated with clinically symptomatic stages, whereas in the terminal stages 5 and 6, the pathologic process reaches the neocortex, with the high-order sensory association cortex and prefrontal areas being affected first and later progressing to the primary sensory and motor areas or involving the entire neocortex (Fig. 74-2).

Recent studies have only partly confirmed this staging by showing that all brains of individuals with clinical PD reveal α-Syn–positive inclusions and neuronal loss in the medullary and pontine nuclei and SN and additional lesions in the NBM (90% to 98.5%), olfactory bulb (70%), limbic cortex (50% to 60%), cingulate area (32% to 46%), frontal cortex (29% to 31%), and amygdala (25%), which corresponds to LB stages 4 to 6.[156] Although one study revealed significant interrater and intrarater reliability and supported the suitability of the staging procedure for application in routine neuropathology and brain banking,[157] more recent studies have shown that some early PD symptoms may occur in rare patients with LB stage 2 (e.g., autonomic and bladder dysfunction, sleeping disorders, constipation, orthostatic hypotension, and depression) and more often in stage 3, in which most patients clinically manifested stiffness, asymmetric rigidity, and mild hypomimia but no tremor.[153] In one study, only 6.3% of PD brains diverged from the hypothetic staging scheme of α-Syn pathology,[61] whereas others revealed that between 17% and 47% of all cases of autopsy-proven PD did not follow the predicted spread of α-Syn inclusions and that in 7% to 8.3% of cases, the DMX was not involved despite definite α-Syn inclusions in the higher brainstem or even cortical regions.[53,156,158,159] In contrast, in large autopsy samples, 49% to 55% of individuals with widespread α-Syn pathology were neurologically intact and lacked clinical symptoms or were not classifiable.[53,160]

Therefore, the predictive validity of these concepts was suggested to be doubtful because there was no relationship between Braak stage and the clinical severity of PD,[161] and their relationships to coincidental other pathologies are unclear.[61,62] A new unifying system for LB disorders was proposed recently that correlates with nigrostriatal degeneration, cognitive impairment, and motor dysfunction.[163] Although the previous classifications left 42% to 50% of elderly individuals unclassified, all were classifiable into one of the following stages: I, olfactory bulb only; IIa, brainstem predominant; IIb, limbic predominant; III, brainstem and limbic; and IV, neocortical (Fig. 74-3). Progression of individuals through these stages was accompanied by stepwise deterioration in terms of striatal TH concentration, SN pigmented cell loss, Mini-Mental Status Examination (MMSE) score, and Unified Parkinson's Disease Rating Scale (UPDRS) part 3. There were significant correlations between these measures and LB-type α-Syn pathology. If validated in a greater proportion of patients, the proposed staging system would improve on its predecessors by allowing classification of a greater proportion of patients.

Early brainstem cell loss in PD is mainly confined to A9 neurons in the SN and is associated with more widespread formation of LBs that rapidly infiltrate the brain, particularly in patients with short survival, whereas those with disease onset at a younger age and longer survival usually have a typical clinical course consistent with the Braak PD staging scheme, which is not consistent with the unitary concept of the pathogenesis of LB pathology.[164]

Incidental LB disease (iLBD) is the term used when LBs are found in the nervous system in individuals without clinically documented parkinsonism. The distribution of LBs is similar to that in PD, with one or multiple brain areas involved, and some also have sparing of LBs in the limbic or temporal cortex (average Braak PD stage of 2.7), whereas in definite PD cases, more numerous LBs are found in all regions and the Braak PD stage is significantly higher (4.4). Decreased TH immunoreactivity was shown in the striatum and epicardial nerve fibers in comparison to normal controls, but not to the same extent as in PD.[165,166] These findings suggest that iLBD is probably a precursor to or a preclinical form of PD and that the lack of symptoms is due to subthreshold pathology.

Single clinicopathologic case reports suggested that random eye movement (REM) sleep behavior disorder (RBD) may represent iLBD or an early clinical manifestation of PD[167] or may precede or coincide with Parkinson's disease dementia (PDD).[168]

Neuronal Vulnerability

The neurodegenerative lesions in PD show a selective vulnerability of SN neurons rich in NM and caspase-3, which have high expression of DAT mRNA, unrelated to their intrinsic capacity for DA synthesis.[143] The majority of midbrain neurons severely affected in PD are melanized cells located in the densely packed ventral tier of the SNc; they contain CAB and glycolytic enzymes but are poor in DAT and arborize profusely in the extrastriatal components of the BG and sparsely in the striatum. Dopaminergic neurogenesis, intracellular and extracellular substances, and interactions among these factors have been discussed as essential causes of selective death of dopaminergic neurons in PD.[169] The susceptibility of nigral dopaminergic neurons may further lie within the transcription profile of these cell populations.[170] Neurons in the STN and GABAergic cells in the SNr, rich in calcium-binding proteins (calcineurin and parvalbumin) are either not affected or involved only in the terminal stages of PD. A close relationship among SN cell loss, α-Syn accumulation, and decreased TH immunoreactivity was seen, whereas the majority of pigmented SN but not LC neurons bearing α-Syn aggregates lacked TH reactivity, which leads to a decrease in cytotoxic α-Syn oligomeres. The decreased TH immunoreactivity in pigmented neurons can be considered a cytoprotective mechanism in PD,[123] but it can also be preserved in neurons with early α-Syn accumulation.[122]

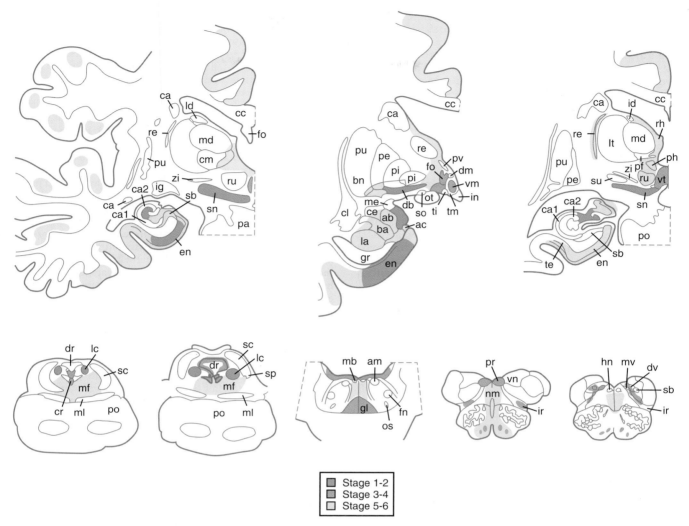

Stage 1-2
Stage 3-4
Stage 5-6

FIGURE 74-2 Progress and pattern of distribution of Parkinson's disease–related neuronal pathology. ab, accessory basal nucleus of the amygdala; ac, accessory cortical nucleus of the amygdala; ad, anterodorsal nucleus of the amygdala; am, anteromedial nucleus of the thalamus; an, abducens motor nucleus; ba, basal nucleus of the amygdala; bn, basal nucleus of Meynert; ca, caudate nucleus; ca1, first Ammon's horn sector; ca2, second Ammon's horn sector; cc, corpus callosum; ce, central nuclei of the amygdala; cg, central gray of the mesencephalon; cl, claustrum; co, cortical nuclei of the amygdala; cr, central nucleus of the raphe; db, nucleus of the diagonal band; dm, dorsomedial hypothalamic nucleus; dr, dorsal nucleus of the raphe; ds, decussation of the superior cerebellar peduncles; dv, dorsal nuclear complex of the vagal nerve; en, entorhinal region; fn, facial motor nucleus; fo, fornix; gi, gigantocellular reticular nucleus; gr, granular nucleus of the amygdala; hn, hypoglossal motor nucleus; in, infundibular nucleus; ir, intermediate reticular zone; lc, locus caeruleus; ld, laterodorsal nucleus of the thalamus; lg, lateral geniculate body; li, nucleus limitans thalami; lt, lateral nuclei of the thalamus; md, mediodorsal nuclei of the thalamus; me, medial nuclei of the amygdala; mf, medial longitudinal fasciculus; mg, medial geniculate body; ml, medial lemniscus; mm, medial mamillary nucleus; ms, medial septal nucleus; mt, mamillothalamic tract; mv, dorsal motor nucleus of the vagal nerve; oi, oliva inferior; os, oliva superior; ot, optic tract; pe, external pallidum; pf, parafascicular nucleus; ph, posterior hypothalamic nucleus; pi, internal pallidum; po, pontine gray; pr, nucleus prepositus; pu, putamen; pv, paraventricular nucleus; re, reticular nucleus of the thalamus; rm, nucleus raphes magnus; ru, nucleus ruber; sb, subiculum; sc, superior cerebellar peduncle; sf, solitary fascicle; sn, substantia nigra; so, supraoptic nucleus; sp, subpeduncular nucleus; st, nucleus of the stria terminalis; su, subthalamic nucleus; te, transentorhinal region; tl, lateral tuberal nucleus; tm, tuberomamillary nucleus; tp, tegmental pedunculopontine nucleus; vl, ventrolateral nuclei of the thalamus; vm, ventromedial hypothalamic nucleus; vn, vestibular nuclei; vt, dopaminergic nuclei of the ventral tegmentum (paranigral nucleus and pigmented parabrachial nucleus); zi, zona incerta.

In the midbrain A9 area, the region of greatest vulnerability in PD, intracellular NM lipid changes, increased concentrations of α-Syn, and interactions with increased iron make dopaminergic nigral neurons susceptible to oxidative stress.[171-175] Dysfunction of the BG circuitry in PD may affect the iron content not only in the SN but also in other BG as well.[176] In the later stages of degeneration, SN neurons show a significant reduction in intracellular pigment, whereas those of normal morphologic appearance exhibit increased pigment density associated with an increased concentration of α-Syn with respect to its lipid com-

ponent and loss of cholesterol. No such changes were observed in other NM-containing neurons in the A2, A6, and A10 areas in early PD, which emphasizes the selectivity of the early NM changes in A9 neurons.[20]

Symptom-Related Specific Lesion Patterns in Parkinson's Disease

The major clinical subtypes of PD show specific morphologic patterns of pathophysiologic importance.

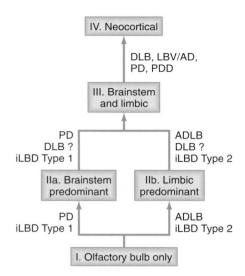

```
        IV. Neocortical
              ↑
        DLB, LBV/AD,
          PD, PDD
              ↑
        III. Brainstem
         and limbic
              ↑
  PD                    ADLB
  DLB ?                 DLB ?
  iLBD Type 1           iLBD Type 2
  ┌──────────────┐  ┌──────────────┐
  │ IIa. Brainstem│  │ IIb. Limbic  │
  │ predominant   │  │ predominant  │
  └──────────────┘  └──────────────┘
       ↑                    ↑
  PD                    ADLB
  iLBD Type 1           iLBD Type 2
  ┌──────────────────────────────┐
  │   I. Olfactory bulb only      │
  └──────────────────────────────┘
```

FIGURE 74-3 Scheme of the hypothetic progression pathways and stages of Lewy body (LB) disorders. The pathway for Parkinson's disease (PD) is suggested to proceed through stage IIa (brainstem predominant), and that for dementia with LBs (DLB) and Alzheimer's disease (AD) with LBs probably passes through stage IIb. For incidental LB disease (iLBD), both pathways seem possible, whereas only PD/PD dementia (PDD), DLB, and the LB variant of AD (LBV/AD) progress to the neocortical stage. (Modified from Beach TG, Adler CH, Lue LF, et al. Unified staging system for Lewy body disorders: correlation with nigrostriatal degeneration, cognitive impairment, and motor dysfunction. *Acta Neuropathol.* 2009;117:613-634.)

In the *rigid-akinetic type*, which occurs in about 50% of all patients, the ventrolateral SNc projecting to the dorsal putamen degenerates more severely than the medial parts projecting to the CN and anterior putamen. There is ventromedial gradient loss of TH- and DAT-immunoreactive fibers and endings from the dorsal to the ventral putamen, with prominent involvement of the met-ENK and SP-rich acetylcholinesterase-poor striosomes of the putamen projecting to the severely involved ventrolateral SNc. DA loss in the GPe and GPi does not match the more severe DA loss in the putamen.[138] Preservation of the CAB-positive somatostatin-rich matrix, which shows increased somatostatin mRNA expression and projects to the GABAergic neurons of the SNr and motor thalamus, suggests that the endings richest in DAT are most sensitive to degeneration.[177] Dopaminergic denervation of the striatum causes severe loss of dendrites on type I MSNs, the principal targets of dopaminergic input from the SN,[178] and loss of convergent nigrostriatal DA and corticostriatal glutamate axon integrity, and the abundant α-Syn pathology in the neostriatum,[125,179] dystrophic neurites in the CN, progressive loss of TH- and DAT-immunoreactive nigrostriatal fibers, and reduced met-ENK immunostaining suggest transsynaptic degeneration as a substrate for the severe motor deficits and decreased efficacy of DA-mimetic treatment in the late stages.[180,181] Reduced dopaminergic input to the putamen causes increased activity of the GABAergic indirect striatal efferent loop via the SNr and GPi to the ventrolateral thalamus projecting to the cortex (Fig. 74-4; also see Fig. 74-1). Excessive excitatory glutamatergic drive from the STN and Gpi/SNr leads to an akinetic-rigid syndrome through reduced cortical activation. The increased GABAergic activity is reduced by levodopa treatment and disappears in the course of the disease, and changes in *N*-methyl-D-aspartate (NMDA) receptors and glutamatergic synapses may be generated, events favoring drug resistence and motor complications.[182,183] Free endogenous DA may induce a relative hyperstimulation of dopaminergic receptors, which may account for the develoment of motor fluctuations and dyskinesias after levodopa treatment (see Fig. 74-4); it has also been related to increased pro-ENK mRNA levels in the striatum.[184,185] Dyskinesia is critically related to the levodopa dosage via loss of synaptic depotentiation.[186]

The *tremor-dominant* type of PD occurs in about 25% of patients and shows less severe total cell loss and less severe depletion of the lateral SNc, but damage to the retrorubral A8 field, which is usually preserved in rigid-akinetic PD. It projects to the matrix of the dorsolateral striatum and ventromedial thalamus and influences striatal efflux via the SNc and thalamus to the prefrontal cortex (see Fig. 74-1).[187] In contrast to rigid-akinetic PD, DA levels in the ventral GPi were normal in PD with prominent tremor, a finding suggesting functional disequilibrium between GABAergic and dopaminergic influences in favor of DA in the caudoventral parts of the GPi, which may contribute to the resting tremor.[138] Functional neuroimaging of patients with resting tremor suggests increased activity of the ventral intermediate thalamus and dysfunction of cerebellar connections,[188] and recent morphometric magnetic resonance imaging (MRI) studies have for the first time demonstrated volume reduction in the cerebellum of PD patients with rest tremor, thus documenting involvement of the cerebellar-thalamic-cortical circuit in the pathogenesis of PD rest tremor,[189] which has considerable implications for stereotactic treatment of tremor (deep stimulation of the ventral intermediate thalamus).[190]

Involvement of Extranigral Systems

PD is a multisystem disorder with involvement of many extranigral systems.[22,25,59,151] The extranigral lesions in PD correlate well with early premotor symptoms, later nonmotor fluctuations, and advanced non–DA-responsive nonmotor features.[191] The olfactory bulb has a special vulnerability for LB–α-Syn pathology, and early involvement has been reported in patients with PD, DLB, iLBD, and AD with LBs.[151,163,192-197] Recent studies have found differences in the severity of LB pathology across the olfactory cortex: more severe involvement of the temporal than the frontal division of the piriform cortex, the olfactory tubercle, and the anterior entorhinal cortex.[198] Most lesions are region specific and do not affect all neurons containing a specific transmitter or harboring LBs, which may explain the complex pattern of deficits of the disorder seen in PD. Both LBDs and PSP are associated with marked neuronal loss (40% to 55%) in the glutamatergic center median (CM) and parafascicular (PF) thalamic nuclei, which together with involvement of dopaminergic SN and cholinergic pedunculopontine neurons, may contribute to the movement and cognitive dysfunctions in both disorders.[199,200] Both diseases further include the mesocortical dopaminergic system, fibers originating from the medial SNc, the ventral tegmental area, and the retrorubral area, and lesions in these areas are related to cognitive and behavioral impairment; the noradrenergic system, with loss of 40% to 50% of LC neurons, is more severely affected in PD patients with depression and dementia, whereas the dorsal vagal nucleus shows little but severe SP-positive neuronal loss and early involvement by α-Syn pathology. The adrenergic nuclei A1 and A2 in the medulla remain intact, whereas noradrenaline-synthesizing cells in the C11 area are depleted. The serotoninergic system suffers loss of TH-immunoreactive neurons in the central raphe nucleus and a 50% reduction in PH-8 serotonin-synthesizing neurons in the caudal midbrain and pons, which causes a reduction in serotonin transporters in both the striatum and midbrain, regions that are not affected in the early stages of PD.[201,202] In the cholinergic system, the magnocellular part of the NBM shows a 30% to 40% reduction that does not correlate with age or disease duration; the reduction is less severe in patients with PD without dementia

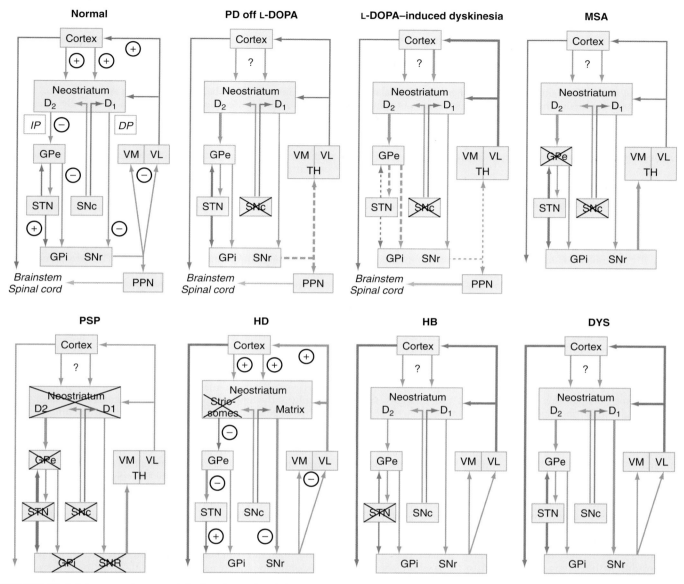

FIGURE 74-4 Schematic diagram of the basal ganglia–thalamocortical circuitry under normal conditions and in hypokinetic and hyperkinetic movement disorders. The *width of lines* represents the relative change in activity versus normal. *Disrupted lines* represent altered patterns with an increase or decrease in neuronal activity; *dashed arrow*, reduced activity; *solid arrow*, increased activity. D_1 and D_2, dopamine 1 and 2 receptor subtypes; DYS, dystonia; GPe and GPi, external and internal segment of the globus pallidus; HB, hemiballism; HD, Huntington's disease; IP/DP, indirect/direct pathway; MSA, multisystem atrophy; Normal, normal conditions; PD, Parkinson's disease; PPN, pedunculopontine nucleus; PSP, progressive supranuclear palsy; SNc and SNr, substantia nigra pars compacta and reticulata; STN, subthalamic nucleus; TH, thalamus; VL and VM, ventrolateral and ventromedial thalamic nuclei.

and in control individuals than in patients with PDD or AD. It is associated with a decrease in cortical and hippocampal cholinergic innervation, but its character as primary or secondary (retrograde) degeneration is under discussion.[59,203] The nucleus tegmentalis pedunculopontinus (PPNc), a cholinergic loop nucleus in the caudal mesencephalic tegmentum, suffers 36% to 57% cell loss, which is strongly correlated with SN cell depletion but not with the duration of illness and LB counts, as well as unaltered parameters in the thalamus and STN, thus suggesting retrograde rather than primary degeneration of the nucleus. Overactivity of the PPNc in 1-methyl-4-phenyl-1,2,3,6-tetrahydropyridine (MPTP)-induced parkinsonism indicates dysfunction of the tegmentonigrosubthalamocortical loops, which contributes to disorders of gait, locomotion, posture, and cogni-

tion.[204] The Westphal-Edinger nucleus, a cholinergic subdivision of the oculomotor complex that regulates pupillary constriction, suffers 55% neuronal loss in PD, which together with damage to the periaqueductal gray matter and nucleus interstitialis of Cajal, explains the neuro-ophthalmic and REM sleep dysfunctions. Pathologic lesions of the amygdala affect mainly the accessory cortical and lateral nuclei,[205] which are involved in endocrine and autonomic dysfunctions. Other systems involved in PD are the reticular brainstem nuclei controlling the somatomotor and autonomic systems,[151,206] the posterolateal hypothalamus, the CM-PF thalamus,[207] the intralaminar thalamic nuclei,[208] and the intermediolateral nuclei and Clark's column in the spinal cord. The GABAergic system suffers a reduction in the activity of glutamate decarboxylase (GAD) in the BG, a decrease in GAD mRNA in the GPe, and a decline in GABA receptors because of degeneration of dopaminergic neurons, which increases GABAergic activity in the early stages of PD but disappears in the course of the disease and with the introduction of levodopa therapy. The peptidergic system shows a reduction in ENK, somatostatin, and neuropeptide receptors in the BG, an increase in somatostatin and mRNA expression, and a reduction of SP in the thalamus and NMDA receptors in the CN, whereas increased phosphorylation of NMDA receptors in striatal neurons is related to levodopa-induced complications.[182] There is early involvement of the autonomic plexuses and nerves by α-Syn pathology,[49] but the cutaneous nerves are affected in rather late stages of the disease.[56]

ETIOLOGY AND PATHOGENESIS OF PARKINSON'S DISEASE

The etiology of PD has long been thought to involve both genetic and environmental factors, but until recently there has been no direct evidence to support either one as a causative factor.[209,210] A molecular interaction between environmental risk factors and genetic factors has been implicated in the etiology of sporadic PD.[211] The pathogenesis of the neurodegeneration in PD and other LBDs has been related to a cascade of multiple noxious factors, including misfolded aggregated α-Syn, the formation of free radicals, lipid peroxidation, oxidative and proteolytic stress, mitochondrial dysfunction and nuclear RNA deficits, protein-iron and NM-iron interactions, excitotoxicity, iron and transcriptional dysregulation, disorders in calcium homeostasis, neuroinflammation, impaired bioenergetics, inhibition or loss of neuroprotective mechanisms, perturbation of protein degradation systems such as the UPS and ALP, excitotoxicity from increased glutamatergic input, and interaction between these and other factors.[84,112,209,210,212-216] The demonstration that α-Syn is degraded by both proteasome and autophagy pathways indicates a possible linkage between the UPS and ALP, and the fact that mutated α-Syn inhibits ALP functioning by binding to the receptor on the lysosomal membrane for the autophagy pathway further supports the assumption that the ALP may be related to the development of PD.[83] Recent microarray analyses of dopaminergic SN neurons in PD patients revealed downregulation of members of the PARK gene family and dysregulation of multiple genes associated with programmed cell death (PCD), providing a "molecular fingerprint identity" of late-stage PD.[217] All possible pathogenetic factors need to be carefully analyzed and are consistent with the multiple-hit hypothesis of PD.[218,219]

PATHOLOGY OF DEMENTIA IN PARKINSON'S DISEASE

PDD, which has an incidence rate of 95 to 112.5 per 1000 patient-years, a point prevalence close to 30%, and a cumulative prevalence of 48% to 83% after 15 to 20 years of follow-up, respectively, is suggested to have a lifetime incidence rate that is increased four to six times over that of age-matched controls.[106,220] CNS lesions contributing to the cognitive impairment in PD are dysfunction of the subcorticocortical networks as a result of neuronal loss in the brainstem and limbic areas, cholinergic deficits in the cortex and thalamus associated with neuronal loss in the NBM and decreased striatal dopaminergic function,[25,59,221] decreased nicotinic acetylcholine receptors (nAChRs),[222] and degeneration of the medial SN and nuclei of other ascending pathways causing dysfunction of the striatosubfrontal and mesocorticolimbic loops. The cognitive deficits in early PD are associated with impaired nigrostriatal dopaminergic function, which results in abnormal processing in the cortico-BG circuit with reduced prefrontal and parietal metabolism, whereas mesocortical DA transmission initially appears to be preserved.[223] Frequent lesions are cortical and hippocampal LBs and AD pathology with

loss of synapses and neurons, presynaptic α-Syn aggregates,[89] or variable combinations of these changes. They may have a common origin with mutual triggering because of synergistic reactions between α-Syn, amyloid-β, and tau protein, with frequent morphologic overlap or co-occurrence of lesions.[101,103,104,224-226] However, epidemiologic, neuroimaging, and neuropathologic data support PDD as being distinct from AD.[227]

Although a few cortical LBs are found in virtually all cases of sporadic PD, the impact of cortical LBs and AD pathology on cognitive impairment is a matter of discussion. Some studies have demonstrated that the number of LBs in the frontal cortex or the number of LB densities in the limbic cortex is a better predictor of dementia in PD than AD pathology is.[228-231] Cognitive impairment is often correlated with the density of LNs and neuritic degeneration in the hippocampus and periamygdaloid cortex, which causes disruption of the limbic loop and "disconnection" from key areas, as described in AD,[232] and is a major basis for the dementia and visual hallucinations.[233,234] The density of both limbic LBs and neuritic plaques correlated well with the severity of the dementia,[235] although hippocampal atrophy and cell loss are not necessarily involved in the memory impairment in PD.[236] The increasing cognitive decline with increasing pathologic LB stages from 3 to 6 secondary to progression of α-Syn pathology[237] was not confirmed by others.[224,238,239] PD patients without dementia may have AD pathology largely restricted to the limbic system (neuritic Braak stages <4), whereas patients with PDD often have severe AD lesions, with or without neocortical atrophy. However, quantitative stereologic studies found no global loss of neocortical neurons but could not exclude local neuronal loss in specific subpopulations in small but essential subregions in PD.[240] In PDD, increased atrophy of the hippocampal head and amygdala is observed.[241]

In a large autopsy series of elderly patients with clinical parkinsonism (37.6% with dementia), only 3.2% of patients with dementia had LB Braak stages 3 to 5, whereas 7% of PDD patients had LB stages 4 or 5 with additional severe AD pathology (neuritic Braak stages 5 and 6). More than half of them showed a strong relationship between the severity of α-Syn and tau pathology. Other degenerative disorders with superimposed AD or vascular pathology accounted for 7% and 17%, respectively, and more than 31% had DLB with or without AD. Mild cerebrovascular lesions (lacunar state, few microinfarcts) were almost never associated with PDD. PDD patients had significantly more severe AD lesions than did patients without dementia, but LB Braak scores were only moderately increased in PDD.[224] In the Sydney Multicenter Study of PD, 47% of 17 PDD brains had diffuse LBs as the only cause of dementia, whereas the others had mixed pathology.[220] ^{11}C-PIB PET studies showed cortical Aβ deposits comparable to AD in some PDD patients, and fluorescence microscopy in postmortem sections revealed binding of PIB to LBs and NM in the SN of both PD and PDD brainstem, which was not seen in controls.[242] The association among cognitive impairment, moderate LB scores, and AD lesions suggests an influence of AD-related pathology on the progression of neurodegeneration and on cognitive decline in PD.[159]

GENETIC FORMS OF PARKINSON'S DISEASE

Although familial parkinsonism with clear mendelian inheritance is rare (5% to 10%), the importance of genetic factors is increasingly being recognized.[243] Molecular analysis of familial PD has identified point mutations and abnormalities in gene copy number in multiple genes, including *SNCA* (on chromosome 4q21), *RKH*, *UCHL-1*, *DJ-1*, the more common PTEN-induced kinase 1 (*PINK1*), *LRRK2*, and *MAPT*, many of them coding for proteins found in LBs or implicated in mitochondrial function, or both.[22,244,245] To date, 15 genetic loci, *PARK1* to *PARK15* ("Park loci"), have been linked to familial forms of parkinsonism.[246,247] Mutations in other genes have been linked to parkinsonism in small numbers of families or in individual cases but have not (yet) been assigned a *PARK* locus number.[248] Several genes in which mutations have been linked to familial PD have been implicated as possible risk factors for sporadic PD.[249,250] Genetic models contributed to understanding of the pathomechanisms of PD.[251-253] In pathologically proven PD, glucocerebrosidase (*GBA*) gene mutations have been suggested to be the most common genetic factor for this disease.[254]

Different mutations in a single gene exhibit considerable clinical and neuropathologic variables both within and between kindreds. Neuropathologic studies of brains with α-Syn/*SNCA* mutations showed cell loss in pigmented brainstem nuclei with widespread LBs, many individuals with cerebral cortex A53T mutations (e.g., in the Contursi family) had conspicuous α-Syn neuritic pathology, tau-positive neuritic and perikaryal inclusions, and some had both tau and α-Syn pathology.[96,255,256] Pathologically confirmed LBD with progressive parkinsonism and dementia caused by *SNCA* duplication results in hyperaccumulation of phosphorylated α-Syn in the brain.[257] A recent neuropathologic study of a patient with familial PD secondary to A30P mutant α-Syn showed findings identical to those of idiopathic PD (IPD).[258] Individuals with *SNCA* gene triplication have unusual neuronal loss and gliosis in the hippocampus, with pleomorphic LBs, α-Syn–positive glial inclusions, and widespread severe neuritic pathology.[259] Autosomal recessive juvenile parkinsonism related to mutations in the *PRKN* gene on chromosome 6q25.2-27 shows severe cell loss in the nigrostriatal tract and LC with remarkable absence of LBs or α-Syn pathology but occasional cortical tau pathology.[260] In compound heterozygous cases, LB pathology or NFTs have been identified.[259,261] A Japanese family with autosomal dominant parkinsonism (*PARK7*) showed nigral neuronal lesions without LBs,[262] reminiscent of some cases of familial juvenile PD caused by mutations of the *PARK2* gene.[260] One autopsy case with a UCH-L1 (*PARK5*) gene mutation had α-Syn pathology similar to IPD.[263] Three patients with heterogeneous mutation of *PARK6* have shown LB pathology, although this may be coincidental. No histopathologic studies of brains of homocygotic DJ1 (*PARK7*) mutation and of ATP13A2 (*PARK9*) carriers have been reported. Other autosomal dominant forms of PDD, with or without dystonia, may pathologically resemble PD with neuronal loss in the SN and striatum, with or without subcortical or cortical LBs, amyloid plaques, and NFTs.[264-266] LRRK2 mutations (*PARK8*), a major cause of late-onset parkinsonism, and patients with multiple mDNA deletions have pathology comparable to sporadic PD[247,250,263,267,268] but display variable neuropathology, including α-Syn and tau inclusions,[252,269,270] thus suggesting an upstream role of LRRK2 in protein aggregation.[90] LRRK2 is considered a key player in the pathogenesis of PD.[271] The pathology in Japanese patients demonstrated nigral degeneration without LBs.[272] Others have shown disparate pathologies such as nonspecific neuronal loss and gliosis in the SN to LBs and LNs or tau-positive pathology similar to PSP.[273-276] Thus, PARK9 seems to be a form of MSA. Recent studies have raised the possibility of a role of TDP-43—which has been reported in FTLD-U, amyotrophic lateral sclerosis (ALS), some AD cases,[277,278] and in familial LB disorders[279]—that is potentially analogous to the association of tau pathology in LB disorders. The combination of autosomal dominant parkinsonism, hypoventilation, depression, and severe weight loss (Perry's syndrome[280]) is an early-onset (40 to 56 years of age), rapidly progressing disease morphologically characterized by massive neuronal loss in the SN without LBs and involvement of putative respiratory neurons in the ventral medulla.[281] Recent studies have found TDP-43–positive, highly pleomorphic neuronal inclusions, dystrophic neurites, and axonal spheroids in a predominantly pallidonigral distribution. The pathologic forms of TDP-43 were neurochemically similar to those found in FTLD-U, and there were no mutations in progranulin (GRN)

or TDP-43 (TARDBP) genes. These data indicate that Perry's syndrome is a unique TDP-43 proteinopathy selective to the extrapyramidal system, with sparing of the neocortex and motor neurons.[282] Mutations of the *DCTN1* gene coding for the large subunit of dynactin, which is involved in microtubule-associated intracellular transport, have been found to be associated with Perry's syndrome.[283] The phenotypic variablity observed in familial PD reflects genetic interactions arising from differences in genetic backgrounds.

Dementia with Lewy bodies

DLB describes a progressive syndrome in the elderly with the core neuropsychiatric features of fluctuating levels of consciousness, visual hallucinations, and cognitive impairment associated with parkinsonism. The pathologic features include a variable burden of α-synucleinopathy with widespread cortical LBs and various degrees of AD-type pathology. Based on current clinical diagnostic criteria[23,24,284,285] that have low sensitivity, early discriminatory diagnosis of DLB has been discussed,[286] but there are still no generally accepted biomarkers to distinguish DLB from other dementias. In population-based clinical studies of people older than 65 years, its prevalence was reported to be 0.3%, which suggests that it could account for up to 10% of all dementia cases, consistent with DLB rates of 10% to 15% from hospital-based autopsy series. In a community-based study of individuals older than 65 years, 5% met consensus criteria for DLB (3.3% probable, 1.3% possible) and represented 22% of all dementia cases,[287] which is consistent with estimates of LB prevalence in a dementia register confirmed by autopsy.[288] In recent autopsy series, DLB was the second most frequent cause of dementia in the elderly after AD and accounted for 7% to 30%, with a mean incidence of 15%.[289] Other population-based autopsy studies have found that LBs were evenly distributed between individuals with dementia and those without or showed no relationship between α-Syn–positive lesions and clinical findings.[53] No classic epidemiologic studies for DLB have been reported.

No single gene determinant of DLB has been described, although a few families with autosomal dominant inheritance have been reported[290-292] and patients with autopsy-confirmed DLB have an increased frequency of a familiy history of dementia.[293] There is evidence that DLB and familial PD are related to an E46K mutation of α-Syn with autopsy findings of diffuse DLB without AD-type pathology,[294] which has recently also been associated with *GBA* mutations.[295] Mutations in the α-Syn gene may predispose to familial DLB.[296] In a Belgian DLB family, a novel locus at 2q35-q36 has been identified,[297] and in a family with pathologically confirmed early-onset DLB with extensive tauopathy, mutations in known genes were absent.[298] Twin pairs may be discordant for neuropathologically confirmed DLB.[299] The fact that many members of kindreds with mutations in the *SNCA* gene have some features of DLB, as well as the frequent occurrence of LBs in familial and sporadic AD, may suggest an overlap in the genetic factors of these disorders, but its pathogenesis is unknown.

NEUROPATHOLOGY OF DEMENTIA WITH LEWY BODIES

The macroscopic appearance of the brain in patients with DLB is usually similar to that in PD, including some degrees of diffuse cerebral atrophy and variable pallor of the SN and LC. The histologic hallmark is α-synucleinopathy manifested as LBs of the classic and cortical type and neuritic degeneration with or without AD-type pathology according to three main patterns: (1) widespread LBs associated with (sometimes numerous) cortical diffuse Aβ plaques and low Braak NFT stages, (2) widespread

TABLE 74-6 Consensus Pathologic Guidelines for Scoring Cortical Lewy Body Deposition

CORTICAL REGION	BRODMANN AREA	ANATOMY	SCORE		
Entorhinal cortex	29	Medial flank of the collateral sulcus	0	1	2
Cingulate gyrus	24	Whole gyral cortex	0	1	2
Midfrontal cortex	8/9	Lateral flank of the superior frontal sulcus	0	1	2
Midtemporal cortex	21	Inferior surface of the superior temporal sulcus	0	1	2
Inferior parietal lobule	40	Lateral flank of the parietal sulcus	0	1	2

Cortical Lewy body score: 0 to 2, brainstem predominant; 3 to 6; limbic or "transitional"; 7 to 10, neocortical. For each region, Lewy bodies are counted from the depth of the sulcus to the lip. Counts are not made over the crest of the gyri except for the cingulate gyrus. Lewy bodies are predominantly located in deeper cortical layers (layers 5 and 6). In each region a count of up to five Lewy bodies in the cortical ribbon gives a score of 1 in the table. Counts greater than five score as 2. The sum of the five areas is used to derive the category of cortical spread (maximum score of 10).

LBs with sufficient neuritic plaques and NFTs for an independent diagnosis of AD, and (3) "pure" LB disease involving widespread cortical areas without significant AD-type pathology.[300] According to the revised consensus pathologic guidelines, LB density is assessed semiquantitatively, based on α-Syn immunohistochemistry, in five cortical regions (Tables 74-6 and 74-7). This protocol has been simplified by excluding the frontal region as the common occurence of occasional LBs in this region in patients with PD in the absence of dementia.[235] According to the severity and anatomic distribution of LBs, patients are allocated to the brainstem-predominant (PD), limbic (or transitional), and neocortical type with widespread cortical LBs.[23,301] These guidelines did not provide definite diagnostic criteria as is sometimes mistakenly assumed, and they were not included in the protocol of the Consortium to Establish a Registry for Alzheimer's Disease (CERAD), which is used for the semiquantitative evaluation of neuritic plaques and NFTs.[302] For revised neuropathologic criteria of DLB see Fujishiro and colleagues.[303]

Cortical involvement by α-Syn pathology varies in DLB. In some cases, LBs are relatively restricted to the limbic structures ("transitional" LBD), whereas in others they are widespread in the cortical areas ("diffuse" or "neocortical" LBD); most numerous in the limbic structures, deep layers of the temporal and frontal lobe, and anterior cingulate cortex; less frequent in the parietal and occipital cortex; and absent in the primary sensory or motor cortex. The anatomic distribution of LBs in DLB does not follow the hierarchical spread of NFTs,[303] although in some cases, clusters of LBs appear to be more closely related spatially to clusters of senile plaques than to NFTs. They affect various groups of neurons, including pyramidal cells and GABAergic interneurons, whereas cortical neurons expressing calcium-binding proteins are spared.[304] The upper cerebral cortex and amygdala frequently show spongiform changes with loss of neurons and apical dendrites.

AD-type pathology of variable intensity and extent is frequent (see Table 74-7). Thirty-two percent to 89% (depending on the criteria used to define AD) of neuropathologically defined DLB

cases have concomitant Alzheimer changes; in the Hisayama study, for example, about 60% of autopsy-confirmed DLB cases had severe AD pathology.[305] Approximately 80% have numerous diffuse plaques and few or no neuritic plaques, around 60% have NFTs in the entorhinal cortex in moderate to severe intensity and rare neocortical NFTs, and about 30% have advanced AD-type changes with Braak NFT stages 5 to 6; a subgroup with minimal diffuse Aβ deposition and no neuritic AD lesions or lesions restricted to the hippocampus is referred to as "pure" DLB. They may show a preponderance of diffuse plaques with different proportions of Aβ subtypes (DLB with less Aβ-40 and AD with more frequent Aβ-40 than Aβ-42 deposits).[306,307] In a personal series of 103 autopsy-proven DLB cases, 62% were classified as "pure" DLB without considerable neuritic AD lesions (68% transitional, 22% diffuse cortical forms), and 38% were associated with severe AD-type pathology (Braak stages 5 and 6). Reclassification of 51 Japanese autopsy cases gave similar results: 66.7% fulfilled the definition of DLB with Braak AD stages 1 to 4, whereas 33.3% had AD criteria (Braak stages 4 to 6; CERAD C) that did not meet these LB stages.[308] Although the Aβ load and plaque density are consistently higher in patients with AD and DLB than in controls, the Aβ pathology of DLB patients with frequent single large clusters of diffuse plaques differs from that in "pure" AD.[309] Neuritic plaques are frequently present at a burden equivalent to that in definite AD according to the CERAD protocol,[310] and many patients have diffuse Aβ plaques with few neuritic elements[228] or only minimal cerebral Aβ deposition. LBD and the LB variant of AD (LBV/AD) were found to differ from "pure" AD in that neuritic plaques generally do not contain paired helical filaments (PHFs) unless they are accompanied by neocortical NFTs.[311] Patients with significant neuritic AD pathology sufficient for the diagnosis of definite AD with LBs can be divided into those with the clinical features of DLB, in whom LBV/AD should be diagnosed,[312,313] and those with more prominent AD pathology and minor α-Syn pathology limited to the amygdala, which is considered a distinct form of α-synucleinopathy.[314] Most DLB brains have an excess of AD-typical phosphorylated tau protein in the hippocampus and are considered to have higher Braak stages of AD pathology than seen in PD patients without dementia and age-matched controls but lower LB stages than those with "pure" AD.[315,316] Biochemical evalution of tau, Aβ, and α-Syn overlap in sporadic DLB cases showed that all brains were associated with important deposits of all three proteins that were similar in quality to those in AD, thereby confirming less severe NFT pathology in DLB versus AD. Tau pathology was less severe in DLB (+AD) than in "pure" AD.[317] Recent studies have shown co-occurrence of abnormal deposition of α-Syn, tau, and TDP-43 in AD, specific subtypes of FTLD-U, and DLB, which suggests common pathogenic pathways, probably triggered by genetic factors.[318,319] Clinical diagnostic accuracy was higher for DLB cases with low Braak AD

TABLE 74-7 Neuropathologic Diagnosis of Dementia with Lewy Bodies

	ALZHEIMER-TYPE PATHOLOGY		
Braak stage	0-2	3-4	5-6
Lewy body disease			
Brainstem predominant	Low	Low	Low
Limbic (transitional)	High	Intermediate	Low
Diffuse (neocortical)	High	High	Intermediate

stages but only 15% to 39% in those with severe AD pathology.[239,320] These data indicate that in DLB, AD pathology has more influence than the cortical LB distribution on both phenotype and diagnostic accuracy.[320,321] Cortical PIB binding in DLB is associated with AD-like characteristics.[322]

"Pure" DLB cases usually show no significant differences in neocortical synapse density and synaptophysin reactivity versus controls, whereas severe synapse protein loss comparable to AD is seen in LBV/AD.[310,311,323] Despite comparable neocortical LB counts and choline acetyltransferase (ChAT) losses, the DLB patients had significantly less dementia than did the LBV/AD patients.[324] There are differences in the expression of α-Syn and 20S proteasome isoforms in DLB, AD, and aged controls.[325,326] DLB cortex does not show overexpression of α-Syn, but there may be a primary defect in clearance of the protein,[327] and insoluble α-Syn did not correlate with the number of LBs but did correlate strongly with the expression of several heat shock proteins.[328]

Hippocampal pathology in DLB is usually less prominent than in AD, and neuronal loss in the perforant pathway is milder and more variable than that in AD.[329] Diffuse neuritic lesions in the CA2/3 region of the hippocampus were initially regarded as a means to discriminate diffuse DLB from PD,[330] but recent studies have shown more frequent involvement of the CA2/3 subareas by α-Syn deposits in DLB than in PD/PDD (79% versus 36%).[25,159] These data suggest a specific involvement of hippocampal projections in DLB.[331]

The cerebellum in DLB and PD shows Aβ-positive inclusions in the white matter, with most being located in Purkinje cell axons and not observed in MSA.[332] Loss of cholinergic pedunculopontine tegmental neurons occurs in DLB but is less severe than in MSA, probably because it does not represent the primary mechanism of RBDs in these conditions.[333] In DLB, LBs, Lewy neurites, and dystrophic axons were observed in the ventrolateral medulla (VLM), which controls the sympathetic output maintaining arterial pressure, but the number of catecholaminergic and serotoninergic neurons was not significantly depleted, thus suggesting that the orthostatic hypotension in DLB is due to involvement of sympathetic ganglia neurons rather than VLM neurons.[334]

Glial lesions in DLB include α-Syn–positive, tau-negative, thorn-shaped astrocytes or coiled bodies,[118,335] but the glial cytoplasmic inclusions (GCIs) of MSA are not seen. The role of microglia in the evolution of DLB is unresolved,[336] but neuroinflammatory reactions have been implicated in the neuronal damage, including LB formation.[337]

Dementia with Lewy Bodies versus Parkinson's Disease/ Parkinson's Disease Dementia

The question whether DLB and PD/PDD are different disorders or represent distinct phenotypes in a continuum within the spectrum of LBDs and their relationships to AD have been a matter of controversy.[25,285,338-340] Their neuropathologies show both similarities and slight differences. Morphology, molecular isoforms, and immunohistochemistry of cortical and subcortical LBs and the ascending spreading pattern of α-Syn pathology do not significantly differ between both phenotypes, with the late stages 5 and 6 of LB pathology suggesting a transition between PD and DLB, although DLB has a higher density of cortical LBs and AD lesions than PDD does.[341] The SN and other subcortical nuclei in DLB show variable neuronal loss that is often indistinguishable from sporadic PD, except for the occasionally more severe loss in the ventrolateral or dorsolateral tier as opposed to the predominant cell loss in the medioventral parts of the SNc in PD/PDD. A major morphologic difference is the significantly more frequent and severe load of diffuse amyloid plaques in the striatum in DLB, dissociated from cortical and limbic AD-type lesions, than that seen in PD patients without dementia, who are virtually free of Aβ pathology.[341-344] Tau pathology in the striatum is also more frequent in DLB. No correlations have been found between LB density in any brain area of DLB patients with cognitive changes or parkinsonism, between LB density and Braak AD stages or the frequency of neuritic plaques,[224] or between LBs in the cortex and SN, thus suggesting that DLB should not be considered a severe form of PD. Although LB densities, in general, cannot separate DLB from PDD, there is more frequent involvement by α-Syn deposits in the limbic system in DLB, in particular the CA2/3 subareas of the hippocampus.[159] The severity and duration of dementia appear to be related to both increased parahippocampal LB density and neuritic plaque grade. A screening algorithm suggesting that LB density thresholds in the parahippocampus may distinguish PD with dementia from PD without dementia independent of other pathologies[205] awaits further confirmation. However, individuals can show significant cognitive disturbances with minimal cortical LBs and, conversely, widespread cortical LB pathology without cognitive decline.[237,238]

Differences in the proportion of Aβ-40 deposits and LB pathology in AD and DLB, the lack of relationship of LB formation to the number of AD lesions, variation in the distribution of tau pathology and cholinergic biochemistry, and genetic differences in apolipoprotein ε4 and ε2 frequency[345,346] argue for separation of DLB and AD. However, both PD and cortical LBD manifested the same seven α-Syn isoforms but with changes in expression.[347] Conversely, more severe LB pathology is found in DLB with severe AD than in diffuse forms, and the various biochemical and morphologic overlapping between PD, DLB, and AD, including colocalization of tau and α-Syn epitopes in LBs, suggests that the process of LB formation is triggered, at least in part, by AD pathology.[25,348,349] This collision of two processes may occur in the same brain region or even within single cells in the human brain, for example, in *LRRK2* mutations,[273] in animal models of PD,[350] and in rare familial forms of DLB,[298] with association of phospho-tau and α-Syn in both NFTs and LBs[351] and in vitro promotion of tau aggregation by α-Syn and vice versa.[352] Others have suggested that amyloid rather than tau enhances α-Syn pathology in the human brain and tg mice.[225,353] These interactions highlight the interface between these and other misfolded proteins,[354] which may represent molecular mechanisms in the overlapping pathology of AD and PD/DLB,[103,104] and together with recent biochemical data on tau and Aβ[317] challenge the view of DLB as a distinct entity. The global cortical amyloid burden is high in DLB but low in PDD, thus suggesting that Aβ may contribute to the cognitive impairment in DLB.[355]

The frequency of associated cerebrovascular pathology in DLB is lower than in both PD and AD but higher than in age-matched controls, which suggests less susceptibility to stroke in the DLB population. Conversely, as in PD and AD, the cognitive impairment appears to be independent of coexisting vascular pathology and is related mainly to AD or cortical LB pathology, or a combination of both.[224] In conclusion, the pathology underlying the cognitive impairment in PDD and DLB is heterogeneous, but there are some differences in the topography and severity of lesions between both phenotypes that need further elucidation.

BIOCHEMISTRY OF DEMENTIA WITH LEWY BODIES

In addition to nigrostriatal degeneration with disruption of dopaminergic input to the striatum and low DAT in DLB in comparison to AD, the cholinergic system is abnormal[356] as a result of NBM pathology.[357] Although neuronal loss in the cholinergic basal forebrain is commonly found in these disorders, early and more widely spread cholinergic losses (reduced neocortical ChAT levels and ChAT-immunoreactive neurons as a result of

NBM pathology) differentiate DLB from AD.[358] Muscarinic M_1 and M_2 receptors in DLB are affected differently from those in AD,[359] thus indicating differences in the underlying extent of pathology in the cholinergic projection from the basal forebrain. Deficits in neuronal nAChRs in the thalamus, CN, and putamen related to the loss of dopaminergic neurons[360] may contribute to the neuropsychiatric features in DLB.[361] Involvement of different cholinergic nuclei in the amygdala in DLB and AD may be due to involvement of both the basal forebrain and brainstem nuclei,[362] although the cholinergic projective neurons are intact in DLB and provide a rationale for cholinergic therapy.[363] Reduction of nAChR binding in the putamen did not correlate with α-Syn expression in both PD and DLB[364] or with plaques and NFTs in AD and DLB, so it is not a reliable marker of cognitive loss in these disorders[365]; however, other researchers have shown a different pattern of nAChR loss in AD and DLB.[366] The striatum in DLB exhibits a variable reduction (more than in AD, less than in PD) in TH immunoreactivity and loss of DA markers, findings reflecting the degeneration of DA neurons in SN.[367]

Multiple System Atrophy

This adult-onset, progressive neurodegenerative disorder of unknown etiology is clinically characterized by autonomic failure and motor impairment with variable combinations of poorly levodopa-responsive parkinsonism, cerebellar ataxia, and corticospinal tract dysfunction. Diagnostic consensus criteria recommend classification into MSA-P (predominant parkinsonism, 80% in the western world) and MSA-C (predominant cerebellar features associated with olivopontocerebellar atrophy [OPCA], around 20%),[21] and red flag categories had a specificity of 98.3% and sensitivity of 84.2%.[368] These criteria were simplified recently.[369] Autonomic dysfunction (urogenital dysfunction, orthostatic hypotension) is common in both variants and reflects degeneration of the central and peripheral autonomic pathways.[370] MSA is less common than PD, with a prevalence of 1.9 to 4.9 per 100,000 and an incidence of 3 per 100,000 individuals.[371] Familial clustering is uncommon, but familial forms with autosomal recessive inheritance may occur,[372] and a single patient with MSA-C had an abnormal expansion in one of the two spinocerebellar ataxia 3 (SCA3) alleles.[373,374] No mutation in the α-Syn gene or effect of genetic variation in other genes related to PD and no clearly established environmental risk factors have been identified,[373] but in the rostral pons of MSA patients, significant changes in the expression of 254 genes (180 downregulated, 74 upregulated) were found, some similar to those in the SN of patients with PD and others related to oligodendrocyte function. SNCA variants have been shown to be associated with increased risks for MSA.[376]

The brain grossly reveals atrophy and green-gray discoloration of the putamen in MSA-P and atrophy of the cerebellum, middle cerebellar peduncles, and pons in MSA-C. The pigmented brainstem nuclei are pale, and cerebral cortical atrophy may be present. The histologic hallmark is cytoplasmic α-Syn–immunoreactive oligodendroglial inclusions (GCIs) within oligodendroglial cells, demonstration of which is required for the diagnosis of definite MSA.[22,377] Less frequent are neuronal cytoplasmic inclusions (NCIs), neuronal intranuclear inclusions, astroglial cytoplasmic inclusions of similar composition, rare Ub-positive nuclear or cytoplasmic inclusions (or both) within neurons resembling those in motor neuron diesease, and Ub-positive neuritic dystrophy reminiscent of neuropil threads but lacking tau immunoreactivity. These changes are associated with neuronal cell loss, reactive gliosis, iron deposition, and demyelination; they occur in an antomically selective manner and affect the pons, medulla, putamen, cerebellum, SNc, and preganglionic autonomic structures.[22,370,378,379] Degeneration of the striatonigral system is most severe in the dorsolateral caudal putamen

and lateral SN, thus suggesting transsynaptic degeneration of striatonigral fibers. Additional damage to the GP and STN leads to dysfunction of these inhibitory nuclei projecting to the motor thalamus, a mechanism similar to that in PSP (see Fig. 74-4). Microglial proliferation and the nonheme iron (Fe^{3+}) content in the SNc and GP are more prominent than in LBD and controls, similar to PSP.[380] Neuronal loss in the hypothalamus, catecholaminergic and noradrenergic groups in the VLM arcuate nucleus, and the intermediate zone of the anterior spinal horn and vagal autonomic nuclei contributes to parkinsonism and the autonomic and endocrine dysfunction in MSA,[377,381] whereas mesopontine cholinergic neuron involvement (PPTNc, laterodorsal tegmental nuclei) may contribute to REM behavior disorders (RBDs).[333] In the cerebellum, the Purkinje cells are more severely affected in the vermis, with atrophy of the olivary nucleus, cerebellopontine fibers, and basis pontis. The degree and pattern of striatonigral and olivopontocerebellar degeneration correlate with the density and distribution of GCIs, the duration of illness, and the clinical subtype of MSA,[382,383] but there is no clear correlation between α-Syn glial burden and neuronal disease. Based on semiquantitative assessment of neuronal loss, astrocytosis, and GCIs in various brain areas, four degrees of severity were distinguished for both striatonigral degeneration and OPCA.[383] Both grading systems were shown to reflect the initial symptoms, disease progression, and clinical key features, but a low correlation between involvement of the two major systems and the natural history of the disorder was observed. Postmortem MRI changes in the putamen (type 1, mild atrophy and isointensity; type 2, atrophy and diffuse hyperintensity with a hyperintense putaminal rim [HPR]; type 3, putaminal atrophy and isointensity or hypointensity with HPR) reflect various degrees of histologic changes.[384] Fluorodeoxyglucose (FDG)-PET studies showed a stable metabolic brain network characterized by decreased metabolism in the putamen and cerebellum, significantly different from healthy controls.[385] These changes range from "minimal-change MSA" with degeneration restricted to the SN[386,387] to fully developed lesions. Widespread occurrence in the initial stages with a short disease duration underlines the multisystem character of "glial degeneration" of the disease.[388] Involvement of other neuronal populations may be linked to frontal lobe dysfunction and cortical motor involvement,[389,390] but AD-type lesions were less frequent in MSA than in age-matched control brains.[25] LBs were seen in 10.7% to 22.7% of autopsy-proven MSA cases,[25,373] whereas AD-type lesions were rare.[391] Patients with MSA-P show more severe and more widespread cognitive dysfunctions than do those with MSA-C, which may be associated with prefrontal involvement.[392] Loss of mesopontine cholinergic neurons in MSA is more severe than in DLB but may not be associated with RBD.[333]

The GCIs are argyrophilic, triangular, sickle- or half moon–shaped, oval or conical cytoplasmic aggregates composed of fibrillary α-Syn, Ub, and a large number of multifunctional proteins, including 14-3-3 protein and LRRK2[347,393,394]; they form a meshwork of loosely packed filaments or tubules 15 to 30 nm in diameter with a periodicity of 70- to 90-nm and straight filaments, both consisting of polymerized α-Syn, granular material, and variable types of filaments.[36,375] Tau protein appears not to be a principal component.[395] The soluble α-Syn in GCIs differs from the insoluble form in LBs, probably because of different processing of α-Syn.[396] An early change is the accumulation of p25α (tubulin polymerization–promoting protein [TPPP]), with its localization and pattern being virtually identical to that of α-Syn.[397-399] TPPP is a potent stimulator of α-Syn agregation[400] and may decrease myelin basic protein, thereby favoring both the deposition and fibrillation of α-Syn and altering myelin metabolism.[397,400] Myelin lesions are well documented in MSA and are most frequent in the external capsule, striatopallidal fibers, cerebellar white matter, middle cerebellar peduncle, and transverse pontine tracts, but they can be identified in otherwise apparently normal areas.[401] GCIs and microglial burden are greatest in mild to moderate white matter lesions and decrease with progression of myelin damage, but they showed no correlation with the severity of gray matter damage in the putamen and SN, which is in line with previous findings of decreased GCIs in severely affected areas.[402] Oligodendroglial changes are more widespread than α-Syn–positive GCIs, thus suggesting that primary oligodendroglial pathology is the main engine that drives the disease process, with secondary degeneration of the oligodendroglia-myelin-axon-neuron complex.[403] MSA can be considered a primary oligodendrogliopathy and is a unique entity associated with synucleinopathy, early myelin dysfunction, and axonal damage leading to secondary neurodegeneration.[404] Incidental MSA showing widespread GCIs without clinical neurological disease is rare,[386,405,406] as is the coexistence of MSA and PSP.[407]

TAUOPATHIES

Tau abnormalities are increasingly common in the neurodegenerative disorders known as tauopathies, with filamentous neuronal and glial tau inclusions associated with the degeneration of affected brain areas being morphologic hallmarks.[408,409] Human tau proteins are encoded by a single gene consisting of 16 exons on chromosome 17q21. The adult human brain has six tau isoforms that differ by the presence of either three (3R) or four (4R) carboxy-terminal tandem repeat sequences of 31 to 32 amino acids that are encoded by exons 9 to 12. The triplets of 3R- and 4R-tau isoforms differ as a result of alternative splicing to generate isoforms with or without 29– or 58–amino acid inserts.[410] The splice site mutations result in increased inclusion of exon 10, which causes a relative release of tau isoforms containing 4R domains over those containing 3R domains. This could be a central mechanism in several tauopathies.[411] Western blot binding has distinguished patterns of soluble and insoluble tau different from those of other disorders, and these patterns have formed the basis for biochemical classification of the major tauopathies.[221] In contrast to AD, postencephalitic parkinsonism (PEP), and Guamanian ALS-Parkinson's disease complex (ALS-PDC) (which have 3R and 4R triplets of 68, 64, and 60 kD), PSP and CBD contain predominantly 4R-tau doublets with two 68- and 64-kD insoluble tau bands at exon 10; they are the most common sporadic tauopathies and are often manifested as atypical parkinsonism. The morphology of the neuronal and glial inclusions is distinctive (see Table 74-2), but there is frequent overlap between different disorders; DJ-1 protein is present in neuronoglial inclusions in tau diseases and is associated with both 3R- and 4R-tau isoforms.[412] It is suggested that the isoform composition of sporadic tauopathies may have a spectrum of findings in individual cases and that the cellular isoform composition may differ in various brain regions.[413]

Progressive Supranuclear Palsy

PSP, or Steele-Richardson-Olszewski syndrome, a predominantly sporadic progressive movement disorder, is the most common atypical parkinsonian disease,[371,414] with incidence rates increasing with age from 0.3 to 14 per 100,000 per year and a prevalence between 1.4 and 6 per 100,000.[415] The mean age at disease onset is around 60 years, and mean survival is 5 years. PSP is clinically manifested by progressive postural instability and falls, supranuclear vertical gaze palsy, and frontal cognitive disturbances,[416,417] but the presence of atypical cases with a variety of clinical syndromes is indicative of the heterogeneity of PSP.[418,419] Two clinical phenotyes have been termed *Richardson's syndrome* (RS) for typical expression of the disease with a rapid course and *PSP-parkinsonism* (PSP-P), which often mimics PD.[420,421] Given these variants, it is not surprising that overall

diagnostic accuracy is just 70% to 75%.[422] The clinical syndrome of PSP may arise through several pathologic processes: RS, PSP-P, FTDP-17, FTLD-U, FTLD-MND (FTLD with motor neuron disease), CBD, progressive subcortical gliosis, and MSA.[22] Research pathologic criteria for PSP have been proposed.[20,421,423]

Typical cases show atrophy of the STN, midbrain, and pontine tegmentum, loss of pigment from the SN, and atrophy of the superior cerebral peduncle[424]; in addition, there may be mild cortical atrophy. Histologically, PSP is characterized by MSA, globose tangles (different from the flame-shaped cortical NFTs), neuronal threads, and tau deposits in glia in specific BG, diencephalon, and brainstem regions, including the SNc, SNr, LC, STN, pallidum, striatum, periaqueductal gray matter, red nucleus, raphe nuclei, oculomotor complex, trochlear nuclei, pontine tegmentum and basis, dentate and inferior olivary nuclei, and spinal gray matter.[22] They differ ultrastructurally and biochemically from those in AD or PEP in that they overexpress 4R-tau with a polymorphous tandem repeat allele located in the intron of the tau gene and are composed of 12- to 15-nm straight tubules/filaments containing 4R-tau with a sequence encoded on exon 10.[425] Swollen achromatic neurons in the cortex and BG contain tau aggregates with straight filaments, which are also present in "tufted" or thorn-shaped astrocytes (stellate with fine radiation processes and straight, irregular 22-nm filaments, in contrast to the "astrocytic plaques" of CBD) and in oligodendroglia as "coiled bodies" (straight 14-nm filaments with a relatively smooth surface) throughout the neuraxis, in particular, the white matter. Only few tangle-bearing neurons but many tau-positive oligodendrocytes are seen in the brainstem tegmentum and pontine nuclei, but not in the SNc, and they exhibit DNA fragmentation and may express caspase-3.[426] The astrocytic tau pathology and microglial activation in PSP correlate with NFT density and neuronal loss.[427,428] Cortical pathology predominates in the precentral gyrus, entorhinal cortex, hippocampus, dentate granule cells, and extranigral A10 midbrain cell groups[429]; the distribution of NFTs is similar to that in PEP and Guamanian ALS/PDC. Severe damage to the GPi, GPe, SNr, and STN causes dysfunction of striatal efflux to the motor thalamus, thereby accounting for akinesia-rigidity and its resistance to dopaminergic treatment (see Fig. 74-4). There are significant morphologic and biochemical differences between the two clinical phenotyes: PSP-P has a significantly lower tau pathology score with more restricted involvement of the SN, STN, and Gpi and a mean 4R-tau/3R-tau ratio of 2.8, whereas RS has more severe and more widely distributed tau pathology, the score of which correlates negatively with disease duration,[430,431] and a mean 4R-tau/3R-tau ratio of 1.6. The cortical tau pathology in PSP differs from that in AD, with the highest density seen in the prefrontal and limbic areas and the major location being in the deeper cortical layers, as compared with a bimodal distribution in AD. In patients with PSP and cortical symptoms, tau pathology is more excessive in the cortex because of loss of synapses.[432] Hippocampal and amygdala pathology is usually minimal, but 20% of patients have ballooned neurons and argyrophilic grains (AGs) in the limbic region.[433] LBs and cerebrovascular lesions are rare,[425,430,434] although vascular PSP has been described as a multi-infarct disorder.[435] The LBs in PSP are suggested to represent an independent disease process.[436] The major genetic risk factor for sporadic PSP, which represents around 85% of all cases, is a common variant in the gene encoding tau protein, with a prevalence of A0/A0 genotypes and the presence of the H1/H1 genotype being a genetic predisposition marker.[437] Recent studies have suggested that this may result in altered expression for specific tau protein isoforms.[425] In PSP-P patients, no mutations of microtubule-associated protein (MAP) tau in exons 1 and 10 were found.[438] Most, but not all cases of familial PSP are considered to be part of the spectrum of disorders of FTDP-17, which is associated with *MAPT* mutations, whereas small kindreds of PSP are linked to chromosome 1.[439]

Neurochemically, nigrostriatal dysfunction in PSP is associated with an 80% to 90% reduction in DA and a 40% to 50% reduction in homovanillic acid (HVA) in the CN and putamen, whereas the mesocortical and mesolimbic dopaminergic systems remain intact in comparison to PD. FDG-PET studies showed a specific metabolic brain network characterized by metabolic decreases in the brainstem and medial frontal cortex that is significantly different from healthy controls.[385] Cell loss from the cholinergic NBM, striatum, and thalamus is less severe than in AD, but the cholinergic systems are severely affected, with a 40% to 80% reduction in ChAT activity, which may play a role in the motor and cognitive dysfunction in PSP, and the 60% loss of neurons in the PPNc may correlate with disequilibration in PSP.[440,441] Mental decline is often ascribed to subcortical pathology related to dysfunction of the striatofrontal or prefrontal circuits as a result of degeneration of the BG and brainstem tegmental nuclei affecting the hippocampal and prefrontal structures,[442] but there is no difference in subcortical tau pathology between PSP patients with and without cognitive impairment.[432] Loss of postsynaptic DA D$_2$ receptors from the BG accounts for the failure of response to levodopa treatment.[443]

Corticobasal Degeneration

CBD, previously described as corticodentatonigral degeneration with neuronal achromatism,[444] is a rare, sporadic, late-onset progressive disorder of unknown etiology that is clinically manifested as non–levodopa-responsive rigidity with focal asymmetric cortical signs (apraxia and aphasia; "alien hand syndrome") and frontal lobe dementia.[445] The clinical syndrome is not specific for CBD, and clinical features of pathologically proven CBD, PSP, Pick's disease (PiD), and FTLD overlap.[446] Neuropathologic evaluation reveals depigmentation of the SN and asymmetric atrophy of the posterior frontal, parietal, and perirolandic cortex along with neuronal loss, superficial laminar spongiosis, and gliosis, with the temporal and occipital lobes being unaffected. The histologic hallmarks of CBD are prominent neuronal and glial cytoplasmic tau inclusions (ballooned/achromatic neurons) in the cortex, BG, brainstem, and cerebellum and extensive accumulation of tau-positive thread-like processes throughout the brain, which are more widespread than in PSP. The ballooned neurons are similar to those seen in PiD and contain phosphorylated neurofilament protein and αB-crystallin. The aggregates of CBD are composed of predominantly 4R-tau isoforms with exclusively exon 10 isoforms,[447] identical to PSP and certain forms of FTDP-17, and they do not stain with antibodies to 3R isoforms and Ub.[19,448,449] Ultrastructurally, they consist of 10- to 15-nm filaments, with fewer 25- to 30-nm filaments, granular material, and lipofuscin, resembling those seen in PSP.[450] The twisted ribbons in CBD are different from the PHFs in AD. In the white matter, "astroglial plaques" and numerous inclusions involve both astrocytes and oligodendroglia ("coiled bodies"). They do not stain for α-Syn or Ub and thus differ from the GCIs in MSA. Astrocytic plaques, typical for and of significant diagnostic value in CBD,[19] resemble the neuritic plaques in AD, but instead of clustering around amyloid cores, the tau-positive processes surround unstained neuropil. They are frequent in the prefrontal and orbital regions and can be found throughout the striatum, but are uncommon in the brainstem.[451] AGs, which also have a predominance of 4R-tau[452,453] and show no differences in frequency of the extended haplotype between PSP and CBD, occur in both disorders more frequently than in controls without dementia and patients with AD.[433] Although the tau isoforms in CBD may differ from those in PSP, they share as a common risk factor the extended H1 tau haplotype, which is overrepresented in both disorders, thus reinforcing molecular commonality of the two conditions.[416,454] Cases described in the literature as familial CBD are now regarded as FTDP-17 associated with tau gene mutation.[455] Minimal research pathologic criteria for CBD are cortical and striatal tau-positive neuronal and glial inclusions, particularly astrocytic plaques and thread-like lesions in both the gray and white matter, as well as neuronal loss from the SN,[19] but these criteria alone do not allow distinction from familial tauopathies (FTDP-17, PiD), so additional genetic and molecular information is necessary. An increased apparent diffusion coefficient of the putamen (by diffusion-weighed brain imaging) provides good discrimination between PD and atypical parkinsonism (e.g., Richards' PSP syndrome and CBD and involvement of the superior cerebellar peduncle in PSP).[456]

Postencephalitic Parkinsonism

This progressive neurodegenerative disorder, a sequela of encephalitis lethargica and other viral encephalitides, is clinically featured by rigid parkinsonism, oculomotor lesions (ocular palsy and oculogyric crises), and cognitive impairment.[457] Sporadic cases have been reported.[458,459] In addition to depigmentation of the SN, neuropathologic evaluation reveals marked neuronal loss and astrocytosis in the brainstem—particularly in the SN (diffuse and more marked than in PD)—and widespread occurrence of tau-positive globose NFTs, neuropil threads, and glial inclusions in the brainstem, BG, NBM, and amygdaloid complex but less severe occurrence in the striatopallidum, thalamus, hypothalamus, and cerebellum. NFTs and neutrophil threads, composed of 22-nm twisted tubules with occasional straight filaments showing 3R- plus 4R-tau and Ub immunoreactivity, are identical to those in AD. Tau-immunoreactive astroglia are seen in affected areas, whereas tufted astrocytes, oligodendroglial inclusions, astrocytic plaques, and ballooned neurons (all typical of CBD) or Pick bodies are absent. Perivascular aggregates of lymphocytes and plasma cells can be found in the midbrain for many years after the initial encephalitic illness, although they are sparse in long-surviving patients. Microglial activation may be striking. Cortical pathology is common, with NFTs mainly in the hippocampus and less often in layers II and III of other cortical areas, different from that in AD.[460] Neither LBs nor α-Syn pathology was detected in PEP.[461] The distribution of lesions shows similarities and overlapping with PSP, and it is extremely difficult to distinguish the two disorders by histopathology alone,[457,458] although there are distinctive clinical differences and subtle deviations in the distribution of lesions, with rare involvement of the red nucleus, cranial nerves IV and XII, inferior olivae, and striatopallidum, different cortical involvement, and less tau pathology in the white matter in PEP. Lesions in the cholinergic subcortical supranuclear centers of gaze movement in some cases of PEP cause gaze palsy and lid apraxia similar to that in PSP.[459] There is total absence of α-Syn–positive deposits in any brain areas of patients with PEP, thus classifying it as a "pure" tauopathy.[457,461,461a] Despite epidemiologic evidence of a viral infection, the etiology and pathogenesis are unknown, and recent molecular-biologic studies have failed to identify influenza virus in archival material from PEP brain.[462,463]

Pick's Disease

This progressive dementia with personality deterioration and signs of frontal disinhibition exhibits rare extrapyramidal symptoms. Most cases are sporadic, but familial cases, usually with autosomal dominant inheritance as a result of *MAPT* mutations, have been reported.[464] Gross inspection shows frontotemporal atrophy, often with a "knife blade" appearance of the cortical gyri, dilated ventricles, and degeneration of the striatum and SN. Histologic examination shows loss of neurons, astrocytosis, and extensive spongiosis of the outer cortical layers; swollen neurons

("Pick cells"), indistinguishable from the swollen achromatic (ballooned) neurons in other conditions; and characteristic argyrophilic intraneuronal cytoplasmic inclusions (Pick bodies), abundant in the granule neurons of the dentate fascia and pyramidal neurons of the hippocampus. Their major component is 3R-tau,[411,465] but some patients have a mixture of 3R-tau and 4R-tau.[453] Ultrastructurally, they have loosely arranged, 10- to 16-nm straight filaments and 22- to 24-nm twisted filaments with a periodicity either longer or similar to the PHFs of AD.[466] Some patients have extensive loss of pigmented neurons in the SN,[467] whereas in others the SN is preserved.

Frontotemporal Dementia with Parkinsonism Linked to Chromosome 17-Tau

This group, linked to chromosome 17 associated with mutations of the *MAPT* gene for tau protein, referred to as FTDP-17, includes a variety of cases characterized by disturbances in behavior and personality with parkinsonian features.[221,468] The gross features are focal temporal atrophy with rust-colored appearance of the GP as a result of increased iron pigment and depigmented SN.[469] The dominant histologic feature is diffuse tau immunoreactivity of the pretangles in neurons, with some patients also having NFTs resembling those in AD, globose tangles and astrocytic lesions similar to those in PSP or CBD, and tau-positive glial inclusions also resembling those in PSP, CBD, and argyrophilic grain disease. Ultrastructurally, the filaments found in different mutations vary in structure and appearance, with PHFs, 15- to 27-nm-wide twisted ribbons, and 12- to 15-nm or 15- to 20-nm straight tubules. Neuronal loss in the cortical and subcortical gray matter is associated with astrogliosis. The hippocampal lesions resemble those of hippocampal sclerosis.[221] Despite significant pathologic heterogeneity between different mutations, some broad correlations have been suggested, including tau pathology resembling AD, PSP, CBD, or PiD. There are similarities and differences between cases of FTDP linked to mutations in *MAPT* and progranulin (*PGRN*).[468] A recent report of a tau S305S mutation in a family with autopsy-proven FTDP-17 provides further evidence of the clinical and pathologic variability in patients with mutations in the tau gene.[470] There is no relationship to TDP-43, the signature protein of FTLD-U.[471]

Guamanian and Other Forms of Western Pacific Parkinsonism

A high incidence of ALS and PDC was recognized in three regions of the western Pacific, the Mariana islands of Guam and Rota, the Muro district on the Kii peninsula in Japan, and western New Guinea. The incidence of ALS/PDC in Guam has declined since the 1960s.[472] Guamanian PDC and ALS-PDC of the Chamorro population may appear clinically similar to FTLD-U and ALS. Neuropathologic evaluation shows cerebral and BG atrophy, depigmentation of the SN and LC, and widespread loss of neurons and gliosis in the hippocampus, amygdala, NBM, brainstem tegmentum, and dentate nucleus, accompanied by abundant NFTs, granulovacuolar degeneration, and Hirano bodies in the hippocampus.[473-475] The severe atrophy of the frontal and temporal cortices and base of the brainstem differs from the brainstem lesions in PSP and AD. The loss of large neurons in neostriatum and nucleus accumbens in Guamanian PDC is more severe than in PSP and may be linked to marked degeneration of the limbic areas. The NFTs in the cortex show a predilection for layers II and III, similar to that in PSP.[460] Ultrastructural and biochemical analysis of NFTs in both the Japanese and Guamanian forms of PDC shows similarities to AD, including all six tau isoforms.[474] Glial pathology is prominent in the PDC of Guam and includes granular astrocytes, coiled inclusions in the oligodendroglia, and tau-positive

fine granules in the frontal white matter that are composed of 4R-tau isoforms.[476] α-Syn–positive aggregates in the amygdala in the PDC of Guam often colocalize with neurons harboring NFTs, and spherical α-Syn–positive structures occur in the molecular layer of the cerebellar cortex.[476,477] The cortex in PDC is distinguished from that in AD and PSP by accumulation of α-Syn, thus suggesting that PDC should be considered a synucleinopathy, as well as a tauopathy.[478] Guamanian PDC was associated with cortical TPD-43–positive dystrophic neurites and neuronoglial inclusions in the gray and white matter. Biochemical analysis showed the presence of FTLD-U–like insoluble TPD-43, and the spinal cord exhibited tau-positive tangles and TDP-43–positive inclusions. These results indicate that Guamanian PDC and ALS are associated with pathologic TDP-43, the major disease protein in FTLD-U.[479] The western Pacific clusters of neurodegenerative disease may reveal factors similar to the cause of AD and other tauopathies, but genome-wide analysis has failed to identify a single gene locus for Guamanian PDC, thus supporting the hypothesis of a mixed genetic/environmental or pure environmental etiology,[480] but the cause remains enigmatic. The cycad hypothesis suggests that dietary consumption of cycad toxins or sterol glucosides is causative but has not been substantiated.[481]

SECONDARY PARKINSONISM

About 10% of all patients with parkinsonism have secondary forms caused by certain drugs and toxins, metabolic disorders, viral infections, multiple infarcts, brain tumors, trauma, or hydrocephalus (see Table 74-5).

Vascular Parkinsonism (Pseudoparkinsonism)

The term *vascular parkisonism* (arteriosclerotic pseudoparkinsonism)[482] implies a rare akinetic-rigid syndrome resulting from cerebrovascular disease, but with a variety of clinical and pathologic features distinct from those of sporadic PD. It accounts for 3% to 6% of all parkinsonian syndromes and is difficult to diagnose with clinical certainty. Symptoms include bilateral symmetrical rigidity, bradykinesia predominantly involving the lower limbs ("lower body" parkinsonism), postural instability, shuffling gait, falls, dementia, and corticospinal disorders, but resting tremor is unusual.[483] Neuropathologic evaluation shows multiple ischemic lesions secondary to small-vessel disease in the striatum, pallidum, white matter, and less often the SN that involve the corticostriatopallidal (nigral), thalamocortical, and other loops in the absence of coexisting pathologic lesions linked to neurodegenerative disease.[484-486] The postmortem demonstration of LBs in 13% of patients with multi-infarct encephalopathy, an incidence that is twice as common as in age-matched controls, suggests subclinical PD, whereas vascular lesions in the BG and white matter are observed in 44% to 58% of individuals without dementia and in up to 94% of individuals with dementia.[224] The vascular damage should be evaluated as a possible additional, but independent, pathogenic factor.[487]

Drug- and Toxin-Related Parkinsonism

Drug-induced parkinsonism (DIP), which can be clinically confused with rigid-akinetic IPD, is most often associated with neuroleptic drugs, calcium channel blocking agents, and other substances causing DA depletion, blockage of postsynaptic D_1 and D_2 receptors, or transient loss of striatonigral TH immunoreactivity.[488,489] DIP affects 15% to 60% of patients treated with typical neuroleptics, depending on their type, dose, and the underlying susceptibility of the patients.[490-492] It is a common form of parkinsonism that is under-recognized, especially in the elderly.[493] Many of them show age-related SNc cell loss and iLBD and are predisposed to adverse drug effects as a result of relative DA deficiency.

The pathology of parkinsonism resulting from carbon monoxide and carbon disulfide intoxication or postnarcotic encephalopathy consists of anoxic lesions or necrosis of the pallidum and SN.[494] Methanol intoxication causes bilateral putaminal necrosis and variable necrosis of the subcortical white matter.[495] Chronic lead intoxication causes SN damage, and manganese encephalopathy is characterized by widespread neuronal loss and gliosis in the pallidum, particularly the GPi, and in the striatum with little or no SN damage and absence of LBs, which contrasts with the typical findings in PD.[496,497] Severe parkinsonism was reported after poisoning with potassium cyanide and was due to neuronal loss and gliosis in the GP, putamen, and SNr, but the SNc was spared.[498] Individuals in whom severe levodopa-responsive parkinsonism developed after exposure to MPTP—a synthetic heroin drug that leads to mitochondrial damage and neuronal death—show diffuse neuronal loss and gliosis in the SN along with extracellular NM and activated microglia but without typical LBs.[499] Eosinophilic inclusion bodies resembling LBs have been seen in the SN and LC of MPTP-treated aged monkeys, but their ultrastructure differed from that of typical human LBs.[500] Other toxins that may cause parkinsonism include paraquat, rotenone, and other herbicides and pesticides.[501-504]

Other Lesions Causing Parkinsonism

Parkinsonism has been observed in a wide variety of disorders involving the brainstem or SN, or both, that affect the dopaminergic projections; it can occur after conditions such as head trauma with direct destruction of the SN by bullet injury, after direct traumatic impact, or after herniation-contusion of the upper brainstem or secondary damage to the midbrain caused by vascular compression.[505] *Pugilistic encephalopathy*, or boxer's dementia, which is often accompanied by parkinsonian symptoms, is characterized by diffuse cortical atrophy; degeneration of the corpus callosum and cerebellum; severe cell loss in the SN, LC, and striatum with widespread NFTs in the superficial cortical layers that are often absent in the hippocampus; and widely distributed Aβ deposits. In contrast to AD, however, only sparse or absent neuritic plaques are present,[506,507] although the NFTs show the same tau isoform profile and phosphorylation state as in AD.[508] Parkinsonism has also been obsrved in rare cases of tuberculoma, tumors of the brainstem, solid tumors causing brainstem compression, calcification of the BG (Fahr's disease), viral encephalitis, subacute sclerosing panencephalitis, multiple sclerosis, and normal-pressure hydrocephalus.[509]

HYPERKINETIC MOVEMENT DISORDERS

Conditions characterized by excessive movement are grouped together as hyperkinetic disorders, in contrast to the poverty of movements seen in akinetic-rigid movement disorders. The clinical range includes chorea, myoclonus, ballism, dystonia, and tics (see Table 74-1).

Chorea

Chorea is typified by nonrhythmic, rapid, involuntary movements. It may be divided into two main groups: hereditary and sporadic (Table 74-8).

Huntington's Disease

This autosomal dominant disorder, clinically manifested as chorea, involuntary movements, dystonia, emotional disturbances, and psychiatric symptoms progressing to dementia and cachexia,[510] is caused by an unstable expansion of CAG (trinucle-

TABLE 74-8 Causes of Chorea

HEREDITARY

Huntington's disease
Neuroacanthocytosis
Huntington's disease–like syndromes
Benign hereditary chorea
Dentatorubral-pallidoluysian atrophy
Paroxysmal choreoathetosis
Wilson's disease
Lesch-Nyhan syndrome
Hallervorden-Spatz disease (pantothenate kinase–associated neurodegeneration)
Ataxia-telangiectasia
Lesch-Nyhan syndrome
Hereditary ferritinopathy
Spinocerebellar ataxia (especially SCA-17)

SPORADIC

Sydenham's chorea
Chorea gravidarum
Autoimmune disease (systemic lupus erythematosus)
Antiphospholipid syndrome
Behçet's syndrome
Metabolic derangements
Drug induced (dopamine receptor blocking drugs, stimulants, levodopa, anticonvulsants)
Focal lesions (vascular)
Infectious (human immunodeficiency virus, abscesses in the basal ganglia, Creutzfeldt-Jakob disease)
Paroxysmal chorea (paroxysmal nonkinesigenic/kinesigenic dyskinesia)

otide) repeats in the coding region of the gene *IT15* (for "interesting transcript," referred to as HD-IT15 CAG repeats) on chromosome 4p16.3. It encodes the 350-kD protein huntingtin, which has important functions in healthy brain.[511,512] The disease occurs when the critical threshold of 37 polyQ is exceeded.[513] The age at onset is inversely related to CAG repeat length. Middle-aged and late-onset patients are seen with a hyperkinetic disorder, whereas juvenile or early-onset ones have bradykinesia and rigidity.

Macroscopic changes in the brain vary with the duration and stage of the disease. Early stages show no gross changes, whereas the late stages are characterized by severe cerebral atrophy, gyral shrinkage, and bilateral atrophy in the neostriatum with enlargement of the frontal horns of the lateral ventricles and atrophy of other brain areas, thus suggesting that HD is a polytypic disorder. Histologically, there is loss of neurons with astrocytosis and microgliosis in the striatum, and increased oligodendrocytic density may precede the onset of symptoms by years.[514] The striatal degeneration involves stereotypic neuronal loss progressing in a caudal to rostral direction, dorsomedially to ventrolaterally in the CN, and dorsally to ventrally in the putamen with sequential involvement of the striatum, GPe, and GPi. The severity of anatomic lesions correlates with clinical severity and has been classified into five grades.[515,516] Grade 0 (<1% of all HD brains) is assigned to individuals with clinical signs and normal-appearing brains but dysfunction of vulnerable striosomal spiny neurons and gliosis in the neostriatum preceding neuronal loss. Grade 1 (4% of all HD brains) shows atrophy of the CN tail with neuronal loss and gliosis; the bodies of the CN and putamen appear grossly normal but may show focal variations. Grade 2 (16% of HD brains) is associated with atrophy of the head of the CN (still slightly convex and bulging into the ventricle) and mild to moderate gross atrophy of the putamen. Grade 3 (52% of all HD brains) exhibits severe atrophy of the head of the CN and putamen. The microscopic changes in grades 2 and 3 are more severe than those in grade 1. In grade 4, severe atrophy of the total neostriatum (95% loss of CN volume) and pallidum occurs along with involvement of the striosomes and matrix in a dorso-ventral progression[517] and a concave contour of the head of the CN. In at least 50% of grade 4 HD brains, the nucleus accumbens remains relatively preserved.

In grades 1 and 2, nonstriatal structures of the brain show no or mild atrophy, whereas in grades 3 and 4, the GP, neocortex, thalamus, STN, white matter, and cerebellum show atrophy with neuronal loss. The GPe is more involved than the GPi. Neuronal loss with or without astrocytosis is seen in the center median of the thalamus,[199] in the SNr without involvement of the SNc, and in the STN with little gliosis. The cerebellar and hippocampal atrophy, often reported in patients with juvenile onset, is probably due to hypoxia resulting from seizures. Cortical degeneration is variable, depending on the stage of the disease, and requires morphometric evaluation.[516] Cell type–specific vulnerability correlates with triplet repeat mutation gains. Neostriatal pathology starts with the loss of ENK- and GABA-containing medium and spiny neurons projecting to the GPe, with relative sparing of the large cholinergic interneurons and medium-sized aspiny neurons and interneurons containing NO synthase, nicotinamide adenine dinucleotide phosphate (NADPH) diaphorase, and various neuropeptides.[516,517] This is consistent with current models of BG function in which hyperkinesia results from interruption of the indirect pathway involving the striatal GPe, STN, and GPi as a result of increased glutamatergic stimulation of the cortex secondary to the reduced inhibitory effects of the GPi and SNr (see Fig. 74-4).[518] In the later stages of HD, the decreased motor activity (bradykinesia) and rigidity are the result of damage extending to the nucleus accumbens, GP (showing loss of SP- and calcineurin-immunoreactive fibers and neurons), amygdala, ventrolateral thalamus, lateral hypothalamus, STN, and SNc (with 40% to 50% cell loss), disappearance of corticostriatal neurons from cortical layer V, and additional loss of striatal GPi efferents (direct pathway).[519] In juvenile cases, corresponding to early rigid Westphal variants, the striatal GPe and GPi efferents degenerate, thus suggesting that degeneration of the direct pathway is responsible for the rigidity (see Fig. 74-4). The differences between rigid and choreiform HD are not related to presynaptic SN damage but to involvement of striatal GABA- and SP-containing neurons projecting to the GPi that inhibit increased dopaminergic activity of the neostriatum. The coexistence of hyperkinetic and hypokinetic movement disorders in HD may be explained by involvement of the direct and indirect pathways in the BG-thalamocortical circuit, but the models of striatal connectivity and pathology are insufficient to explain the nonmotor features often seen in early HD.[520] The cognitive changes in HD are related to diffuse cortical atrophy with cell loss in the deep layers and loss of corticostriatal neurons in frontal layer V and in the entorhinal cortex and subiculum, which causes disorders of the striatofrontal and limbic circuitry. There is an increasing prevalence of non-neuritic tau pathology in the limbic areas and Aβ deposits in the neocortex in young patients with early stages of HD but less rapid progress in advanced age, thus explaining a rare coexistence of HD and AD.[521]

Neuronal intranuclear inclusions composed of aggregates of abnormal huntingtin protein have been demonstrated by immunohistochemistry studies with antibodies against huntingtin protein and Ub in both humans and tg mouse models.[522,523] They are present in the cerebral cortex, hippocampus, and to a lesser extent, the neostriatum, amygdala, and dentate and red nuclei.

Dystrophic neurites with similar immunohistochemical properties in the cortex, medial temporal lobe, and striatum are more common than nuclear inclusions. The frequency of cortical intranuclear inclusions correlates with the extent of CAG expansion and is inversely related to the age at onset and death, whereas no such relationships were detected for the striatum, which reflects the advanced neuronal loss accrued by the time of death.[524] In earlier stages of HD, accumulation of N-terminal huntingtin protein occurs in the cytoplasm together with dystrophic neurites inducing degeneration of the corticostriatal pathway.[525] The role of mutant huntingtin protein in neuronal degeneration and the pathogenic mechanisms of HD are not yet fully understood, but it is presumed that huntingtin protein is cleaved by caspases, with toxic gain of function leading to cytoskeletal defects, synaptic dysfunction, and reduced brain-derived neurotrophic factor and neurotrophic receptor signaling.[526] Evidence suggests that conformational changes in the expanded polyglutamine induce a cascade of cellular mechanisms, including excitotoxicity; altered proteasome degradation, cell signaling, and regulation of transcription; increased free radical and oxidative damage products; early mitochondrial calcium defects; impaired energy metabolism; transport dysfunctions; and apoptosis.[22,516,527,528] Recent studies showed that a protein called *Rhes*, which is specific to the stratum, mediates the neurotoxic effect of mutant-huntingtin.[529]

Other Hereditary Choreas

Neuroacanthosis

This rare, genetically heterogeneous condition shows an association of erythrocytic acanthocytosis with chorea, dystonia, and the later development of akinetic-rigid parkinsonism, the severity of which is not correlated with the degree of acanthosis. The most prevalent form is autosomal recessive with mutation of the *CHAC* gene on chromosome 9q21,[530] but there are various genetic and clinical subtypes. Neuropathologic data are sparse and not well correlated with genetics. Neuroacanthosis is characterized by gross atrophy of the neostriatum with loss of small and medium-sized neurons, severe pallidal involvement, and less consistent lesions in the thalamus, SN, and spinal anterior horns. The absence of changes in the cerebral cortex, STN, and cerebellum may help in differetiating this condition from HD.[22] Peripheral nerves may show chronic axonal neuropathy.[531]

Huntington's Disease–Like Syndromes

Approximately 1% of patients with a clinicopathologic picture of HD have no mutation of the *huntingtin* gene, and three separate mutations or linkages have been identified. Autosomal dominant HD-like type 1 (HDL-1), caused by an expanded octapeptide repeat in the prion gene at chromosome 20pter-p12, with valine at codon 129, shows atrophy of the BG, variable cortical atrophy, and prion-specific changes, including typical prion plaques.[532]

Autosomal dominant HDL-2 occurs in patients of African ancestry and exhibits features similar to HD: frontal inhibition with parkinsonism but absence of choreoathetosis. It is due to a CAG/CTG repeat expansion in the juntophilin-3 gene on chromosome 16q243. Degeneration of the dorsal and lateral CN and putamen and the neocortices is associated with Ub- and TATA box binding protein–immunoreactive neuronal intranuclear inclusions. Its neuropathologic similarity to HD suggests partial pathogenetic overlap of both disorders.[533]

Autosomal recessive HDL-3, linked closely to the HD locus on chromsome 4p, is characterized by chorea, dystonia, ataxia, spasticity, and cognitive defects with onset in the first decade of life, as well as progressive frontal cortical atrophy and bilateral CN atrophy on MRI, but no autopsy studies have been reported.

Benign Hereditary Chorea

Benign hereditary chorea is clinically and genetically heterogeneous. A number of kindreds with autosomal dominant inheritance, related to mutations in the *TTF1* (thyroid transcription factor 1) gene on chromosome 14q,[534] have an onset of chorea in childhood with little progression and without mental deterioration. Functional imaging studies reveal changes in the BG similar to HD, but the neuropathology of benign hereditary chorea is not well documented.

Sporadic Chorea

Nongenetic forms include those of autoimmune pathogenesis, such as Sydenham's chorea, which occurs after streptococcal infection and is frequently linked to classic rheumatic fever or systemic lupus erythematosus (antiphospholipid syndrome). Affected patients have unilateral involuntary movements and other symptoms, but the neuropathology is uncertain.[535] Other forms include polycythemia vera or vascular chorea caused by small strokes in the striatum, toxoplasmosis in patients with acquired immunodeficiency syndrome,[536] herpes simplex encephalitis,[537] and paraneoplastic chorea.[538]

Hereditary Striatal Necrosis

This rare, autosomal dominant or recessive progressive disorder with gait disturbance, dystonia, rigidity, ataxia, and optic atrophy morphologically shows bilateral necrosis of the neostriatum and GP with vascular proliferation, as well as similar lesions variably involving the thalamus, SN, and brainstem tegmentum, but rarely the cerebral cortex. Pathologic evaulation shows overlap with mitochondrial encephalopathies such as Leigh's disease and Leber's optic neuropathy.[539] In childhood, however, bilateral striatal lesions may occur in a variety of disorders.[22]

Dentatorubral-Pallidoluysian Atrophy

This rare autosomal dominant disorder, largely confined to populations with Japanese ancestry, is caused by an abnormally expanded CAG triplet in the gene for atrophin-1 secondary to a CTG-B37 mutation on chromosome 12p13.31.[540] The pathogenic range of CAG repeats is 54 to 79, with normal alleles having fewer than 26 repeats. The diverse clinical picture includes chorea, athetosis, ataxia, myoclonus, epilepsy, and dementia, with considerable intrafamilial variations. Early-onset patients with larger CAG repeat expansions tend to have prominent myoclonic epilepsy. Adult-onset cases may be mistaken for HD and other types of SCA. Neuropathologic examination reveals MSA with neuronal loss and gliosis involving the cerebellar dentate nucleus, GPe, STN, and red nucleus, with disruption of the dentatorubral, pallidofugal, spinocerebellar, and motor systems. Milder changes involve the striatum, thalamus, SN, inferior olivae, midbrain tegmentum, spinocerebellar tracts, and posterior spinal columns, often associated with neuroaxonal dystrophy, but the cerebral cortex is largely spared.[22] Patients with the Haw River syndrome have smaller expansions of the *atrophin-1* gene with calcification of the pallidum, demyelination of cerebral white matter, and atrophy of the dentate nucleus and pallidum.[541] The intranuclear and cytoplasmic inclusions in the neurons and oligodendroglia of various brain sites are immunoreactive for Ub and *atrophin-1* and have expanded polyglutamine tracts.[542,543] Their density correlates with CGA repeat length, thus suggesting that these protein aggregates may be a common feature in the pathogenesis of glutamine repeat neurodegenerative disorders.[544]

Machado-Joseph Disease

Machado-Joseph disease/SCA3 is a fatal, autosomal dominant progressive ataxia in Europe and Japan that results from CAG expansion in the *MJC1* gene and toxic overexpression of ataxin-3, which maps to chromosome 14q.32.1.[545] It was subdivided into different clinical types. Type 1, the least common, has an onset from 5 to 20 years of age and features spasticity, rigidity, and bradykinesia but little ataxia. Type 2, the most frequent, is characterized by progressive ataxia and spasticity. Type 3 (late onset) is typified by ataxia, distal amyotrophy, and areflexia. Type 4 shows prominent parkinsonism. There is involvement of the cerebellar afferent and efferent pathways, extrapyramidal structures, and lower motor neurons, with cell loss in the SN, STN, dentate and red nuclei, Clark's column, raphe nuclei, cranial nerve motor nuclei, and anterior horns; the striatum and cerebral cortex are less affected. The degenerative changes are often accompanied by intranuclear neuronal inclusions immunoreactive with ataxin-3 and Ub.[22] Its pathogenesis is related to aggregation of ataxin-3, which causes selective neuronal loss.

Progressive Pallidal Degeneration

These rare, autosomal recessive or sporadic disorders are manifested as dystonia, choreoathetosis, rigid akinesia, oculomotor and gait disorders, and pseudobulbar palsy secondary to atrophy of the pallidoluysionigral system and are defined purely morphologically. It is not clear whether they represent distinct diseases.

Pallidal degeneration is characterized by isolated bilateral atrophy of the GP with gliosis and degeneration of the efferent pallidal fibers and *pallidoluysian atrophy* by bilateral atrophy and gliosis of the GPe and STN. *Pallidonigral* and *pallidonigroluysian degeneration*, which may be associated with levodopa-resistent akinesia, is typified by degeneration of the GP, STN, and SN and occasional involvement of the ventromedial thalamus and iron deposition in the affected nuclei.[546] In single cases with progressive choreiform or dystonic disorders or nonprogressive cerebral palsy, autopsy has revealed symmetrical degeneration of the GPe or status marmoratus of the BG associated with polyglucosan bodies in neuronal perikarya, axons, and dendrites (Bielschowsky bodies).[22] The combination of recessive early-onset parkinsonism and pyramidal tract signs is known as pallidopyramidal syndrome and has recently been discussed critically.[547]

Hallervorden-Spatz Disease

NBIA-I or PKAN defines a group of genetic autosomal-recessive degenerative disorders with progressive dystonia, akinetic rigidity, optic atrophy, retinitis pigmentosa, seizures, and dementia.[548,549] The majority of classic cases are caused by mutations in the pantothenate kinase 2 (*PANK2*) gene linked to chromosome 20p12.3-13 (Online Mendelian Inheritance in Man [OMIM] 234200),[550] whereas others bear mutations in the *PLA2G6* gene on chromosome 22.[551] Classic PKAN with infantile onset consists of dystonia, early pyramidal signs, cognitive decline, and retinal changes; the atypical juvenile form features neurobehavioral involvement and slower progress; and adult forms are typically extrapyramidal disorders with dementia. Different subtypes can be reliably distinguished by T2* and T2 fast spin-echo brain MRI, which provides an accurate clinical and subsequent molecular diagnosis.[552] Neuropathologic evaluation reveals a rust-brown discoloration of the GP and SN, loss of neurons, gliosis, and iron pigment deposits; histologic markers are axonal spheroids (dystrophic 20- to 120-µm swellings) immunoreactive for neurofilament and Ub in many areas of the CNS and peripheral nervous system. Ultrastructurally, the terminal axons and presynaptic endings are filled with granulovesicular and tubulomembranous material with a paracrystalline appearance and a central cleft. Detection in biopsy material as the method of choice for in vivo diagnosis of the disorder[553] was replaced by genetic studies to detect mutations in the *PANK2* gene,[554] the relationships of which to neurodegeneration and iron deposition in the brain are obscure. Although the pathogenic cascade involving PANK2 deficiency, iron deposition, and accumulation of insoluble α-Syn remains to be delineated, dysregulation of neuronal lipid metabolism appears to play a key role in PKAN. *PANK2* is one of four human genes that encode PANK activity, which catalyzes the rate-controlling first step in the pathway of coenzyme A synthesis—and thereby fatty acid metabolism—by phosphorylation of pantothenate (vitamin B$_5$) to phosphopantothenate. In addition to PD and DLB, PKAN is likely to be the third human synucleinopathy that is associated with dysregulation of fatty acid metabolism. Widespread α-Syn–immunoreactive inclusions and extensive tau pathology with NFTs often coexisting with LBs have been observed in juvenile- and adult-onset Hallervorden-Spatz disease and have been related to disturbances caused by axonal damage.[555,556] Atypical adult forms of cortical α-Syn and tau pathology are considered a distinctive clinicopathologic entity.[557]

The disease is thought to be part of a widespread spectrum of neuroaxonal dystrophies that include infantile, late infantile, juvenile, adult, and senile forms, all of which share the presence of axonal spheroids; however, there are neuroimaging and ultrastructural differences between the infantile and other forms.[549,552] Mutations in the *PLA2G6* gene cause both infantile neuroaxonal dystrophy and, more rarely, an atypical neuroaxonal dystrophy that overlaps clinically with other forms of NBIA.[558]

Neuroferritinopathy

This hereditary multisystem disorder is caused by mutations in the gene encoding ferritin light chain (FTL) in various pedigrees. Its clinical features include choreoathetosis, parkinsonism, focal dystonia, cerebellar signs, and cognitive impairment.[559] The distribution of its hallmark cytoplasmic lesion, the iron/ferritin body, which is probably formed in oligodendrocytes, depends on the underlying genetic subtype. It involves the BG and is associated with cystic degeneration, particularly of the GP. A tg mouse model expressing a pathogenic FTL mutation shows pathology similar to the disease in humans, but its pathogenesis is not fully understood.[22] It may be diagnosed by muscle or nerve biopsy.[560]

Neuronal Intranuclear Inclusion Disease and Basophilic Inclusion Body Disease

Both neuronal intranuclear inclusion disease (NIID) and basophilic inclusion body disease (BIBD) are rare, progressive, fatal sporadic and rarely familial neurodegenerative conditions whose heterogeneous clinical phenotype includes motor neuron, extrapyramidal, and cerebellar signs, as well as choreoathetosis, tremor, levodopa-responsive dystonia, rigidity, dysarthria, behavioral changes, cognitive impairment, and autonomic dysfunctions. Patients with infantile or juvenile onset have cardiomyopathy, and adult-onset cases exhibit dementia with parkinsonism and autonomic dysfunction.[22,561-563] The neuropathology of both NIID and BIBD is quite similar: the brain shows various degrees of generalized atrophy that is accentuated in the frontotemporal and frontoparietal regions. The striking morphologic feature in both disorders is the presence of neuronal and glial intracytoplasmic and intranuclear inclusions in many areas of the central, peripheral, and visceral nervous systems and in parenchymal cells of the adrenal medulla.[22] The intraneuronal eosinophilic inclusions in NIID are immunopositive for Ub, neurofilament, α-internexin, and ataxin-3 but negative for tau, amyloid precursor protein, Aβ, and TPD-43, whereas the basophilic inclusions in BIBD are positive for α-internexin and p62 protein but negative for tau, α-Syn, polyglutamine, and TPD-43. These disorders are associated with multisystemic degeneration with neuronal loss and gliosis in the neocortices, hippocampus, basal ganglia, SN, cerebellum, and spinal cord, often accompanied by pyramidal tract degeneration.[22,563] NIID or neuronal intermediate filament inclusion disease (NIFID) was recently classified as a new entity of frontotemporal lobar degeneration.[564] Familial cases are well documented, but no causative gene has been identified; polyglutamine extension is unlikely in the pathogenesis of NIID. The differential diagnosis includes various types of FTLD, atypical parkinsonism, and trinucleotide repeat disorders. The etiology of both disorders is unclear, but an unknown protein besides α-internexin and neurofilament may play a pivotal pathogenic role, at least in some NIID cases.

Wilson's Disease (Hepatolenticular Degeneration)

Wilson's disease (WD), an autosomal recessive disorder characterized by liver disease (cirrhosis) and cerebral degeneration along with abnormal hepatic copper metabolism and excretion, is caused by mutation of the *ATP7B* gene on chromsome 13q14.3, which encodes a copper-transporting P-type adenosine triphosphatase (ATPase).[565] The protean clinical manifestations of WD vary with pediatric or adult onset. A constant, diagnostically important sign in the eye is the Kayser-Fleischer ring, which is caused by deposition of copper in the limbus of the cornea. Its clinical features include tremor, dystonia, parkinsonism, abnormal behavior, and schizophrenia-like symptoms.[566] Neuropathologic studies show copper deposition, especially in the basal ganglia, with cavitation, neuronal loss, gliosis, and occasionally subcortical myelin degeneration and neuronal loss in the deep frontal cortex.[22,567] Many mutations have been described in the *WD* gene, which is expressed primarily in the liver.[568] The most common mutation (H1069Q) replaces a histidine residue in a cytoplasmic loop adjacent to the adenosine triphosphate–binding domain, which is essential for normal function of both the *WD* gene product and the related gene mutated in Menkes' disease.[569]

Menkes' Disease

The X-linked recessive disorder known as Menkes' disease (MD) is due to mutations of the *ATP7A* gene, which encodes a copper-transporting P-type ATPase and shows more than 75% homology with the *WD* gene.[570] *ATP7A* has a dual function: incorporation of copper into copper-dependent enzymes and maintenance of intracellular copper levels by removing excess copper from the cytosol.[571] The reduced activity of these enzymes results in systemic copper deficiency, which accounts for most of the features of MD: abnormal hair, mental retardation, hypotonia, and cerebellar degeneration.[572] MRI shows brain atrophy and abnormal myelination. Neuropathologic evaluation reveals diffuse cerebral atrophy, multilocal neuronal degeneration, and abnormal Purkinje cell dendritic arborization with axonal swellings.[22] Clinical differences from WD probably arise from the tissue-specific functions of the gene products, with the *MD* gene being expressed predominantly in the placenta, gastrointestinal tract, and blood-brain barrier; mutation of *ATP7A* results in failure of copper transport through the placenta with resultant deficiency of brain-specific cuproenzymes.

Myoclonus and Startle Syndromes

Myoclonus, defined as brief, electric shock–like jerks caused by rapid, involuntary contraction of a single muscle or muscle group, is a nonspecific sign of CNS disease that occurs in a wide range of degenerative disorders, including advanced AD, Creutzfeldt-Jakob disease, dentorubral-pallidoluysian degeneration (DRPLD), LBD, CBD,[573] and other CNS conditions, including those induced by hypoxia, trauma, and drugs. Distinction should be made between cortical and subcortical forms. Cortical forms are related to hyperexcitability of the somatosensory and primary motor cortex and are due to point mutations in the gene encoding GLRA1, which causes abnormalities in channel gating. Subcortical forms are associated with lesions in the brainstem, such as palatal myoclonus secondary to lesions in the central tegmental tract and dentate nucleus. Opsoclonus (ocular myclonus) is seen in children with neuroblastoma or in adults with CNS infections, but the pathogenic mechanisms are unknown.[574]

Ballism and Hemiballism

Ballism is a severe form of chorea characterized by involuntary, violent flinging movements of the limbs. When unilateral, it is called *hemiballism*. Most cases are caused by damage to the STN or its outflow tracts as a result of vascular disease (infarct or hemorrhage). Rarely, other focal lesions are caused by metastases, demyelination, infections, or tumors. Bilateral ballism is rare.[575] Experimental lesions in monkeys showed that more than 20% of the STN must be destroyed to produce hemiballism. Lesions of the STN reduce the normal inhibitory output from the GPi and SNr and result in reduced activity of the inhibitory GABAergic STN-pallidal pathway to the thalamic nuclei. The increased glutamatergic drive in the cortex produces ballism through enhanced synchronization of neuronal activity (see Fig. 74-4).

Dystonia

Dystonia, a syndrome of sustained muscle contractions that frequently causes abnormal posture or twisting and repetitive movements, comprises a heterogeneous group of phenotypes that may be due to different hereditary degenerative, metabolic, or genetic diseases.[576,577] It is classified by age of onset, severity, distribution of abnormal movements, and cause, and one must distinguish between primary, generalized, focal or segmental, and mixed dystonias, dystonia-plus syndromes, and hereditary degenerative and paroxysmal dystonias.[578,579]

Primary dystonias include predominantly generalized and focal ones. Seventeen different types have been differentiated according to genetic aspects.[16,22,580,581,581a] Predominantly generalized dystonias include autosomal dominant early-onset or primary (idiopathic) torsion dystonia (PTD/*DYT1*), autosomal recessive dystonia (*DYT1*), and dominant (*DYT4*) forms. Most PTD cases are caused by mutations in the *DYT1* gene on chromosome 9q32.q34, which encodes the protein torsin A,[582] familial-onset dystonia is due to deletion of the torsin A gene in exon 5 or mutation of the gene encoding ε-sarcoglycan, and a minority of patients have no abnormalities in the torsin A gene. Other adult-onset familial forms of torticollis have been mapped to *DYT7* on chromosome 18p, to *DYT6* on chromosome 8p21.q22, or to other loci. Neuroimaging studies show increased metabolism of the presupplementary motor and parietal association cortices in *DYT1*- and *DYT6*-associated dystonia and increased metabolism in the striatum, anterior cingulate gyrus, and cerebellum of carriers.[583] Evidence suggests that dystonia results from functional BG disturbances, particularly those involving striatal control of the GPi and SNr, which causes altered thalamic control of cortical motor planning in the supplementary motor area and abnormal regulation of the brainstem and spinal inhibitory intraneuronal mechanism,[584] as shown by thalamo-frontal disinhibition and abnormal central sensorimotor processing (see Fig. 74-4).[585] Recent neuroimaging studies showing reduction of axons in the pontine brainstem and white matter of the sensorimotor region suggested disturbances in the cerebellothalamocortical pathways,[586] and genotype-phenotype interaction in PTDs were revealed by different changes in brain structures.[589a] Earlier neuropathologic studies reported no abnormalities in dystonia 1 and 5, nor cell loss or gliosis in the striatum SN, LC, and PPNc; a patchy pattern of neuronal loss and gliosis in the CN and putamen; and infrequent NFTs and LBs in the brainstem nuclei, all of which are obviously independent of the genotype.[587] Analysis of patients with *DYT1* frontotemporal dementia revealed neuronal inclusions and immunoreaction for torsin A, Ub, and lamin A/C in brainstem nuclei, findings not present in late-onset focal forms, which show normal brain structures in most patients.[588,589]

Focal or *segmental dystonias* include autosomal dominant focal dystonia (*DYT7*) and adult-onset PTD; 25% of patients have a family history, including blepharospasm, writer's cramp, and other focal dystonias. Patients with blepharospasm associated with oromandibular dystonia (Meige's syndrome) may be inclined to the development of parkinsonism, and LB pathology has been reported.[590] An unusual familial phenotype showed an association of focal dystonia and cerebellar atrophy.[591] For *mixed dystonia* (adult-onset primary type [*DYT6*] and PTD with craniocervical or upper limb onset [*DYT13*]), no neuropathologic data are available.[22] Spasmodic dystonia (SD) is a primary task-specific focal dystonia characterized by involuntary spasms in the laryngeal muscles during speech, frequently related to brainstem intraneuronal excitability and probably caused by modulation of descending input from higher brain centers such as the BG.[592] No neuropathologic data are available. Recent studies have found small clusters of microglia in the reticular formation surrounding the solitary tract nucleus, spinal trigeminal nucleus, nucleus ambiguus, inferior oliva, and pyramids, along with mild neuronal degeneration and depigmentation in the SN and LC, but no abnormal protein deposits or signs of demyelination or axonal degeneration were found. These subtle abnormalities of the brainstem in patients with SD may represent changes secondary to abnormalities in the supramedullary regions.[593]

Dystonia-plus syndromes include dopa-responsive dystonia (DRD) (*DYT5*), inherited myoclonus-dystonia-parkinsonism (*DYT12*), and rapid-onset dystonia-parkinsonism, which may be focal or generalized. Autosomal dominant DRD (Segawa's syndrome) is associated with mutations in *GCH1* on chromosome 14q, which encodes guanosine triphosphate cyclohydrolase I, the rate-limiting enzyme in the biosynthesis of tetrahydrobiopterin, a cofactor of TH that regulates DA synthesis. Neuropathologic evaluation reveals hypopigmentation of the SN and LC without neuronal loss and absence of LBs.[587] A new locus, *DYT16*, shows phenotypic similarities to *DYT12*.

Myoclonus-dystonia is a rare autosomal dominant disorder characterized by a combination of myoclonic jerks and dystonia, with onset in the first or second decade of life. A major culprit gene, the ε-sarcoglycan gene (*SGCE*), is located on chromosome 7q21 (*DYT11*, OMIM 604140), but mutations or deletions of *SGCE* are detected in less than 40% of patients with a typical course, thus suggesting that the disorder is genetically heterogeneous; its neuropathology and pathogenesis are unclear.[581]

Complicated recessive dystonia-parkinsonism syndromes with overlapping features include conditions that have been classified under the *PARK* and *DYT* genes and the NBIA disorder.[594]

Heredodegenerative dyskinesias include X-linked dystonia-parkinsonism (*DYT3* with the gene locus at X13.1), also known as "Lubag's disease"; it is prevalent in the Philippines and is characterized by segmental or generalized focal dystonia and the later development of parkinsonism as a result of reduced expression of the D$_2$ receptor gene (*DRD2*) in neurons.[595] CN atrophy and a patchy pattern of neuronal loss and gliosis, with preferential loss of striosome projections to the GP and SN, suggest that this dystonia may result from an imbalance in activity between the striosomal and matrix pathways.[596]

Paroxysmal dyskinesias are classified as kinesigenic or nonkinesigenic (*DYT8*) with episodes of dystonia, chorea, and athetosis lasting minutes to hours; these disorders are associated with mutation of the myofibrillogenesis regulator 1 gene (*MR1* on chromosome 2q33-35; no pathologic abnormalities are seen in the brain). Hypogenic and exercise-induced forms (*DYT9* and *DYT10* mapping to 16p12-q2; no reported mutations) have also been described, but there are few neuropathologic data.[22]

Secondary dystonias can be caused by a variety of neurological disorders, including PD, parkinsonism syndromes, HD, lysosomal storage and mitochondrial disorders, organic amino-acidurias, and others.[580] They are rarely associated with ponto-mesencephalic lesions.[597] Primate models have revealed that in brainstem areas, various affected BG nuclei of the thalamus causing disruption of sensory receptive fields in the supplementary motor area (SMAp) may lead to dystonia.[598]

Tic Disorders

Tics are involuntary, brief, stereotyped movements or vocalizations that can be suppressed at the expense of mounting inner tension. They are classified as motor tics (brief movements), vocal tics (uttering brief sounds), and sensory tics (brief sensations).[599] Tics may be simple or complex and may appear semipurposeful (e.g., obscene gestures). They may be associated with several neurodegenerative disorders or may be complications of drug therapy or CNS infection. Transient tics are the most common and mild form. Chronic tic disorders are severe and include Tourette's syndrome, which is clinically defined by the presence of motor and vocal tics. Those not meeting the criteria are known as "secondary tic disorders" and can be due to infections, drugs, toxins, stroke, or trauma. Genetic studies have shown links to chromosomes 2, 8, and 11. Imaging studies indicate a reduction in CN volume and increased density of type 2 vesicular monoamine transporter (VMAT2).[600] No specific anatomic CNS lesions have been observed, except reduced dynorphin-like staining in the GPe and SN, decreased parvalbumin-positive GABAergic interneurons in the striatum, and increased parvalbumin-positive projection neurons in the GPi.[601]

Tremor Syndromes

Tremor is a common disorder characterized by rhythmic involuntary oscillatory movements of the body. For currently proposed phenomenology and syndrome classification of tremors and their pathophysiology, see other sources.[16,190,602] *Essential tremor* (ET), one of the most common neurological disorders, may occur at any age and is occasionally associated with rest and intention tremor. In addition to environmental agents, genetic factors may contribute to its onset. Three gene loci (*ETMI1* and *ETMI2* on 3q.13 and 2p24.1 and a locus on 6p23) have been identified in families with this disorder.[603] Functional MRI found overactivity in the cerebellum, red nucleus, and GP without activation of the inferior olivary nucleus.[604] Until recently, no consistent morphologic abnormalities have been identified, but postmortem studies have demonstrated a reduction in Purkinje cell number and the occurrence of torpedo bodies (early axonal swellings indicating neuronal degeneration) in the cerebellar cortex without LBs in the majority of patients with ET; a small proportion have brainstem LBs. Others have observed cerebellar gliosis and LC depletion, thus suggesting that ET seems to be a heterogeneous degenerative disorder.[605-608] Determination of the clinical differences between patients with and without LBs and elucidation of the pathophysiology of ET require further study.

CONCLUSION

Despite considerable clinical and pathologic overlapping, most types of movement disorders, particularly those of neurodegenerative origin, show characteristic pathologic pictures. The depo-sition of pathologic fibrillary proteins or the distribution patterns of CNS lesions may or may not be typical cytoskeletal signposts pointing to the correct dignosis and to their pathophysiology (see Table 74-2). Because in vivo markers for most of these disorders (except those with known molecular genetic backgrounds) are lacking, the diagnosis usually depends on clinicomorphologic features. Specific identification and correct diagnosis of some of these disorders may be difficult because they share clinical and morphologic phenotypes with other neurodegenerative diseases or have considerable intrafamilial, interfamilial, and interindividual differences. Therefore, comprehensive morphologic studies using modern methods of neurobiology are needed to distinguish the different disease entities. Consensus data on clinical and neuropathologic criteria, together with molecular genetic and biochemical data, will aid in correctly classifying and diagnosing neurodegenerative movement disorders and provide further insight into their pathophysiology and pathogenesis as a basis for future preventive and therapeutic strategies.

SUGGESTED READINGS

Beach TG, Adler CH, Lue LF, et al. Unified staging system for Lewy body disorders: correlation with nigrostriatal degeneration, cognitive impairment and motor dysfunction. *Acta Neuropathol.* 2009;117:613-634.

Bernheimer H, Birkmayer W, Hornykiewicz O, et al. Brain dopamine and the syndromes of Parkinson and Huntington. Clinical, morphological and neurochemical correlations. *J Neurol Sci.* 1973;20:415-455.

Beyer K, Ariza A. Protein aggregation mechanisms in synucleinopathies: commonalities and differences. *J Neuropathol Exp Neurol.* 2007;66:965-974.

Braak H, Del Tredici K, Rub U, et al. Staging of brain pathology related to sporadic Parkinson's disease. *Neurobiol Aging.* 2003;24:197-211.

Deramecourt V, Bombois S, Maurage CA, et al. Biochemical staging of synucleinopathy and amyloid deposition in dementia with Lewy bodies. *J Neuropathol Exp Neurol.* 2006;65:278-288.

Dickson D, Rademakers R, Hutton ML. Progressive supranuclear palsy: pathology and genetics. *Brain Pathol.* 2007;17:74-82.

Dickson DW, Bergeron C, Chin SS, et al. Office of Rare Diseases neuropathologic criteria for corticobasal degeneration. *J Neuropathol Exp Neurol.* 2002; 61:935-946.

Forno LS. Neuropathology of Parkinson's disease. *J Neuropathol Exp Neurol.* 1996;55:259-272.

Galvin JE. Interaction of α-Synuclein and dopamine metabolites in the pathogenesis of Parkinson's disease: a case for the selective vulnerability of the substantia nigra. *Acta Neuropathol.* 2006;112:115-126.

Gilman S, Low PA, Quinn N, et al. Consensus statement on the diagnosis of multiple system atrophy. *J Neurol Sci.* 1999;163:94-98.

Hardy J, Lewis P, Revesz T, et al. The genetics of Parkinson's syndromes: a critical review. *Curr Opin Genet Dev.* 2009;19:254-265.

Hauw JJ, Daniel SE, Dickson D, et al. Preliminary NINDS neuropathologic criteria for Steele-Richardson-Olszewski syndrome (progressive supranuclear palsy). *Neurology.* 1994;44:2015-2019.

Holton JL, Schneider SA, Ganesharajah T, et al. Neuropathology of primary adult-onset dystonia. *Neurology.* 2008;70:695-699.

Ince PG, Clark B, Holton J, et al. Disorders of movement and system degenerations. In: Love S, Louis DN, Ellison DW, eds. *Greenfield's Neuropathology*, 8th ed. London: Hodder Arnold; 2008:889-1030.

Jellinger KA. A critical evaluation of current staging of alpha-synuclein pathology in Lewy body disorders. *Biochim Biophys Acta.* 2009;1792:730-740.

Jellinger KA. Vascular parkinsonism. *Therapy.* 2008;5:237-255.

Jellinger KA. Lewy body disorders. In: Youdim MBH, Riederer P, Mandel SA, et al, eds. *Degenerative Diseases of the Nervous System.* New York: Springer Science; 2007:267-343.

Josephs KA, Petersen RC, Knopman DS, et al. Clinicopathologic analysis of frontotemporal and corticobasal degenerations and PSP. *Neurology.* 2006; 66:41-48.

Kreitzer AC. Physiology and pharmacology of striatal neurons. *Annu Rev Neurosci.* 2009;32:127-147.

Kuusisto E, Parkkinen L, Alafuzoff I. Morphogenesis of Lewy bodies: dissimilar incorporation of α-Synuclein, ubiquitin, and p62. *J Neuropathol Exp Neurol.* 2003;62:1241-1253.

Lees AJ, Hardy J, Revesz T. Parkinson's disease. *Lancet.* 2009;373:2055-2066.

Lippa CF, Duda JE, Grossman M, et al. DLB and PDD boundary issues: diagnosis, treatment, molecular pathology, and biomarkers. *Neurology.* 2007;68:812-819.

Litvan I, ed. *Atypical Parkinsonian Disorders—Clinical and Research Aspects.* Totowa, NJ: Humana Press; 2005:512.

Louis ED, Faust PL, Vonsattel JP, et al. Neuropathological changes in essential tremor: 33 cases compared with 21 controls. *Brain.* 2007;130:3297-3307.

McKeith IG, Dickson DW, Lowe J, et al. Diagnosis and management of dementia with Lewy bodies: third report of the DLB Consortium. *Neurology.* 2005; 65:1863-1872.

McNaught KS, Jackson T, JnoBaptiste R, et al. Proteasomal dysfunction in sporadic Parkinson's disease. *Neurology.* 2006;66:S37-S49.

Moore DJ, West AB, Dawson VL, et al. Molecular pathophysiology of Parkinson's disease. *Annu Rev Neurosci.* 2005;28:57-87.

O'Brien J, Ames D, McKeith I, et al, eds. *Dementia with Lewy Bodies and Parkinson's Disease Dementia.* London: Taylor & Francis; 2006.

Parkkinen L, Pirttila T, Alafuzoff I. Applicability of current staging/categorization of α-Synuclein pathology and their clinical relevance. *Acta Neuropathol.* 2008;115:399-407.

Perl DP, Olanow CW. The neuropathology of manganese-induced parkinsonism. *J Neuropathol Exp Neurol.* 2007;66:675-682.

Schiesling C, Kieper N, Seidel K, et al. Review: familial Parkinson's disease—genetics, clinical phenotype and neuropathology in relation to the common sporadic form of the disease. *Neuropathol Appl Neurobiol.* 2008;34:255-271.

Schlossmacher MG. alpha-Synuclein and synucleinopathies. In: Growdon JH, Rossor MN, eds. *The Dementias 2.* Oxford: Butterworth Heinemann; 2007:184-213.

Spillantini MG, Crowther RA, Jakes R, et al. α-Synuclein in filamentous inclusions of Lewy bodies from Parkinson's disease and dementia with lewy bodies. *Proc Natl Acad Sci U S A.* 1998;95:6469-6473.

Trojanowski JQ, Revesz T. Proposed neuropathological criteria for the post mortem diagnosis of multiple system atrophy. *Neuropathol Appl Neurobiol.* 2007;33:615-620.

Utter AA, Basso MA. The basal ganglia: an overview of circuits and function. *Neurosci Biobehav Rev.* 2008;32:333-342.

Vonsattel JP. Huntington disease models and human neuropathology: similarities and differences. *Acta Neuropathol.* 2008;115:55-69.

Full references can be found on Expert Consult @ www.expertconsult.com

PART 3

Neurology of Movement Disorders

CHAPTER 75

Clinical Overview of Movement Disorders

Ihtsham ul Haq ■ Kelly D. Foote ■ Michael S. Okun

Movement disorders are a group of conditions that arise from functional aberrations in the motor and the nonmotor basal ganglia pathways.[1] Movement disorders are common and affect all age groups. A list of the most common movement disorders and their reported incidences are presented in Table 75-1.[2-12] The early signs and symptoms of movement disorders may be subtle and easily hidden by conscious or unconscious incorporation by the patient into common daily gestures. The key to diagnosing a movement disorder is careful study of its phenomenology, as well as its associated nonmotor features. In this chapter we provide an overview of movement disorders for practicing neurosurgeons, a topic that has also been covered by other authors.[13-15]

PHENOMENOLOGY: DEFINING SYMPTOMS THROUGH OBSERVATION

Patients with syndromes arising from dysfunction of the basal ganglia typically have a combination of motor and nonmotor manifestations. A thorough history and examination will avoid unnecessary tests and reduce subspecialty referrals. Once the history and general neurological examination have established the context for an abnormal movement, the movement should be characterized by visual inspection. Movements are classified on the basis of speed, anatomy, character, intentionality (i.e., voluntary, involuntary, or unvoluntary), triggers, and relieving factors.

First, the anatomic region involved should be defined. Focal disorders affect one region of the body, regional disorders affect two contiguous body parts, and generalized disorders affect both sides of the body or the axis, or both. Regarding a specific appendage, the movement may be further classified as being proximal or distal. Next, the disorder should be characterized as hyperkinetic or hypokinetic. Hyperkinetic disorders are typified by excessive movement (e.g., tremor), whereas hypokinetic disorders are typified by reduced movement (e.g., bradykinesia in Parkinson's disease [PD]). The quality of the movement should also be described. Is the movement *rhythmic* like a tremor or jerky and *irregular* as in myoclonus? Does it alter when the patient is at *rest*, maintaining a *posture*, or performing an *action*? Does it persist during sleep? Does the movement travel smoothly from body part to body part, as in chorea? Are opposing muscle groups co-contracting, as occurs in dystonia? Is it preceded by a

premonitory urge and followed by a sense of relief, as with tics? Does the patient have difficulty with skilled movements, as in apraxia?

The patient should also be asked whether the movement is *voluntary* or *involuntary*. Movements may be referred to as "*unvoluntary*" when it is unclear which category applies.[19] Triggers and relieving factors should be identified. Does the movement worsen with action or is it relieved? Do particular positions precipitate the abnormality? Is there specific sensory input that relieves the symptoms?

Finally, the presence of specific nonmotor symptoms can lead the clinician to the proper diagnosis. Table 75-2 lists common features of movement disorders and the specific diagnoses that they may suggest.

HYPERKINESIAS

Tremor

In tremor a body part oscillates rhythmically about a set point. The tremor may be regular or irregular, unilateral or bilateral, symmetrical or asymmetric, and present in one or several body regions. The frequency and amplitude of a tremor depend heavily on its underlying cause.

Tremor is classified according to its appearance or its cause.[20,21] If the tremor occurs during movement, it is referred to as *action or kinetic tremor*. A tremor occurring in the absence of activity is classified as *rest tremor*. *Postural tremor* is manifested when a specific position is maintained (e.g., holding the arm extended). Finally, *physiologic tremor* is the term applied to nonpathologic postural tremor, which typically has a frequency of 8 to 12 Hz. *Drug-induced tremors* are usually due to an enhancement of physiologic tremor.

Tremor may be triggered by synchronized oscillatory signals arising from one of several locations. These signals may originate centrally, from circuits in either the basal ganglia or cerebellum that are involved in sensorimotor integration, motor timing, muscle coordination, or sympathetic control.[21] One common example of centrally driven tremor is *essential tremor* (ET). ET has been ascribed to overactive central oscillators in the thalamus[22,23] and to thalamocortical loop overactivity. In contrast, cerebellar and rubral tremors, which may occur after stroke or traumatic brain injury, are thought to result from motor

TABLE 75-1 Prevalence of Selected Movement Disorders in the United States

SYNDROME	PREVALENCE (PER 100,000)	COMMON AGE GROUP
Parkinson's disease	295.6	60-70
Progressive supranuclear palsy	0.4-6.4	60-70
Multiple system atrophy	2.2-4.4	50-60
Essential tremor	415	>40
Huntington's disease	2-6.3	<20 or >35
Tourette's syndrome	1850-2990	<18
Cervical dystonia	5.7-8.9	40
Restless legs syndrome	4200-9800	>45
Friedreich's ataxia	1.2-2	5-15

Data from references 2-12, 16-18.

dysregulation (i.e., from unbalanced feedforward or feedback systems, or from both).

Weighting a tremoring limb can help determine whether the tremor is physiologic or a pathologic tremor of central origin. Tremors predominantly of central origin will decrease in frequency when loaded, whereas the 8- to 12-Hz oscillation of physiologic tremor typically does not.[22]

Although it can be difficult to differentiate among subtypes of tremor solely on the basis of their frequency, it may be helpful to note that tremors of the hands greater than 11 Hz or less than 6 Hz are almost always pathologic.[24] Pathologic tremors also seem to have a "floor" frequency. PD tremor and ET are among the lower frequency tremors and typically do not oscillate at less than 4 Hz.[24] Tremors with frequencies in this range are usually due to malfunction of the brainstem or cerebellum. The frequency of a tremor may decrease slightly over time,[25] in one series by approximately 2 to 3 Hz over a period of 4 to 8 years.[26] This small degree of change does not usually lead to diagnostic confusion.

Amplitude cannot be used effectively to differentiate tremor types[27] because it may vary widely within a particular tremor subtype. Generally, tremor subtypes with the lowest frequency can be expected to have the highest amplitude and vice versa, but this

TABLE 75-2 Examples of Features, Categories, and Syndromes Helpful in Diagnosis

FEATURES	CATEGORIES	EXAMPLES OF SPECIFIC SYNDROMES
Speed	Hyperkinetic	Tremor, chorea, myoclonus, tics, restless legs syndrome
	Hypokinetic	Apraxia, blocking tics, parkinsonism: bradykinesia, primary progressive freezing of gait
Region	Whole body	Hyperekplexia, generalized dystonia
	Hemibody	Hemiparkinsonism, hemidystonia
	Segmental	Segmental myoclonus
	Multifocal	Polyminimyoclonus
	Focal	Writer's cramp
	Proximal	Rubral tremor
	Distal	Painful legs when moving toes
	Oral	Tardive dyskinesia, neuroacanthocytosis
Character	Rhythm	Rhythmic: Parkinson's disease, essential tremor
		Arrhythmic: myoclonus, dystonic tremor
	Frequency	Faster: essential tremor, orthostatic tremor
		Slower: rubral tremor
	Amplitude	Large: essential tremor, rubral tremor
		Fine: orthostatic tremor, physiologic tremor
	At rest	Parkinsonism: tremor
	During posture	Physiologic tremor, drug-induced tremor, essential tremor, some cerebellar and dystonia tremors
	With action	Cerebellar tremor, essential tremor, dystonic tremor
	Accompaniment	Tics: premonitory urge
Intentionality	Voluntary	Tics
	Involuntary	Tardive dyskinesia, stereotypies, tics
	Unvoluntary	Tic disorders
Triggers	Action	Musician's dystonia
	Position	Orthostatic tremor
	Sensory stimulation	Catalepsy, hyperekplexia, stimulus-sensitive myoclonus
Relieving factors	Sleep	Improves: dystonia, tremor, not essential palatal tremor
	Sensory tricks (gestes antagoniste)	Improves: dystonia
Nonmotor features	Autonomic	Multiple system atrophy: orthostasis, parkinsonism: drooling
	Psychiatric	Huntington's disease, Parkinson's disease: depression

rule is not absolute. Emotional distress, exercise, and fatigue may exacerbate tremors of any subtype. Stressors tend to increase the amplitude of a tremor but have less effect on tremor frequency.

Common tremor conditions include ET, PD, dystonic tremor, cerebellar/outflow tremor, Holmes' tremor, physiologic tremor, palatal tremor, neuropathic tremor, drug/toxin-induced tremors, task-specific tremor, primary writing tremor, and psychogenic tremor.[21] The characteristics of these tremors are presented in Table 75-3.[21,22,27-36]

Specific Tremor Disorders

Physiologic Tremor

Physiologic tremor is a term applied to the 8- to 12-Hz tremor seen in any healthy person who is intentionally sustaining a posture. More proximal regions of the body oscillate at a lower frequency, more distal ones at a higher frequency. For example, physiologic tremor has a frequency of 3 to 5 Hz at the elbow, whereas metacarpophalangeal tremor usually ranges from 17 to 30 Hz.[22] When this tremor impairs motor performance, it is referred to as *enhanced physiologic tremor*.[30]

Physiologic tremor is typically symmetrical. As with other tremor types, the amplitude is reported to decrease with age, particularly after the age of 50,[20,27] although some authors have found otherwise.[27] Age has not been shown to affect the frequency of physiologic tremor.[27,37]

It is unclear whether mild forms of the syndrome can be distinguished from ET. Both ET and physiologic tremor can be elicited by posture, both are fairly symmetrical, and both occur predominantly in the arms.[27] Observing the progression of a tremor over time will eventually reveal whether a given patient has ET or physiologic tremor.

Essential Tremor

ET is the most common tremor disorder. It is generally manifested as a low-amplitude, bilateral action and postural tremor with a frequency of 6 to 8 Hz. The tremor usually has its onset in adulthood and worsens over time, but it may begin in childhood and can coexist with other movement disorders.[38] The overall prevalence of ET is similar between genders,[39] although women with ET seem to be more prone to head tremor than men.[40]

ET involves the upper limbs in more than 90% of patients.[41] It less commonly involves the head, legs, or voice. It rarely affects the face or trunk. ET often has a postural component that may be reported as a rest tremor by patients. Patients commonly first complain of difficulty with tasks requiring fine coordination, such as threading a needle, tying knots, or writing. Later, more gross activities are also affected. In severe cases, basic activities of daily living may become impossible to perform.

Cognitive dysfunction[42] and gait abnormalities[43] may also be features of ET. Set shifting, verbal fluency, and other frontal cortex functions are impaired in patients with ET relative to age-matched controls. This cognitive impairment has been reported to not correlate with tremor severity.[42]

Several features of ET point to an underlying cerebellar or brainstem pathology. Patients with ET frequently have an end point tremor and difficulty with tandem gait. There are case reports of ipsilateral improvement in symptoms after cerebellar infarction,[44] and inducing lesions of the cerebellothalamic receiving area (the ventral intermediate nucleus of the thalamus) is an

TABLE 75-3 Tremors and Their Characteristics

TREMOR DISORDER	REST	POSTURAL	ACTION	FREQUENCY	AVERAGE AGE AT ONSET	FAMILY HISTORY	FEATURES
Cerebellar tremor	−	+	+++	2-5 Hz	Variable	Variable	May be severe with action
Drug-induced tremor	+/−	++	+		Variable	None	Improves with drug discontinuation
Dystonic tremor	+	++	++	Irregular, 3-8 Hz	Adulthood	Variable	Irregular
Essential tremor	+	++	+++	6-8 or 8-12 Hz	Early adult	Common	Usually slightly asymmetric, involves the hands most commonly
Orthostatic tremor	−	++	−	10 or 14-16 Hz	Late	Rare	Occurs only on standing still
Palatal tremor	++	−	++	1-4 Hz	Variable	Rare	EPT may be accompanied by a click; SPT may persist in sleep
PD tremor	+++	+	+/−	4-9 Hz	Middle age	Occasional	Variable in appearance; improves with levodopa in 60% of individuals
Physiologic tremor	−	++	+	8-12 Hz	Childhood	Common	Present in all individuals
Posttraumatic tremor	+/−	++	++		Variable	None	Appearance varies with the site of trauma; myoclonus is frequently present
Rubral tremor	++	+++	+++	2-5 Hz	Variable	None	Large amplitude
Task-specific tremor	−	−	++	4-7 Hz	Adulthood	Occasional	Tremor with task or task-associated position

EPT, essential palatal tremor; PD, Parkinson's disease; SPT, symptomatic palatal tremor.
Data from references 21, 22, 27-36.

effective treatment of ET. Although positron emission tomography has shown increased olivary glucose utilization and cerebellar blood flow,[45] the brains of ET patients appear to be structurally normal.[46]

A family history of tremor is common in patients in whom ET is diagnosed. A positive family history has been reported in as many as 96% of patients[47] and as few as 17%,[48] depending on the sample. A survey of New York City residents showed a 5- to 10-fold increase in risk for ET in first-degree relatives, as well as an increase in the likelihood of ET developing in family members with earlier onset of symptoms in the patient.[49]

Several inherited forms of ET have been identified, including the gene loci *EMT1* (on chromosome 3q13), *EMT2* (on 2p24), and an unnamed gene locus on 6p23.[48,50] ET has been reported in fragile X syndrome, Kennedy's syndrome,[51] XXYY syndrome,[52] and Klinefelter's syndrome.[53] Sex chromosome–related tremors often have associated ataxia and may represent a separate tremor type.

The presence of a rest tremor in a patient who otherwise meets the criteria for ET can be confusing. Current opinion among movement disorder neurologists favors the diagnosis of ET when the action and postural components of a tremor greatly outweigh the rest component and the rest component is bilateral. New-onset unilateral rest tremor should always bring PD to mind. Although isolated head tremor is often diagnosed as ET, if upper extremity tremor is absent, it is better that it be referred to as *dystonic tremor*.

The question of whether ET predisposes patients to the later development of PD is also a perplexing one. There are some cases in which families appear to be prone to both PD and ET. Jankovic's group reported that the same locus yielded pure ET and ET-PD-dystonia in different families.[54] As of this writing, the exact association between ET and PD remains a topic of discussion.

Parkinsonian Tremor

The tremor of PD was described by James Parkinson in 1817 in his historic *Essay on the Shaking Palsy*[55] and further characterized by Charcot in the 1860s in his lectures at the Salpetriere.[56] PD tremor is a 4- to 9-Hz low-amplitude rest tremor. The tremor often has a prominent proximal thumb component that gives it a "pill-rolling" quality. Nevertheless, the presence of a pill-rolling tremor is not diagnostic.

Although there is some thought that PD tremor may dampen or "burn out" over time, others have observed the opposite. Parkinson himself wrote that "as the debility increases … the tremulous agitation becomes more vehement [and] the motion becomes so violent as not only to shake the bed-hangings, but even the floor and sashes of the room."[55]

Unlike typical ET, PD hand tremor may worsen in the ipsilateral lower limb before affecting the contralateral hand. A typical pattern of spread is for the dominant hand to be affected first, followed by the dominant foot and then the nondominant hand. Although different extremities exhibit the same frequency of tremor, they need not shake simultaneously. When tremor is bilateral in onset without involving the legs, causes other than PD should be considered.

Re-emergent tremor occurs while sustaining a prolonged position and most likely represents a rest tremor that has been reset by the relative stasis of a persistent position.[57] Postural tremor that begins immediately on adopting a position is seen in as many as 93% of patients with PD and correlates with the degree of functional disability.

The pathogenesis of PD tremor is not well understood.[58] In monkeys with 1-methyl-4-phenyl-1,2,3,6-tetrahydropyridine (MPTP)-induced parkinsonism, basal ganglia neurons begin to fire synchronously. Some authors have suggested that PD tremor originates from loss of segregation of these information channels and subsequent synchronization of adjacent circuits.[59] Loss of

dopamine in the basal ganglia may unmask pacemaker-like properties of the basal ganglia.[60] It should be noted that the severity of PD tremor does not correlate with the severity of dopamine neuronal loss[21] and that treatment with levodopa improves bradykinesia and rigidity more reliably than it does tremor.

The central origin of PD tremor is demonstrated by the observation that afferent denervation affects the amplitude and frequency of the tremor but does not abolish it.

Cerebellar Tremor

Cerebellar tremor is characterized as a jerky, low-frequency (2 to 5 Hz), high-amplitude action tremor. This tremor may be accompanied by other cerebellar signs such as ataxia, dysdiadochokinesia, dysarthria, dysmetria, and telegraphic speech. The normal pattern of cerebellar ballistic control, as described by Hallett and associates, consists of sequential agonist-antagonist–second agonist activation.[61] Research into the tremor-generating mechanism is ongoing.

Rubral Tremor (Holmes' Tremor)

Patients with lesions in the region of the red nucleus may be disposed to the development of what is referred to as a *rubral tremor*, first described by Holmes in 1904.[61a] Although predominantly an action tremor, rubral tremor frequently has a significant resting component. The amplitude of movement tends to be large and it can sometimes adopt a "wing-beating" appearance. Rubral tremors are among the slowest tremors, with frequencies often less than 4 Hz.[24]

As with cerebellar and symptomatic palatal tremor, rubral tremor arises from damage to the cerebellar and brainstem motor pathways and from dysregulation of motor control during movement.

Posttraumatic Tremor

The motor coordination control centers and their connections are situated deep in the brain, and to damage them generally requires substantial injury. Consequently, posttraumatic tremor is rarely an isolated finding. The character of the tremor depends on the region of the brain that is damaged. Damage to the brainstem may produce rest tremor if it affects the substantia nigra and related pathways. Damage to the cerebellum may result in a low-frequency action tremor. Because multiple regions are usually damaged, posttraumatic tremors are generally mixed in character. In one series of severe posttraumatic tremors, all patients displayed both action and postural tremors, whereas rest tremor was seen in just 56% of cases.[62] Posttraumatic tremor is often accompanied by myoclonus. As noted by Obeso and Narbona, this apparent myoclonus appears in some cases to be an exaggeration of a beat of the ongoing tremor rather than true myoclonus.[63]

Drug-Induced Tremor

Drug-induced tremors are united by a common cause rather than a common appearance. The onset of tremor should be temporally related to drug ingestion.[20,64]

Drugs most commonly associated with tremor include alcohol, amiodarone, antidepressants, antiepileptic medications, beta-agonist bronchodilators, caffeine, immunosuppressive agents, lithium, neuroleptics, nicotine, steroids, and sympathomimetics.[65] Alcohol intoxication (acute or chronic) and immunosuppressive agents may produce cerebellar tremors.[66] Sympathomimetics, serotonin reuptake inhibitors, nicotine, and other centrally acting agents typically produce an enhanced physiologic tremor. Because the physiologic effects of an offending drug are rarely limited to tremor, the causative agent may also be recognized by associated non-neurological symptoms.

There are numerous less commonly encountered tremor types that one must consider in the differential diagnosis of tremor.

 Additional material can be found on Expert Consult @ www.expertconsult.com.

Chorea

Chorea consists of random and complex involuntary movements that flit from body part to body part. Chorea may resemble exaggerated fidgetiness. The movements can be focal or generalized and are usually absent during sleep. The word *chorea* is derived from the Greek *khoreia* or "to dance." Chorea may be among the first defined movement disorders. Chorea Sancti Viti (St. Vitus' dance) was described in the Middle Ages. It was one term among several (*St. John's dance, tarantism*) used to refer to the independent outbreaks of "dancing mania" that occurred in central Europe, most notably around the time of the plague.[79] "St. Vitus' dance" is now used predominantly to refer to Sydenham's chorea. Choreas can be further classified by their appearance. *Athetosis* refers to a slow, sinuous, undulating movement, usually of the hands or feet. Sudden and large-amplitude movements are referred to as *ballistic*, derived from the Greek word meaning "to throw."

Multiple chorea syndromes have been described (Table 75-4), including Huntington's chorea, Sydenham's chorea, Wilson's disease, neuroacanthocytosis, Friedreich's ataxia, dentatorubral-pallidoluysian atrophy (DRPLA), McLeod's syndrome, benign hereditary chorea (BHC), spinocerebellar ataxia (SCA types 2, 3, or 17), chorea gravidarum, drug-induced chorea, metabolic chorea (i.e., secondary to accumulation of toxins or liver, kidney, or endocrine disease), tardive dyskinesia, paraneoplastic syndromes, polycythemia vera, and psychogenic chorea.[80-89]

Chorea Syndromes

Huntington's Disease

Huntington's disease (HD) is the most common form of inherited chorea. Symptoms usually begin during the third to fifth decades of life. Although chorea is the most common initial symptom,[90] unsteadiness of gait, dystonia, myoclonus, loss of bulbar control, and cognitive changes also occur and may appear before chorea does. Bradykinesia usually develops as the disease progresses, but it may be underappreciated in the presence of more obvious symptoms.

The chorea of HD is typically symmetrical and tends to increases in amplitude over time. The first manifestation of chorea may be a slight flicking of the fingers seen while walking.[80] Patients are frequently unaware of their movements and may continue to treat their gyrations with indifference, even when made aware of them. Early symptoms include an impairment of rapid saccades,[91,92] psychiatric and mood changes, and tics.[93] Ataxia is unusual and should raise concern for another syndrome, such as neuroacanthocytosis, SCA, or Friedreich's ataxia.[80]

Impersistence of movement is a classic feature of HD. Patients typically have difficulty maintaining tongue protrusion. They also tend to have difficulty keeping their gaze fixed on an object. Paradoxically, they may have trouble switching their attention from the examiner's face. This has been referred to as a *visual grasp reflex* and is not specific for HD.[94]

HD is defined as being of juvenile onset if symptoms occur by the age of 20. It is more often associated with stiffness, eye

---

TABLE 75-4 Chorea Syndromes

GENETIC CHOREA SYNDROMES	GENE (CHROMOSOME)*	GENE DEFECT (SYMPTOMATIC RANGE)	PROTEIN PRODUCT	AGE AT ONSET	INHERITANCE
Benign hereditary chorea	TITF1 (14q)	Variable	Thyroid transcription factor-1	<5	Autosomal dominant
DRPLA	ATN1 (12p12)	CAG repeat (>49)	Atrophin-1	<20 or >40	Autosomal dominant
Huntington's chorea	IT15/HD (4p16)	CAG repeat (>35)	Huntingtin	<20 (juvenile) or 35-50	Autosomal dominant
HDL1	PRNP (20p12)	Octapeptide repeat	Prion protein	20-40	Autosomal dominant
HDL2	JPH3 (16q24)	CTG-CAG repeat (>44)	Junctophilin-3	25-45	Autosomal dominant
HDL3	(4p15)	Unknown	Unknown	3-4	Autosomal recessive
HDL4/SCA17	TBP (6q27)	CAA-CAG repeat (>42)	TATA-box binding protein	25-40	Autosomal dominant
Neuroferritinopathy	FTL (19q13)	Variable	Ferritin light-chain polypeptide	40	Autosomal dominant
Choreoacanthocytosis	CHAC/VPS13A (9q21)	Variable	Chorein	20-30	Autosomal recessive
McLeod's syndrome	XK (Xp21)	Variable	Xk antigen	40-60	X-linked recessive
PKAN/NBIA	PANK2 (20p13)	Variable	Pantothenate kinase-2	3-5	Autosomal recessive
Wilson's disease	ATP7B (13q14)	Variable	ATP7B protein	20-30	Autosomal recessive
PKD	EKD2 (16q13)	Variable	Unknown	10-20	Autosomal dominant (25% sporadic)
PNKD	MR1, FPD (2q34)	Variable	Unknown	5-20	Autosomal dominant

*These gene and chromosome linkages were identified in smaller cohorts. Other genes may be implicated in a given individual.
DRPLA, dentatorubral-pallidoluysian atrophy; HDL, Huntington's disease like; NBIA, neurodegeneration with brain iron accumulation; PKAN, pantothenate kinase–associated neurodegeneration; PNKD, paroxysmal nonkinesogenic dyskinesia; PKD, paroxysmal kinesogenic dyskinesia; SCA, spinocerebellar ataxia.
Data from references 79-89.

movement difficulties, and bradykinesia than adult-onset HD is. Seizures are also more frequent in juvenile-onset HD.[95] Adult-onset HD is occasionally manifested as this phenotype.[96]

The cognitive and behavioral features of HD are both prominent and disabling. They are similar to those seen after frontal lobe damage. Grasp, snout, and other primitive reflexes may be prominent. Scores on psychomotor tests such as the Trail Making B and Stroop Interference Test show declines earlier in the course of HD than do tests of memory. Worsening scores correlate with the degree of striatal atrophy present.[97] Dementia occurs in the majority of patients, although exceptions may occur when the chorea is of late onset.[98] Other psychiatric symptoms include apathy, depression, lability, impulsivity, outbursts of anger, mania, and paranoia.[79,80] Physicians should always inquire about substance abuse and suicidality.[65]

The genetic defect responsible for HD is a CAG repeat on chromosome 4 in a region that encodes the protein huntingtin, whose function is unknown.[99] The number of copies of this repeat determines the presence or absence of clinical HD; patients with 29 to 35 repeats are expected to be asymptomatic.[79,100] The number of CAG repeats may increase in transmission and result in *anticipation*: earlier onset and increasing severity in successive generations. Paternal inheritance of HD has been correlated with a higher number of triplet repeats in the next generation,[101,102] probably because of gene expansion during spermatogenesis.[103] An increased number of triplet repeats correlates with both earlier disease onset and the degree of functional decline.[104]

The diagnosis of HD is based on clinical features and confirmed by genetic testing for the huntingtin gene. Striatal atrophy is the classic finding on imaging studies, but frontal lobe atrophy is also seen. Physicians may encounter the HD phenotype in the absence of the HD genotype. In one large series, approximately 7% of patients displaying the HD phenotype proved not to have a mutation in the huntingtin gene.[105]

Four Huntington's disease–like (HDL) syndromes have been identified. All are rare. HDL1 is an inherited prion disorder. HDL2 is caused by a CAG/CTG expansion in the junctophilin-3 protein and is more common in patients of African, Mexican, Spanish, or Portuguese descent. HDL2 is the most HD-like of the HDLs in its symptomatology. It may be accompanied by erythrocyte acanthocytosis.[88] An early childhood–onset HDL variant, HDL3, has been identified in isolated cohorts.[88] Its genetic basis remains unknown. HDL4 is synonymous with SCA type 17 (SCA17). SCA17 has a variety of phenotypes, one of which closely mimics the symptoms of HD. HDL4 arises from a CAA-CAG repeat in chromosome 6.

Sydenham's Chorea

Sydenham's chorea is a delayed complication of infection with group A β-hemolytic streptococci that usually develops 4 to 8 weeks after the infection,[79] but it may develop as long as 6 months afterward. Sydenham's chorea may be the sole manifestation of rheumatic fever in as many as 20% of patients[106,107] and remains the most common cause of acute childhood chorea in the world.

The typical age at onset of Sydenham's chorea is 8 to 9 years; it is rarely seen in children younger than 5 years.[79,108] The chorea usually generalizes but there are exceptions, and 20% of patients remain hemichoreic. Sydenham's chorea may be accompanied by tics and psychiatric symptoms. Obsessive-compulsive disorder (OCD) and attention-deficit/hyperactivity disorder (ADHD) occur in 20% to 30% of patients and may precede or follow the onset of chorea.[109] The disease is self-limited and spontaneously remits after 8 to 9 months in a large percentage of patients, but up to 50% may still have chorea 2 years after infection.[110]

Antineuronal antibodies are present in a majority of patients with Sydenham's chorea.[109] Antistreptolysin (ASO) titers are typically elevated but are nonspecific for infection with group A streptococci; this test is not useful in diagnosing Sydenham's chorea. However, elevated ASO titers may be of help in distinguishing a recurrence of Sydenham's chorea from a chorea from some other cause.[111,112] Magnetic resonance imaging (MRI) in patients with Sydenham's chorea has been reported to show transient swelling in the striatum and globus pallidus and increased signal on T2-weighted images.[113,114]

Tardive Chorea/Dyskinesia

Tardive dyskinesia results from treatment with dopamine receptor blocking agents. Tardive syndromes are less frequently caused by atypical than by typical neuroleptics. Dopamine-depleting medications have not been definitively associated with tardive dyskinesia.[65] Some common antiemetics (e.g., metoclopramide) and some antitussives (e.g., Phenergan) are dopaminergic blockers whose use may lead to the development of tardive movements.

The most common pattern of tardive dyskinesia is stereotyped and repetitive movement of the face. Tongue-thrusting and involuntary chewing movements reminiscent of those seen in choreoacanthocytosis may be seen. Tardive dyskinesia is often accompanied by a feeling of restlessness. This akathisia may be localized and reported as a "burning" sensation, often of the genitals or mouth.[115]

Although tardive chorea has been reported after treatment with atypical antipsychotics, it occurs infrequently in this setting. Of the neuroleptics, clozapine appears least likely to induce tardive disorders.[116] Large clinical trials have recently suggested that although atypical antipsychotics produce tardive dyskinesia less often than first-generation antipsychotics do, the difference may not be as great as was thought.[116,117]

Other less common forms of chorea are discussed in detail on Expert Consult @ www.expertconsult.com.

Myoclonus

Myoclonus is a sudden, arrhythmic, involuntary movement that is "shock-like" in its rapidity. When multiple, these movements do not flow into one another, which distinguishes them from chorea. True myoclonus is due to brief synchronous firing of agonist and antagonist muscles that typically lasts 10 to 50 msec and rarely more than 100 msec.[135,136]

Myoclonus can be classified by either phenomenology, extent, or trigger. *Positive myoclonus* occurs with active muscle contraction, of which *hypnic jerks*, a sudden body-wide contraction that occurs as a person drifts between sleep and wakefulness, are a commonly experienced example. *Negative myoclonus* is manifested as brief inhibition of a given muscle group. *Asterixis* is an example of negative myoclonus and consists of sudden and involuntary relaxation of a dorsiflexed hand or other body part. The EMG pattern of negative myoclonus is distinctive, with aperiodic electrophysiologic silences ranging from 0.05 to 0.5 second in the antagonist muscle groups.[15,24] When frequent, these signs can be mistaken for postural tremor.

Alternatively, myoclonus may be defined by the portion of the nervous system deemed responsible for the symptoms, such as *cortical myoclonus*, *subcortical myoclonus*, or *spinal myoclonus*. Finally, myoclonus can be classified as simply *epileptic* or *nonepileptic*. When myoclonus is triggered by movement, it is referred to as *action-induced myoclonus*. When myoclonus occurs in response to a touch or loud noise, the term *stimulus sensitive* applies. The phenomenon of *hyperekplexia*—an exaggerated startle response to a sudden, unexpected stimulus—is an example of stimulus-sensitive myoclonus.

 Myoclonus is most often encountered as one of a collection of symptoms rather than as a pathology's primary manifestation. Symptomatic myoclonus may be a feature of any process involving cortical, basal ganglionic, or cerebellar degeneration, such as Creutzfeldt-Jakob disease or PD. Hepatic, renal, endocrine, and other metabolic derangements may variably be manifested as myoclonus. Primary myoclonic syndromes include the myoclonic epilepsies, essential hereditary myoclonus, palatal myoclonus, nocturnal myoclonus (also referred to as *periodic leg movements of sleep*), minipolymyoclonus, and physiologic myoclonus.[137]

> A detailed discussion of the myoclonus syndromes can be found on Expert Consult @ www.expertconsult.com.

Dyskinesia

Dyskinesia refers to any disordered and involuntary movement. It is a broad term that encompasses movements that may also be referred to as *choreic* or *dystonic*. Dyskinesias are typically arrhythmic and not suppressible. The sufferer may be unaware of these movements, even when severe. The limbs, neck, and face are the most frequently affected, but axial symptoms may also occur. When dyskinesia occurs in the face, the features may appear wry or overanimated. Head bobbing, blinking, lip smacking, and tongue protrusion are common. When dyskinesia occurs in the limbs, the movements may be proximal or distal and of either high or low amplitude. The limbs may tap, whirl, or writhe. Low-amplitude dyskinesias of the hands can resemble tremor. Axial dyskinetic movements may consist of rocking, arching, and twisting and rarely occur in the absence of facial or appendicular symptoms.

The designation "dyskinesia" is most commonly used to describe the movements observed in patients receiving chronic dopaminergic therapy for PD; however, dyskinesia may also be *tardive* (i.e., a delayed side effect of dopamine-blocking medications). Although usually secondary to prolonged medication use, there have been reports of tardive dyskinesia developing after only a month's exposure to neuroleptic medications.[162,163]

 Dyskinesia syndromes include abdominal (belly dancer's) dyskinesia, levodopa-induced dyskinesia, tardive dyskinesia, and the paroxysmal dyskinesias.[164]

> A detailed discussion of specific dyskinesia syndromes can be found on Expert Consult @ www.expertconsult.com.

Tics

Tics are brief movements that are commonly preceded by a feeling of discomfort that builds until the tic appears, followed by a temporary feeling of relief. These preceding "premonitory urges" may consist of a feeling of itching or tension in the affected body part.[173] These sensations are also referred to as *sensory tics*.[174] One of the hallmarks of tics is that they are temporarily suppressible, although they typically rebound with increased frequency and severity after conscious suppression. Tics occupy a middle ground between voluntary and involuntary movements. They are usually described by those who have them as being purposefully executed but performed out of a feeling of need.[175] This mix of volition and compulsion has led some to refer to these movements as "semivoluntary" or "unvoluntary."[19]

Tics can be *clonic* (i.e., brief), *dystonic* (i.e., sustained), or *phonic* (vocal). These subtypes can in turn be *simple* or *complex*. Simple tics consist of isolated actions, such as throat clearing or winking. Complex tics consist of speech or coordinated actions. They

sometimes include obscene gestures, in which case they are termed *copropraxia*. When the obscenity is verbal, the complex phonic tic is referred to as *coprolalia*. Tics can also be manifested as interruptions in or slowing of ongoing motion. Jankovic has also described *blocking tics*, or abrupt interruptions of activity preceded by a premonitory urge.[14]

Tic disorders include transient tourettism, Tourette's syndrome, chronic tic disorder, tardive tourettism, and drug-induced tourettism. Adult onset of a primary tic disorder is highly unusual. Any adult with a first manifestation of tics should be carefully examined for secondary causes such as infection, neuroleptic exposure, cocaine use, or trauma.[176]

Tic Disorders

Tourette's Syndrome

Tourette's syndrome is defined by the onset of motor and vocal tics before adulthood (<18 years) that cannot be ascribed to another medical condition. The full definition, as set out by the Tourette Syndrome Classification Study Group, adds that the tics must occur multiple times throughout a period of at least a year and that the tics must evolve over time.[177] Findings on neurological examination in a patient with Tourette's syndrome are generally normal.

The first tics are usually observed around the age of 5 or 6, and tic severity peaks 4 to 5 years later.[178] Only 4% of Tourette patients fail to manifest tics by the age of 11.[179] Tic frequency is lowest in patients' early 20s, coincident with frontal lobe maturation.[178] In addition to this long-term variation, tics also wax and wane on a day-to-day basis. Tics are worsened by heightened emotional states, stress, and fatigue.

The tics of Tourette's syndrome are commonly accompanied by ADHD and OCD.[180] ADHD has been reported to precede tic onset by a mean of 2 years,[181] whereas OCD is reported to be manifested in adolescence.[182] The phenotype of Tourette-related OCD differs from that of primary OCD. In primary OCD, patients' obsessions often focus on fears of contamination or a need for checking. In Tourette's syndrome, obsessions center on concerns with symmetry, fear of violent thoughts, and a need to perform activities in a particular manner.[183] These obsessions may lead to self-injurious behavior. Patients have been reported to hit themselves in the eyes or throat or bite and scratch themselves.[184,185] Such behavior may be seen in as many as 53% of patients with Tourette's syndrome.[179]

A growing body of research suggests that Tourette's syndrome has a strong hereditary component.[186-188] The syndrome appears to follow a sex-influenced but autosomal dominant mode of transmission.[189] In Tourette kindreds, men appear more likely to manifest a typical tic-predominant syndrome and women are more likely to have OCD without tics.[190] When obtaining a family history, it should be recalled that mild symptoms may be ascribed to idiosyncrasies of personality by family members.

The pathology of the disorder has been attributed to dysfunction of the corticostriatal-thalamocortical pathway,[182] and further localization remains speculative. The striatum has been a past focus of research. Evidence of frontal cortex involvement has also been increasing.[191,192]

The *Diagnostic and Statistical Manual of Mental Disorders*, fourth edition, lists *chronic tic disorder* and *transient tourettism* (*transient tic disorder of childhood*) alongside Tourette's syndrome as the primary tic disorders. Chronic tic disorder differs from Tourette's syndrome in that the patient need not have both phonic and motor tics. Transient tourettism differs from Tourette' syndrome in that symptoms last less than 1 year. This syndrome is the mildest and most common tic disorder. Tics can be seen transiently in 20% of children younger than 10 years.[193]

Both transient tourettism and chronic tic disorder probably represent points on a continuum of tic-causing pathology, of which Tourette's syndrome is the most severe expression.

Other Causes of Tics

Drug-induced tourettism is also well described. Although antiepileptic drugs and dopamine-blocking medications have been used to treat tics, both classes of drug have also been reported to lead to Tourette-like symptoms.[194,195] Of the drugs of abuse, cocaine has been implicated most frequently in tic production.[176] Secondary tourettism may also be seen with HD,[93] autism spectrum disorders,[196] and choreoacanthocytosis[197] and sometimes after trauma.[198]

Akathisia

Akathisia refers either to an uncomfortable sensation of inner restlessness or to the voluntary activity performed to relieve that restlessness. It is often manifested by an inability to remain seated, crossing and uncrossing the legs, or pacing.[199] Akathisia usually occurs after the administration of neuroleptic medications. It may occur shortly after exposure (acute akathisia) or as a late complication of treatment (tardive akathisia).

Akathisia can be difficult to distinguish from tics[200] and restless legs syndrome (RLS).[201] All three of these disorders are characterized by movements that are performed to relieve an unpleasant internal sensation. Akathetic patients do not typically report the feeling of building tension that tic sufferers do. Akathisia also differs from both tic disorders and RLS in that the movements that akathetic patients perform feel neither compelled nor involuntary.

Akathetic Disorders

Restless Legs Syndrome

RLS may be defined as a feeling of unease or dysesthesia that is referred specifically to the lower limbs and is improved by movement.[202] The symptoms of RLS are usually bilateral and diurnal. Symptoms may be worse during the nighttime hours, even when patients remain awake.[203]

RLS is the most common of the movement disorders. Large population surveys have found that it affects 3% to 19% of adults, depending on their age.[12,204] RLS is typically a disease of patients' middle years, although it should be noted that in one patient series, up to a third of patients experienced their first symptoms before the age of 10.[205]

The underlying cause of RLS may be idiopathic or secondary. There is good evidence that familial inheritance accounts for at least some of the secondary cases of RLS. Iron deficiency anemia is responsible for RLS in a subset of patients. In this subgroup, treating the deficiency seems to relieve the symptoms. Therefore, iron deficiency should be ruled out in patients with RLS symptoms.

Drug-Induced Akathisia

Dopamine-blocking agents may lead to either acute or delayed feelings of restlessness, and it may be included among the tardive syndromes as *tardive akathisia*.[35] Less commonly, serotonin reuptake inhibitors,[206] calcium channel blockers,[207] and tricyclic antidepressants[208] have also been associated with akathisia.

Stereotypies

Stereotypies are repetitive movements or vocalizations that mimic a purposeful action, are performed outside that action's normal context, and are involuntary or "semivoluntary."[210] The hand wringing of Rett's syndrome is one example of stereotyped behavior.[210] Stereotypies should be differentiated from *automatisms*. Automatisms, such as the odd behavior that can occur during partial complex seizures, are sudden in onset, occur in the background of a clouded sensorium, are time limited, do not reliably occur after periods of stress, may take place during sleep, may be followed by a postictal behavioral change, and occur randomly.

Stereotypies should also be distinguished from repetitive *perseverative* behavior, or behavior that represents "a restriction of behavioral possibilities without excessive production."[211] A *mannerism* is "a bizarre way of carrying out a purposeful act which usually occurs as the result of the incorporation of a stereotypy into a goal directed behavior."[14,212]

Stereotypies may be triggered by an inability to adopt competing motor patterns when faced with an environmental cue,[211] as opposed to compulsive behaviors and tics, which are thought to be triggered by internal cues.

As outlined by Jankovic, the most common stereotypies are facial grimacing, staring at lights, waving objects before the eyes, repetitive sounds, arm flapping, body rocking, repetitive touching, feeling and smelling objects, jumping, toe walking, and hand and body gesturing.[213] Stereotypies can be seen in patients with autism, Asperger's syndrome,[214] schizophrenia, and mental retardation and after exposure to neuroleptic medications (*tardive stereotypy*).[215] Although it is common to find stereotypies in any of these syndromes, stereotypies are most typical of autism.[216,217]

A detailed discussion of specific stereotypy syndromes can be found on Expert Consult @ www.expertconsult.com.

HYPOKINESIAS

Bradykinesia

Bradykinesia refers to a decrease in movement velocity. This phenomenon should be distinguished from the reduction in amplitude that is termed *hypokinesia*. Patients may report bradykinesia as a nonspecific feeling of fatigue. The term *akinesia*, when properly used, refers to a complete lack of movement or an inability to initiate movement. Although *akinesia*, *bradykinesia*, and *hypokinesia* are distinct, clinicians should be aware that these terms are frequently used interchangeably.

Bradykinesia Syndromes

Gait Freezing

Freezing is a situation-specific akinesia: a sudden arrest of or inability to initiate gait. Freezing is most common during initiation of movement, when approaching an obstacle, or when attempting to turn. It is often seen in advanced PD and can be life altering; a significant number of patients who freeze restrict their social activity to avoid exacerbating situations. Freezing may also occur in patients with OCD, primary progressive gait apraxia, and progressive supranuclear palsy (PSP).

A detailed discussion of other less common bradykinesia syndromes can be found on Expert Consult @ www.expertconsult.com.

DISORDERS WITH MIXED HYPOKINESIA AND HYPERKINESIA

Parkinsonian Disorders

James Parkinson eloquently described what we now know as PD in his *Essay on the Shaking Palsy* in 1817,[55] in which he identified rest tremor, stooped posture, excessive salivation, and festination as features of the disease. Little was added to this description until Charcot's lectures of the 1860s,[240] in which he added rigidity and akathisia to the list of PD symptoms. By 1893, physicians were distinguishing patients' "fixity of feature and of limb" from their "slowness of movement"[241] as they realized that bradykinesia and rigidity were separable symptoms.

Four cardinal features dominate the current description of PD: rest tremor, bradykinesia, rigidity, and postural instability. *Parkinsonism* is a nonspecific term used to describe situations in which some, but not necessarily all of these four signs are present.

Parkinson's Disease

PD is defined as a parkinsonism characterized by the aforementioned cardinal features. PD is not always responsive to dopaminergic medications. Although improvement after the administration of levodopa or dopamine agonists is suggestive, it is neither necessary nor sufficient for the diagnosis of PD.[242]

The first symptoms of PD usually manifest in the fifth decade of life.[243] Rest tremor is the first symptom in 70% of PD patients.[244] Young-onset PD is defined as beginning in the second through fourth decades of life. Patients with this type of PD are more likely to have dystonia and levodopa-induced dyskinesias early in their disease course.[245,246] Juvenile-onset PD (first symptom before the age of 20) is rare and suggests genetic or secondary parkinsonism.[246] Individuals with young-onset PD constitute approximately 5% of referred patients in western countries.[245]

PD tremor has a frequency of approximately 5 Hz and variable amplitude. The tremor is typically more distal than proximal. It may be intermittent and is almost always asymmetric.[60] Like most tremors, it is worsened by distraction—either cognitive tasks (e.g., performing arithmetic) or motor tasks (e.g., walking). Strong emotion also tends to exacerbate PD tremor.

Postural and gait instability is the least specific of the cardinal features of PD. The parkinsonian gait is characterized by shuffling of the feet, decreased arm swing on one or both sides of the body, and flexion of the neck and spine. Patients are typically unable to turn in a single step and instead break their turns into multiple small increments. The body characteristically remains aligned with the feet during these maneuvers ("en bloc turns"). Patients are unstable and may be unable to recover from a backward tug. Both *festination* and *retropulsion* may be seen. Festination arises from an inability to return to an erect posture once leaning forward. Patients appear to chase their center of gravity as a result and are "thrown on the toes and forepart of the feet; being … irresistibly impelled to take much quicker and shorter steps, and thereby to adopt unwillingly a running pace."[55] Retropulsion is an analogous behavior that occurs as a result of patients' inability to recover from a backward-leaning posture.

The pathogenesis of PD probably involves both environmental and genetic factors.[247] Environmental factors that have been linked to PD include pesticide exposure, living in a rural area, and drinking well water.[248,249] Interestingly, tobacco use is inversely associated with risk for PD.[250] MPTP, a by-product of meperidine synthesis, caused parkinsonism in drug users exposed to it in the in the late 1970s and early 1980s.[251] Nonhuman primates injected with MPTP display levodopa-responsive akinesia, rigidity, and tremor, as well as levodopa-induced dyskinesias.[252]

MPTP exposure results in selective death of dopaminergic cells of the substantia nigra, the same abnormality observed in the autopsied brains of patients with PD. Based on cadaveric studies, PD is believed to be clinically manifested only after approximately 80% of striatal dopamine and 50% of nigral neurons have been lost.[253]

Approximately 10% to 15% of patients with PD also report PD in a first-degree relative.[254-256] Common environmental exposure probably accounts for a proportion of these cases,[257] but the fact that individuals with similar exposure vary in their expression of parkinsonian symptoms, coupled with the identification of multiple susceptibility genes,[258,259] supports the idea that the pathogenesis of PD involves both genetic predisposition and environmental exposure. Several genetic defects have been implicated in inherited PD, including alterations in the *parkin*,[260] *LRRK2*,[261] phosphatase and tensin homolog (PTEN)-induced kinase (*PINK1*),[262] and α-synuclein (*PARK1* or *SNCA*) genes.[263] Although the list of familial forms of PD continues to lengthen, PARK1, LRRK2, and PINK1 are the most common forms currently identified and together account for 3% of all patients with parkinsonism.[264] Genetic forms of PD tend to have a younger onset than sporadic PD does.

Of the cardinal features of PD, bradykinesia has the best correlation with disease severity. Bradykinesia and rigidity are also the symptoms best explained by current models. According to the Alexander, DeLong, and Strick model, bradykinesia arises from excessive inhibition of the thalamus by the globus pallidus (pars) interna (GPi), either directly by GPi overactivity or indirectly by overactivation of the GPi by an overactive subthalamic nucleus.[1] This model does not perfectly account for all observed PD phenomena (for example, lesions in the GPi reduce dyskinesias rather than increasing them).[265] Models that emphasize the role of aberrant motor plan selection, neuronal oscillation, and neuronal synchrony have been proposed and continue to evolve.[266-268]

Parkinsonian rigidity is a function of enhanced static or postural reflexes and should be differentiated from bradykinesia,[269] in the same way that stiffness and slowing are not identical. The rigidity may be of either a "lead pipe" or "cogwheel" quality and is typically asymmetric.

Care should be taken to exclude cases of parkinsonism caused by the administration of phenothiazine antiemetics or dopamine-depleting neuroleptics.[60] Suspicion of a Parkinson's plus syndrome should be raised by the presence of cerebellar deficits, corticospinal tract signs, or vertical gaze restriction. Autonomic dysfunction or postural instability early in the disease course are also atypical for idiopathic PD.[270]

Dementia with Lewy Bodies

Dementia with Lewy bodies (DLB) is the second most common cause of dementia after Alzheimer's disease.[271,272] It is characterized by progressive parkinsonism, hallucinosis, and dementia.[273] In the parkinsonism of DLB, tremor is commonly minimal or absent. Hallucinations and delusions may occur spontaneously or be provoked by dopaminergic medications, even at low doses. Patients' hallucinations tend to be visual, vivid, complex, and well formed. Interestingly, patients usually have good insight into the unreality of their visions.[274] A fluctuating level of attention and alertness is also typical of DLB, and patients may vary dramatically in their alertness from hour to hour or day to day.[60] Unlike PD, myoclonus frequently appears early in the course of DLB. Supranuclear ophthalmoparesis has also been reported.[275]

Differentiating DLB from Alzheimer's disease can be difficult, but the presence of hallucinosis, gait impairment, rigidity, or tremor early in the disease course should strongly suggest the diagnosis of DLB.[276]

Progressive Supranuclear Palsy

PSP was first described by Steele, Richardson, and Olszewski in 1964.[277] It is characterized by progressive and symmetric parkinsonism, gait instability, and gaze palsies.[277] Frequent falls are the most common initial symptom and arise from a combination of gait freezing and loss of postural reflexes. Patients typically lack insight into this impairment, thereby compounding their difficulties.[279] As with DLB, tremor is not a prominent part of the clinical picture of PSP.

Downgaze paralysis is the classic manifestation of PSP, but it is usually preceded by a slowing of vertical saccades.[280] Convergence failure and square-wave jerks may be seen. Patients may progress to complete ophthalmoparesis. Initially, doll's eye maneuvers can overcome this problem, but the vestibulo-ocular reflex is often lost over time.[281]

Bulbar symptoms are prominent in PSP. The increased muscular tone of the face and throat produces a characteristic "startled face" and a low-pitched dysarthria. Eyelid-opening apraxia is a frequent complicating factor, as is dysphagia. Dysphagia is the most frequent cause of death; most PSP patients die of aspiration-related complications within a decade of the diagnosis.[282]

Patients may also display behavior that is not congruent with their subjective emotional state. This *pseudobulbar affect* is manifested as displays of tearfulness without the feeling of sadness or laughter without the sensation of amusement. PSP may also lead to *emotional incontinence*, in which patients respond disproportionately but congruently to an emotional stimulus.

Several pathologic series have suggested that the syndrome of *pure akinesia with gait freezing*, a disorder of gait interruption and akinesis on gait initiation, is sufficiently similar in its pathology to PSP to be considered a variant.[283,284]

Corticobasal Degeneration

Corticobasal degeneration (CBD) is manifested as asymmetric parkinsonism with cortical symptoms. Asymmetric hand "clumsiness" is the most common initial complaint and was seen in 50% of patients in one series.[285] Other motor symptoms include asymmetric rest tremor, limb dystonia, rigidity, and cortical myoclonus. The alien hand phenomenon (AHP), in which the patient's limb performs uncontrolled movements and is thought of as "other," is also seen in CBD.[286] Although it aids in the diagnosis, AHP is not specific. AHP may also be seen after vascular lesions,[287] gunshot wounds,[288] seizures,[289,290] and Alzheimer's disease.[291]

The dementia of CBD is characterized by progressive aphasia, frontal lobe symptoms, dyscalculia, mild memory difficulty, and apraxia. The apraxia is most often of an ideomotor type and is detected during neurological examination by patients' inability to pantomime tool-using actions. Although aphasia was once thought to be rare in CBD, it is common and may be the initial feature.[292]

Multiple System Atrophy

Multiple system atrophy (MSA) is subdivided into two syndromes based on whether parkinsonism (MSA-P) or cerebellar ataxia (MSA-C) predominates.[293,294]

MSA-P, or striatonigral degeneration, most resembles PD. The combination of rapid disease progression, symmetrical symptoms, absence of rest tremor, and a paucity of levodopa response suggests a diagnosis of MSA.[295,296] Patients with MSA-C, or olivopontocerebellar atrophy, display progressive cerebellar ataxia and parkinsonism. Gaze-evoked or positional nystagmus occurs more frequently in MSA-C than in MSA-P. Square-wave jerks may be seen in both subtypes.[297]

Dysautonomia eventually develops in most patients with MSA. Many authors no longer consider dysautonomia-predominant MSA (Shy-Drager syndrome) to be a distinct category. The autonomic symptoms of MSA include impotence, diaphoresis, orthostatic hypotension, and incontinence. Incipient orthostatic hypotension may be unmasked by treatment with dopaminergic medications.[298]

Normal sphincter EMG findings are rare in patients with MSA of any subtype, as long as the symptoms have been present for at least 5 years.[299] Whether sphincter EMG is useful in differentiating MSA from other parkinsonisms earlier in the course of the disease remains a topic for research. MSA of any subtype can be difficult to distinguish from either PD or PSP on a patient's first visit. Litvan and coauthors[300] reported that the presence of at least six of the following eight features at the patient's first visit—sporadic adult onset, lack of levodopa response, cerebellar signs, dysautonomia, parkinsonism, pyramidal signs, no downward gaze palsy, and no cognitive dysfunction—was predictive of MSA with a median sensitivity of 59% and positive predictive value of 67%. MRI abnormalities such as the "hot cross bun sign" (cross-shaped T2-weighted hyperintensity of the pons because of the degeneration of transverse pontine fibers) and putaminal enhancement may be seen in as many as 65% of patients with MSA.[301,302]

Dystonia

Dystonia is defined as an abnormal simultaneous co-contraction of agonist and antagonist muscle groups. This contraction may be brief or sustained or focal or generalized. Common locations include the neck (cervical dystonia, or *torticollis*), eyelids (*blepharospasm*), or vocal cords (*spasmodic dysphonia*).

Dystonia is almost always worsened by voluntary movement. Conversely, relaxation or sleep can ameliorate or abolish the symptoms. Dystonias can be posture or action dependent. Some patients with gait restrictions as a result of leg dystonia improve dramatically when asked to walk backward. Other patients find that their hands cramp painfully only when attempting to play a particular musical instrument. Some patients display "sensory tricks," or *geste antagonistes*: they find that touching a particular body part temporarily relieves their dystonia.

Dystonias may be classified according to their anatomic distribution (focal, general, or segmental), their underlying cause (primary, secondary, or genetic), or young (i.e., <26 years) versus older age at the onset of symptoms. Focal dystonias are most common, but many dystonias with a focal onset generalize later (Table 75-5).[303-315,319] The younger the age at the onset of symptoms, the more likely it is for the dystonia to generalize.

Dystonic Syndromes

Primary Dystonia

Primary dystonias are "pure" dystonias that cannot be ascribed to another disease process. They may be either sporadic or genetic. Most sporadic primary dystonias are focal (e.g., torticollis, blepharospasm, lingual dystonia, spasmodic dysphonia, or task-specific dystonia).[316] The numerous heritable dystonias are subclassified into dystonia-torsion (DYT) categories and are summarized in Table 75-5.

The most common cause of early-onset generalized dystonia is DYT1 dystonia (Oppenheim's dystonia). It occurs relatively frequently in the Ashkenazi Jewish population, with a prevalence of 1 in 2000. DYT1 is inherited in an autosomal dominant fashion with a penetrance of 30% to 40%.[317] The onset of symptoms is usually in late childhood/early adolescence, and they generally begin in one leg and later generalize.

DYT7, or adult-onset focal dystonia, is another autosomal dominant dystonia.[311] Onset is typically in middle age. Symptoms are focal or multifocal and involve predominantly the upper part of the body.

TABLE 75-5 Inherited Dystonia Syndromes

	EPONYM	EXTENT	FEATURES	ONSET	INHERITANCE	GENE (CHROMOSOME)
DYT1	Oppenheim's dystonia	Generalized	Early limb onset	Childhood to adolescence	Autosomal dominant	Torsin A (9q34)
DYT2	—	Generalized or segmental	Early onset	Childhood to adolescence	Autosomal recessive	—
DYT3	Lubag: X-linked dystonia-parkinsonism	Initially focal, then generalizes	Seen in Filipino patients, in whom generalized parkinsonian and dystonic features develop	Adulthood	X-linked recessive	(Xq13)
DYT4	—	Focal: dysphonia and torticollis	Single Australian kindred	Adolescence to adulthood	Autosomal dominant	—
DYT5	Dopa-responsive dystonia (Segawa's disease)	Limb onset, generalized	Usually limb onset, levodopa responsive, diurnal; may have parkinsonian features	Infancy or childhood	Autosomal dominant (childhood) Autosomal recessive (infantile)	GTP cyclohydrolase I (14, childhood), tyrosine hydroxylase (11, infant)
DYT6	—	Segmental (craniofacial and limb)	Seen in Mennonite kindreds	Adulthood	Autosomal dominant	(8p)
DYT7	Adult-onset focal dystonia	Focal or multifocal	Seen in large German kindred	Adulthood-elderly	Autosomal dominant	(18)
DYT8	Paroxysmal nonkinesigenic dyskinesia	Episodic and focal	Paroxysms of dystonia or chorea precipitated by caffeine, stress	Variable	Autosomal dominant	Myofibrillogenesis (2q)
DYT9	Paroxysmal dyskinesia with episodic ataxia and spasticity	Episodic and focal	Paroxysms of dystonia or chorea	Childhood-adolescence	Autosomal dominant	(1p)
DYT10	Paroxysmal kinesigenic dyskinesia	Episodic and focal	Paroxysms of dystonia or chorea precipitated by movement	Childhood-adolescence	Autosomal dominant	(16p)
DYT11	Myoclonus-dystonia	Variable	30% positive for ε-sarcoglycan; improves with alcohol; associated with OCD, panic	Variable	Autosomal dominant	ε-Sarcoglycan (7q21, 11q23)
DYT12	Rapid-onset dystonia-parkinsonism	Generalized	Acute to subacute onset of generalized dystonia and parkinsonism	Childhood to adolescence	Autosomal dominant	ATP1A3 (19q13)
DYT13	—	Segmental (craniofacial and upper body)	Seen in single Italian kindred	Childhood to adulthood	Autosomal dominant	KCNA1 (1p)
DYT15	—	Limb onset	Alcohol-responsive myoclonic and limb dystonia	Childhood to adolescence	Autosomal dominant	(18p11)

OCD, obsessive-compulsive disorder.
Data from references 303-315, 319.

Dystonia Plus Syndromes

Dystonia plus syndromes are conditions in which parkinsonism, tremor, or myoclonus develop in addition to dystonia. Dystonia plus can be divided into dystonia-parkinsonism (DYT3 and DYT12), dopa-responsive dystonia (DYT5), paroxysmal dystonia (DYT8, DYT9, and DYT10), and myoclonus-dystonia (DYT11).

These syndromes are discussed in greater detail on Expert Consult @ www.expertconsult.com.

Secondary Dystonias

Any insult to the sensorimotor circuitry can lead to dystonia, and thus secondary dystonias have a variety of causes. Dystonia has been reported after ischemia, hypoxia, infection, neoplasm, drug

TABLE 75-6 Causes of Secondary Dystonia

Infection	Creutzfeldt-Jakob disease
	Reye's syndrome
	Subacute sclerosing panencephalitis
	HIV infection
	Viral encephalitis
Drugs	Anticonvulsants
	Dopamine receptor blocking agents
	Ergots
	Fenfluramine
	Flecainide
	Some calcium channel blockers
Toxins	Carbon disulfide
	Carbon monoxide
	Cyanide
	Disulfiram
	Manganese
	Methanol
	3-Nitropropionic acid
	Wasp sting toxin
Metabolic	Hypoparathyroidism
	PKAN
Brain/brainstem lesions	AVM
	Central pontine myelinolysis
	Multiple sclerosis
	Paraneoplastic brainstem encephalitis
	Primary antiphospholipid syndrome
	Stroke
	Trauma
	Tumors
Spinal cord lesions	Syringomyelia
Peripheral lesions	Electrical injury

AVM, arteriovenous malformation; HIV, human immunodeficiency virus; PKAN, pantothenate kinase–associated neurodegeneration.
Used with permission from Fernandez HH, Rodriguez RL, Skidmore FS, et al. *A Practical Approach to Movement Disorders: Diagnosis and Medical and Surgical Management.* New York: Demos Medical; 2007.

or toxin exposure, metabolic derangement, inflammatory disease, and trauma. In evaluating a patient with dystonia, it is important to identify any treatable conditions, such as Wilson's disease or drug exposure. Tardive dystonia results from exposure to neuroleptics. The many causes of secondary dystonia are summarized in Table 75-6.

DISORDERS OF COORDINATION

Ataxia

The term *ataxia* refers to clumsy or poorly organized movements. Ataxia stems from deficits in the cerebellar, vestibular, or proprioceptive pathways. It may affect speech, manual dexterity, or gait. Ataxic patients often complain of feeling as though they are inebriated; alcohol's cerebellar coordination–impairing effects produce a picture of ataxia with which the lay public is immediately familiar. Pure ataxia is not associated with deficits in strength or motor planning.

Ataxic movements are poorly aimed or timed; patients have difficulty properly estimating the distance required to reach a target or terminating an action at the proper moment. For example, patients might fail to release a ball when they desire to do so and throw it to the ground instead of forward. Similarly, ataxic patients might knock over a glass when trying to lift it or strike their teeth when trying to drink. Speech may sound poorly formed or take on an arrhythmic and staccato quality.

Any process that damages the cerebellar system may produce ataxia, including trauma, neoplasm, infarction, infection, or genetic mutation. For reasons of scope, this section will focus on the inherited ataxia syndromes.

The inherited ataxia syndromes are most easily classified by their pattern of inheritance: autosomal dominant, autosomal recessive, and X-linked. These disorders are summarized in Table 75-7.[122,323-327]

A detailed discussion of these syndromes can be found on Expert Consult @ www.expertconsult.com.

MOVEMENT DISORDERS CAUSED BY METABOLIC OR SYSTEMIC DISEASE

Toxic/Metabolic Syndromes

Wilson's Disease

Wilson's disease is an autosomal recessive disorder of copper metabolism that causes both liver and basal ganglia damage. For this reason, Wilson's disease is also referred to as *hepatolenticular degeneration*. The disease is well known for manifesting a variety of symptoms. The initial symptom may be a tremor, dystonia, or chorea. The findings may differ substantially even within the same kindred.[331] Given this fact and the potentially treatable nature of the syndrome, all patients with a movement disorder before the age of 50 should be checked for the presence of Wilson's disease.

Wilson's disease causes neurological symptoms in roughly 40% of patients, with liver disease in 40% and psychiatric disease in the remainder.[332] The age at onset varies, but the first symptoms usually appear between the ages of 11 and 25. Patients with liver impairment tend to be affected at a younger age than those with neurological symptoms.[333,334]

The neurological symptoms of Wilson's disease are typically a parkinsonian akinetic-rigid syndrome, generalized dystonia, or a proximal postural/action tremor with ataxia and dysarthria. Although pure chorea may be seen in Wilson's disease, it is an unusual manifestation of the syndrome. Psychiatric findings include pseudobulbar affect, impulsivity, and depression. Frank psychosis is rare. If the disease is untreated, symptoms worsen and result in death from liver failure or severe neurological compromise.

Based on epidemiologic studies in Europe and the United States, the prevalence of Wilson's disease is estimated to be about 15 to 30 cases per 1,000,000 people. Heterozygous carriers are present in the general population at a rate of 1 in 100 to 150 individuals.[335,336]

The underlying pathology is accumulation of copper in the liver and basal ganglia as a result of impaired copper excretion secondary to mutations in an adenosine triphosphatase (ATPase) that aids in transmembrane copper transportation and binding of copper to the carrier protein ceruloplasmin. This ATPase is encoded by the gene *ATP7B*, located on chromosome 13.[87] *ATP7B* defects result in accumulation of copper within hepatocytes, which eventually spills over into other tissues, including the brain. Copper accumulation leads to increased, but insufficient urinary copper excretion and high serum levels of free copper.